**Dedication**

I would like to dedicate this book to my family: to a Father and Mother who, as a team, demonstrated a passion for medicine in a lifetime of love and dedication to their family and community; and to my wife, Cheri, and two wonderful daughters, Lanier and Virginia, who make life a fascinating experience worth it all. Through their sacrifices and steadfast encouragement, they have participated not only in the editing of this work, but the care of each and every patient.

My family and I wish to acknowledge the commitment and medical expertise provided by my colleagues at the Cleveland Clinic in the Departments of Cardiothoracic Anesthesia, Cardiovascular Medicine, and Thoracic & Cardiovascular Surgery throughout our medical encounter in 2001. This textbook would not be a reality were it not for their remarkable care and support. It is a privilege and honor to be a part of this Cleveland Clinic family.

*Robert M. Savage, MD*

I would like to thank my colleagues and teachers over the years for helping me understand how to shape and reshape a sphere of possibilities, and my family Leena, Rebecca, and Benjamin for teaching me how to savor each moment.

*Solomon Aronson, MD*

# CONTENTS

# CONTRIBUTORS

**Ahmad Adi, MD**
Staff Anesthesiologist
Department of Cardiothoracic Anesthesia
The Cleveland Clinic Foundation
Cleveland, Ohio

**John Apostalakis, MD**
Staff Anesthesiologist
Department of Cardiothoracic Anesthesia
The Cleveland Clinic Foundation
Cleveland, Ohio

**Maged Argalious, MD**
Staff Anesthesiologist
Department of General Anesthesia
The Cleveland Clinic Foundation
Cleveland, Ohio

**Solomon Aronson, MD, FACC**
Chicago, Illinois

**Daryl Atwell, MD**
Staff Anesthesiologist
Department of Cardiothoracic Anesthesia
The Cleveland Clinic Foundation
Cleveland, Ohio

**Erik A. K. Beyer, MD**
Department of Thoracic and Cardiovascular Surgery
The Cleveland Clinic Foundation
Cleveland, Ohio

**Bruce Bollen, MD**
Department of Anesthesiology
International Heart Institute of Montana
St. Patrick's Hospital
Missoula, Montana

**Michael K. Cahalan, MD**
Professor and Chair, Department of Anesthesiology
University of Utah School of Medicine and
University of Utah Hospital and Clinics
Salt Lake City, Utah

**Michelle Capdeville, MD**
Associate Professor
Chief, Cardiothoracic Anesthesia
Department of Anesthesiology
University Hospitals of Cleveland and
Case Western Reserve University School of Medicine
Cleveland, Ohio

**Ivan Casserly, MD, FACC**
Advance Interventional Fellow
Department of Cardiovascular Medicine
The Cleveland Clinic Foundation
Cleveland, Ohio

**Mark A. Chaney, MD**
Associate Professor
Director of Cardiac Anesthesia
Department of Anesthesia and Critical Care
University of Chicago
Chicago, Illinois

**Alexander N. Chapochnikov, MD, PhD**
Rockford Anesthesiologist Association
Swedish-American Hospital
Rockford, Illinois

**Jacek Cywinski, MD**
Staff Anesthesiologist
Department of General Anesthesia
The Cleveland Clinic Foundation
Cleveland, Ohio

**Indu Deglurkar, MD**
Department of Thoracic and Cardiovascular Surgery
The Cleveland Clinic Foundation
Cleveland, Ohio

**Ellise Delphin, MD**
Chair, Department of Anesthesia
University of Medicine and Dentistry of New Jersey
Newark, New Jersey

**Pierre Devilliers, MD**
Staff Anesthesiologist
Department of Cardiothoracic Anesthesia
The Cleveland Clinic Foundation
Cleveland, Ohio

**Andra Duncan, MD**
Staff
Department of Cardiothoracic Anesthesia
The Cleveland Clinic Foundation
Cleveland, Ohio

**Frank W. Dupont, MD**
Assistant Professor of Anesthesiology
Department of Anesthesiology
Tufts University School of Medicine
Boston, Massachusetts
Baystate Medical Center
Springfield, MA

**Carlos Duran, MD, FACC**
President and CEO
Department of Cardiovascular Surgery
International Heart Institute of Montana
Missoula, Montana

**Christiano N. Faber, MD**
Department of Thoracic and Cardiovascular Surgery
The Cleveland Clinic Foundation
Cleveland, Ohio

**Elyse Foster, MD, FACC**
Professor of Medicine and Anesthesia
Director, Adult Echocardiography Laboratory
University of California, San Francisco
San Francisco, CA 94143-0214

**Mario J. Garcia, MD, FACC**
Director of Echocardiography
Department of Cardiology
The Cleveland Clinic Foundation
Cleveland, Ohio

**A. Marc Gillinov, MD, FACC**
Staff Surgeon
Surgical Director
Center for Atrial Fibrillation
Department of Thoracic and Cardiovascular Surgery
The Cleveland Clinic Foundation
Cleveland, Ohio

**Gonzalo Gonzalez-Stawinski, MD**
Department of Thoracic and Cardiovascular Surgery
The Cleveland Clinic Foundation
Cleveland, Ohio

**Katherine A. Grichnik, MD**
Associate Professor
Department of Anesthesiology
Duke University Medical Center
Durham, North Carolina

**Alina Grigore, MD**
Assistant Clinical Professor of Anesthesiology
Director of Cardiovascular Anesthesia Echocardiography
Department of Cardiovascular Anesthesia
Texas Heart Institute
Houston, Texas

**Lori B. Heller, MD**
Clinical Instructor of Cardiac Anesthesia
Department of Anesthesia
University of Washington
Swedish Medical Center
Seattle, Washington

**Kathy J. Hoercher, RN**
Director of Research
Department of Kaufman Center for Heart Failure
The Cleveland Clinic Foundation
Cleveland, Ohio

**Steven Insler, DO**
Staff Anesthesiologist
Department of Cardiothoracic Anesthesia
The Cleveland Clinic Foundation
Cleveland, Ohio

**David Jayakar, MD**
Director of Cardiac Surgery
Cardiovascular Surgery Network
801 Mac Arthur Boulevard, Suite 205
Munster, IN 46321

**Randall R. Joe, MD**
Professional Staff
Department of Cardiovascular Anesthesiology
Texas Heart Institute
Houston, Texas

**Brian Johnson, MD**
Fellow
Department of Cardiothoracic Anesthesia
The Cleveland Clinic Foundation
Cleveland, Ohio

**Marc Kanchuger, MD**
Associate Professor
Chief of Cardiothoracic and Transplant Anesthesia
Department of Anesthesia
New York University School of Medicine
Tisch Hospital of New York University Medical Center
New York, New York

**Colleen Gorman Koch, MD, MS**
Staff Anesthesiologist
Department of Cardiothoracic Anesthesia
The Cleveland Clinic Foundation
Cleveland, Ohio

**Steven Konstadt, MD, MBA, FACC**
Professor of Anesthesiology
The Mount Sinai School of Medicine
New York, New York

**Eric Kraenzler, MD**
Staff Anesthesiologist
Director, Section of Thoracic Anesthesia
Department of Cardiothoracic Anesthesia
The Cleveland Clinic Foundation
Cleveland, Ohio

**Nhung T. Lam, MD**
Staff Physician
Department of Anesthesia
Southwest Washington Medical Center
Vancouver, Washington

**Michael G. Licina, MD**
Staff Anesthesiologist
Department of Cardiothoracic Anesthesia
The Cleveland Clinic Foundation
Cleveland, Ohio

**Jia Lin, MD**
Staff Anesthesiologist
Department of General Anesthesia
The Cleveland Clinic Foundation
Cleveland, Ohio

**Bruce W. Lytle, MD, FACC**
Chair
Department of Thoracic and Cardiovascular Surgery
The Cleveland Clinic Foundation
Cleveland, Ohio

**Jonathan B. Mark, MD**
Professor and Vice Chairman
Department of Anesthesiology
Veterans Affairs Medical Center
Duke University Medical Center
Durham, North Carolina

**Joseph P. Mathew, MD**
Associate Professor of Anesthesiology
Chief, Division of Cardiothoracic Anesthesiology
Department of Anesthesiology
Duke University Medical Center
Durham, North Carolina

**Patrick McCarthy, MD, FACC**
Chief, Division of Cardiothoracic Surgery
Northwestern Medical Faculty Foundation, Inc.
Co-Director, Northwestern Cardiovascular Institute
    Northwestern Memorial Hospital
Professor of Surgery
Northwestern University Feinberg School of Medicine
Chicago, Illinois

**Glenn S. Murphy, MD**
Assistant Professor, Department of Anesthesiology
Director, Cardiac Anesthesia
Northwestern University Feinberg School of Medicine
    Academic Institution
Evanston Northwestern Healthcare
Evanston, Illinois

**Kim J. Payne, MD**
Assistant Professor
Department of Anesthesiology and Perioperative
    Medicine
Medical University of South Carolina
Charleston, South Carolina

**Albert C. Perrino, Jr., MD**
Associate Professor
Department of Anesthesiology
Yale University School of Medicine
New Haven, Connecticut

**Greg Pitas, MD**
Assistant Staff
Department of Cardiothoracic Anesthesia
The Cleveland Clinic Foundation
Cleveland, Ohio

**Mihai V. Podgoreanu, MD**
Assistance Professor
Department of Anesthesiology
Duke University Medical Center
Durham, North Carolina

**Dominique Prud'homme, MD**
Staff Anesthesiologist
Department of Cardiothoracic Anesthesia
The Cleveland Clinic Foundation
Cleveland, Ohio

**James Ramsay, MD**
Professor of Anesthesiology
Emory University School of Medicine
Atlanta, Georgia

**Scott T. Reeves, MD, MBA, FACC**
Professor, Vice Chair Research
Department of Anesthesia and Perioperative Medicine
Medical University of South Carolina
Charleston, South Carolina

**Alexander Rovner, MD, FACC**
Advanced Imaging Fellow
Cardiovascular Imaging
Department of Cardiovascular Medicine
The Cleveland Clinic Foundation
Cleveland, Ohio

**Isobel A. Russell, MD, PHD, FACC**
Professor, Department of Anesthesia and Perioperative
    Care
Chief, Cardiac Anesthesia
Moffitt-Long Hospitals
University of California
San Francisco, California

**Robert M. Savage, MD, FACC**
Co-Director Intraoperative Echocardiography Service
Departments of Cardiothoracic Anesthesia and
    Cardiovascular Medicine
The Cleveland Clinic Foundation
Cleveland, Ohio

**Rebecca A. Schroeder, MD**
Associate Professor and Anesthesiologist
Department of Anesthesiology
Duke University School of Medicine
Durham, North Carolina

**Jack S. Shanewise, MD, FACC**
Director of Cardiothoracic Anesthesiology
Columbia University College of Physicians and Surgeons
New York, New York

**Stanton K. Shernan, MD, FACC**
Director of Cardiac Anesthesia
Assistant Professor of Anesthesia
Department of Anesthesiology, Perioperative and Pain
    Medicine
Brigham & Women's Hospital
Boston, Massachusetts

**Takahiro Shiota, MD, FACC**
Associate Professor of Medicine
Department of Cardiovascular Medicine
Lerner College of Medicine of Case Western Reserve
    University
The Cleveland Clinic Foundation
Cleveland, Ohio

**Gardar Sigurdsson, MD, FACC**
Advanced Imaging Fellow
Cardiovascular Imaging
The Cleveland Clinic Foundation
Cleveland Ohio

**Nicholas G. Smedira, MD, FACC, FACS**
Surgical Director, Cardiac Transplantation and
    Mechanical Assist Devices
Surgical Director, Kaufman Center for Heart Failure
Department of Thoracic and Cardiovascular Surgery
The Cleveland Clinic Foundation
Cleveland, Ohio

**Kirk T. Spencer, MD, FACC**
Associate Professor
Department of Medicine Section of Cardiology
University of Chicago
Chicago, Illinois

**Gautam M. Sreeram, MD**
Assistant Professor
Department of Anesthesiology
Duke University School of Medicine
Durham, North Carolina

**William J. Stewart, MD, FACC**
Associate Professor of Medicine
Co-Director Intraoperative Echocardiography Service
Department of Cardiovascular Medicine
The Cleveland Clinic Foundation
Cleveland, Ohio

**James D. Thomas, MD, FACC**
Charles and Loraine Moore Chair of Cardiovascular
    Imaging
Professor of Medicine and Biomedical Engineering
Department of Cardiovascular Medicine
The Cleveland Clinic Foundation
Cleveland, Ohio

**Daniel M. Thys, MD, FACC, FAHA**
Chairman and Professor
Department of Anesthesiology
St. Luke's - Roosevelt Hospital Center
College of Physicians and Surgeons of Columbia
    University
New York, New York

**Christopher A. Troianos, MD**
Chair and Program Director
Department of Anesthesiology
Mercy Hospital of Pittsburgh
Pittsburgh, Pennsylvania

**Murat Tuzcu, MD, FACC**
Director, Intravascular Ultrasound Lab
Department of Cardiovascular Medicine
The Cleveland Clinic Foundation
Cleveland, Ohio

**Daniel P. Vezina MD, MSC, FRCPC**
Assistant Professor
Department of Anesthesiology
Department of Internal Medicine, Division of Cardiology
Director of Perioperative Echocardiography
University of Utah
Salt Lake City, Utah

**David F. Vener, MD**
Staff Anesthesiologist
Department of Congenital and Cardiothoracic Anesthesia
The Cleveland Clinic Foundation
Cleveland, Ohio

**Lee K. Wallace, MD**
Associate Staff Anesthesiologist
Director of Intraoperative Echocardiography Education
Department of Cardiothoracic Anesthesia
The Cleveland Clinic Foundation
Cleveland, Ohio

**Jay Weller, MD**
Staff Anesthesiologist
Department of Cardiothoracic Anesthesia
The Cleveland Clinic Foundation
Cleveland, Ohio

**Patrick L. Whitlow, MD, FACC**
Director, Interventional Cardiology
Department of Cardiovascular Medicine
The Cleveland Clinic Foundation
Cleveland, Ohio

**James B. Young, MD, FACC**
Chair and Professor
Department of Medicine
The Cleveland Clinic Lerner College of Medicine
The Cleveland Clinic Foundation
Cleveland, Ohio

The introduction of transesophageal echocardiography in the operating room represented a major advance for cardiovascular surgery of all types. It provides easily accessible information about the anatomy of the heart under physiologic conditions, as well as being able to demonstrate the pathophysiology. TEE has taught cardiologists, anesthesiologists, and cardiac surgeons the nuances of anatomy and pathophysiology, which has led to improved surgical results. Currently, this modality is the standard for intraoperative evaluation of surgical interventions and is a valuable monitoring method during surgical procedures.

The *Comprehensive Textbook for Intraoperative Transesophageal Echocardiography* brings together an enormous amount of information in a readily accessible manner and will be an excellent reference for anesthesiologists, cardiologists, and cardiac surgeons. The illustrations are plentiful and extremely helpful in providing understanding of the written text. The text is thoughtful, timely, and practical. This textbook represents a significant contribution to the dissemination of knowledge regarding this important diagnostic modality.

*Delos M. Cosgrove*
President and CEO
Cleveland Clinic Foundation

During my training in internal medicine at University of California, San Francisco, in the late 1970s I was extremely fortunate to be among the first to see esophageal echocardiography performed in the United States. This had an indelible impact on my career, with the excitement of a pioneering imaging modality that provided exquisite, real-time insights about cardiac anatomy and physiology. Indeed, one of the first things that I did after arriving at Johns Hopkins in 1982 for cardiology training was to push for the use of transesophageal echocardiography in the operating room. My first grant and research project used intraoperative TEE to detect regional wall motion of the left ventricle immediately after surgical coronary revascularization. With the exceptional support of the cardiac anesthesia team, and particularly Dr. Tom Blanck, we performed systematic intraoperative TEE in

over 100 patients and showed, for the first time with two-dimensional echocardiographic imaging, confirmation of regional wall motion improvement directly following bypass grafting. Even some segments that were thinned, with significant hypokinesia, could be seen to rapidly exhibit restoration of function. The term "hibernating" myocardium, reflecting chronic, subclinical ischemic myocardial dysfunction, had been vividly demonstrated, which we reported in our TEE study in 1985. We also were among the first to demonstrate the value of intraoperative TEE in tracking microbubbles, and could envision a useful application to make cardiac surgery potentially safer from the standpoint of limiting systemic or cerebral embolization.

Early on a critical lesson was so apparent. The work took the collective input of the cardiac surgeon, the cardiac anesthesiologist, and cardiologist in order for images to be acquired, interpreted, and executed. Perhaps there is no better model in the cardiovascular arena today for these three disciplines to come together around a patient and imaging modality—one that is extremely powerful for telling us what is going on "inside," right in the midst of a major operation. Little did we know at that time how important this field was to become.

In the two decades that have passed since that juncture this field has gone through unparalleled, explosive growth. Now, intraoperative TEE is the state-of-the-art choice for imaging during multiple types of surgery. In this phenomenal textbook, a panoramic and complete assessment of intraoperative TEE is presented. The fundamental principles are laid out, a full review of all aspects of the TEE cardiovascular exam is provided, and virtually all of the ways TEE can influence the decision process are presented. The experts who have come together to contribute are exceptional, not only for having built this important field, but also for representing many diverse disciplines within the cardiovascular domain.

While intraoperative TEE has become a mature and widely accepted imaging modality to improve patient outcomes, there will always be room for refinement in the years ahead. Setting the limits on who should have this technique in a world of resource restraints, while at the same time improving the output of data represent different types of challenges. The use of intraprocedural TEE has been an integral part of the first percutaneous mitral valve repairs that have been performed, and it remains to be seen whether this technique will be a suitable alternative for some patients compared with surgical repair.

Accordingly, the organization of the TEE field by Savage and Aronson represents a welcome addition to the knowledge base in cardiovascular medicine, anesthesiology, and surgery. It has been a veritable joy to see the blossoming of the field over the years, and I hope a monograph such as this will serve as the foundation for even more enhancement in the future.

*Eric J. Topol,* MD
Chief Academic Office
Cleveland Clinic

When told about this book, I got excited. Two greater rascals or better teachers, I've never met. Bob and Sol were there in the beginning as we sought to establish standards of excellence in perioperative TEE with our colleagues in cardiology. But what was the best way to take those wanting to incorporate TEE into the care of their patients to this higher plane? As they contributed to many of the initial courses incorporating TEE, they watched. But they didn't just watch; they dreamed, they created. They engaged the leadership of the cardiovascular disciplines and developed a comprehensive TEE program. Year after year, they continually made it better. That is what they've done in this book; they have taken the best in echocardiographic education and made it better.

Transesophageal echocardiography was always exciting. Bill Hamilton assigned one of Nelson Schiller's fellows to Mike Cahalan and me in 1980. He brought a noisy machine and a funny looking black snake with him. The first time we wheeled that Diasonics into an OR, the heart appeared in a way I'd never imagined it before. Mike and I shared another fellow, and John Smith and Peter Kremer became constant soul mates teaching us the joys of knowing what was really going on with the patient's volume status and myocardial contractility. I immediately predicted that machine would be in every OR within five years at a cost of $5,000 or less, and be integrated into the ECG monitor. We invited and grabbed Hewlett Packard

and GE, but neither seemed to go for this OR application. However, our excitement could not be contained.

We loved the knowledge, and doctors Wylie, Stoney, and Ehrenfeld (in vascular surgery) and Paul Ebert (in cardiac surgery) started changing operations and care for the patient. We presented the 2-D ECHOs for the first time at the Society of Cardiovascular Anesthesiologist's meeting the next year. Fawzy Estafanous saw it and the rest—as they say—is history. He and Bill Stewart moved it to the Cleveland Clinic (and I to the University of Chicago). Bob and Sol are the natural offspring of these efforts, but like many children, they did better than their parents did.

This book exhibits the best in care buttressed by the best teachers who support it. Examining the figures of the book is exciting. Bob and Sol have had their pick of the best teachers because they have watched each of them lecture; they've looked at their slides, critiqued their performances, and condensed the material into one masterful text. If this sounds like an endorsement—it is. The pictures and figures are masterful, magnificent, and illuminating examples of the points the authors are trying to make.

While the playfulness of these editors does not come through fully in this book, you can imagine, if you have attended one of their courses, the wonderful communication and excitement of watching perioperative transesophageal echocardiography come alive for the patient. What really comes through from reading this book isn't just the art of doing transesophageal echocardiography but the joy and the responsibility of helping the patient. One can't help but to share that joy and responsibility just by having this book on the shelf.

I can't help but wonder if this textbook will join Harrison's in Internal Medicine, Nelson's in Pediatrics, Goodman & Gilman's in Pharmacology, and Sabiston's in Surgery as a recurring classic. I get the feeling after reading this first edition, that it has a real chance of making that grade. I feel honored to write this foreword. This work represents the accumulated knowledge of a 25-year period concisely presented and brilliantly organized. I hope all who read it will benefit from it, and most importantly, I hope your patients are lucky enough to benefit from the wisdom this masterful volume shares.

*Michael F. Roizen*

# PREFACE

Since the first reported use of intraoperative echocardiography in 1972, which demonstrated the success of an open mitral commissurotomy using epicardial m-mode, clinical application of intraoperative TEE has rapidly developed (1). Frazin and Talano subsequently demonstrated the ability to accurately measure valve size and flow velocities in 1975, using a transducer passed into the esophagus on a thin cable (2). In the early 1980s, Kremer, Hanrath, and Roizen managed patients undergoing abdominal aortic aneurysm resections with TEE guidance, and Topol et al. first demonstrated the diagnostic ability of intraoperative TEE to detect immediate and sustained changes in regional myocardial function following coronary artery bypass grafting (3,4).

With modified application of real-time, two-dimensional imaging with color flow mapping in patients with cardiovascular disease and demonstrations of its intraoperative clinical impact on the patient, the 1990s saw an expansion of intraoperative TEE from predominantly clinical reports and research to the mainstream of clinical practice. It was clear that intraoperative evaluation of structural cardiac anatomy and function influenced the management of patients and improved outcomes. Today it is the rule rather than the exception that expertise in perioperative TEE is expected from perioperative physicians in order to fully support either a cardiovascular surgical program or noncardiac surgical program with higher risk patients. As the 1990s saw the widespread adaptation of perioperative TEE into clinical practice, it also saw a growing interest in establishing standards for its use. Collaborative interdisciplinary practice guidelines were published (and updated) along with training recommendations (5,6). The National Board of Echocardiography (NBE) was founded and established that perioperative TEE was deserving of its unique certification and pathway for diplomacy. To insure quality of care for their patients, hospitals began to consider requirements for clinical TEE credentialing of physicians who were interested in adding this diagnostic technology to their practices.

We have already witnessed the extension of perioperative TEE from traditional cardiac surgery applications to noncardiac surgical interventions, including its expanded use in the intensive care unit. The benefits of TEE utilization in noncardiac surgery will no doubt be explored and advanced further. In addition, advances in ultrasound technology, such as contrast, three-dimension, tissue Doppler, and dobutamine stress echocardiography has made it possible to perform sophisticated intraoperative evaluations of cardiac function, valve anatomy, and flow dynamics with increasing ease. New instruments have been developed that are more affordable, smaller, and easier to use, thereby enabling application of ultrasound diagnostics to a wider and more diverse group of patients. Ultrasound utilization has expanded into pre-op clinics, post-surgery recovery rooms, and pain clinics with increasing frequency. Indeed, the last two decades have witnessed many changes related to the introduction of TEE into the operating room. However important these changes may have been, the future challenges facing healthcare will require changes that promise to be even more exciting.

We find ourselves in the midst of a growing cardiovascular pandemic in the United States and throughout the world (7). Due to the aging of our population, cardiovascular disease is expected to remain the leading cause of death and disability for men and women worldwide. The number of individuals over the age of 65 years is projected to increase from 420 million to 973 million by the year 2030 (20–24) (8). In the United States alone, this number will increase from 35 to 71 million by the year 2030 (9). This age group has an increasing incidence of atherosclerotic vascular disease, degenerative valve disease (aortic, mitral, and tricuspid), and congestive heart failure, in addition to comorbidities associated with other chronic diseases (10–12). These demographic trends dictate that the future practice of medicine will involve progressively older and higher risk patients with clinically significant cardiovascular disease. With healthcare cost for patients over 65 being up to five times greater, cardiovascular disease will remain the leading cause of healthcare expense throughout the world when coupled with advances in biotechnology. We are faced with the challenges predicated by this patient population undergoing more sophisticated procedures coupled with similar expectations of steadily declining morbidity and mortality. If we are to realize similar outcomes for this emerging patient population, it will require novel perioperative man-

*xiii*

agement strategies, cost-effective developments in the treatment of cardiovascular disease, and an expansion of the collective volume of cardiovascular centers capable of providing such sophisticated care. In meeting this growing challenge, all potential solutions will require a greater availability of expertise in perioperative transesophageal echocardiography.

Perioperative ultrasound has been transformed from an uncommon to a required care option in the perioperative management of our patients. We can recognize that the practice of perioperative medicine has continued to make important contributions to the advancement of medicine overall. Of course, adaptation of new technologies into clinical practice requires education and training to stay abreast of the ongoing advances in innovative technology. It is the purpose of this text to fulfill this requirement by providing the perioperative clinician with an up-to-date understanding of the current state-of-the-art transesophageal echocardiography and its potential applications.

This book has been structured for the novice as well as the more experienced echocardiographer. For the novice, it provides a gradual progression to the more advanced applications. For the more experienced echocardiographer, the introductory chapters will serve to reinforce their previous understanding. The subject is approached by laying a foundation of the principles of ultrasound and the fundamentals of the intraoperative examination. The text builds on this foundation by exploring the potential clinical applications of this technology in the perioperative management of patients undergoing cardiovascular and noncardiac surgical interventions.

Redundancy has purposely been incorporated within the structural progression of the textbook and within the individual chapters. Each chapter is concluded with a distinct synopsis of the Key Points to reinforce the principles covered in the text. Comprehensive tables of the most frequently required reference measurements of cardiovascular structures, hemodynamic formulas, valve severity assessment criteria, aortic pathology classification of atheromatous disease, and ventricular dysfunction are included in the appendix. To encourage their use in the clinical arena, these tables and graphs are provided on a heavier quality of paper with perforated inner margins to encourage their posting in more convenient settings and reproduction. While reproduction is encouraged for your convenience, please maintain the reference copyright notation when reproducing these tables.

This textbook should be recognized as the cumulative knowledge of a collaborative team of leading surgeons, cardiologists, and anesthesiologists who have witnessed and advanced the transformation of a once novel tool in clinical practice to its current conventional application. Moreover, the authors of this text have extensive experi-

ence with these applications and will offer their insights into perioperative TEE and how it may be applied when one stretches the sphere of possibilities.

It is our hope that the collective labors of our efforts will enhance the ability of the perioperative community to improve the daily care of their patients as we test the limits of the innovations. Ultimately these will provide the solutions leading to affordable, high quality medical care in an environment that challenges the very foundations of health-care delivery (13,14).

*Robert M. Savage*
*Solomon Aronson*

## REFERENCES

1. Johnson ML, Holmes JH, Spangler RD, et al. Usefulness of echocardiography in patients undergoing mitral valve surgery. J Thorac Cardiovasc Surg 1972;64:922–8.
2. Frazin L, Talano JV, Stephanides L. Esophageal echocardiography. Circulation 1975;54:102–4.
3. Kremer P, Roizen MT, Gutman J, et al. Cardiac monitoring by transesophageal 2-D echocardiography during abdominal aortic aneurysmectomy. Circulation 1982;66:II-17(abst).
4. Topol EJ, Weiss JL, Guzman PA, et al. Immediate improvement of dysfunctional myocardial segments after coronary revascularization: detection by intraoperative transesophageal echocardiography. J Am Coll Cardiol 1984;4:1123–34.
5. Thys DA (chair): Practice Guidelines for Perioperative Transesophageal Echocardiography: A Report by the American Society of Anesthesiologists and the Society of Cardiovascular Anesthesiologists Task Force on Transesophageal Echocardiography. Anesth Analg 1996;84:986.
6. Cheitlin MD. Armstrong WF, Aurigemma GP, et al. ACC/AHA/ASE 2003 guideline update for the clinical application of echocardiography—summary article: a report of the American College of Cardiology/American Heart Association Task Force on Practice guidelines (ACC/AHA/ASE Committee to Update the 1997 Guidelines for the Clinical Application of Echocardiography). J Am Coll Cardiol 2003;42(5):954–70.
7. Bonow RO, Smaha LA, Smith SC, et al. World Heart Day 2002: the international burden of cardiovascular disease: responding to the emerging global pandemic. Circulation 2002; 106(13):1602–05.
8. Murray C, Lopez AD. Alternative projections of mortality and disability by cause 1990–2020: global burden of disease study. Lancet 1997;394(9064):1498–1504.
9. Center for Disease Control, Public health and aging: trends in aging-United States and worldwide, JAMA 2003;289(11): 1371–73.
10. Singh JP, Evans JC, Levy D, et al. Prevalence and clinical determinants of mitral, tricuspid, and aortic regurgitation (the Framingham Study). Am J Cardiol 1999;83:897–902.
11. Aronow WS, Ahn C, Kronson I. Echocardiographic abnormalities in African-American, Hispanic, and white men and women aged > 60 years. Am J Cardiol 2001;87(9)1131–33.
12. Supino PG, Borer JS, Yin A. The epidemiology of valvular heart disease: an emerging public health problem. Advances in Cardiology 2002;39:1–6.
13. Poretr ME, Teisberg E, Brown G. Innovation: medicine's best cost cutter. NY Times 1994 Feb 27.
14. Bonow R, Smith SC Jr. Cardiovascular manpower: the looming crisis, Circulation 2004;109(7):817–20.

# ACKNOWLEDGEMENTS

This textbook reflects only a small portion of the valuable contributions made by so many to the science of perioperative echocardiography. The practice of perioperative echocardiography is the result of a remarkable collaboration between colleagues in cardiovascular anesthesia, cardiovascular medicine, and cardiovascular surgery to develop educational opportunities and establish standards of excellence. This collaboration has allowed us to achieve our ultimate goal—to promote the highest traditions of our respective disciplines and ultimately the interests of the patients we serve.

The editors gratefully acknowledge the long hours of diligent work of our contributing authors and editors. We are also grateful for the valuable assistance of our secretarial support (Jan McCann, Angie Geller and Glenada Brooks) in helping us meet deadlines and arranging overnight mail pickups. We acknowledge the tireless work of our friends at Lippincott Williams & Wilkins including Joyce Murphy (Managing Editor), Adam Glazer (Senior Marketing Manager) and Craig Percy and Brian Brown (Acquisition Editors). Finally, we wish to express our gratitude to our many colleagues who have encouraged and supported us throughout the course of this project.

SECTION I

# Principles of Echocardiography

# Physics of Echocardiography

## *James D. Thomas, Michael G. Licina, and Robert M. Savage*

Echocardiographic imaging relies on the reflection of ultrasound waves from structures within the cardiovascular system. This chapter will outline the physical principles of sound wave mechanics, ultrasound generation, transmission, reflection, and reconstruction, along with applications of Doppler echocardiography. Important concepts will be reinforced through repetition of principles fundamental to a practical understanding of clinical ultrasound. It is hoped that by understanding the basics behind image production, the intraoperative echocardiographer will have a better understanding of how to apply this technology in a variety of clinical settings.

## KEY CONCEPTS

*Echocardiography* is the use of sound waves to produce an image of the heart and/or surrounding structures. *Sound* is a mechanical vibration in a physical medium, such as air, water, or tissue, which when stimulating the auditory apparatus produces the sensation of hearing. Sound travels through a medium in the form of a propagating wave. In this wave, there are areas in which the particles in the medium are either compressed or widened (areas of rarefaction). Sound can be expressed graphically as a sine wave (Fig. 1.1).

The height above or below the baseline represents the degree of particle compression and rarefaction, respectively. *Amplitude* (A) is the maximal compression of the particles above this baseline and is described in terms of decibels (dB). Amplitude equates to the loudness of the sound wave. It is the changes in amplitude that produce the gray, 2-D echocardiographic images.

*Decibels* are logarithmic units based on a ratio of the measured value (MV) to a reference value (RV) so dB = 20 log (MV/RV). Thus, a ratio of 10,000 to 1 is 80 dB and a ratio 2 to 1 is 6 dB. The advantages of using the decibel scale are that a very large range can be compressed into a smaller number of values and that low amplitude (weak) signals can be displayed alongside high amplitude (strong) signals. This compression, using the dB scale, is important in echocardiographic signal processing because amplitude measurements are the basis for 2-D echocardiography views.

*Intensity* refers to the level of sound energy in an area of tissue. This concept is represented as

$$\text{Intensity (I) (watts / cm}^2) = \text{Power (watts) / beam area (cm}^2)$$

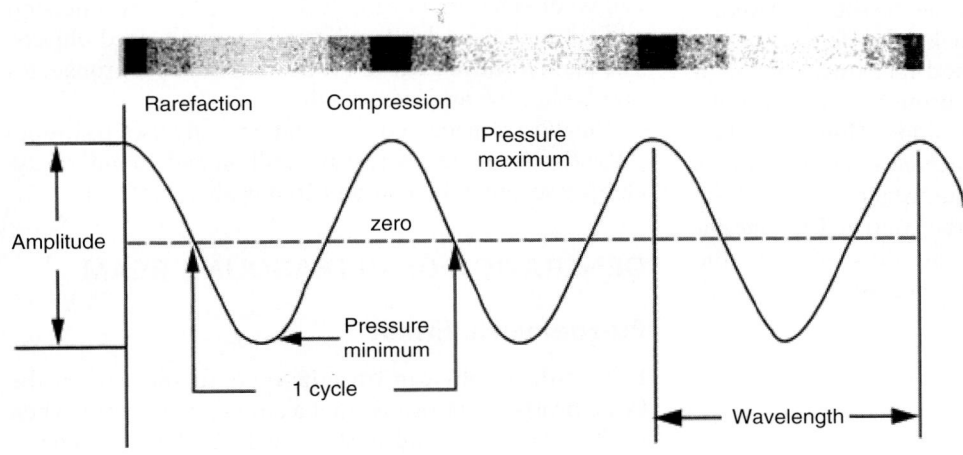

**FIGURE 1.1.** Schematic Diagram of a Sound Wave

Intensity is proportional to the amplitude of the ultrasound wave squared.

$$I \sim A^2$$

A higher ultrasound wave amplitude will cause greater intensity and thus a greater chance of tissue injury. Remember that lithotripsy uses high-intensity ultrasound waves to destroy renal calculi, whereas echocardiography uses low-intensity ultrasound waves.

*Wavelength* ($\lambda$) refers to the distance between two adjacent areas of maximal compression. The number of wavelengths per unit time is the *frequency* of the wave (f). Frequency may be expressed as cycles per second also called *hertz* (Hz). *Wavelength* ($\lambda$) times the *frequency* (f) is equal to the *propagation velocity* (c) of the wave as expressed by the formula:

$$c = f \times \lambda$$

where c = propagation velocity

$\lambda$ = wavelength

f = frequency

Because the propagation velocity of sound waves in human tissues of the heart is relatively constant—1540 meters/second or $1.5 \times 10^3$ meters/sec—the wavelength is inversely related to the frequency of the sound wave and may be calculated as:

$$\lambda = c/f = \frac{1.54 \times 10^3 \text{ meters/sec}}{f \text{ (Mhz)}}$$

*Resolution* is the ability to distinguish two points in space and is determined by wavelength. Wavelength is important in echocardiography because image resolution is no greater than 1 or 2 wavelengths and the depth of penetration of the ultrasound wave is directly proportional to its wavelength. The longer the wavelength, the lower the resolution and the greater the tissue penetration. It is the changes in frequency that form the basis for Doppler echocardiography.

*Acoustic impedance* is the process of sound traveling through a medium; it is defined by the density of the medium times the velocity of sound that travels through that medium. As sound passes through a homogenous substance, it travels in a linear fashion. However, when the sound wave reaches an interface between two tissues with differing densities (acoustic impedances), part of the sound beam is reflected back to the source. The amount of reflection is dependent upon the differences in the acoustic impedances of the two tissues. Acoustic impedance is represented as

$$z = \rho \times v$$

where $\rho$ is the density

$v$ is the velocity

*Reflection* occurs when an ultrasound wave reaches a boundary between two surfaces of differing acoustic impedances and a proportion of the wave is reflected back along the ultrasound beam path to the transducer. A greater acoustic impedance causes a greater amount of the ultrasound beam to be reflected. Reflections off a smooth surface, such as a mirror, are called *specular*. With specular reflections, most of the ultrasound waves are reflected and very little of the wave continues distal to this interface.

*Refraction* is the change in direction, or bending, of an ultrasound wave as it travels through mediums of differing acoustic impedances. It occurs when there are different propagation speeds and an oblique angle between the ultrasound beam and the surface interface. These changes in ultrasound beam direction by refraction can lead to the formation of imaging artifacts. Changing the ultrasound transducer angle to allow a 90° angle between the ultrasound beam and the surface interface can minimize the possible formation of artifacts; this minimizes the refraction.

*Scattering* is a type of reflection that occurs when ultrasound waves strike small or irregularly shaped objects, such as red blood cells. The reflected waves are dispersed in many different directions and are much weaker than specular reflections.

*Attenuation* is the loss of the ultrasound wave as it travels through tissues. It is the loss of intensity and amplitude. It is directly related to the distance the wave front travels.

*Absorption* occurs when ultrasound wave energy is converted to another energy form, such as heat or mechanical vibrations. Absorption is directly related to ultrasound frequency—the greater the frequency the better the absorption. In soft tissue, absorption is the primary cause of attenuation.

*Sound* can be classified as subsonic or infrasonic, audible sound, and ultrasound.

*Ultrasound* is sound with a frequency greater than 20,000 cycles per second. The principal advantages of using ultrasound for diagnostic imaging are that ultrasound can be directed in a beam, it obeys the laws of reflection and refraction, and it is reflected by small-sized objects. The main disadvantage of ultrasound is that it propagates poorly through a gaseous medium.

Diagnostic medical ultrasound typically uses transducers with a frequency between 1 million and 20 million cycles per second (Hz) or 1 and 20 megahertz (MHz).

## GENERATION OF ULTRASOUND BEAM

### Piezoelectric Effect

Echocardiography can trace its roots to 1880, when the Curie brothers discovered that a cut plate of quartz, when subjected to a mechanical stress, will develop an electrical

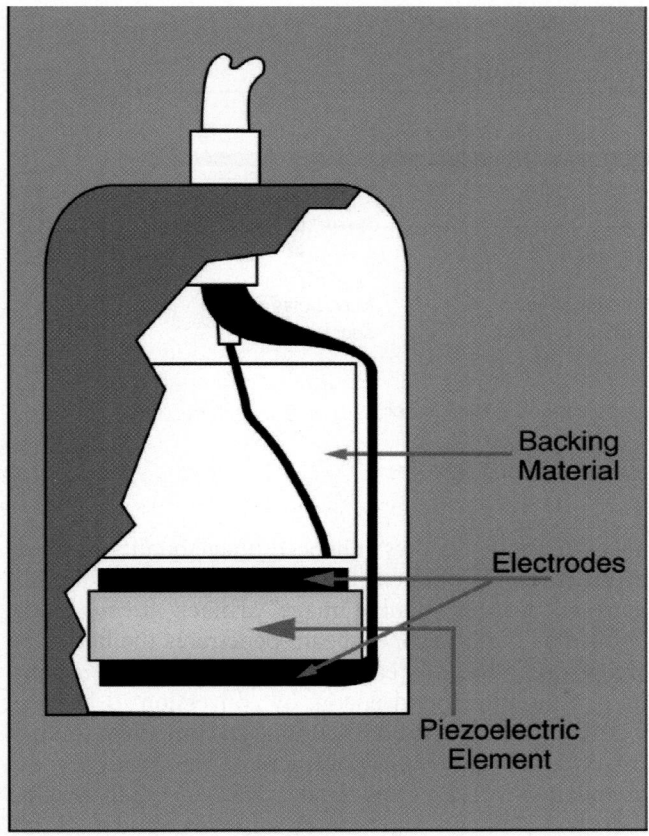

**FIGURE 1.2.** Piezoelectric Plate Construction. An electrical charge results when a cut plate of quartz crystal is subjected to ultrasonic mechanical stress. Conversely, the piezoelectric plate vibrates, producing ultrasonic sound waves, when it is subjected to an alternating electrical current.

charge on its surface (Fig. 1.2). The use of mechanical stress on a crystal to produce electrical energy is known as the pressure electric effect or *piezoelectric effect* (Fig. 1.3). The following year, the brothers discovered the re-

verse of this principle—that is, if this crystal is placed in an alternating electrical field, the crystal will change shape or vibrate in a characteristic fashion (1–5). This formed the basis of ultrasonography.

Ultrasound is generated by the piezoelectric effect. For certain types of crystals and ceramics, the molecules within the material are highly polarized, demonstrated by the ovals labeled positive and negative. When an electric charge is placed across the crystal, these dipoles attempt to line up with the electric field and their movement distorts the crystal slightly, causing it to vibrate. This vibration is transmitted into the body in the form of ultrasonic waves. The ultrasound transducer also serves as a receiver, in that reflected ultrasonic waves impacting on the crystal face cause minuscule movements of these individual dipoles, inducing an electric field that can be detected by electrodes and then amplified for processing and display in the ultrasound machine.

## IMAGING WITH ULTRASOUND

All ultrasonic imaging is based on a predictable relationship between time and distance for ultrasound propagation within the body (Fig. 1.4). When an ultrasound pulse is generated, it travels at approximately 1,540 m/sec. This pulse will travel 20 cm to the object and its echo will travel 20 cm back to the ultrasound transducer. The total distance is 40 cm. The time required is approximately 267 $\mu$sec. Now if an ultrasound pulse is sent out and you know the time echo pulse returns, it is easy to calculate the distance the object is from the ultrasound transmitter. The ultrasound machine then translates this echo time interval into a distance for display on the screen. If the echo return time is t msec, then the depth (in cm) of a returning echo will be given approximately by d = 77t (5–7). An important limitation of ultrasound is that for unambiguous visualization of structures, a second ultrasound pulse cannot

**Piezoelectric Effect**

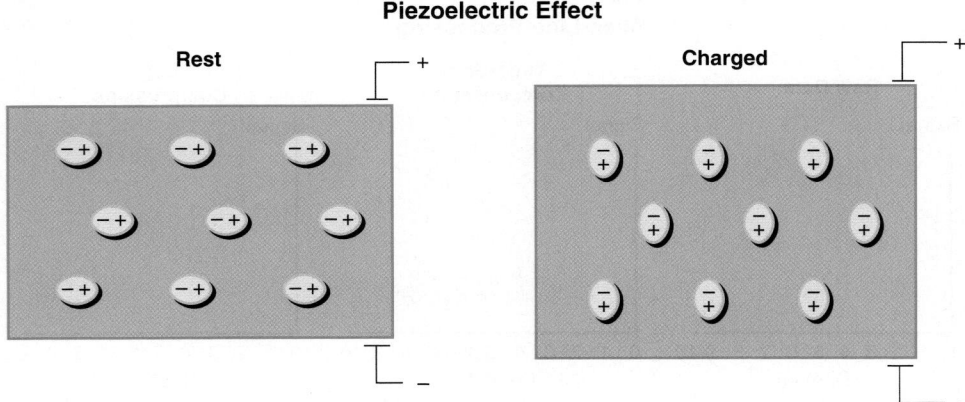

- On transmit, electricity vibrates the crystal, emitting ultrasound
- On receive, ultrasound vibrations generate an electric signal

**FIGURE 1.3.** Piezoelectric Effect. For certain crystals and ceramics, highly polarized molecules can be made to vibrate in the presence of an electrical signal, producing an ultrasonic wave. Similarly, when such a crystal is hit by ultrasound, the vibrating molecules will generate an electrical signal at the same frequency.

**Time = Depth**

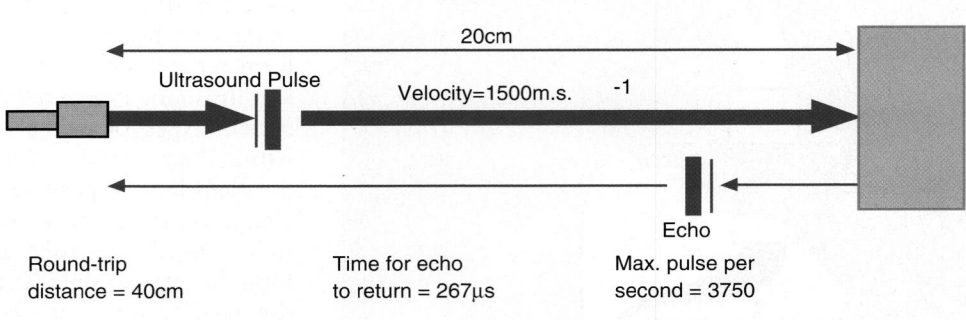

**FIGURE 1.4.** Imaging with Ultrasound. Because of the fairly constant speed of ultrasound in tissue (1,500–1,540 m/sec), the delay between transmission and receipt of an echo indicates the depth of the structure causing the echo. For an echo delay for t msec, the depth of centimeters is given by 77t; similarly, the maximal pulse repetition frequency (in kHz) available at depth d is given by 77/d.

- For depth d, time t, and speed of sound c (1500 – 1540 m/sec):
- $d = ct/2 \approx 77t$ (d in cm, t in ms)
- Maximal pulse repetition frequency: $PRF = c/2d \approx 77/d$

be emitted until echoes have returned from the deepest structures of interest. This pulsed repetition frequency (PRF, in kHz) is therefore given approximately by 77/d.

The interaction of the ultrasonic wave with the tissues and organs of the body can be described in terms of reflection, scattering, refraction, and attenuation. *Reflection* is the basis of all ultrasonic imaging and is where the beam is reflected at tissue boundaries and interfaces. The amount of the beam reflected is dependent on the relative change in *acoustic impedance* between the two tissues. Smooth tissue boundaries with lateral dimensions greater than one wavelength of the beam act as specular (mirror-like) reflectors. Optimum return of the reflected ultrasound beam occurs at a perpendicular angle to the transducer. With less than or greater than a 90-degree angle, *dropout* (this appears as a poor echo image) may occur. *Scattering* occurs when the ultrasound beam strikes small structures (less than 1 wavelength) and the ultrasonic energy is scattered in all directions. Refraction is where ultrasound waves are deflected from a straight path as they pass through a medium with different acoustic imped-

ance. Refraction allows enhanced image quality by using acoustic "lenses" to focus the beam, but can lead to problems, such as the "double image" artifact. *Attenuation* is defined as the ultrasound beam penetrates the body; the signal strength is decreased or attenuated due to *absorption* of the ultrasound energy by conversion to heat, as well as by reflection and scattering. Overall attenuation is frequency dependent; as you increase the frequency, the attenuation increases and the depth for adequate imaging decreases. Air has a high acoustic impedance and markedly attenuates the ultrasound signal.

It is important to realize that as ultrasound propagates through the body, it is continuously attenuated and dispersed as it passes through blood and tissue, especially lung tissue. The signals returning to the transducer may vary in strength by as much as a millionfold, a variation that would overwhelm the display possibilities of the machine and the interpretive abilities of the viewer. Therefore, this raw data is logarithmically compressed to turn this exponential decay in signal strength into a linear decrease in signal strength as shown in Figure 1.5.

**Scan-Line Processing**

| Raw Data | Time-Gain Compensation | Log Compression |
|---|---|---|

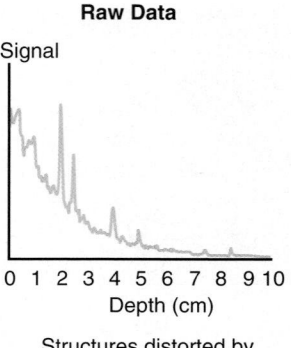

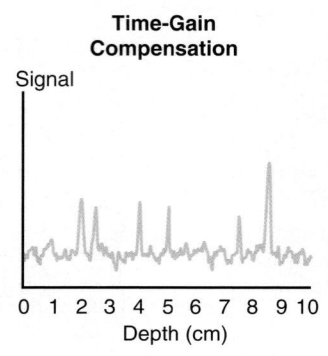

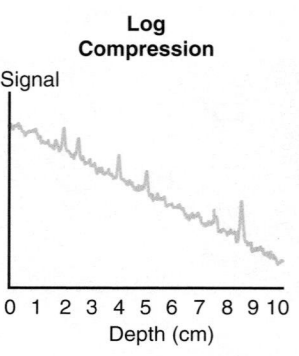

**FIGURE 1.5.** Scan Line Processing. Because the exponential attenuation in signal strength varies up to a millionfold with imaging depth, it is necessary to logarithmically compress the signal to make its decay linear. Differential amplification is then applied based on depth (time-gained compensation) to flatten out the background signal and allow the true ultrasound reflections to emerge.

Structures distorted by attenuation and 1,000,000-fold variation in signal strength

Compresses signal so it can be displayed to the viewer. Adjusted by "Dynamic Range"

Preferentially amplifies deeper signals to adjust for attenuation

This adjustment is termed *compression* and is altered by a knob on the ultrasound machine labeled either compression or dynamic range. This compressed signal still requires differential amplification so that deeper signals are brought up to the same level as more shallow echoes. This time gain compensation is typically adjusted by a series of slide controls on the machine to differentially amplify various depths of the image. By flattening out the background signal in this way, the true returning echoes can be seen with their actual echocardiographic reflectance.

## TRANSDUCERS

The transducer is made up of the piezoelectric element, electrodes (matching layer, faceplate, and acoustic lens), case with insulation, and backing material.

Ultrasound transducers utilize piezoelectric crystals to generate and receive ultrasound waves (Fig. 1.3). These crystals have the ability to expand and compress when an electrical current is administered. Conversely, when a piezoelectric crystal receives an ultrasound wave, a high frequency electrical current is generated. Even though the crystal may function as both a transducer and receiver of ultrasound, it is referred to as a transducer even though it is in the receiver mode approximately 99% of the time (3–5). Currently available transducers are quite sensitive and can detect a received wavelength signal that is less than 1% of the initially transduced signal (7,8). Knowing the velocity of ultrasound in tissue and the time between the ultrasound transmission and reception, the image distance from the transducer is determined.

The transducer contains the electrodes that, when an electric current is applied to them, stimulate the piezoelectric element. These same electrodes conduct an electric current from the piezoelectric element when the reflected ultrasound beam strikes the piezoelectric element. This current travels to the ultrasound system for further processing and image production.

The matching layer or faceplate is the interface with the piezoelectric element and the esophagus in the case of transesophageal echocardiography. This layer has an acoustic impedance between the piezoelectric element and the esophagus that causes less ultrasound energy to be reflected from the esophagus and more of the ultrasound wave to be transmitted. This is further enhanced by the use of ultrasound gel between this matching layer and the esophagus. The matching layer also contains an acoustic lens to help focus the ultrasound beam. The case and insulator surround the transducer as a plastic or metal housing that functions as protection from electric noise and prevents electrical shock to the patient. The backing material or damping element acts to dampen or "ring down" the piezoelectric crystals quickly. It shortens the pulse duration and spatial pulse length. The damping material improves the picture quality. Continuous wave Doppler uses a pair of piezoelectric crystals, one continuously in the transducer mode and one in the receiver mode. Pulse wave Doppler employs a single crystal that transmits and waits to receive the return signal before transmitting again.

## WAVE FRONT CHARACTERISTICS

The signal formed by multiple piezoelectric crystals is referred to as a beam and may be either unfocused or focused (Fig. 1.6). The unfocused beam travels initially in a columnar fashion in its near field zone, then spreads out in the far field. The near field's length is directly proportional to the diameter of the transducer and inversely related to the wavelength. This is represented by this equation:

$$F_n = D^2 / 4\lambda$$

$F_n$ = length of the near field

$D$ = diameter of the transducer

$\lambda$ = wavelength

This near field is also called the *Fresnel zone* (Fig. 1.6). Images obtained in the near field are superior to the far field in image resolution (remember the inverse relationship between $\lambda$ and f), and beam manipulation is better.

A 5 MHz transducer with a 5 mm diameter has a near field distance equal to 20.8 cm (4,7,8).

$$\lambda = c / f = \frac{1.54 \times 10^3 \text{ meters/sec}}{f \text{ (Mhz)}}$$

$$\lambda = c / f = \frac{1.54 \times 10^3 \text{ meters/sec}}{5 \text{ (Mhz)}} = 0.3 \text{ mm}$$

$$F_n = D^2 / 4\lambda$$

$$F_n = D^2 / 4\lambda = 25mm^2 / 4 \times 0.3 \text{ mm} = 20.8 \text{ cm}$$

Distal to the near field, the beam diverges in a manner that is directly proportional to the wavelength and inversely related to the transducer diameter (divergence angle = 1.22 $\lambda$ / D) (3,4,7). This is the far field, also called the *Fraunholfer zone*. The resulting beam has both a lateral width and height. The dispersion of the beam beyond the near field results in "side lobes," with reflected signals being interpreted as originating from within the main beam.

Beams can be focused by either making the transducer surface concave or electronically focusing the beam by the crystal activation sequence. Focusing allows for better image resolution at the focused area, but the far field diverges greatly. Thus, images from the far field are poor in quality. The focal zone can be manipulated on the echocardiography machines to improve image resolution (Fig. 1.6).

The ability to distinguish two points in space is referred to as *resolution*. Such distinction may be either in the axial dimension (oriented along the length of the ultrasound beam), lateral (side-to-side resolution), or eleva-

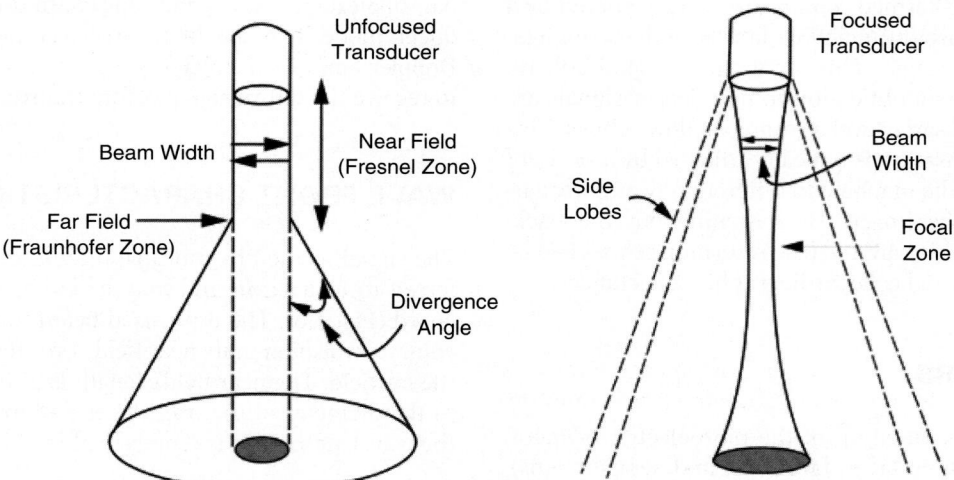

**FIGURE 1.6.** Unfocused versus Focused Beam. The unfocused transducer beam travels columnar in the near field (Fresnel) zone and spreads out in the far field (Fraunhofer) zone. *Near field* length is directly proportional to the diameter of the transducer and inversely related to the wavelength ($Fn = D2 / 4\lambda$). The *far field* transducer beam diverges in a manner proportional to the wavelength and inversely related to the transducer diameter (divergence angle ($\lambda$) = $1.22 \lambda / D$). Focused beams are made by either electronic activation sequencing or physically by transducer surface concavity focusing. Focusing allows for better near field image resolution. The focal zone may be altered to improve image resolution.

tional (resolution along the beam thickness). Of the three different types of resolution, axial is the most precise. Lateral resolution is dependent on the width of the generated beam. The narrow beams have better lateral resolution. Far distances from the transducer lead to a wider beam width. This wider beam width decreases the lateral resolution. Thus, there will be image blurring at greater depths of field.

## REVIEW OF CONCEPTS

Ultrasonic waves propagate through the body as longitudinal traveling waves, displacing the tissue to and from by microscopic amounts in the direction parallel to the sound production, and alternately compressing and expanding the tissue as it passes. Wave energy exists as kinetic energy in the form of particle motion and potential energy in the form of tissue compression and rarefaction. Typical ultrasound waves used in medical imaging have frequencies between 1.5 and 15 MHz. The velocity of propagation of these waves is specific to the tissue in which the waves are traveling, but for typical soft tissue, this speed is approximately 1540 m/sec. All waves are characterized by an inverse relationship between wavelength ($\lambda$) and frequency (f), with wavelength ($\lambda$) × frequency (f) = speed of propagation (c).

$$\lambda \times f = 1.54 \text{ m / sec}$$
$$\lambda = 1.54 / f$$

Remember the *inverse* relationship between wavelength and frequency. Therefore, a 1.5 MHz frequency transducer wave will have approximately a 1 mm wavelength, whereas a 15 MHz frequency transducer will have a wavelength of 0.1 mm. The image resolution can be no more than 1 or 2 wavelengths; therefore, the greater the frequency the better the resolution. The depth that the ultrasound wave will penetrate is dependent on the wavelength. The longer wavelength will have the greater penetration. There is a trade off in selecting transducer frequency—penetration versus resolution. A high frequency transducer will provide better resolution close to the probe. A lower frequency transducer will provide better penetration.

The size of the ultrasonic wave is clearly critical to determining the *axial resolution* of the image. To take maximal advantage of this potential resolution, an imaging ultrasound pulse must be extremely short—just one or two wavelengths in duration—whereas a Doppler ultrasound pulse, where frequency fidelity is more important, is typically longer in duration.

### Resolution

*Axial resolution* is the ability to distinguish two structures that are close to each other and front to back. It is often called longitudinal, radial, range, or depth resolution. It is dependent on transducer frequency (higher frequency more resolution), transducer bandwidth (wider bandwidth improves resolution by allowing a shorter pulse—less overlap of reflected signals from adjacent reflectors), and short pulse duration/length.

*Lateral resolution* is the minimal distance two side-by-side structures can be separated and still produce two distinct echoes. It is approximately equal to beam diameter, since beam diameter varies with depth (think of near field, focus, and far field) the lateral resolution will vary with depth. Lateral resolution is the best at the focus, because the beam is the narrowest here.

*Temporal resolution* is resolution pertaining to time. It is the ability to accurately locate moving structures at a particular instant in time. The higher the frame rate (images per unit of time) the better the temporal resolution. The factors that affect temporal resolution (for color Doppler) include the number of pulses per scan line, the imaging depth, the sector size, and the line density (lines per angle of sector). Remember, anything that requires more time will decrease the temporal resolution.

## ULTRASOUND INSTRUMENTS AND IMAGING MODALITIES

### A-, B-, or M-mode Echocardiography

Cardiac ultrasound imaging modalities may be thought of in terms of one-dimensional (A-, B-, or M-mode) or two-dimensional echocardiography. More recently, three-dimensional echo has been introduced into the clinical setting. Single-dimension echo A- or B-mode echocardiography has the capability to determine the distance between the transducer and the reflective interface and the intensity of the reflected ultrasound. In the A-mode, this intensity is noted by the height of the electric signal on the oscilloscope, whereas the B-mode (brightness) echo depicts the intensity of reflection by varying degrees of brightness of the reflected point. M-mode echo provides a time or motion mode so that the B-mode is provided with a time reference (Fig. 1.7). In the B- or M-modes, only a single crystal is used. The depth of imaging is determined by only the time it takes for the ultrasound to travel from the transducer to the object and back to the ultrasound crystal. The frequency with which a transmission may be repeated is referred to as the pulse repetition frequency (PRF). The typical M-mode pulse generation frequency is up to 3,800 times per second (pulse repetition frequency) (7–9). Such a pulse repetition frequency permits the evaluation of rapidly moving structures, such as valve leaflets or small vegetations, on cardiac structures. This allows for superior temporal resolution.

### Two-Dimensional Echocardiography

In two-dimensional echo, image generation results from rapid and repetitive scanning along multiple B-mode

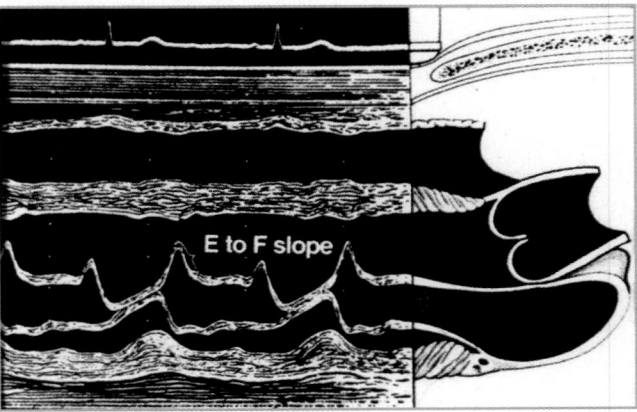

**FIGURE 1.7.** M-mode Display. By repetitively sweeping a single scan line across an oscilloscopic display, it is possible to obtain a time-motion display along a single scan line.

lines in a fan-shaped sector. The transducer crystals send out an ultrasound wave and waits for the wave's return. The transducer sends out another wave at a slightly different angle. This process is repeated for about 100 scan lines. This information is then processed to obtain the two-dimensional image. This results in a sweeping of the ultrasound beam across an image plane, and occurs at a rate of up to 60 times/sec resulting in a real-time, life-like image of the heart and its internal structures (4,7). The beam may be steered or swept along an imaging plane either mechanically or electronically as used in current phased array transducers.

The earliest echocardiographic imaging machines simply showed a display similar to an oscilloscopic display. For moving structures, this became almost impossible to interpret, so engineers developed the M-mode display, where the strength of returning echoes is displayed vertically on the screen and the temporal variation is spread out horizontally across the screen. Although largely superseded by subsequent developments, M-mode displays are still helpful for making precise measurements and for observing precise temporal relationships between events inside the heart. This is due to the high sampling rate of M-mode imaging (> 1,000 per second) versus two-dimensional imaging (30 to 60 per second) (7–9).

The earliest successor to the M-mode display was the mechanical sector scanner (Fig. 1.8), where single or multiple crystals were swept across the echocardiographic image and the resulting scan lines drawn on an oscilloscope for interpretation. This crude sector scanner was characterized by sparse imaging in the depths of the image.

To overcome the limitations of mechanical scanners, virtually all modern ultrasound machines use phased array transducers (Fig. 1.9), in which a linear array of tiny ceramic crystals emit ultrasound in a specific order as guided by timed electrical impulses. Each of these crystals emits spherical waves, but when added together, they

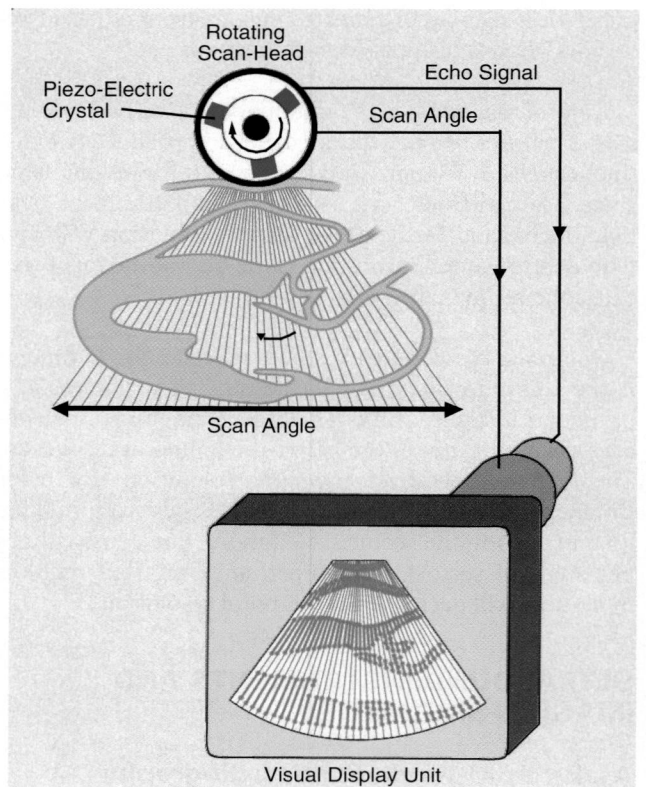

**FIGURE 1.8.** Two-Dimensional Sector Scan. By sweeping an M-mode crystal across a sector, it was possible to build up a two-dimensional image of the heart.

## Phased Array Transducer

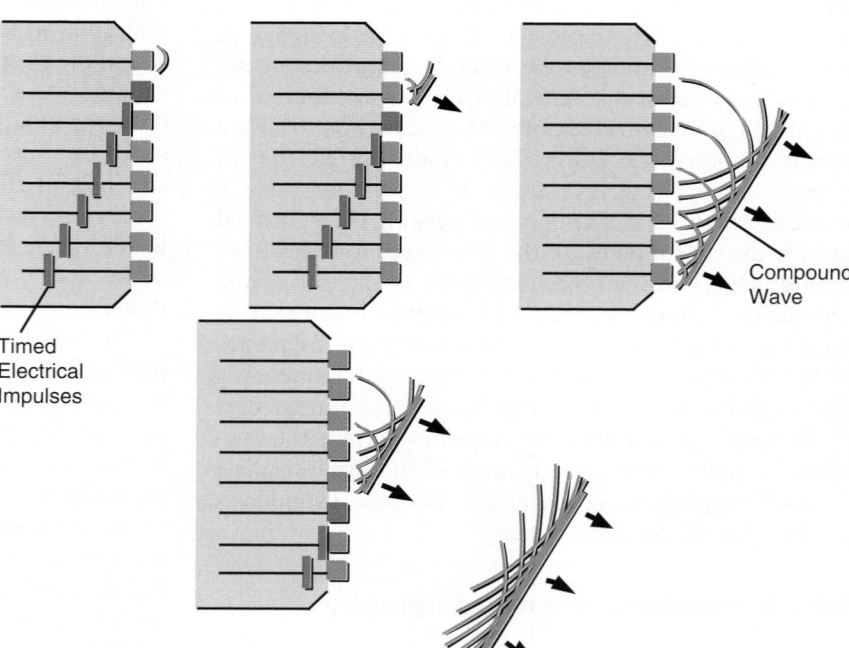

**FIGURE 1.9.** Phased Array Transducer. By precisely timing the discharge of multiple tiny crystals, it is possible to direct a wave front in an arbitrary direction within the sector scan, allowing two-dimensional imaging to be performed without any parts.

**Focused Transmission**

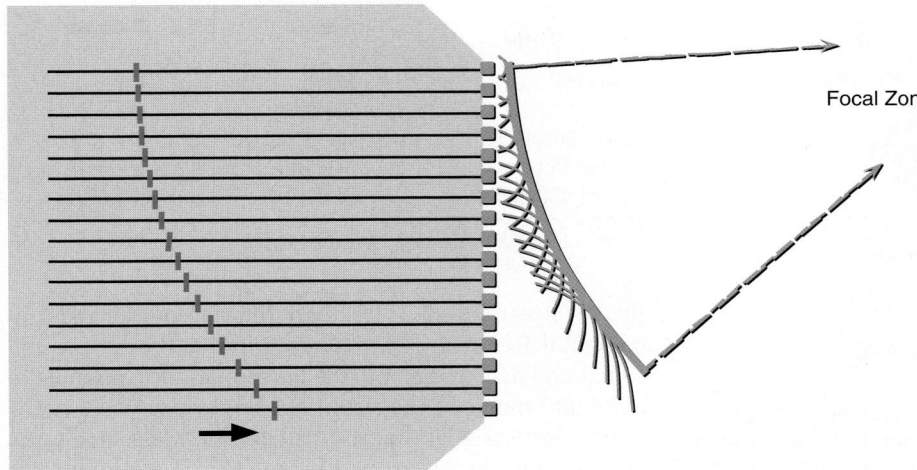

Focal Zone

**FIGURE 1.10.** Focusing the Echo Beam. By adjusting the delay in crystal firing, it is possible to produce a curved wave front that comes to a focus at a specific region of interest within the image.

produce a compound wave that is planar, and propagates into the body in a direction determined by the timing of the electrical impulses. The ability to precisely order the timing of these impulses allows one to produce waves that have specific characteristics that allow them to be focused at a specific point within the body (Fig. 1.10). This focusing is possible both on transmission and reception, so that by delaying the receipt of specific ultrasound signals from each crystal, one can focus attention at various points within the ultrasound image (Fig. 1.11).

As previously discussed, the finite speed of sound and tissue limits the maximum number of pulses that can be emitted in one second. This causes a fundamental limitation in the frame rate possible in two-dimensional imaging, since the number of scan lines per frame multiplied by the number of frames per second cannot exceed the pulse repetition frequency. As we will see, the problem is compounded in color Doppler flow imaging, as there is an additional requirement for multiple pulses per scan line to determine the velocity along that line.

Figure 1.12 demonstrates the tradeoff between these parameters in spatial and temporal resolution. Recently, however, it has been possible to apply parallel computer processing with the reception of ultrasound, allowing

**Focused Transmission and Reception**

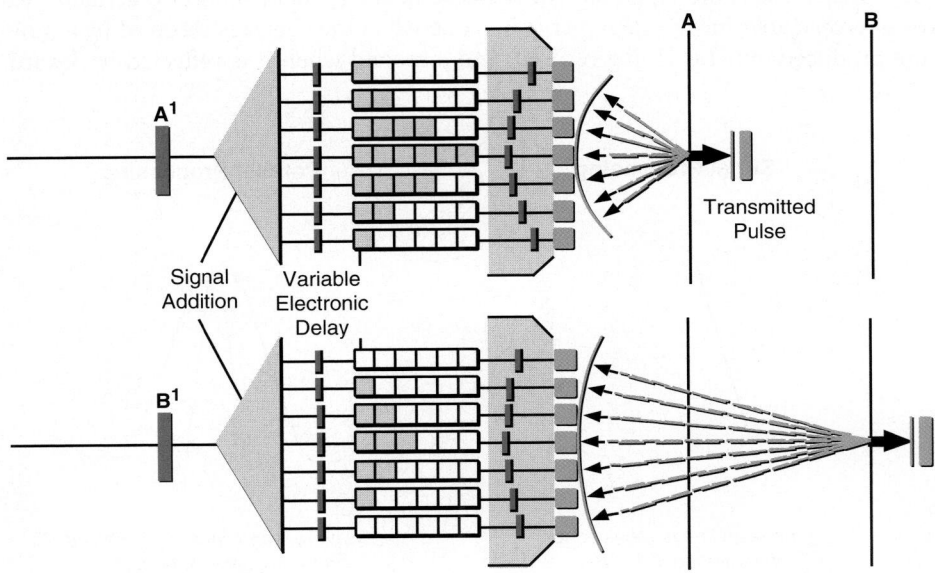

**FIGURE 1.11.** Focused Reception of Ultrasound. Delay lines may be introduced to allow dynamic focusing on reception of ultrasound as well as transmission.

**Temporal, Spatial, and Velocity Trade-offs in Doppler Flow Mapping**

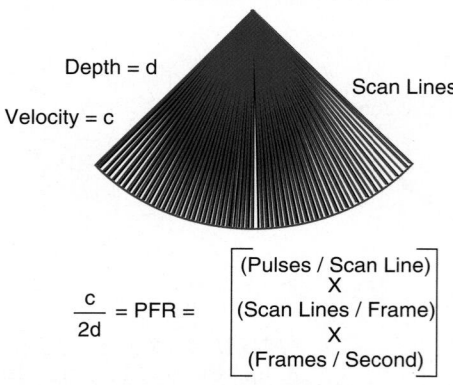

$$\frac{c}{2d} = PFR = \begin{array}{c} \text{(Pulses / Scan Line)} \\ \times \\ \text{(Scan Lines / Frame)} \\ \times \\ \text{(Frames / Second)} \end{array}$$

**FIGURE 1.12.** Relationship between Imaging Resolution, Frame Rate, and Pulse Repetition Frequency. In the absence of parallel processing, the product of frame rate, scan lines per frame, and pulses per scan line (in color Doppler) cannot exceed the pulse repetition frequency.

▶ **TABLE 1.1 Echocardiographic Frame Rates Serial vs. Parallel Processing**

|  | *Serial* | *Parallel* |
|---|---|---|
| M-mode: | 200 Hz | 400 Hz |
| 2-D: | 30–40 Hz | 120–400 Hz |
| Color Doppler: | 10–15 Hz | 40–120 Hz |
| Tissue Doppler: | 7–12 Hz | 30–90 Hz |
| Spectral Doppler: | 50–200 Hz | 50–400 Hz |

the strongest echoes (11,12). By filtering out all the fundamental frequency on the reception of the ultrasound signal and displaying only the harmonics, it is possible to eliminate much of the near-field artifact, as well as the cavity clutter signal that results from the weak side lobes arising from the ultrasound beam (13). This process has resulted in dramatic improvements in transthoracic image quality, particularly in technically difficult subjects, although it has not proven to be necessary in transesophageal echo imaging.

## Doppler Echocardiography

The Doppler principle is used to determine the velocity of blood or tissue motion inside the body. As shown in Figure 1.15, when a source of sound is moving toward an observer, its frequency is shifted upward, whereas, if the sound source is moving away from the observer, it is shifted downward in frequency. This is described mathematically in Figure 1.16. For sound transmitted from a moving object, the shift in frequency is roughly proportional to the velocity relative to the speed of sound in that medium. Thus, if blood were moving at 1% the speed of sound, there would be a 1% shift in the frequency of that sound. In the case of ultrasound, there are actually two Doppler shifts, one when the sound is received by a moving red cell, and a second when it is reflected backward,

multiple scan lines to be processed simultaneously. This has allowed a sudden increase in two-dimensional and color Doppler frame rate as shown in Figure 1.13 and Table 1.1.

Another dramatic improvement in ultrasound image quality in recent years has been the result of tissue harmonic imaging. As shown in Figure 1.14, there is a gradual change in the shape of the ultrasound wave as it propagates through the body, due to the fact that the crest of the wave propagates faster than troughs, ultimately producing more of a saw-tooth shape (9,10). The only way to generate such an altered shape in the wave form is by injecting energy into it at harmonics (or multiples) of the fundamental frequency. These harmonics have two important characteristics: 1) They are not present near the skin, but only develop after the wave is propagated into the region of the heart; and 2) they are produced only by

**Serial Processing**

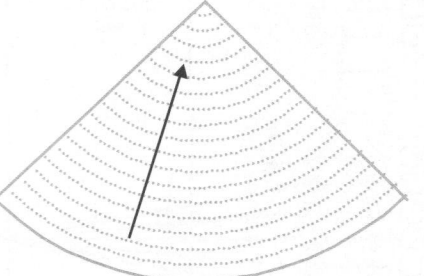

*One scan line is received for each ultrasound pulse.*

**Parallel Processing**

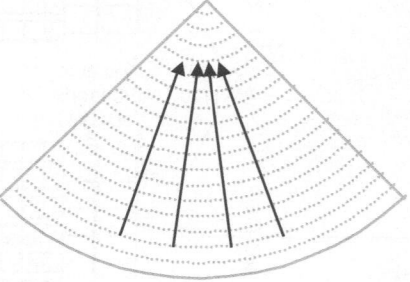

*Several scan lines are received for each ultrasound pulse.*

**FIGURE 1.13.** Serial versus Parallel Processing. By simultaneously processing multiple scan lines, it is possible to increase frame rate dramatically over the prior limitations of single scan line processing.

**Harmonic Generation**
*Harmonics Emerge as Wave Travels*

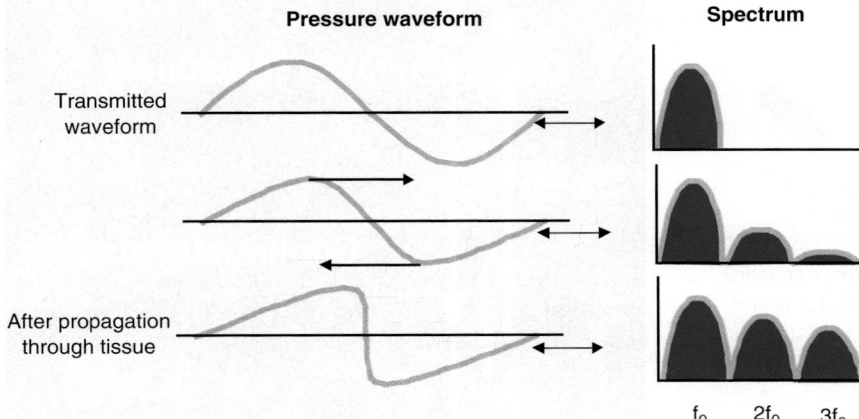

**FIGURE 1.14.** Harmonic Generation. Because of the nonlinear propagation of ultrasound in tissue, harmonic energy appears in the waves as they propagate deeper into the chest.

so that blood moving at 1% of the speed of sound will shift the frequency by 2. An additional complicating factor is that the frequency shift is only proportional to the component of velocity that is moving towards the transducer, given by the cosine of $\theta$ where $\theta$ is the angle of blood movement relative to the ultrasound beam. By taking all of these factors into account, it is possible to take an observed frequency shift and calculate a velocity as demonstrated in Figure 1.16. Doppler echocardiography is based on the principle that a moving object will alter the frequency of the reflected ultrasound. The change in frequency due to the scattering of ultrasound signals after contacting moving cellular blood components is the Doppler shift.

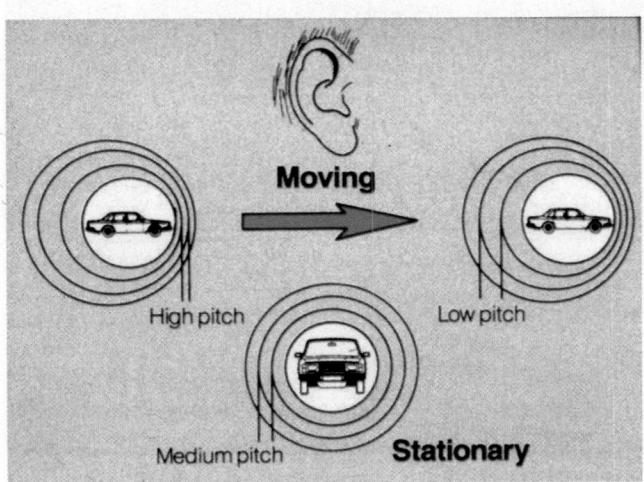

**FIGURE 1.15.** The Doppler Principle. For sound transmitted from a moving object, the shift in frequency is roughly proportional to the velocity relative to the speed of sound in that medium.

*Doppler Effect*

*Nonmoving Object: $f_t = f_r$*

Transmitting ultrasound probe at frequency $f_t$

Receiving ultrasound probe at frequency $f_r$

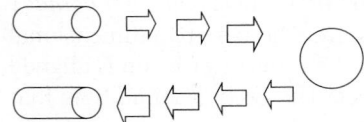

*Object Moving toward Probe: $f_r > f_t$*

*Object Moving Away from Probe: $f_t > f_r$*

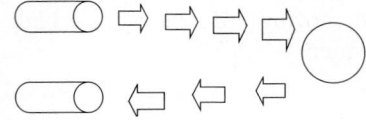

Thus, the blood flow can be determined using the Doppler effect of the reflected ultrasound frequency from the red blood cells.

The mathematical relationship between the change in frequency of the reflected signal and the velocity of the red cell is:

$$V = \frac{f_r - f_t \times c}{\cos \theta \times 2 f_t}$$

where $\Delta f = f_r - f_t$ = Doppler frequency shift

$\theta$ = the angle of incidence between the Doppler transducer and the velocity vector.

### The Doppler Principle

- *Sound transmitted from a moving object:*

$$\frac{\Delta f}{f} = \frac{v}{c}$$

- *Sound reflected from a moving object*

$$\frac{\Delta f}{f} = \frac{2v}{c}$$

- *....from an object moving at angle*

$$\frac{\Delta f}{f} = \frac{2v \cos \theta}{c}$$

- *Rearranging........*

$$v = \frac{c \, \Delta f}{2f \cos \theta}$$

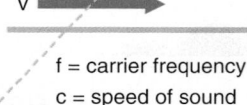

f = carrier frequency
c = speed of sound

**FIGURE 1.16.** The Doppler Principle. Mathematical derivation of the Doppler equation.

Remember, as the angle $\theta$ approaches 90°, the cos $\theta$ is zero. Whereas at an angle $\theta$ of 0°, the cos $\theta$ is one. C = the velocity of sound in tissue (1540 m/s) constant. $f_t$ = the frequency of the transmitted signal. This number is known because you set the frequency. Two represents that it is the reflected signal (travel to and then travel from). $f_r$ is the reflected signal frequency.

Based on the above assumptions, the best Doppler measurements are made when the Doppler probe is aligned parallel to the blood flow. This is the *First Paradox* of Doppler echocardiography. The best two-dimensional images are obtained when the transducer beam is aligned perpendicular to the object. The *Second Paradox* is that high resolution two-dimensional images are obtained with high ultrasound frequencies but high quality Doppler signals require low Doppler frequencies (< 2MHz). This is because the equipment used can't accurately pick up the reflected signals from fast moving red cells with a high transmitted transducer frequency (4,5,7).

### Continuous Wave Doppler

The simplest Doppler principle to understand is that of continuous wave Doppler. In this modality, ultrasound is continually transmitted by one crystal and continually received by another. Figure 1.17 demonstrates this principle along with a typical display of aortic stenosis velocity. Continuous wave Doppler allows the quantification of arbitrarily high velocities, but does not give information on where along the scan line that velocity is originating. This is termed *range ambiguity*. The most common application of continuous wave Doppler is application of the Bernoulli equation to quantify pressure drop across a stenosis. The fundamental principle of the Bernoulli

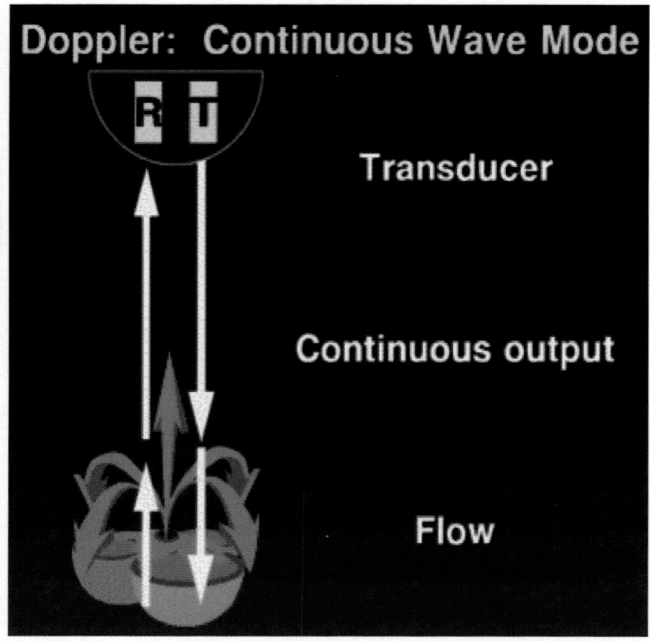

**A**

**B**

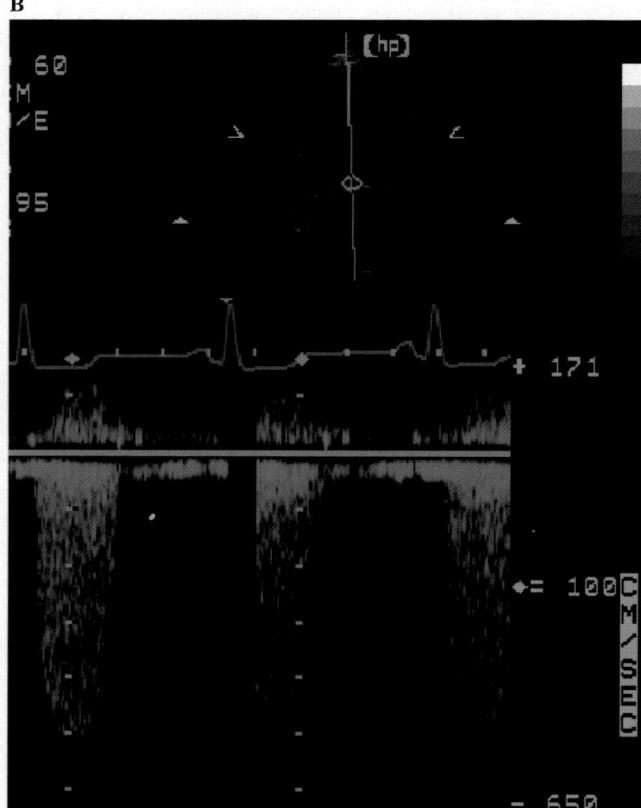

**FIGURE 1.17.** Continuous Wave Doppler. By using two crystals to continuously send and receive ultrasound, it is possible to quantify velocities of any speed in the heart, though at the price of not knowing where that velocity originates along the scan line.

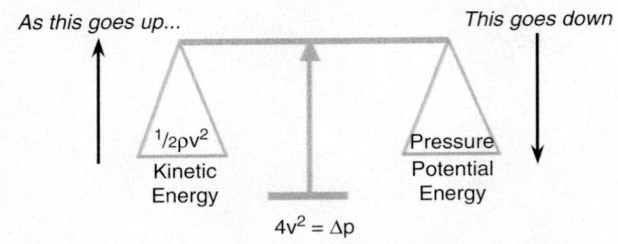

**Bernoulli Equation**
*Balancing Potential and Kinetic Energy*

As this goes up...          This goes down

$^1/_2\rho v^2$
Kinetic
Energy

Pressure
Potential
Energy

$4v^2 = \Delta p$

**FIGURE 1.18.** Bernoulli Equation. By accounting for the balance between potential and kinetic energy, it is possible to qualify the pressure drop across a valvular stenosis.

equation is conservation of energy, whereby an increase in kinetic energy as blood accelerates through a stenosis must be accompanied by a concomitant fall in potential energy, represented by pressure across that stenosis (Fig. 1.18). For sufficiently abrupt and severe stenosis, with pressure drop measured in mmHg and velocity in meters per second, the pressure drop $\Delta p$ is given quite simply by $\Delta p = 4v^2$. This will cause range ambiguity but eliminate aliasing. Thus, the CW Doppler can measure high velocity flows (in excess of 7 m/sec) as in stenotic valves. The processing of the continuous wave Doppler uses fast Fourier Transformation (14–17). The ultrasound system's computers perform fast Fourier Transformation. It uncovers the returning complex frequency shift signals and transforms them into the individual velocities.

### Pulsed-Wave Doppler

The second major type of Doppler processing is pulsed-wave Doppler, where the Doppler interrogation is at a particular depth rather than across the entire line of the ultrasound beam, as in continuous wave Doppler. The pulsed wave (PW) transducer is used as both a receiver and transmitter of ultrasound waves. In pulsed-wave Doppler, the transducer emits a burst of ultrasound and then turns off. The reflected waves from different distances return at different times. The receiver mode in the same transducer is then gated open corresponding to a particular depth of interrogation. A complete cycle of transmission waiting and receiving is called the pulse repetition frequency (PRF). The greater the depth of interrogation of the pulsed ultrasound beam the longer the waiting period. Therefore, the deeper the interrogation, the lower the PRF, and the lower the maximal velocity that can be measured. To interrogate at a certain depth (D), time must be permitted for the ultrasound burst to travel to and from the depth or equal to 2(D). The time gate (delay) between transmission and reception is expressed in the relation $T_d = 2D/Vc$ (4). As the depth increases, eventually the frequency of sampling will be insufficient to measure the particular Doppler shift. When the Doppler frequency shift is less than half the sampling frequency shift, an ambiguous signal will appear to be going in the opposite direction (3,5,7). This is referred to as aliasing and occurs when Doppler shifts above the Nyquist limit are obtained. A similar phenomenon is seen in western movies when the frame rate of the movie camera is exceeded by the velocity of the movement of the wagon wheels, resulting in the appearance of a wheel rotating in reverse direction.

The pulse repetition frequency (PRF) is the amount of short bursts of ultrasound at a particular frequency per second. The maximal velocity that can be quantified by pulsed-wave Doppler systems is limited to one-half of the PRF. This maximal frequency shift is known as the *Nyquist limit*. At frequency shifts above this limit the returning signal becomes distorted and the velocity is indeterminable. This distortion above the Nyquist limit is called *aliasing*. Pulsed-wave Doppler is useful to determine blood flow at a precise location. However, the receiving circuitry is turned on only for a brief interval, corresponding to a depth of specific interest, as shown in Figure 1.19. This process is repeated, allowing a whole series of Doppler-shifted signals to accumulate before being processed by a fast Fourier transformation to yield the specific velocity at that point (11–14). A new set of pulses is then begun, which will be accumulated and analyzed to detect the next point in time in the Doppler spectrum.

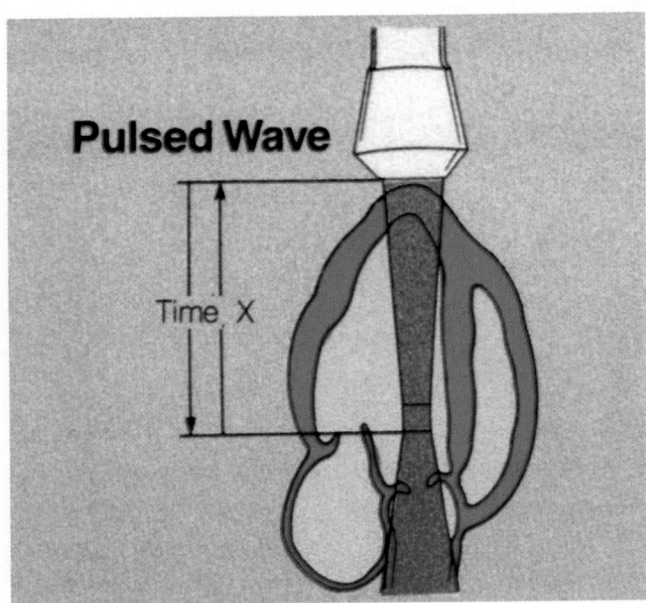

**FIGURE 1.19.** Pulsed-wave Doppler. A brief burst of ultrasound is allowed to propagate into the chest and then the receiver circuitry is activated to receive Doppler-shifted information from a specific depth.

There is a tradeoff between the fidelity to velocity (which is improved by having multiple pulses per time-point) and the temporal resolution of the Doppler (which is improved by having short pulse trains to allow more rapid sampling in time). It is also important to recognize that the pulsed-Doppler sample volume is not infinitesimally small, but instead has a certain length, width, and thickness, as shown in Figure 1.20. Thus, it is important to consider whether an observed signal may actually arise from an adjacent structure rather than the one that is thought to be interrogated.

The major problem with pulsed-wave Doppler is that of aliasing. Signal processing theory dictates that to fully resolve a signal of frequency $f$, it is necessary to sample it at twice that frequency ($2f$) (3,4,7). For example, in Figure 1.21, the solid white waveform is fully determined by the samples represented by the white dots. In contrast, if the underlying signal is in fact the dotted waveform, then the samples are too sparsely spaced to determine what the true frequency of that waveform is. What this means in pulsed-Doppler examinations is that there is a maximum velocity detectable by pulsed-wave Doppler, which is given by the depth of the sample volume and the frequency of interrogation. Figure 1.22 indicates that above this aliasing velocity, the pulsed-wave signal will wrap around, appearing to come from the opposite direction, whereas continuous wave Doppler is capable of resolving velocities of any magnitude, although at the sacrifice of having no range resolution to localize where along the scan line the signal arose. In order to eliminate aliasing from a pulsed-Doppler interrogation, continuous wave Doppler can be used (range ambiguity is an issue): use a low frequency transducer, decrease the depth of

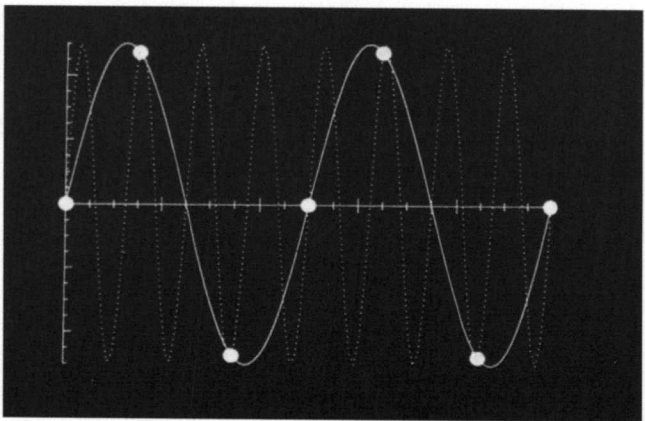

**FIGURE 1.21.** Aliasing: Understanding Doppler Waveform. To fully resolve a waveform, it must be sampled at least twice per cycle.

interrogation by changing the view (increases the PRF), use high PRF Doppler, and change the baseline scale to shift the wrapped around signal in to the right position.

### Color Doppler Echocardiography

Color flow Doppler is based on pulsed-wave (PW) Doppler in that multiple sample volumes are evaluated along each individual sampling line. Usually up to eight ultrasound bursts along each sample or scan line are used to determine the frequency shifts (velocities) being

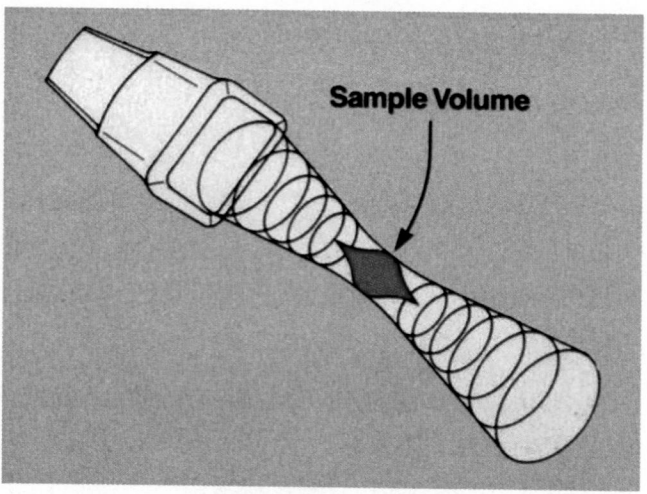

**FIGURE 1.20.** Pulsed-Doppler Sample Volume. The sample volume is not infinitesimally small, but can be adjusted in its length, width, and thickness. The larger the sample volume, the stronger the Doppler signal, but also the greater potential for detecting extraneous signals around the area of interest.

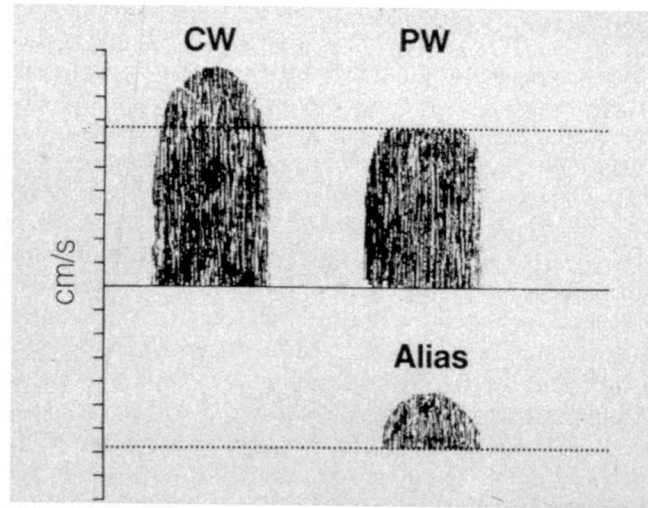

**FIGURE 1.22.** Continuous-wave versus Pulsed-wave Doppler. Because of the limited sampling interval (pulse repetition frequency) pulsed-wave Doppler can only detect velocities up to a certain magnitude before they wrap around and appear to be coming from the opposite direction. In contrast, continuous-wave Doppler, with its continuous sampling, is able to resolve velocities that are arbitrarily high, though at the cost of range resolution.

encoded in color (red indicating flow toward the transducer and blue indicating flow away from the transducer). Each burst is called a *packet* and the packet size is eight (4,7). Because color Doppler echocardiography is based on PW technology, it is subject to the limitations of PW Doppler as aliasing. As with PW Doppler, if the sampling velocity exceeds one-half the pulse repetition frequency for that particular depth, aliasing of the color signal will occur. This is visualized as an immediate change from red to blue, or color aliasing, as the interface where the blood flow velocity exceeds the established maximal measurable velocity. Decreasing each of the following parameters may decrease the Nyquist limit or the maximal measurable velocity of flow: 1) depth of interrogation sector, 2) width of interrogation sector, 3) scan line density, and 4) density of ultrasound bursts per scan line. Shifting each of these parameters in addition to shifting the baseline away from the flow will optimize the signal and reduce aliasing. In color Doppler flow mapping, an entire sector screen is encoded in color representing the velocity of blood or tissue motion within that sector. It uses a fundamentally different manner of signal processing from the fast Fourier transformations used by pulsed- and continuous-wave Doppler. This is due to the amount of data that must be processed by color flow mapping. As shown in Figure 1.23, a brief burst of ultrasound is emitted, but then the entire returning sound train for the whole sector of interest is received, amplified, and stored in memory. Then a second pulse is emitted and likewise is stored in digital memory. Then using a mathematical method called *autocorrelation,* the wave fronts in pulse 1 and 2 are compared with each other. In regions where blood flow is moving toward the transducer, the waves of pulse 2 tend to be shifted forward relative to the signal in

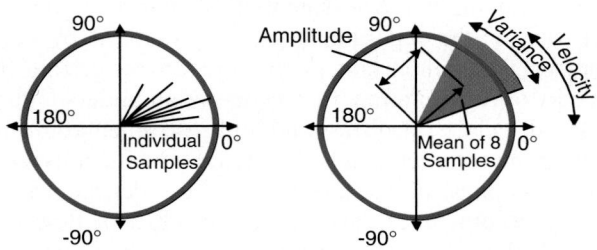

**Color Doppler Processing**
*Calculation of Velocity (Phase),*
*Variance and Amplitude*

**FIGURE 1.24.** Color Doppler Processing. By averaging the phase and amplitude of multiple color Doppler pulses together, it is possible to obtain a more precise estimate of color flow velocity.

pulse 1; whereas when blood is going away from the transducer, the pulse 2 signal lags a bit behind pulse 1. This permits the machine to determine velocity all along the scan line. If only two pulses were emitted, then about all that could be determined from the autocorrelation would be whether the blood was moving toward or away from the transducer. Instead, multiple pulses are emitted and all compared with each other, generating a family of velocity estimates as shown in Figure 1.24. These velocity estimates have characteristic phase (the angle around the circle, proportional to the velocity), amplitude (the strength of the signal), and variance (the degree of scatter between successive estimations related to turbulence). By averaging these together, it is possible to obtain a more precise estimate of velocity for every point along the scan line.

With color flow mapping, as with two-dimensional echocardiography, there is a tradeoff between temporal resolution and the accuracy of the information in the image (Fig. 1.12). If the packet size is increased the velocity accuracy is increased but the temporal, or real-time, resolution is decreased. Most packet sizes are between 3 and 20 pulses (4,7). If there are too few pulses the velocity determinations will be inaccurate. If there are too many pulses the frame rate will be low. The same is true for the line density (the number of scan lines per frame). Velocity mode of color flow mapping is the representation of the average of the packet velocities along a scan line. Variance mode of color flow mapping is a continuation of the velocity mode. The packet velocities are averaged, then the variability between the individual velocity estimates in the packet is examined. If the packet contains a broad band of velocities, then another color is introduced into the color map. These colors are typically green or yellow. If the range of these velocities is small, then only a small amount of variance color is introduced. If the range is large, then a large amount of variance color is introduced.

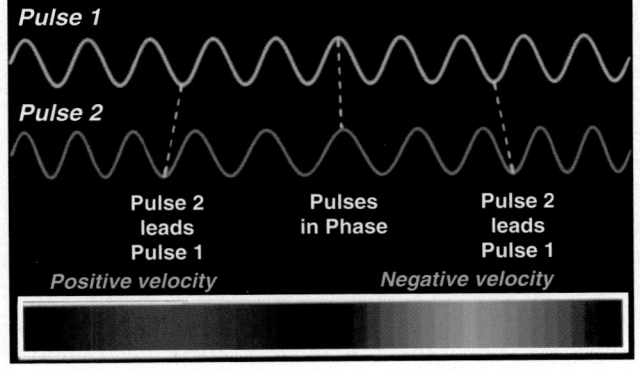

**FIGURE 1.23.** Color Doppler Processing by Autocorrelation. By comparing the phase shift in successive pulses of ultrasound, it is possible to determine the velocity all along the sector of interest.

### Instrumentation Factors in Color Doppler Imaging

One of the most important applications of color Doppler echocardiography is assessment of valvular regurgitation. The size of the regurgitant jet, as visualized by color Doppler, is an important method for characterizing the severity of regurgitation. Consequently, an understanding of the principles of ultrasound and instrumentation impacting the color jet area is essential. First, one must consider the physical parameter that best determines jet size—jet momentum, given by the product of flow rate through the regurgitant orifice and the driving velocity. Thus, for the same amount of flow going through a valve, a high-pressure jet will appear larger than a low-pressure jet, explaining why blood pressure should be measured at the time of any echocardiographic examination. There also is an important issue of jet constraint and distortion by adjacent walls. As shown in Figure 1.25, eccentrically directed wall jets tend to flatten out along the wall and are considerably smaller than the equivalently sized central jets, by a factor of more than half (Coanda effect) (17). Finally, there are a host of instrumentation factors than can impact the appearance of the jet. Figure 1.26 shows the impact of color gain on a mitral regurgitant jet as visualized by transesophageal echo. Clearly, as gain is increased, the jet appears larger, and ultimately (gain = 56) there is extraneous color in the tissue, indicating excessive gain. In general, the color gain should be advanced until color pixels just begin to appear within the tissue, and then reduced slightly to eliminate these. Output power has a similar effect on jet size, and should generally be set at levels that are well within the FDA standards for output power. Figure 1.27 demonstrates the impact of pulse repetition frequency or scale on the size of the jet. For color Doppler, there is a finite number of velocity bins that are represented on the screen, typically about 16 forward and 16 backward. Thus, the lowest velocity that is visible is approximately 1/16 of the maximal velocity (4). Because maximal velocity is determined by the pulse repetition frequency (PRF) and the transducer frequency, reducing PRF can make the jet larger by encoding lower velocities within the jet. When the scale is set at the maximum value (69 cm/sec), the instrument displays all velocities greater than about 4 cm/sec. Reducing the scale to 39 now encodes velocities greater than 2 cm/sec, with a larger jet, while reducing it still further to 17 encodes velocities greater than 1 cm/sec with a clearly larger jet size.

Transducer frequency has a dual effect on the size of the regurgitant jet. The primary effect of increasing transducer frequency is to encode lower velocities within the jet, making the jet appear larger. However, higher frequency ultrasound is attenuated more by intervening tissue, so this may make the jet appear smaller. Typically, the frequency effect dominates in transesophageal echo, where there is little attenuation, whereas the attenuation effect is dominant in transthoracic echocardiography (Figure 1.28). There are many other ways to alter color Doppler display, but in general, it is recommended that a standard setup be established for a given laboratory, and that this standard be adhered to unless there are special circumstances. In this way, the eye may become trained to assess regurgitant jets in a consistent manner based upon the local paradigm for setting up instruments.

## High Frame Rate Doppler

Some of the newer ultrasound platforms provide a high PRF mode. In high PRF Doppler, a pulsed-Doppler signal is sent to a structure at a specific depth. Some of that pulse penetrates further. If you set the sample volume to 0.5, 2, 3, or 4 times the structure's depth, these additional wave fronts will add (return in the same phase). In high PRF mode, sampling does not wait for a specific distance gate. If the sample volume is placed at one-half the distance from the structure to be analyzed, aliasing can be eliminated. Thus with high PRF Doppler, higher velocities may be measured but with the potential artifact of ambiguity or image appearance at multiples or fractions of the true depth (18).

## Contrast Echocardiography

*Myocardial contrast echocardiography* (MCE) is a diagnostic technique that utilizes an ultrasound contrast agent and adapted ultrasound systems to enhance ultrasound imaging. Early MCE applications employed contrast solutions containing relatively large bubbles, which were injected into the venous circulation to demonstrate gross anatomic abnormalities. Currently contrast solutions are available containing smaller and more stable microbubbles approximately the size of red blood cells. Presently, several commercially produced *contrast agents* are undergoing evaluation (Table 1.1). In general, the mean diameter of the microsphere is smaller than red blood cells (10 μm) (19–21). These enabling agents behave as intravascular tracers. The ultrasound technology available for contrast agent detection and quantitation has evolved greatly in the past few years. Contrast echocardiography is a diagnostic tool used for assessing intracardiac structures. When contrast is employed to image intracardiac shunts, right heart valvular incompetence, and/or pericardial effusions then hand-agitated saline (or blood or both) is used. The agitated solution, which serves to produce as ultrasound reflectors, creates relatively large microcavitations (40–50 microns in diameter). These microbubbles are unstable and do not last long after mixed in solution. More recently, microbubbles produced by commercial processes have resulted in smaller, more stable tracer agents (20,21). When these agents are injected intravenously, they cross the pulmonary circulation and allow enhancement of left-sided structures. In addition to

*(text continues on page 21)*

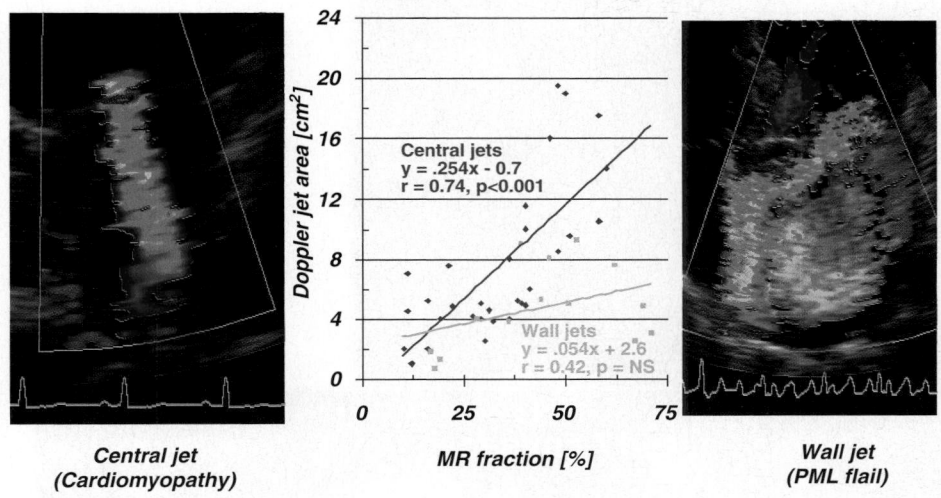

### Determinants of Jet Size
*Wall jets are 58% smaller than equivalent central jets*

**Central jets**
y = .254x - 0.7
r = 0.74, p<0.001

**Wall jets**
y = .054x + 2.6
r = 0.42, p = NS

Doppler jet area [cm²] (y-axis)

MR fraction [%] (x-axis)

**Central jet
(Cardiomyopathy)**

**Wall jet
(PML flail)**

**FIGURE 1.25.** Impact of Wall Impingement on Jet Size. Jets that are directed eccentrically against a chamber wall are less than half the size of centrally directed jets.

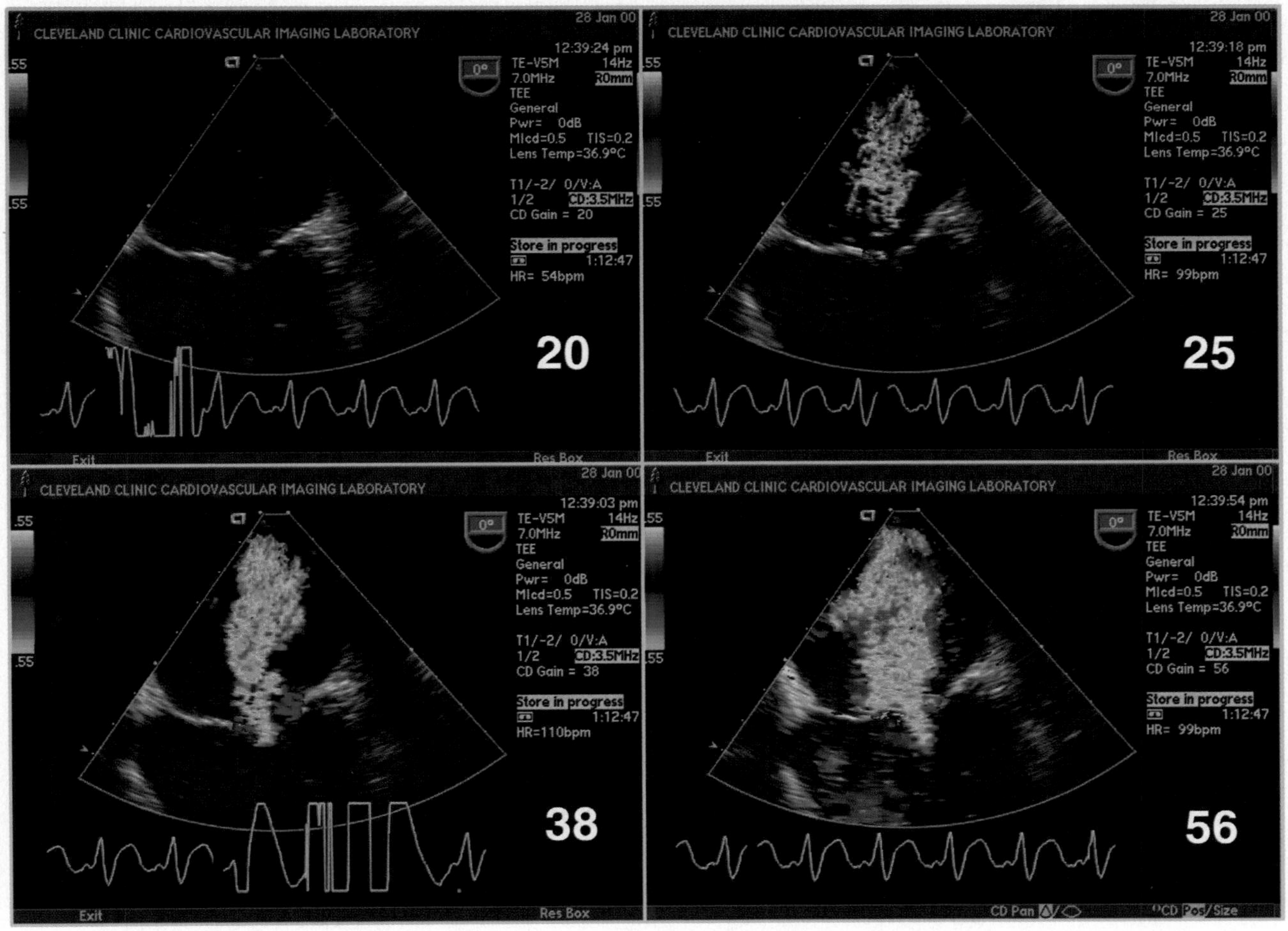

**FIGURE 1.26.** Impact of Color Gain on Jet Size. By highlighting weaker Doppler signals, color gain (and the corresponding transmission parameter, output power) critically impacts jet size.

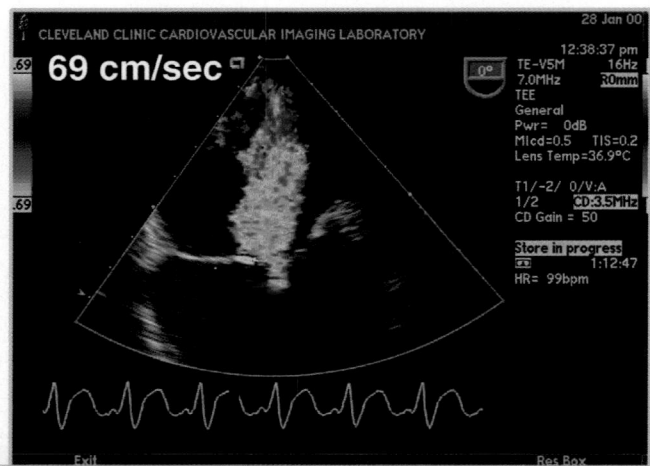

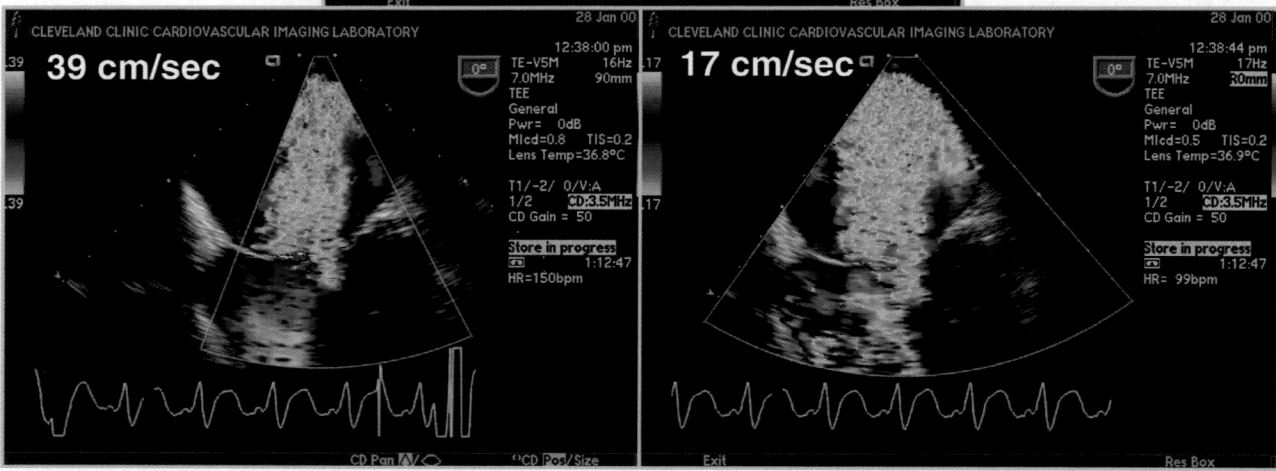

**FIGURE 1.27.** Impact of Color Scale on Jet Size (Velocity Effect). Reducing the pulse repetition frequency (PRF) lowers the minimal velocity displayed by color Doppler, thus making jets appear larger.

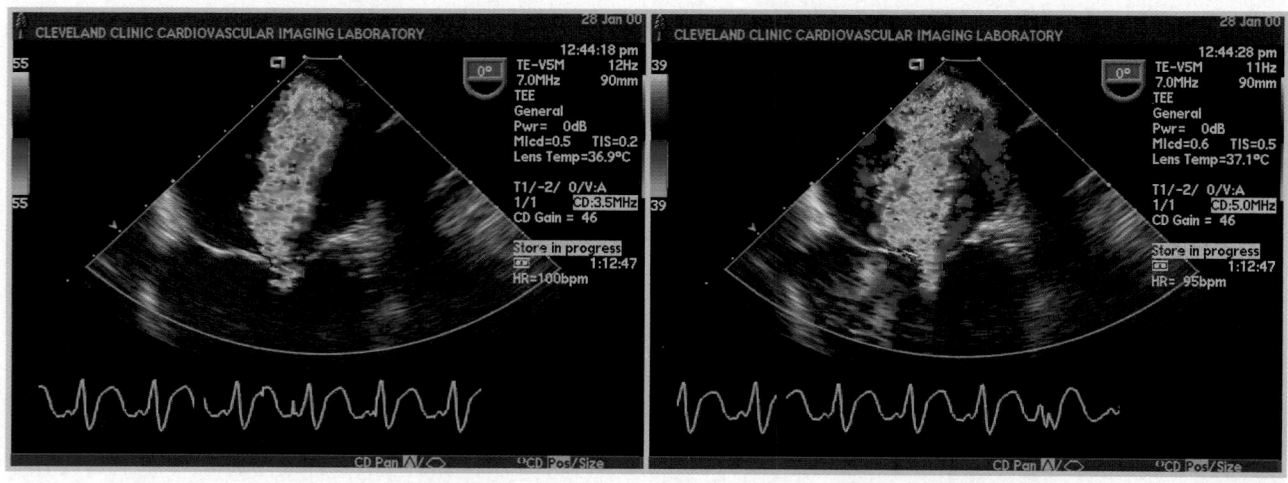

*Frequency = 3.5 MHz*          *Frequency = 5 MHz*
*Nyquist Limit = 55 cm/sec*     *Nyquist Limit = 39 cm/sec*
*Vmin ≈ 3.5 cm/sec*             *Vmin ≈ 2.5 cm/sec*

**FIGURE 1.28.** Impact of Transducer Frequency on Jet Size. Increasing the transducer frequency lowers the minimal velocity displayed by color Doppler, thus making jets appear larger by TEE. For transthoracic echo, the increased attenuation of higher frequency ultrasound generally makes the jet appear smaller.

left-sided valvular incompetence, their use has been shown to be valuable for enhancing endocardial borders and therefore regional wall motion assessment. It has been shown that despite increased resolution afforded by higher frequency TEE transducers, approximately 5% to 10% of the time, during surgical imaging, adequate wall motion abnormality interpretation is not possible. Erb et al. demonstrated that the use of contrast intraoperatively with TEE enables visualization 70% of the time when regions were not visualized without contrast (22). MCE will also enhance Doppler interrogation when inadequate spectral envelopes are problematic. Since the ultrasound contrast agents behave as surrogate RBC, they create an excellent Doppler signal enhancer. Finally, the direct, real-time interpretation of cardioplegic distribution and myocardial function reserve are applications of contrast combined with stress echo that enable the echocardiographer and surgeon to assess the adequacy of myocardial protection and surgical revascularization (23,24).

## CONCLUSIONS

The purpose of this chapter is to enable the reader to be more comfortable with the terminology and concepts that serve as the foundation for the daily use of ultrasound technology in the management of patients. A more thorough understanding of the physical principles of ultrasound effectively permits the acquisition of higher quality echocardiographic data on which the perioperative team may base their clinical decisions.

### KEY POINTS

- *Sound* can be classified as subsonic or infrasonic (less than 20 cycles/s), audible sound (20–20,000 cycles/s), and ultrasound (greater than 20,000 cycles/s).
- Echocardiography is based on the electrical conversion (by piezoelectric crystals) of reflected ultrasound waves (greater than 20,000 cycles/s frequency) from structures and blood flow within the cardiovascular system.
- Sound waves are characterized by the properties of properties of frequency (f) or number of cycles / sec, amplitude (A or loudness), and wavelength (λ) or distance between two adjacent ultrasound cycle.
- Using the average propagation velocity of ultrasound through tissue (c) or 1,540 m/s, the relation between frequency (f) and wavelength (λ) is characterized as:

$$c \ (1540 \ m/s) = f \ (cycles/s) \times \lambda \ (mm)$$

or

$$\lambda \ (mm) = c \ (1540 \ m/s) \ / \ f \ (cycles/s)$$

- *Resolution* is the ability to distinguish two points in space and is inversely related to wavelength and directly related to frequency. It follows that the longer the wavelength, the less the frequency, the less the resolution, but the greater the tissue penetration. Ultrasound waves that are reflected from structures and blood moving toward the transducer compress the wavelength and increase the frequency. The magnitude of this difference is referred to as the *Doppler shift* and is determined by the velocity and direction of the structure reflecting the ultrasound beam. Processing of this Doppler shift information by the ultrasound platform results in the two-dimensional image, as well as color flow, pulsed-wave, and continuous wave Doppler information.

## REFERENCES

1. Saxon D. Elementary quantum mechanics. San Francisco: Holden-Day, 1968:1–16.
2. Wells PNT. Biomechanical ultrasonics. New York: Academic Press, 1977.
3. Hatle L, Angelsen B. Doppler ultrasound in cardiology: Physical Principles and clinical application. Philadelphia: Lea & Febiger, 1982.
4. Thomas JD. Principles of imaging. In Fozzard HA, Haber E, Jennings RB, Katz AM. The heart and cardiovascular system, 2nd ed., New York: Raven Press, 1996:625–68.
5. Wells PN. Physics and engineering: milestones in medicine. Medical Engineering & Physics. 2001;23(3):147–53.
6. Coulam CM, Erickson JJ, Rollo FD, James AE. The physical basis of medical imaging. New York: Appelton-Century-Crofts, 1981.
7. Weyman AE, Cross-sectional echocardiography, 2nd ed. Philadelphia: Lea & Febiger, 1994.
8. Deserranno D, Greenberg NL, Thomas JD, Garcia MJ. A new automated method for the quantification of mitral regurgitant volume and dynamic regurgitant orifice area based on a normalized centerline velocity distribution using color M-mode and continuous wave Doppler imaging. Journal of Biomechanical Engineering. 2003;125(1):62–9.
9. Thomas JD, Griffin BP, White RD. Cardiac imaging techniques: which, when, and why. Cleveland Clinic Journal of Medicine. 1996;63(4):213–20.
10. Prior DL, Jaber WA, Homa DA, Thomas JD, Mayer Sabik E. Impact of tissue harmonic imaging on the assessment of rheumatic mitral stenosis. American Journal of Cardiology. 2000;86(5):573–6, A10.
11. Rubin DN, Yazbek N, Garcia MJ, Stewart WJ, Thomas JD. Qualitative and quantitative effects of harmonic echocardiographic imaging on endocardial edge definition and side-lobe artifacts. Journal of the American Society of Echocardiography. 2000;13(11):1012–8.

12. Desser TS, Jeffrey RB. Tissue harmonic imaging techniques: physical principles and clinical applications. Seminars in Ultrasound, CT & MR. 2001 Feb.;22(1):1–10.
13. Prior DL, Jaber WA, Homa DA, Thomas JD, Mayer Sabik E. Impact of tissue harmonic imaging on the assessment of rheumatic mitral stenosis. American Journal of Cardiology. 2000;86(5):573–6, A10.
14. Bracewell RN. The Fourier transform and its applications. New York: McGraw Hill, 1978.
15. Application of Fourier processing in echocardiography. In Weyman AE. Cross-sectional echocardiography, 2nd ed. Philadelphia: Lea & Febiger, 1994:1299–1306.
16. Chandra S, Garcia MJ, Morehead A, Thomas JD. Two-dimensional Fourier filtration of acoustic quantification echocardiographic images: improved reproducibility and accuracy of automated measurements of left ventricular performance. Journal of the American Society of Echocardiography. 1997;10(4):310–9.
17. Chao K, Moises V, Shandas R, Elkadi T, Sahn DJ, Weintraub R. Influence of the Coanda effect on color Doppler jet area and color encoding. In vitro studies using color Doppler flow mapping. [Journal Article] Circulation. 1992;85(1):333–41.
18. Giesler M, Goller V, Pfob A, et al. Influence of pulse repetition frequency and high pass filter on color Doppler maps of converging flow in vitro. International Journal of Cardiac Imaging. 1996;12(4):257–61.
19. Main ML, Asher CR, Rubin DN, et al. Comparison of tissue harmonic imaging with contrast (sonicated albumin echocardiography and Doppler myocardial imaging for enhancing endocardial border resolution. American Journal of Cardiology. 1999;83(2):218–22.
20. Rubin DN, Thomas JD. New imaging technology: measurement of myocardial perfusion by contrast echocardiography. Coronary Artery Disease. 2000;11(3):221–6.
21. Pasquet A, Greenberg N, Brunken R, Thomas JD, Marwick TH. Effect of color coding and subtraction on the accuracy of contrast echocardiography. International Journal of Cardiology. 1999;70(3):223–31.
22. Erb JM, Shanewise JS. Intraoperative contrast echocardiography with intravenous optison does not cause hemodynamic changes during cardiac surgery. Journal of the American Society of Echocardiography. 14(6):595–600, 2000.
23. Aronson S, Savage R, Lytle B, Albertucci M, Karp RB, Loop F. Identifying the etiology of left ventricular dysfunction during coronary bypass surgery: The role of myocardial contrast echocardiography. J Cardiovasc Thorac Anes 1998;12:512–18.
24. Aronson S, Jacobsohn E, Savage R, Albertucci M. The influence of collateral flow on distribution of cardioplegia in patients with an occluded right coronary artery. Anesthesiology 1998;89:1099–107.

## QUESTIONS

1. Changing the image depth in echocardiography will change the _____.
   A. frequency of the ultrasound wave
   B. the pulse repetition frequency
   C. amplitude
   D. propagation velocity
   E. pulse duration

2. Axial resolution is improved by _____.
   A. decreasing bandwidth
   B. increasing wavelength
   C. decreasing pulse duration
   D. decreasing frequency
   E. increasing beam width

3. Lateral resolution is dependent on _____.
   A. amplitude
   B. propagation velocity
   C. acoustic impedance
   D. beam width
   E. reverberations

4. Which of the following modalities should be used to obtain the mitral inflow time velocity interval?
   A. Color M-mode
   B. Continuous wave Doppler
   C. Pulsed-wave Doppler
   D. Color Doppler
   E. Amplitude-modulated echocardiography

5. Which of the following can be used to improve the temporal resolution using color Doppler?
   A. Increasing line density
   B. Increasing color sector
   C. Decreasing depth
   D. Decreasing amplitude
   E. Decreasing interrogation angle

# Chapter 2

# Digital Echocardiography

## *Mario J. Garcia*

Over the last two decades, echocardiography has created a tremendous impact in health care. Much of the success of echocardiography is due to its ability to provide "live" moving images that can be reviewed and easily understood by all types of health-care providers and patients. This ability has been only minimally exploited in the past, given the limitations of analog technology. Meanwhile, other areas of medical imaging have adopted digital recording as the standard.

The first efforts in digital echocardiography occurred in the early 1980s. Given storage capacity and processing speed limitation, digital echo was limited to stress testing and evaluation of coronary artery disease, using a quad-screen format and grayscale images (1). New technological advances in echocardiography today permit registering moving images in digital format, allowing logical archival; rapid data retrieval, copy, and transfer; off-line quantitative analysis; and side-by-side comparison with superior image resolution (2).

The American Society of Echocardiography established a task force in 1992 to educate the echocardiographic community on the promise and pitfalls of digital echocardiography and advise the Digital Images and Communications in Medicine (DICOM) committee on a standard image format for echocardiography (3).

## ANALOG VERSUS DIGITAL IMAGING

In order to appreciate the advantages of digital echocardiography, we first need to understand the fundamental principles of analog and digital imaging. The principal feature of analog representations is that they are continuous. In contrast, digital representations consist of values measured at discrete intervals. Analog technology refers to electronic transmission accomplished by adding signals of varying frequency or amplitude to carrier waves of a given frequency of alternating electromagnetic current. Analog data is typically represented as a series of sine waves. Television, radio, and telephone transmission mostly use analog technology, although more recently, the use of digital technology in these fields is rapidly expanding. A theoretical advantage of analog data is its ability to provide in theory an infinite spectrum of data. This is most easily appreciated when analyzing the fidelity of signals that are "naturally" analog, such as audio or video signals. In order to transform this data into a digital format, an electronic process known as analog-to-digital conversion needs to be implemented. The input to any analog-to-digital converter consists of a signal with a theoretically infinite number of values that has been transformed to an electrical voltage, and the output is a multi-level signal that has defined levels, typically a power of two (e.g., 2, 4, 8, 16, 32). Thus, the most basic digital signal has only two states and is called a binary signal, whereas the only possible values are 0 and 1. Any number can then be represented in binary form as sequences of zeros and ones. Because we are primarily interested in images in echocardiography, let's analyze how a picture can be converted into digital data.

A rectangular image of theoretically unlimited resolution is first limited to a matrix of finite dimensions, e.g., 800 horizontal × 600 vertical lines (VGA resolution). This matrix then has 480,000 pixels (smallest distinct geographical square zone). In a picture each pixel may contain color information within a scale. The number of color values is given by a number of bits that are contained in each pixel, and is equal to two to the power of the number of bits; e.g., if there are three bits per pixel, then eight different values could be encoded (000, 001, 010, 100, 011, 101, 110, and 111). In a typical grayscale echocardiographic image, there are 256 shades of gray (8-bits per pixel, or $2^8 = 256$). Thus, the size of the raw binary digital file that encodes the information contained in this picture is $400 \times 600 \times 8 = 384,000$ bits (or 48,000 bytes, since 1 byte = 8 bits). If higher color definition is required, the number of bits per pixel may be increased. A 32-bit per pixel resolution provides $2^{32} = 4,294,967,296$ colors and will require $400 \times 800 \times 32 = 1,920,000$ bits = 240,000 bytes. Regardless of its resolution, digital data has a finite limitation, and that is why, in theory, an audio signal recorded in analog format (vinyl record) may be reproduced with higher fidelity than a digital recording (compact disc). If this is the case, what is the advantage of digital media?

Digital signals travel more efficiently than analog signals, mainly because digital impulses, which are well defined, are easier for electronic circuits to distinguish from noise, which is chaotic. Noise can occur naturally or by electrical interference and is incorporated randomly to analog data during transmission, recording, processing, and display. In an audio recording, noise can be appreciated as background "hissing." Once noise is introduced, it cannot be separated from the original signal and is compounded with more noise introduced during each additional process. Thus, every time that analog data is transferred and/or copied, signal-to-noise ratio decreases. For that reason, second copies of video or music analog recordings are never identical to their originals. Here lies one of the main advantages of digital media—it is capable of identically reproducing the original set of data.

## COMPONENTS OF A DIGITAL LABORATORY

### Data Acquisition

Cardiac ultrasound imaging equipment initially obtains analog data from the imaging transducer, where ultrasonic reflections stimulate a piezoelectric crystal to produce electrical impulses (Fig. 2.1). In order to convert these electrical impulses into images, they need to be processed by a computer that analyzes time delay, signal intensity, and frequency shifts in order to determine the location, density, and velocity of each cardiac structure. Because most computers can only process digital data, the original analog signals need to be transformed to dig-

ital signals. A process known as analog-to-digital conversion performs this task, during which continuous data is converted into discrete values. For example, color Doppler usually displays 32 velocity values (16 for each direction). Thus, for a Nyquist velocity of 64 cm/sec, each discrete velocity represents a multiple of 4 cm/sec, and the original analog input is rounded to the nearest digital value (e.g., 7 cm/sec to 8 cm/sec). At the time of digital processing, other pertinent data are added to the images (time and date, equipment settings, calibration data, patient demographics, etc.). However, binary digital impulses, all by themselves, appear as long strings of ones and zeros, and have no apparent meaning to a human observer. In order to display still or moving ultrasound images in a video monitor, they need to be converted to analog signals. The circuit that performs this function is a *digital-to-analog converter*.

Basically, digital-to-analog conversion is the opposite of analog-to-digital conversion. Although this process is required as a final step in order to provide meaningful information to a human observer, it introduces noise and results in loss of the other pertinent data described above. Thus, the most efficient method to obtain true digital echocardiographic data requires direct output of digital images from an ultrasound machine, before digital-to-analog conversion. Selected cine-loops of fixed (temporal interval) or variable length (e.g., ECG-triggered, single or multiple cardiac cycles) may be then stored to disk or transmitted through a standard network. Most modern ultrasound systems provide digital output, though their implementation details may differ. With direct digital output, maximal fidelity is maintained, and calibration information is retained, facilitating quantitation on an off-line review workstation. An alternative to direct digital output is digitalization of video output data. This method per-

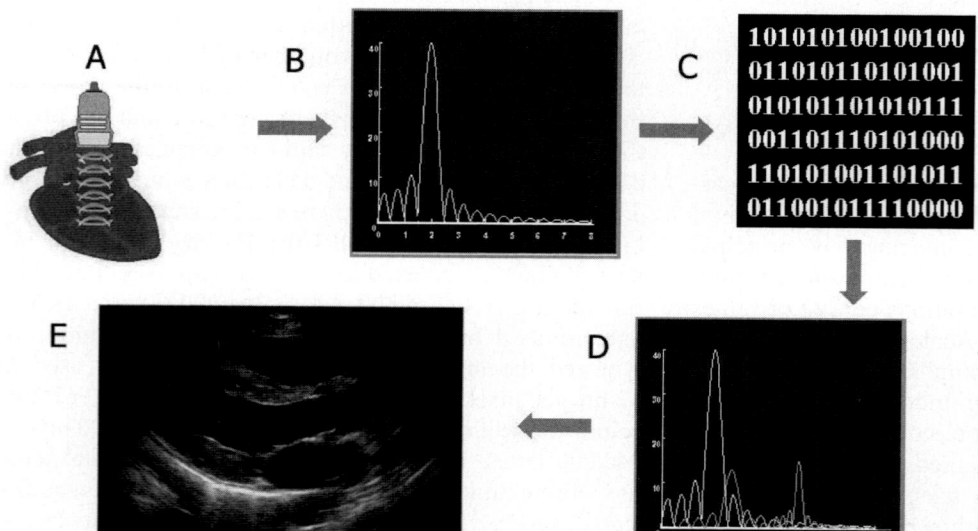

**FIGURE 2.1.** Generation of an echocardiographic image. **A:** Ultrasound pulses. **B:** Analog electrical impulses. **C:** Analog-to-digital conversion. **D:** Digital-to-analog conversion. **E:** Video output. Notice the distortion of the original signal by added noise (**D**).

mits retrofitting of older ultrasounds systems, however, at the expense of some introduction of noise and without calibration information. Nevertheless, for legacy systems this is a quite acceptable way of integrating them into a digital laboratory. Most medium and large laboratories are familiar with the use of digitizing equipment used for stress echocardiography. Over recent years, several manufacturers have developed computer systems equipped with acquisition cards and dedicated software suitable for echocardiography. These systems take the direct video output used by the video recorder and monitor and reconvert the analog input to digital data. While virtually any generic product can be used to capture images, variable resolution adjustment, trimming, ECG triggering, labeling, and formatting capabilities are only available through dedicated commercially available systems.

## Data Compression

In order to efficiently store and transfer digital echocardiographic studies, some form of data compression is required. A single-frame echocardiographic image has a resolution of 640 horizontal × 480 vertical pixels × 24-bits per pixel, equalling 922 KB. Thus, at an average frame rate of 30 Hz, a 15 min uncompressed echocardiography study requires about 25 GB. Handling uncompressed data therefore becomes impractical, given current storage and transfer speed limitations.

One way of reducing the size of a digital echo study is by implementing clinical or "intelligent" compression. In a conventional echocardiographic study, a sonographer records 2-D and color Doppler images, as well as several M-Mode and spectral Doppler still frames obtained from multiple windows, angulations, and depths. Each segment recorded comprises several cardiac cycles. Using "intelligent" compression, representative video loops of a more limited length are acquired instead, either based on ECG-triggered cardiac cycles or on segments of fixed one- or two-second durations. A typical echocardiographic study may be reduced in this manner to about 30 loops of approximately one second each. A complete study, therefore, could consist of 30 seconds instead of 15 min of data, reduced to 0.8 GB, or in other words, achieving 30:1 compression. Intelligent compression works well most of the time, with minimal loss of diagnostic content, because single cardiac cycles contain mostly the same information that multiple repeated cardiac cycles obtained from the same view, angle, and depth do. There are pitfalls and limitations of intelligent compression, however, which will be discussed later in this chapter.

An alternative or complementary way to reduce the size of a digital echocardiographic study is the implementation of digital compression. Digital compression is obtained by specific mathematical algorithms that seek to summarize data redundancy within one image or over consecutive images in a temporal sequence. Two general forms of digital compression exist, *lossless* and *lossy compression*.

Lossless compression algorithms, such as run length encoding (RLE), reduce only redundant information. For example, in an echo image, the pixels of the nonimage portion of the 640 × 480 matrix outside the scan sector always has the same value and thus can be reduced to a simple mathematical expression. Converting the gray-scale areas of a color Doppler image to an 8-bit depth (256 shades of gray per pixel) can also reduce image size, without content loss. Most lossless compression algorithms, however, can achieve only modest reductions in file size, typically 2:1 to 3:1.

Conversely, lossy compression can achieve 20:1 or greater data reduction. Lossy compression algorithms, such as the LZW used for Target Image File Format (TIFF) images or the Joint Photography Expert Group (JPEG) format, are commonly used for still-frame images and have been adopted by DICOM. The JPEG compression format includes 29 distinct coding processes and provides adjustable compression quality; the greater quality factor corresponding to the lesser compression (Fig. 2.2). Therefore, a tradeoff can be made between image quality and file size. The JPEG compression algorithm uses a frequency-based transform (Discrete Cosine Transform or DCT), a quantization technique for losing selective information that can be acceptably lost from visual information and Huffman coding, a technique of lossless compression that uses code tables based on statistics about the encoded data. The JPEG compression scheme has demonstrated in clinical studies to be usable in echocardiography at compression ratios of 20:1 or higher (4–6). Additionally, clinical studies have shown that interpretations made by digital acquisitions are accurate in comparison to the traditional videotape review (7–9).

Other lossy compression algorithms are specifically designed for motion sequences. The MJPEG algorithm applies JPEG compression to each individual image in a sequence. The Moving Picture Experts Group (MPEG) format also employs temporal compression, exploiting the redundancies in the temporal domain. MPEG is the current motion picture industry standard for digital video (DVD) and digital audio compression. There are multiple MPEG formats, each designed for a different purpose. MPEG-1 was originally designed for encoding video for broadcasting at a transmission rate of about 1.5 Mbps (millions of bits per second). MPEG-1 audio layer-3 (MP3) is a variation of this format used for compressing digital audio. MPEG-2 can encode interlaced images at transmission rates over 4 Mbps and is used for digital TV broadcast via cable or satellite. MPEG-1 and -2 can compress digital video by factors varying from 25:1 to 50:1. Both MPEG-2 and MPEG-3 may be used to broadcast

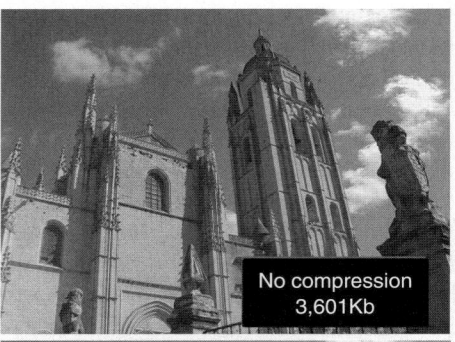
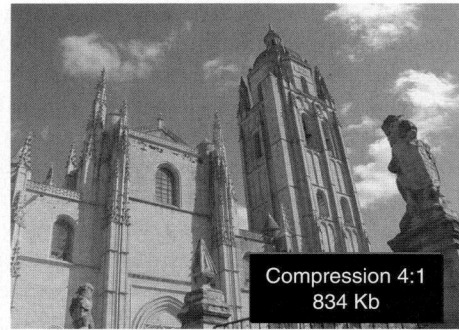
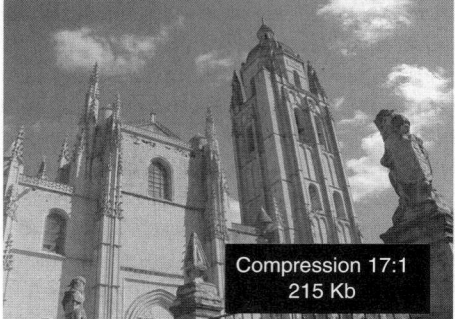
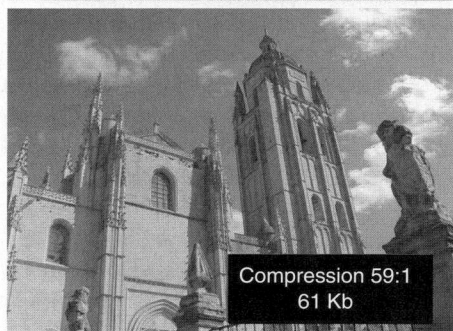

**FIGURE 2.2.** Impact of JPEG image compression on image quality and file size.

High Definition Television (HDTV) signals. MPEG-4 is the newest standard developed and used for Direct Video Disc (DVD). In addition to the techniques used for JPEG compression, MPEG uses motion-compensated predictive coding, in which the differences in what has changed between an image and its preceding image are calculated and only the differences are encoded, as well as bidirectional prediction, in which some images are predicted from the pictures immediately preceding and following the image. MPEG-1 (10–13) and MPEG-2 (14) have been shown to be useful transfer syntaxes in echocardiography, and have been clinically validated at compression ratios up to 100:1. In a recent multicenter study, we demonstrated the clinical capability of MPEG-recorded echocardiograms (15). We have continued to investigate the use of MPEG compression and its effect on quantitative measures (16). Six reviewers performed blind measurements from still-frame images selected from 20 echocardiographic studies simultaneously acquired in s-VHS and MPEG-1 format. Measurements were obtainable in 1,401 of 1,486 (95%) MPEG-1 variables versus 1,356 of 1,486 (91%) sVHS variables (p < 0.001). There was excellent agreement between MPEG-1 and sVHS two-dimensional linear (r = 0.97, MPEG-1 = 0.95 sVHS + 1.1 mm, p < 0.001, $\Delta$ = 9 ± 10%), two-dimensional area measurements (r = 0.89), color jet areas (r = 0.87, p < 0.001), and Doppler velocities (r = 0.92, p < 0.001). Interobserver variability was similar for both sVHS and MPEG-1 readings. Our results indicate that quantitative off-line measurements from MPEG-1 digitized echo studies are feasible and comparable to those obtained from sVHS. However, as of today, MPEG formats have not been incor-

porated by DICOM. Ultrasound equipment manufacturers have not adopted this technology due to the high cost of the hardware required for MPEG encoding. Nevertheless, independent companies have developed and marketed systems that can be adapted to existing ultrasound machines.

Future compression schemes, such as wavelet compression, promise even more efficiency (quality-to-file size ratio). *Wavelets* are mathematical functions similar to Fourier analysis, which make recovery of weak signals from noise possible. Wavelet-compressed images can further reduce file size by a factor of 4:1 compared to JPEG. In wavelet compression, images are converted into a set of mathematical expressions. We have investigated the application of the wavelet transform to two-dimensional sequences of image data derived from digital subtraction of consecutive frames. Images were divided into primary (P) and delta ($\Delta$) frames, with the image content of each $\Delta$ frame defined as the difference from the previous P frame. A wavelet-compression algorithm utilizing difference image data (1P:4$\Delta$) results in a CR of nearly 100:1 and an improved SNR (P: 36.5 ± 0.05, $\Delta$: 32.4 ± 0.13 dB) compared with JPEG (31.96 ± 0.10 dB, CR = 20:1). More recently this approach has been extended using a three-dimensional wavelet transform for the compression of echocardiographic sequences (17, 18).

## Data Transfer

Network transfer is the most efficient method for delivering echocardiographic studies from the acquisition to the interpretation and to the final storage location. A network is a series of nodes (input and output devices) interconnected by communication paths. Networks can be characterized in terms of spatial distance as local area networks (LAN), metropolitan area networks (MAN), and wide area networks (WAN). A LAN is a group of computers and associated devices that share a common communications line and typically share the resources of a single main computer or server within a small geographic area (such as the ones used in a medical office building or hospital setting within an office building). Usually, the server has specific applications and data storage that are shared by multiple computer users. Individual users needing applications can download and upgrade them as frequently as needed, and run them from their local computers. Networks permit the sharing of common resources, such as viewer stations and printers. Thus multiple people can simultaneously access the same data—an important advantage of the digital echocardiographic laboratory that cannot be matched with analog video technology. A user can share files with others on the LAN server; but read and write privileges can be restricted at multiple levels by a LAN administrator. Thus, other unique advantages of the digital echo lab are data redundancy and tight data security. A network can be characterized by the type of data transmission in use (TCP/IP or System Network Architecture); by the usual nature of its connections (dial-up or switched, dedicated or non-switched, or virtual connections); and by the types of physical links. All these variables in turn determine data-transfer speed.

Ethernet is the most widely installed LAN technology. An Ethernet LAN can use different types of physical links, such as twisted pair wires, coaxial cable, or optical fiber. The most commonly installed Ethernet systems are 10BASE-T, and provide transmission speeds up to 10 Mbps (Megabits or million bits per second). "BASE" indicates baseband signaling, which means that only Ethernet signals are carried on the medium, and "T" represents twisted-pair. In addition to 10BASE-T, 10-megabit Ethernet can be implemented with other media types: 10BASE-2, using thin-wire coaxial cable, provides a maximum segment length of 185 meters; 10BASE-5, using thick-wire coaxial cable, maintains a signal up to 500 meters; 10BASE-F, using optical fiber, which carries much more information than conventional copper wire, is in general not subject to electromagnetic interference; and 10BASE-36, using broadband coaxial cable, carries multiple baseband channels for a maximum length of 3.6 kilometers. Fast Ethernet provides transmission speeds up to 100 megabits per second (100BASE-T) and can also have different types of physical connection: 100BASE-T4 (four pairs of copper-twisted wire), 100BASE-TX (two pairs of data-grade twisted-pair wire), and 100BASE-FX (two-strand optical fiber cable). Gigabit Ethernet provides 1 gigabit (or 1 billion bits) per second and it uses primarily optical fiber cable. Other technology available that can transfer data at even higher speeds, such as ATM (asyn-

chronous transfer mode) and 10-Gigabit Internet, are not so practical for internal implementation but will likely play a significant role in the future of digital echocardiography in telemedicine.

A network is built in a manner similar to the building of a road system: many smaller one-lane country roads lead to two-lane roads that lead to a few multiple-lane highways as one approaches areas of major traffic. Thus, in a network, 10BASE-T Ethernet may be used to connect individual users (such as physicians' offices) to the server, while 100BASE-T is used to connect areas of higher traffic (ultrasound machines and central reading stations for the server), and Gigabit Ethernet may serve as the system backbone (connecting the server to storage devices). LAN Devices (ultrasound machines, viewing stations, etc.) are connected to the cable with 10BASE-T or 100BASE-T network cards. A network card or adapter is a circuitry designed to provide expanded capability to a computer. It is provided on the surface of a standard-size rigid material and then plugged into one of the internal ultrasound machine computer's expansion slots in its motherboard. A network card can control a device (such as a hard disk drive) from a remote connection. LAN devices may compete for access at any given time, thus a protocol using carrier sense multiple access with collision detection (CSMA/CD) is implemented, which acts as a "traffic light." A large network operates more efficiently with the implementation of network switches. A switch is a device that selects a path or circuit for sending a unit of data to its next destination. A switch may also include the function of a router, a device or program that can determine the route and specifically what adjacent network point the data should be sent to. Network switches, also known as layer-three switches or IP switches, control traffic among LAN devices that have specific IP addresses. A network connection can be used exclusively for a given time interval by two or more LAN devices and then switched for use to another set of parties. This type of all-or-nothing switching is known as circuit-switching and is primarily used for telephone communications. Alternatively, using packet-switching, multiple LAN devices can share the same paths at the same time and the particular route a data unit travels can be varied as traffic conditions change in the network. In packet-switching, a file is divided into packets, which are units of a certain number of bytes. The network addresses of the sender and of the destination are added to each packet. Packets from the same file may travel different routes and arrive at different times, but at their destination, these are reassembled into the original file. Packet-switching is the preferred method implemented in computer network communications.

Having the ultrasound machine connected to the hospital network at the time of the examination allows you to send complete studies at once or incrementally, loop by loop as images are obtained. A complete adult echo study may contain 50 to 100 MB (megabytes or millions of bytes) of data. This volume of data must be moved across the network when the exam is first conducted and then again every time the exam is reviewed. Therefore, a single examination can generate several hundred megabytes of network traffic. It is clear that high-speed connections (at least 100 Mbps) are necessary in order to make data transfer fast and efficient (Fig. 2.3). Even more important than the basic speed of the network is having the proper architecture. Networks may use either routers or switches in moving packets of data around. The advantage of a switch is that it establishes an isolated connection between the two computers that are transferring the echo data at a given time, thus limiting the impact on other network traffic.

An alternative to the use of a network connection is the use of removable media, commonly referred as "sneaker net." Studies may be temporarily stored in the ultrasound device hard drive and later transferred or directly recorded into removable optical media and then transferred to the review workstation. Most modern ultrasound machines provide an optional magneto-optical recording device, capable of recording from 120 MB to more than 1 GB (giga or billion bytes) per disk. Internal or external readers installed in the reading stations can then be used to read the contents of these disks. Although this last method is considerably slower, it may be feasible for small-volume labs, in the absence of an existing digital network. It may also be easier to implement when the same ultrasound machine is used at multiple locations (e.g., performance of bedside ultrasound studies) without a physical network connection. Another disadvantage of the sneaker net approach is the lack of a standard format for removable media, resulting in the need to use multiple media types and devices in echo laboratories that carry multiple ultrasound systems from different vendors.

## Data Storage

Once a digital echocardiographic study is acquired and transferred, it will require some type of storage (Fig. 2.4). In general terms, it is best to think of storage at different levels. Storage for immediate review of current studies needs to be rapidly accessible, while long-term storage for older studies that have already been reviewed and interpreted requires higher capacity and not necessarily fast speed. There is an inverse relationship between capacity and access speed and a direct relationship between speed and cost.

The fastest access storage media is random access memory (RAM). RAM is the physical medium where the operating system, application programs, and data in current use (e.g., an open echocardiographic study) reside, so that they can be quickly reached by the computer's microprocessor. RAM has the physical form of discrete microchips or modules containing multiple chips that are plugged directly into the computer's motherboard and are directly connected to the microprocessor. RAM is much faster to read (in the order of nanoseconds) than the computer's hard disk (in milliseconds); however, the data only resides in RAM temporarily and is replaced with new data every time a new task is performed (such as opening a second study), and is erased every time the computer is turned off. RAM primarily focuses on work at hand, but can only keep a limited amount of data at a time. If the capacity of RAM is exceeded (e.g., by opening a very long echocardiographic study), the microprocessor needs to access the hard disk (virtual memory), slowing down the

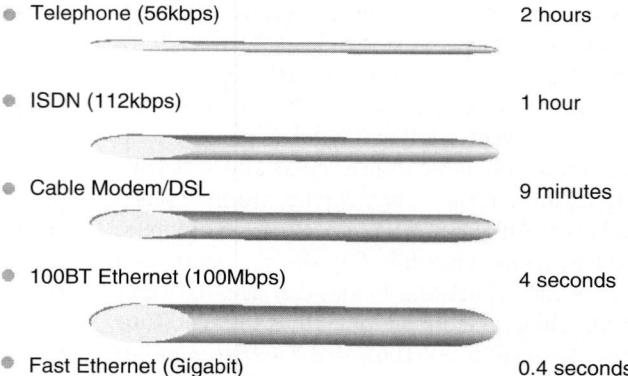

| | |
|---|---|
| Telephone (56kbps) | 2 hours |
| ISDN (112kbps) | 1 hour |
| Cable Modem/DSL | 9 minutes |
| 100BT Ethernet (100Mbps) | 4 seconds |
| Fast Ethernet (Gigabit) | 0.4 seconds |

**FIGURE 2.3.** Average transmission time for a 50-megabyte echocardiographic file for various types of transmission lines.

* Network speed increases efficiency but at a price. T1 or T100 are reasonable.
* Installing a network switch isolates your sub-network from external traffic, also increasing transfer speed.

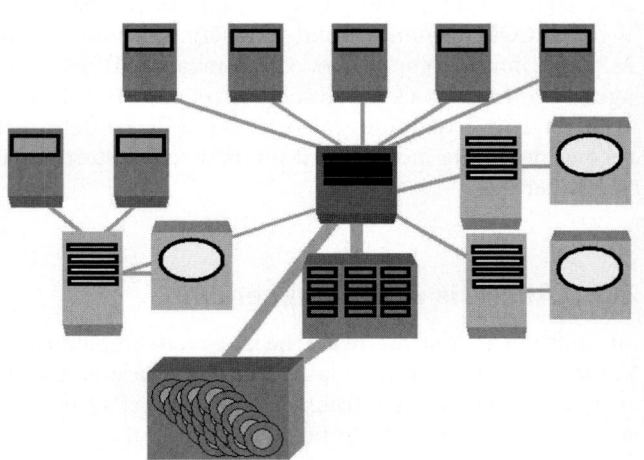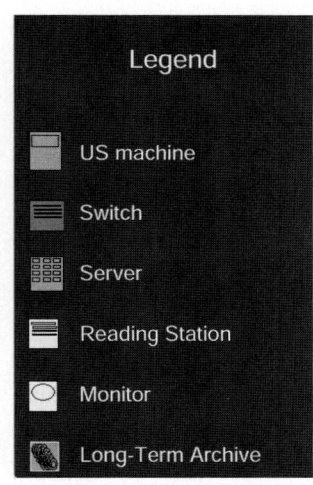

**FIGURE 2.4.** Typical architecture of a large digital echocardiographic laboratory.

computer's operation. Fortunately, the cost of RAM has dramatically decreased over the years, and today's midrange personal computers have anything from 64 to 256 MB standardly available. In order to operate efficiently, however, a viewing/reading station requires a minimum 1GB of RAM, since the operating system, the viewer application software and at least one echocardiographic study, will be loaded at a time. It must be emphasized that the size of an echo study file loaded into RAM is the size of the study fully decompressed. This is typically 10 to 20 times larger than the original compressed file, so that a typical 30 MB compressed file can require up to 600 MB of RAM space. If multiple studies need to be loaded and reviewed simultaneously, or if multiple applications need to run simultaneously (word processor, web browser, spreadsheet, virus protection software) these requirements will increase, otherwise, the microprocessor will need to access the hard disk and the process will be significantly slower. Therefore, in order to maximize performance, the following basic principles should be observed: 1) install more RAM than the minimum anticipated need; 2) limit the size of each echocardiographic study—for example, save a pre- and postintraoperative study for the same patient as two separate smaller files; and 3) avoid the use of multiple applications, e.g., isolate your laboratory subnetwork from any other internal or external networks whenever possible and then turn off virus protection software.

The second hierarchical level of storage is within the main computer server. Here enough space should exist to store all studies that have been acquired and reviewed. Depending on the anticipated volume, this device may be a high-end PC or a dedicated high-capacity hard disk RAID array (redundant array of independent hard disks). The size of the local storage can be tailored to fit the data generation and particular requirements of a given lab. Storage capacity should include not only current studies,

but also older studies performed in patients who are currently active (outpatients with scheduled echo exams and inpatients). These are desirable for serial comparisons. A system that communicates with the hospital information service may search and retrieve ahead of time selected studies from long-term storage devices for online comparisons. A RAID array also permits storing the same files on a different hard disk. Because the use of multiple disks increases the mean time between failures, storing data redundantly also increases fault-tolerance. Thus data stored in a given disk will not be lost in the event of an individual disk failure. A RAID array appears to the operating system as a single logical hard disk. In a RAID array each hard drive is partitioned into units (stripes) ranging from a sector (512 bytes) up to several megabytes. The stripes of all the disks are interleaved and addressed in order. In a single-user system, such as an echocardiographic laboratory server, where large records are stored, the stripes may be intentionally configured small so that the parts of a single file are stored in multiple disks and can be accessed quickly by reading all disks simultaneously. RAID arrays can be configured in at least nine different manners, allowing the system to be optimally configured for a specific application. Probably, the most suitable configuration for a dedicated digital echo lab server is RAID-3. This type uses striping and dedicates one drive to detect errors and recover data. Data recovery is accomplished by calculating the exclusive object recognition (XOR) of the information recorded on the other drives. Local RAID array servers can store up to about 1 TB (terabyte or trillion bytes) of data, but eventually reach a physical storage limitation, particularly for a large volume laboratory. At our institution, our dedicated echo lab RAID array server stores $1/2$ TB. Given our volume of about 160 studies at 40 MB per file, it permits local storage of about two months of current data. Thus, it is clear that a third device dedicated to long-term storage is required.

The third hierarchical level dedicated to long-term storage requires the highest capacity at the lowest cost. Because retrieval of these files is performed infrequently, access speed is not a priority. Long-term storage devices can take the physical form of jukeboxes that contain different types of removable or fixed media. These can be multiple sequential hard drives, CD-ROM, DVD-ROM, digital linear tape (DLT), or Advanced Intelligent Tape (AIT). The capacity is greater with the latter, whereas each magneto-digital tape may store several gigabytes of data at a cost of less than 5 cents/GB, reaching up to 1 or more PB (pedabytes or quadrillion bytes) for the entire system. At the Cleveland Clinic, we share a digital tape archive (PowderHorn, StorageTek, Louisville, Colorado) with the cardiac catheterization laboratory and the department of radiology. The library will hold up to 6,000 20 GB cartridges. An archive utility from Problem Solving Concepts performs a scheduled backup of daily studies to the tape archive. This can currently be performed using the standard file transfer protocol (FTP) or through a network file system (NFS) connection. The utility also automatically removes studies from local storage that have been previously archived. Average access time to retrieve a study from the digital tape archive is 2 minutes 20 seconds, although the range for access is between 1.5 and 4.5 minutes. The mean transfer rate (including tape mounting and data transfer) is 0.40 MB/s. Nevertheless, this time delay still compares very favorably with the time that it would take to find an individual videotape in a library and to locate a single study within a tape. Optical media, such as a CD, can also hold content in digital form. These disks are written and read by laser and include several CD and DVD formats. Optical disc capacity ranges from 0.6 to 6 GB. One optical disk holds about the equivalent of 500 floppies worth of data. Durability is an important advantage of optical media; lasting up to seven times as long as traditional magnetic storage media. CD-R disks usually hold between 650 and 700 MB. Using packet-writing software and a compatible CD-R drive, it is possible to save data to a CD-R in the same way data is saved to a floppy disk; however, each part of the disk can only be written once. It is not possible to delete files and then reuse the space. Re-writeable disks (CD-RW) use an alloy layer that can be transformed to and from a crystalline state repeatedly so that files can be deleted and the disk reused. Given the lower cost and higher reliability of CD-R disks, these are probably a better option for long-term storage. DVDs (digital versatile disks) are higher capacity optical disks and are expected to eventually replace CD-R technology. A DVD with two layers on each side can store up to 17 gigabytes of data. This technology is relatively in its infancy and current costs of removable media and hardware are still high compared to other long-term storage options. Neverthe-

less, DVDs could become more widespread in the future if the DICOM committee and ultrasound vendors adopt MPEG-2 image compression as a standard. MPEG-2 images have four times the resolution of MPEG-1 images and can deliver real-time video at 60 interlaced fields per second providing more than 2 hours of video storage capacity per DVD.

## Data Analysis and Management

In addition to the hardware necessary to implement a digital echocardiographic laboratory, software is needed to manage the storage, transfer, and archival of data as well as the connectivity to hospital information systems, including scheduling, reporting, and billing. This software in general continuously runs in the background over the network, interacting with each of the echo machines, and viewing stations. It manages the image transfers from the network echo machines or computer disk to the local storage, and then migrates that data onto the archive. This software may be part of an integrated hardware–software-network solution or a stand-alone piece of software to be used on third-party hardware purchased separately. Integrated solutions are usually more expensive but easier to implement. In general, they are also easier to service, since any problem that may occur falls into the responsibility of a single manufacturer and service contract. Software solutions are less expensive and offer the advantage of allowing unlimited future hardware upgrades, running separate applications within the same hardware. Maintenance issues, however, may become more complex because problems need to be troubleshot in order to determine if they are caused by software, hardware, or the network itself, which may be covered by separate contracts and manufacturers. Either integrated or separate software solutions for the digital echo lab can provide similar functionality. At the most basic level, they may serve as an image viewer, be able to open different file formats, and perform image decompression and display. At the most advanced level they can provide integration with a hospital information system, automatic billing, off-line measurements, report generation, and export functions to multiple databases and even a web browser (Fig. 2.5). These solutions require the installation of management software in the server and client software at each reading/viewing terminal. Each client and the server are related in a manner that when the client makes a service request from the server, the latter fulfills the request. In a network, the client/server model provides a convenient way to interconnect programs that are efficiently distributed across different locations. It permits each client to access the full database of studies archived in the server, and automatically distributes upgrades from

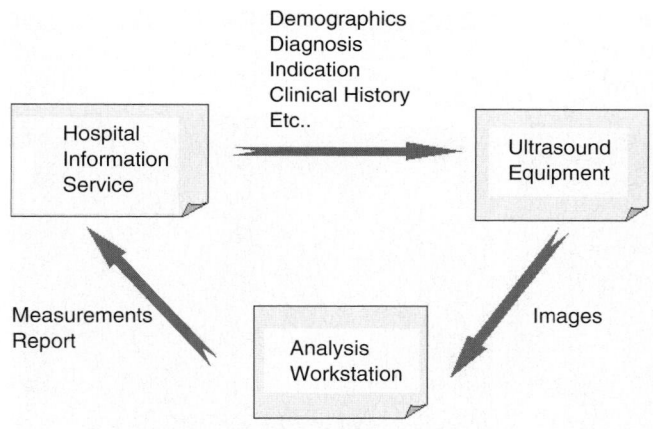

**FIGURE 2.5.** Diagram illustrating the process of integration of the echocardiogram into the hospital information network and electronic medical record.

the server, to each client. TCP/IP (Transmission Control Protocol/Internet Protocol) is the basic communication language used in client/server relationships. TCP/IP is a two-layer program. The higher layer, TCP, manages the assembling of a message or file into smaller packets that are transmitted over the network and received by a TCP layer that reassembles the packets into the original message. The lower layer, IP, handles the address part of each packet so that it gets to the right destination. Packets from the same message may travel through different paths and in different orders, they are reassembled correctly at the destination. TCP/IP and applications that use TCP/IP are stateless because each client request is considered a new request unrelated to any previous one, allowing multiple clients to implement communications with the server independently and simultaneously. Different application protocols that use TCP/IP include the Internet Hypertext Transfer Protocol (HTTP), the File Transfer Protocol (FTP), Telnet for remote communications, and the Simple Mail Transfer Protocol (SMTP).

Studies acquired at the ultrasound machine are sent to the server using TCP/IP protocols, where each machine has a unique IP address. Once the complete study is received, it appears in the server's archive. A significant difficulty in some environments may be the inability for some echocardiographs to dynamically obtain a network address. Dynamic Host Configuration Protocol (DHCP) services are often used with PC hardware to allow connections in various locations, and maintain order with the control and uniqueness of network addresses. Unfortunately, current DICOM configurations on several manufacturers' machines require fixed network addresses for communication. As echocardiographic labs expand with variable hospital infrastructures, the need for echocardio-

graphic devices to have network connections in multiple locations grows, particularly during portable studies.

A database that includes the patient's name, medical record number, date and time of the study, and study type, as well as any other desired information, is then available to the review workstations. This database maintains the list of all files stored at either the RAID array or at the long-term storage device. The server software can monitor the capacity of the server's RAID array and can be automatically set up to erase old studies to accommodate new ones and to transfer studies to the long-term archive. These maintenance functions can occur transparently at times when network traffic is lower (such as at night). If the server is connected with the hospital information system, it can identify patients that appear in the active hospital list (in-patients or out-patients) and automatically retransfer their preexisting studies from the long-term archive to the RAID array, making them immediately available for review, if desired.

Client software at each reviewing station permits query of the server's database. Once single or multiple studies are called for review, they need to be transferred over the network. Upon arrival, they are stored in the client's hard disk and partially or fully loaded into RAM. A series of thumbnails appear in the viewer's screen, indicating each specific video clip or still-frame image. The user can navigate through each thumbnail or at random, calling each one of the images available in any desired sequence, a unique advantage of digital echocardiography not available through videotape. Once they are selected, these images appear at their full resolution in the screen. Multiple controls permit contrast and brightness adjustment, play speed control, trimming, and magnification. Side-by-side comparison of different clips within a study, or from different studies, is also an extremely useful feature that is unique to digital echocardiography (Fig. 2.6). A complete and customizable measurement package is often available, permitting the performance of almost any measurement and calculation that is commonly performed directly in the ultrasound machine. In contrast to videotape, calibration is not necessary because the calibration information is already included in the digital file. This feature is not available, however, for digitized studies. The results of these measurements and calculations can be transferred into a database and used to generate a report at the end of the review (Fig. 2.7). This feature can save time and eliminate human error. Moreover, measurements can be compared with tables of normalcy, and thus used to generate automatic interpretation. Once a report is completed, it can be electronically signed, transferred to the electronic medical record, and sent to a network printer at a specific location—as an e-mail attachment to the referring physician or posted as a web page—with a single keystroke.

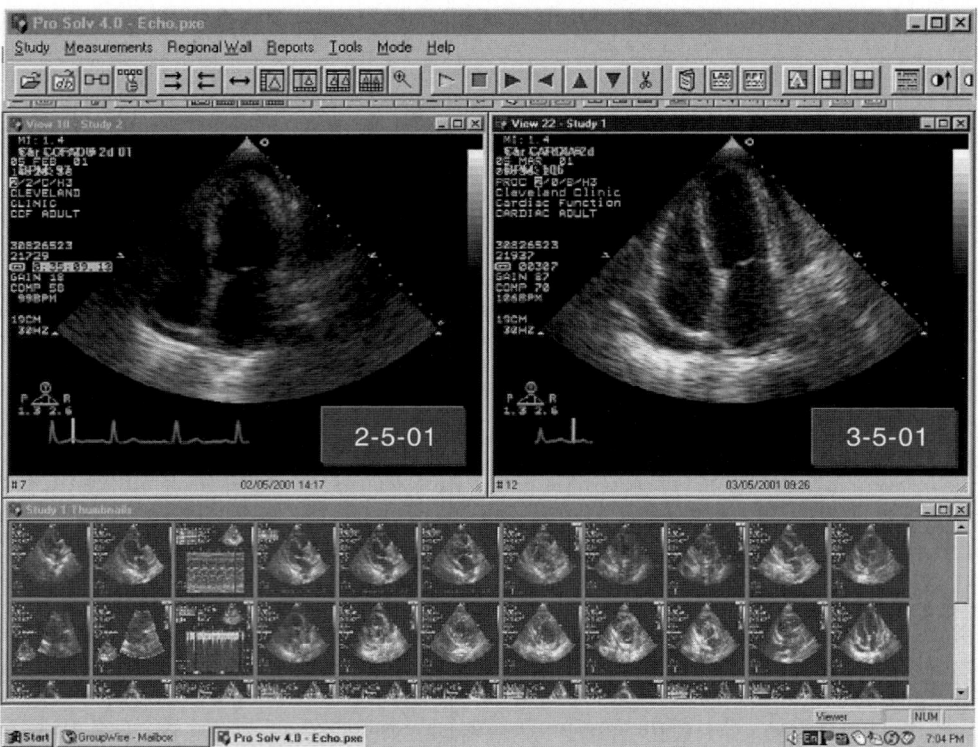

**FIGURE 2.6.** Side-by-side display of studies performed in the same patient on different days demonstrated a progression in size of a pericardial effusion.

## Remote Access

One useful feature of the digital echo lab is remote access capability. In theory, a client can be located at any remote location as long as an Internet location is in place. There are, however, two practical limitations: remote access speed and data confidentiality. Data encryption should be implemented for data transmission outside the hospital "firewall" in order to protect patient confidentiality and to comply with state and federal regulations.

Remote access can be implemented through various types of wire or wireless connections. Traditional phone service (plain old telephone service or POTS) can provide a connection between two points, such as a server and a remote access client at home over twisted-pair copper wires. Telephone services are designed for analog transmission, where an audio signal is converted to electrical impulses of varying amplitude and frequency and sent over a twisted-pair wire. A modem is a device that

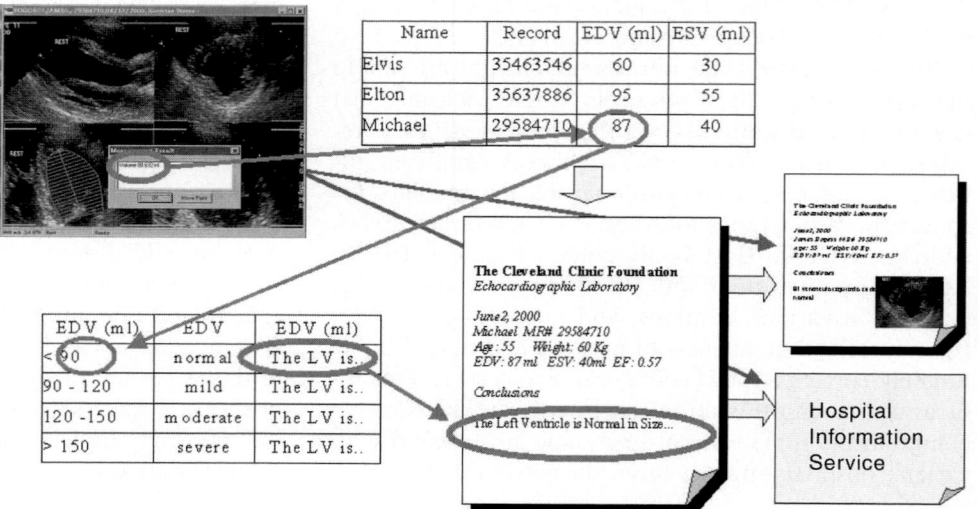

**FIGURE 2.7.** Intelligent interpretation and direct generation of a report based on direct image measurements using preestablished rules.

converts digital-to-analog signals and vice versa, therefore adapting telephone lines for the transmission of digital data. The maximum data transfer speed that can be implemented using regular modems is about 56 Kbps (thousand bits per second). At this limited speed, a 30 MB digital echo study would take 71 minutes to download (transfer from the server to the remote client). This limitation is in part due to the time that is required for the digital-to-analog data conversion at the server's modem and for the analog-to-digital conversion at the remote client's modem. ISDN (integrated services digital network) can provide digital transmission over ordinary telephone copper wire with the installation of an ISDN adapter provided that the telephone company, the server, and the remote client have an installed ISDN adapter. Using ISDN transmission, transfer speed increases to 128 Kbps, reducing the transmission time of the 30 MB file to less than 31 minutes—improved, but still impractical for routine implementation. ISDN in concept is the integration of both analog and digital data over the same network. Although the ISDN you can install is integrating these on a medium designed for analog transmission, broadband ISDN is a service that could eventually extend the integration of both services using fiber optic and radio wave transmission. Broadband ISDN incorporates the use of frame relay for high-speed data transmission, a fiber-distributed data interface, and the synchronous optical network (SONET), supporting transmission at 2 Mbps (megabits or millions of bits per second) or higher. At this speed, the transmission of our 30 MB example file will require less than two minutes.

DSL (digital subscriber line) can also provide high-bandwidth data transfer over ordinary telephone lines. A DSL service requires close distance to a telephone that offers the service. With DSL, data can be downloaded from 1 to 6 Mbps. The speed depends on the physical distance between the telephone company and the subscriber and the thickness of the copper wire line in use. On the other hand, data can only be uploaded at about 128 Kbps, thus DSL is adequate for receiving, but not for sending, digital echo studies. This is not an issue if the sender (echo lab) is connected to the telephone company through an asynchronous transfer mode (ATM) network. DSL also provides continuous (not dialed-in) connection independent of telephone communications that can be carried simultaneously through the same line. In DSL, data travels in digital format, as in ISDN.

Cable modem allows Internet access through the cable TV coaxial line, with an average download speed of about 1.5 Mbps. Access speed, however, depends on the number of users connected simultaneously, who share the bandwidth. Cable modems are attached to the computer using a 10BASE-T Ethernet adaptor card. Cable modem also provides continuous connection.

We have recently validated the process of using Internet technology to transfer digital echo images, without any loss of image quality, to our center. This process is much more cost and time efficient—factors particularly important when critical patient care decisions need to be made (19).

Remote transmission of echocardiographic images has multiple potential civilian and noncivilian applications. We have recently demonstrated the feasibility of performing *live* transmission of echocardiographic images (20). For this demonstration, a sonographer and cardiologist were present at the NASA Lewis facility in Cleveland, performing an echocardiographic study and playing it over the NASA Research and Education Network (NREN), using ATM protocol and MPEG-2 encoding. At cell loss and cell error ratios of $10^{-5}$, performance was nominal, with image quality far superior to videotape. When cell loss and cell error ratios rose to $10^{-3}$, the system froze, but this represents an extreme degree of network noise. Using a two-way audio link, a staff echocardiographer in California was able to guide the acquisition of a study in Cleveland, a model for future remote guidance of acquisition by nontrained personnel. In collaboration with the NASA Ames Research Center (ARC) for Bioinformatics, a virtual hospital demonstration was performed between NASA Ames, Stanford University, Salinas Community Hospital, the Navajo Indian Reservation, and the Cleveland Clinic showing feasibility for high bandwidth (50–622 Mbps) telemedicine between remote clinics and tertiary care hospitals. This includes real-time transmission of three-dimensional echocardiograms acquired at the Cleveland Clinic and rendered in the Biocomputation Laboratory at Ames. The "Virtual Collaborative Clinic" application combines highly sophisticated medical imaging with high-performance, high-speed networking. Doctors can receive and rotate three-dimensional, high-resolution, 24-bit color stereomedical images, working online from their desktops. They can collaborate in near real time with remote colleagues for consultation, diagnosis, and treatment planning. Using a "CyberScalpel," doctors can also "cut" into images and move "bone" around for surgical simulation.

### Data Exchange Format

The format or language that is used to manage digital information may be generic or proprietary. The proprietary format may be designed to manage best the data produced by an individual vendor, but may not necessarily permit universal application. DICOM established the major elements of the echocardiographic format in 1993, which are universally applicable. There is thus a great deal of familiarity with this standard, and all the major echo vendors are now supporting it. It should be emphasized that the DICOM standard is a communications protocol designed to facilitate exchange of images between echo machines, archives, and reviewing stations, as well as from other imaging modalities in radiology. When properly implemented, DICOM should allow images to be taken from any echo machine, transmitted over any network, viewed and analyzed on any computer, and stored on any archive. One of the key issues that DICOM addresses is digital image compression (Fig. 2.8).

DICOM (Digital Imaging and Communications in Medicine) is an application layer network protocol for the transmission of medical images, waveforms, and ancillary information. It was originally developed by the National Electrical Manufacturers Association (NEMA) and the American College of Radiology (ACR) for computed tomographic (CT) and magnetic resonance imaging (MRI) scan images. It is now controlled by the DICOM Standards Committee, and supports a wide range of medical images across the fields of radiology, cardiology, pathology, and dentistry. DICOM uses TCP/IP as the lower-layer transport protocol. The DICOM standard is a communications protocol designed to facilitate exchange of images between echo machines, archives, and reviewing stations. When properly implemented, DICOM should allow images to be taken from any echo machine, transmitted over any network, viewed and analyzed on any computer, and stored on any archive (21).

## Converting from Analog to Digital Echocardiography

Despite the feasibility and advantage of digital echocardiography (22–24), a recent review of the Laboratory Data Project of the *American Society of Echocardiography* revealed that only 3% of echo labs currently consider themselves predominately digital in their data handling. Implementing the transition to a digital echocardiographic laboratory requires a gradual process that involves educa-

tion and training of cardiac sonographers and physicians interpreting the studies, in addition to completing the installation steps described above. Sonographers must be familiarized with the details of digital echo acquisition on each machine, so that they can easily adapt to changing circumstances and perform basic troubleshooting that can correct the vast majority of problems that arise in the digital echo lab. They must be taught how to quickly switch from a single beat protocol to one with multiple beats that they may wish to implement if the patient has atrial fibrillation or other arrhythmias. Familiarity with network cable connections and troubleshooting is also a necessary part of this education process. Equally important to this technical education is developing strategies for conducting the digital echo examination. In general, the standard acquisition sequence used in analog echocardiography may be implemented using digital storage (serial and logical acquisition of different views). Because deletion and editing can be performed with relative ease after data acquisition, it is preferable to start with redundant number of views. Similar education is needed for the staff reviewing and interpreting the study. This is, however, a very brief transition period, because the manifest efficiencies of digital echocardiography in terms of reading time, ease of comparisons with previous studies, and easy quantification from built-in calibration are far superior compared with videotape.

### Advantages of Digital Echocardiography

The advantages of digital echocardiography are demonstrated in improved image review and quantification.

Videotape cassettes contain 2-h recordings of multiple consecutive studies, making the search of an individual study time consuming. In contrast, digital echo studies are organized in a digital archive, which permits instantaneous search and retrieval. This archival system also al-

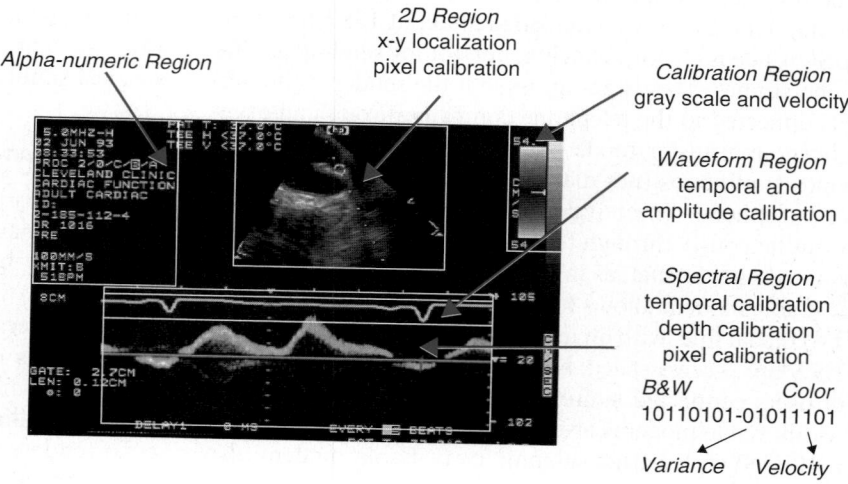

**FIGURE 2.8.** Constituents of a typical DICOM file, including the image, displayed and hidden calibration, and demographic data.

lows query by date, name, medical records, specific diagnosis, and individual demographics, making it a powerful research tool. Exam review is improved by higher/stable image quality, random access to images/views in a study, and rapid comparison with prior studies. Videotape studies contain redundant information and frequently segments of suboptimal image recordings, thus requiring 15–20 min for review. Conversely, digital studies can be edited easily and off-axis and poor quality images deleted, allowing extra time for more in-depth review of important findings. Navigation from specific point to specific point is difficult in videotaped studies, and requires repeated rewinding and replays. Because finding a given view can take a long time, the reader needs to rely primarily on images retained in memory. Digital echocardiography permits quick point-to-point navigation by clicking on the desired image thumbnails.

Review of older patient studies is often important, but requires significant time and effort and is rarely done in a busy laboratory. Videotape libraries may be far away, tapes are often misplaced or missing, and then tapes need to be scanned until the study of interest is found. In digital echo, an older study can be found with a click of a button and retrieved within seconds or minutes. Several studies can be reviewed easily and even compared side by side. This is particularly important when comparing subtle abnormalities, such as change in size of a pericardial effusion, wall motion abnormalities, etc.

Quantification is simpler with DICOM calibration information, allowing direct measurements that, in turn, promote generation of electronic reports and databases (25). Digital echocardiography also facilitates meaningful telemedicine consultation and research applications. With the development of a large database, users can search records for unique combinations of findings or measured parameters easily, not only deriving quantitative information, but also the raw data and images for subsequent review and extended analysis.

Remote diagnosis and consultation via telemedicine is a great potential advantage of digital echocardiography. Studies performed at a primary care hospital, in an ambulance, or in an emergency department can be sent to a tertiary referral center for interpretation. The accuracy of digital compared with videotape echo studies has been previously demonstrated (26). The feasibility of teleconsultation has been demonstrated (27) from remote communities to a tertiary facility. In this series, 83% of studies provided accurate diagnostic information, with most inaccuracies caused by the selection and transmission of a reduced number of images containing incomplete information. Although no significant morbidity was attributed to inconclusive transmission, this study highlights the importance of appropriate selection of diagnostic and complete digital studies.

Other advantages of digital echocardiography include the ability for multiple readers to review the same study simultaneously from multiple locations, such as during case conferences, sending selected views to referring physicians and patients on disk or via e-mail.

### Implementing Digital Echocardiography in the Operating Room

The operating environment is unique, and therefore requires appropriate planning prior to the implementation of digital echocardiography. Ideally, a network attachment should exist, connecting the server to ultrasound machines and viewers installed in the operating rooms. Transthoracic and/or transesophageal studies previously performed can then be brought in and reviewed in the operating room. This function is very useful when the findings in the operating room appear to disagree with those previously reported, often due to differences in loading conditions and the effects of general anesthesia. Studies performed in the operating room can also be stored, transferred, and displayed in the viewer, for the surgeon to review at a later time, thus liberating the ultrasound machine for use at another location.

Establishing a comprehensive protocol is essential in order to standardize the performance of digital studies. This protocol can be tailored to the specific type of pathology and the institutional needs. It is important to ensure the acquisition of an adequate ECG signal for triggering, and to monitor the quality of this signal during the entire time of the study acquisition, because electrical signals from the cautery and other equipment often interfere. Storing pre- and postoperative studies as a separate file is often more practical for side-by-side comparison and prevents the creation of studies that are too large to handle.

Practice makes perfect, and this is particularly true when implementing digital echocardiography. Early mistakes are common during the implementation of digital echocardiography. Videotape backup is always recommended until the new system is adequately implemented and all users are familiar with its use. However, the numerous advantages of digital echocardiography outweigh by far the growing pains.

### KEY POINTS
- The principal feature of analog representations is that they are continuous. In contrast, digital representations consist of values measured at discrete intervals.
- Digital signals travel more efficiently than analog signals, mainly because digital impulses,

which are well defined, are easier for electronic circuits to distinguish from noise, which is chaotic.

- In order to efficiently store and transfer digital echocardiographic studies, some form of data compression is required.
- Network transfer is the most efficient method to deliver echocardiographic studies from the acquisition to the interpretation and to the final storage location.
- The fastest access storage media is random access memory (RAM). RAM is the physical medium where the operating system, application programs, and data in current use (e.g., an open echocardiographic study) reside so that these can be quickly reached by the computer's microprocessor.
- DICOM (Digital Imaging and Communications in Medicine) is an application layer network protocol for the transmission of medical images, waveforms, and ancillary information.
- Quantification is simpler with DICOM calibration information, allowing direct measurements that, in turn, promote generation of electronic reports and databases.
- Remote diagnosis and consultation via telemedicine is a great potential advantage of digital echocardiography.

## REFERENCES

1. Feigenbaum H. Exercise echocardiography. J Am Soc Echocardiogr 1988;1:161–6.
2. Feigenbaum H. Digital recording, display, and storage of echocardiograms. J Am Soc Echocardiogr 1988;1:378–83.
3. Thomas JD, Khandheria B. Digital formatting standards in medical imaging: A primer for echocardiographers. J Am Soc Echo 1994;7:100–4.
4. Karson TH, Chandra S, Morehead AJ, Stewart WJ, Nissen SE, Thomas JD. Compression of digital echocardiographic images: Impact on image quality. J Am Soc Echo 1995;8:306–18.
5. Thomas JD, Chandra S, Karson TH, Pu M, Vandervoort PM. Digital compression of echocardiograms: Impact on quantitative interpretation of color Doppler velocity. J Am Soc Echocardiogr 1996;9:606–15.
6. Karson TH, Zepp RC, Chandra S, Morehead A, Thomas JD. Digital storage of echocardiograms offers superior image quality to analog storage even with 20:1 digital compression: Results of the Digital ERA (Echo Record Access) study. J Am Soc Echocardiogr 1996;9:769–78.
7. Segar DS, Skolnick D, Sawada SG, et al. A comparison of the interpretation of digitized and videotape recorded echocardiograms. J Am Soc Echocardiogr 1999;12(9):714–19.
8. Lambert AS, Miller JP, Foster E, Schiller NB, Cahalan MK. The diagnostic validity of digitally captured intraoperative transesophageal echocardiographic examinations compared with analog recordings: A pilot study. J Am Soc Echocardiogr 1999;12(11):974–80.
9. Haluska B, Wahi S, Mayer-Sabik E, Roach-Isada L, Baglin T, Marwick TH. Accuracy and cost- and time-effectiveness of
10. digital clip versus videotape interpretation of echocardiograms in patients with valvular heart disease. J Am Soc Echocardiogr 2001;14:292–8.
11. Soble JS, Yurow G, Brar R, et al. Comparison of MPEG digital video with super VHS tape for diagnostic echocardiographic readings. J Am Soc Echocardiogr 1998;11:819–25.
12. Garcia MJ, Thomas JD, Greenberg NL, et al. Comparison of MPEG-1 digital video with S-VHS tape for quantitative echocardiographic measurements. J Am Soc Echocardiogr 2001;14:144–221.
13. Spencer K, Weinert L, Mor-Avi V, et al. Electronic transmission of digital echocardiographic studies: effects of MPEG compression. International J Cardiol 2000; 75(2–3):141–5.
14. Spencer K, Solomon L, Mor-Avi V, et al. Effects of MPEG compression on the quality and diagnostic accuracy of digital echocardiography studies. J Am Soc Echocardiogr 2000;13(1):51–7.
15. Main ML, Foltz D, Firstenberg MS, et al. Real-time transmission of full-motion echocardiography over a high-speed data network: Impact of data rate and network quality of service. J Am Soc Echocardiogr 2000;13(8):764–70.
16. Soble JS, Yurow G, Brar R, et al. Comparison of MPEG digital video with super VHS tape for diagnostic echocardiographic readings. J Am Soc Echocardiogr 1998;11:819–25.
17. Garcia MJ, Thomas JD, Greenberg NL, et al. Comparison of MPEG-1 digital video with S-VHS tape for quantitative echocardiographic measurements. J Am Soc Echocardiogr, accepted.
18. Hang X, Greenberg NL, Thomas JD. Compression of echocardiographic data using the Wavelet Packet Transform. IEEE Computer Society, Los Alamitos, CA; Computers in Cardiology, 1998;329–31.
19. Hang X, Greenberg NL, Garcia MJ. Compression of high frame rate echocardiographic sequences using 3D-wavelet transform. Circulation 1999;100(18):I-571.
20. Firstenberg MS, Greenberg NL, Garcia MJ, et al. Internet-based transfer of cardiac ultrasound images. J Telemedicine and Telecare, 2000;6(3):168–71.
21. Main ML, Foltz D, Firstenberg MS, et al. Real-time transmission of full motion echocardiography over a high speed data network: impact of data rate and network quality of service. J Am Society Echo, 2000;13(8):764–70.
22. Thomas JD. The DICOM image formatting standard: what it means for echocardiographers. J Am Soc Echocardiogr 1995;8:319–27.
23. Ehler D, Vacek JL, Bansal S, Gowda M, Powers KB. Transition to an all-digital echocardiography laboratory: a large, multi-site private cardiology practice experience. J Am Soc Echocardiogr 2000;13(12):1109–16.
24. Mathewson JW, Perry JC, Maginot KR, Cocalis M. Pediatric digital echocardiography: a study of the analog-to-digital transition. J Am Soc Echocardiogr 2000;13(6):561–9.
25. Feigenbaum H. Digital echocardiography. [Review] [19 refs] Am J Cardiol 2000;86(4A):2G–3G.
26. Thomas JD. Digital storage and retrieval: the future in echocardiography. Heart 1997; 78(suppl 1):19–22.
27. Mohler ER, Ryan T, Segar DS, et al. Comparison of digital with videotape echocardiography in patients with chest pain in the emergency department. J Am Soc Echocardiogr 1996;9:501–8.
28. Sobezyk WL, Solinger RE, Rees AH, et al. Trans-telephonic echocardiography: successful use in a tertiary pediatric referral center. J Pediatr 1993;122:S84–S88.

## QUESTIONS

1. The following are characteristic advantages of digital versus analog images, except:
   A. Digital images can incorporate calibration data
   B. Digital signals have a continuous range

C.  Digital images are easier to compress
D.  Copies of digital images can be identical to the original

2.  The size of a noncompressed color digital image that has a spatial resolution of 1,200 × 800 pixels and a color resolution of 65,536 values is approximately:
    A.  62 Gb
    B.  62 Mb
    C.  2 Mb
    D.  15 Mb
    E.  15 Kb

3.  The ultrasound transducer transmits information to the system board in the form of:
    A.  Electrical analog signals
    B.  Electrical digital signals
    C.  Acoustic analog signals
    D.  Acoustic digital signals

## Chapter 3

# Imaging Artifacts and Pitfalls

## Lori B. Heller and Solomon Aronson

An *artifact* can be defined as any structure in an ultrasound image that does not have a corresponding anatomic tissue structure. Artifacts are a common occurrence in an ultrasound display because they are often the result of the physical properties of ultrasound itself. Recognizing artifacts is essential to proper ultrasound interpretation, because not identifying an artifact as such may lead to unwarranted clinical intervention or concern. Similarly, pitfalls may also cause improper diagnoses. *Pitfalls* are normal anatomic structures that are often erroneously interpreted as pathologic. This chapter will discuss the detection and avoidance of artifacts, as well as the identification of common echocardiographic pitfalls.

## ARTIFACTS

Artifacts may be classified into four main categories: missing structures, degraded images, falsely perceived objects, and structures with a misregistered location.

## MISSING STRUCTURES

The absence of an object or area that should be projected on the ultrasound display is considered an artifact. *Missing structures* occur for several reasons and can be related to the resolution of the ultrasound image. *Resolution* is defined as the ability to distinguish between two distinct structures that are in close proximity. Lateral resolution, or the ability to distinguish between two objects in a horizontal plane, is related to the bandwidth of the ultrasound beam. If two structures are closer together than the width of the lateral resolution, they will appear as a single image; in essence, the display is missing images. The best lateral resolution occurs at the focal zone, where the near field meets the far field and where the beam width is the narrowest (Fig. 3.1). Longitudinal, or axial, resolution is the ability to distinguish between two structures in the longitudinal direction. Longitudinal resolution is determined by the spatial pulse length. Because the smallest resolvable distance between two reflectors is

one wavelength, higher frequency (and therefore shorter wavelength) transducers have greater axial resolution (1). It follows, then, that lower frequency transducers are less able to distinguish two separate objects in the vertical plane.

*Acoustic shadowing* may also create missing images. It occurs when the ultrasound beam reaches a strong reflector. This reflector decreases the beam intensity to distal structures, essentially blocking the beam to that area. Therefore, any image that lies deep to the strongly reflecting item cannot be seen. It places a shadow (or anechoic) area distal to the original structure. This commonly occurs with high-density structures, such as prosthetic valves, and heavily calcified objects (2). When shadowing occurs, an alternate acoustic window is required to view the objects or areas of interest (Fig. 3.2).

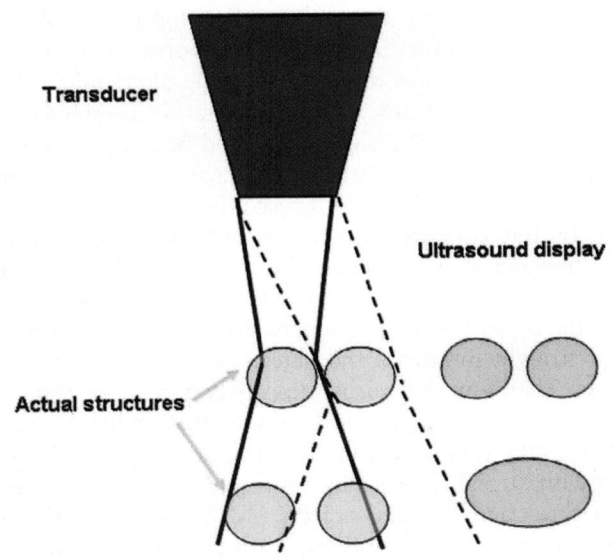

**FIGURE 3.1.** As the depth increases away from the focal zone, lateral resolution is decreased. Even as the scan line moves laterally, noted by the dotted lines, the two separate objects seen in the far field are unable to be viewed as distinct entities.

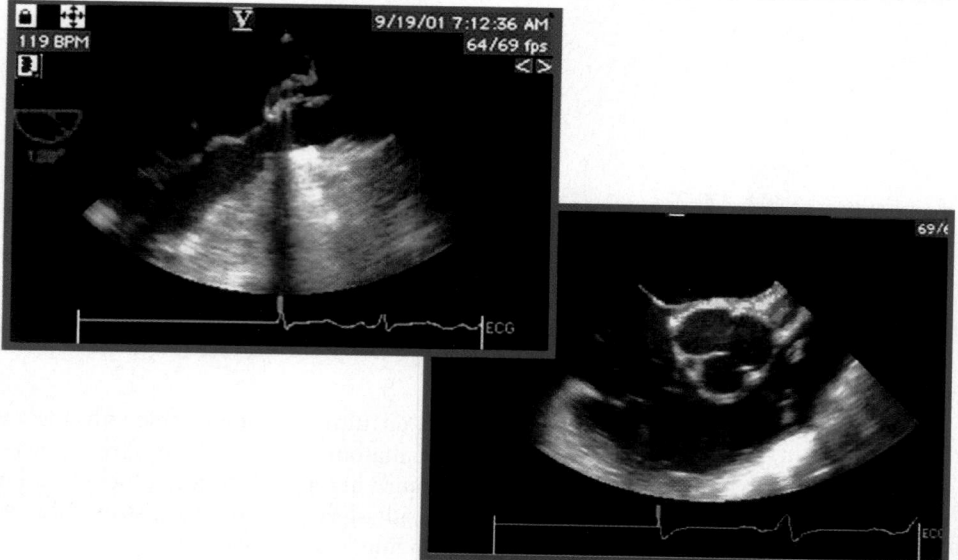

**FIGURE 3.2.** Shadowing. Left, long axis view of the left ventricle and LVOT demonstrating shadowing through the center of the image. This resulted from a suture line of a bioprosthetic valve. Right, to image the aortic annulus in its entirety, a change in imaging plane from 120 degrees to 30 degrees was required.

## DEGRADED IMAGES

An image of imperfect or poor quality is referred to as degraded and is often due to artifact phenomena. *Reverberations* are a type of image degradation. They are secondary reflections that occur along the path of a sound pulse and are a result of the ultrasound "bouncing" in between the structure and another reflecting surface. Reverberations appear as parallel yet irregular lines extending from the object away from the transducer. They occur when either the near side of the object, a second object, or the transducer itself functions as another reflecting surface. When the transducer functions as this additional reflector, an image is displayed as expected after the ultrasonic beam is returned to the transducer. However, this same beam is then sent back to the object, reflected back again to the transducer, strikes the transducer face, and is reflected back to the target (Fig. 3.3). These repeated journeys traveled by the same beam produce additional signals that are interpreted as the same object at twice the distance from the primary target. This can occur multiple times, and the result is multiple images displayed on the screen in a straight line from the object away from the transducer. Therefore, a reverberation is two or more equally spaced echo signals at increasing depths, twice the distance as the original signal. Reverberations generally occur with strong, superficial reflectors, such as calcified structures and metallic objects (3). A common site for this is in the descending thoracic aorta and is known as a linear reverberation. More commonly, reverberations are merged together and appear as a solid line directed away from the transducer. This is called *comet tail* or *ring down* (Fig. 3.4).

*Enhancement* is another type of image degradation and is the reciprocal of acoustic shadowing. If a structure is a weak reflector or the medium through which the ultrasound travels has a lower attenuation rate than soft tissue, the beam is attenuated less than normal. The echoes below the weak reflector are then enhanced and these structures appear to be brighter than normal, or hyperechoic (Fig 3.5). This can be adjusted in the vertical plane by decreasing the time-gain compensation on the console.

*Noise* can also degrade the quality of an image. Noise has many etiologies, including excessive gain and other changes in settings, but in the operating room arena it is most commonly from electrical interference such as electrocautery. Noise appears as very small amplitude echoes on the scan. It is most likely to affect low-level echolucent areas rather than bright echogenic areas (Fig 3.6).

## FALSELY PERCEIVED OBJECTS

*Falsely perceived objects* may occur as a result of *refraction*. Refracted ultrasound waves are beams that have been deflected from their original uniform path and occur as a result of the waves passing with a different acoustic impedance. The transducer assumes the reflected signal originated from the initial scan line and the image is displayed as such (Fig. 3.7). Objects may therefore appear laterally or otherwise displaced from their true position and a side-by-side double image is created. A mirror image can also be created as a result of the ultrasound wave bouncing in between the near and the far side of the structure before returning to the transducer, similar to a reverberation. This mirrored image is

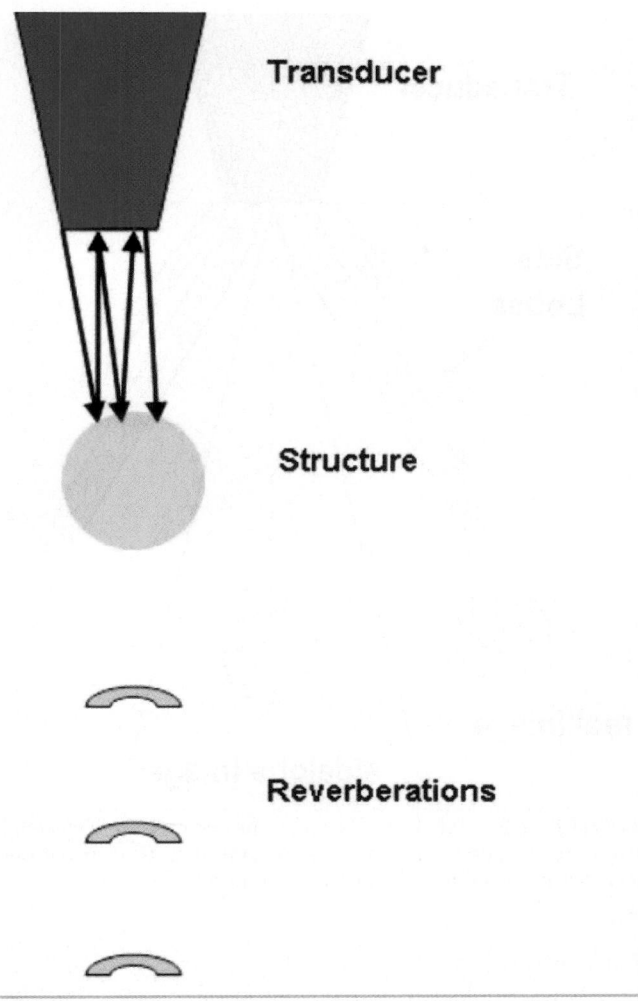

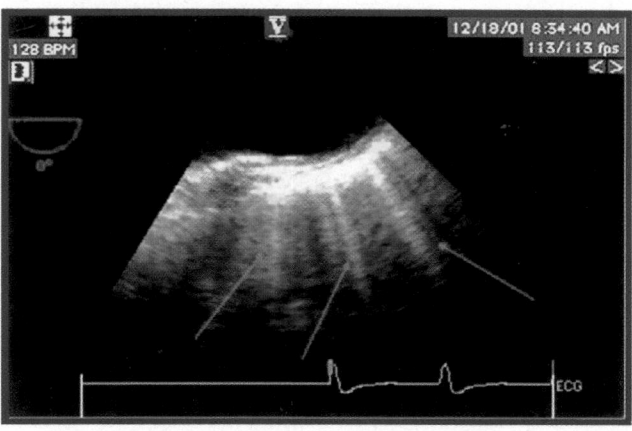

**FIGURE 3.4.** Reverberation. Merged reverberations form a single line away from the transducer and are called *ring-down* or *comet tail*.

**FIGURE 3.3.** Reverberation. When the transducer functions as an alternate reflecting source, reverberations appear as parallel yet irregular lines away from the structure.

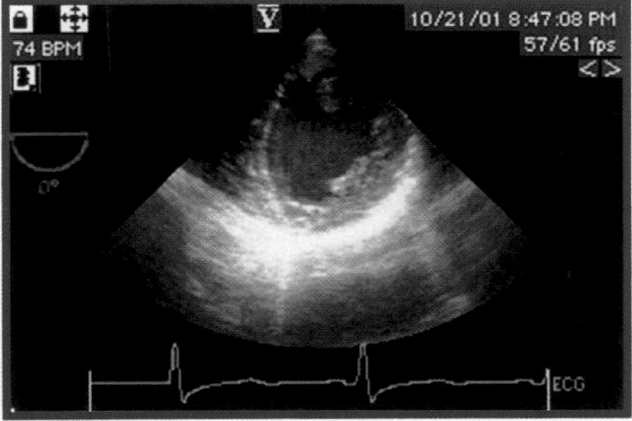

**FIGURE 3.5.** Enhancement. In this transgastric, short-axis view, enhancement is seen along the anterior wall and anterior pericardium. This can be improved by adjusting the time gain compensation or vertical gain.

always located on a straight line between the transducer and the artifact and is always deeper than the true reflector. A common place of occurrence for this is the descending aorta and is often referred to as a double-barrel aorta (3) (Fig. 3.8). Falsely perceived objects due to refraction and mirror images can often be overcome by altering the scanning angle.

## MISREGISTERED LOCATIONS

Although the main ultrasound beam is central, multiple beams are projected out from the transducer in a diverging manner (Fig. 3.9). These beams are referred to as *side lobes* and can result in images being placed in the wrong location on the displayed image. Generally, the energy in these extraneous beams is much less than the main beam and therefore produces no effect or image. However, if

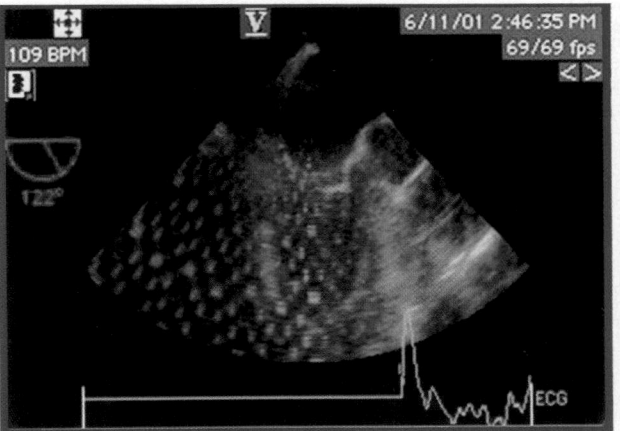

**FIGURE 3.6.** Noise. Artifact from the electrocautery degrades this midesophageal, long-axis view.

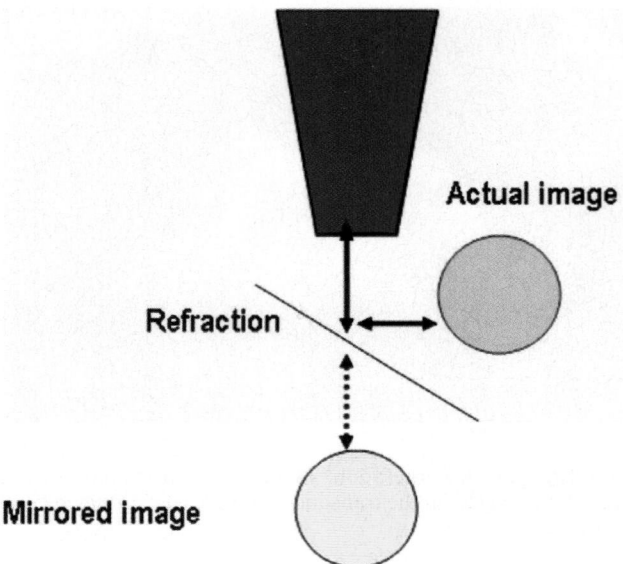

**FIGURE 3.7.** Refraction. As a result of a change in acoustic impedance of the tissue, some of the sound waves are refracted from their original courses. A false mirror image is then placed distal to the actual object.

these beams, or side lobes, reach a strong specular reflector, the reflected energy will be added to the reflected energy of the main beam. Side-lobe artifacts usually become apparent when they do not conflict with real, more intense echoes. An enlarged cardiac chamber often provides this setting. If the emitted echo beam is rapidly oscillating, then multiple side-lobe artifacts may be displayed as a curved line at the level of the true object with the brightest area corresponding to the original structure (Fig. 3.10) (1). In the ascending aorta, a side-lobe artifact may create the appearance of a false dissection (Fig. 3.11) (although more commonly, false dissections in the ascending aorta are a

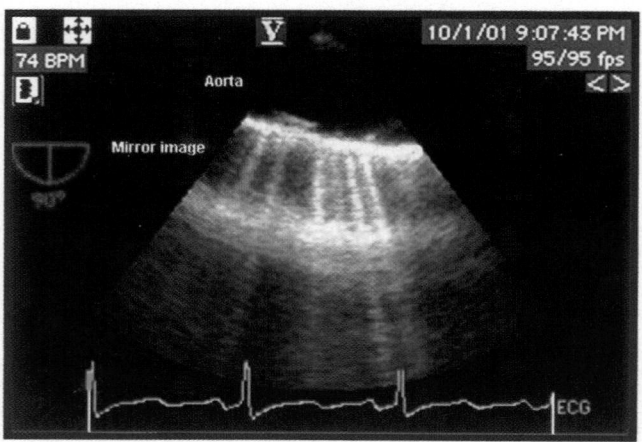

**FIGURE 3.8.** Double-Barrel Aorta. A mirror image is created in the descending thoracic aorta. This is a common artifact.

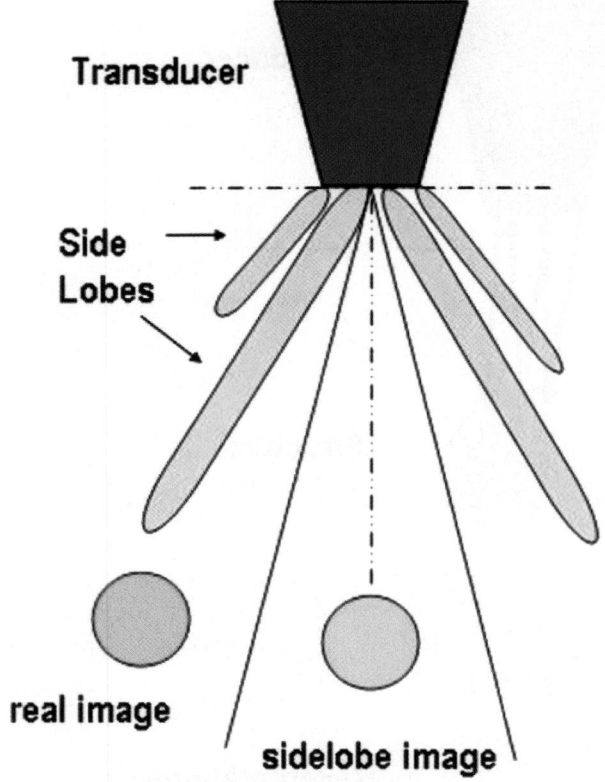

**FIGURE 3.9.** Side Lobes. Extraneous beams are projected from the transducer. Information is relayed as though the objects are in the path of the main ultrasound beam.

reflection artifact related to the left atrium) (4). Identification is accomplished by recognition of the fact that the side-lobe artifacts cross anatomical walls and cavities without regard for natural borders, and always have a common radius from the transducer. They may disappear with adjustment of the depth or angle of the transducer.

*Range ambiguity* can also result in the display of structures in false locations and occurs with high pulse-repetition frequency (PRF). With a high PRF, a second Doppler pulse is sent out before the first Doppler signal along the same scan line is received. Therefore, the machine is unable to recognize the returning signal as originating from the first, second, or even a subsequent pulse. This results in deep structures appearing closer to the transducer than their true locations. When an unexpected object is observed in a cardiac chamber, it is often due to range ambiguity. This can be differentiated from a real structure by changing the depth setting of the image (and therefore the pulse repetition frequency) (Fig. 3.12) (5).

## Pitfalls

Pitfalls are normal structures that are often erroneously interpreted as pathologic. It is important for an echocardiographer to review and become familiar with these

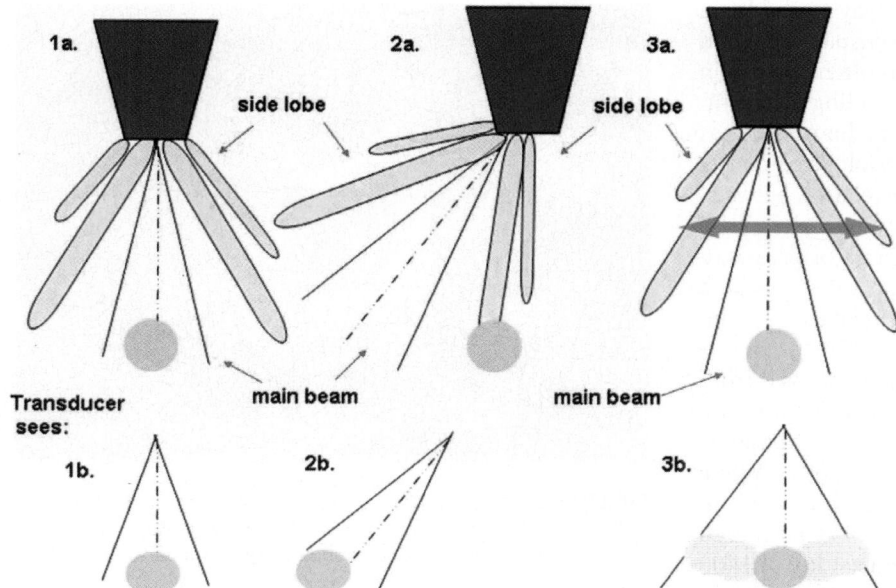

**FIGURE 3.10.** Side Lobes. The oscillation of the transducer may cause the side lobe artifact to appear curved.

entities in order to avoid advocating unnecessary clinical intervention. These structures can be organized according to the cardiac chambers and are reviewed here in order of the right atrium, right ventricle, left atrium, left ventricle, aortic valve, and pericardium.

## Right Atrium

In the right atrium, the *eustachian valve* is often visualized. It is an embryological remnant of the right valve of the sinus venosus, and serves to divert the blood flow from the inferior vena cava (IVC) through the fossa ovalis into the left atrium in utero. It is a thin, elongated structure located at the junction of the IVC and the right atrium and seen in approximately 57% of individuals (7).

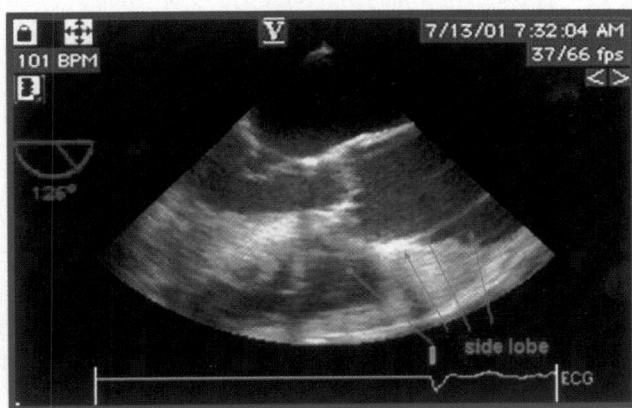

**FIGURE 3.11.** Side Lobe. Side lobes can create the appearance of an ascending aortic flap or false dissection.

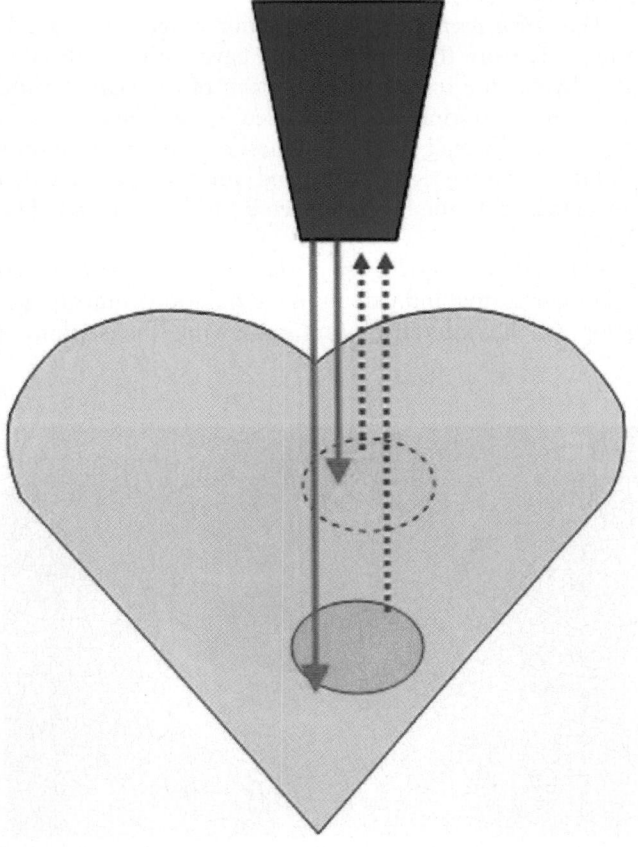

**FIGURE 3.12.** Range Ambiguity. When there is range ambiguity, it is not clear which pulse is being received back by the transducer. As a result, some objects can be placed falsely close to the transducer.

It can be quite large and extend all the way to the fossa ovalis; however, it does not cross the tricuspid valve and enter into the right ventricle (6–8). It can often be seen in multiple views of the right atrium, including the four-chamber and bicaval view. While the eustachian valve has long been considered to be of no physiological consequence, a recent study found a strong correlation between persistent eustachian valve and patent foramen ovale, thus predisposing these patients to increased risk of paradoxical emboli (8). In addtion, the eustachian valve can be a source of infective endocarditis (9) and mistaken for intracardiac turmor or thrombus (10).

Another right atrial structure most likely derived from the sinus venosus is the *Chiari network*. It is a thin, mobile, web-like structure that can be seen in 2% of patients undergoing transesophageal echocardiography. While this structure is benign, there is a high likelihood of an associated patent foramen ovale (83% v. 28%) with a high degree of right to left shunting (11). In one study of 1400 patients Chiari's network was found significantly more in patients with unexplained arterial embolic events than those being evaluated for other reasons. Atrial septal aneurysms also occur at a higher frequency in these patients (24%) (11).

The *crista terminalis* is a muscular ridge that extends anteriorly from the superior vena cava (SVC) to the IVC and divides the trabeculated portion of the right atrium from the posterior smooth-walled sinus venarum segment. It is formed by the junction of the sinus venosus and the primitive right atrium and can be confused with a thrombus or tumor. It is best seen in the bicaval view (Fig. 3.13).

*Lipomatous hypertrophy of the interatrial septum* also occurs in normal individuals. Accumulation of fat can develop in the interatrial septum, giving the septum a

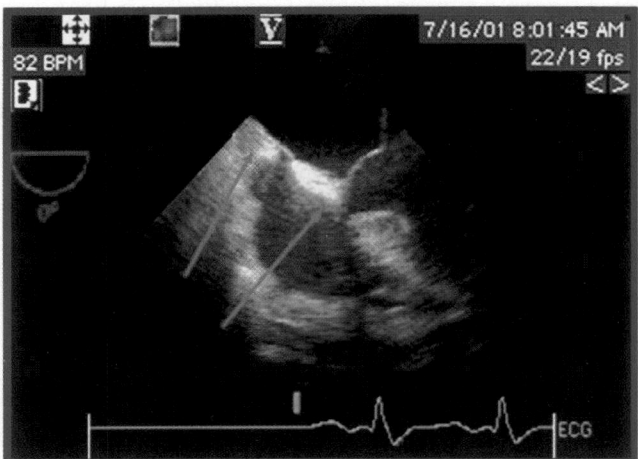

**FIGURE 3.14.** Lipomatous Hypertrophy of the Interarterial Septum. The fatty infiltration of the atrial septum spares the fossa ovalis and gives it a dumbbell-shaped appearance.

dumbbell appearance as the fat infiltrates the septum but spares the fossa ovalis (Fig. 3.14).

## Right Ventricle

Trabeculations are part of the normal ventricular chamber musculature and are seen as muscle bundles on the endocardial surface. While located on both sides of the heart, they are often more frequently visualized on the right. Right ventricular hypertrophy may accentuate trabeculations. The *moderator band* is the most prominent muscular ridge in the right ventricle. It appears as a linear structure in the apical third of the right ventricle extending from the free wall to the septum (Fig. 3.15). The moderator band corresponds to part of the electrical con-

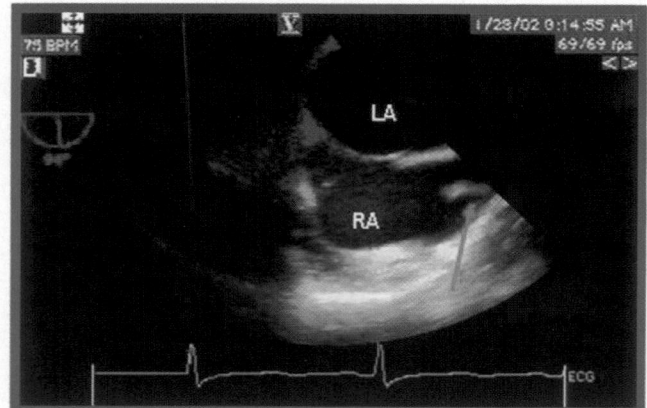

**FIGURE 3.13.** Crista Terminalis. This structure, seen in the bicaval view, divides the trabeculated anterior wall of the right atrium from the smooth-walled posterior portion. It can sometimes be confused with thrombus.

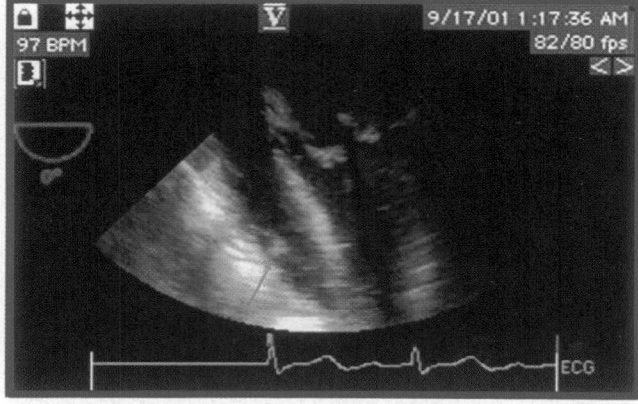

**FIGURE 3.15.** Moderator Band. The most prominent muscular bundle in the right ventricle. It extends from the RV free wall to the septum.

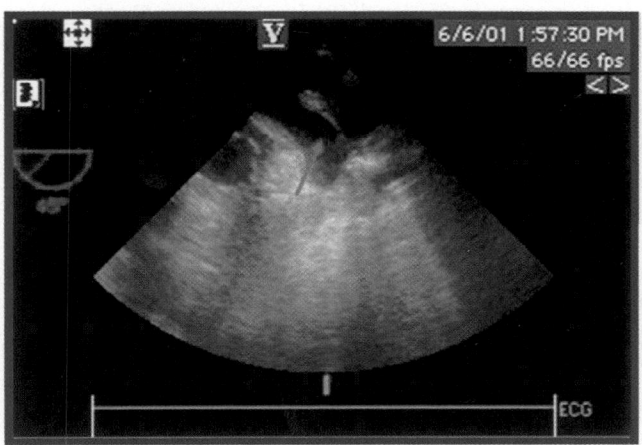

**FIGURE 3.16.** Coumadin Ridge. The atrial tissue between the left upper-pulmonary vein and the atrial appendage can be mistaken for an atrial thrombus.

duction system, housing some Purkinje fibers. It sometimes can be confused with thrombus.

## Left Atrium

There is a distinct raphé between the left superior pulmonary vein and the atrial appendage. This area extends into the left atrium and often has a "Q-tip"-like appearance. It is normal atrial tissue, but its appearance can result in unnecessary anticoagulation in those suspected of having an atrial clot. For this reason, it is often referred to as the "Coumadin ridge." A two-chamber image (midesophageal at 90 degrees) usually provides the view required to visualize this raphé (Fig. 3.16).

## Left Ventricle

The left ventricular papillary muscles, where the chordae from the mitral valve attach, are much more prominent than in the right ventricle on transesophageal echocardiography. The papillary muscles identify the midventricular level. Rarely, one of the papillary muscles may be bifid, resulting in an appearance of three separate papillary muscles, and can sometimes be confused with a left ventricular mass. If rupture of the papillary muscle occurs as a complication of acute myocardial infarction, the entire muscle or a portion of the muscle can be seen as a prolapsing mass in the left atrium during systole.

The left ventricle is characterized as having a smooth endocardial surface, but may occasionally have trabeculations, usually finer than those seen in the right ventricle. Similar to the moderator band on the right, the left ventricle may have a prominent band in the apical third of the chamber and is referred to as a *false tendon* (Fig. 3.17). This structure is thought to represent false chordae tendonae and is not pathologically significant (8).

## Aortic Valve

Some normal variants of the aortic valve can be confused with valvular vegetations. The *nodules of Arantius* are the normal leaflet thickening seen at the central portion of the leaflets of the aortic valve. These nodules tend to enlarge with age. *Lambl's excrescences* are small mobile densities consisting of connective tissue. They protrude out linearly from the coaptation point of the aortic valve and are up to 5 mm in length. These also occur with increasing frequency with age. They can sometimes be confused with vegetations; however, repeat exam revealing densities that are unchanged often assists in ruling out the diagnosis of endocarditis. There is no evidence that Lambl's excrescences are associated with strokes (12). This is in contrast to papillary fibroelastomas, previously referred to as giant Lambl's excrescences, which are lobulated masses on the valve leaflet. These tumors can be found on either side of the valve and range in size from a few millimeters to 4 cm. Unlike Lambl's excrescences, they are associated with embolic events and often warrant excision.

In the five-chamber view at the level of the aortic valve, only the right and noncoronary cusps are visualized. The left coronary cusp is imaged on end and may appear to be a valvular vegetation as it moves in and out of the imaging plane. Confirmation of the nonpathologic nature of this structure can be achieved by imaging this area from a different angle, thus transecting the valve in a plane more parallel to its axis (13).

## Pericardium

When a pericardial effusion occurs, the echo-free space between the pericardium and the myocardium becomes more apparent. Sometimes this space may mimic an abscess or false chamber. The transverse sinus is an example of such a space. It is the pericardial reflection between

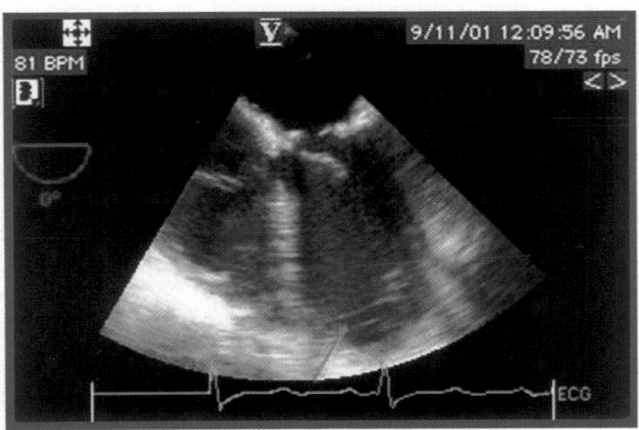

**FIGURE 3.17.** False Tendon. A prominent band seen in the apical third of the left ventricle. It is thought to represent a false chordae.

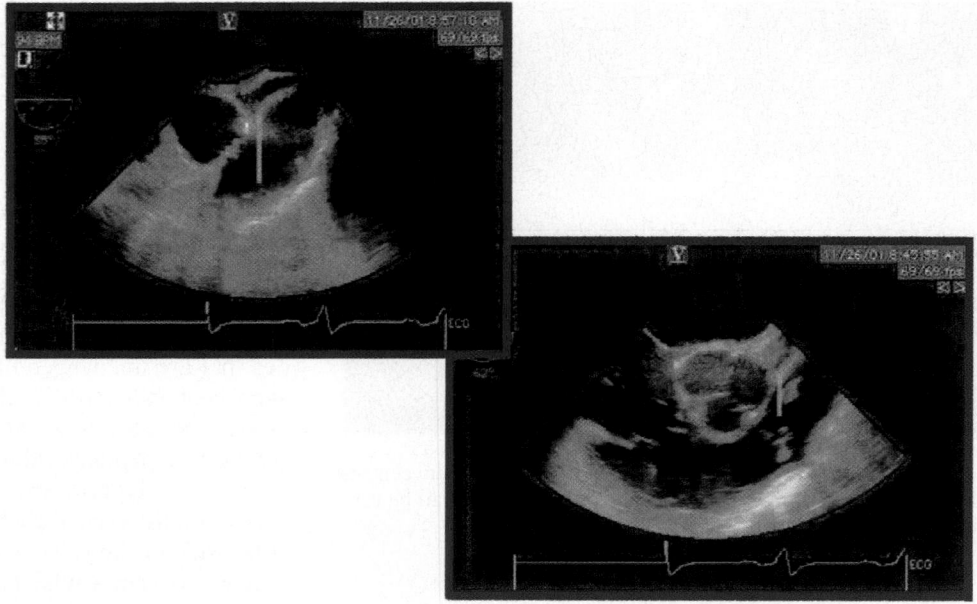

**FIGURE 3.18.** Transverse Sinus. This echo-free space between the posterior descending aorta and the left atrial appendage is the reflection of the pericardium. It indicates a pericardial effusion. Fibrinous material can collect in the space (**right**).

the posterior ascending aorta and the anterior left atrium, and can be seen in the short- and long-axis views of the aortic valve (Fig. 3.18). Depending on the plane of the echo, the atrial appendage may be seen floating in the space, giving the illusion of an intracardiac mass (13,14).

When chronic pericardial disease occurs, fibrinous material can be seen in the sac (Fig. 3.18). If the stranding

has a more nodular appearance, the presence of a malignant effusion with metastases must be considered.

## CONCLUSION

Recognizing imaging artifacts and mastering the diagnosis of common echocardiograph pitfalls are essential

**▶ TABLE 3.1.   Transesophageal Imaging Pitfalls**

| | | |
|---|---|---|
| **Right Atrium** | Eustachian Valve | Embryologic remnant. Thin, elongated structure located at the junction of the IVC and the LA |
| | Chiari Network | Embryologic remnant. Thin, web-like structure located in lower third of RA |
| | Crista Terminalis | Muscular ridge that extends from the SVC to the IVC |
| | Lipomatous Hypertrophy of the Interatrial Septum | Fatty infiltration of the IAS |
| | Pacing Wires/Catheters | Also seen in other chambers. Cause of multiple artifacts and extraneous echoes. |
| **Right Ventricle** | Moderator Band | Prominent muscular trabeculation in apical third of chamber |
| | Papillary Muscles | Chordal attachment of tricuspid valve |
| **Left Atrium** | Persistent Left Superior Vena Cava | Echo-free space between LUPV and LAA. Suspected with dilated CS; confirmed with injection of agitated saline into upper extremity. |
| | Coumadin Ridge | Atrial tissue between LUPV and LAA. Can have Q-tip–like appearance |
| | Interatrial Septal Aneurysm | Bulging fossa ovalis greater than 1.5 cm. Associated with PFO. |
| **Left Ventricle** | Papillary Muscles | Chordal attachment of mitral valve |
| | False Tendon | Band in apical third of chamber. Thought to represent false chordae tendonae. |
| **Aortic Valve** | Nodules of Arantius | Thickening at central coaptation point of leaflets |
| | Lambl's excrescences | Fibroelastic densities that protrude from the leaflets toward the ventricular side |
| **Pericardium** | Transverse Sinus | Pericardial reflection between posterior descending aorta and left atrium. Most notable when pericardial fluid is present. |

parts of echocardiography. Many artifacts are based on the physical properties of ultrasound itself and require at least a basic understanding of these concepts. While the pitfalls of ultrasound imaging require some amount of memorization or recall, many artifacts can be distinguished from true structures by noting their characteristics or by altering the imaging settings.

## KEY POINTS

* Artifacts are any structure in a display that does not have a corresponding anatomic tissue structure.
* Artifacts can be classified as missing structures, degraded images, falsely perceived objects, and structures in the wrong location.
* Artifacts occur as a result of limitations in detail resolution, the properties of ultrasound itself, or equipment malfunction.
* Resolution is the ability to distinguish between two distinct structures. Decreased resolution can result in missing structures.
* Two common artifacts are acoustic shadowing and reverberation.
* Acoustic shadowing occurs when a strong reflector blocks the interpretation of the ultrasound images below it. An alternate window is required to see these structures.
* Reverberations are equally spaced image artifacts that appear at increasing depths from the strong reflector being imaged.
* Pitfalls are errors in interpretation of normal structures. It is important to be able to identify these normal structures or variants to prevent unnecessary clinical intervention.

## REFERENCES

1. Feigenbaum H. Echocardiography. 5th ed. Feigenbaum H, ed. Philadelphia: Lea and Febiger, 1993.
2. Bach DS. Transesophageal echocardiographic (TEE) evaluation of prosthetic valves. Cardiol Clin 2000;18(4)751–71.
3. Kremkau FW, Taylor KJW. Artifacts in ultrasound imaging. J Ultrasound Med 1986;5:227–37.
4. Flachskampf FA, Daniel WG. Transesophageal echocardiography. Aortic Dissection. Cardiol Clin 2000;18(4)807–17.
5. Losi MA, Betocchi S, et al. Determinants of aortic artifacts during transesophageal echocardiography of the ascending aorta. Am Heart J 1999;137(5)967–72.
6. Otto, CM. Textbook of clinical echocardiography. 2nd ed. Philadelphia: W.B. Saunders Company, 2000.
7. Limacher MC. Echocardiographic anatomy of the eustachian valve. Am J Cardiol 1986;57(4)363–5.
8. Schuchlenz HW, Saurer G, Weihs W, Rehak P. Persisting eustachian valve in adults: relation to patent foramen ovale and cerebrovascular accidents. J Am Soc Echocardiogr 2004;17(3):231–33.
9. San Roman JA, Vilacosta I, Sarria C, Garcimartin I, Rollan MJ, Fernandez-Aviles F. Eustacian valve endocarditis: is it worth searching for? Am Heart J 2001;142(6):1037–40.
10. Carson W, Chiu SS. Image in cardiovascular medicine: eustachian valve mimicking intracardiac mass. Circulation 1998;97:2188.
11. Schneider B, Hofmann T, Justen MH, Meinertz T. Chiari's network: normal anatomic variant or risk factor for arterial embolic events? J Am Coll Cardiol 1995;26(1)203–10.
12. Goldman JH, Foster E. Transesophageal echocardiographic (TEE) evaluation of intracardiac and pericardial masses. Cardiol Clin 2000;18(4)849–60.
13. Shively B. Transesophageal echocardiographic (TEE) evaluation of the aortic valve, left ventricular outflow tract, and pulmonic valve. Cardiol Clin 2000;18(4)711–29.
14. Aronson S, Ruo W, Sand M. Inverted left atrial appendage appearing as a left atrial mass with TEE during cardiac surgery. Anesthesiology 1992;76:1054–55.

## QUESTIONS

1. Increasing frequency
   A. creates more reverberations
   B. improves resolution
   C. increases penetration
   D. causes shadowing

2. The following can cause structures to be displayed in a false location
   A. acoustic shadowing
   B. noise
   C. refraction
   D. reverberation

3. Range ambiguity results in structures being placed in the wrong location. The actual location can be determined by:
   A. changing the omniplane
   B. harmonic imaging
   C. decreasing the gain
   D. changing the depth setting

4. The following is an embryologic remnant that has no pathological significance
   A. Eustachian valve
   B. Moderator band
   C. Transverse sinus
   D. Lambl's excrescence

## Chapter 4

# Optimizing Two-Dimensional Echocardiographic Imaging

*Stanton K. Shernan*

The operator of an echocardiographic console is not only responsible for accurately interpreting the information displayed on the ultrasound monitor, but like an artist, must be skillful and knowledgeable in assisting with the creation and development of the actual desired image. Ultrasound image acquisition requires an in-depth understanding of ultrasound physical principles and echocardiographic technology, in addition to an appreciation of cardiac anatomy and physiology. A thorough integration of these important variables is necessary before the clinician can utilize echocardiographic data to make correct diagnoses, and effectively influence perioperative anesthesia and surgical decision making. Without this knowledge the ultrasonographer may not be able to delineate important details of the generated image, and can misinterpret artifacts. Consequently, the inexperienced ultrasonographer is actually vulnerable to exposing patients to increased morbidity by either missing important pathology, or providing erroneous information that leads to unnecessary therapeutic intervention. This chapter will review the important concepts for optimizing the acquisition, processing, and display of real-time, two-dimensional transesophageal echocardiographic (TEE) images.

## THE IMPACT OF ULTRASOUND PHYSICAL PROPERTIES ON IMAGE ACQUISITION

### Ultrasound Physics

Echocardiography involves the generation of images of the heart and surrounding structures using reflected ultrasound. Generally speaking, a sound wave is a mechanical vibration in a physical medium. As the sound beam propagates, vibrations in the path of the beam result in compression and rarefaction of particles in the medium. A sound wave can be described by the following characteristics (Fig. 4.1):

| | |
|---|---|
| Amplitude | The magnitude of the peak or trough of the generated sound wave measured in pascals (Pa) |
| Cycle | The combination of one compression and one rarefaction |
| Wavelength ($\lambda$) | The length of a complete cycle between one compression and one rarefaction |
| Frequency ($f$) | The number of cycles per second measured in hertz (Hz) |
| Velocity ($v$) | Propagation of sound in a medium measured in meters/second (m/s). |

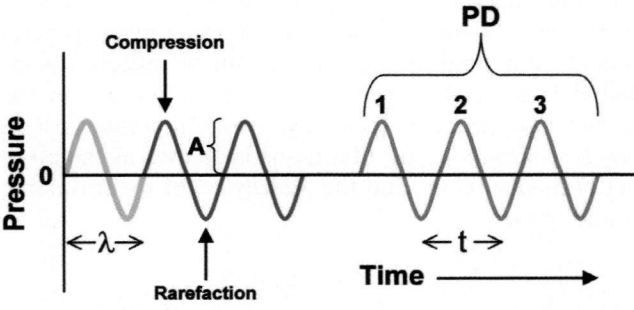

**FIGURE 4.1.** Characteristics of an ultrasound wave. The *amplitude* of a sound wave (*A*) is defined as the magnitude of the peak or trough of the generated sound wave measured in units of acoustic pressure called *pascals* (Pa). Amplitude is often described in terms of decibels (dB), which are logarithmic units describing the ratio of a measured value of acoustic pressure to a reference value. A *cycle* is a sequence of changes in amplitude that recur at regular intervals. The *wavelength* ($\lambda$) is the length of one complete cycle between one *compression* and one *rarefaction*. The *frequency* ($f$) is the number of cycles per second. The *pulse duration* (*PD*) is the product of the number of cycles (Nc = 3) within a packet of ultrasound, and its duration. The period of one cycle is *t*, time.

*Ultrasound* is defined as sound waves with a frequency above 20,000 Hz, and is therefore inaudible to the human ear, which has a range of 20 Hz to 20 kHz. Ultrasound, however, is a practical and ideal source of energy because it obeys the laws of transmission, reflection, and refraction; can be directed in a beam; and is relatively safe in the quantities used for medical diagnostic purposes. In clinical practice, diagnostic ultrasound transducers typically use frequencies in the range of 1–20 MHz.

According to the formula for the velocity of sound propagation (*v*):

$$v = f \times \lambda$$

the ultrasound *wavelength* ($\lambda$) is dependent upon both the *frequency* (*f*), which is determined by properties of the selected transducer, and the *velocity* (*v*), which is determined by the medium through which the beam is directed. Because the velocity in a given biological tissue is relatively constant at 1540 m/sec, the wavelength is primarily determined by the frequency.

## Interaction of Ultrasound with Biological Tissues

A thorough understanding of the variables involved in optimizing the acquisition and display of ultrasound images requires an appreciation for the interaction between ultrasound and biological tissues, during transmission and reception. Sound-wave propagation is affected by the density and homogeneity of the interacting medium. When a wave propagates through an inhomogeneous medium, such as a biological tissue, only a portion is reflected back to the transducer for eventual image generation. To a certain extent, the amount of reflected ultrasound is directly proportional to the difference in the acoustic impedance between two different tissues. *Acoustic impedance* (Z) of a tissue is defined as the product of its *density* (p) and the *velocity* (v) of the traversing sound waves:

$$Z = p \times v$$

As sound passes across the boundary of two tissues with different acoustic impedance, part of the sound wave is reflected back from the tissue interface. The remainder of the wave is absorbed, scattered, and refracted. Structures of greater density, such as calcified tissue or prosthetic material, will reflect ultrasound waves to a greater extent and thus appear more strongly echogenic.

Ultrasound reflection is also dependent upon several other factors, including the angle of impact, interface surface irregularities, the size of the interface relative to the ultrasound wavelength, and attenuation of the sound wave. When ultrasound encounters an interface at an an-

gle, part of the wave is reflected off the interface with an angle of reflection equal to the angle of incidence. Images generated from contact of the ultrasound beam with a large, smooth, and perpendicular interface are referred to as *specular echoes* and result in a greater reflection of sound back to the transducer, thus producing better quality images. Conversely, less sound is reflected back towards the transducer as the angle of incidence becomes increasingly more acute. Consequently, when the ultrasound beam is parallel to a target, reflection is significantly limited and creates an area of echo lucency (echo dropout). Most structures have minor surface irregularities that create radiating *scattered echoes* with amplitudes 100 to 1,000 times less than specular reflectors. Small structures (< 1 wavelength in lateral dimension) also create scattered echoes (1). For example, red blood cells are sometimes called Rayleigh scatterers because of the scattered echoes they produce due to their small size (8 μm) compared to the wavelength of an ultrasound beam (300 μm for a 5 MHz transducer) (2). Thus, higher frequencies (shorter wavelengths) are required to visualize smaller objects, although scattered echoes may still be produced by inhomogeneities of the medium.

As an ultrasound wave traverses through tissues, it becomes weakened or *attenuated*, resulting in loss of the signal due to reflection, scattering, and absorption of sound energy with conversion to heat. *Refraction* of an ultrasound wave can also occur as it traverses an interface of two media in which the velocity of sound is different. Attenuation increases with higher frequencies and greater image depths. Thus, lower frequency (longer wavelength) transducers with greater penetration may be required to improve the evaluation of structures in the far field at the expense of near-field resolution (Fig. 4.2). Biological tissues with different acoustic impedances also have varying effects on attenuating ultrasound waves. For example, the distance a 2 MHz ultrasound wave can travel in blood before attenuating to one-half its amplitude is 200 times greater than the distance the same ultrasound wave can travel in air before weakening to a similar degree (3). This variability in the effect of different biological tissues on the propagation of ultrasound waves accounts for some of the difficulty in visualizing an air-filled lung (Fig. 4.3). In addition, the difficulty in imaging the aortic arch and great vessels with TEE is due to the presence of the interposing, air-filled, right mainstem bronchus (4). In attempting to obtain optimal images, an experienced ultrasonographer can compensate for some ultrasound physical limitations. For example, the aortic arch and great vessels can be seen in > 90% of patients using an appropriate probe-tip flexion and multiplane angle rotation (5). Alternatively, an epiaortic surface probe can be utilized to improve the quality of ascending aorta and aortic arch images. Loss of the TEE probe-tip-tissue-contact interface is also a signi-

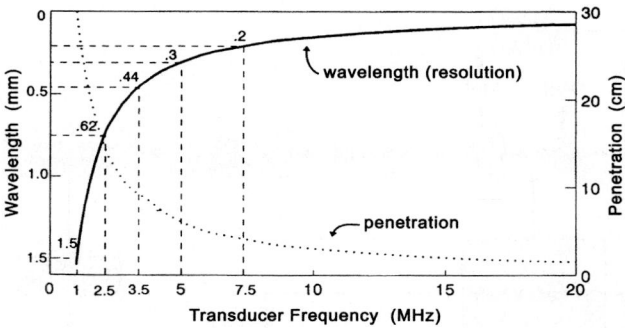

**FIGURE 4.2.** Graph of transducer frequency (horizontal axis) versus wavelength (*solid line*) and penetration (*dotted line*) of the ultrasound signal in soft tissue. Although higher frequency transducers (shorter wavelength) offer improved axial, lateral, and temporal resolution, the depth of penetration is greater with lower frequencies (longer wavelengths) and thus may permit better visualization of distant structures in the image scan. *mm*, millimeters; *cm*, centimeters; *MHz*, megahertz. From Otto C. Principles of echocardiographic image acquisition and Doppler analysis. In: Otto C, ed. *Textbook of clinical echocardiography.* 2nd ed. Philadelphia: W.B. Saunders Company, 2000, with permission.

ficant source of compromised image quality when imaging from the transgastric depth. However, ultrasound image quality can be improved at this depth by removing gastric air with orogastric suctioning and using a generous amount of ultrasonic lubrication immediately prior to TEE probe insertion, to maintain an airless contact between the probe tip and the gastroesophageal interface.

A thorough understanding of how two-dimensional TEE image acquisition and display can be optimized begins with an appreciation of ultrasound physical properties and its interaction with biological tissues during transmission and reception.

## THE IMPACT OF ULTRASOUND INSTRUMENTATION ON IMAGE GENERATION AND DISPLAY

The conversion of reflected ultrasound signals into real-time, two-dimensional echocardiographic images is a complex process, involving numerous electronic and digital manipulations. The basic technological requirements for diagnostic medical ultrasound imaging include instrumentation capable of beam generation, reception of the returning echoes, signal processing and display (Fig. 4.4). Optimizing the generation of cardiac images requires an appreciation for the contributions of each essential component of this elaborate circuitry.

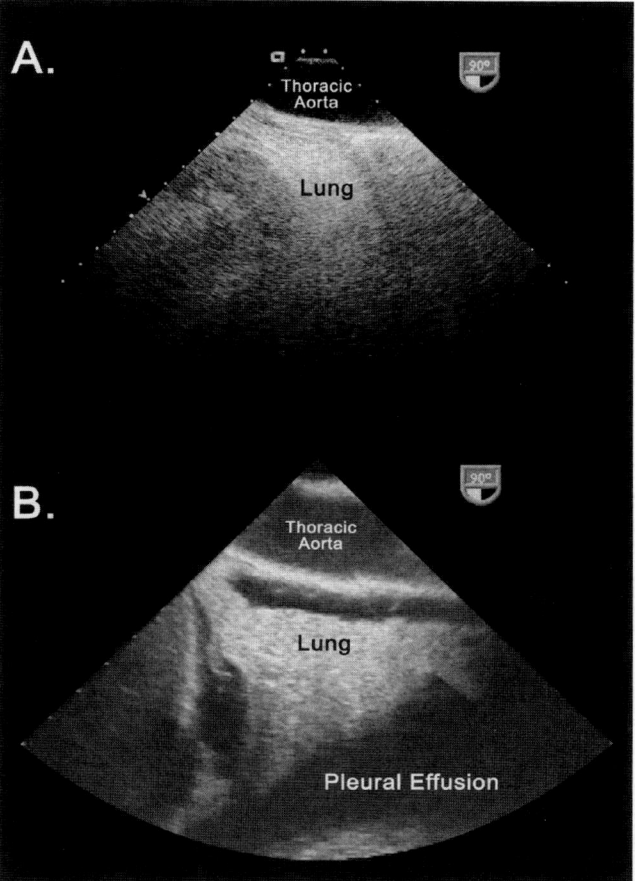

**FIGURE 4.3.** Effect of air on ultrasound wave propagation. **A:** Long-axis, transesophageal echocardiographic (TEE) view of the descending thoracic aorta and adjacent normal left lung. The propagation of an ultrasound wave is markedly attenuated by air-filled structures, such as the normal lung. In addition, most of the ultrasound wave is reflected at the air-tissue interface due to significant acoustic impedance mismatch. **B:** Long-axis, TEE view of the descending thoracic aorta and adjacent left lung, in the presence of a pleural effusion. The low attenuation coefficient of the serous fluid in the left thorax permits circumferential visualization of the partially collapsed lung.

## Master Synchronizer

The master synchronizer coordinates the elapsed time interval between electronic signal emission from the transmitter that results in the generation of the pulsed ultrasound beam from the transducer, and the electronic conversion of the received ultrasound signal (Fig. 4.4). This time interval is important for correlating the signal amplitude to the depth of the tissue interface. The returning sound wave amplitude ultimately determines pixel brightness, while the time for the sound to return determines the image depth. The synchronizer also assists with the introduction of any special amplification based on elapsed time (6). Decreasing the voltage amplitude

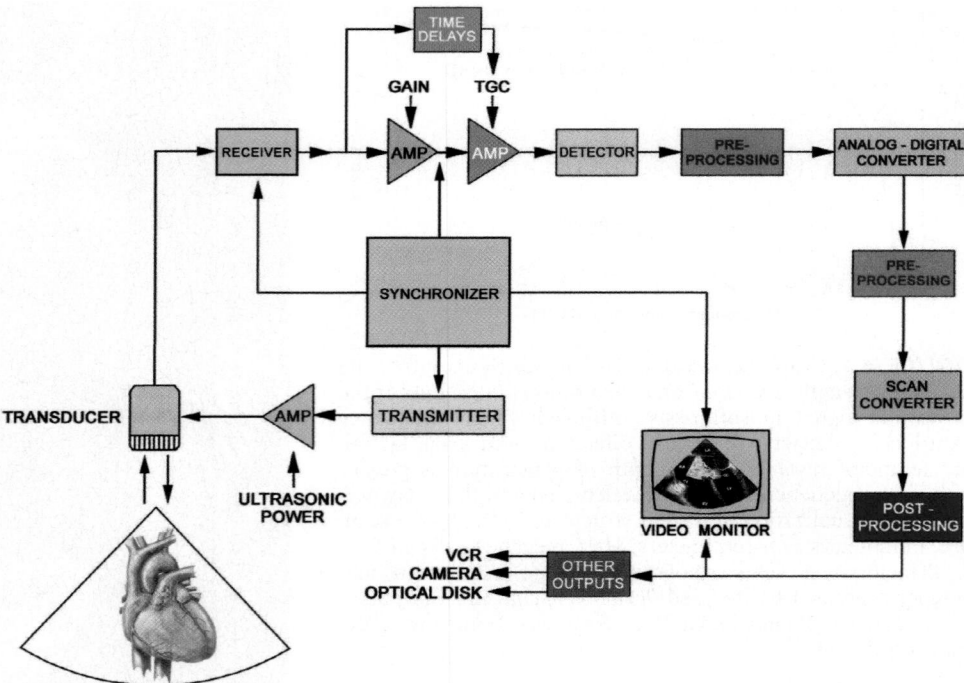

**FIGURE 4.4.** A basic block diagram of the essential ultrasound system components that are required to generate, transmit, receive, process, and display two-dimensional echocardiographic images. *AMP,* amplifier; *TGC,* time gain compensation; *VCR,* video cassette recorder.

produced by the transmitter (power) results in a decrease in the amplitude of the ultrasound pulse produced by the transducer and a decrease in the corresponding amplitude of the returning signal.

## Transducers

The transducer serves as an electroacoustic conversion device composed of multiple piezoelectric crystals, which are capable of generating, transmitting, and receiving ultrasound waves. In response to an alternating electrical current from the transmitter, the crystal alternately compresses and expands, thereby generating an ultrasound wave. Conversely, when a returning ultrasound signal contacts a piezoelectric crystal, an electric current is generated that is eventually amplified and processed before being displayed on the ultrasound console monitor for interpretation. A transducer's *fundamental resonance frequency* is inversely proportional to the thickness of the piezoelectric material. The pulse of ultrasound, however, is actually composed of a range of frequencies, called the *frequency bandwidth.*

In generating an ultrasound image the piezoelectric crystals of the transducer emit a short burst of ultrasound, which is followed by a passive period of "listening" for returning echoes. Ideally, all echoes from one pulse must be received before the next pulse is emitted. Emission of a pulse prior to the reception of all echoes from greater depths would result in range ambiguity. The

number of times the crystal is pulsed or electrically stimulated per second is coordinated through the synchronizer and is called the *pulse repetition frequency* (PRF). The *pulse repetition period* is the amount of time required to transmit a pulsed ultrasound wave plus the time devoted to listening. The PRF is limited by the maximum sampling depth and the velocity of ultrasound in the medium. Because the velocity of ultrasound is nearly constant for most interacting tissues, the PRF will increase if the depth of interest is decreased.

The *pulse duration* is the product of the number of cycles within a burst or packet of ultrasound ($N_c$) and its duration (Fig. 4.1). The pulse duration (PD) can also be calculated using transducer frequency:

$$PD = \frac{Nc}{f}$$

The length of the pulse (*spatial pulse length*) and pulse duration directly affect *axial resolution,* which is the ability to distinguish two structures that are close to each other along the direction of beam propagation as two separate structures (Fig. 4.5). One way for the ultrasonographer to optimize axial resolution is to increase the transducer frequency, which decreases the wavelength and therefore shortens the pulse duration. It is important to remember, however, that increasing the ultrasound frequency decreases the depth of penetration and may compromise far-field imaging. The pulse duration can also be shortened by

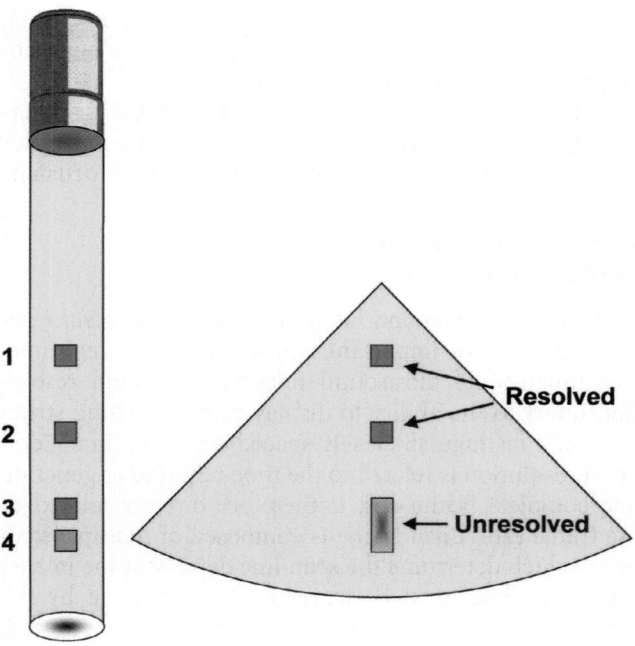

**FIGURE 4.5.** Axial resolution refers to the minimum distance between two structures oriented parallel to the ultrasound beam axis that permits visualization of the structures as separate, distinct reflectors on the monitor screen. The structures (*squares 1 & 2*) closest to the transducer are spaced far enough apart to be distinguished as separate reflectors. The two distant structures (*squares 3 & 4*) are too closely spaced along the direction of the ultrasound beam to be resolved and, therefore, appear merged on the monitor screen. From Zagebski J. Properties of ultrasound transducers. In: Zagebski J, ed. *Essentials of ultrasound physics*. St. Louis: Mosby, 1996, with permission.

using transducers with broad frequency bandwidths, which include a greater mixture of high and low frequencies compared to narrow bandwidths. Consequently, broad bandwidth transducer pulses are more likely to preserve higher frequencies as ultrasound waves penetrate through tissue, and therefore have greater sensitivity than narrow frequency bandwidths (6). Finally the use of damping material in the construction of transducers minimizes piezoelectric crystal ringing and vibration thereby producing a shorter pulse duration. Thus, axial resolution can be improved by assuring a short pulse duration through the use of an appropriately dampened transducer with a high-frequency and broader frequency bandwidth (Fig. 4.6).

Ultrasound beam geometry is also an important factor for determining image quality and is dependent upon several factors. For a nonfocused transducer, the near field is columnar-shaped and nondivergent. The length of the near field, also known as the Fresnel zone, is determined by the diameter of the transducer face aperture (D) and the wavelength (λ) according to the equation:

$$\text{Length} = (D)^2 / 4\lambda$$

The beam begins to diverge beyond the focal point into the far field known as the Fraunhofer zone. Objects are generally better imaged when they are in the Fresnel zone because the beam is comprised of more parallel waves, and reflecting surfaces in the zone tend to be more perpendicular (7). *Lateral resolution* is one of the most significant variables in determining ultrasound image quality and tends to deteriorate in the far-field region because of beam divergence. Lateral resolution describes the ability of a transducer to resolve two objects that are adjacent to each other and perpendicular to the beam axis (Fig. 4.7). Lateral resolution also refers to the ability of the beam to detect single small objects across the width of the beam (6). In general, lateral resolution is most optimal when the ultrasound beam width is narrow. Lateral resolution may therefore be improved by increasing the frequency (shortening the wavelength), although tissue penetration will be compromised (Fig. 4.8). Increasing the transducer aperture diameter may also improve lateral resolution by lengthening the near-field depth at the expense of a wider proximal near field. Furthermore, unlike transthoracic probes, the size of the transducer is somewhat limited by

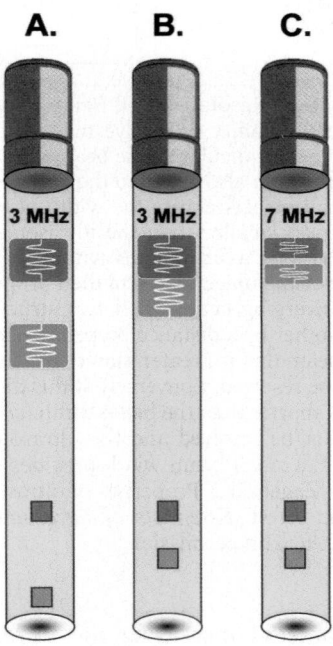

**FIGURE 4.6.** Axial Resolution and Pulse Duration. **A:** The two reflectors (*squares*) are far enough apart to permit resolution by the separately returning echo pulses. **B:** The two reflectors (*squares*) are too close to prevent the returning echo pulses from merging. **C:** Increasing the transducer frequency from 3 MHz to 7 MHz shortens the pulse duration and spatial pulse length, thus permitting resolution by preventing merging of the returning echo pulses (*squares*). From Zagebski J. Properties of ultrasound transducers. In: Zagebski J, ed. *Essentials of ultrasound physics*. St. Louis: Mosby, 1996, with permission.

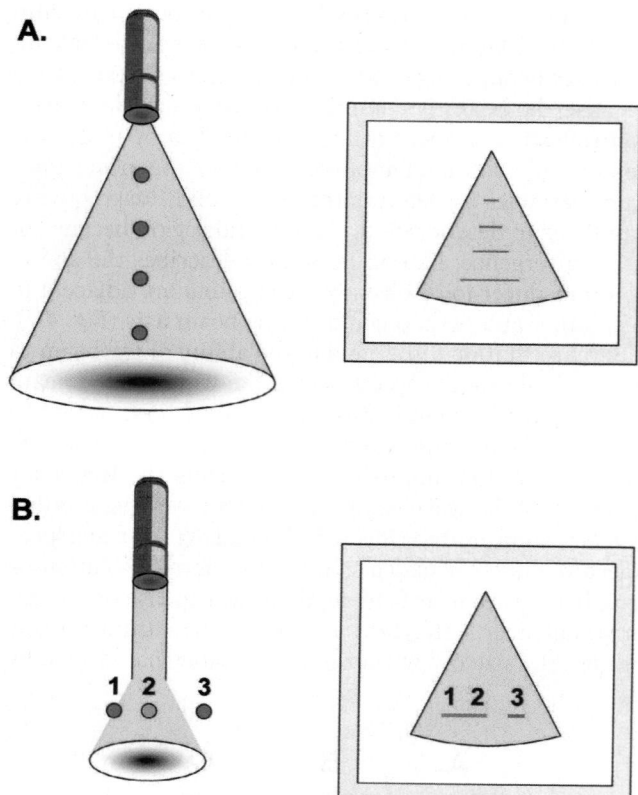

**FIGURE 4.7.** Lateral Resolution and Beam Width. Lateral resolution refers to the ability to resolve two adjacent structures that are oriented perpendicular to the beam axis as separate entities. Lateral resolution also refers to the ability of the beam to detect single small objects across the width of the beam. **A:** A single object (*circle*) smaller than the ultrasound beam width will be imaged as long as it remains within the beam. Consequently, the size of the object will lengthen proportionally with the width of a diverging beam. **B:** If two structures are separated from each other by a distance perpendicular to the axis of the ultrasound beam that is greater than the beam width (*circles 2 & 3*), they can be resolved. Conversely, if this distance between two structures is shorter than the beam width (*circles 1 & 2*), the structures will not be resolved and the ultrasound image will merge. Therefore, a small beam width provides optimal lateral resolution. From Zagebski J. Properties of ultrasound transducers. In: Zagebski J, ed. *Essentials of ultrasound physics*. St. Louis: Mosby, 1996, with permission.

esophageal diameter. Increasing the ultrasound signal amplitude increases the detection of echoes at the beam margins thus effectively increasing beam width and decreasing lateral resolution (7,8).

Lateral resolution can also be improved by focusing the transducer (Fig. 4.8). The focal depth can be altered by adding an acoustic lens or mirror (external focusing), making the surface of the piezoelectric crystal concave (internal focusing), or via direct manipulation by the ultrasonographer through the use of electronic focusing methods (6). With increasing degrees of focusing, the beam width narrows at the focal point, thus optimizing

image quality by increasing the beam intensity. Focusing, however, limits the near-field depth because the beam diverges rapidly beyond the focal zone.

Lateral resolution is an important variable in determining ultrasound image quality, and is ultimately influenced by transducer size, shape, frequency, and focusing.

## Real-Time Imaging and Temporal Resolution

In addition to axial and lateral resolution, *temporal resolution* is also an important consideration for real-time, two-dimensional ultrasound imaging. Temporal resolution refers to the ability to display rapidly moving structures and distinguish closely spaced events in time. Temporal resolution is related to the time required to generate one complete frame and is therefore directly related to the frame rate. Each frame is composed of multiple scan lines, which determine the scan-line density of the image. Each scan line must be traversed in round trip by the ultrasound pulse before the next pulse can be emitted. The PRF, which is dependent upon the speed of sound in tissue and the depth, is therefore limited by the transmit time for the signal to reach the designated target and return (8).

The frame rate and temporal resolution will be affected by how quickly the scan lines in a given image sector can be traversed. Assuming that the velocity of sound in tissue is 1540 m/s, the round-trip time for an individual scan line to be traversed back and forth is 13 µs/cm. The time ($T_{line}$) required to scan a single line of length (D) can therefore be calculated from the following formula (9):

$$T_{line} = 13 \ \mu s/cm \times D \ (cm)$$

The time required to scan a frame ($T_{frame}$) consisting of a given number of scan lines (N), can also be calculated:

$$T_{frame} = NT_{line}$$

The maximum frame rate ($FR_{max}$) can then be calculated from the reciprocal of $T_{frame}$:

$$FR_{max} = 1/T_{frame}$$
$$FR_{max} = \frac{77,000/s}{N \times D \ (cm)}$$

Therefore, assuming preservation of scan-line density and spatial resolution, the temporal resolution and frame rate can be improved only by reducing depth or sector size (Figs. 4.9 and 4.10). Alternatively, for a given depth and sector size, using a higher frequency transducer with decreased tissue penetration will also permit an increased frame rate and improved temporal resolution. Temporal resolution is dependent upon depth, sector scan angle, scan-line density, and the transducer frequency.

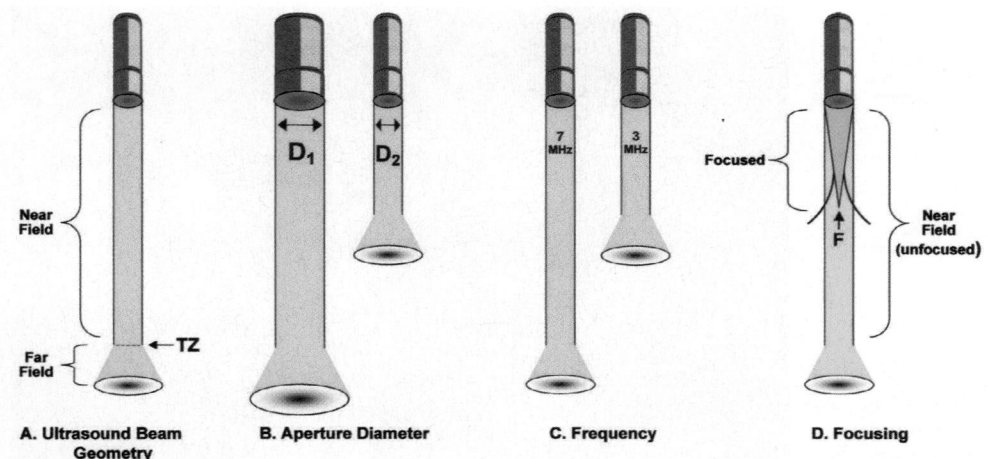

**FIGURE 4.8.** Lateral Resolution and Ultrasound Beam Geometry. **A:** An unfocused ultrasound beam is composed of a near field, which ends at the transition zone (*TZ*) before diverging into the far field. Lateral resolution is most optimal in the near field where the ultrasound beam remains narrow. **B:** Increasing the diameter of the transducer aperture (*D1* > D2) produces a longer near field. **C:** Increasing the transducer frequency (7 MHz vs. 3 MHz), produces a longer near-field length at the expense of decreased penetration. **D:** A focused transducer produces a focal point (*F*) that is closer to the transducer thus creating a narrower and shorter near field.

## Amplification and Time Gain Compensation

Signal processing can be initiated once the returning ultrasound wave is received by the transducer and converted back into an electrical form. Amplifiers increase the small voltage amplitudes received from the transducer to allow further signal processing prior to storage (Fig. 4.4). The gain control determines the amplification of the returning signal and is similar to the volume control on an audio system. Increasing the gain can compensate for signal loss due to attenuation, however excessive

gain can cause saturation and interfere with lateral resolution (7). Time Gain Compensation provides selective depth-dependent amplification, by increasing receiver gain with increasing echo arrival time (Fig. 4.11). Consequently, amplification can be progressively increased from the *near to far field* to compensate for attenuation-associated decreases in the signal amplitude of echoes returning from distant structures. Alternatively, Lateral Gain Compensation allows for compensation of nonuniformities in image brightness caused by different amounts of attenuation along individual scan lines from *side to side* within the image sector (9).

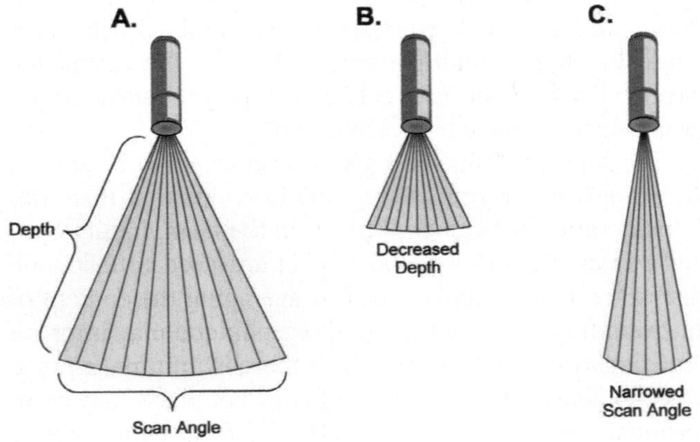

## Preprocessing

Signal processing involves numerous complex manipulations of the electrical signal prior to its display. Preprocessing refers to modifications of the signal that determine the specific numeric values assigned to the echo intensities. Because preprocessing occurs prior to storage in the computer memory, these functions cannot typically be performed on "frozen" images (Fig. 4.4). Preprocessing begins with signal amplification and includes other complex manipulations such as *filtering*, *demodulation*, and *differentiation*. Initial signal preprocessing involves filtering the noise from returning echoes by eliminating frequencies outside the desired echo bandwidth. The signal can be further processed through *detection* or *demodulation*, which converts echo voltages from radio frequency form to video form, thereby displaying only the positive components of the signal (10). Differentiating the signal accentuates the leading edge, shortening the signal dura-

**FIGURE 4.9.** Temporal Resolution, Depth, and Scan Angle. For a given scan-line density **(A)** the frame rate and temporal resolution can be improved by **(B)** decreasing depth, **(C)** narrowing the scan angle, or increasing the transducer frequency.

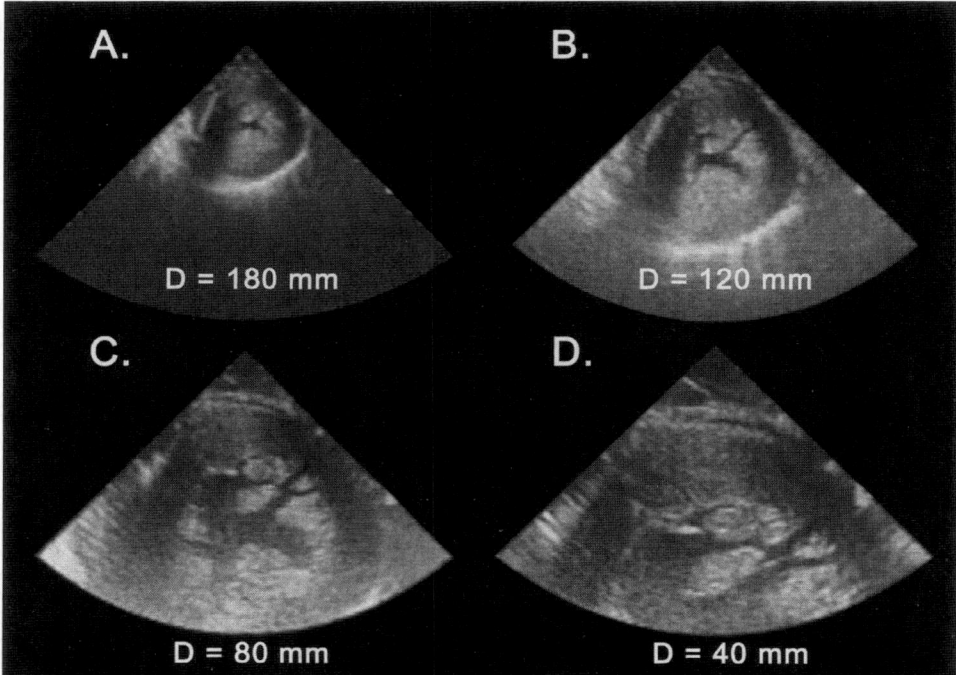

**FIGURE 4.10.** The effect of changing depth on temporal and spatial resolution. Decreasing the scan depth (**A:** 180 mm; **B:** 120 mm; **C:** 80 mm; **D:** 40 mm) allows for a balance of improved temporal resolution (maximum frame rate) by decreasing the time required to scan all the lines within the sector, while maintaining or improving spatial resolution. *mm*, millimeter

tion and making the width of the echo less gain sensitive (7). Edge enhancement is responsible for improved resolution and easier quantitative measuring during M-mode scanning, although it is not commonly utilized for two-dimensional imaging (11).

Dynamic-range manipulation is also a preprocessing option within limited control of the ultrasonographer. *Dynamic range* refers to the range of useful ultrasound signals that can be identified and used by a given component of the ultrasound system (9). The displayed dynamic range includes the range of ultrasound signals remaining after excessively strong signals falling beyond the saturation level are eliminated along with weak signals below the reject and noise levels (Fig. 4.12). A compromise must still exist, however, between the desire to maintain a wide dynamic range for optimal gray-scale recording, and the advantage that a narrow range offers in facilitating the discrimination between true image signals and noise (11). Although a broad dynamic range may increase the detection of weaker signals, this may occur at the expense of noise amplification. The displayed dynamic range can be controlled by the operator by adjusting the *compression*. Logarithmic compression of the linear scale representing the breadth of echo intensities, can be altered to reassign the values of some weak echo amplitudes to zero (black) or some of the strongest to maximum (white) (Fig. 4.12) (10). Increasing compression generally reduces the dynamic range to produce a higher contrast image.

Additional preprocessing functions may be introduced later in image processing, yet still prior to actual memory storage. For example, increasing the *persistence* provides a smoother image of a slower moving structure by averaging and updating sequential frames. Although temporal resolution may be compromised by the requirement for increased sampling time, the image quality of slower moving structures improves because variations in signal levels from regions of comparable strength echoes are reduced (12). Persistence should be kept to a minimum to preserve temporal resolution when visualizing cardiac structures, which tend to be moving relatively rapidly. Increasing persistence also reduces the grainy appearance in the image associated with *speckle*, which represents the constructive and destructive interference pattern of scattered (nonspecular) reflections. Speckle is further reduced by *spatial compounding*, which averages frames obtained from scan lines directed at multiple angles, thereby increasing the probability that specular echoes will be produced from a perpendicular angle of incidence (10).

The numeric value of a given pixel can also be altered by employing preprocessing modifications that take into consideration the values of pixels in the near vicinity. *Spatial processing* and *smoothing* (12) are used to calculate the value of a particular pixel by averaging the content of surrounding pixels. Although this technique may improve the display of an image in which there is minimal change in echo density, the averaging of adjacent pixels may compromise some spatial detail (10,11). *Edge enhancement* utilizes a convolution or filtering process that alters the magnitude or number of weighting factors to change signal levels across an interface in order to detect subtle changes in echo density (12). Finally, *write zoom* or

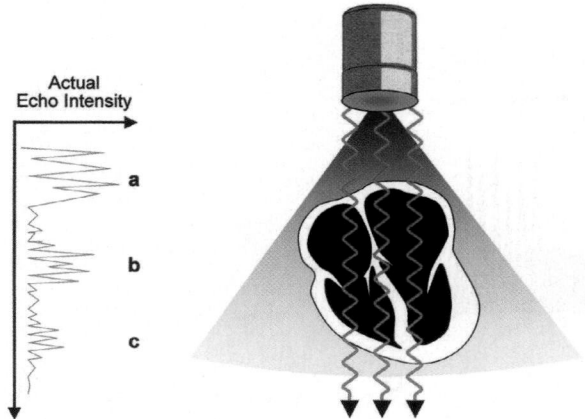

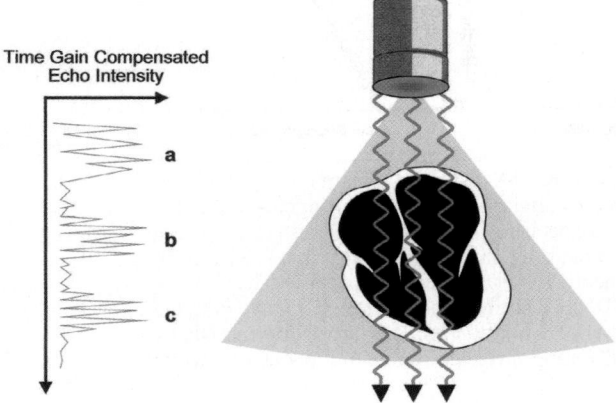

**FIGURE 4.11.** Time Gain Compensation (TGC) provides selective depth-dependent amplification, by increasing receiver gain with increasing echo arrival time. Increasing the amplitude of signals arriving from reflectors at greater depths compensates for attenuation associated with greater traveling distances. When TGC is optimally increased from the near to far field ($a \rightarrow b \rightarrow c$), echoes from similar reflectors are displayed with uniform brightness regardless of their depths in the image scan. From Thys M, Hillel Z. How it works: Basic concepts in echocardiography. In: Bruijn N, Clements F, eds. *Intraoperative use of echocardiography.* Philadelphia: JB Lippincott, 1991, with permission.

regional expansion selection (RES) is a preprocessing magnification technique applied during data collection that actually increases the number of pixels within the expanded region thus improving spatial resolution at the expense of a smaller field of view (Fig. 4.13).

## Analog-to-Digital Converters

In analog form, voltage amplitudes are continuously variable and proportional to the echo amplitude. The analog-to-digital converter (ADC) converts an analog signal to a digitized format by assigning it discrete numeric values

▶ **TABLE 4.1.  Bits, Bytes, and Binary Numbers**

| Number of Bits | Number of Levels Using the Binary System |
|:---:|:---:|
| 1 | 2 |
| 2 | 4 |
| 3 | 8 |
| 4 | 16 |
| 5 | 32 |
| 6 | 64 |
| 7 | 128 |
| 8 | 256 |
| 9 | 512 |
| 10 | 1024 |

8 bits, 1 byte; 1024 bytes, 1 kilobyte

(Fig. 4.14). The ADC conversion can occur at a variety of sites along the circuit, although there appears to be a trend among industries to move this process closer to the front end. For example, some array instruments employ digital beam formers, which require echo signals to be digitized from each element of the transducer before they are combined into a single reflector along each beam line (9). Digital signals offer some advantages over their analog counterparts, including longer-term stability of the displayed image. In addition, digital signals facilitate quantitative manipulation, processing, and analysis of received echoes (12).

Digital signals are stored in random access memory (RAM) as a series of binary bits, which can only exist in either a 1 or 0 ("on" or "off") state. Further precision is acquired by using the binary system to generate large numbers from individual bits (Table 4.1). Thus, in the binary system, eight-bit resolution corresponds to a precision of one part in $2^8$ or 256 levels. At least eight- to ten-bit resolution is commonly employed for acquiring video signals (10,13).

## Scan Conversion and Storage in Computer Memory

The initial ultrasound sector scan is represented by approximately 100 scan lines containing thousands of digitized coordinates. The scan converter locates each series of echoes corresponding to the scan line representing pulses from the transducer (Fig. 4.4). Digital scan conversion converts information obtained within these radial sector scan lines into a rectangular, checkerboard matrix of picture elements or pixels (usually 512 × 512) suitable for storage in memory and eventual video display (14). During the construction of an ultrasound image, the echo signals are oriented into corresponding pixel locations or addresses, which are determined from the echo delay

*(text continues on page 59)*

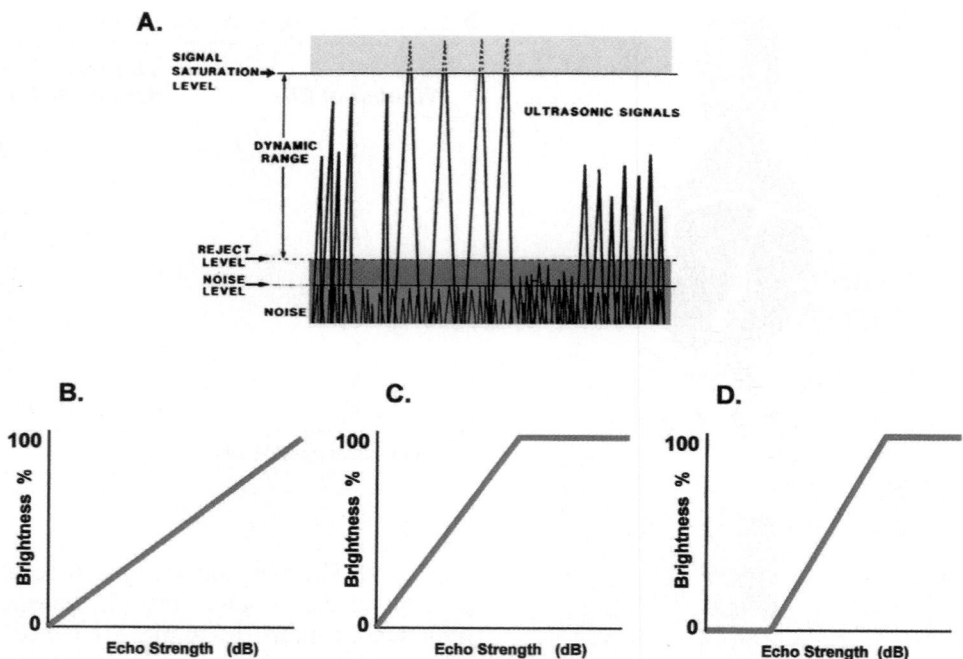

**FIGURE 4.12.** Displayed Dynamic Range and Compression. **A:** The displayed dynamic range includes the ultrasound signal range measured in decibels that remains after excessively strong signals falling beyond the saturation level are eliminated along with weak signals below the reject and noise levels. From Thys M, Hillel Z. How it works: Basic concepts in echocardiography. In: Bruijn N, Clements F, eds. Intraoperative use of echocardiography. Philadelphia: JB Lippincott, 1991, with permission. **B–D:** The effect of compression on narrowing the displayed dynamic range (DR): **(B)** fully displayed DR; **(C)** narrowing the DR by compressing stronger ultrasound signals to white (100% brightness); **(D)** narrowing the DR by compressing both weaker ultrasound signals to black (0%) and stronger ultrasound signals to white (100%), respectively.

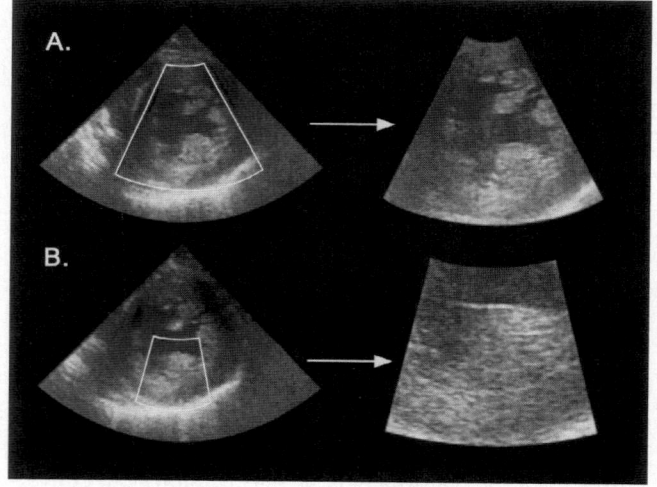

**FIGURE 4.13.** Write zoom or regional expansion selection is a preprocessing function that permits magnification while improving spatial resolution. **A:** The area of interest is first selected by positioning a box *(outlined quadrangular box)* within the image scan. Activating the write zoom function (⇒) provides magnification and improved spatial resolution of the outlined area. **B:** Decreasing the size of the initial outlined quadrangular box results in further magnification and spatial resolution at the expense of a smaller field of view.

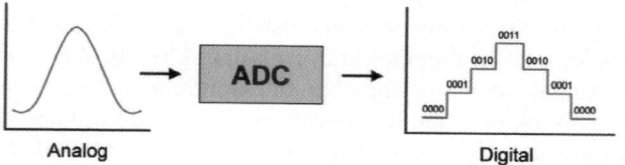

**FIGURE 4.14.** The analogue-to-digital converter (ADC) converts an analog signal to a digitized format by assigning it discrete numeric values, using a binary number system. Digital signals offer some advantages over their analog counterparts, including longer-term stability of the displayed image, and facilitation of quantitative manipulation, processing and analysis of received echoes.

time and transducer beam coordinates (Fig. 4.15). Each pixel is assigned the digitized value representing the echo intensity of the ultrasound signal returning from a specific anatomic site. The combination of a binary storage system and multiple layered matrices allows up to 1024 shades of gray to be stored for a ten-bit system, far exceeding the 32–64 shades of gray that a monitor can display for each pixel, and the 50–100 shades of gray that can be differentiated by human vision.

## Postprocessing

Following scan conversion and storage in memory, the signal can be further modified. In contrast to preprocessing, postprocessing refers to image processing performed after data is retrieved from memory (Fig. 4.4). Postprocessing primarily determines the particular shade of gray assigned to a pixel depending on the signal amplitude versus brightness level relationship selected by the operator (Fig. 4.16). Furthermore, because the range of echo amplitudes in stored memory far exceeds the number of brightness levels that can be displayed on the monitor, a range of pixel values may be assigned to a single brightness level. The translation of the range of pixel values

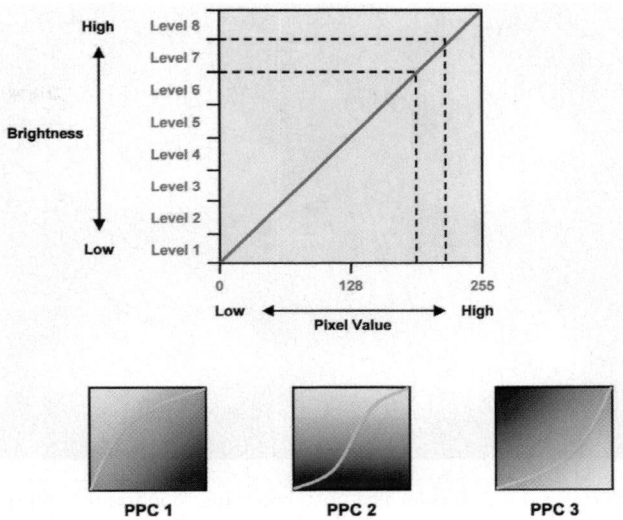

**FIGURE 4.16.** Postprocessing (gray-scale mapping) determines the range of pixel values assigned to a particular brightness level (**upper figure**). This linear relationship can be further altered (**lower figure**) by selecting one of several postprocessing curves (*PPC*) that suppress gray levels at either end of the spectrum of pixel values (*PPC₁, PPC₂, PPC₃*). The assignment of a particular gray-scale map only affects the brightness of the displayed pixel and not its original stored value.

stored in RAM to brightness levels is called *gray-scale mapping*. The assignment of a particular gray-scale map only affects the brightness of the displayed pixel and not its original stored value. Consequently, in comparison to preprocessing, a postprocessing function can generally be performed on a frozen image. Black-and-white inversion reverses the gray-scale assignments, such that white represents low-echo intensity and black represents higher-echo intensity.

B color is another postprocessing function that represents echo intensity in various colors rather than shades of gray (Fig. 4.17). B color may improve contrast resolution by facilitating the ability to distinguish subtle differences in echo intensity between adjacent tissues (10). Read zoom is a postprocessing magnification function. In comparison to write zoom the spatial resolution is not improved during read zoom magnification because the number of pixels representing the original scanned area remains the same.

## Image Display, Recording, and Storage

Following final postprocessing modification of the signal, a digital-to-analog converter converts the digitized data stored as discrete numbers in memory, back into analog format as continuously variable voltages that control the brightness of the monitor for display (Fig. 4.4). A typical

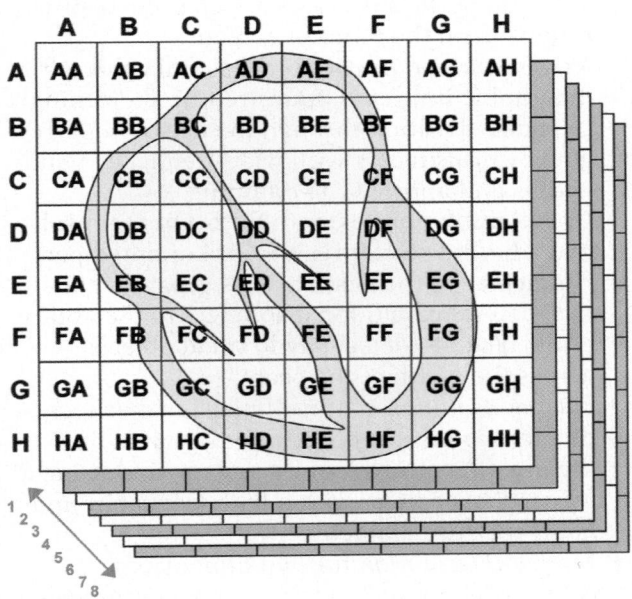

**FIGURE 4.15.** Scan conversion involves the orientation of echo signals into corresponding pixel locations (*AA, AB, AC, etc.*) on a matrix. The pixel locations are determined from the echo delay time and transducer beam coordinates. Each pixel is assigned a discrete digitized value representing the echo intensity of the ultrasound signal returning from a specific anatomic site. The combination of a binary storage system and multiple layered matrices (at least *8 to 10 layers*) allows for a greater number of gray shades.

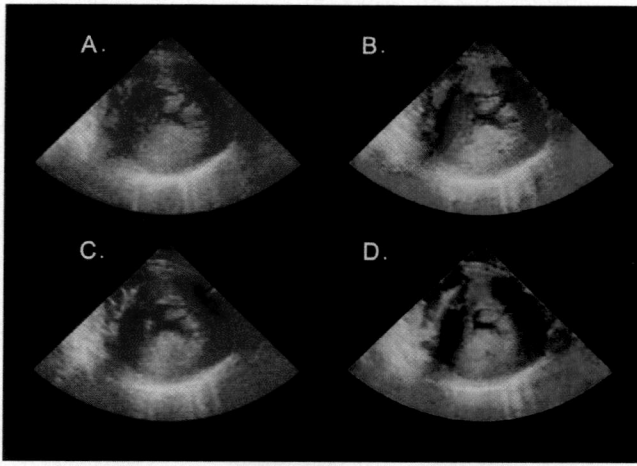

**FIGURE 4.17.** B color is a postprocessing function that represents echo intensity in various colors rather than shades of gray. A variety of B color maps can be selected **(A–D).**

television monitor uses an interlaced scan-line system in which each video frame is composed of two fields. One field contains the even-numbered, horizontal scan lines (raster lines) while the other includes the odd raster lines. Consequently, an interlaced scan-line system provides 60 video fields/sec, resulting in a 30 Hz frame rate. In contrast, a noninterlaced computer monitor provides improved temporal resolution with frame rates of at least 75–80 Hz (Fig. 4.18). The brightness and contrast controls of the computer monitor should also be adjusted accordingly. In addition, it may be necessary to diminish the brightness of the ambient lighting in order to optimize the visualization of ultrasound images. Resolution, the ability to distinguish two point targets as separate entities, is better preserved by recording and storing ultrasound images on an optical disk in comparison to video tape, which requires further compression of the data.

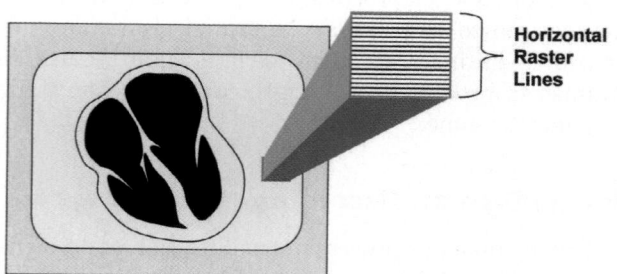

Horizontal
Raster
Lines

**FIGURE 4.18.** Ultrasound images are displayed on a monitor screen as a composition of horizontal raster lines (525 lines/frame).

## SUMMARY

Echocardiographic images are actually "created" through a complex series of manipulations involved in the generation of sound waves and electrical signals. Many of these manipulations are within the control of the echocardiographic console operator. Axial, lateral, and temporal resolution must be optimized to limit the interference associated with artifacts. In addition, appropriate signal processing and display of ultrasound images is necessary before this information can be accurately interpreted. Ultimately, the accurate diagnosis of cardiac pathology using echocardiography requires a thorough understanding of all the variables that affect acquisition and display of ultrasound images.

### KEY POINTS

- Ultrasound waves become weakened or *attenuated* as they traverse through biological tissues, especially with the use of high-frequency transducers and greater image depths.
- *Axial resolution* refers to the minimum distance between two structures oriented parallel to the ultrasound beam axis that permits visualization of the structures as separate, distinct reflectors on the monitor screen.
- *Axial resolution* of two-dimensional echocardiographic images is optimized by shortening the pulse duration through the use of high-frequency transducers with wide-frequency bandwidths and appropriate damping.
- *Lateral resolution* refers to the ability to resolve two adjacent structures that are oriented perpendicular to the beam axis as separate entities. Lateral resolution also refers to the ability of the beam to detect single small objects across the width of the beam.
- *Lateral resolution* of two-dimensional echocardiographic images is optimized by avoiding the use of excessive power or gain, and using a focused transducer with a high frequency and large aperture diameter.
- *Temporal resolution* for two-dimensional echocardiographic imaging can be optimized while maintaining line density by minimizing depth, minimizing the sector angle, and using high-frequency transducers.
- *Preprocessing* refers to modifications of the signal that determine the specific numeric values assigned to the echo intensities prior to storage in the computer memory.

- *Postprocessing* (gray-scale mapping) determines the range of pixel values assigned to a particular brightness level after retrieval from computer memory, and only affects the brightness of the displayed pixel rather than its original stored value.
- The *analog-to-digital converter* converts an analog signal to a digitized format by assigning it discrete numeric values, using a binary number system.

## REFERENCES

1. Otto C. Principles of echocardiographic image acquisition and Doppler analysis. In: Otto C, ed. Textbook of clinical echocardiography. 2nd ed. Philadelphia, W.B. Saunders Company, 2000:1–28.
2. Zagebski J. Physics of diagnostic ultrasound. In: Zagebski J, ed. Essentials of ultrasound physics. St. Louis: Mosby, 1996: 1–19.
3. Goss S, Johnston R, Dunn F. Comprehensive compilation of empirical ultrasonic properties of mammalian tissue. J Acoust Soc Am 1978;64:423.
4. Konstadt S, Reich D, Quintana C, Levy M. The ascending aorta: how much does transesophageal echocardiography see? Anesth Analg 1994;78:24–244.
5. Orihashi K, Matsuura Y, Sueda T, et al. Aortic arch branches are no longer a blind zone for transesophageal echocardiography: a new eye for aortic surgeons. J Thorac Cardiovasc Surg 2000;120:466–72.
6. Hedrick W, Hykes D, Starchman D. Basic ultrasound instrumentation. In: Hedrick W, Hykes D, Starchman D, eds. Ultrasound physics and instrumentation. 3rd ed. St. Louis: Mosby, 1995:31–70.
7. Weyman A. Physical principles of ultrasound. In: Weyman A, ed. Principles and practice of echocardiography. 2nd ed. Philadelphia: Lea & Febiger, 1994:3–28.
8. Feigenbaum H. Instrumentation. In: Feigenbaum H, ed. Echocardiography. 5th ed. Baltimore: Williams & Wilkins, 1993:1–67.
9. Zagebski J. Pulse-echo ultrasound instrumentation. In: Zagebski J, ed. Essentials of ultrasound physics. St. Louis: Mosby, 1996:46–68.
10. Kremkau F. Imaging instruments. In: Kremkau F, ed. Diagnostic ultrasound: principles and instruments. 6th ed. Philadelphia: W.B. Saunders Company, 2002:101–66.
11. Thys M, Hillel Z. How it works: Basic concepts in echocardiography. In: Bruijn N, Clements F, eds. Intraoperative use of echocardiography. Philadelphia: JB Lippincott, 1991: 13–44.
12. Hedrick W, Hykes D, Starchman D. Digital signal and image processing. In: Hedrick W, Hykes D, Starchman D, eds. Ultrasound physics and instrumentation. 3rd ed. St. Louis: Mosby, 1995:208–38.
13. Thomas J. Digital image processing. In: Weyman A, ed. Principles and practice of echocardiography. 2nd ed. Philadelphia: Lea & Febiger, 1994:56–74.
14. Zagebski J. Image storage and display. In: Zagebski J, ed. Essentials of ultrasound physics. St. Louis: Mosby, 1996:69–86.

## QUESTIONS

1. Axial resolution can be optimized by employing which one of the following characteristics of an ultrasound transducer?
   A. Decreased damping
   B. Lower frequency
   C. Decreasing the focal depth
   D. Wider bandwidth

2. Lateral resolution can be optimized by employing which one of the following variables?
   A. Lower transducer frequency
   B. Narrower transducer aperture diameter
   C. Focused transducer
   D. Increased power

3. Temporal resolution can be improved by which one of the following variables?
   A. Decreasing depth
   B. Increasing scan angle
   C. Decreasing transducer frequency
   D. Increasing scan-line density

# Intraoperative Examination

# Surgical Anatomy of the Heart: Correlation with Echocardiographic-Imaging Planes

## Bruce Bollen, Carlos Duran, and Robert M. Savage

A familiarity with cardiovascular anatomy is fundamental to understanding the standard imaging planes commonly utilized in daily clinical applications of ultrasound in the perioperative environment. This is especially true for intraoperative transesophageal and epicardial echocardiography where anatomic localization of pathology is required to answer specific surgical questions. In addition, pathologic processes, such as endocarditis, dilatation of cardiac chambers and vascular structures, and congenital abnormalities may result in distortion of normal relational anatomy making it challenging even for experienced echocardiographers to recognize the structural anatomy of the heart. Understanding the three-dimensional anatomic relation of the cardiac fibrous skeleton, cardiac chambers, valves, and vascular structures provides a greater ability to recognize resulting distortions of normal anatomy. It will be the purpose of this discussion to introduce the novice echocardiographer to basic cardiac anatomy, yet challenge the experienced echocardiographer to develop a greater understanding of cardiac anatomy in relation to their practice.

## FIBROUS SKELETON OF THE HEART

The fibrous skeleton of the heart is formed by the U-shaped cords of the aortic annulus and their extensions forming the right trigone, left trigone, and a smaller fibrous structure from the right aortic coronary cusp to the root of the pulmonary artery (1). This "skeleton" plays a primary function of supporting the heart within the pericardium. A continuum of fibrous tissue extends from the fibrous skeleton providing attachments for the atriums, ventricles, and valve leaflets (Fig. 5.1).

Three U-shaped cords of the aortic annulus join to each other at the commissures of the aortic valve, forming a scalloped fibrous crown-like skeleton of the aortic

valve. The right fibrous trigone extends from the base of the noncoronary cusp, and is more substantial than the left fibrous trigone. The left fibrous trigone extends from the base of the left coronary cusp. A scalloped area is formed between the right and left trigones and the annular attachment of the left and noncoronary cusp. This is called the *intertrigonal space* and has no proper skeletal structure. A broad membranous curtain extending from the aortic annulus to the mitral annulus covers this space.

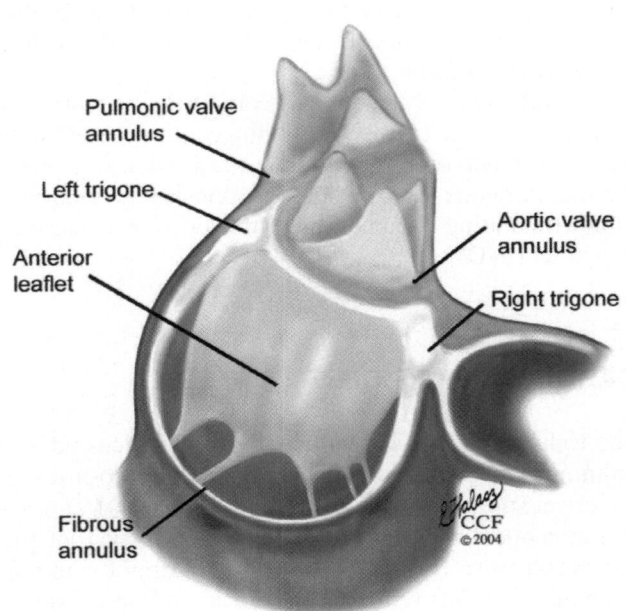

**FIGURE 5.1.** Fibrous skeleton of the heart consisting of three U-shaped cords of the aortic annulus, the right and left trigones, and the fibrous structure from right coronary cusp to the root of the pulmonary artery. Extensions from skeleton include the aortic curtain, mitral and tricuspid annulus, and anterior leaflet of the mitral and pulmonic valves.

This broad membrane is often referred to as the aortic curtain and the space as the mitral aortic interstitial fibrosis or intervascular space. This membrane merges with the anterior third of the mitral annulus becoming the middle portion of the anterior leaflet of the mitral valve.

From the left and right fibrous trigones a fibrous tissue continuum extends around the left and right atrioventricular orifices, forming the annuli fibrosi of the mitral and tricuspid annuli. The mitral annulus is the transition area where the left atrium, mitral valve leaflets, and left ventricle come together. The mitral valve leaflets form a membranous curtain attaching to the mitral annulus. The anterior circumferential portion of the mitral annulus associated with the left trigone, intertrigonal space, and right trigone area is the attachment point of the anterior leaflet of the mitral valve. This anterior portion of the mitral annulus has minimal shape change during the cardiac cycle and is less prone to dilation because of its rigid structure. Its margins are defined surgically by two dimples raised at the border of the right and left trigones when lifting the anterior leaflet.

The annuli fibrosi of the mitral annulus becomes thinner and poorly defined as it extends posteriorly from the left and right trigones. This portion of the annulus is poorly supported and is prone to dilation in pathologic states. The posterior leaflet of the mitral valve attaches to this portion of the annulus. Dilation of the annular attachment of the posterior leaflet creates increased tension on the middle scallop of the posterior leaflet, explaining the 60% occurrence of chordal tears in the middle scallop of the posterior leaflet (2).

From the base of the annular cord of the noncoronary cusp a membrane extends becoming continuous with the interventricular septum. Its downward extension forms the membranous septum. This relationship is important in understanding the anatomy of the left ventricular outflow tract (LVOT).

## CARDIAC VENTRICLES

The right ventricle has two openings—the tricuspid and pulmonic valves—separated by a band of myocardium, the crista supraventricularis. The left ventricle (LV) has a common opening at its base shared by the aortic root and the mitral valve (Fig. 5.2). Although sharing a common opening in the left ventricle, the aortic and mitral valves are set at an angle to each other (Fig. 5.3). The changing of this angle during valve repair has been reported to influence the likelihood of postrepair systolic anterior motion (SAM) of the mitral valve (2).

The left ventricular outflow tract (LVOT) is defined anteriorly by the membranous and the muscular portions

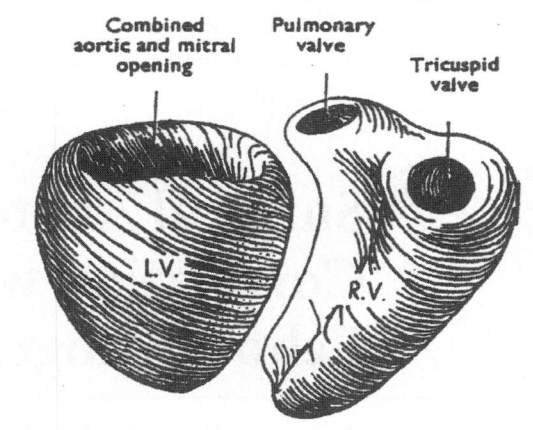

**FIGURE 5.2.** Diagram showing that the tricuspid and pulmonary valves occupy separate openings within the right ventricle, whereas the mitral and aortic valves share a common opening in the base of the left ventricle.

of the interventricular septum (3,4). The superior part of the membranous septum is directly continuous with the right wall of the aortic root. The membranous septum is beneath the noncoronary cusp. The posterior portion of the LVOT is defined by the anterior leaflet of the mitral valve.

To facilitate reporting of left ventricular function the ventricle is divided into segments. Various segmental classifications have been utilized. The Society of Cardiovascular Anesthesiologists and the American Society of Echocardiography have developed a 16-segment model of the LV based on the recommendations of the Subcommittee on Quantification of the ASE Standards Committee. This model divides the LV into three levels: basal, mid, and apical. The basal and mid levels are each divided circumferentially into six segments and the apical into four (Figs. 5.4 and 5.5) (5).

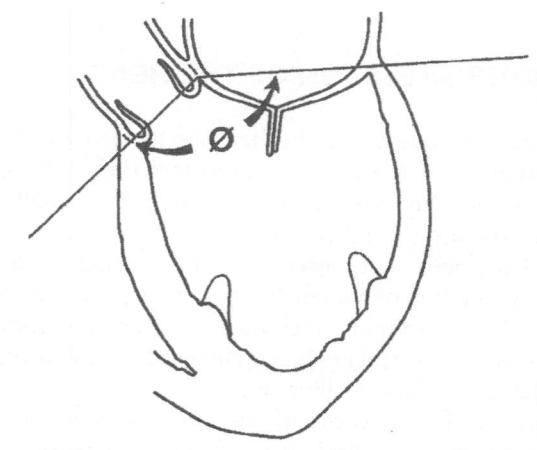

**FIGURE 5.3.** Diagram of the mitroaortic angle (Ø).

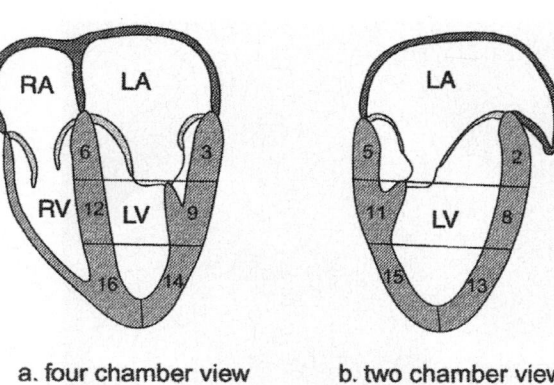
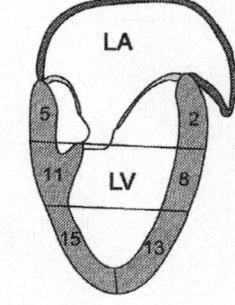

a. four chamber view    b. two chamber view

| Basal Segments | Mid Segments | Apical Segments |
|---|---|---|
| 1=Basal Anteroseptal Anterior | 7=Mid Anteroseptal | 13=Apical |
| 2=Basal Anterior | 8=Mid Anterior | 14=Apical Lateral |
| 3=Basal Lateral | 9=Mid Lateral | 15=Apical Inferior |
| 4=Basal Posterior | 10=Mid Posterior | 16=Apical Septal |
| 5=Basal Inferior | 11=Mid Inferior | |

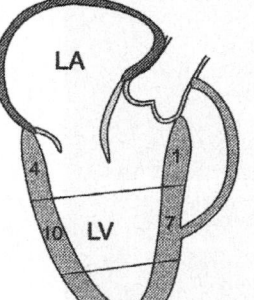

c. long axis view

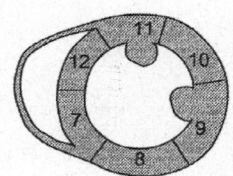

d. mid short axis view

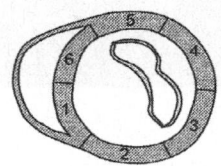

e. basal short axis view

**FIGURE 5.4.** Sixteen-segment model of the left ventricle. **A:** Four-chamber views show the three septal and three lateral segments. **B:** Two-chamber views show the three anterior and three inferior segments. **C:** Long-axis views show the two anteroseptal and two posterior segments. **D:** Mid short-axis views show all six segments at the mid level. **E:** Basal short-axis views show all six segments at the basal level.

## TRICUSPID VALVE

The tricuspid valve of the right ventricle has three leaflets. Its orifice viewed from the right ventricle is triangular with anterior, posterior, and septal sides. The tricuspid annulus is relatively indistinct especially in the septal region. The tricuspid valve has three leaflets: anterior, posterior, and septal. The anterior leaflet, the largest of the three, is semicircular to quadrangular in shape. Chordae attaching to the anterior leaflet arise from the anterior and medial papillary muscles. The posterior leaflet is usually the smallest. The leaflet has several indentations or clefts that give it a scalloped appearance. Its chordae arise from the posterior and anterior papillary muscles. The septal leaflet is primarily attached to the septum, the remainder attaching to the posterior wall of the right ventricle (Fig. 5.6). Part of its basal attachment is to the posterior wall of the right ventricle but most of its attachment is to the septal wall. Its chordae arise from the posterior and septal papillary muscles.

Silver et al. defined three commissures: anteroseptal commissure, anteroposterior commissure, and posteroseptal commissures (8). These commissures define the margins of the leaflets of the tricuspid valve. The anteroseptal commissure is defined by a deep indentation in the membranous interventricular septum where the anterior and septal walls of the right ventricle join. The anteroposterior commissure is defined by fan-shaped chorda at the acute margin of the right ventricle and the anterior papillary muscle pointing to the commissure. The posteroseptal commissure is defined by attaching fan-shaped chordae, the most medially placed posterior papillary muscle, and a fold of tissue on the septal leaflet.

The basal attachments of the leaflets to the annulus are at different levels in the heart. The posterior leaflet and the posteroseptal half of the septal leaflet are roughly horizontal and about 15 mm lower than the highest part of the valve's attachment, which occurs at the anteroseptal commissure near the midpoint of the membranous interventricular septum.

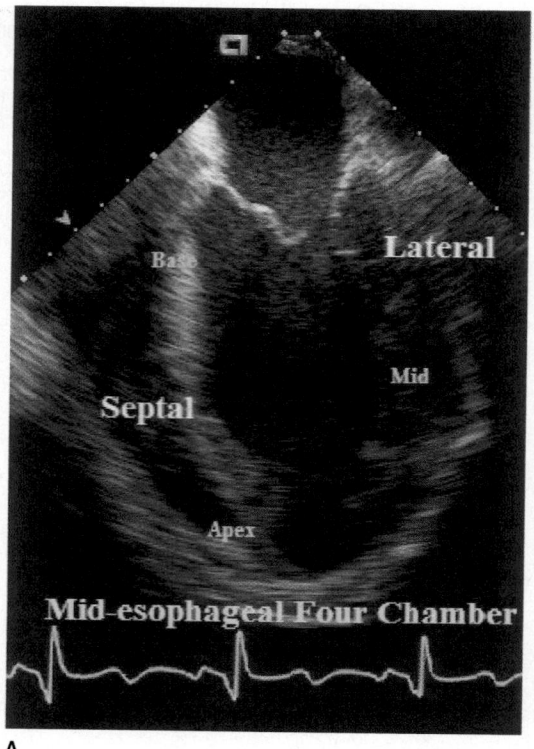

A

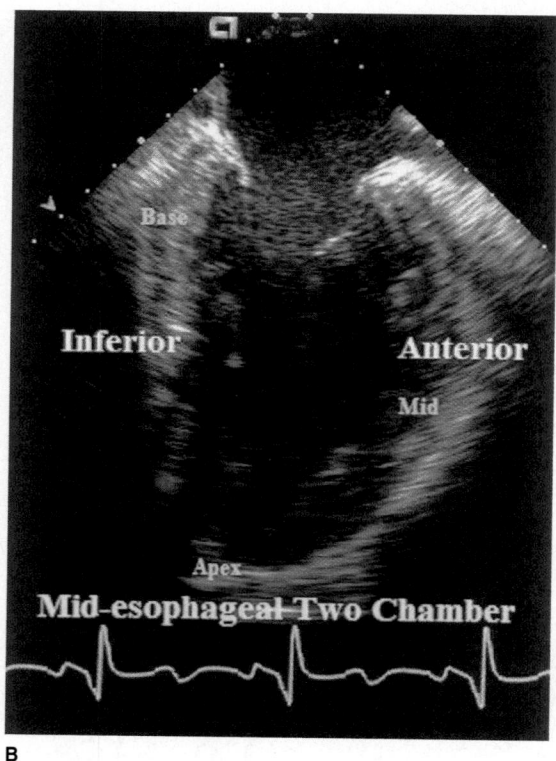

B

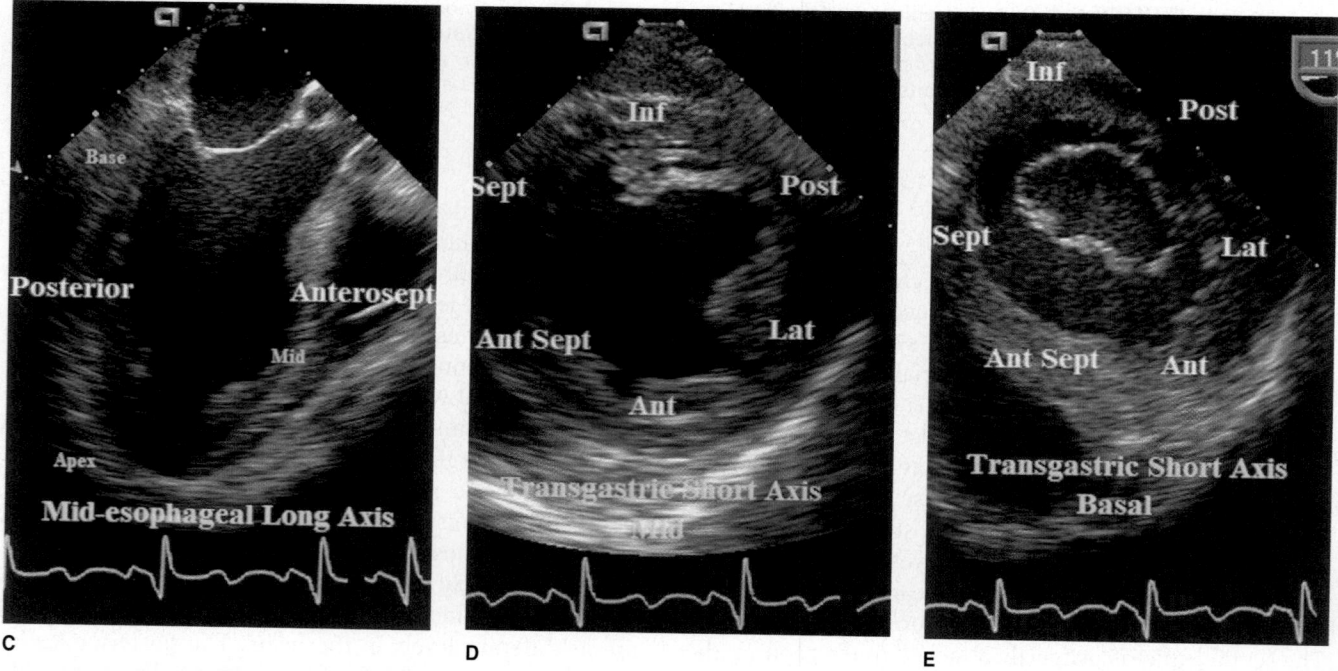

C

D

E

**FIGURE 5.5.** Sixteen-segment model of the left ventricle. **A:** Midesophageal four-chamber imaging plane showing the three septal and three lateral segments. **B:** Midesophageal two-chamber showing the three anterior and three inferior segments. **C:** Midesophageal long-axis views showing the two anteroseptal and two posterior segments. **D:** Transgastric mid short-axis views showing all six segments. **E:** Transgastric basal short-axis views show all six segments at the basal level.

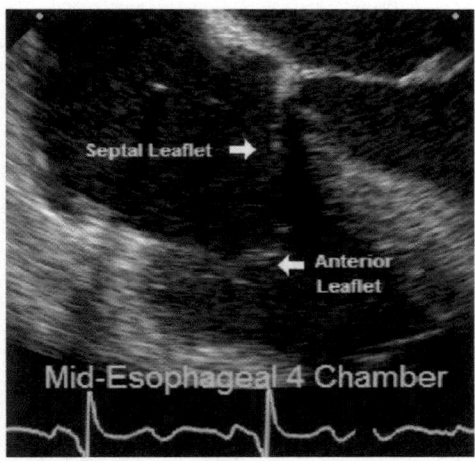

FIGURE 5.6. Midesophageal, four-chamber, two-dimensional image plane with focus on tricuspid valve.

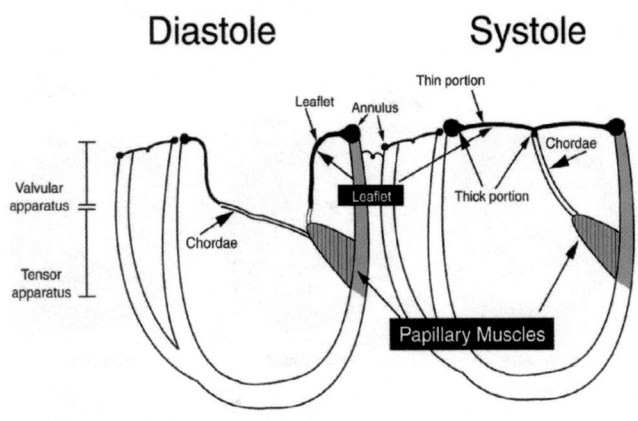

FIGURE 5.8. The valve apparatus consisting of the mitral valve leaflets, chordae, papillary muscles, free wall of the left ventricle, and the mitral annulus.

The chordae of the tricuspid valve originate from papillary muscles or directly from the muscle of the posterior or septal walls of the right ventricle. Silver et al. defined chordae as being rough zone, fan-shaped, basal, free edge, and deep chordae (8).

## PULMONIC VALVE

The pulmonic annulus is not part of the fibrous skeleton as is the aortic annulus. It is attached to the base of the aorta by a flimsy fibrous extension of the aortic root

called the *tendon of conus*. The rest of the pulmonic valve has muscular attachments to the right ventricle and interventricular septum (Fig. 5.7). The pulmonic valve normally has three cusps with a nodule at the midpoint of each free edge. The pocket behind the cusp is the sinus.

## MITRAL VALVE APPARATUS

The mitral valve apparatus is an anatomical term describing structures of the left ventricle associated with mitral valve function (Fig. 5.8) (See also Chapters 14 and 28). These structures consist of the fibrous skeleton of the heart, the mitral annulus, mitral leaflets, mitral chordae, and the papillary muscle-ventricular wall complex. This anatomic description oversimplifies the complex mechanical interaction of the heart, which makes the left ventricular chamber functional.

The important role of TEE in mitral valve repair makes it imperative that the echocardiographer understands mitral valve anatomy. This understanding of anatomy is then used to define the mitral valve anatomy visualized by multiplane TEE imaging of the mitral valve. The echocardiographer must be able to communicate important anatomic/pathological findings to the surgeon performing a mitral valve repair. In addition to the anatomical terms for portions of the mitral valve, there are two surgical nomenclatures used: the Carpentier terminology (adopted by ASE/SCA) (5,7) and the Duran terminology (8,9). Ideally, the echocardiographer should be familiar with all of these terminologies (Fig. 5.9). Intraoperative echocardiographic identification of the different segments of the anterior and posterior mitral valve leaflets is dependent on understanding this terminology and their relation to the standard imaging planes (Figs. 5.10 and 5.11).

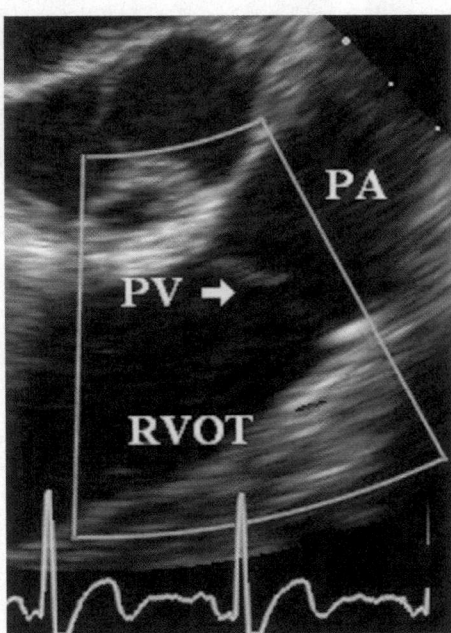

FIGURE 5.7. Midesophageal RV inflow-outflow two-dimensional imaging plane with focus on pulmonic valve.

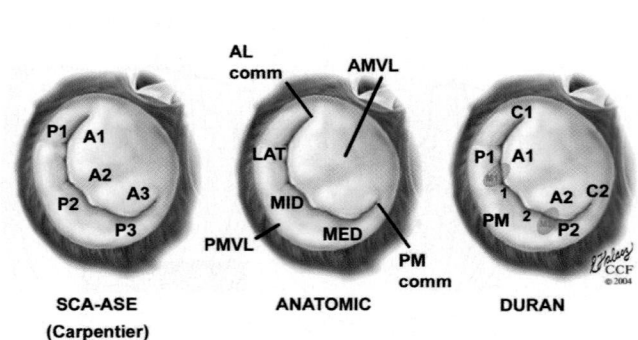

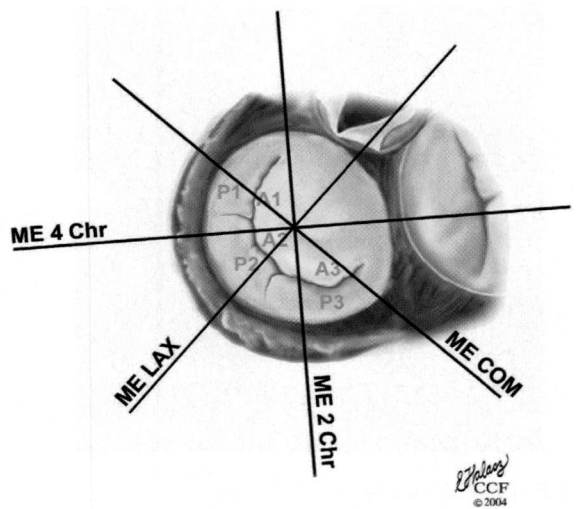

**FIGURE 5.9.** Comparison of SCA/ASE terminology with the anatomic nomenclature and Duran terminology.

**FIGURE 5.10.** Standard imaging planes and mitral valve anatomy. Imaging planes depicted above: Midesophageal four-chamber (ME 4Chr), midesophageal commissural, midesophageal two-chamber (ME 2Chr), midesophageal long axis (ME LAX).

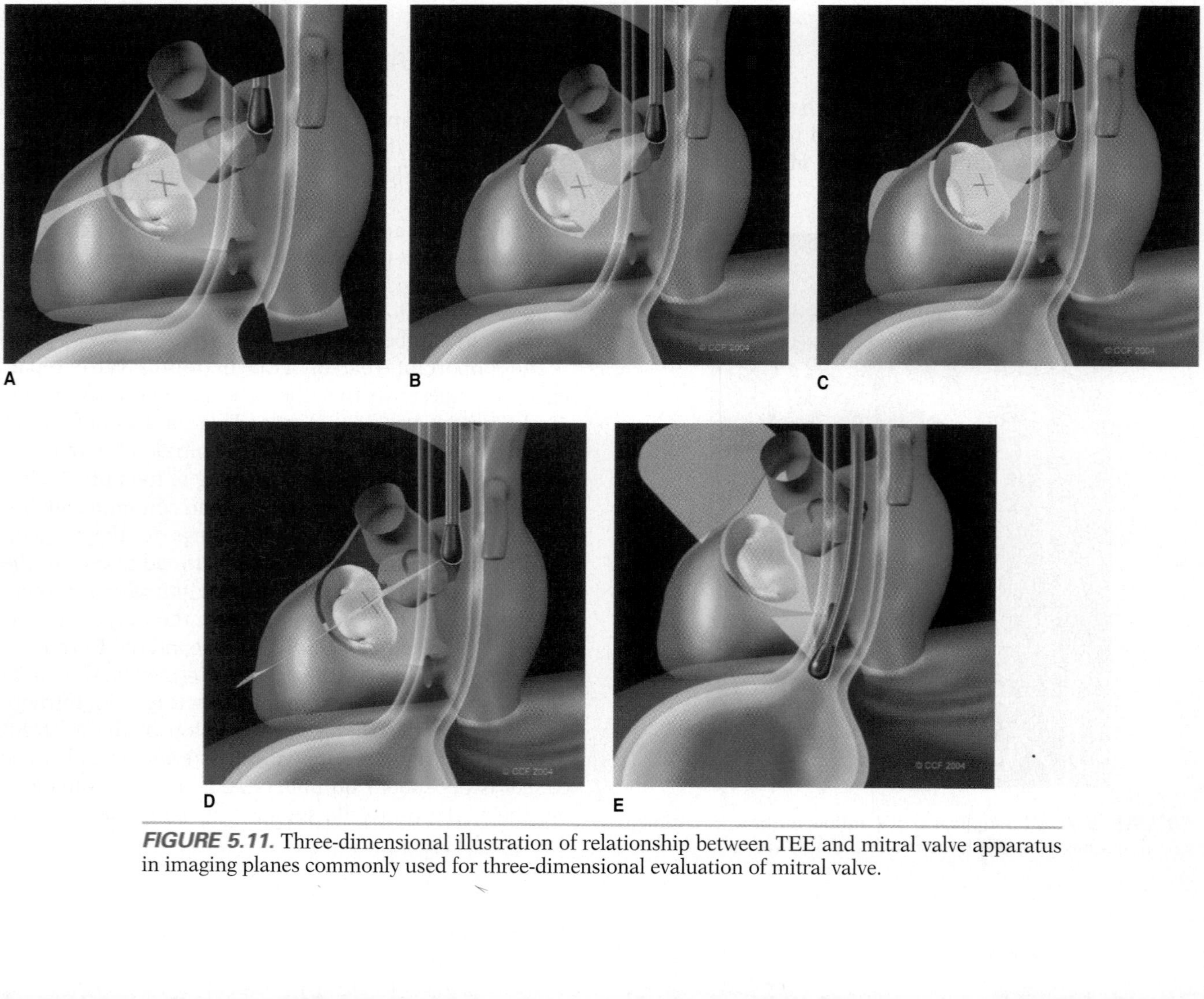

A

B

C

D

E

**FIGURE 5.11.** Three-dimensional illustration of relationship between TEE and mitral valve apparatus in imaging planes commonly used for three-dimensional evaluation of mitral valve.

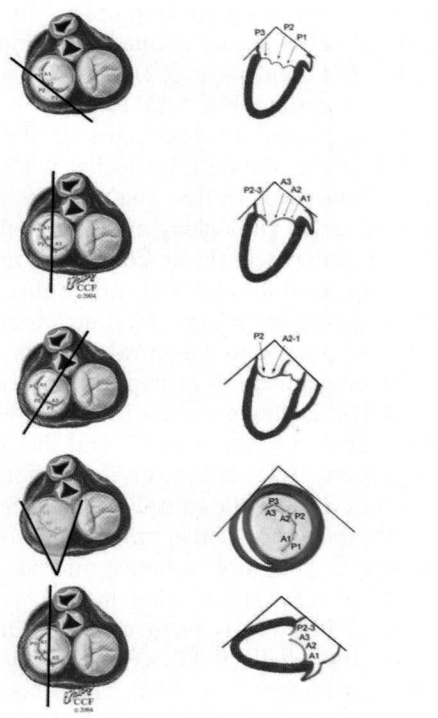

**FIGURE 5.12.** TEE-imaging planes and segmental mitral valve leaflet identification using SCA-ASE nomenclature.

## MITRAL VALVE LEAFLETS: CARPENTIER-SCA TERMINOLOGY

The Carpentier terminology is solely a terminology of the mitral leaflets and does not involve naming chordae or papillary muscles (7). The lateral scallop of the posterior leaflet is named P1, middle scallop named P2, and medial scallop named P3. The anterior leaflet is divided into A1,

A2, A3 based upon the portion of the anterior leaflet making contact with P1, P2, and P3 during systole (Figs. 5.12, 5.13, and 5.14 and Table 28.2). The SCA/ASE terminology does not in fact define chordal attachment to the leaflets. However, it is important for the echocardiographer to understand the orientation of chordae as related to this terminology. For this purpose, their attachments are explained and related to the Carpentier terminology (Figs. 5.12, 5.13, and 5.14 and Table 28.2). The chordae tendineae are fibrous strings radiating from the left ventricular papillary muscles or the ventricular free wall (posterior leaflet only) and attaching to the mitral leaflets in an organized manner (10). Chordae from the papillary muscles radiate upward attaching to the corresponding halves of the anterior and posterior leaflets. Chordae arising from the anterior papillary muscle attach to A1, P1, (AC), and the lateral half of P2 and A2. Chordae arising from the posterior papillary muscle attach to A3, P3, (PC), and the medial half of P2, and A2 (Figs. 5.12, 5.13, and 5.14 and Table 28.2). This relation aids in defining the portion of the mitral valve that is echocardiographically visualized.

There are two chordae attaching to the ventricular surface of the anterior leaflet that are by far the thickest and largest of the chordae to the mitral valve. They have been called strut or stay chordae. One arises from the anterior papillary muscle and attaches to the A1/A2 area of the anterior leaflet; the other arises from the posterior papillary muscle and attaches to the A2/A3 portion of the anterior leaflet (Fig. 5.14).

## MITRAL VALVE APPARATUS—DURAN TERMINOLOGY

The Duran mitral valve nomenclature is based on dividing the structures of the mitral valve into what is seen by the surgeon observing the valve through a left atriotomy.

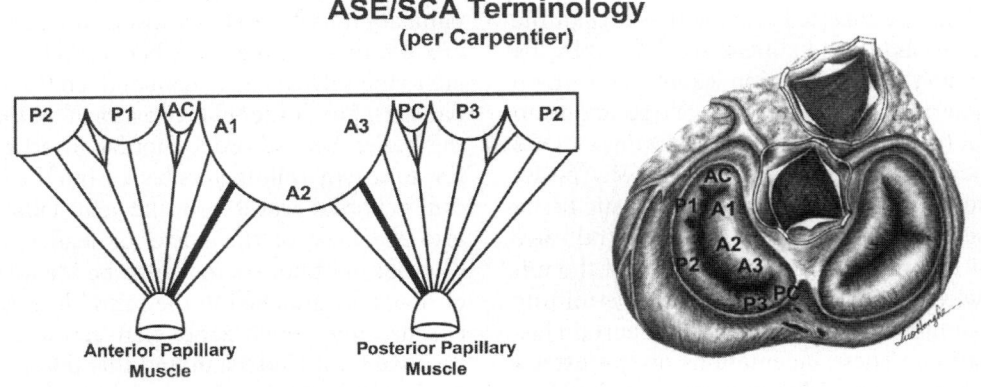

**FIGURE 5.13.** Chordal relationships—ASE/SCA terminology. Anterior leaflet divided into A1, A2, and A3. Posterior leaflet divided into P1 (anterolateral scallop), P2 (middle scallop), and P3 (posteromedial scallop). Commissural clefts not named anterior or posterior. Chordae arising from the anterior papillary muscle attach to A1, AC, and P1, and the lateral half of P2 and A2. Chordae arising from the posterior papillary muscle attach to A3, PC, and P3, and the medial half of P2 and A2.

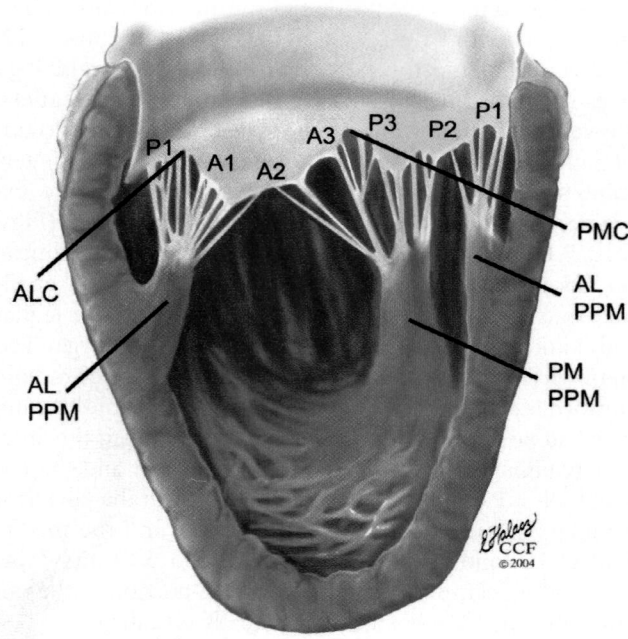

**FIGURE 5.14.** Chordal relationships—ASE/SCA terminology. The anterior mitral valve leaflet is shown in *yellow*. The posterior mitral valve leaflet is shown in *blue*. Chordae arising from the anterior papillary muscle attach to A1–P1, and the lateral half of P2 and A2. Chordae arising from the posterior papillary muscle attach to A3–P3 and the medial half of P2 and A2. Depicted above: Anterior leaflet divided into A1, A2, and A3. Posterior leaflet divided into P1 (anterolateral scallop), P2 (middle scallop), and P3 (posteromedial scallop). Anterolateral commissure (ALC), posteromedial commissure (PMC), posteromedial papillary muscle (PM PPM), anterolateral papillary muscle (AL PPM).

The structures of the mitral apparatus in this orientation are defined as being anterior (A) or posterior (P) and being left or right as viewed by this surgical view. Left-sided structures are noted by the numeral 1 and right-sided by the numeral 2. The chordae tendineae are named by the area of the leaflet into which they are inserted, independent of whether they are inserted into the free edge or the ventricular surface. Chordae tendineae are defined by the location of attaching to the anterior leaflet based upon the area of attachment and right and left orientation to their related strut (stay) chords. The papillary muscles are defined as M1 (anterior papillary muscle) and M2 (posterior papillary muscle) (11). A curtain of fibroelastic tissue extends from the mitral annulus forming the mitral valve leaflets (12,13,14). The combined surface area of the mitral leaflets is twice that of the mitral orifice, permitting large areas of coaptation. The free edge of this curtain has multiple indentations. These indentations do not extend to the annulus. The commissural area between the anterior and posterior leaflets is in fact a small leaflet and is delineated by the attachment of the commissural fan chordae. These chordal attachments define the commissural area attaching to the commissural scallops, which

have variable size but great importance for the function of the mitral valve. Duran defines the commissural scallops as left (C1) and right (C2) as seen by the surgeon through an atriotomy (Fig. 5.15) (8).

The anterior leaflet is semicircular in shape. The base-to-apical height of the anterior leaflet is almost twice as great as the posterior leaflet. The annular attachment of the anterior leaflet runs along approximately 30% of the annular circumference. Duran defines the anterior leaflet as A, and divides it into left (A1) and right (A2) halves as seen by the surgeon through a left atriotomy. The posterior leaflet is attached to the mitral annulus along the free wall of the left ventricle. It extends from the anterior commissure (C1) attachment of the LV free wall to the junction of the posterior left ventricle and the muscular ventricular septum (C2). The posterior leaflet attachments involve about 70% of the mitral annulus. Small indentations in the posterior leaflet most commonly give it a three-scallop appearance: a larger middle scallop (PM), lateral scallop (P1), and smaller medial scallop (P2) on either side of PM. PM is further divided into a left half (PM1) and right half (PM2) as viewed by the surgeon through an atriotomy (Fig. 5.15). The echocardiographer performing TEE is able to measure the height of the anterior leaflet and the three scallops of the posterior leaflet. Anatomic measurements of normal heights of these leaflets are given in Tables 5.2 and 5.3 (12).

The chordae tendineae are fibrous strings radiating from the left ventricular papillary muscles or the ventricular free wall (posterior leaflet only) and attaching to the mitral leaflets in an organized manner (11). Chordae from the papillary muscle radiate upward attaching to the corresponding halves of the anterior and posterior leaflets. Chordae arising from M1 (anterior papillary muscle) attach to A1, C1, P1, and PM1. Chordae arising from M2 (posterior papillary muscle) attach to A2, C2, P2, and PM2. This relation aids in defining the portion of the mitral valve visualized echocardiographically. The majority of chordae branch either soon after leaving the papillary muscle or before insertion into the leaflet. There are also cross-connections between chordae as they radiate to the valve leaflets. Lam defined three orders of chordae (12). First-order chordae attach on the free margin of the leaflet. Second-order chordae insert anywhere from a few to several millimeters back from the free edge. Third-order chordae travel from the ventricular wall and insert into the base of the posterior leaflet only (Fig. 5.16). Chordal morphology may also be identified on the basis of how they attached to the mitral leaflet. Lam classified chordae into rough zone, cleft, basal, and commissural chordae (13). Understanding this different chordal morphology is helpful to the surgeon in defining the scallops of the mitral valve. There are two chordae attaching to the ventricular surface of the anterior leaflet that is by far the thickest and largest of the chordae to the mitral valve. They have been called "strut" or "stay chordae." One

▶ TABLE 5.1.  **Height and Spread of the Anterolateral and Posteromedial Commissures of the Mitral Valve**

| | Present study | | | Rusted, Scheifley, and Edwards (1952) | | | | Cheichi and Lees (1956) | | |
|---|---|---|---|---|---|---|---|---|---|---|
| Commissural Area | Male (26) | Female (24) | Commissure | | Male (25) | Female (25) | Junctional Tissue | | Male (60) | Female (45) |
| | **Anterolateral** | | | **Anterior** | | | | **Anterior** | | |
| Height (cm) | 0.8 (0.5–1.3) | 0.7 (0.5–1.0) | Height (cm) | | 0.8 (0.5–1.3) | 0.7 (0.4–1.1) | Height (cm) | | 0.8 (0.6–1.2) | 0.7 (0.6–1.1) |
| Spread (cm) | 1.2 (0.6–1.9) | 0.9 (0.3–1.5) | — | | — | — | Breadth (cm) | | 1.7 (0.7–2.4) | 1.5 (0.7–2.1) |
| | **Posteromedial** | | | **Posterior** | | | | **Posterior** | | |
| Height (cm) | 0.8 (0.6–1.2) | 0.8 (0.4–1.1) | Height (cm) | | 0.8 (0.5–1.3) | 0.7 (0.3–1.0) | Height (cm) | | 0.7 (0.5–0.9) | 0.6 (0.4–0.8) |
| Spread (cm) | 1.8 (1.2–2.6) | 1.5 (0.9–2.2) | — | | — | — | Breadth (cm) | | 1.3 (0.7–1.8) | 1.2 (0.7–1.6) |

Note: Measurements of the commissures given by Rusted, Scheifley, and Edwards (1952) and of the junctional tissues given by
Cheichi and Lees (1956) are added for comparison.

arises from M1 and attaches to A1 of the anterior leaflet; one arises from M2 and attaches to the A2 portion of the anterior leaflet.

The papillary muscles are large trabeculae carnae originating from the junction of the middle and apical third of the left ventricular wall in a plane posterior to the intercommissural plane in diastole. Rusted et al., suggested the nomenclature anterior (anterolateral) and posterior (posterolateral) based upon the consistent relationship that each papillary muscle bears with its respective commissural area (C1, C2) (16). According to Duran's surgical classification, the anterior papillary muscle is termed M1 and the posterior termed M2. The anterior papillary muscle (M1) is located on the anterior-lateral free wall of the left ventricle. The posterior papillary muscle (M2) originates at the junction of the posterior left ventricular free wall and the muscular ventricular septum (8). They extend into the upper third of the ventricular cavity below the commissural tissue (C1, C2) of the left ventricle. The papillary muscles most commonly have one head, but may have double, triple, or multiple heads. The M1 papillary muscle is more commonly supplied by two separate

## Duran Terminology

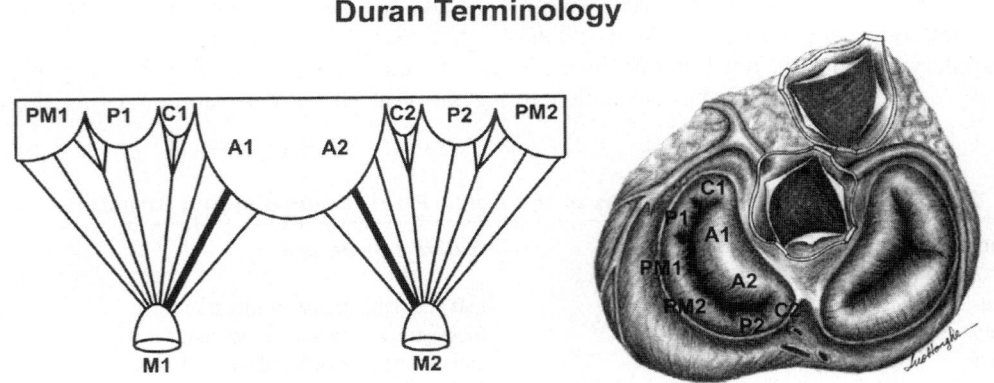

**FIGURE 5.15.** Duran terminology. Diagram of the mitral valve apparatus. Anterior leaflet is divided into A1 and A2. Posterior leaflet is divided into P1, PM, and P2. PM is further divided into PM1 and PM2. Anterior papillary muscle M1 and posterior papillary muscle M2. Commissural scallops are labeled C1 and C2. Observe that all leaflets with a numerical 1 are held by chordae arising from M1 and those leaflets with a numerical 2 are held by chordae arising from M2. Darkened chordae from M1 to A1 and M2 to A2 represent strut or stay chordae.

▶ TABLE 5.2. **Height and Width of the Anterior and Posterior Leaflets of the Mitral Valve, Comparing the Data of Rusted, Scheifley, and Edwards (1952) and of Cheichi and Lees (1956)**

| | *Present study* | | *Rusted, Scheifley, and Edwards (1952)* | | *Cheichi and Lees (1956)* | |
|---|---|---|---|---|---|---|
| *Height and Width* | *Male (26)* | *Female (24)* | *Male (25)* | *Female (25)* | *Male (60)* | *Female (25)* |
| | **Anterior Cusp** | | **Anterior Cusp** | | **Aortic Leaflet** | |
| Height | 2.4 | 2.2 | 2.3 | 2.1 | 2.1 | 2.2 |
| (cm) | (2.0–3.0) | (1.8–3.5) | (1.6–2.9) | (1.6–2.5) | (1.9–3.2) | (1.8–2.7) |
| Width | 3.6 | 2.9 | — | — | 3.7 | 3.3 |
| (cm) | (2.5–4.8) | (1.8–4.2) | | | (2.5–4.5) | (2.4–4.2) |
| | **Posterior Leaflet Middle Scallop** | | **Posterior Cusp** | | **Ventricular Leaflet** | |
| Height | 1.4 | 1.2 | 1.3 | 1.2 | 1.4 | 1.2 |
| (cm) | (0.9–2.0) | (0.7–1.8) | (0.8–1.8) | (0.7–2.4) | (1.8–2.5) | (0.8–2.4) |
| Width | 2.3 | 1.8 | — | — | 3.3 | 3.0 |
| (cm) | (1.3–3.8) | (0.6–2.6) | | | (2.5–4.1) | (2.3–3.6) |
| | **Anterolateral Commissural Scallop** | | | | **Anterior Leaflet Accessory** | |
| Height | 1.1 | 1.0 | — | — | 1.1 | 1.0 |
| (cm) | (0.9–2.0) | (0.8–1.4) | | | (0.8–1.8) | (0.7–1.3) |
| Width | 1.6 | 1.4 | | | 1.5 | 1.2 |
| (cm) | (0.9–4.0) | (0.9–2.0) | | | (1.1–1.8) | (1.0–1.6) |
| | **Posteromedial Commissural Scallop** | | | | **Posterior Accessory Leaflet** | |
| Height | 1.0 | 0.8 | — | — | 0.9 | 0.9 |
| (cm) | (0.6–1.7) | (0.5–1.1) | | | (0.6–1.2) | (0.7–1.0) |
| Width | 1.5 | 1.1 | | | 1.1 | 0.8 |
| (cm) | (0.9–3.1) | (0.5–2.2) | | | (0.8–1.5) | (0.7–1.2) |

arteries: the first obtuse marginal arising from the left circumflex and the first diagonal arising from the left anterior descending artery (15–17). A single artery, usually from the right coronary artery or the third obtuse marginal of the left circumflex, most commonly perfuses the M2 papillary muscle. The greater incidence of M2 papillary muscle dysfunction or rupture in myocardial ischemia has been associated with the single artery supply to it versus the common dual supply to the M1 papillary muscle. The papillary muscles do not function in isolation from the left ventricular wall and chordae/leaflets to

which they attach. The whole mitral valve apparatus interaction is important for proper ventricular function.

## AORTIC ROOT

The aortic root is the portion of the ventricular outflow that supports the leaflets of the aortic valve. The superior boundary of the aortic root is the sinotubular junction and the inferior boundary is the plane defined by the bases of the aortic semilunar valves attaching to the

▶ TABLE 5.3. **Relationship of Various Portions of the Aortic Root to Surrounding Structures**

| *Portion of Aortic Root* | *Related Structure* |
|---|---|
| Noncoronary sinus | Left and right atriums, transverse sinus |
| Right coronary sinus | Right atrium, free pericardial space |
| Left coronary sinus | Left atrium, free pericardium |
| Non-/right coronary interleaflet triangle (membranous septum) | Right atrium, conduction system, septal leaflet of tricuspid valve, right ventricle |
| Right/left coronary interleaflet triangle | Potential space between aorta and pulmonary trunk or infundibulum |
| Left/noncoronary interleaflet triangle (subaortic curtain) | Left atrium, makes up large portion of the aortic leaflet of the mitral valve |

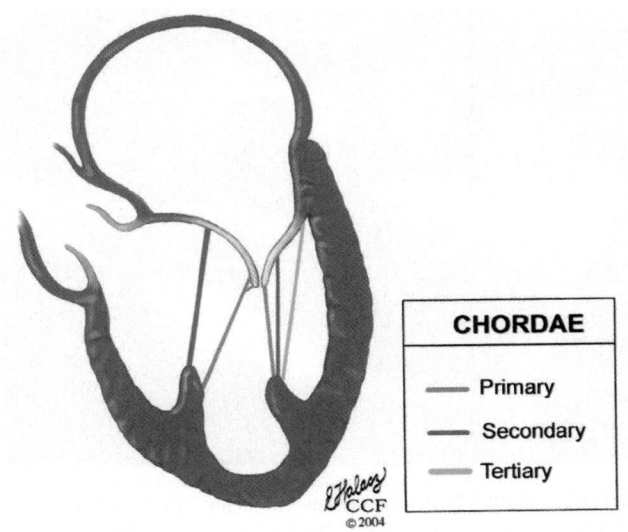

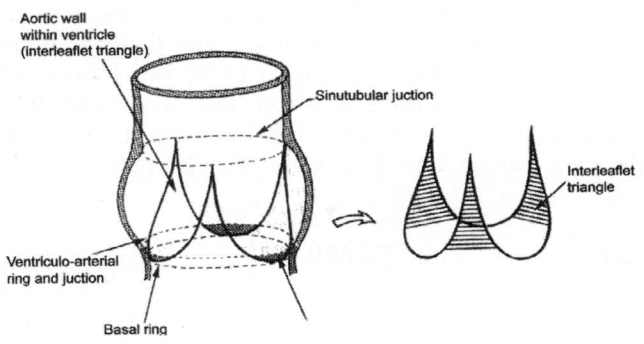

**FIGURE 5.17.** Diagram of the aortic root. **Inset:** The coronet-like arrangement of the valvar attachments.

**FIGURE 5.16.** There are three orders of chordae. First-order chordae attach on the free margin of the leaflet. Second-order chordae insert anywhere from a few to several millimeters back from the free edge. Third-order chordae travel from the papillary muscle and ventricular wall and insert into the base of the posterior leaflet only.

crown-shaped aortic annulus. Within these boundaries the aortic root is composed of the aortic valve leaflets, the sinuses of Valsalva, and the interleaflet triangles (Fig. 5.17) (16).

There are three functional semilunar leaflets of the normal aortic valve. Each leaflet has

1. A functional hinge point where it attaches to the aortic root
2. A body of the semilunar valve
3. A coaptation surface of the leaflet with a thickened central nodule (nodule of Arantii)

The hinge point of the aortic leaflets attaches to the aortic root in a semilunar fashion along the crown-shaped aortic annulus (annulus fibrosus). The superior apex of each leaflet attaching to the annulus fibrosus, attaches to the sinotubular junction. The bases of the aortic leaflets attach to the annulus at or below the anatomic ventricular arterial junction. The three cusps are referred to as right coronary, left coronary, and noncoronary cusps based on the coronary ostium associated with the cusp (Fig. 5.18). The cusps are of similar but not equal sizes. Corresponding with each cusp of the aortic valve, the aortic root is expanded forming the three sinuses of Valsalva. The sinuses of Valsalva are defined inferiorly by the attachments of the aortic valve leaflets and superiorly by the sinotubular junction (Figs. 5.19, 5.20, and 5.21). The sinotubular junction is thicker than the adjacent sinuses and is circular, defining the beginning of the aorta proper. The thickness and circular nature of the sinotubular junction

play an important role in supporting the aortic valve leaflets. Dilation of the sinotubular junction can cause aortic insufficiency and may be a contraindication for placing a stentless aortic valve. The interleaflet triangles are the portion of the aortic root between the attachments of the aortic valve leaflets along the annulus fibrosus and the plane defined by the three bases of the aortic annulus (18). These interleaflet triangles, although part of the aortic root, are exposed to left ventricular pressures in that they lay below the basal attachment of the aortic leaflets. Understanding the anatomic relationships of the

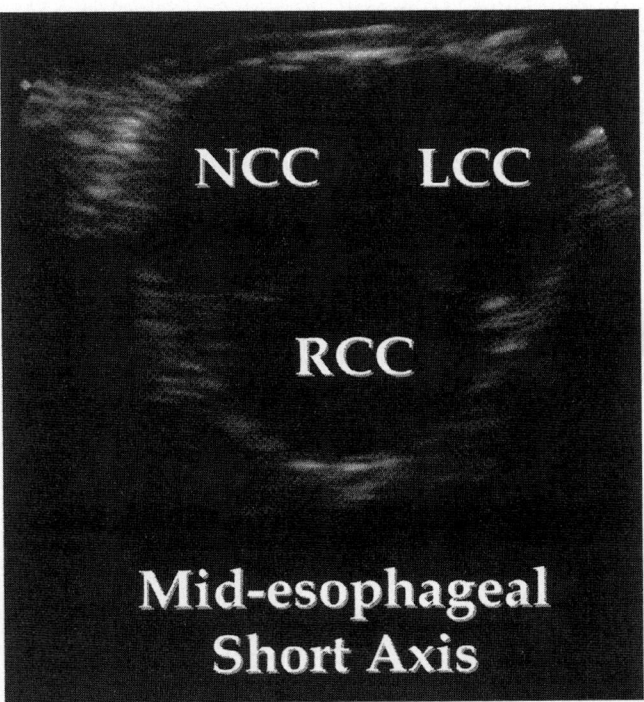

**FIGURE 5.18.** Midesophageal short-axis imaging plane demonstrating the three coronary cusps: right coronary cusp (RCC), noncoronary cusp (NCC), and left coronary cusp (LCC).

aortic root to other cardiac structures is critical when evaluating abnormal cardiac shunts and fistulas (Table 5.3). Measurement of the diameter of the annular base of the aortic valve, sinus of Valsalva, sinotubular junction, and ascending aorta provides important data for surgical decision making (Figs. 5.19, 5.20, and 5.21) (18).

## CORONARY ANATOMY

The left main and right coronary arteries (RCA) supplying the heart arise from ostia in the left sinus of Valsalva and right sinus of Valsalva, respectively. The left main coronary artery then divides into the left anterior descending (LAD) coronary artery and the circumflex coronary artery. At the base of the heart the RCA and circumflex artery form a circle around the heart in the atrioventricular groove. A long-axis loop is formed by the LAD and the posterior descending coronary artery (Fig. 5.22) (19). The posterior descending artery originates as a termination of the right coronary and/or circumflex coronary artery. The term *dominance* in regards to the coronary circulation defines which of these two vessels terminate to form the posterior descending artery. A right dominant circulation is one in which the PDA is formed as a termination of the RCA. A left dominant coronary circulation is one where the PDA is formed as a branch of the circumflex coronary artery. Right dominance occurs in 85% of hearts, whereas left dominance occurs in about 10%–15% of hearts. Vessels may be codominant if the right coronary gives rise only to the posterior descending artery and the circumflex to vessels supplying the posterior left ventricle. The left main coronary artery originates from an ostium in the left sinus of Valsalva. The left main coronary artery bifurcates into the left anterior descending artery and the circumflex coronary artery. Occasionally an additional branch comes off that parallels the diagonal arteries of

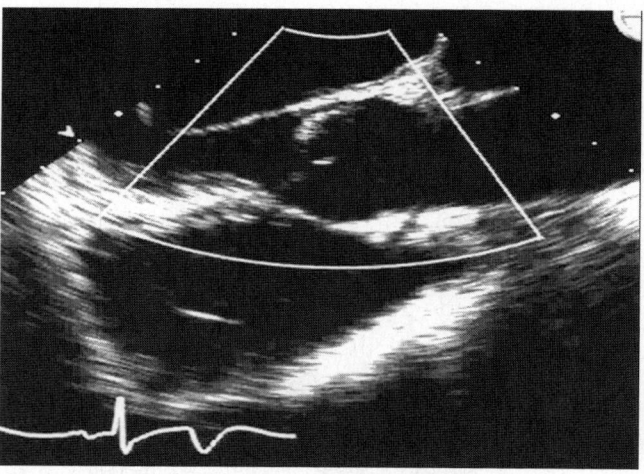

**FIGURE 5.20.** The midesophageal long-axis imaging plane demonstrating the aortic root consisting of the aortic valve annulus, aortic valve leaflets, coronary sinuses, sinotubular junction, and ascending (tubular) aorta.

the left anterior descending artery. Such a branch off the left main is called the *ramus intermedius*.

The left anterior descending coronary artery originates from the left main and travels along the anterior interventricular sulcus to the apex of the heart. In most cases the artery extends to the posterior aspect of the heart communicating with the posterior descending artery. The LAD sends large septal perforating arteries perpendicularly into the interventricular septum. Diagonal branches of the LAD course obliquely between the LAD and circumflex artery supplying the left ventricular free wall anteriorly and laterally. The LAD supplies a few small branches to the right ventricular free wall. The left circumflex coronary artery originates from the left main coronary artery and then travels along the left atrial ventricular groove on the left, coursing posteriorly, and supplies the posterior segment of the LV. Obtuse marginal branches of the circumflex anterior supply

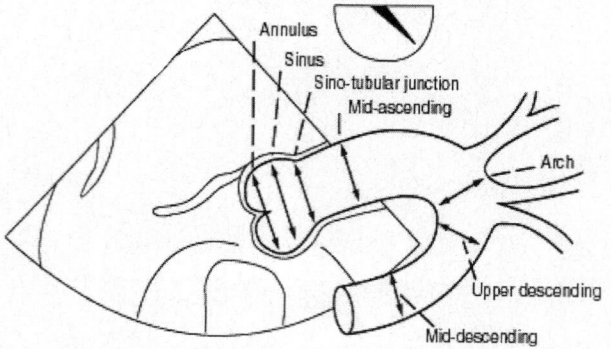

**FIGURE 5.19.** Schematic representation of the midesophageal long-axis imaging plane demonstrating the aortic root. Measurements are taken at the annulus (hinge point of the aortic valve), sinus of Valsalva, sinotubular junction, and ascending aorta.

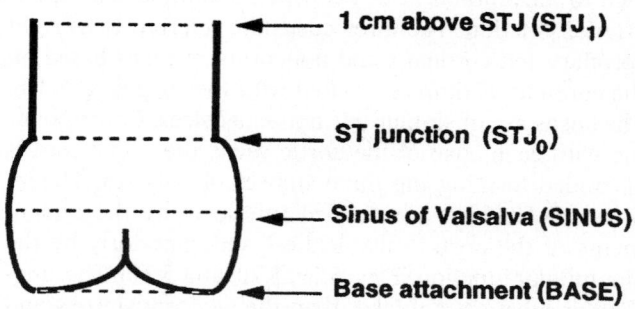

**FIGURE 5.21.** Schematic representation of four levels of aortic root where measurements are taken.

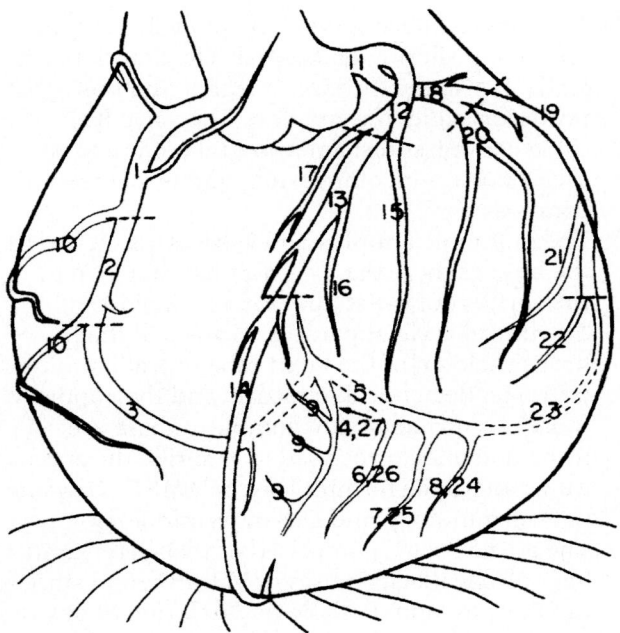

**FIGURE 5.22.** Diagram of the anatomic segments of the coronary arteries for use in locating lesions in individual patients. Proximal, mid, and distal portions of the right coronary artery (*1, 2, 3*). Posterior descending coronary artery, which, as the dotted segments proximal to it indicate, may arise from the right (*4*) or left (*27*) system (*4, 27*). Right posterolateral segment (*5*), an extension of the right coronary artery in association with right dominant systems (*6, 7, 8*). From it come several inferior surface (marginal) branches, called right posterolateral arteries, to the back of the left ventricle. Left dominant systems have a comparable left posterolateral segment, leading to the posterior descending artery. Inferior septal branches of the posterior descending artery (*9*). Acute marginal branches of the coronary artery (*10*). Left main coronary artery (*11*). Proximal, mid, and distal portions of the left anterior descending coronary artery (*12, 13, 14*). First and second diagonal branches (*15, 16*). The first diagonal may originate almost from the bifurcation of the left main coronary artery, and was formerly called a ramus intermedius. Additional diagonal branches may be present. First septal branch of the anterior descending artery (*17*). The proximal and distal portions of the left circumflex coronary artery (*18, 19*). The first, second, and third obtuse marginal branches of the circumflex artery, the first is usually the largest vessel (*20, 21, 22*). An extension of the circumflex artery, called the left AV artery, present only in patients with a left dominant system (*23*). In such patients, this vessel gives off further inferior surface ("marginal") branches to the back of the left ventricle, now called left posterolateral arteries (*24, 25, 26*), before terminating in the left posterior descending coronary artery (*27*). From the National Heart, Lung, and Blood Institute Coronary Artery Surgery Study (CASS), and the American Heart Association, Inc., with permission.

the obtuse margin of the left ventricle. In left dominant circulation, the circumflex provides left posterolateral (marginal) arteries to the inferior portion of the left ventricle.

The right coronary originates from an ostium in the right sinus of Valsalva. Traveling in the right atrioventricular groove, the RCA gives off branches to the anterior right ventricular free wall. Traveling in the region of the acute margin of the right ventricle the RCA gives off acute marginal branches, which course to the apex of the heart. In right dominant circulations the RCA courses posteriorly, terminating by bifurcating into the posterior descending and right posterolateral segment artery. The posterior descending artery travels in the posterior interventricular sulcus, giving rise to septal, right ventricular, and left ventricular branches. The right posterolateral segment artery gives rise to marginal branches supplying the inferior surface of the left ventricle.

The general areas of the left ventricular wall supplied by the coronary arteries have been summarized in the standard ASE/SCA Guidelines for Performing Intraoperative TEE according to the standardized 16 segmental views (Fig. 5.23) (5). The LAD supplies the basal, mid, and apical septal segments; basal and mid anteroseptal segments; basal, mid, and apical anterior segments. The LAD provides blood to the anterior two-thirds of the septum. The LAD supplies conduction tissue, including the bundle of His, the right bundle branch, and the anterior fascicle of the left bundle.

The circumflex artery supplies the basal, mid, and apical lateral segments and the basal and mid posterior segments. In hearts that have a left dominant circulation, the circumflex gives rise to the posterior descending artery supplying both the inferior wall, the inferior third of the septum, and the atrioventricular node. In addition, it provides blood supply to the posteromedial papillary muscle and portions of the posterior fascicle of the left bundle. The proximal left circumflex supplies the sinoatrial node in 65% of hearts.

The RCA in right dominant circulations provides basal, mid, and apical inferior segments of the left ventricle (Fig. 5.23). In addition, in right dominant systems (85% of patients), the RCA provides blood supply for the inferior one-third of the septum and is the origin of the atrioventricular (AV) node artery.

## CONCLUSION

It has been the purpose of this discussion to familiarize the echocardiographer with the cardiovascular anatomy, which is essential for utilizing ultrasound in the perioperative management of patients. We have reviewed cardiac structure from the fibrous skeleton to a detailed examination of the cardiac valves. This discussion will serve as the basis for a fuller understanding of three-dimensional cardiac structure and enable a more capable provision of the critical information that will guide the management of the patient's clinical course.

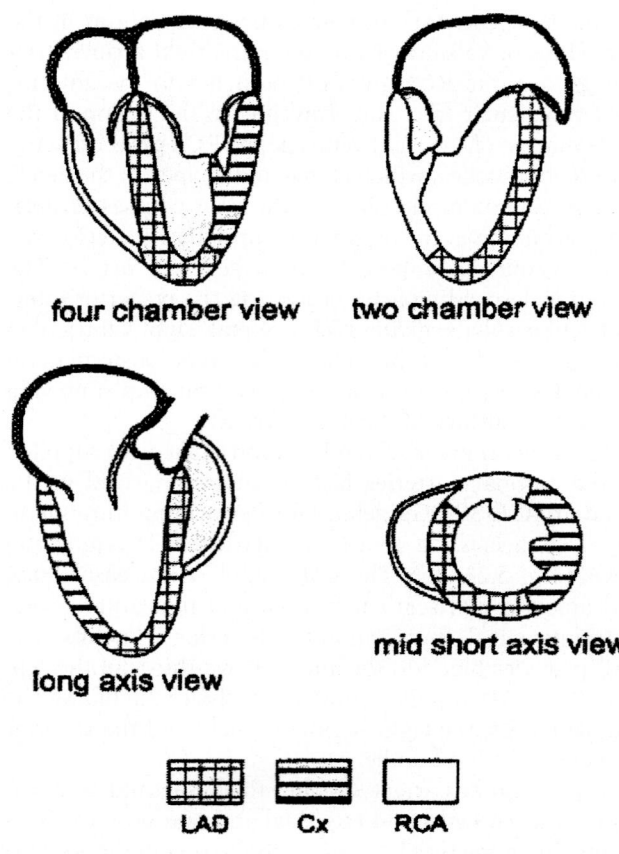

four chamber view          two chamber view

long axis view

mid short axis view

LAD          Cx          RCA

**FIGURE 5.23.** Typical regions of myocardium perfused by each of the major coronary arteries to the left ventricle. Other patterns occur as a result of normal anatomic variations or coronary disease with collateral flow. LAD, left anterior descending; Cx, circumflex; RCA, right coronary artery.

## KEY POINTS

- The fibrous skeleton of the heart is formed by the U-shaped cords of the aortic annulus forming the right and left trigones. From the left and right trigones, a fibrous tissue continuum extends around the left and right atrioventricular orifices, forming the annuli fibrosi of the mitral and tricuspid annuli. The mitral annuli fibrosi thins posteriorly, permitting pathologic annular dilatation and increased tension on the middle scallop of the PMVL.
- The Society of Cardiovascular Anesthesiologists and American Society of Echocardiography have jointly developed a sixteen-segment model of the LV based on the recommendations of the Subcommittee on Quantification of the ASE Standards Committee, which divides the LV into three levels (basal, mid, and apical). The base and mid levels are divided into six segments and the apex into four.

- The three leaflets of the tricuspid valve are the anterior, posterior, and septal. The anterior leaflet is usually the largest leaflet and the posterior leaflet the smallest. The valve has three commissures: anteroseptal commissure, anteroposterior commissure, and posteroseptal commissure.
- The pulmonic annulus and valve are attached to the base of the aorta by a fibrous extension of the aortic root called the *tendon of conus*.
- The mitral valve apparatus consists of the fibrous skeleton of the heart , the mitral annulus, mitral leaflets, mitral chordae, and the papillary muscle-ventricular wall complex. There are three nomenclatures used to describe the apparatus: anatomic terminology, SCA/ASE (Carpentier) terminology, and Duran terminology.
- The aortic root is comprised of the aortic annulus, valve leaflets, sinuses of Valsalva, and sinotubular junction. Pathologic distortion of any of these components may result in aortic-valve dysfunction.
- The aortic valve has three coronary cusps (right, left, and noncoronary) with corresponding expanded sinuses inferiorly defined by attachment of the leaflet and the sinotubular junction.
- The heart is supplied by three coronary arteries: the left anterior descending (LAD), the circumflex (LCx), and the right coronary artery (RCA). The LAD supplies the anterior two-thirds of the interventricular septum, anterolateral free wall of the LV, and the infranodal conduction system (Bundle of His, right bundle branch, and left anterior fascicle). The LCx supplies the posterior and inferior (7% of patients) wall of the LV and portions of the posterior fascicle of the LBB. It also supplies the posteromedial papillary muscle. The RCA supplies the right ventricle and the inferior LV (in 85% of patients) in addition to the AV node. Myocardial ischemia produces regional wall-motion abnormalities and dysrhythmias that may be predicted on the basis of coronary circulation.

## REFERENCES

1. Zimmerman J, Bailey CP. The surgical significance of the fibrous skeleton of the heart. J Thorac Cardiovasc Surg 1962;44:701–712.
2. Kunzelman KS, Reimink MS, Cochran RP. Annular dilation increases stress in the mitral valve and delays coaptation: a finite element computer model. Cardiovasc Surg 1997; 5(4):427–24.
3. Lee KS, Stewart WJ, Lever HM, Underwood PL, Cosgrove DM. Mechanism of outflow tract obstruction causing failed mitral valve repair. Circulation 1993;88(Part 2):24–29.

4. Mihaileanu S, Mariono JP, Chauvaud S, et al. Left ventricular outflow obstruction after mitral repair (Carpentier's technique): proposed mechanism of disease. Circulation 1988;78(Suppl 1):I-78–I-84.
5. Maslov AD, Regan MM, Haering JM, Johnson RG, Levine RA. Echocardiographic predictors of left ventricular outflow tract obstruction and systolic anterior motion of the mitral valve after mitral valve reconstruction for myxomatous disease. J Am Coll Cardiol 1999;34:2096–2104.
6. Walmsley R, Watson H. The outflow tract of the left ventricle. Brit Heart J 1966;28:435–47.
7. Shanewise JS, Cheung AT, Aronson S, et al. ASE/SCA for performing a comprehensive multiplan transesophageal echocardiography council for intraoperative echocardiography and the Society of Cardiovascular Anesthesiologist task force for certification in perioperative transesophageal echocardiography. J Am Soc Echocardiogr 1999;12:884–900.
8. Silver MD, Lam JHC, Ranganathan N, Wigle ED. Morphology of the human tricuspid valve. Circ 1971;43:33–48.
9. Carpentier AF, Lessana A, Relland JYM, Belli E, Loulmet DF, et al. The "physio-ring": An advanced concept in mitral valve annuloplasty. Ann Thorac Surg 1995;60:1177–86.
10. Kumar N, Kumar M, Duran CMG. A revised terminology for recording surgical findings of the mitral valve. The Journal of Heart Valve Disease 1995;4:70–75.
11. Bollen BA, Hong He Lou, Oury JH, Rubenson DS, Savage RM, Duran C. A systematic approach to intraoperative transesophageal echocardiographic evaluation of the mitral valve with anatomic correlation. J Cardiothorac and Vasc Anest 2000;14,No.3 (June):330–8.
12. Lam JHC, Ranganathan N, Wigle ED, Silver MD. Morphology of the human mitral valve. II. The valve leaflets. Circulation 1970;41:459–67.
13. Lam JHC, Ranganathan N, Wigle ED, Silver MD. Morphology of the human heart valve. I. Chordae Tendineae: A new classification. Circulation 1970;41:449–58.
14. DePlessis LA, Marchand P. The anatomy of the mitral valve and its associated structures. Thorax 1964;19:221–27.
15. Silverman, ME, Hurst JW. The mitral complex. Interaction of the anatomy, physiology, and pathology of the mitral annulus, mitral valve leaflets, chordae tendineae, and papillary muscles. Amer Heart Journal 1968;3:399–418.
16. Rusted IE, Schiefly CH, Edwards JE. Studies of the mitral valve. I. Anatomical features of the normal mitral valve and associated structures. Circulation 1952;6:825–31.
17. Voci P, Bilotta F, Caretta Q, Mercanti C, Marino B. Papillary muscle perfusion pattern: A hypothesis for ischemic papillary muscle dysfunction. Circulation 1995;91:1714–18.
18. Kirkland JW, Barratt-Boyes BG. Cardiac Surgery. 1986 John Wiley and Sons; 1986:19.
19. Principal investigators of CASS and their associates: The National Heart, Lung, and Blood Institute Coronary Artery Surgery Study (CASS). Circulation June 1981;62(Suppl 1).

## QUESTIONS

1. The left fibrous trigone is adjacent to which anatomic structure?
   A. The middle scallop of the PMVL
   B. The septal leaflet of the tricuspid valve
   C. The posteromedial commissure
   D. The base of the lateral AMVL

2. Which portion of the mitral annulus has the least shape change during the cardiac cycle?
   A. Anterolateral annulus
   B. Posteromedial annulus
   C. Anterior annulus
   D. Posterior annulus

3. The thinnest portion of the annulus fibrosa is located:
   A. Anteriorly
   B. Anterolaterally
   C. Posteromedially
   D. Posteriorly

4. The SCA and ASE standard nomenclature divides the apex into each of the following segments, *except:*
   A. Anterior
   B. Posterior
   C. Inferior
   D. Lateral

5. Strut or stay chordae are thicker and originate from the anterior and posterior muscles and attach to which of the following segments of the mitral valve?
   A. Lateral base of the AMVL
   B. Medial midportion of the AMVL
   C. Lateral base of the PMVL
   D. Middle edge of the PMVL

# Comprehensive and Abbreviated Intraoperative TEE Examination

## Jack S. Shanewise, Daniel P. Vezina, and Michael K. Cahalan

Since its first use assessing cardiac function in the operating room over 20 years ago (1–3), transesophageal echocardiography (TEE) has come to play a critical role in the anesthetic management of patients undergoing surgery that involves the heart and great vessels. It is used as a diagnostic tool during cardiac surgery as well as a monitor of cardiac function, and many studies have shown that it has a significant impact on both the surgical care and anesthetic management these patients receive (4–7). This chapter will review an approach to performing a comprehensive intraoperative TEE examination using a multiplane probe.

There are several good reasons to complete a comprehensive TEE examination whenever possible. One important aspect of learning TEE is to become familiar with normal and abnormal anatomy of the heart and great vessels as imaged with echocardiography. The more complete exams performed, the more exposure there is to normal and abnormal pathology. Complete examinations also maximize exposure to the various TEE views, allowing one to become familiar with these more quickly. Performing and recording a comprehensive TEE examination at the beginning of an operation establishes a set of baseline findings. Should unexpected problems arise later in the case, this baseline record can be reviewed to determine whether subsequently noted findings are new or were preexisting. Finally, there is a small but important percentage of patients in which the comprehensive TEE examination reveals an unexpected incidental finding, which often can have an important impact on the care a patient receives. There may be situations in which the patient is unstable and a complete examination cannot be performed; in this situation, the main purpose of the TEE examination should be accomplished first so that the important issue for the case is addressed. Then, the remainder of the comprehensive examination may be completed as the situation allows.

## PREVENTION OF TEE COMPLICATIONS

Although generally a very safe procedure when performed in appropriately selected patients with proper technique, TEE can, on rare occasions, result in serious complications (8,9). Therefore, every comprehensive TEE examination begins with a search for contraindications to the procedure (Table 6.1). Symptomatic esophageal stricture, esophageal diverticulum, recent esophageal surgery, and esophageal tumor are generally considered absolute contraindications to TEE. Assessment before the procedure includes a review of the medical record and an interview with the patient whenever possible. Specific questions are asked regarding the presence of dysphagia, hematemesis, and a history of esophageal disease. When a history of esophageal disease or symptoms is discovered, the relative risk of performing TEE must be balanced against the potential benefit of the procedure. The decision to proceed despite such symptoms should be documented in the medical record with an acknowledgement of the increased risk, including informed consent from the patient. Evaluation by a gastroenterologist with

▶ TABLE 6.1. **Contraindications for Transesophageal Echocardiography**

| |
|---|
| I Absolute |
|     Recent esophageal or gastric surgery |
|     Symptomatic esophageal stricture |
|     Esophageal diverticulum |
|     Esophageal tumor or abscess |
| II Relative |
|     History of mediastinal radiation |
|     Symptomatic hiatal hernia |
|     Coagulopathy |
|     Unexplained UGI bleed |
|     Esophageal Varices |
|     Cervical spine disease |

esophagoscopy can be helpful in assessing the risk of performing TEE.

Excessive force must never be used to insert or manipulate the probe within the esophagus. Perforation of the pharynx by TEE probe insertion and of the esophagus from TEE examination have been reported (10,11) and may be more likely in elderly women, possibly due to more delicate tissue and smaller body size. Less catastrophic complications of TEE include dental and oropharyngeal trauma, mucosal injuries causing GI bleeding, and laryngeal dysfunction, possibly increasing the risk of aspiration postoperatively (12,13). One case report also documented the displacement of an esophageal stethoscope into the stomach occurring during a TEE examination. The dislodged device was retrieved several weeks later using endoscopy (14).

## INTRAOPERATIVE TEE INDICATIONS

There are three categories of indications for intraoperative TEE described by the ASA/SCA Practice Guidelines (15). Category one indications are supported with the strongest evidence in the literature and expert opinion and include hemodynamic instability and valve repair surgery. Category two indications are supported by weaker evidence in the literature and expert consensus. These include patients at risk for myocardial ischemia during surgery and operations to remove cardiac tumors. Category three indications have little scientific evidence or expert support for their use and include monitoring for emboli during orthopedic procedures and intraoperative assessment of graft patency. In judging whether intraoperative TEE is indicated in a particular situation, three factors must be considered. First are patient characteristics—specifically the presence and nature of cardiovascular disease and risk factors for complication due to TEE. Second, the surgical procedure and the role that TEE could play in facilitating its accomplishment must be considered. Finally, the availability of appropriate echocardiographic equipment and expertise in the institution where the procedure is to be formed must be considered.

## OPTIMIZING IMAGE QUALITY

The settings of the echocardiography system have an important impact on the quality of the images obtained. One of the challenges of learning TEE is to know when the image has been optimized, even if of poor quality, and when further efforts to improve it are a waste of time. There is a fair amount of variation in the quality of echo images from patient to patient. The depth of the image is adjusted so that the entire structure of interest is included

and centered in the image. General image gain and dynamic range (compression) are adjusted so that the blood in the chambers is nearly black but distinct from the gray scales of the soft tissues. Time gain controls are adjusted so that there is a uniform level of overall brightness from the near field to the far field of the image. Most TEE probes can provide images on several frequencies. Higher frequencies have better resolution but less penetration than lower frequencies, so the highest frequency with adequate penetration to provide a clear image of the structure being examined is selected. Color flow Doppler is adjusted by increasing the gain until background noise appears in the color sector, and then decreasing it until the noise is just no longer visible. The size and position of the color sector are set to be as small as possible still including the entire area of interest. This helps increase the frame rate, or temporal resolution of the image.

## COMPREHENSIVE TEE EXAMINATION

The American Society of Echocardiography (ASE) and the Society of Cardiovascular Anesthesiologists (SCA) jointly published guidelines for performing a comprehensive intraoperative TEE examination (16,17). The guidelines describe 20 views of the heart and great vessels that include all four chambers and valves of the heart as well as the thoracic aorta and the pulmonary artery (Fig. 6.1). The order in which these views are acquired during a TEE examination may vary from person to person. The following is a description of an approach to performing a comprehensive intraoperative TEE. It is merely one example of many equally valid ways to proceed. It is usually most efficient to complete all of the midesophageal views first, proceed to the transgastric views, and then finish up with an examination of the thoracic aorta.

### General Considerations

The process of examining cardiac structures with TEE begins with moving the transducer into the desired location, and then pointing the imaging plane in the proper direction by manipulating the probe to obtain the desired image. This is accomplished primarily by watching the image develop as the probe is manipulated rather than by relying on the depth markers of the probe or the multiplane angle icon on the screen. These markers and orientation guides can provide a general indication of the transducer location and imaging plane orientation, but final development of the image is always based on the appearance of the structures displayed in the image. There is individual variation in the anatomic relationship of the esophagus to the heart, and this relationship must be taken into consideration when performing a TEE examination. In some patients the esophagus is lateral to the

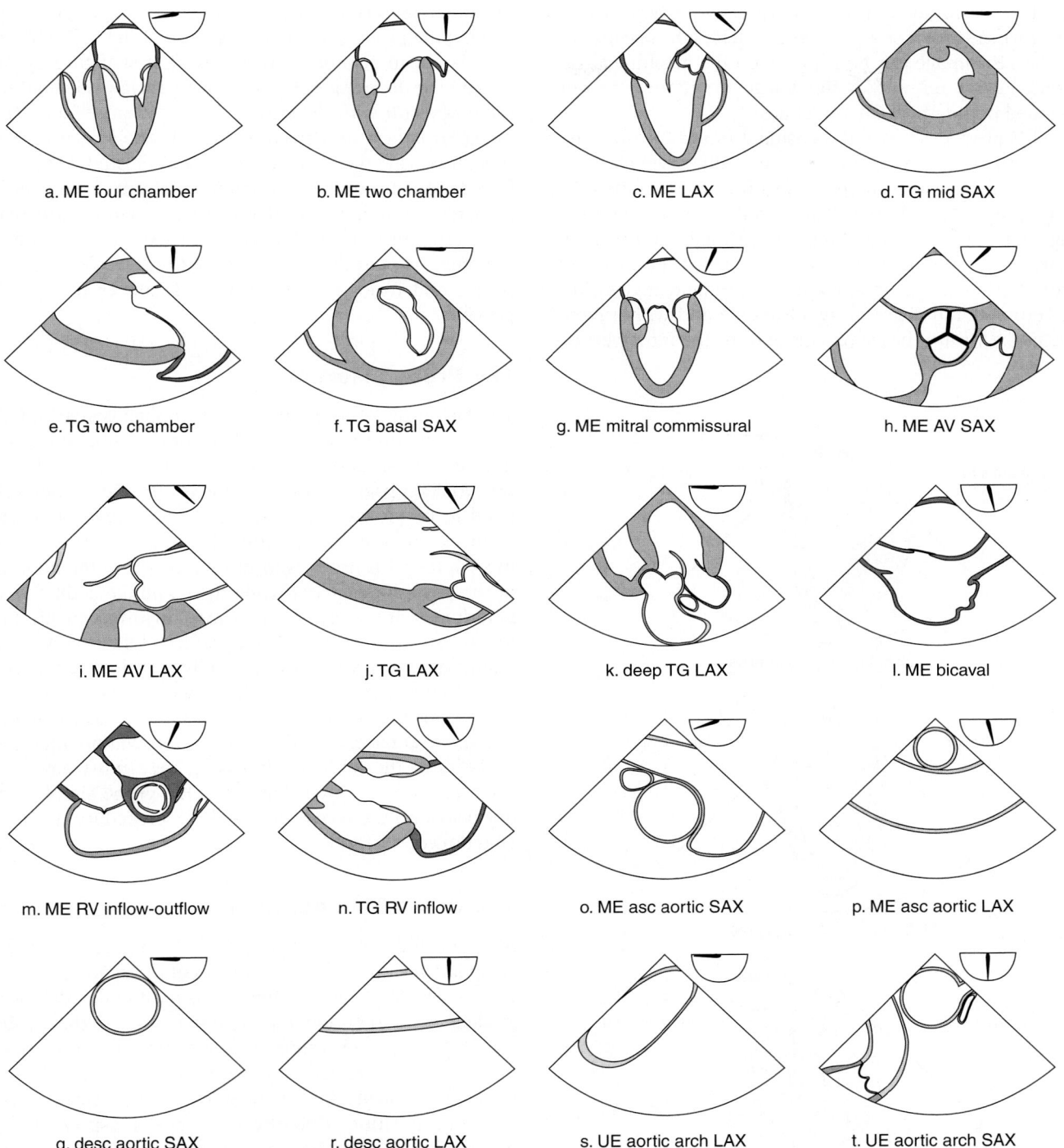

**FIGURE 6.1.** Twenty cross-sectional views comprising the recommended comprehensive TEE examination. Approximate multiplane angle is indicated by the icon adjacent to each view. ME, midesophageal; TG, transgastric; UE, upperesophageal; SAX, short axis; LAX, long axis; AV, aortic valve; RV, right ventricle; asc, ascending; desc, descending.

heart, while in others it is more directly posterior to the left atrium (LA). The up-down and left-right orientation of the TEE image can be adjusted on the machine as desired. Figure 6.2 shows the image orientation recommended in the ASE/SCA guidelines.

TEE produces a two-dimensional image or cross section through the structure being examined, which exists in three dimensions in space. In order to examine each structure in its entirety it is necessary to move the imaging plane through the three-dimensional extent of the structure by manipulating the probe. This is done for the more horizontal imaging planes (multiplane angles close to zero and 180 degrees) by advancing and withdrawing the probe within the esophagus and for the more vertical

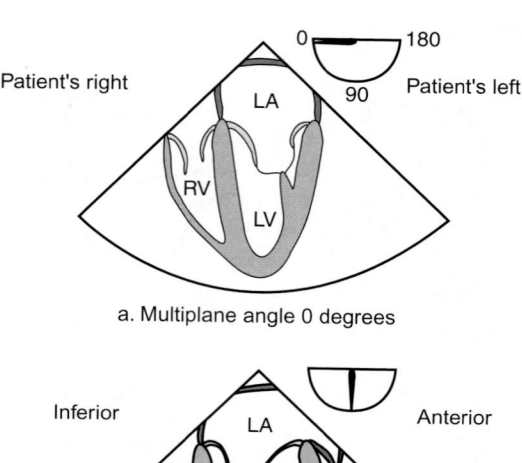

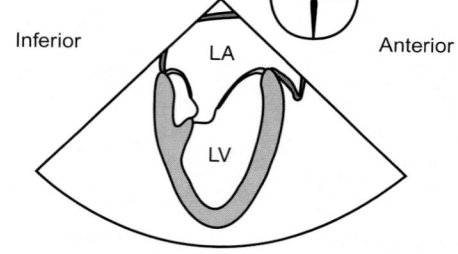

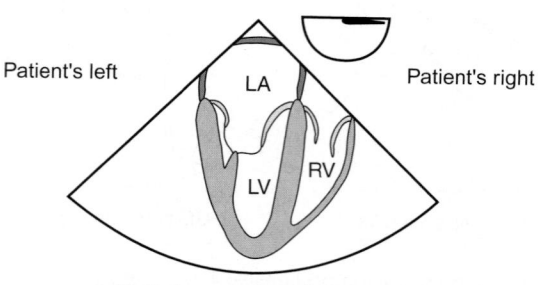

**FIGURE 6.2.** Conventions of image display followed in the guidelines. Transducer location and the near field (vertex) of the image sector are at the top of the display screen and far field at the bottom. **A:** Image orientation at multiplane angle zero degrees. **B:** Image orientation at multiplane angle 90 degrees. **C:** Image orientation at multiplane angle 180 degrees. LA, left atrium; LV, left ventricle; RV, right ventricle.

imaging planes (multiplane angles close to 90 degrees) by turning the probe to the patient's left and right. The imaging plane can also be moved through a structure by increasing or decreasing the multiplane angle while holding the probe still with the structure in the centerline of the image. It is best to focus attention on one structure at a time, following the same sequence in each study. The preferred sequence of the examination will vary from person to person, but if followed routinely it will ensure that each structure is checked on each examination. Each structure should be examined with multiple imaging planes and from more than one transducer position if possible.

## TEE Probe Insertion

The TEE probe is inserted into the esophagus after induction of general anesthesia and tracheal intubation when used during surgery. An orogastric tube is inserted into the stomach prior to inserting the probe and suction applied to remove air or fluid that may be present in the stomach and esophagus. After the orogastric tube is removed, the TEE probe is inserted gently into the midline of the posterior pharynx while the mandible is displaced anteriorly with a jaw lift or thrust in order to lift the tongue and the glottis off the posterior pharynx. Gentle attempts to insert the probe blindly may be tried. However, if after a few attempts the probe does not pass into the esophagus, a laryngoscope is used to displace the mandible anteriorly and provide visualization that the probe is in the midline. Excessive force must never be used, and on rare occasions the TEE probe simply will not pass into the esophagus, and the procedure must be abandoned.

## TEE Probe Manipulation

After the TEE probe is inserted, it is manipulated to develop and acquire a series of images of the heart and great vessels. The following terminology is used in the ASE/SCA guidelines to describe the manipulation of the probe (Fig. 6.3). These terms are made assuming that the imaging plane is directed anteriorly from the esophagus through the heart in a patient in the standard supine anatomic position. Rotating the anterior aspect of the probe within the esophagus toward the patient's right is called "turning to the right," and rotating it toward the left is called "turning to the left." Pushing the tip of the probe more distal into the esophagus or the stomach is called "advancing the transducer," and pulling the tip more proximally is called "withdrawing." Flexing the tip of the probe with the large control wheel anteriorly is called "anteflexing," and flexing it posteriorly "retroflexing." Flexing the tip of the probe with the small control wheel to the patient's right is called "flexing to the right,"

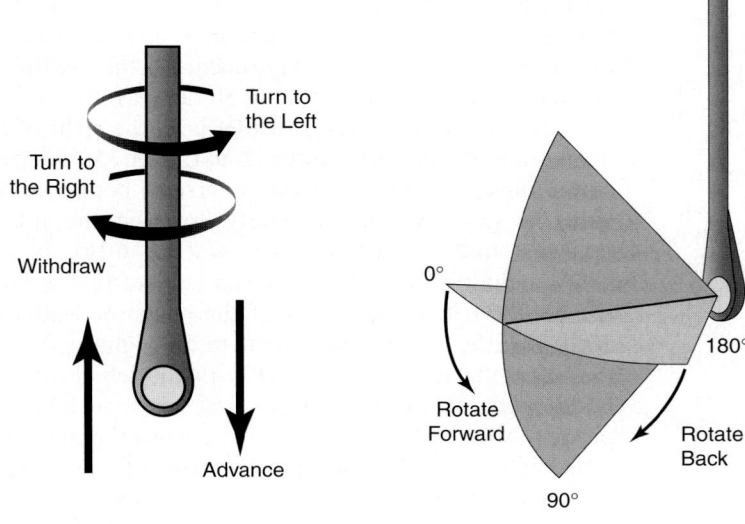

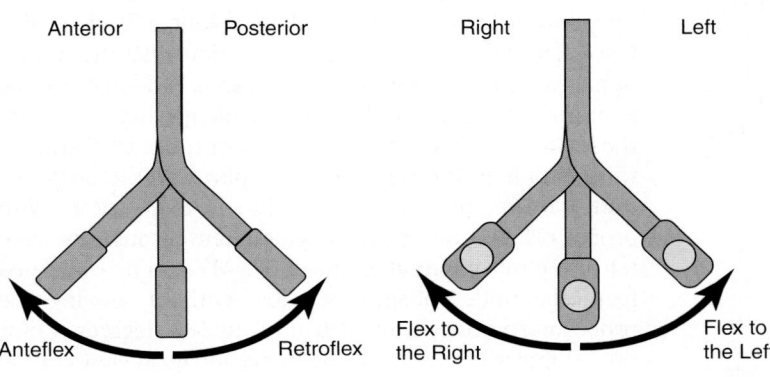

**FIGURE 6.3.** Terminology used to describe manipulation of the probe and transducer during image acquisition.

and flexing it in the opposite direction is called "flexing to the left." Finally, increasing the transducer multiplane angle from zero degrees towards 180 degrees is called "rotating forward," and decreasing in the opposite direction towards zero degrees is called "rotating back."

## Left Atrium and Pulmonary Veins

The comprehensive TEE examination is started by locating the transducer at the midesophageal level posterior to the LA. The LA is then examined from top to bottom with the multiplane angle at zero degrees (horizontal plane) by advancing the probe until the plane passes through the floor of the LA and then withdrawing until the dome of the atrium is reached. The multiplane angle is then increased to about 90 degrees and the probe turned to the left. Near the lateral and superior aspect of the LA, the base of the left atrial appendage (LAA) is seen opening into the atrium. The LAA is examined carefully for throm-

bus by increasing and decreasing the multiplane angle while holding the LAA on the centerline of the image. Turning the probe to the left and withdrawing slightly identifies the left upper pulmonary vein (LUPV), which enters the LA from an anterior to posterior direction just lateral to the LAA. Pulsed wave Doppler is used to examine the LUPV flow velocity profile by placing the sample volume at least 1 cm within the vein. Advancing 1 to 2 cm and turning slightly further to the left will identify the left lower pulmonary vein (LLPV). In some patients the LUPV and LLPV enter the LA as a single vessel. Adjusting the multiplane angle up and down will often open up the veins in the image. The right upper pulmonary vein (RUPV) is next examined by turning the probe to the right at the level of the LAA beyond the interatrial septum (IAS). Like the LUPV, the RUPV can be seen to enter the superior aspect of the LA in an anterior to posterior direction. The right lower pulmonary vein (RLPV) is then seen by turning the probe slightly to the right and advancing 1 to 2 cm.

## Mitral Valve Midesophageal Views

Attention is now turned to the mitral valve (MV), which is examined with several midesophageal views. The MV apparatus includes the anterior and posterior leaflets, annulus, chordae tendinae, papillary muscles, and LV walls. The two leaflets meet at the anterolateral and posteromedial commissures, each of which is related to a corresponding papillary muscle with a similar name. The posterior leaflet anatomically consists of three scallops: lateral (P1), middle (P2), and medial (P3). For descriptive purposes, the anterior leaflet is divided into thirds: lateral third (A1), middle third (A2), and medial third (A3) (Fig. 6.4).

The first step in developing the midesophageal views of the MV is to position the transducer posterior to the midlevel of the LA and direct the imaging plane through the middle of the mitral annulus parallel to the transmitral flow. Retroflexion of the probe tip is often necessary to achieve this because the MV annulus is located inferior to the base of the heart in many patients. The multiplane angle is then increased just until the aortic valve (AV) disappears to develop the midesophageal four-chamber view (Fig. 6.1a), usually around 10 to 20 degrees. In this view the posterior mitral leaflet is to the right of the image display, and the anterior mitral leaflet is to the left. Because the midesophageal four-chamber view transects the MV

obliquely, it is difficult to be sure exactly which portion of the anterior and posterior leaflets are seen in a particular image. A transition in the image occurs as the multiplane angle is increased to about 60 to 80 degrees. Beyond the transition point the anterior leaflet is to the right of the display and the posterior leaflet is to the left. At this transition angle, the imaging plane intersects both commissures of the MV simultaneously, forming the midesophageal mitral commissural view (Fig. 6.1g). In this view the middle third of the anterior leaflet (A2) is seen in the middle between portions of the posterior leaflet on each side; the lateral scallop (P1) to the right of the display, and the medial scallop (P3) to the left. From the midesophageal mitral commissural view turning the probe to the right moves the plane toward the medial or right side of the MV through the base of the anterior leaflet, and turning the probe to the left moves the plane toward the lateral side through the posterior leaflet. Next, the multiplane angle is rotated forward to between 120 to 160 degrees until the left ventricular outflow tract (LVOT), AV, and proximal ascending aorta line up in the image to develop the midesophageal long-axis view (Fig. 6.1c). The midesophageal long-axis view, like the midesophageal mitral commissural view, is oriented to the anatomy of the MV and useful for identifying regions of the leaflets. In this view the anterior mitral leaflet (middle third, A2) is to the right of the display and the posterior mitral leaflet (middle scallop, P2) is to the left. With proper orientation of the imaging plane through the center of the mitral annulus, the entire MV can be examined from the midesophageal window without moving the probe by rotating forward from 0 to 180 degrees. Color flow Doppler is applied to the midesophageal views of the MV to detect flow disturbances such as mitral regurgitation or mitral stenosis. This is easily accomplished by rotating the multiplane angle backwards from the midesophageal long-axis view through the mitral commissural and four-chamber views. The transmitral inflow velocity profile is examined with pulsed wave Doppler in the midesophageal four-chamber view or midesophageal long-axis view by placing the sample volume between the open tips of the mitral leaflets. This is useful for assessing mitral stenosis and diastolic function of the LV.

## Aortic Valve Midesophageal Views

Following examination of the MV with midesophageal views, attention is turned to the AV, which is a semilunar valve located close to the center of the heart and with three cusps. The midesophageal AV short-axis view (Fig. 6.1h) is developed from the midesophageal window by advancing or withdrawing the probe until the AV comes into view and then turning the probe until the AV is centered in the display. The image depth is adjusted to between 10 to 12 cm until the AV is at the midlevel of the display. The multiplane angle is then rotated forward un-

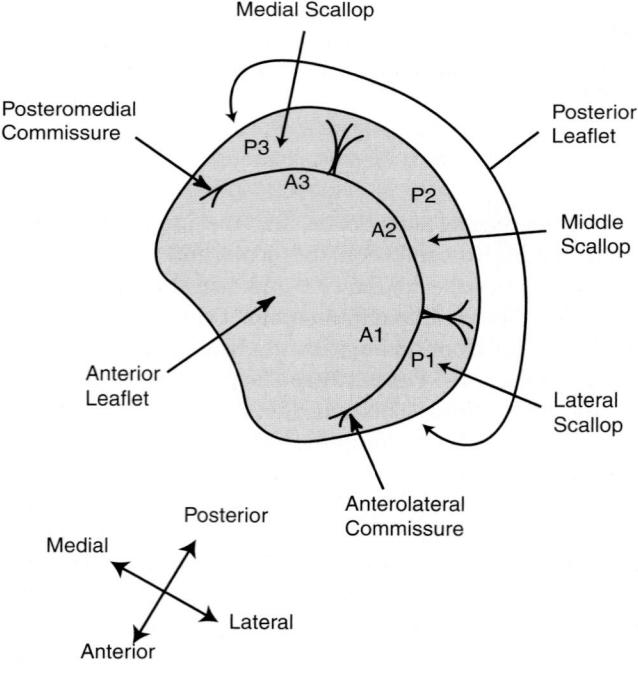

**FIGURE 6.4.** Mitral Valve Anatomy. A1, lateral third of the anterior leaflet; A2, middle third of the anterior leaflet; A3, medial third of the anterior leaflet; P1, lateral scallop of the posterior leaflet; P2, middle scallop of the posterior leaflet; P3, medial scallop of the posterior leaflet.

til a symmetrical image of all three cusps of the aortic valve is seen, approximately 30 to 60 degrees. The cusp adjacent to the atrial septum is the noncoronary cusp, the cusp farthest from the probe is the right coronary cusp, and the remaining is the left coronary cusp. The imaging plane is moved superiorly through the sinuses of Valsalva by withdrawing and anteflexing the probe slightly to bring the right and left coronary ostia and then the sinotubular junction into view. The probe is then advanced by moving the imaging plane through and then under the AV annulus showing a short-axis view of the LVOT. Color flow Doppler is applied to the midesophageal AV short-axis view to detect flow disturbances such as aortic regurgitation and aortic stenosis.

The midesophageal AV long-axis view (Fig. 6.1i) is developed by rotating the multiplane angle forward to 120 to 160 degrees while keeping the AV in the center of the display until the LVOT, AV, and proximal ascending aorta line up in the image. The proximal ascending aorta appears towards the right of the display and the LVOT to the left. The right coronary cusp is always toward the bottom of the display, but the cusp that appears posteriorly in this view may be the left or the noncoronary cusp depending on exactly how the imaging plane passes through the valve. This view is similar to the midesophageal long-axis view in that it shows where both left sided valves come together, but has less depth to include only the AV. The midesophageal AV long-axis view is the best view for measuring the size of the aortic root. The diameters of the AV annulus, sinuses of Valsalva, sinotubular junction, and proximal ascending aorta may be measured, adjusting the probe from side to side to maximize the internal diameter of these structures. The diameter of the aortic valve annulus is measured during systole where the aortic valve cusps attach to the ventricle and is normally between 1.8 and 2.5 cm. Color flow Doppler is applied to the midesophageal AV long-axis view to detect flow abnormalities through the LVOT, AV, and proximal ascending aorta. It is particularly useful for detecting and quantifying the severity of aortic regurgitation.

## Left Ventricle Midesophageal Views

Following examination of the MV and AV with the midesophageal views, attention is turned to the LV. Figure 6.5 illustrates the segmental model recommended in the

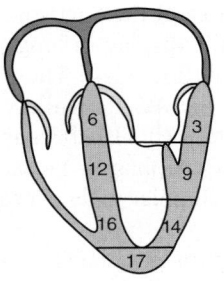

a. four chamber view

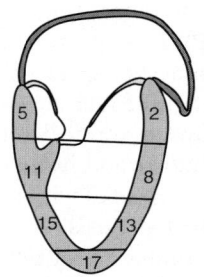

b. two chamber view

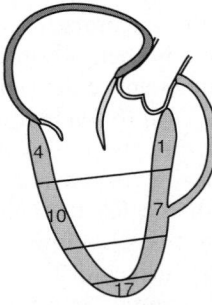

c. long axis view

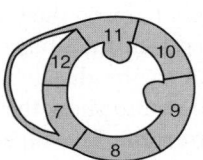

d. mid short axis view

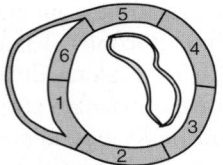

e. basal short axis view

| Basal Segments | Mid Segments | Apical Segments |
|---|---|---|
| 1= Basal Anteroseptal | 7= Mid Anteroseptal | 13= Apical Anterior |
| 2= Basal Anterior | 8= Mid Anterior | 14= Apical Lateral |
| 3= Basal Anterolateral | 9= Mid Anterolateral | 15= Apical Inferior |
| 4= Basal Inferolateral | 10= Mid Inferolateral | 16= Apical Septal |
| 5= Basal Inferior | 11= Mid Inferior | 17= Apex (Apical Cap) |
| 6= Basal Inferoseptal | 12= Mid Inferoseptal | |

*FIGURE 6.5.* Seventeen-segment model of the left ventricle. **A:** Four-chamber view shows the 3 inferoseptal and 3 anterolateral segments and the apex (apical cap). **B:** Two-chamber view shows the 3 anterior and 3 inferior segments and the apex (apical cap). **C:** Long-axis view shows the 2 anteroseptal and 2 inferolateral segments and the apex (apical cap). **D:** Mid short-axis views show all 6 segments at the midlevel. **E:** Basal short-axis views show all 6 segments at the basal level.

guidelines for describing regional wall motion abnormalities as modified to comply with standards adopted by the American Heart Association in 2002 (18). Currently in clinical practice, analysis of LV regional function is based on a qualitative visual assessment of the motion and thickening of a segment during systole. The recommended qualitative grading scale for wall motion is: 1 = normal (> 30% thickening), 2 = mildly hypokinetic (10% to 30% thickening), 3 = severely hypokinetic (< 10% thickening), 4 = akinetic (does not thicken), 5 = dyskinetic (moves paradoxically and thins during systole). The apex (apical cap, segment 17) does not include endocardium and is not usually assigned a wall motion score. All 17 segments can be examined by obtaining the three midesophageal views of the LV. To obtain these, the transducer is again positioned behind the midlevel of the LA and the imaging plane aimed through the center of the mitral annulus and the apex of the LV. The apex is usually somewhat more inferior than the MV annulus, so the tip of the probe may need to be retroflexed to direct the imaging plane through the apex. Excessive force should never be applied, and in some patients it may not be possible to align the imaging plane in this manner. The depth of the image is increased to include the entire apex, usually to 16 cm. Rotating the multiplane angle forward from 0 degrees to between 10 and 20 degrees until the diameter of the tricuspid annulus is maximized and the aortic valve is no longer in view develops the midesophageal four-chamber view (Fig. 6.1a), which shows the basal, mid, and apical segments in the anterolateral wall and the inferoseptal wall. Rotating the multiplane angle forward until the right atrium (RA) and right ventricle (RV) disappear, usually about 80 to 100 degrees, develops the midesophageal two-chamber view (Fig. 6.1b), which shows the basal, mid, and apical segments in the inferior wall and the anterior wall. Finally, by rotating the multiplane angle forward until the LVOT, AV, and the proximal ascending aorta come into view and are aligned, usually between 120 and 160 degrees, the midesophageal long-axis view (Fig. 6.1c) is developed. This view shows the basal and midanteroseptal segments and the basal and midinferolateral segments. As with the MV, the entire LV can be examined by simply rotating forward from 0 to 180 degrees without moving the probe, if the imaging plane is properly oriented through the center of the mitral annulus and the LV apex.

## Right Heart Midesophageal Views

Following examination of the left ventricle, attention is directed to the right ventricle (RV). Examination of the RV begins with the midesophageal four-chamber view. From there the probe is turned to the right until the tricuspid valve (TV) is in the center of the display. The image depth is adjusted to include the tricuspid annulus and

RV apex. In this view the apical portion of the anterior RV free wall is to the right of the display and the basal anterior free wall to the left. Next the midesophageal RV inflow-outflow view (Fig. 6.1m) is obtained by increasing the multiplane angle to between 60 and 90 degrees while keeping the TV visible until the right ventricular outflow tract (RVOT), pulmonic valve (PV), and main pulmonary artery (PA) come into view and are aligned. This view shows the RVOT to the right side of the display and the inferior (diaphragmatic) portion of the RV free wall to the left. The TV apparatus includes three leaflets (anterior, posterior, and septal), annulus, chordae tendinae, papillary muscles, and RV walls and is examined with the views used to examine the RV. In the midesophageal four-chamber view the TV is seen with the septal leaflet to the right of the display and the posterior or anterior leaflet to the left, depending on the exact orientation of the imaging plane. The probe is advanced and withdrawn to move the imaging plane through the tricuspid annulus from its inferior to superior extent. Next, the multiplane angle is rotated forward keeping the tricuspid annulus in the center of the display to develop the midesophageal RV inflow-outflow view. In this view the anterior leaflet of the TV is to the right side of the display and the posterior leaflet to the left. Color flow Doppler is applied to these views to detect flow abnormalities of the tricuspid valve. The PV is seen to the right of the display in long axis in the midesophageal RV inflow-outflow view. The PV is a trileaflet, semilunar valve, like the AV. Its leaflets, however, are more difficult to image with TEE because they are thinner and farther from the esophagus. Views of the PV are repeated with color flow Doppler to detect regurgitation or stenosis.

Examination of the right atrium (RA) begins with the midesophageal four-chamber view, which allows direct comparison of its size to the LA. The probe is turned to the right to bring the RA into the center of the display and the depth of the image adjusted to maximize the size of the RA in the display. The probe is then advanced and withdrawn to show the atrium in its entire inferior to superior extent. The superior vena cava (SVC) and inferior vena cava (IVC) are examined from the midesophageal four-chamber view by withdrawing or advancing the probe from their junctions with the RA to their more proximal portions. The coronary sinus is shown next by identifying it along the posterior surface of the heart in the atrioventricular groove as it empties into the RA at the most inferior and posterior extent of the atrial septum adjacent to the septal leaflet of the TV. A long axis of the coronary sinus may be developed from the midesophageal four-chamber view by slightly advancing or retroflexing the probe to move the imaging plane through the floor of the left atrium.

Increasing the multiplane transducer angle forward until the IVC in the left side of the display and the SVC appears in the right side (usually between 80 and 110 degrees), develops the midesophageal bicaval view (Fig. 6.11). The right atrial appendage, extending superiorly from the anterior aspect of the RA is seen in this view (Fig. 6.1l). The right atrial appendage, extending from the anterior, superior aspect of the RA is also seen in this view. The imaging of the RA is completed by turning the probe to the left and the right through the lateral to the medial extent of the atrium.

The interatrial septum (IAS) is shown through its entire medial-lateral extent with the midesophageal bicaval view by turning the probe to the right and left. The IAS has a thin region centrally called the "fossa ovalis" and thicker regions called the "limbus," anteriorly and posteriorly. To detect interatrial shunts color flow Doppler is applied to the IAS. Low velocity flow through an atrial septal defect or a patent foramen ovale may be more easily detected if the scale (Nyquist limit) of the color flow Doppler is decreased to about 30 cm/sec. Another way to detect right to left interatrial shunting is to inject agitated saline into the RA as positive airway pressure is released. The appearance of contrast in the LA in less than five cardiac cycles indicates the presence of an interatrial shunt.

## Left Ventricle Transgastric Views

The transgastric views of the LV are developed by advancing the probe into the stomach and anteflexing the tip until the heart comes into view. At a multiplane angle of 0 degrees the short-axis view of the LV will be seen, and the probe is then turned as needed to the left or right to center the LV in the display. The depth of the image is set to include the entire LV, usually 12 cm. Next, to facilitate final positioning of the probe the multiplane angle is increased to 90 degrees to show a view of the LV with the apex to the left and the mitral annulus to the right of the display. The probe is advanced or withdrawn as needed to position the transducer at the midpapillary level and the anteflexion of the probe adjusted until the long axis of the LV is horizontal in the display. The multiplane angle is decreased to between 0 and 20 degrees until the circular symmetry of the chamber is maximized to obtain the transgastric mid short-axis view (Fig. 6.1d). This view is the most popular view for monitoring LV function because it simultaneously shows regions of the LV supplied by the right, circumflex, and left anterior descending coronary arteries. It can be used to measure LV chamber size and wall thickness at end diastole. Normal LV wall thickness is less than 1.2 cm and LV short-axis diameter less than 5.5 cm. Calculation of fractional area change as an index of LV systolic function may be performed in this view by measuring the end diastolic and end systolic areas of the chamber. Rotating the multiplane angle forward to approximately 90 degrees until the apex and the mitral annulus come into view develops the transgastric

two-chamber view (Fig. 6.1e). The length of the displayed LV image is maximized by turning the probe as needed to the left or right. This view displays the basal and mid segments of the inferior and anterior walls. The apex of the LV is often not visible in the transgastric two-chamber view. It is useful for examining the chordae tendinae, which are perpendicular to the ultrasound beam in this view. The chordae to the anterolateral papillary muscle are at the bottom of the display and those to the posteromedial papillary muscle are at the top.

## Mitral Valve Transgastric Views

Withdrawing the probe from the transgastric mid short-axis view until the MV appears develops the transgastric basal short-axis view (Fig. 6.1f), which shows all six basal segments of the LV. The transgastric basal short-axis view shows a short-axis view of the MV. Advancing the transducer slightly deeper into the stomach with more anteflexion in order to align the imaging plane as parallel as possible to the mitral annulus may improve the short-axis view of the MV. If the cross section obtained is not perfectly parallel to the annulus, which is often the case, the probe may be withdrawn to image the posteromedial commissure, then advanced to image the anterolateral commissure. In these views of the MV the anterolateral commissure is in the far field to the right of the display, the posteromedial commissure in the near field to the left. The anterior leaflet is to the left of the display and the posterior leaflet to the right. These views of the MV are very useful for localizing leaflet abnormalities. Color flow Doppler applied to the transgastric basal short-axis view can be used to determine the location of a regurgitant orifice in patients with MR.

## Right Heart Transgastric Views

In the transgastric mid short-axis view the RV is seen to the left side of the display from the LV. The transgastric RV inflow view (Fig. 6.1n) is developed by turning the probe to the right to center RV cavity in the display and then rotating the multiplane angle forward to between 100 and 120 degrees until the apex of the RV appears in the left side of the display. This view provides good views of the inferior (diaphragmatic) portion of the RV free wall, located in the near field. In some patients images of the RVOT and PV can be developed from the transgastric RV inflow view by decreasing the multiplane angle towards zero degrees and anteflexing the probe. The TV is also seen in the transgastric RV inflow view with the RA to the right of the display and the RV to the left, and color flow Doppler is applied to detect flow abnormalities. It also usually shows the best images of the tricuspid chordae tendinae because they are perpendicular to the ultrasound. A short-axis view of the TV can be developed by withdrawing the probe slightly towards the base of the heart until the tricuspid annulus is

centered in the display and decreasing the multiplane angle to about 30 degrees. In this view the posterior leaflet of
the TV is in the near field to the left, the anterior leaflet is
in the far field to the left, and the septal leaflet to the right
side of the display. Color flow Doppler is applied to these
views to detect flow disturbances.

## Aortic Valve Transgastric Views

The primary use of the two transgastric views of the AV is
to make Doppler measurements of the flow through the
LVOT and AV. Midesophageal views cannot be used for
this purpose because this flow is perpendicular to the
Doppler beam from the midesophageal window. Transgastric views of the AV also provide images of the ventricular aspect of the valve in some patients. The transgastric
long-axis view (Fig. 6.1j) is obtained from the transgastric
mid short-axis view by rotating the multiplane angle forward to 90 to 120 degrees until the AV comes into view in
the far field to the right side of the display. Turning the
probe slightly to the right may help to bring the AV and
LVOT into view in some cases.

To develop the deep transgastric view of the AV, the
probe is advanced deep into the stomach from the transgastric mid short-axis view and positioned adjacent to the
LV apex. The probe is then anteflexed until the imaging
plane is oriented towards the base of the heart producing
the deep transgastric long-axis view (Fig. 6.1k). Deep in
the stomach the exact position of the probe and transducer is more difficult to determine and control, but
some trial and error turning, flexing, withdrawing, advancing, and rotating of the probe develops this view in
most patients. The AV is located at the bottom of the display in the far field in the deep transgastric long-axis
view, with the LV outflow directed away from the transducer. Doppler quantification of flow velocities through
the LVOT and the AV is usually possible with one or the
other of these views in most patients, but detailed images
of the valve anatomy are difficult to obtain because it is
so far from the transducer. Flow velocity through the AV
is measured by aiming the continuous wave Doppler
beam through the LVOT across the valve. Normal peak
AV flow velocity is less than 1.5 meters/second. Positioning the pulsed wave Doppler sample volume just proximal
to the AV in the center of the LVOT allows the blood flow
velocity in the LVOT to be measured. Normal peak LVOT
flow velocity is less than 1.2 meters/second. Using color
flow Doppler to image the flow through the LVOT and AV
may facilitate directing the Doppler beam through the
area of maximum flow.

## TEE EXAMINATION OF THE THORACIC AORTA

After finishing the transgastric views of the heart, the thoracic aorta is examined. The probe is withdrawn to the
level of the diaphragm and turned to the patient's left at

zero degrees multiplane angle until the distal descending
thoracic aorta is seen developing the descending aorta
short-axis view (Fig. 6.1q). The descending thoracic aorta
is examined from the diaphragm to the arch by withdrawing the probe to the aortic arch. At the level of the diaphragm, the esophagus is located anterior to the aorta.
It winds around within the thorax until at the level of the
distal arch it is posterior to the aorta, so as the probe is
withdrawn, it is turned to the right (anteriorly) keeping
the descending aorta centered in the image. It is difficult
to maintain contact between the transducer and the aorta
within the stomach, so the mid and distal abdominal
aorta are difficult to see with TEE. The multiplane angle
is rotated forward to 90 degrees to obtain the descending
aorta long-axis view (Fig. 6.1r), and the probe is withdrawn and advanced to examine the entire descending
thoracic aorta.

It is difficult to determine anterior and posterior or
right to left orientations related to the descending thoracic aorta in the TEE images because of the lack of internal anatomic landmarks and the variable relationship between it and the esophagus. One approach describing
lesion locations is to record probe depth from the incisors. The presence of an adjacent structure, such as the
LA or the base of the LV, may also be used to determine
the level of the descending aorta being shown.

Next the probe is withdrawn to the upper esophageal
window about 20 to 25 cm from the incisors at zero degrees multiplane angle to develop the upper esophageal
aortic arch long-axis view (Fig. 6.1s). The probe is turned
to the right (anterior) as it is withdrawn to keep the aorta
in view because the midaortic arch lies anterior to the
esophagus. The distal arch is to the right of the display
and the proximal arch to the left. Withdrawing the transducer above the upper esophageal aortic arch long-axis
view produces images of the left carotid artery and proximal left subclavian artery in some individuals. Because
the trachea often lies between the proximal aorta and the
esophagus, the right brachiocephalic artery is more difficult to image. The left brachiocephalic vein is also often
seen anterior to the arch in these views.

Next, the upper esophageal aortic arch short-axis view
(Fig. 6.1t) is developed by increasing the multiplane forward to 90 degrees. With this view the probe turned to the
right (anteriorly) to image the arch more proximally and
to the left (posteriorly) to image distally. In many patients
images of the main PA and the PV can be obtained in the
left side of the display by turning the probe back and
forth until these structures are seen. Retroflexing the
probe will often improve this view of the PV. If the PA and
the PV are seen in this view, blood flow velocities through
each of these structures can be measured using Doppler
echocardiography. The origin of the branches of the aortic arch is often seen to the right of the display.

Finally, the comprehensive TEE examination is completed by advancing the probe to a depth of about 30 cm

from the incisors placing the transducer at the level of the right pulmonary artery to image the proximal and midascending aorta. The ascending aorta is positioned in the center of the image and the multiplane angle adjusted until the vessel is a circle, usually between 0 and 60 degrees, developing the midesophageal ascending aortic short-axis view (Fig. 6.1o). The probe is advanced and withdrawn to see different portions of the ascending aorta. The midesophageal ascending aortic long-axis view (Fig. 6.1p) is then developed by increasing the multiplane angle until the anterior and posterior walls of the aorta appear as two parallel, curved lines, usually between 100 and 150 degrees. The inside diameter of the ascending aorta at the sinotubular junction and the midlevel may be measured from these long-axis and short-axis images.

This completes the acquisition of the images for the comprehensive intraoperative TEE examination. Another abbreviated examination is usually performed immediately after cardiopulmonary bypass to check the results of the surgery and again after the chest is closed. It is important that the results of the TEE examination be reported to the surgeon and other subsequent caregivers, such as the ICU team. It is best to speak directly with the surgeon to avoid any confusion about what was and was not seen on the TEE examination. The findings should also be documented in the medical record.

## ABBREVIATED TEE EXAMINATION

Because of time constraints and relatively narrow diagnostic goals, anesthesiologists often perform a more limited intraoperative examination than described in the ASE/SCA's task force recommendation for a comprehensive TEE examination (see previous section) (16,17). However, even when time is critical, the examination performed should allow at least the basic applications of TEE as outlined in the 1996 guidelines for perioperative TEE: to detect markedly abnormal ventricular filling or function, extensive myocardial ischemia or infarction, large air embolism, severe valvular dysfunction, large cardiac masses or thrombi, large pericardial effusions, and major lesions of the great vessels (15). A minimum of eight different cross sections drawn from the 20 cross sections delineated in the comprehensive examination are required to meet these diagnostic goals. Four of the cross sections are imaged in both two-dimensional and color Doppler to assess valvular function. The next paragraph will describe the probe manipulations required to achieve these cross sections. The reader should review Figure 6.1 to understand the terms used in this description (16).

### Probe Manipulations and Examination Sequence

After the TEE probe is introduced safely into the esophagus, it is advanced to the midesophageal (ME) level (28–32 cm measured at the upper incisors), and the aortic valve (AV) is imaged in the short-axis (SAX) by turning the probe, adjusting its depth in the esophagus, and rotating the multiplane transducer to 25–45 degrees until the three cusps of the valve are seen as approximately equal in size and shape (Fig. 6.1h). Image depth is set to 10–12 cm as required to position the AV in the center of the video screen. This cross section is ideal for detection of aortic stenosis. The videotape is activated at this point and kept running throughout the rest of the examination. Videotape is very inexpensive relative to the cost of a missed diagnosis. Next, the probe is turned slightly to position the AV in the center of the video screen, and then the multiplane angle is rotated forward to 110–130 degrees to bring the long axis (LAX) of the AV in view (Fig. 6.1i). This cross section is best for detection of ascending aortic abnormalities including type I aortic dissection. Color Doppler is used for assessment of aortic valve competence. For detection of valvular stenosis and regurgitation, the maximum possible Nyquist limit is used (ideally above 50 cm/sec). Next, the color Doppler is discontinued and the probe is turned rightward until the ME bicaval cross section comes into view (Fig. 6.1l). This cross section is seen best usually at a multiplane angle between 90 and 110 degrees and is ideal for assessing caval abnormalities, as well as compression of the right atrium from anteriorly located masses or effusions and the left atrium from posteriorly located masses or effusions. In addition, the bicaval cross section may reveal collections of air located anteriorly in the left or right atrium, as well as the structure of the interatrial septum including the foramen ovale. Next, the multiplane angle is rotated back to 60–80 degrees and the probe is turned leftward just past the aortic valve to bring the ME right ventricular (RV) inflow and outflow cross section into view (Fig. 6.1m). Usually, an image depth of 12–14 cm is required to position the RV outflow track in the center of the video screen. This cross section reveals the contractile function of the RV, the outflow tract, as well as the pulmonary valve function with the application of color Doppler. Next, the transducer is rotated back to 0 degrees, the probe advanced 4–6 millimeters into the esophagus, and gently retroflexed it until all four cardiac chambers are visualized (ME four-chamber) (Fig. 6.1a). Often, rotating the transducer 10–15 degrees will enhance the view of the tricuspid annulus. Usually, an image depth of 14–16 cm is required to include the LV apex in the sector scan. In two-dimensional imaging, the free wall of the RV and the anterolateral and inferoseptal wall segments are evaluated for contractile function. With color Doppler, both the mitral and tricuspid valves are assessed. Stenotic and regurgitant lesions can be diagnosed accurately. During this assessment, the image depth is decreased to 10–12 cm to afford a magnified view of the valves and maximization of the Nyquist limits (above 50 cm /sec). Next, color Doppler is discontinued, the left ventricle is positioned in the center of the screen, and the multiplane angle is rotated forward to 90 degrees to bring into view the ME two-chamber cross section (Fig. 6.1b). The image depth is returned to 14–16 cm. This cross section is best for revealing the function of the basal and apical segments of the anterior and inferior LV walls as well as anterior and inferior pericardial collections. When air emboli collect in the left ventricle, they can be seen best usually in this view as very echogenic areas located along the anterior apical endocardial surface. Then, the transducer is rotated forward to 135 degrees to reveal the ME LAX cross section that is best for assessment of the anteroseptal and inferolateral wall segments for contractile LV function (Fig. 6.1c). Together, the ME four-chamber, two-chamber, and LAX cross sections reveal all 17 segments of the left ventricle (Fig. 6.5). However, the next and last of the basic cross sections provide a second look at the mid-ventricular segments as well as other benefits. To achieve this cross section, the transducer is rotated back to 0 degrees, the left ventricle centered in the screen and the probe advanced 4–6 cm into the stomach. Then, it is flexed gently anteriorly to reveal the transgastric (TG) SAX cross section (Fig. 6.1d). This cross section is ideal for monitoring LV filling and contractile function. All major coronary arteries supplying the myocardium are viewed in this cross section. Moreover, changes in preload cause greater changes in the LV short-axis than in the long-axis dimension, and movement of the probe from this cross section is readily apparent because the papillary muscles provide prominent landmarks. Since this cross section is used to judge filling and ejection, image depth is consistently set to 12 cm so that the size and function of the heart is judged easily relative to previously examined hearts.

## Limitations

The abbreviated examination has significant limitations that must be appreciated. Clearly, it is an insufficient examination for the quantitative evaluation of hemodynamics, comprehensive valvular assessment, detection of flawed cardiac repairs, and other advanced TEE applications. Advanced applications of perioperative TEE should not be provided based on the abbreviated examination alone. Instead, the abbreviated examination is viewed best as serving two needs: first, as an emergency tool for the very rapid detection of life-threatening cardiac problems not diagnosed readily with other less invasive perioperative techniques; and second, as the minimum examination of basic perioperative TEE practitioners, who recognize the limitations of this examination and seek appropriate consultation when advanced TEE applications are required.

## KEY POINTS

- The comprehensive perioperative TEE exam recommended by the SCA/ASE guidelines consists of 20 views.
- Develop a consistent, systematic approach to performing the comprehensive exam.
- Performing a comprehensive TEE exam whenever possible rapidly increases knowledge and skill, provides a baseline for later comparison, and is more likely to detect previously undiagnosed abnormalities.
- Screen for esophageal disease BEFORE inserting the TEE probe.
- NEVER apply excessive force when inserting or manipulating the TEE probe.
- Adjust image depth, overall gain, dynamic compression, time delay gain, focus, and frequency to optimize two-dimensional image quality.
- Determine the location of the TEE transducer in relation to the heart, then the orientation of the imaging as it passes through the heart.
- The imaging plane can be moved through the structure being examined by advancing and withdrawing the probe, turning (rotating) the probe to left and right, or increasing and decreasing the multiplane angle.
- The centerline of the image stays the same if the probe is not moved as the multiplane angle is changed.
- Examine each structure with multiple views.
- An abbreviated exam of eight views can achieve the basic applications of perioperative TEE more rapidly than the comprehensive.

## REFERENCES

1. Matsumoto M, Oka Y, Strom J, Frishman W, Kadish A, Becker RM, Frater RW, Sonnenblick EH. Application of transesophageal echocardiography to continuous intraoperative monitoring of left ventricular performance. Am J Cardiol 1980;46(1):95–105.
2. Cahalan MK, Kremer P, Schiller NB, et al. Intraoperative monitoring with two-dimensional transesophageal echocardiography. Anesth 1982;57(3):A153.
3. Dubroff JM, Clark MB, Wong CY, Spotnitz AJ, Collins RH, Spotnitz HM. Left ventricular ejection fraction during cardiac surgery: a two-dimensional echocardiographic study. Circulation 1983;68(1):95–103.
4. Stevenson JG, Sorensen GK, Gartman DM, Hall DG, Rittenhouse EA. Transesophageal echocardiography during repair of congenital cardiac defects: identification of residual problems necessitating reoperation. J Am Soc Echocardiogr 1993;6(4):356–65.
5. Hartman GS, Yao FS, Bruefach M 3rd, et al. Severity of aortic atheromatous disease diagnosed by transesophageal

echocardiography predicts stroke and other outcomes associated with coronary artery surgery: a prospective study. Anesth Analg 1996;83(4):701–8.

6. Sheikh KH, Bengtson JR, Rankin JS, de Bruijn NP, Kisslo J. Intraoperative transesophageal Doppler color flow imaging used to guide patient selection and operative treatment of ischemic mitral regurgitation. Circulation 1991;84(2):594–604.

7. Grigg LE, Wigle ED, Williams WG, Daniel LB, Rakowski H. Transesophageal Doppler echocardiography in obstructive hypertrophic cardiomyopathy: clarification of pathophysiology and importance in intraoperative decision making. J Am Coll Cardiol 1992;20(1):42–52.

8. Daniel WG, Erbel R, Kasper W, et al. Safety of transesophageal echocardiography. A multicenter survey of 10,419 examinations. Circulation 1991;83(3):817–21.

9. Kallmeyer IJ, Collard CD, Fox JA, Body SC, Shernan SK. The safety of intraoperative transesophageal echocardiography: a case series of 7200 cardiac surgical patients. [Journal Article] Anesth Analg 2001;92(5):1126–30.

10. Spahn DR, Schmid S, Carrel T, Pasch T, Schmid ER. Hypopharynx perforation by a transesophageal echocardiography probe. Anesthesiology 1995;82(2):581–3.

11. Brinkman WT, Shanewise JS, Clements SD, Mansour KA. Transesophageal echocardiography: not an innocuous procedure. Ann Thorac Surg 2001;72(5):1725–6.

12. Hogue CW Jr, Lappas GD, Creswell LL, et al. Swallowing dysfunction after cardiac operations. Associated adverse outcomes and risk factors including intraoperative transesophageal echocardiography. J Thorac Cardio Surg 1995;110(2):517–22.

13. Rousou JA, Tighe DA, Garb JL, Krasner H, et al. Risk of dysphagia after transesophageal echocardiography during cardiac operations. Ann Thorac Surg 2000:69(2):486–9; discussion 489–90.

14. Humphrey LS. Esophageal stethoscope loss complicating echocardiography J Cardiothoracic Anesth 1988;2:356.

15. Practice guidelines for perioperative transesophageal echocardiography. A report by the American Society of Anesthesiologists and the Society of Cardiovascular Anesthesiologists Task Force on Transesophageal Echocardiography. Anesthesiology 1196;84(4):986–1006.

16. Shanewise JS, Cheung AT, Aronson S, et al. ASE/SCA guidelines for performing a comprehensive intraoperative multiplane transesophageal echocardiography examination: recommendations of the American Society of Echocardiography Council for Intraoperative Echocardiography and the Society of Cardiovascular Anesthesiologists Task Force for Certification in Perioperative Transesophageal Echocardiography. AnesthAnalg 1999;89(4):870–84.

17. Shanewise JS, Cheung AT, Aronson S, et al. ASE/SCA guidelines for performing a comprehensive intraoperative multiplane transesophageal echocardiography examination: recommendations of the American Society of Echocardiography Council for Intraoperative Echocardiography and the Society of Cardiovascular Anesthesiologists Task Force for Certification in Perioperative Transesophageal Echocardiography. J Am Soc Echocardiogr 1999;12(10):884–900.

18. Cerqueira MD, Weissman NJ, Dilsizian V, et al. Standardized myocardial segmentation and nomenclature for tomographic imaging of the heart: a statement for healthcare professionals from the Cardiac Imaging Committee of the Council on Clinical Cardiology of the American Heart Association. [Review] [11 refs] [Consensus Development Conference. Journal Article. Review] Circulation 2002;105(4):539–42.

19. Miller JP, Lambert AS, Shapiro WA, Russell IA, Schiller NB, Cahalan MK. The adequacy of basic intraoperative transesophageal echocardiography performed by experienced anesthesiologists. Anesth Analg 2001;92:1103–10.

## QUESTIONS

1. What is the major use of the deep transgastric long-axis view?
   A. Measure velocities in the LVOT and AV
   B. Obtain detailed two-dimensional images of the AV
   C. Assess global LV function
   D. Measure the size of the LVOT
   E. Examine the mitral chordae tendinae

2. The basal posterior segment of the left ventricle is in which of the following TEE views?
   A. Midesophageal four-chamber
   B. Midesophageal two-chamber
   C. Transgastric two-chamber
   D. Transgastric mid short-axis
   E. Transgastric basal short-axis

3. Which two midesophageal TEE views are aligned with the anatomy of the mitral valve?
   A. Four-chamber and two-chamber
   B. Two-chamber and long-axis
   C. Mitral commissural and long-axis
   D. Four-chamber and mitral commissural
   E. Two-chamber and mitral commissural

4. What is the minimum number of views needed to achieve the basic perioperative TEE applications described in the 1996 guidelines?
   A. 6
   B. 8
   C. 10
   D. 15
   E. 20

# Chapter 7

# Updated Indications for Intraoperative TEE

*Daniel M. Thys*

In the United States, intraoperative echocardiography (IOE) has become integral to the care of many cardiac surgical patients (1). In a recent survey of all active members of the Society of Cardiovascular Anesthesiologists (SCA) residing in the United States or Puerto Rico, Morewood et al. documented that 94% of respondents practice at institutions that use IOE (2). Furthermore, 72% of anesthesiologists working at such institutions responded that they personally employed transesophageal echocardiography (TEE) during anesthetic care.

Intraoperative echocardiography is widely used because it is thought to provide information that significantly influences clinical management and improves patient outcome. Although there is limited scientific evidence to substantiate such perception, several recent case series have documented the usefulness of IOE in adult cardiac surgery (3–8). Investigators have usually examined whether IOE yielded new information and how frequently the new information had an impact on anesthetic or surgical management. In adult cardiac surgery, the total number of patients included in these reports was 11,444 (Table 7.1). The incidence of new information ranged from 12.8% to 38.6%, while the impact on treatment ranged from 9.7% to 48.8%.

As in adult cardiac surgery, the use of IOE has become routine in many pediatric cardiac surgery centers. While

**TABLE 7.1. The Usefulness of IOE in Adult Cardiac Surgery**

| Number of Patients | New Information | Change in Management |
|---|---|---|
| 3,245 (3) | 15 % | 14 % |
| 851 (4) | — | 14.6 % |
| 203 (5) | 12.8 % | 10.8 % |
| 5,016 (6) | 22.9 % | — |
| 238 (7) | 38.6 % | 9.7 % |
| 1,891 (8) | — | 48.8 % |

**TABLE 7.2. The Usefulness of IOE in Pediatric Cardiac Surgery**

| Number of Patients | Residual Defects |
|---|---|
| 86 (9) | 12.8 % |
| 200 (10) | 10.5 % |
| 667 (11) | 6.6 % |
| 1,000 (12) | 4.4 % |
| 532 (13) | 8 % |
| 104 (14) | 14.4 % |

epicardial echocardiography was used most commonly in the early years, the use of TEE has increased with the development of smaller TEE probes. Several recent studies have documented the utility of intraoperative TEE, particularly for the detection of residual defects after cardiopulmonary bypass (CPB) (9–14). These reviews reported on a total of 2,589 cases. The detection of significant residual defects after CPB ranged from 4.4% to 14.4% (Table 7.2).

Because of their retrospective nature, most of these reports do not withstand rigorous scientific scrutiny. Nonetheless, they confirm the clinical opinion that IOE provides new information on cardiac pathology in a significant number of patients and that the new information results in frequent management changes. Most physicians who care for cardiac surgical patients believe these benefits to be real and have adopted the technique in their clinical practice.

## PRACTICE GUIDELINES

In 1996, a task force of the American Society of Anesthesiologists/Society of Cardiovascular Anesthesiologists (ASA/SCA) published practice guidelines for perioperative transesophageal echocardiography (15). The recommendations of the task force address *indications*, the clinical settings in which TEE should be considered, and *proficiency*, the cognitive and technical skills expected of anesthesiologists who perform perioperative TEE. The guidelines are evidence-based and focus on the effectiveness of perioperative transesophageal echocardiography (TEE) in improving clinical outcomes. A literature search conducted at that time retrieved 1,844 articles of which 588 were considered relevant to the perioperative setting.

The recommendations were divided into three categories based on the strength of supporting evidence or expert opinion that the technology improves clinical outcomes (Table 7.3). *Category I* indications are supported by the strongest evidence or expert opinion; TEE is frequently useful in improving clinical outcomes in these settings and is often indicated, depending on individual circumstances (e.g., patient risk and practice setting). *Category II* indications are supported by weaker evidence and expert consensus; TEE may be useful in improving clinical outcomes in these settings, depending on individual circumstances, but appropriate indications are less certain. *Category III* indications have little current scientific or expert support; TEE is infrequently useful in improving clinical outcomes in these settings, and appropriate indications are uncertain. The lack of supporting evidence for Category III indications is often due to the absence of relevant studies rather than to existing evidence of ineffectiveness. Thus, many Category III indications are worth investigating and future research and technological developments may enhance their role in routine practice.

The recommendations refer to clinical problems rather than to individual patients, who often have more than one potential reason for performing TEE. Thus, although patients may not necessarily require perioperative TEE because they have a cardiomyopathy (Category III), the same patients may need TEE because of coexisting hemodynamic problems (Category I). Similarly, physicians must integrate multiple variables in assessing a patient's need for TEE. Factors associated with the patient, procedure, and clinical setting each contribute to the overall risk of perioperative complications and cumulatively alter the benefit-harm ratio of using TEE. Physicians should consider each of these variables when calculating the appropriateness of using TEE.

In 1997, the American Heart Association (AHA) and American College of Cardiology (ACC) published guidelines for the clinical application of echocardiography (16). In 2000, the AHA/ACC task force was reconvened to update the guidelines. The American Society of Echocardiography was invited to participate in the development of the guidelines. The task force also decided to include a section on intraoperative echocardiography. In the preparation of this section, a literature search was conducted

that identified an additional 118 articles related to the intraoperative use of echocardiography. The current text includes information that was retrieved in the most recent search and includes new recommendations for the clinical application of IOE. The indications for IOE provided in the new guidelines are based on the initial ASA/SCA guidelines as well as the newer information (Table 7.4).

The AHA/ACC guidelines utilize the following classification system for indications.

**Class I:** Conditions for which there is evidence and/or general agreement that a given procedure or treatment is useful and effective.

**Class II:** Conditions for which there is conflicting evidence and/or a divergence of opinion about the usefulness/efficacy of a procedure or treatment.

 **IIa:** Weight of evidence/opinion is in favor of usefulness/efficacy.

 **IIb:** Usefulness/efficacy is less well established by evidence/opinion.

**Class III:** Conditions for which there is evidence and/or general agreement that the procedure/treatment is not useful/effective and in some cases may be harmful.

## INDICATIONS FOR SPECIFIC LESIONS OR PROCEDURES

### Adult Cardiac Surgery

#### Mitral Valve Repair

Two recent studies from Japan have confirmed the usefulness of intraoperative transesophageal echocardiography (TEE) for the assessment of residual regurgitation after mitral valve repair (17,18). Kawano et al. observed that 5 of 34 patients had 1+ regurgitation on postoperative ventriculography. Four of these patients demonstrated a maximal mosaic area > 2 cm² on color flow Doppler by TEE immediately after cardiopulmonary bypass (CPB). They all developed rapidly progressing mitral regurgitation (MR) in the postoperative period. In a study by Saiki et al. (18), 40 of 42 patients with no or trivial MR (mosaic area ≤ 2 cm²) also had no or trivial MR early and late postoperatively (12). The other two patients in whom moderate MR was detected intraoperatively by TEE, evolved to moderate regurgitation three months later.

Aklog et al. have recently examined the role of intraoperative TEE in the evaluation of ischemic mitral regurgitation (19). They studied 136 patients with a preoperative diagnosis of moderate ischemic MR, without leaflet prolapse or pathology, who underwent isolated coronary artery bypass grafting (CABG). They observed that intraoperative echocardiography downgraded MR in 89% of patients and that CABG alone leaves many patients with

▶ TABLE 7.3. Indications for Perioperative TEE

*Category I*

Intraoperative evaluation of acute, persistent, and life-threatening hemodynamic disturbances in which ventricular function and its determinants are uncertain and have not responded to treatment
Intraoperative use in valve repair
Intraoperative use in congenital heart surgery for most lesions requiring cardiopulmonary bypass
Intraoperative use in repair of hypertrophic obstructive cardiomyopathy
Intraoperative use for endocarditis when preoperative testing was inadequate or extension of infection to perivalvular tissue is suspected
Preoperative use in unstable patients with suspected thoracic aortic aneurysms, dissection, or disruption who need to be evaluated quickly
Intraoperative assessment of aortic valve function in repair of aortic dissections with possible aortic valve involvement
Intraoperative evaluation of pericardial window procedures
Use in intensive care unit for unstable patients with unexplained hemodynamic disturbances, suspected valve disease, or thromboembolic problems (if other tests or monitoring techniques have not confirmed the diagnosis or if patients are too unstable to undergo other tests)
Intraoperative assessment of repair of cardiac aneurysms
Intraoperative evaluation of removal of cardiac tumors

*Category II*

Perioperative use in patients with increased risk of myocardial ischemia or infarction
Perioperative use in patients with increased risk of hemodynamic disturbances
Intraoperative assessment of valve replacement
Intraoperative detection of foreign bodies
Intraoperative detection of air emboli during cardiotomy, heart transplant operations, and upright neurosurgical procedures
Intraoperative use during intracardiac thrombectomy
Intraoperative use during pulmonary embolectomy
Intraoperative use for suspected cardiac trauma
Preoperative assessment of patients with suspected acute thoracic aortic dissections, aneurysms, or disruption
Intraoperative use during repair of thoracic aortic dissections without suspected aortic valve involvement
Intraoperative detection of aortic atheromatous disease or other sources of aortic emboli
Intraoperative evaluation of pericardiectomy, pericardial effusions, or evaluation of pericardial surgery
Intraoperative evaluation of anastomotic sites during heart and/or lung transplantation
Monitoring placement and function of assist devices

*Category III*

Intraoperative evaluation of myocardial perfusion, coronary artery anatomy, or graft patency
Intraoperative use during repair of cardiomyopathies other than hypertrophic obstructive cardiomyopathy
Intraoperative use for uncomplicated endocarditis during noncardiac surgery
Intraoperative monitoring for emboli during orthopedic surgery
Intraoperative assessment of repair of thoracic aortic injuries
Intraoperative use for uncomplicated pericarditis
Intraoperative evaluation of pleuropulmonary disease
Monitoring placement of intraaortic balloon pumps, automatic implantable cardiac defibrillators, or pulmonary artery catheters
Intraoperative monitoring of cardioplegia administration

Practice Guidelines for perioperative transesophageal echocardiography. A report by the American Society of Anesthesiologists and the Society of Cardiovascular Anesthesiologists Task Force on transesophageal echocardiography. Anesthesiology 1996;84:986–1006.

significant residual MR. A reduction in the severity of mitral regurgitation when assessed by IOE was also reported by Grewal et al. (20). They studied 43 patients with moderate to severe MR and observed that MR improved by at least one grade in 51% of patients when assessed under general anesthesia.

### Valve Replacement

Nowrangi et al. reviewed the impact of intraoperative TEE in patients undergoing aortic valve replacement (AVR) for aortic stenosis (21). They reviewed the clinical data of 383 patients and observed that 54 patients had mitral valve replacement (MVR) at the time of the AVR. In

▶ TABLE 7.4. **Updated Indications for Intraoperative Echocardiography***

*Class I*

1. Evaluation of acute, persistent, and life-threatening hemodynamic disturbances in which ventricular function and its determinants are uncertain and have not responded to treatment
2. Surgical repair of valvular lesions, hypertrophic obstructive cardiomyopathy, and aortic dissection with possible aortic valve involvement
3. Evaluation of complex valve replacements requiring homografts or coronary reimplantation such as the Ross procedure
4. Surgical repair of most congenital heart lesions that require cardiopulmonary bypass
5. Surgical intervention for endocarditis when preoperative testing was inadequate or extension to perivalvular tissue is suspected
6. Placement of intracardiac devices and monitoring of their position during port-access and other cardiac surgical interventions
7. Evaluation of pericardial window procedures in patients with posterior or loculated pericardial effusions

*Class IIa*

1. Surgical procedures in patients at increased risk of myocardial ischemia, myocardial infarction, or hemodynamic disturbances
2. Evaluation of valve replacement, aortic atheromatous disease, the Maze procedure, cardiac aneurysm repair, removal of cardiac tumors, intracardiac thrombectomy, and pulmonary embolectomy
3. Detection of air emboli during cardiotomy, heart transplant operations, and upright neurosurgical procedures

*Class IIb*

1. Evaluation of suspected cardiac trauma, repair of acute thoracic aortic dissection without valvular involvement, and anastomotic sites during heart and/or lung transplantation
2. Evaluation of regional myocardial function during and after off-pump CABG procedures.
3. Evaluation of pericardiectomy, pericardial effusions, and pericardial surgery
4. Evaluation of myocardial perfusion, coronary anatomy, or graft patency
5. Dobutamine stress testing to detect inducible demand ischemia or to predict functional changes after myocardial revascularization

*Class III*

1. Assessment of residual duct flow after interruption of patent ductus arteriosus
2. Surgical repair of uncomplicated secundum ASD

*Cheitlin MD, Armstrong WF, Aurigemma GP et al. ACC/AHA/ASE 2003 guideline update for the clinical application of echocardiography—summary article: a report of the American College of Cardiology/American Heart Association Task Force on Practice Guidelines (ACC/AHA/ASE Committee to Update the 1997 Guidelines for the Clinical Application of Echocardiography). Published simultaneously in J Am Soc Cardiol 2003;2(5):954–70 and Circulation.

six patients, MVR was not planned but was performed on the basis of the IOE findings. In 25 patients, MVR was cancelled because of the IOE findings, while the surgical plan was altered in an additional 18 patients.

The clinical impact and cost-saving implications of routine IOE were studied prospectively in 300 patients by Ionescu et al. (22). In two patients undergoing AVR, significant MR detected by IOE resulted in MVR and in one patient undergoing MVR, aortic regurgitation resulted in AVR. The authors calculated that the extension of an existing TEE service to routine IOE resulted in savings of $109 per patient per year.

Morehead et al. have studied the significance of paravalvular jets detected by IOE after valve replacement (23). In 27 patients, multiple jets were detected after valve replacement. They were more common and larger in the mitral position and after insertion of mechanical valves. Reversal of anticoagulation with protamine reduced the incidence and size of the jets in all patients.

The outcome of mild periprosthetic regurgitation identified by IOE was also studied by O'Rourke et al. (24). Of 608 patients undergoing isolated aortic or mitral valve replacement, 113 were found to have trivial or mild periprosthetic regurgitation at surgery. While the observation was benign in most patients, four patients were found to have progression of the regurgitation by late transthoracic echocardiographic examination.

### Coronary Artery Surgery

Bergquist et al. studied how TEE guides clinical decision-making in myocardial revascularization (25). For the 584 intraoperative interventions that were recorded, TEE was the single most important guiding factor in 98 instances (17%). TEE was the single most important monitor influencing fluid administration; antiischemic therapy; and vasotrope, inotrope, vasodilator, or antiarrhythmic administration. In two patients, critical surgical interventions were made solely on the basis of TEE. In high-risk coronary artery bypass grafting (CABG), Savage et al. observed that in 33% of patients at least one major surgical management alteration was initiated on the basis of TEE, while in 51% of patients, at least one major anesthetic/hemodynamic change was initiated by a TEE finding (26).

Arruda et al. evaluated the role of power Doppler imaging to assess the patency of CABG anastomosis (27). In 11 of 12 patients, the flow in the left anterior descending coronary artery (LAD) could be visualized before and after the anastomosis. In one patient, the graft was revised because of worsened flow after CPB.

### Minimally Invasive Cardiac Surgery

With the growing interest in minimally invasive cardiac surgery, the role of IOE in these procedures has been evaluated. Applebaum et al. reported that TEE facilitated the placement of intravascular catheters during port-access surgery, thereby avoiding the use of fluoroscopy (28). Fluoroscopy was only helpful as an aide to TEE for placement of the coronary sinus catheter. Falk et al. observed that TEE was particularly useful for monitoring the placement and positioning of the endoaortic clamp that is used in these procedures (29). Similar benefits were reported by Schulze et al. (30).

In minimally invasive valve surgery, Secknus et al. noted intracardiac air in all patients (33). New left ventricular dysfunction was more common in patients with extensive air by IOE. Second CPB runs were required in 6% of patients. Kort et al. examined the role of IOE in 153 patients undergoing minimally invasive aortic valve replacement (31). Postbypass mild aortic regurgitation was observed in two patients. On follow-up, moderate regurgitation was observed in 4 patients, mild-to-moderate in 2, and mild in 18 patients. The regurgitation was paravalvular in eight of these patients.

In patients undergoing coronary bypass without CPB, Moises et al. detected 31 new regional wall motion abnormalities (RWMA) during 48 coronary artery clampings (32). At the time of chest closure, 16 segments had partial recovery and 5 of these had not recovered. Seven days later, the RWMA persisted in the five without recovery and in two with partial recovery. These patients had more clinical problems postoperatively.

### Air Embolization

In a study of 20 patients undergoing CABG, Yao et al. observed intraluminal aortic air emboli in all patients (34). While embolization was unevenly distributed throughout the procedure, 42% were detected within 4 minutes of aortic cross-clamp release and 24% after partial occlusion clamp release. Tingleff et al. studied two groups of 15 patients: group I consisted of patients undergoing true "open heart" procedures, while patients in group II underwent CABG (35). Air embolism was detected in all patients in group I with episodes occurring up to 28 minutes after termination of CPB. In most cases, TEE clearly

demonstrated that the air originated in the lung veins and was not retained in the heart. For patients in group II, air embolism was noted in only half the patients and was seen only in the period between cross-clamp removal and termination of CPB.

### Aortic Atheromatous Disease

The relationship between the severity of aortic atheromatous disease and postoperative dysfunction has been established previously. Choudhary et al. documented severe atheromatous disease in 12 of 126 patients undergoing CABG (36). Protruding atheromas were significantly more common in patients over 60 years of age. Out of four patients with grade V atheromas, two developed right hemiplegia postoperatively. To determine the optimal method to detect ascending aortic atheromas intraoperatively, manual palpation, TEE, and epiaortic scanning were compared in 100 patients (37). Age greater than 70 years and hypertension were significant risk factors for severe ascending atheromas. Epiaortic scanning was found superior to both manual palpation and TEE.

## Pediatric Cardiac Surgery

### Mitral Regurgitation

Lee et al. studied the validity of intraoperative TEE for predicting the degree of MR at follow-up in 47 patients with atrioventricular defects (38). Intraoperative TEE was useful in detecting severe MR that required further repair at the same time. In 21 patients, however, there was a discrepancy between the intraoperative and follow-up grades of MR. The authors noted that blood pressures were significantly lower and heart rates significantly higher intraoperatively.

### Aortic Regurgitation

Fourteen patients who underwent repair of ventricular septal defect with aortic regurgitation were studied by intraoperative TEE (39). The severity of prolapse of each aortic cusp and its adjacent sinus was assessed. The valvular regurgitation was quantitated by Doppler-derived regurgitant indices. TEE detected prolapse of the aortic valve and its sinus in all patients. On the basis of the TEE findings, an aortic valve exploration was executed in 12 patients. No residual aortic regurgitation was observed post-CPB, but a residual VSD was detected in five patients.

### Transposition of the Great Vessels

Less than perfect coronary artery translocation accounts for the majority of perioperative deaths after the arterial switch procedure for transposition of the great vessels. Shankar et al., using epicardial echocardiography, studied four neonates with a failing left ventricle or difficulty of weaning from CPB (40). In two patients, coronary arterial problems in the form of kinking of the proximal left coronary artery and extrinsic compression of the artery by the neopulmonary trunk were identified and corrected. In two other patients, supravalvar aortic stenosis was recognized leading to prompt revision.

### *Patent Ductus Arteriosus Interruption*

The efficacy of intraoperative TEE in reducing the incidence of residual ductal flow after video-assisted thoracoscopic (VATS) patent ductus arteriosus (PDA) interruption was studied by Lavoie et al. (41). In 2 of 30 consecutive patients (mean age 2.4 yrs; mean weight 11.2 kg), intraoperative TEE detected residual flow after placement of the vascular clip, requiring placement of a second clip. At one-month follow-up, three patients presented with residual duct flow.

## MISCELLANEOUS NEW APPLICATIONS

### Three-Dimensional Echocardiography

With the development of three-dimensional echocardiography, several investigators have explored its incremental value for the intraoperative detection of valvular lesions (42–44). In many instances, 3D-echocardiography provided complementary morphologic information that explained the mechanisms of abnormalities seen on conventional echocardiography. Three-dimensional echocardiography also allowed direct visualization and planimetry of regurgitant orifice areas and measurement of regurgitant volumes. Vogel et al. used 3D-echocardiography to image congenital cardiac lesions as they would be visualized by a surgeon (45). This approach yielded additional information in the diagnosis of supravalvular mitral membranes, doubly committed subarterial ventricular septal defects, and subaortic stenoses caused by restrictive ventricular septal defects in double inlet left ventricles.

### Intraoperative Stress Echo

Intraoperative dobutamine stress echocardiography has been utilized to detect inducible demand ischemia in patients with severe coronary artery disease and to predict functional changes after myocardial revascularization (46,47). In 75 of 80 anesthetized patients with severe coronary artery disease scheduled for noncardiac surgery, inducible ischemia was detected after a standard dobutamine-atropine stress protocol. None of the patients suf-

fered significant complications. The diagnostic value of intraoperative dobutamine stress echocardiography in this patient population remains to be determined. In CABG surgery, changes in myocardial function after low-dose dobutamine were highly predictive for early and late changes in myocardial function from baseline function. When improvement in function was noted after dobutamine, the odds ratios for early and late improvement were 20.7 and 34.6, respectively.

## COMPLICATIONS

Intraoperative TEE is not without risks. Hogue et al. studied independent predictors of swallowing dysfunction after cardiac surgery (48). In addition to age and length of intubation after surgery, intraoperative use of TEE was a highly significant ($p < 0.003$) predictor of swallowing dysfunction. In another study of 838 consecutive cardiac surgical patients, significant factors causing postoperative dysphagia were studied by multiple logistic regression (49). After controlling for other significant factors such as stroke, left ventricular ejection fraction, intubation time, and duration of operation, the patients with intraoperative TEE had 7.8 times greater odds of dysphagia than those without.

In a recent review of 7,200 adult cardiac surgical patients, Kallmeyer et al. reported on the safety of intraoperative transesophageal echocardiography (50). They observed no mortality and a morbidity of only 0.2%. Most complications were related to probe insertion or manipulation that resulted in oropharyngeal, esophageal, or gastric trauma. In seven patients, diagnostic esophagogastroduodenoscopy (EGD) was indicated because of postoperative odynophagia. Acute upper gastrointestinal bleeding occurred in two patients. In one of these patients, EGD revealed several linear esophageal tears while in the other only erythema and diffuse oozing were observed. Esophageal perforation occurred in one elderly female patient. The patient suffered from dyspnea two days after the surgical procedure. The perforation resulted in a hydropneumothorax and required surgical repair. One esophageal perforation was also reported by Schmidlin et al. in a series of 2,296 intraoperative TEE examinations (8).

Greene et al. evaluated the safety of TEE in pediatric cardiac surgery by performing an endoscopic examination of the esophagus following TEE (51). In 50 patients undergoing repair of congenital cardiac surgery, the endoscopic examination was performed after removal of the TEE probe. In 32 patients, mild mucosal injury was observed, but none resulted in long-term feeding or swallowing difficulties.

## KEY POINTS

* Although intraoperative TEE is widely utilized during cardiac surgery because it is perceived to be useful, scientific evidence demonstrating its usefulness is generally lacking.
* Practice guidelines developed by professional organizations classify indications for perioperative TEE on the basis of the strength of supporting evidence or expert opinion that the technology improves outcomes.
* In the ACC/AHA guidelines for perioperative echocardiography, new Class I indications include the evaluation of complex valve replacements and the placement of intracardiac devices.
* In the ACC/AHA guidelines for perioperative echocardiography, new Class IIb indications include the evaluation of regional myocardial function during off-pump coronary bypass procedures, intraoperative dobutamine stress testing, and assessment of residual duct flow after interruption of patent ductus arteriosus.
* While the incidence of complications after perioperative transesophageal echocardiography is low, probe insertion and manipulation may result in oropharyngeal, esophageal, or gastric trauma.

## REFERENCES

1. Thys DM. Echocardiography and anesthesiology: Successes and challenges. Anesthesiology 2001;95:1313–4.
2. Morewood GH, Gallagher ME, Gaughan JP, Conlay LA. Current practice patterns for adult perioperative transesophageal echocardiography in the United States. [See comment.] [Journal Article] Anesthesiology. 2001;95(6):1507–12.
3. Click RL, Abel MD, Schaff HV. Intraoperative transesophageal echocardiography: 5-year prospective review of impact on surgical management. Mayo Clin Proc 2000;75: 241–7.
4. Couture P, Denault AY, McKenty S, et al. Impact of routine use of intraoperative transesophageal echocardiography during cardiac surgery. Can J Anaesth 2000;47:20–6.
5. Michel-Cherqui M, Ceddaha A, Liu N, et al. Assessment of systematic use of intraoperative transesophageal echocardiography during cardiac surgery in adults: a prospective study of 203 patients. J Cardiothorac Vasc Anes 2000;14:45–50.
6. Mishra M, Chauhan R, Sharma KK, et al. Real-time intraoperative transesophageal echocardiography—how useful? Experience of 5,016 cases. J Cardiothorac Vasc Anesth 1998; 12(6):625–32.
7. Sutton DC, Kluger R. Intraoperative transesophageal echocardiography: impact on adult cardiac surgery. Anaesth Intensive Care 1998;26:287–93.
8. Schmidlin D, Bettex D, Bernard E, et al. Transesophageal echocardiography in cardiac and vascular surgery: implications and observer variability. Br J Anaesth 2001;86 (4): 497–505.
9. Rosenfeld HM, Gentles TL, Wernovsky G, et al. Utility of intraoperative transesophageal echocardiography in the assessment of residual cardiac defects. Pediatr Cardiol 1998;19: 346–51.
10. Sheil ML, Baines DB. Intraoperative transesophageal echocardiography for pediatric cardiac surgery by an audit of 200 cases. Anaesth Intensive Care 1999;27:591–5.
11. Stevenson JG. Role of intraoperative transesophageal echocardiography during repair of congenital cardiac defects. Acta Paediatr Suppl 1995;410:23–33.
12. Ungerleider RM, Kisslo JA, Greeley WJ, et al. Intraoperative echocardiography during congenital heart operations: experience from 1,000 cases. Ann Thorac Surg 1995;60(6 Suppl):S539–42.
13. Sloth E, Pedersen J, Olsen KH, et al. Transesophageal echocardiographic monitoring during paediatric cardiac surgery: obtainable information and feasibility in 532 children. Paediatr Anaesth 2001;11:657–62.
14. Durongpisitkul K, Soongswang J, Sriyoschati S, et al. Utility of intraoperative transesophageal echocardiogram in congenital heart disease. J Med Assoc Thai 2000;83 Suppl 2: S46–53.
15. Practice Guidelines for perioperative transesophageal echocardiography. A report by the American Society of Anesthesiologists and the Society of Cardiovascular Anesthesiologists Task Force on transesophageal echocardiography. Anesthesiology 1996;84:986–1006.
16. Cheitlin MD, Alpert JS, Armstrong WF, et al. ACC/AHA guidelines for the clinical application of echocardiography. Circulation 1997;95:1686–1744.
17. Kawano H, Mizoguchi T, Ayoagi S. Intraoperative transesophageal echocardiography for evaluation of mitral valve repair. J Heart Valve Dis 1999;8:287–93.
18. Saiki Y, Kasegawa H, Kawase M, et al. Intraoperative TEE during mitral valve repair: does it predict early and late postoperative mitral valve dysfunction? Ann Thorac Surg 1998; 66:1277–81.
19. Aklog L, Filsoufi F, Flores KQ, et al. Does coronary artery bypass grafting alone correct moderate ischemic mitral regurgitation? Circulation 2001;104 (Suppl 1):I68–75.
20. Grewal KS, Malkowski MJ, Piracha AR, et al. Effect of general anesthesia on the severity of mitral regurgitation by transesophageal echocardiography. Am J Cardiol 2000;85(2): 199–203.
21. Nowrangi SK, Connolly HM, Freeman WK, et al. Impact of intraoperative transesophageal echocardiography among patients undergoing aortic valve replacement for aortic stenosis. J Am Soc Echocardiogr 2001;14: 863–6.
22. Ionescu AA, West RR, Proudman C, et al. Prospective study of routine perioperative transesophageal echocardiography for elective valve replacement: clinical impact and cost-saving implications. J Am Soc Echocardiogr 2001;14:659–67.
23. Morehead AJ, Firstenberg MS, Shiota T, et al. Intraoperative echocardiographic detection of regurgitant jets after valve replacement. Ann Thorac Surg 2000;69 (1):135–9.
24. O'Rourke DJ, Palac RT, Malenka DJ, et al. Outcome of mild periprosthetic regurgitation detected by intraoperative transesophageal echocardiography. J Am Coll Cardiol 2001;38: 163–6.
25. Bergquist BD, Bellows WH, Leung JM. Transesophageal echocardiography in myocardial revascularization. Influence on intraoperative decision making. Anesth Analg 1996;82: 1139–45.
26. Savage RM, Lytle BW, Aronson S, et al. Intraoperative echocardiography is indicated in high-risk coronary artery bypass grafting. Ann Thorac Surg 1997;64:368–73.
27. Arruda AM, Dearani JA, Click RL, et al. Intraoperative application of power Doppler imaging: visualization of myocardial perfusion after anastomosis of left internal thoracic artery to left anterior descending coronary artery. J Am Soc Echocardiogr 1999;12(8):650–4.
28. Applebaum RM, Cutler WM, Bhardwaj N, et al. Utility of transesophageal echocardiography during port-access minimally invasive cardiac surgery. Am J Cardiol 1998; 82:183–8.

29. Falk V, Walther T, Diegeler A, et al. Echocardiographic monitoring of minimally invasive mitral valve surgery using an endoartic clamp. J Heart Valve Dis 1996;5:630–7.
30. Schulze CJ, Wildhirt SM, Boehm DH, et al. Continuous transesophageal echocardiographic (TEE) monitoring during port-access cardiac surgery. Heart Surg Forum 1999;2:54–9.
31. Kort S, Applebaum RM, Grossi EA, et al. Minimally invasive aortic valve replacement: echocardiographic and clinical results. Am Heart J 2001;142:391–2.
32. Moises VA, Mesquita CB, Campos O, et al. Importance of intraoperative transesophageal echocardiography during coronary artery surgery without cardiopulmonary bypass. J Am Soc Echocardiogr 1998;11:1139–44.
33. Secknus MA, Asher CR, Scalia GM, et al. Intraoperative transesophageal echocardiography in minimally invasive cardiac valve surgery. J Am Soc Echocardiogr 1999;12:231–6.
34. Yao FS, Barbut D, Hager DN, et al. Detection of aortic emboli by transesophageal echocardiography during coronary artery bypass surgery. J Cardiothorac Vasc Anesth 1996;10:314–7.
35. Tingleff J, Joyce FS, Pettersson G. Intraoperative echocardiographic study of air embolism during cardiac operations. Ann Thorac Surg 1995;60:673–7.
36. Choudhary SK, Bhan A, Sharma R, et al. Aortic atherosclerosis and perioperative stroke in patients undergoing coronary artery bypass: role of intraoperative transesophageal echocardiography. Int J Cardiol 1997;67:31–8.
37. Sylivris S, Calafiore P, Matalanis G, et al. The intraoperative assessment of ascending aortic atheroma: epiaortic imaging is superior to both transesophageal echocardiography and direct palpation. J Cardiothorac Vasc Anesth 1997;11:704–7.
38. Lee HR, Montenegro LM, Nicolson SC, et al. Usefulness of intraoperative transesophageal echocardiography in predicting the degree of mitral regurgitation secondary to atrioventricular defect in children. Am J Cardiol 1999;83:570–3.
39. Leung MP, Chau KT, Chiu C, et al. Intraoperative TEE assessment of ventricular septal defect with aortic regurgitation. Ann Thorac Surg 1996;61:854–60.
40. Shankar S, Sreeram N, Brawn WJ, et al. Intraoperative ultrasonographic troubleshooting after the arterial switch operation. Ann Thorac Surg 1997;67:445–8.
41. Lavoie J, Javorsky JJ, Donahue K, et al. Detection of residual flow by transesophageal echocardiography during video-assisted thoracoscopic patent ductus arteriosus interruption. Anesth Analg 1995;80(6):1071–5.
42. Abraham TP, Warner JG, Jr, Kon ND, et al. Feasibility, accuracy, and incremental value of intraoperative three-dimensional transesophageal echocardiography in valve surgery. Am J Cardiol 1997;80(12):1577–82.
43. Breburda CS, Griffin BP, Pu M, et al. Three-dimensional echocardiographic planimetry of maximal regurgitant orifice area in myxomatous mitral regurgitation: intraoperative comparison of proximal flow convergence. J Am Coll Cardiol 1998;32(2):432–7.
44. De Simone R, Glombitza G, Vahl CF, et al. Three-dimensional color Doppler for assessing mitral regurgitation during valvuloplasty. Eur J Cardiothorac Surg 1999;15(2):127–33.
45. Vogel M, Ho SY, Lincoln C, et al. Three-dimensional echocardiography can simulate intraoperative visualization of congenitally malformed hearts. Ann Thorac Surg 1995;60(5):1282–8.
46. Seeberger MD, Skarvan K, Buser P, et al. Dobutamine stress echocardiography to detect inducible demand ischemia in anesthetized patients with coronary artery disease. Anesthesiology 1998;88(5):1233–9.
47. Aronson S, Dupont F, Savage R, et al. Changes in regional myocardial function after coronary artery bypass graft surgery are predicted by intraoperative low-dose dobutamine echocardiography. Anesthesiology 2000;93(3):685–92.
48. Hogue CW, Jr, Lappas GD, Creswell LL, et al. Swallowing dysfunction after cardiac operations. Associated adverse outcomes and risk factors including intraoperative transesophageal echocardiography. J Thorac Cardiovasc Surg 1995;110(2):517–22.
49. Rousou JA, Tighe DA, Garb JL, et al. Risk of dysphagia after transesophageal echocardiography during cardiac operations. Ann Thorac Surg 2000;69(2):486–9.
50. Kallmeyer IJ, Collard CD, Fox JA, et al. The safety of intraoperative transesophageal echocardiography: A case series of 7,200 cardiac surgical patients. Anesth Analg 2001;92:1126–30.
51. Greene MA, Alexander JA, Knauf DG, et al. Endoscopic evaluation of the esophagus in infants and children immediately following intraoperative use of transesophageal echocardiography. Chest 1999;116:1247–50.

## QUESTIONS

1. Practice guidelines for perioperative echocardiography:
   A. Define the allowed usage of echocardiography
   B. Are based on proven indications only
   C. Refer to clinical problems rather than to individual patients
   D. Determine the level of reimbursement for the procedure

2. In the AHA/ACC/ASE guidelines, the meaning of a class I indication is that TEE:
   A. Should be used whenever the condition is present
   B. Is useful and effective
   C. Is not associated with harmful effects
   D. Will guarantee reimbursement for the procedure

3. In minimally invasive cardiac surgery, intraoperative echocardiography has been found useful for all of the following *except*:
   A. Placement of intracardiac and intravascular catheters
   B. Assessment of postcardiopulmonary bypass valvular function
   C. Assessment of regional wall motion during coronary artery clamping
   D. Evaluation of intracardiac air after valvular surgery
   E. Prediction of long-term outcome after coronary artery bypass surgery

4. In cardiac surgical patients, the reported morbidity after intraoperative transesophageal echocardiography is approximately:
   A. 1 per 10,000 patients
   B. 1 per 5,000 patients
   C. 1 per 1,000 patients
   D. 1 per 500 patients
   E. 1 per 100 patients

# Organization of an Intraoperative Echocardiographic Service: Personnel, Equipment, Maintenance, Safety, Infection, and Continuous Quality Improvement

*Glenn S. Murphy, Joseph P. Mathew, and Stanton K. Shernan*

Since the mid-1980s, transesophageal echocardiography (TEE) has been used with increasing frequency in both cardiac and noncardiac operating rooms. Intraoperative TEE services are provided at nearly all of the institutions in North America where cardiac anesthesiologists practice (1,2). Echocardiography provides the clinician in the operating room with real-time information about cardiac function, cardiac anatomy, and hemodynamics. Immediate access to this data may improve outcomes in high-risk surgical patients.

Developing an intraoperative TEE service requires a considerable investment in equipment and training of personnel. Close, collaborative relationships between anesthesiologists, cardiologists, and TEE support staff must be developed in order to assure safe patient care. A significant expense is involved in the purchase and maintenance of TEE probes and machines. Space must be dedicated for the sterilization and storage of probes. This chapter reviews several essential components involved in the organization of a successful intraoperative TEE service.

## PERSONNEL

Outside of the operating room setting, cardiologists have traditionally performed and interpreted TEE exams. Since the introduction of monoplane probes into clinical practice nearly 20 years ago, anesthesiologists have assumed an integral role in the development of intraoperative TEE. Anesthesiologists quickly recognized the utility of TEE as an accurate and sensitive monitor of left ventricular filling and global and regional systolic function. The development of advanced Doppler imaging techniques greatly enhanced the monitoring and diagnostic capabilities of the clinician caring for the high-risk surgical patient.

In North America, the majority of intraoperative TEE studies are performed by cardiovascular anesthesiologists or cardiologists. Poterack et al. conducted a survey of anesthesiology training programs in 1992 to determine who uses TEE in the operating room (3). Fifty-four percent of respondents reported that the anesthesiologist was primarily responsible for interpretation of TEE data, whereas the remaining respondents reported the cardiologist responsible. In 2000, a survey was mailed to the members of the cardiovascular section of the Canadian Anesthesiologists' Society (2). Nearly all respondents (91%) noted that their hospital offered intraoperative TEE services: 13% were provided by cardiologists, 35% by anesthesiologists only, and 52% by both. Similar results were obtained when a survey was distributed to the membership of the Society of Cardiovascular Anesthesiologists in the United States (1). Fifty-two percent of respondents noted that an anesthesiologist performed intraoperative TEE exams, 18% reported that a cardiologist performed the studies, and 29% reported that either physician could be involved. A majority of anesthesiologists (66%) noted that a cardiologist assisted with interpretation of the TEE only upon request (51%) or not at all (15%). One-third of respondents reported that a cardiologist was involved in data interpretation when specific surgical procedures were performed (e.g., valve surgery).

The cognitive and technical skills of anesthesiologists using TEE may vary due to differences in training and clinical experience. In 1996, a Task Force on Practice Guidelines for Transesophageal Echocardiography established by the American Society of Anesthesiologists and the Society of Cardiovascular Anesthesiologists (SCA) recognized two levels of training in perioperative TEE: basic and advanced (4). Anesthesiologists with basic training "should be able to use TEE for indications which lie within the customary practice of anesthesiology," which include assessment of ventricular function, hemodynamics, cardiovascular collapse, and others. Anesthesiologists with advanced training should be able to utilize the full diagnostic potential of TEE. Clinicians with basic training must recognize their limitations and obtain assistance from expert echocardiographers when needed. When presented with complex diagnostic decisions in the operating room, even anesthesiologists with advanced training may require the assistance of a cardiologist. More recently, these training objectives have been updated and modified to include specific cognitive and technical skills required for the basic and advanced levels (5) (Table 8.1). Most importantly, these training guidelines published jointly by the American Society of Echocardiography and the SCA recommend that 150 TEE examinations be completed under appropriate supervision with at least 50 of them personally performed, interpreted, and reported by the trainee as part of "basic" training. At the advanced level of training, 300 complete examinations under appropriate supervision are recommended with at least 150 of these performed, interpreted, and reported by the trainee.

Both task forces have noted that proficiency in TEE could be gradually obtained "on the job" through practice and repetition for physicians unable to participate in a formal training program. However, the same cognitive and technical skills outlined in Table 8.1 are required of these physicians. Anesthesiologists could begin to master the essential cognitive and technical skills by studying standard texts and training videos and by attending TEE workshops and training sessions. In addition, the Task Force recommended that anesthesiologists seeking basic training via this pathway should have at least 20 hours of continuing medical education devoted to echocardiography while physicians seeking advanced training should have at least 50. Finally, a collaborative relationship with an expert in TEE is strongly encouraged. The expert in TEE should be immediately available so that essential intraoperative findings are not missed. Although the presence of the expert echocardiographer would be required less frequently as the expertise of the anesthesiologist increased, a collaborative relationship with the primary echocardiographers in the hospital (cardiologist, radiologist) may be essential for the long-term viability of an intraoperative service.

Qualified TEE support personnel are an important component of the intraoperative TEE team. Support personnel may be responsible for the daily maintenance of the TEE probes to include visual inspection of the probe for defects, cleaning and disinfection following each use, and regular testing for leakage currents. Support staff may improve efficiency in the operating room by entering patient data before each exam and retrieving and storing data (either digital or videotape) when studies are completed. In smaller centers, TEE equipment may be shared between anesthesiologists, cardiologists, and intensivists. The TEE support personnel can assist in transporting and coordinating the use of TEE machines and probes.

## EQUIPMENT AND MAINTENANCE

The cost of purchasing and maintaining an intraoperative echocardiographic system can be considerable. Basic equipment needed for a TEE service includes a standard ultrasound machine, a TEE probe, equipment for cleaning and disinfecting probes, a leakage current tester, a holder for storing the probes between uses, tools to archive data, report and bill generation capacities, and a service contract. A dedicated machine and probe is not necessarily required in every operating room so anesthesia groups must carefully evaluate their needs for intraoperative TEE before investing in equipment. In small hospitals, a single TEE system may be shared by physicians in the echocardiography lab, the operating room, and the ICU (2). Small groups may purchase a single machine and probe to be used in all anesthetizing locations. Even centers caring for a larger volume of high-risk surgical patients may use more than one probe with each ultrasound machine (e.g., four probes are used with two ultrasound machines), with the ultrasound machine transported between operating rooms as needed. In the United States, TEE is largely performed in patients undergoing cardiac surgery (1) and large cardiac centers may devote a single echocardiography system to each cardiac operating room.

The TEE probe is at risk for mechanical damage in the operating room; storage devices that protect the probe in this harsh environment are therefore recommended. Draping the TEE probe over anesthesia carts or ultrasound machines, in particular, is strongly discouraged. The possibility of intraoperative damage is enhanced by the fact that a variety of personnel handle the probe. Dropping the probe or striking it against a hard surface can damage the transducer elements and acoustic lens, the connector, or the control housing. Also, tears and abrasions in the probe can occur as it is advanced and withdrawn against a patient's teeth. After each examination, the probe should be carefully inspected for cracks, abrasions, and perforations. Physical defects in the housing of the probe can expose the patient to infective or electrical hazards. Larger defects can traumatize the esophagus during probe manipulation. In addition, pro-

▶ **TABLE 8.1. Recommended Training Objectives for Basic and Advanced Perioperative Echocardiography**

**Basic Training**

*Cognitive Skills*

1. Knowledge of the physical principles of echocardiographic image formation and blood velocity measurement
2. Knowledge of the operation of ultrasonographs including all controls that affect the quality of data displayed
3. Knowledge of the equipment handling, infection control, and electrical safety associated with the techniques of perioperative echocardiography
4. Knowledge of the indications, contraindications, and potential complications for perioperative echocardiography
5. Knowledge of the appropriate alternative diagnostic techniques
6. Knowledge of the normal tomographic anatomy as revealed by perioperative echocardiographic techniques
7. Knowledge of commonly encountered blood flow velocity profiles as measured by Doppler echocardiography
8. Knowledge of the echocardiographic manifestations of native valvular lesions and dysfunction
9. Knowledge of the echocardiographic manifestations of cardiac masses, thrombi, cardiomyopathies, pericardial effusions, and lesions of the great vessels
10. Detailed knowledge of the echocardiographic presentations of myocardial ischemia and infarction
11. Detailed knowledge of the echocardiographic presentations of normal and abnormal ventricular function
12. Detailed knowledge of the echocardiographic presentations of air embolization

*Technical Skills*

1. Ability to operate ultrasonographs, including the primary controls affecting the quality of the displayed data
2. Ability to insert a TEE probe safely in the anesthetized, tracheally intubated patient
3. Ability to perform a comprehensive TEE examination and to differentiate normal from markedly abnormal cardiac structures and function
4. Ability to recognize marked changes in segmental ventricular contraction indicative of myocardial ischemia or infarction
5. Ability to recognize marked changes in global ventricular filling and ejection
6. Ability to recognize air embolization
7. Ability to recognize gross valvular lesions and dysfunction
8. Ability to recognize large intracardiac masses and thrombi
9. Ability to detect large pericardial effusions
10. Ability to recognize common echocardiographic artifacts
11. Ability to communicate echocardiographic results effectively to health care professionals, the medical record, and patients
12. Ability to recognize complications of perioperative echocardiography

**Advanced Training**

*Cognitive Skills*

1. All the cognitive skills defined under basic training
2. Detailed knowledge of the principles and methodologies of qualitative and quantitative echocardiography
3. Detailed knowledge of native and prosthetic valvular function including valvular lesions and dysfunction
4. Knowledge of congenital heart disease (if congenital practice is planned, then this knowledge must be detailed)
5. Detailed knowledge of all other diseases of the heart and great vessels that is relevant in the perioperative period (if pediatric practice is planned, then this knowledge may be more general than detailed)
6. Detailed knowledge of the techniques, advantages, disadvantages, and potential complications of commonly used cardiac surgical procedures for treatment of acquired and congenital heart disease
7. Detailed knowledge of other diagnostic methods appropriate for correlation with perioperative echocardiography

*Technical Skills*

1. All the technical skills defined under basic training
2. Ability to acquire or direct the acquisition of all necessary echocardiographic data, including epicardial and epiaortic imaging
3. Ability to recognize subtle changes in segmental ventricular contraction indicative of myocardial ischemia or infarction
4. Ability to quantify systolic and diastolic ventricular function and to estimate other relevant hemodynamic parameters
5. Ability to quantify normal and abnormal native and prosthetic valvular function
6. Ability to assess the appropriateness of cardiac surgical plans
7. Ability to identify inadequacies in cardiac surgical interventions and the underlying reasons for the inadequacies
8. Ability to aid in clinical decision-making in the operating room

Reproduced with permission from Cahalan MK, Abel M, Goldman M, et al. American Society of Echocardiography and Society of Cardiovascular Anesthesiologists task force guidelines for training in perioperative echocardiography. Anesth Analg 2002;94:1384–88.

▶ **TABLE 8.2.  Procedures and Chemicals That Damage TEE Probes**

| *Procedures That Damage Probes* |
| --- |
| Autoclaving |
| Immersion in chlorine bleach or alcohol |
| Immersion of the control handle in any liquid |
| Dry heat sterilization |
| Ultraviolet sterilization |
| Gas sterilization |
| Prolonged immersion (several hours) in disinfecting solution |
| *Chemicals That Damage Probes* |
| Iodine |
| Mineral oil |
| Acetone |
| Spray aerosol anesthetics (if applied directly to the probe) |

Adapted from Sequoia Ultrasound System: User and Reference Manuals. Mountain View, CA: Accuson Corp., 2000–2001.

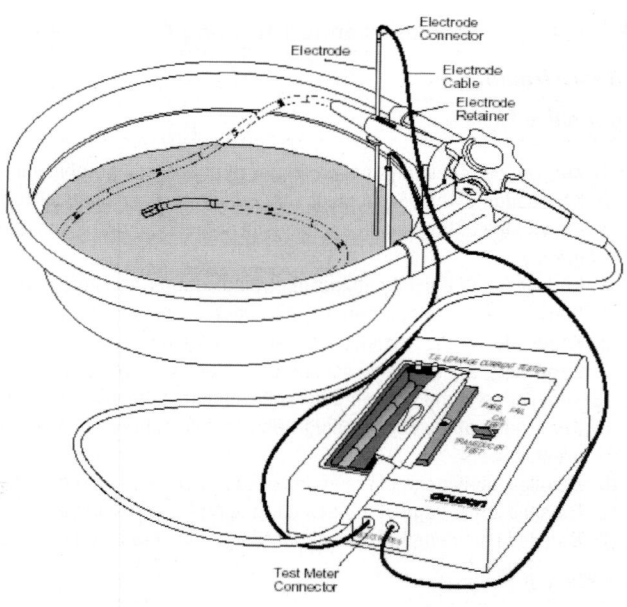

**FIGURE 8.1.** Proper technique for performing a leakage current test.

cedures and chemicals that are used for cleaning and sterilization can damage TEE probes (Table 8.2).

The electrical safety of the TEE system may be compromised if mechanical damage to the probe has occurred. If damage is suspected, the entire probe and cable should be inspected before each use for defects in the housing. A probe should never be used for patient care if obvious defects are present. Since visual inspection may not detect small cracks or perforations, a leakage current test should be performed according to the recommendations of the manufacturer (some require testing following every use of the probe) (Fig. 8.1). Commercially available devices measure the electrical impedance of the system, and provide a warning signal if leakage currents exceed recommended standards (approximately 50 μA) (6). The leakage current test is most often performed during the disinfection process.

Proper storage of the probe will reduce the risk of mechanical damage. For storage between patient exams, the probe should be maintained in a straight rather than flexed position to minimize tension on the cable connections. Commercial wall-mounted racks that protect the transducer in a straight plastic tube can be used in the operating room and cleaning room (Fig. 8.2). Specialized probe holders that stabilize the control housing while the probe is inserted in a patient have been described (7). A probe holder can prevent dropping or mishandling of the control housing, as well as prevent kinking or twisting of cables. During transportation to different sites in the hospital, the probe should be placed in a carrying case, or a protective device should be placed over the transducer elements in the tip of the probe.

## SAFETY

Serious complications associated with the use of TEE are rare (Table 8.3). The largest safety study reviewed data from 10,419 TEE procedures performed in awake patients (8). Morbidity occurred in 0.18% of exams: one death was reported. The safety of intraoperative TEE was

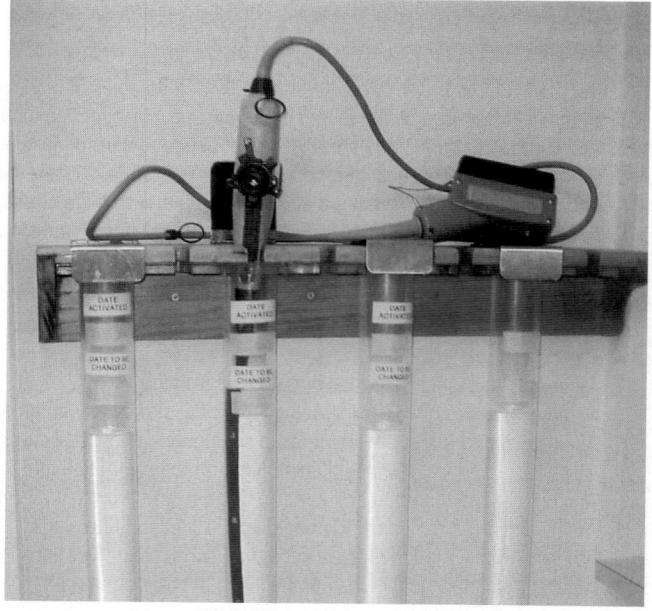

**FIGURE 8.2.** Example of a wall-mounted rack designed to protect transesophageal echocardiography probes during storage.

> **TABLE 8.3.  Complications of Intraoperative TEE**

**Complications Related to the Gastrointestinal System**

Esophageal perforation
Esophageal bleeding
Dysphagia
Odynophagia
Thermal injury
Transient bacteremia
Lip and dental trauma

**Complications Related to Compression of Adjacent Structures**

Tracheal compression
Displacement of the endotracheal tube
Vocal cord paralysis
Cardiac arrhythmias
Hypertension or hypotension
Splenic injury

examined in a case series of 7200 cardiac surgical patients (9). No deaths related to intraoperative TEE were reported in this retrospective study. Morbidity occurred in 14 patients (0.2%); severe odynophagia accounted for half of these complications. In two other large series, morbidity was reported in 0.47% of 1500 ambulatory adult patients and 0% of 5016 cardiac surgical patients (10,11). The safety of TEE appears comparable with upper gastrointestinal (UGI) endoscopy (12).

## Complications Related to the Gastrointestinal System

Several types of trauma to the esophagus and stomach can occur during TEE examinations. Esophageal perforation is a rare but potentially lethal complication. Only one case of esophageal perforation was reported following 7200 intraoperative studies (9). Brinkman et al. described three patients who sustained intrathoracic esophageal perforations over a two-year period at a large academic center (13). This form of trauma may present initially as subcutaneous emphysema, substernal chest pain, hemorrhage, or the appearance of the TEE probe in the surgical field (9,13). Mortality has been reported following esophageal perforation by the TEE probe (14). Trauma to the gastrointestinal system may also produce significant hemorrhage. Injury consistent with a Mallory-Weiss tear has been observed in patients with UGI bleeding following the removal of the TEE probe (9,15).

An association between intraoperative TEE and postoperative swallowing dysfunction has been noted in cardiac surgical patients. In a study of 869 patients undergoing cardiac operations, swallowing dysfunction was identified in 34 subjects (16). Multivariate logistic regression analysis identified intraoperative use of TEE as an independent predictor of this complication. Patients with an impaired swallowing reflex were more likely to develop postoperative aspiration and pneumonia. In a second study of 838 consecutive cardiac surgical patients, TEE use was also significantly related to the development of postoperative dysphagia (17); patients monitored with TEE were 7.8 times as likely to experience dysphagia as those who did not have TEE. In contrast to these studies, two small prospective clinical trials demonstrated no association between intraoperative TEE and postoperative dysphagia (18,19).

Several mechanisms may contribute to esophageal and gastric injuries during TEE examinations. The majority of injuries are likely the result of direct trauma produced by the probe. Extensive manipulation of the probe tip to obtain required images may damage normal tissue. In an animal model, however, no mucosal injury was produced following prolonged and sustained contact of a probe with the esophagus (20). Direct trauma is more likely to occur in the setting of extensive gastric or esophageal pathology. Since all ultrasound transducers generate heat, thermal injury may be produced at the site where the transducer contacts tissue. Theoretically, the risk of thermal injury would be increased during prolonged use or when a significant temperature gradient existed between the transducer tip and the esophagus (during hypothermic cardiopulmonary bypass). Heat-sensing thermistors are now incorporated into the tips of transducers such that when a temperature limit is reached, transmitting power is automatically switched off. Transducers should be inactivated when not in use to reduce the potential for thermal injury. Trauma to the tissue of the esophagus may also occur due to buckling or doubling over of the tip of the TEE probe. This complication can be caused by improper insertion techniques or by excessive mobility in the tip of the probe due to stretching and elongation of the steering cables. The possibility of transducer buckling should be considered whenever difficulty is encountered while withdrawing the probe or adjusting the control knobs. Probe doubling over has been successfully treated by advancing the transducer into the stomach and straightening the tip (21).

## Complications Related to Compression of Adjacent Structures

Several types of airway-related complications have been reported in the literature. Direct compression of the trachea or the endotracheal tube by the TEE probe has been described in infants and small children. In a series of 1,650 pediatric TEE exams, airway obstruction occurred in 14 patients (22). However, a prospective study in pediatric patients demonstrated no changes in pulmonary function variables or gas exchange when a pediatric bi-plane probe was used (23). Airway obstruction associated with intraoperative TEE has been reported in adult patients with aortic pseudoaneurysms and aortic dissections (24,25). Acute hypoxemia secondary to TEE-induced malposition of the endotracheal tube can occur in the operating room. Extensive manipulation of the probe may result in advancement of the oral endotracheal tube into the right mainstem bronchus or inadvertent tracheal extubation (26).

Hemodynamic changes during TEE probe placement are common. Hypertension and tachycardia are frequently observed during passage of the probe and following laryngoscopy-assisted placement. These events are usually brief and self-limited. Hemodynamically significant supraventricular and ventricular arrhythmias have been reported, but significant arrhythmias occur in less than 0.5% of TEE exams performed in awake patients (8,27). The incidence of dysrhythmias is reduced when probe insertion and manipulation occurs in anesthetized patients (4,9). Pharmacologic interventions are rarely required to treat cardiovascular disturbances, since removing the probe can terminate the majority of hemodynamic events.

Vocal cord paralysis is a rare complication of intraoperative TEE. Transient unilateral vocal cord paralysis has been reported in two patients undergoing neurosurgical procedures in the upright position with neck flexion (28,29), with compression of the recurrent laryngeal by the probe being the most likely cause of this injury. Recurrent laryngeal nerve palsy has been observed in 1.9% to 6.9% of cardiovascular surgical patients in the early postoperative period (30,31). Although an association between intraoperative TEE use and recurrent laryngeal nerve injury in cardiac surgical patients has been suggested (32), a prospective study demonstrated that the incidence of recurrent laryngeal nerve palsy was not significantly different in cardiac surgical patients monitored with or without TEE (31). Other factors appear to be responsible for this complication, including surgical manipulation and the duration of cardiopulmonary bypass and tracheal intubation.

## Contraindications

Transesophageal echocardiography examinations should be avoided or performed with great caution in patients with significant esophageal or gastric pathology (Table 8.4). Flexion and extension of the cervical spine is often required during passage of the probe into the esophagus, creating the potential for injury to the spinal cord or esophagus in patients with significant atlantoaxial disease or cervical arthritis. A careful patient examination for any signs or symptoms related to the gastrointestinal system should be conducted prior to each TEE examination. Clin-

▶ **TABLE 8.4. Contraindications to TEE Probe Placement**

***Absolute Contraindications***

Patient refusal
Esophageal strictures, webs, or rings
Esophageal perforation
Obstructing esophageal neoplasms
Cervical spine instability

***Relative Contraindications***

Esophageal diverticulum
Large hiatal hernia
Recent esophageal or gastric surgery
Esophageal varices
History of dysphagia or odynophagia
Cervical arthritis
History of radiation to the mediastinum
Deformities of the oral pharynx
Severe coagulopathy

icians should be aware of any history of dysphagia, odynophagia, upper gastrointestinal bleeding, esophageal or gastric surgery, mediastinal radiation, or esophageal strictures, tumors, varices, or diverticula. Absolute contraindications to the use of TEE include patient refusal, esophageal strictures, webs, rings, esophageal perforation, obstructing esophageal neoplasms, and cervical spine instability. Physicians must weigh the risks and benefits of intraoperative echocardiography in patients with relative contraindications to TEE.

## Infection

### Bacteremia and Endocarditis

Transient bacteremia may occur during any gastrointestinal instrumentation. The incidence of bacteremia during upper gastrointestinal endoscopy without biopsy averages approximately 4% (33). Insertion and manipulation of a TEE probe could induce mild trauma to mucosa and allow the introduction of bacteria from the oral cavity and esophagus into the bloodstream. However, the risk of bacteremia during TEE exams appears low. Several prospective studies have demonstrated that positive blood cultures are obtained in only 0% to 4.2% of patients during and following TEE probe placement (34–36).

In susceptible patients, transient bacteremia can result in bacterial endocarditis. In an analysis of 41 studies of upper endoscopy-induced bacteremia, only two possible cases of endocarditis were noted (33). In both of these patients, factors other than the procedure may have contributed to the development of endocarditis. No cases of endocarditis were reported in the ten studies examining the incidence of bacteremia after TEE (34). A review of the literature reveals only one case report describing a temporal relationship between TEE and endocarditis (37), but a clear cause-and-effect relationship could not be clearly demonstrated.

Antibiotic prophylaxis is not required for procedures with a low risk of induced bacteremia. A position paper from the American Heart Association states that routine antibiotic prophylaxis is not needed before UGI endoscopy (38). Thus, there appears to be little scientific evidence to justify endocarditis prophylaxis for TEE in the perioperative setting. Physicians may choose to administer antibiotics to patients who are considered "high risk" for developing endocarditis (38), including those with a history of valvular heart disease, prosthetic heart valves, congenital heart malformations, or previous endocarditis. Since antibiotics administered to prevent surgical wound infections may not be as effective as endocarditis prophylaxis in susceptible patients, the prophylactic drug regimen recommended by the American Heart Association should be followed (38).

### Cleaning and Disinfection of TEE Probes

Bacterial and viral cross-infection between patients has been documented following upper endoscopy (39). A risk of transmission of infective agents between patients also exists with the TEE probe. At the present time, no formal guidelines have been published that describe recommended techniques for sterilization of the TEE probe. When cleaning the TEE probe, most echocardiographers have adopted guidelines established by gastroenterologists for the disinfection of endoscopes (40).

A space outside of the operating room should be dedicated to the cleaning of the probe immediately following each use. This area must be well ventilated and temperature controlled. Heavy-duty gloves and protective eyewear will protect personnel handling the probe from the caustic effects of glutaraldehyde-based solutions. A sink for washing the probe and a container for holding glutaraldehyde disinfectant solution are the minimal requirements for this area. The establishment of dedicated storage areas for contaminated and clean probes will reduce the risk of transducer damage.

The first step in the decontamination of TEE probes is precleaning. Precleaning is the process of mechanically or chemically removing material from the surface of the probe (6). A variety of precleaning methods can be used to remove blood or other organic matter from the probe. Scrubbing the probe with soap and water or isopropyl alcohol will remove most adherent secretions. Several commercially prepared enzymatic precleaning solutions are also available.

Following precleaning, the probe is immediately placed in a disinfecting solution. Only glutaraldehyde-based solutions approved by the FDA and the manufacturer of the probe should be used. The probe is immersed in the solution only up to the last depth mark since damage to the system will occur if the control handle is submerged in any liquids. The duration of the disinfecting process should be at least 20 minutes to eliminate bacterial and viral contaminants. After removal from the solution, the probe is rinsed in water and allowed to dry for at least 20–30 minutes so that residual glutaraldehyde evaporates.

## ASSESSING QUALITY IN AN INTRAOPERATIVE TEE SERVICE

In the last decade, the use of TEE in the operating room has seen significant technological advances, which have permitted the anesthesiologist to perform a comprehensive examination on every patient but have also heightened the complexity of the procedure. Diagnostic interpretations of these TEE examinations may vary widely, particularly when the anesthesiologist performing the examination is responsible for the anesthetic management of the patient (41). The clinical experience of the examiner conducting a test may also have a favorable or perhaps even a detrimental effect on outcome (42). Continuous quality improvement (CQI) is an educational process used by many physicians and hospitals to assess practice patterns and identify problems in health care delivery, and to develop solutions to those problems. Independent of the mandate from the Joint Commission for the Accreditation of Health Care Organizations that health care providers institute an assessment of quality of care, consensus exists on what should be considered the "proper practice of echocardiography" (4,5), thus making CQI programs a necessary component of every intraoperative TEE service.

Any dialogue on CQI first merits a definition of the word "quality." In the health care field, "quality" has been like love—hard to define (43). Faced with mounting cost pressures in recent years, however, physicians have been forced to adopt more rigorous definitions of quality that have prevailed in the business world for decades. Such definitions emphasize the satisfaction of the customer and not simply whether the product was provided by someone certified and trained to do so. The quality of a product or service may then be defined as "its ability to satisfy the needs and expectations of its customers or the totality of features and characteristics of a product or service that bears on its ability to satisfy stated or implied needs" (44). While these definitions focus our attention on the customer, they also raise an interesting question. Who should be considered as "customers" in the operating room? Is it simply the patient who is undergoing the TEE exam or is it also the surgeon who relies upon the information provided to him to guide the decision-making process? Or perhaps it is also the referring cardiologist who expects the use of TEE to detect and lead to the correction of any residual defects.

In 1995, the American Society of Echocardiography developed a series of recommendations for the application of CQI principles to the field of echocardiography (43). In that document, a CQI process is first defined as continuous—an ongoing process. It is not one that is conducted simply at predetermined times. At times, it may mean that the adequacy of an intraoperative exam may have to be re-evaluated. At other times, educational activities to improve wall motion analysis or ejection fraction estimation may have to be instituted. Quality in the CQI process, as has been discussed above, is focused on the customer. Quality is "doing right things right in echocardiography" (43). It is continuously being redefined and must be judged, in part, by use of a comparative process. Quality is enhanced by repetition Finally, the term "improvement" in CQI implies that attempts are being made to always get better. Change in the practice of echocardiography is ordained as both necessary and desirable.

Eight fundamental principles guide the formation of an intraoperative CQI process (43). To begin with, physicians who perform and interpret intraoperative echocardiographic studies must have adequate primary training. Guidelines for basic and advanced training have been recently published and discussed earlier in this chapter in Table 8.1 (4,5). A certifying examination in perioperative TEE has also been developed and administered with higher overall examination performance associated with longer than 3 months of training and performance and interpretation of at least six examinations a week (45). Beyond primary training and testing, the process of CQI must require that those who perform intraoperative studies maintain a case volume sufficient to maintain their skills and competency. Consensus panels have suggested that continuing competence in echocardiography necessitates the performance of 100 cases per year but similar consensus has not been achieved in the intraoperative arena. It would seem reasonable to assume that a minimum of 1–2 cases per week would be sufficient for a trained echocardiographer to continue to maintain his skills. Third, CQI recognizes that echocardiography is physician supervised and directed. Intraoperatively, a TEE exam may be performed by a resident, fellow, or even a sonographer. In those settings, the supervising physician must always be available to assist in all patient examinations and be capable of performing the study. Fourth, CQI requires periodic impartial review of study performance and interpretation by those at a higher training level. This includes caseload review, performance review, record keeping review, and documentation of proper equipment performance. Storage media for the echocardiograms substantially impact on the ability to

fulfill this requirement. While videotape has been the medium of choice for archiving intraoperative studies primarily because of its low cost, it is cumbersome to retrieve and leads to a time-intensive review process. Digital archives of a sequence of single-beat video loops should therefore be implemented whenever possible.

Fifth, CQI requires formal continuing education at local, regional, and national levels to maintain competence in a rapidly changing field. Sixth, continuing performance, competence, and education must be documented and submitted to a hospital or departmental quality assurance committee. Seventh, CQI requires appropriate utilization review of echocardiographic services. Utilization review should aim to determine if the study was indicated, if the appropriate views were obtained, if the question at hand was answered, and if the study was interpreted and the report distributed in a timely fashion. Finally, CQI requires that the interpretation of echocardiograms be made available in a reasonable period of time. Routine TEE studies should not take longer than 24 hours for interpretive review by a physician and generation of a report to the patient's medical record.

Research into the importance of training and CQI processes for perioperative TEE is limited but a few studies merit discussion. Stevenson recently reported on the outcome of congenital cardiac surgery when TEE was performed by physicians who met training guidelines and compared it to those who did not meet the criteria (41). In his study 219 patients undergoing repair of congenital cardiac defects were included in the study where, in the first year of the study, physicians who met ASE guidelines for pediatric TEE performed intraoperative TEE. In the second year of the study, physicians who performed the exams did not meet the guidelines for training. Despite similar mortality rates for both groups, physicians who did not meet training guidelines had lower rates of adequacy of TEE studies, detection of residual cardiac lesions, and use of TEE in returning to cardiopulmonary bypass for additional surgery. Stevenson concluded that patient outcome is better when physicians who meet published guidelines perform intraoperative TEE and a physician other than the physician providing intraoperative care for the patient should perform the echocardiography exam. In an accompanying editorial, Fyfe further argued that "the conflicting responsibilities of serving as both the intraoperative anesthesiologist and the echocardiographer" might preclude performing either task well (47).

In response, Mathew and colleagues assessed the quality of intraoperative TEE examinations performed by 10 cardiac anesthesiologists participating in a CQI program at a university hospital. The anesthesiologists first interpreted 154 comprehensive TEE examinations from adult patients undergoing cardiac surgery shortly after the examinations were completed in the operating room. A second interpretation of these examinations was then conducted off-line by two primary echocardiographers (a radiologist and cardiologist), and interrater agreement between the three raters was measured using the kappa coefficient ($\kappa$) and percent agreement. Between anesthesiologist and radiologist, the agreement was 83% ($\kappa$: 0.58), between anesthesiologist and cardiologist 80% ($\kappa$: 0.57), and between radiologist and cardiologist 82% ($\kappa$: 0.60). This study demonstrated that an anesthesiologist responsible for the anesthetic management of an adult cardiac patient could in fact function as an intraoperative echocardiographer. Furthermore, the performance and interpretation of the TEE examinations can be conducted at a level comparable to that provided by "experts" evaluating the TEE examinations removed from the demands of the operating room (i.e., off-line). Thus the anesthesiologist and intraoperative echocardiographer need not be mutually exclusive.

Although it appears that the anesthesiologist may be able to simultaneously serve as an echocardiographer, the need for adequate training cannot be minimized. The study by Mathew et al. (48) did reveal that, when compared to the "expert," anesthesiologists with more than five years of experience had higher levels of agreement than those with less than five years of experience. For instance, using bias analysis, they demonstrated that anesthesiologists as a group underestimated fractional area change (FAC) when compared to the off-line assessment of the expert. Much of this underestimation was related to the experience of the user. Similarly, Bergquist et al. (49), in a study evaluating real-time intraoperative interpretation, showed that anesthesiologists can estimate FAC in real time to within $\pm$ 10% of off-line values in only 75% of all cases but to within $\pm$ 20% in 93% of all cases.

Finally, although a CQI process may appear cumbersome, it is a process that can function well in the intraoperative environment. Miller and colleagues (50) reported on a process of providing educational aids and regular TEE performance feedback to eight cardiac anesthesiologists conducting 135 intraoperative TEE studies. The process of education and feedback increased the ability to record a basic TEE examination from 42% to 81%. Furthermore, 79% of the images were interpreted accurately while 15% were not evaluated and only 6% were incorrectly interpreted when compared to the consensus interpretation of up to three experts.

In summary, the demands of the intraoperative environment dictate that a CQI process be implemented as soon as an intraoperative TEE service is established. The prerequisites of this CQI process should not be different from those established for an echocardiography laboratory. A CQI process always seeks to identify problems and fix them without assigning blame. Once problems have been fixed, new ones are identified and the cycle repeats itself endlessly. It is vital that assessments of quality not be directed simply at meeting training requirements or passing tests. Quality is not equivalent to accreditation or certification. It is not exams, tests, or numbers and it is not determined by the user but by the consumer (patient, surgeon, referring cardiologist).

## KEY POINTS

- Physicians performing intraoperative TEE should establish a collaborative relationship with a colleague who has advanced training in TEE.
- After each TEE examination, the probe should be carefully inspected for any cracks or perforations.
- The risks of an electrical injury to a patient will be reduced if a leakage current test is performed after each use of the probe.
- During the preoperative history and physical, patients should be examined for any signs or symptoms of esophageal or gastric disease. The risks and benefits of TEE must be carefully evaluated in patients with relative contraindications to TEE.
- Routine antibiotic prophylaxis to prevent endocarditis is not required prior to TEE except in high-risk patients.
- Transesophageal echocardiography probes must be disinfected for at least 20 minutes in a glutaraldehyde-based solution to eliminate bacterial and viral contaminants.
- Continuous Quality Improvement programs are a necessary component of every TEE service.

## REFERENCES

1. Morewood GH, Gallagher ME, Gaughan JIP, et al. Current practice patterns for adult perioperative transesophageal echocardiography in the United States. Anesthesiology 2001; 95:1507–12.
2. Lambert AS, Mazer CD, Duke PC. Survey of the members of the cardiovascular section of the Canadian Anesthesiologists' Society on the use of perioperative transesophageal echocardiography—a brief report. Can J Anaesth 2002;49:294–6.
3. Poterack KA. Who uses transesophageal echocardiography in the operating room? Anesth Analg 1995;80:454–8.
4. Practice guidelines for perioperative transesophageal echocardiography. A report by the American Society of Anesthesiologists and the Society of Cardiovascular Anesthesiologists Task Force on Transesophageal Echocardiography. Anesthesiology 1996;84:986–1006.
5. Cahalan MK, Abel M, Goldman M, et al. American Society of Echocardiography and Society of Cardiovascular Anesthesiologists task force guidelines for training in perioperative echocardiography. Anesth Analg 2002;94:1384–8.
6. Sequoia Ultrasound System: User and Reference Manuals. Mountain View, CA: Accuson Corp., 2000–2001.

7. Taillefer J, Couture P, Sheridan P, et al. A comprehensive strategy to avoid transesophageal echocardiography probe damage. Can J Anaesth 2002;49:500–2.

8. Daniel WG, Erbel R, Kasper W, et al. Safety of transesophageal echocardiography. A multicenter survey of 10,419 examinations. Circulation 1991;83:817–21.

9. Kallmeyer IJ, Collard CD, Fox JA, et al. The safety of intraoperative transesophageal echocardiography: a case series of 7,200 cardiac surgical patients. Anesth Analg 2001;92:1126–30.

10. Chan KL, Cohen GI, Sochowski RA, et al. Complications of transesophageal echocardiography in ambulatory adult patients: analysis of 1,500 consecutive examinations. J Am Soc Echocardiogr 1991;4:577–82.

11. Mishra M, Chauhan R, Sharma KK, et al. Real-time intraoperative transesophageal echocardiography—how useful? Experience of 5,016 cases. J Cardiothorac Vasc Anesth 1998;12:625–32.

12. Silvis SE, Nebel O, Rogers G, et al. Endoscopic complications. Results of the 1974 American Society for Gastrointestinal Endoscopy Survey. JAMA 1976;235:928–30.

13. Brinkman WT, Shanewise JS, Clements SD, et al. Transesophageal echocardiography: not an innocuous procedure. Ann Thorac Surg 2001;72:1725–6.

14. Massey SR, Pitsis A, Mehta D, et al. Oesophageal perforation following perioperative transesophageal echocardiography. Br J Anaesth 2000;84:643–6.

15. St-Pierre J, Fortier LP, Couture P, et al. Massive gastrointestinal hemorrhage after transesophageal echocardiography probe insertion. Can J Anaesth 1998;45:1196–9.

16. Hogue CW, Jr, Lappas GD, Creswell LL, et al. Swallowing dysfunction after cardiac operations. Associated adverse outcomes and risk factors including intraoperative transesophageal echocardiography. J Thorac Cardiovasc Surg 1995;110:517–22.

17. Rousou JA, Tighe DA, Garb JL, et al. Risk of dysphagia after transesophageal echocardiography during cardiac operations. Ann Thorac Surg 2000;69:486–9; discussion 489–90.

18. Messina AG, Paranicas M, Fiamengo S, et al. Risk of dysphagia after transesophageal echocardiography. Am J Cardiol 1991;67:313–4.

19. Hulyalkar AR, Ayd JD. Low risk of gastroesophageal injury associated with transesophageal echocardiography during cardiac surgery. J Cardiothorac Vasc Anesth 1993;7:175–7.

20. O'Shea JIP, Southern JE, D'Ambra MN, et al. Effects of prolonged transesophageal echocardiographic imaging and probe manipulation on the esophagus—an echocardiographic-pathologic study. J Am Coll Cardiol 1991;17:1426–9.

21. Kronzon I, Cziner DG, Katz ES, et al. Buckling of the tip of the transesophageal echocardiography probe: a potentially dangerous technical malfunction. J Am Soc Echocardiogr 1992;5:176–7.

22. Stevenson JG. Incidence of complications in pediatric transesophageal echocardiography: experience in 1650 cases. J Am Soc Echocardiogr 1999;12:527–32.

23. Andropoulos DB, Ayres NA, Stayer SA, et al. The effect of transesophageal echocardiography on ventilation in small infants undergoing cardiac surgery. Anesth Analg 2000;90:47–9.

24. Arima H, Sobue K, Tanaka S, et al. Airway obstruction associated with transesophageal echocardiography in a patient with a giant aortic pseudoaneurysm. Anesth Analg 2002;95:558–60, table of contents.

25. Nakao S, Eguchi T, Ikeda S, et al. Airway obstruction by a transesophageal echocardiography probe in an adult patient with a dissecting aneurysm of the ascending aorta and arch. J Cardiothorac Vasc Anesth 2000;14:186–7.

26. Ziegeler S, Pulido MA, Hirsch D. Acute oxygen desaturation and right heart dysfunction secondary to transesophageal echocardiography-induced malpositioning of the endotracheal tube. Anesth Analg 2002;95:255–6.

27. Khanderia BK, Tajik AJ, Freeman WK. Transesophageal echocardiographic examination: technique, training, and safety. In: Freeman WK, ed. Transesophageal echocardiography. Boston: Little Brown, 1994:xvi, 599.

28. Gussenhoven EJ, Taams MA, Roelandt JR, et al. Transesophageal two-dimensional echocardiography: its role in solving clinical problems. J Am Coll Cardiol 1986;8:975–9.

29. Cucchiara RF, Nugent M, Seward JIB, et al. Air embolism in upright neurosurgical patients: detection and localization by two-dimensional transesophageal echocardiography. Anesthesiology 1984;60:353–5.

30. Shafei H, el-Kholy A, Azmy S, et al. Vocal cord dysfunction after cardiac surgery: an overlooked complication. Eur J Cardiothorac Surg 1997;11:564–6.

31. Kawahito S, Kitahata H, Kimura H, et al. Recurrent laryngeal nerve palsy after cardiovascular surgery: relationship to the placement of a transesophageal echocardiographic probe. J Cardiothorac Vasc Anesth 1999;13:528–31.

32. Shintani H, Nakano S, Matsuda H, et al. Efficacy of transesophageal echocardiography as a perioperative monitor in patients undergoing cardiovascular surgery. Analysis of 149 consecutive studies. J Cardiovasc Surg (Torino) 1990;31:564–70.

33. Botoman VA, Surawicz CM. Bacteremia with gastrointestinal endoscopic procedures. Gastrointest Endosc 1986;32:342–6.

34. Mentec H, Vignon P, Terre S, et al. Frequency of bacteremia associated with transesophageal echocardiography in intensive care unit patients: a prospective study of 139 patients. Crit Care Med 1995;23:1194–9.

35. Voller H, Spielberg C, Schroder K, et al. Frequency of positive blood cultures during transesophageal echocardiography. Am J Cardiol 1991;68:1538–40.

36. Shyu KG, Hwang JJ, Lin SC, et al. Prospective study of blood culture during transesophageal echocardiography. Am Heart J 1992;124:1541–4.

37. Foster E, Kusumoto FM, Sobol SM, et al. Streptococcal endocarditis temporally related to transesophageal echocardiography. J Am Soc Echocardiogr 1990;3:424–7.

38. Dajani AS, Bisno AL, Chung KJ, et al. Prevention of bacterial endocarditis. Recommendations by the American Heart Association. JAMA 1990;264:2919–22.

39. Birnie GG, Quigley EM, Clements GB, et al. Endoscopic transmission of hepatitis B virus. Gut 1983;24:171–4.

40. Infection control during gastrointestinal endoscopy. Guidelines for clinical application. Gastrointest Endosc 1988;34:37S–40S.

41. Stevenson JG. Adherence to physician training guidelines for pediatric transesophageal echocardiography affects the outcome of patients undergoing repair of congenital cardiac defects. J Am Soc Echocardiogr 1999;12:165–72.

42. Jollis JG, Peterson ED, DeLong ER, et al. The relation between the volume of coronary angioplasty procedures at hospitals treating Medicare beneficiaries and short-term mortality. N Engl J Med 1994;331:1625–9.

43. Recommendations for continuous quality improvement in echocardiography. American Society of Echocardiography. J Am Soc Echocardiogr 1995;8:S1–28.

44. Kisslo J. Reconsidering quality. Heart 1998;80 Suppl 1:S27–9.

45. Aronson S, Thys DM. Training and certification in perioperative transesophageal echocardiography: a historical perspective. Anesth Analg 2001;93:1422–7, table of contents.

46. Popp RL, Winters WL, Jr. Clinical competence in adult echocardiography. A statement for physicians from the ACP/ACC/AHA Task Force on Clinical Privileges in Cardiology. J Am Coll Cardiol 1990;15:1465–8.

47. Fyfe D. Transesophageal echocardiography guidelines: return to bypass or to bypass the guidelines? J Am Soc Echocardiogr 1999;12:343–4.

48. Mathew JIP, Fontes ML, Garwood S, et al. Transesophageal echocardiography interpretation: a comparative analysis between cardiac anesthesiologists and primary echocardiographers. Anesth Analg 2002;94:302–9, table of contents.

49. Bergquist BD, Leung JM, Bellows WH. Transesophageal echocardiography in myocardial revascularization: I. Accu-

racy of intraoperative real-time interpretation. Anesth Analg 1996;82:1132–8.

50. Miller JIP, Lambert AS, Shapiro WA, et al. The adequacy of basic intraoperative transesophageal echocardiography performed by experienced anesthesiologists. Anesth Analg 2001;92:1103–10.

## QUESTIONS

1. Which of the following is an absolute contraindication to the placement of a TEE probe?
   A. Esophageal varices
   B. Esophageal strictures
   C. Cervical arthritis
   D. History of mediastinal radiation

2. All of the following statements about complications related to intraoperative TEE are true *except*:
   A. Compression of the membranous portion of the trachea by the TEE probe can produce airway obstruction.
   B. The ultrasound transducer should be inactivated when not in use to reduce the risk of thermal injury.
   C. Failure to provide antibiotic prophylaxis prior to a TEE exam increases the risk of bacterial endocarditis.
   D. Compression of the recurrent laryngeal nerve by the TEE probe may result in transient vocal cord paralysis.

3. The minimal recommended time required to effectively disinfect a TEE probe in a glutaraldeyde-based solution is:
   A. 10 minutes
   B. 15 minutes
   C. 20 minutes
   D. 30 minutes

# Outcomes in Echocardiography: Statistical Considerations

*Colleen Gorman Koch*

> *To guess is cheap.*
> *To guess wrong is expensive.*
> Old Chinese Proverb

## OUTCOMES RESEARCH

Outcomes research has achieved considerable stature over the last two decades. An increased emphasis on outcomes and assessment of effectiveness has come about in response to a number of factors. Among these factors is the observation of unexplained variation in medical care across geographic areas (1). Variation in practice patterns can, in part, be explained by patient preferences and/or differences in demographics (2). However, variation may also reflect suboptimal care in the low-use areas or needless cost in the high-use areas (3). Considerable variations in practice patterns are likely influenced by physicians' approaches to clinical decision making. Physicians may approach similar medical problems with different theoretical assumptions. Eckman described it in Bayesian terms: Physicians bring differing prior probabilities to the decision making process, which leads to variations in their medical decisions (4). Difficulty incorporating an understanding of disease probabilities into decisions is potentially magnified further by variability in the perceptions of outcomes (2,4). The economics of health care have further driven the increased emphasis on outcomes. The need for cost containment in response to escalating health-care costs (2,3,5), competition within the health-care sector (3), limitations of randomized control trials (6), findings of inappropriate use of medical services (1), and the need for greater accountability have all driven the increased interest in outcomes.

The field of outcomes research distinguishes itself from traditional research in that it can embrace a broader range of endpoints. It may focus on a number of patient-centered outcomes such as measurements of patient satisfaction and quality of life, daily functioning activities, and economics (3,7,8). Another distinguishing feature of outcomes research is its emphasis on effectiveness rather than efficacy. *Efficacy* denotes "usefulness of a medical intervention tested under optimal conditions" (9). Effectiveness can be thought of as the "utility" of a health-care intervention in routine clinical practice (9). An additional factor determining the usefulness of a medical intervention is its *efficiency*, that is, the value of the intervention to the individual patient (9). Johanson summarized these in a practical way: "efficacy addresses the question of whether an intervention can work, effectiveness answers the question of whether it works in a routine practice setting and efficiency determines whether it is worth doing" (9). These concepts figure prominently into the development of practice guidelines from the results of outcomes research. Similar to other research methods, outcomes research focuses on two things: choosing the right variable to study and selecting the data source to make inferences about that specific variable and its relationship to other independent variables (10). Perrin and Mitchell state that "outcomes research gets its name from the choice of the dependent variable." It is the choice of, the definition of, and the development of measures for the dependent variable that has been the focus of research for the last decade. He stressed that current emphasis should be on the inference process: "defining the independent variables and thinking about study design and data sets that allow inferences to be made to set the tone for outcomes research for the future" (10).

A number of goals can be achieved by focusing on outcomes: increased understanding of the effectiveness of various treatment strategies; identifying the most efficient and effective use of limited resources and integrating these into the development of medical standards and practice guidelines; and finally, optimizing the use of resources by third-party payers (3,9). The creation of medical practice guidelines by consensus panels assists physicians in the clinical application of specific diagnostic tests. The American College of Cardiology (ACC) and the American Heart Association (AHA) have developed guidelines for the clinical application of echocardiography. A panel of experts in the field of echocardiography developed the guidelines based on expert opinion and extensive review of the literature. The guidelines serve as a summary of current knowledge on the effectiveness of the imaging test, specifically classifying the clinical utility of echocardiography for specific cardiovascular diseases and common cardiovascular symptoms. Class I reflects evidence or general agreement that the given procedure is effective. Class II reflects conditions where there is conflicting evidence or opinion with regard to the usefulness of echocardiography. Class III reflects conditions for which there is evidence or general agreement that the procedure is not effective or useful (11,12). Recommendations for the use of transesophageal echocardiography (TEE) follow a similar guideline structure, provided by the American Society of Anesthesiologists and the Society of Cardiovascular Anesthesiologists Task Force on Transesophageal Echocardiography (13).

## DATA SOURCES AND METHODS FOR ANALYZING OUTCOMES RESEARCH

Outcomes research may incorporate a variety of methodologies and approaches to collecting, examining, and analyzing data. Data sources include results from randomized clinical trials, quasiexperimental designs, and effectiveness trials (9), cohort or case-control designs, or other retrospective analyses from databases and routine observational data from hospital discharge summaries (3,7,8,14). Data synthesis can be performed in multiple ways, such as metaanalysis, decision analysis, and cross-design synthesis. It is useful to consider the strength of the evidence produced by a study as it relates specifically to a study design; data sources can be listed in descending order of the strength of evidence they produce: randomized controlled trial, nonrandomized trial with contemporaneous controls, nonrandomized trial with historical controls, cohort study, case-control study, cross-sectional study, surveillance (database), descriptive study, and case report (15,16). All of these methods have strengths and weaknesses and can provide valuable information for outcomes research.

## Randomized Controlled Trials

From a design perspective, randomized controlled trials are the strongest for internal consistency (10). The goal of the randomized controlled trial is to reduce variability and bias. Pocock defined variability as "that which deals with imprecision in estimates caused by sampling from non-homogeneous populations" and bias as "any influence which acts to make the observed results non-representative of the true effects of therapy" (17). By the randomization process, randomized controlled trials control for known and unknown confounding variables (3), the end result being comparable groups with regard to comorbid conditions (17). These key design elements are intended to "isolate" or clarify differences in outcome due to treatment assignment rather than specific differences in the patient population (18). Randomization also reduces conscious, as well as unconscious biases, such as those that may occur with patient selection (17). Another strength of randomized controlled trials is their ability to assess efficacy; that is, whether an intervention will produce a desired effect under the best possible circumstances (3). Because of highly specific inclusion and exclusion criteria, randomized controlled trials may not be universally applicable, nor reveal how effective the intervention is for many patients in every day clinical practice (3,18). Finally, not all questions are suitable nor can they all be answered by randomized controlled trials.

## Quasiexperimental Designs

Quasiexperimental designs are studies that manipulate treatment without randomization. Within the control group there is some control over treatment assignment, however, the control group is not randomized. A disadvantage of this experimental design can be a systematic difference between the groups being compared, which can influence outcomes beyond the assigned treatment (19). Quasiexperimental designs can use statistical techniques, such as stratification, matching, and structural modeling to control for known confounding variables (3).

## Effectiveness Trials

Effectiveness trials differ in methodology from randomized controlled trials in that they are population based, often retrospective (1), and are significantly less restrictive. There may be no prescribed protocol, no random assignment of treatment or health-care provider, and there are less stringent exclusion criteria. These trials may include patients with multiple comorbid conditions, occur in office settings and community hospitals, and include an extensive mix of investigators (9). Effectiveness trials can provide practical information about patients seen in routine clinical practice (9). Because of the lack of randomization, risk adjustment strategies are used to control for influential variables in assessing the effectiveness of the health-care intervention (1).

## Cohort Studies

Cohort, or prospective, studies involve two or more groups of "exposed" and "nonexposed" individuals in which groups are followed up to compare the incidence of disease over a period of time. These studies work well when exposure is rare and disease is frequent among the exposed. Cohort studies do not involve a randomization process, in that patients are not randomized to the exposure; therefore, the observed associations between exposure and disease outcome may be influenced by known or unknown variables. A number of potential biases are associated with conducting cohort studies: bias in the assessment of the outcome, information, nonresponse and analytic biases, and patients who are lost to follow-up (20,21).

## Case-Control Studies

Case-control, or retrospective, studies identify groups of patients with a disease—"cases" and comparison groups without disease termed "controls." A determination may then be made as to the proportion of cases and controls that were exposed or not exposed. These studies are optimal when a disease is rare and when exposure is frequent among the population. Since case-control studies require information from past events or exposures, there are potential sources of error with incomplete information about exposure, limitations of recall, and recall bias. Control selection may also be problematic. Matching cases and controls on important variables known to be associated with the disease can help avoid the differences in exposure between the cases and controls being attributable to factors other than exposure status (21,22).

## Databases

Observational data from large databases from which effectiveness outcome studies are reported are primarily compiled for administrative and billing purposes rather than research purposes (18,23). Data acquired for large databases are collected prospectively and therefore not biased by any selection process (9). Database information is obtained from routine clinical practice and therefore may be more reflective of the breadth of medical practice than the randomized trial (64). Observational databases can serve as useful guides to the design of new controlled trials. They can also be useful adjuncts to randomized controlled trials to assess whether efficacy can be translated into effective treatments in routine clinical practice (24). Concato and colleagues reported that well-designed observational studies do not systematically overestimate the magnitude of effects of treatment as compared to randomized controlled trials on the same topic. The popular belief that observational studies are inherently misleading is dispelled by this work (16).

However, methodologies used for large effectiveness outcome studies from databases can lead to erroneous conclusions (9). Data collected for observational studies are uncontrolled observations and, because each person's treatment is chosen rather than randomly assigned, they are prone to selection biases that would be eliminated by the randomization process (9,24). Among other concerns are that there is often a lack of standardized definitions used, medical records may be incomplete, physicians' decisions regarding treatment assignments are not at random, and there may be issues with chart abstraction of data (18,23). Without proper controls, these data sources cannot address specific differences in clinical effectiveness of treatment strategies and therefore, specific treatment comparisons should be interpreted cautiously. Because these large databases rarely contain detailed information on clinical severity, comorbid conditions can be unaccounted for, thus creating potentially important differences in the patient populations (18,23,25). Statistical models can be used to adjust for influential variables between the patient groups being compared that could impact on patient outcome (6,9). However, it is difficult to assume that statisticians know which variables are influential, measure those variables on each patient, and use those measurements to make the appropriate adjustments. Certainly, unknown variables can have important influences on outcome (15). Adjusting for severity may also introduce bias caused by timely changes in severity assessments or by the validity of the adjustment scheme (6).

Propensity modeling represents an advance in statistical techniques as applied to nonrandomized study designs to control for differences in background characteristics among groups under investigation (26). Prior to propensity modeling, multivariable risk factor analysis was the primary methodology used to adjust for baseline differences when examining specific outcomes (29). The propensity score is the conditional probability of assignment to a group given a number of observed covariates (27). It is calculated by predicting group membership from a number of confounding covariates with logistic regression or discriminant analysis (26). The propensity score can be seen as a single confounding covariate representing a collection of confounding covariates. At each given value of propensity score, the distribution of covariates is typically balanced between groups allowing for equivalent comparisons to be made between groups under investigation (28). Particular applications of the propensity score include matching, stratification, or multivariable adjustment on propensity score (26–29).

Difficulties with large databases can be averted by avoiding the use of databases designed for billing or administrative purposes and instead, collecting clinical data according to a specific protocol with a quality assurance program (15).

## DATA SYNTHESIS METHODS

### Metaanalysis

The term *metaanalysis* was first coined by GV Glass in 1976 (30,31) for a quantitative technique that combines the results of multiple studies investigating the same question with roughly the same experimental design or quasiexperimental design (30). Metaanalysis seeks to explore reasons for disparate findings among clinical studies. Many studies are inconclusive, often because of insufficient sample size (30,32,33). By combining the results from a number of studies, metaanalysis can detect patterns across studies, as well as, in some cases, give more precise estimates of treatment effects (30,32). Bangert-Drowns described metaanalysis as each individual study being represented by a data point with its own probabilistic distribution (30). The process of metaanalysis includes: formulating a specific research question, collecting studies through a literature search, and analyzing the quality of the studies. Design characteristics and quality scores for each study are used to develop inclusion and exclusion criteria or for weighing individual study results in a theoretically or mathematically more powerful pooled analysis. The individual study characteristics and outcomes are coded and translated into a common metric and relations between study features and outcomes are statistically tested (30,32,34,35).

### Decision Analysis

Decision analysis, a derivative of operations research and game theory, is a structured step-wise process of combining data to compare treatment strategies by simulation. Two or more treatment strategies are compared in quantitative terms along with potential outcomes of each strategy. These are represented in the form of a decision tree (32,36,37). The concept of decision analysis involves structuring a problem as a decision model, such that alternative therapeutic strategies are specified and the important outcomes selected. Estimates of the probabilities for the outcomes are based upon a systematic search of the literature focusing on those studies with good methodology (20,32). Quantitative values for the outcomes can be expressed in a number of ways: life years, quality-adjusted life years (QALYs), cases of disease, complications prevented, or utilities (20). The product of outcome values and their probabilities of occurrence is the expected value of each clinical strategy (32). A sensitivity analysis is performed to evaluate the degree of uncertainty of the estimates, which is similar to a confidence interval (36). Sensitivity analysis can focus attention on probability estimates that need to be defined more precisely and can provide insight into the "robustness" of the baseline analysis (36).

### Economic Analysis

There are a number of economic analyses: cost-identification, cost-benefit, cost-utility, and cost-effectiveness (38). Cost-effectiveness analysis requires that an intervention be compared to alternatives; implicit with this type of research is the acknowledgement that resources are finite. Economics defines natural units (dollars) that are applicable across all strategies and whose nature is to reflect value. The objective of the analysis may not be so much to limit care or expense, but to limit waste and promote efficiency with the greatest overall benefit (38). The defining principles of cost-effectiveness research include the following: explicitly state the perspective of the analysis; define what benefits are being studied and how they will be measured; define the costs being studied; discount costs and benefits to the extent that costs and benefits occur at different times; and provide a summary statement—a ratio of costs to benefits (39,40). Costs, like risks, may not drive the medical decision-making process, but lend perspective to the pursuit of the best strategy. The importance of the economic assessment and, in particular, the relationship of decision analytical modeling and cost-effectiveness is stressed by Mushlin (41). Decision analytic models can assist in determining those diagnostic procedures that are or are not cost-effective (41). One of the problems with decision analysis is that it may oversimplify medical problems (36). Furthermore, there are particular medical problems that cannot be broken down into a finite set of discrete events with well-defined probabilities (18) or there may not be available data to support the analysis, and there have been methodological problems with measurements such as quality of life (36).

### Cross Design Synthesis

Cross design synthesis is a strategy for effectiveness research that combines observational data from the analysis of databases with results from randomized controlled trials. The inclusion of database information necessitates risk adjustment methods to account for influential patient variables (42).

## MEDICAL TESTS AND PATIENT OUTCOMES

Bossuyt and Lijmer described the relatively indirect relationship between a medical test and patient outcome (Fig. 9.1). Medical tests generate information that can guide the clinician's decision on interventions, such as starting a treatment plan or intervention. Although the relationship between a medical test and patient outcome is primarily an indirect one, complications or side effects from the imaging test may have a direct effect on patient outcome. Bossuyt and Lijmer stress that before introduc-

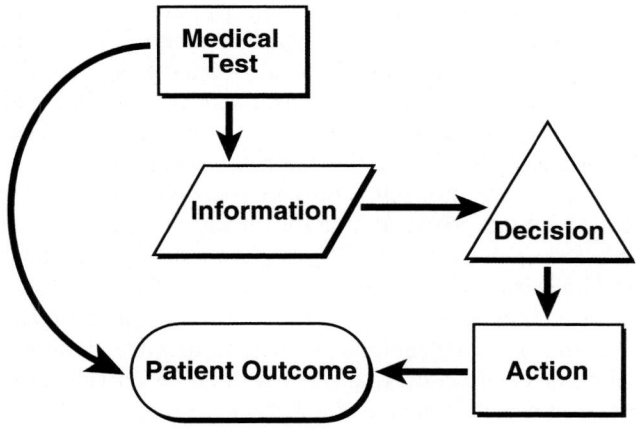

**FIGURE 9.1.** Relationship Between an Imaging Test and Patient Health Outcome. (Modified from Bossuyt P, Lijmer J. Traditional health outcomes in evaluation of diagnostic tests. Acad Radiol 1999;6:577–580, with permission.)

ing an imaging technique, one should address whether the test will do more good than harm, whether the patient will be better off because of the test, and whether the effectiveness of the imaging test has been weighed against the potential increase in resources used (43).

## PERFORMANCE MEASURES OF DIAGNOSTIC IMAGING TESTS

The decision to diagnose is the critical point from which subsequent decisions are predicated (44). Verrilli and Welch studied the relationship between specific diagnostic tests and the therapeutic interventions they triggered. The rates of testing were closely related to the rates of therapeutic interventions. It may be concluded that managing the increase in diagnostic testing may be as important as managing the increase in therapeutic interventions (44). The close link between diagnostic testing and subsequent utilization of therapeutic services has been described by others as well (41). In making decisions to diagnose, clinicians must consider the fundamental principles of diagnostic imaging tests, that is, how they reduce uncertainty, increase diagnostic precision, and affect costs (45). Performance measures utilized to appraise a diagnostic test are the test's sensitivity, specificity, positive and negative predictive values, likelihood ratios, and receiver operating characteristic curves.

## SENSITIVITY AND SPECIFICITY

Sensitivity and specificity were first described in 1947 by Jacob Yerushalmy in the evaluation of the relative effectiveness of identifying tuberculosis cases by various x-ray

techniques (46). The sensitivity of a test is defined as "the proportion of patients with the disease who have a positive test" (47) and is "a measure of how good the test is at detecting disease in patients with the disease" (48). The specificity of a test is defined as "the proportion of patients without the disease who have a negative test" (47), and it is "a measure of how good the test is at ruling out disease in patients who do not have the disease" (48). Henderson stated that there are three purposes of a test: "discovery, confirmation, and exclusion" (49). Tests that seek to exclude or rule out disease and tests that seek to discover disease require high sensitivities. Tests that seek to confirm or rule in a target disorder require a high specificity (49).

Table 9.1 depicts a 2 × 2 contingency table commonly used to describe the relationship between the true diagnosis or "gold standard" of disease status and the test's results. The disease is either present or absent and the test is either positive or negative. Within the four cells there are four possible interpretations of the test results: true positive, true negative, false positive, or false negative among the patients in the sample (50,51).

In general, sensitivity and specificity are test characteristics and should remain constant as long as similar target populations are being examined (47). They are only theoretically independent of prevalence or pretest probability (50,52). A number of factors can influence estimates of a test's sensitivity and specificity: variations in clinical characteristics (53), spectrum of disease severity (52,53), and methods of test performance (52). There is frequently substantial variation in sensitivity and specificity when the patient population used to determine the imaging test's sensitivity and specificity are markedly different from the spectrum of patients in whom the test will be applied in clinical practice (47,50,54). Because the spectrum of diseased patients can vary depending on the severity of disease, a test's sensitivity will tend to be increased in the more severely afflicted patients (47,50). GA Diamond stresses that sensitivity and specificity can vary as a consequence of selection bias and that a test will

▶ TABLE 9.1. The 2 × 2 Contingency Table Depicts the Relationship Between the Disease Status and the Test's Results

| Diagnostic Test Results | Disease Present | Disease Absent |
|---|---|---|
| Positive test result | True positive | False positive |
| Negative test result | False negative | True negative |

From Fletcher RH, Fletcher SW, Wagner EG. Diagnosis. In: Clinical Epidemiology: The Essentials. 3rd ed. Baltimore: Williams and Wilkins, 1996;43–74 with permission.

perform "as advertised" only if it is applied to a similar patient population under comparable conditions (55). There may also be misleading results reported on the performance of a diagnostic test simply by chance if there were small numbers of patients studied and/or if bias is introduced in the interpretation of test results and assignments of diagnoses are not done independently of one another (47). Cecil and colleagues provide the following example of selection bias or work-up bias in reference to patients with coronary artery disease. Bias occurs when the results of a noninvasive test, such as stress thallium imaging, influences whether a subsequent test, such as coronary angiography, is performed. Preferentially performing coronary angiography on patients with positive stress thallium results will result in falsely high test sensitivity and falsely low test specificity. To demonstrate the inaccuracy of sensitivity and specificity in the presence of work-up bias they provided the following example: If only patients with positive stress thallium results were referred for angiography and no patients with normal stress thallium results were referred the observed sensitivity for the detection of coronary artery disease would be 100% and the observed specificity would be 0% (56). Miller and colleagues and Cecil and colleagues provide examples and methods of adjustment for selection bias to yield better estimates of sensitivity and specificity of individual imaging tests (56,57). Hlatky and colleagues describe an interesting concept of sensitivity and specificity in that there is a distribution of sensitivities and specificities across a spectrum of patients versus a previous concept that values of sensitivity and specificity are "averages" of values across the population (53).

## POSITIVE AND NEGATIVE PREDICTIVE VALUES

Predictive value of an imaging test refers to the probability of the patient having or not having disease with a given test result. It is also described as "posttest" or "posterior probability" (50). Hence, positive predictive value is defined as "the proportion of patients with a positive test who are correctly diagnosed and negative predictive value is the proportion of patients with a negative test result who are correctly diagnosed" (58). Unlike sensitivity and specificity, calculated predictive values are conditioned on the prevalence of disease in the population under examination (50,58). Prevalence is defined as " the proportion of persons in a defined population at a given point in time with the condition of question" (50). It is also referred to as a "pretest" or "prior" probability because the probability of disease is known prior to ordering the test (50). The pretest probability of disease in a patient with only demographic information available is the prevalence

of disease in that population (59). The clinician should have a selective approach to ordering diagnostic tests in patients with whom they have a high suspicion for the characteristic disease through available clinical data and specific demographic groups known to be high risk. This will increase the yield of the diagnostic test (50).

The interrelationship between sensitivity, specificity, and prevalence in calculating the positive predictive value of a test is derived from Bayes' theorem of conditional probabilities, first described by Reverend Thomas Bayes in the eighteenth century (50,60). It allows a prior understanding of the likelihood of disease to affect (statistically) the decision-making process. It is the statistical expression of an element in the decision to diagnose: Given a suspicion (pretest probability) of disease in a subject, will a particular test provide data to clarify, confirm, or deny that suspicion (48)? It is known as the inversion theorem by the way it relates the specific probabilities associated with a test to a set of completely different probabilities associated with a diagnosis: given a particular test result, what is the probability of the diagnosis *and* given a particular diagnosis, what is the probability of getting a test result (49)? Bayes' theorem describes the clinician's ability to estimate the chance that a patient has a target disorder based on a particular positive or negative test result and available clinical information (48,50,61).

There is statistical controversy over the use of Bayes' theorem in circumstances where there was no random selection of study patients, where the pretest probability of disease and the particular test results are not conditionally independent, or where a test has variable sensitivity and specificity among groups of patients with varying disease prevalence (61). Multivariate analysis is an alternative approach to estimating performance measures in that there is no assumption of constant sensitivity and specificity over a varying degree of disease prevalence rates nor does it assume that tests are independent of each other (61). Bayes' theorem relating sensitivity, specificity, prevalence, and predictive values is listed below (61).

Positive Predictive Value =

$$\frac{\text{Sensitivity} \times \text{Prevalence}}{(\text{Sensitivity} \times \text{Prevalence}) + (1 - \text{Specificity}) \times (1 - \text{Prevalence})}$$

Negative Predictive Value =

$$\frac{1 - \text{Sensitivity} \times (\text{Prevalence})}{(1 - \text{Sensitivity}) \times \text{Prevalence} + \text{Specificity} \times (1 - \text{Prevalence})}$$

## LIKELIHOOD RATIO

The *likelihood ratio* or likelihood quotient may also describe the diagnostic performance of a test. In their discussion, Radack and colleagues defined the likelihood ratio as "a ratio of two probabilities, the probability of a given test result when the disease is present (the true-positive fraction) divided by the probability of the same test result when the disease is absent (the false-positive fraction)" (52). The likelihood ratio is an expression of the odds that the result of a test or treatment has occurred in a patient who has a disorder, or who has received a benefit, as opposed to a patient without the target disorder, or in whom no benefit occurred (62). When a likelihood ratio is greater than one, it indicates that the probability of disease in a patient with a positive test result is higher. When the likelihood ratio is less than one, the posttest probability of disease is less (62). A likelihood ratio of one, or close to one, means that the posttest probability of disease is unchanged as compared to the pretest probability (62,63). The likelihood ratio provides immediate intuitive sense about the applicability of the test given the result. Sensitivity and specificity measures of diagnostic imaging tests alone cannot provide this relationship between the magnitude and direction of change in the posttest probability of disease (52). One may express a positive likelihood ratio (LR +) or negative likelihood ratio (LR −), characterized as follows (48):

$$LR\,(+) = \frac{\text{Probability of positive test result in diseased patients}}{\text{Probability of positive test result in nondiseased patients}}$$

$$LR\,(-) = \frac{\text{Probability of a negative test result in diseased patients}}{\text{Probability of negative test results in nondiseased patients}}$$

The point of using likelihood ratios is to assess the chance that a test result truly gives a better understanding of risk of disease after the test result is known through the calculation posttest odds (52). It answers the question: What are the odds that a given test result can raise or lower the suspicion (pretest probability) of disease (63)? A modification of Bayes' theorem describes the relationship between a clinician's pretest odds for disease and the likelihood ratio (52). The formulas for converting odds to probability and calculation of posttest odds from pretest odds and likelihood ratios are listed below (50,59,62).

The pretest probability of disease can be converted to pretest odds by the formula listed below (50,59,62,63). Odds are expressed mathematically as the probability of having an event divided by the probability of not having the event (59). For example, a 50% probability would be equivalent to a pretest odds = .50 / .50 = 1 or 1 to 1; a probability of 90% would be equivalent to a pretest odds = .90 /.10 = 9 or 9 to 1.

$$\text{Odds} = \frac{\text{Probability of Event}}{1 - \text{Probability of Event}}$$

Then the product of the pretest odds and the likelihood ratio provides the posttest odds, as follows (52,62,63).

$$\text{Posttest Odds} = \text{Pretest Odds} \times \text{Likelihood Ratio}$$

Posttest odds can then be converted back to probabilities with the use of the formula listed below (52,62,63). To eliminate the need to convert probabilities to odds and back again nomograms can be utilized to carry out the conversions (62,63).

$$\text{Posttest Probability of target disorder} = \frac{\text{Posttest Odds}}{\text{Posttest Odds} + 1}$$

Jaeschke and colleagues provide a general guide to interpretation of actual values of likelihood ratios as the following: "likelihood ratios greater than 10 or less than 0.1 generate large and often conclusive changes from pretest to posttest probability; likelihood ratios of 5–10 and 0.1–0.2 generate moderate shifts in pretest to posttest probability; likelihood ratios of 2–5 and 0.5–0.2 generate small changes in probability; and ratios of 1 to 2 and 0.5 to 1 alter probability to a small degree" (63). One of the advantages of likelihood ratios over sensitivity and specificity measures is the ability to generate multiple likelihood ratios for diagnostic test results that have a range of outcomes. Sensitivity, specificity, and predictive values limit test results to two levels, "positive or negative" whether they are truly ordinal or continuous measures (62). Likelihood ratios can be calculated over different ranges of outcomes without having to lose diagnostic information by collapsing data into binary classifications (50,52).

Jaeschke and colleagues reiterate the concept of variability of test properties depending on the mix of severity of disease and/or different competing conditions. For example, an increase in sensitivity and in the likelihood ratio will occur if patients with the particular disorder all have severe disease. The likelihood ratio will move closer to 1 and the test will appear less useful if patients without the particular disorder have conditions that mimic the test results seen in patients with the target disorder. One may be confident with the results of a test in an individual patient if the practice setting from which the patient comes is similar to that of the study investigation and that an individual meets the inclusion and exclusion criteria reported in the study (63).

Table 9.2 depicts the calculation of various performance measures: sensitivity, specificity, positive and negative predictive values, and likelihood ratios from a 2 × 2 contingency table (50).

Table 9.3 provides a practical application of performance measure calculations using data from a prospective study on two-dimensional (2-D) echocardiographic

▶ **TABLE 9.2.  Listed Are a Number of Performance Measure Calculations from a 2 × 2 Contingency Table**

| Test Results | Disease Present | Disease Absent | |
|---|---|---|---|
| Test result positive | a | b | a+b |
| Test result negative | c | d | c+d |
| Sensitivity = a /a+c | a+c | b+d | a+b+c+d |

Specificity = d /b+d
Positive Predictive Value = a /a+b
Negative Predictive Value = d/ c+d
Prevalence = a+c / a+b+c+d
Likelihood Ratio (+) = $\dfrac{a\,/a+c}{b/\,b+d}$

Likelihood Ratio (-) = $\dfrac{c\,/\,a+c}{d\,/\,b+d}$

Modified from Fletcher RH, Fletcher SW, Wagner EG. Diagnosis. In: Clinical Epidemiology: The Essentials. 3rd ed. Baltimore: Williams and Wilkins, 1996;43–74, with permission.

diagnosis of patients with suspected left ventricular thrombus. The presence or absence of left ventricular thrombus was verified at surgery or autopsy (58). The sensitivity and specificity of 2-D echocardiography for detecting thrombus was 92% and 88%, respectively. The positive predictive value, the probability the patient has a left ventricular thrombus given a positive 2-D echo result, was 83%. The negative predictive value, that is, the probability that the patient does not have a left ventricular thrombus given a negative 2-D echo exam result, was 95%. The likelihood ratio of a positive 2-D echo exam was = 7.6, which tells us that it is 7.6 times more likely to have a positive test in a patient with a left ventricular thrombus than in a patient without. The posttest probability of

disease was 83%. The pretest probability that the patient had left ventricular thrombus increased from 39% without the 2-D echo exam to 83% probability of disease with a positive echo exam result. The pretest probability of disease in this example, 39%, is high. One would be cautious in applying these results to other groups of patients undergoing echocardiography, for example to those in general primary care settings.

## RECEIVER OPERATOR CHARACTERISTIC CURVE

A receiver operator characteristic (ROC) curve is a way to express the relationship between sensitivity and specificity of a diagnostic imaging test with continuous or ordinal results (59). The concept of ROC comes from studies of radar technologists during World War II (47). It derives from a plot of all sensitivity/1-specificity pairs and graphically represents how sensitivity and specificity values change as the "cutoff" or threshold values change (48,65). A plot is made of the sensitivity (true-positive rate) on the y-axis and the 1-specificity (false-positive rate) on the x-axis (47,65), with values on the x and y axes reflecting probability from 0–1.0 (48,59,66). The area under the ROC curve can be thought of as a global summary statistic of a test's diagnostic accuracy or performance (60,61), such that the larger area under the ROC curve, the better the discriminatory power of the test (48,59,66). The higher the overall accuracy of the test, the closer the plot is to the upper left corner of the graph (48,59,66). A test with perfect sensitivity and specificity will have an area under the ROC curve equal to 1 and the "curve" will be rectangular in shape (48). A test that has no discriminating ability results in an area under the curve of 0.5, represented by a 45-degree diagonal line extending from

▶ **TABLE 9.3.  Performance Measure Calculations in an Example of 67 Patients Undergoing Two-Dimensional Echocardiography for Suspected Left Ventricular (LV) Thrombus Formation**

| | LV Thrombus (+) | LV Thrombus (−) |
|---|---|---|
| Echo results (+) | 24 | 5 |
| Echo results (−) | 2 | 36 |
| | 26 | 41 |

Sensitivity = 92%
Specificity = 88%
Pretest probability = 39%
Total patients = 67
Positive predictive value = 83%
Negative predictive value = 95%

Likelihood ratio for a positive test = 7.6
Pretest probability = 39%
Pretest odds of disease = 0.39 / (1 − .39) = 0.64
Posttest odds = 7.6 × .64 = 4.86
Posttest probability = 4.86 / 1 + 4.86 = .829
= 83%

From Bourne R. Con: Some clinical research is not cost-effective—weaknesses of outcomes studies. Spine 1995;20:386–387.

the bottom left to the upper right corner of the graph (47,48,50,65,66). In general, depending on the clinical situation, cut-off points are chosen to provide the best combination of sensitivity and specificity (43). ROC curves are particularly useful when comparing alternative tests for the same diagnosis. The better test will be the one with the larger area under the ROC curve (50,59,66). Figure 9.2 represents an example of a ROC curve. Table 9.4 summarizes key points of diagnostic imaging tests.

## STRATEGIC USE OF DIAGNOSTIC IMAGING TESTS

Patterson and Horowitz have elucidated a strategy for ordering diagnostic testing based on seven sequential queries. This systematic approach to diagnostic test ordering is initially framed by a clinical probability that the patient has the specific disease based on the clinical data. An objective management plan is then based on the overall patient status. Following this, a specific clinical question about the patient is posed prior to ordering the test. The diagnostic test's performance, that is, the sensitivity and specificity of the test is subsequently evaluated in order to judge the reliability of the information provided by the test. The clinician needs to know how to interpret the

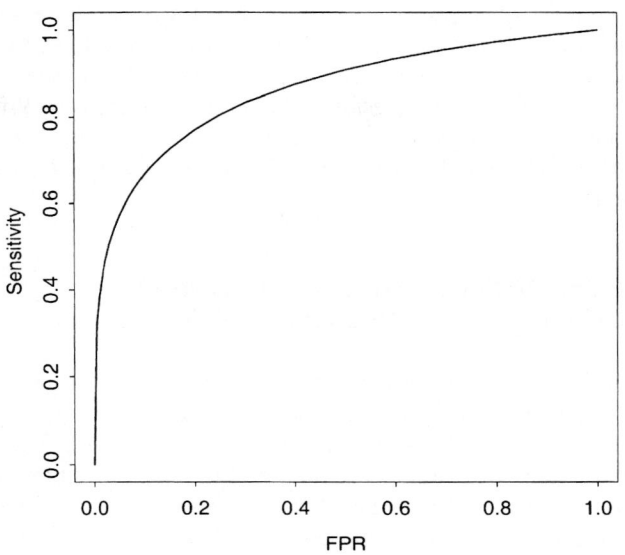

**FIGURE 9.2.** A Receiver Operating Characteristic (ROC) Curve. The sensitivity, true-positive rate, is plotted on the y-axis and 1-specificity, false-positive rate, is on the x-axis. The values on the x and y axes run from a probability of 0–1.0.

▶ TABLE 9.4. **Summary of Key Points**

| Technical Term | Formula | Definition |
|---|---|---|
| Accuracy | (a + d) / (a + b + c + d) | Proportion of people (true positive and true negative) correctly diagnosed |
| Sensitivity | a / (a+c) | Ability of the test to detect disease in individuals who have the disease |
| A sensitive test | | Is a test which is favorable for detecting disease. Produces relatively less false negative, but will lead to more false positive results |
| Specificity | d / (b+d) | Ability of the test to rule out disease in individuals without the condition |
| A specific test | | Is a test that is favorable for ruling out disease. Produces less false positive results, but will lead to more false negative results |
| Prevalence | a+c / a+b+c+d | |
| Positive predictive value | a / (a+b) | Probability that an individual testing positive has disease |
| Negative predictive value | d / (c+d) | Probability that an individual testing negative does not have disease |
| Likelihood ratio of a positive test | Sensitivity / (1-specificity) | How much more likely is a positive test to be found in a patient with disease than without |
| Posttest odds of disease | Pretest Odds × Likelihood Ratio | |
| Posttest probability of disease | Posttest Odds / (posttest odds + 1) | |
| Likelihood ratio of a negative test | (1 − sensitivity) / specificity | How much more likely is a negative test to be found in a patient with disease than without |
| Receiver operating characteristic curve (ROC) | | Graphical representation of sensitivity versus (1 − specificity) over a range of thresholds |
| Area under the curve of a ROC curve | | Overall measure of the discriminatory ability of a test |

Modified from Binder M, Dreiseitl S. The interpretation of test results. Journal of Cutaneous Medicine and Surgery 2000:4;19–25, with permission.

reliability of a positive or a negative test result, knowing the predictive value and predictive error of a test vis-à-vis Bayes' theorem. The clinician can then decide whether to recommend further tests or therapies. Finally, the clinician should consider the trade-off between cost plus patient risk and the data obtained by the diagnostic test (61).

## EVALUATING THE LITERATURE ON DIAGNOSTIC IMAGING TESTS

Fryback and Thornbury have structured a hierarchical model for appraising the efficacy of diagnostic imaging. Because the premise is that, given the significant financial outlay of diagnostic imaging, economy demands fair appraisals of outcomes in a process of accountability. The hierarchical model proposed by Fryback and Thornbury in Table 9.5 provides a framework for evaluating the use of any diagnostic imaging technology. A key feature of this framework is that an imaging technology can be efficacious at a higher level only if it is efficacious at lower levels (68). Level 1, "technical efficacy," addresses the

quality of the images acquired as technical description of image quality. Level 2, "diagnostic accuracy efficacy," is characterized by statistical performance measures, as has been discussed. Level 3, "diagnostic thinking efficacy," focuses on the clinician's diagnostic thinking as it is updated by the results of the test. Level 4, "therapeutic efficacy," describes how the results of the imaging test have affected the patient management plan. Level 5, "patient outcome efficacy," reflects individual patient outcomes as directly related to the results of the test. Level 6, "societal efficacy," analyzes the broad economics of the diagnostic exam (68).

Jaeschke and colleagues provide a structured framework of questions that enable the clinician to approach the assessment and use of articles about diagnostic tests in clinical practice. Table 9.6 summarizes their recommendations on the evaluation and application of results from studies on diagnostic testing (69).

A critical understanding of diagnostic testing and outcomes is complementary to the decision to diagnose. One can rely on data only when the right question has been asked and when the tests performed can answer that question.

▶ **TABLE 9.5. A Hierarchical Model of Efficacy: Typical Measures of Analyses**

| |
|---|
| *Level 1. Technical Efficacy* |
| Resolution of line pairs, modulation transfer function change, gray-scale range, amount of mottle, sharpness |
| *Level 2. Diagnostic Accuracy Efficacy* |
| Yield of abnormal or normal diagnoses in a case series, diagnostic accuracy (percentage correct diagnoses in case series), predictive value of positive or negative examination (in a case series), sensitivity and specificity in a defined clinical problem setting, measures of ROC curve height (d') or area under the curve $A_z$ |
| *Level 3. Diagnostic Thinking Efficacy* |
| Number (percentage) of cases in a series in which image judged "helpful" to making the diagnosis, entropy change in differential diagnosis probability distribution, difference in clinicians' subjectively estimated diagnosis probabilities pre- to posttest information, empirical subjective log-likelihood ratio for test positive and negative in a case series |
| *Level 4. Therapeutic Efficacy* |
| Number (percentage) of times image judged helpful in planning management of the patient in a case series, percentage of times medical procedure avoided due to image information, number or percentage of times clinicians' prospectively stated therapeutic choices changed after test information |
| *Level 5. Patient Outcome Efficacy* |
| Percentage of patients improved with test compared with those without test, morbidity (or procedures) avoided after having image information, change in quality-adjusted life expectancy, expected value of test information in quality-adjusted life years (QUALYs), cost per QUALY saved with image information |
| *Level 6. Societal Efficacy* |
| Benefit-cost analysis from societal viewpoint, cost-effectiveness analysis from societal viewpoint |

ROC, receiver operating characteristic
From Fryback D, Thornbury J. The efficacy of diagnostic imaging. Med Decis Making 1991:11;88–94, with permission.

▶ **TABLE 9.6. Evaluating and Applying the Results of Studies of Diagnostic Tests**

Are the results of the study valid?

**Primary guides:** Was there an independent, blind comparison with a reference standard?

Did the patient sample include an appropriate spectrum of patients to whom the diagnostic test will be applied in clinical practice?

**Secondary guides:** Did the results of the test being evaluated influence the decision to perform the reference standard?

Were the methods for performing the test described in sufficient detail to permit replication?

What were the results?

Are likelihood ratios for the test results presented or data necessary for their calculation provided?

Will the results help me in caring for my patients?

Will the reproducibility of the test result and its interpretation be satisfactory in my setting?

Are the results applicable to my patient?

Will the results change my management?

Will patients be better off as a result of the test?

From Jaeschke R, Gordon G, Sackett D. Users' guides to the medical literature: III How to use an article about a diagnostic test: (A) Are the results of the study valid? JAMA 1994:271;389–391 with permission.

## KEY POINTS

- Efficacy, effectiveness, and efficiency of medical interventions figure prominently in the development of practice guidelines from the results of outcomes research.
- Outcomes research distinguishes itself from traditional research in that it can embrace a broader range of endpoints.
- In the process of medical decision making the clinician should consider the fundamental principles of diagnostic imaging tests.
- There are a number of performance measures for diagnostic imaging tests: sensitivity, specificity, positive and negative predictive values, likelihood ratios, and receiver operating characteristic curves.
- There are organized structural approaches to appraising the literature on diagnostic imaging tests.

## REFERENCES

1. Iezzoni L. Risk adjustment for medical effectiveness research: An overview of conceptual and methodological considerations. J Investig Med 1995;43:136–50.
2. Eddy DM. Medicine, money, and mathematics. American College of Surgeons Bulletin 1991;77:36–49.
3. Epstein A. Sounding board: The outcomes movement—Will it get us where we want to go? N Engl J Med 1990;323:266–70.
4. Sonenberg F, Eckman M. Symposium. Health outcomes research and its interfaces with medical decision making. Med Decis Making 1991;11:S15–S31.
5. Singer AJ, Thode HC, Hollander JE. Research fundamentals: Selection and development of clinical outcome measures. Acad Emerg Med 2000;7:397–401.
6. Davies HT, Crombie I. Interpreting health outcomes. J Eval Clin Pract 1997;3:187–99.
7. Blaiss MS. Why outcomes? Ann Allergy Asthma Immunol 1995;74:359–61.
8. Wennberg JB, Barry MI. Outcomes research. Science 1994;264:758–59.
9. Johanson J. Outcomes research, practice guidelines, and disease management in clinical gastroenterology. J Clin Gastroenterol 1998;27:306–11.
10. Perrin E, Mitchell P. Data. Information and knowledge: Theoretical and methodological issues in linking outcomes and organizational variables: Introduction. Med Care 1997;35:NS84–NS86.
11. Douglas P, Seto T. Outcomes Research Review. J Am Soc Echocardiogr 1998;11:916–20.
12. Ritchie J, Cheitlin M, Eagle K, et al. ACC/AHA guidelines for the clinical application of echocardiography. Circulation 1997;95:1686–1744.
13. American Society of Anesthesiologists and the Society of Cardiovascular Anesthesiologists Task Force on Transesophageal Echocardiography. Anesthesiology 1996;84:986–1006.
14. Bourne R, Keller R. Controversy: Outcomes research. Spine 1995;20:384–87.
15. Moses L. Measuring effects without randomized trials? Options, problems, challenges. Med Care 1995;3:AS8–AS14.
16. Concato J, Shah N, Horwitz R. Randomized, controlled trials, observational studies, and the hierarchy of research designs. N Engl J Med 2000;342:1887–92.
17. Pocock SJ. The justification for randomized controlled trials. In: Clinical Trials: A practical approach. New York: John Wiley & Sons, 1983: 50–65.
18. Simon G, Wagner E, Vonkorff M. Cost-effectiveness comparisons using "real world" randomized trials: The case of new antidepressant drugs. J Clin Epidemiol 1995;48:363–73.
19. Cook TD, Campbell DT. Quasi-experiments: Nonequivalent control group designs. In: Quasi-experimentation: Design and analysis issues for field settings. Boston: Houghton and Mifflin Company, 1979:95–146.
20. Gordis L. Cohort Studies. In: Epidemiology. Philadelphia: WB Saunders Company, 1996:116–23.
21. Gordis L. A pause for review: comparing cohort and case-control studies. In: Epidemiology. Philadelphia: WB Saunders Company, 1996:163–82.
22. Gordis L. Case-control and cross-sectional studies. In: Epidemiology. Philadelphia: WB Saunders Company, 1996:124–40.

23. Bourne R. Con: Some clinical research is not cost-effective—weaknesses of outcomes studies. Spine 1995;20:386–87.

24. Pocock S, Elbourne D. Randomized trials or observational tribulations. N Engl J Med 2000;342:1907–09.

25. Bourne R. Con: Some clinical research is not cost-effective—weaknesses of outcomes studies. Spine 1995;20:386–87.

26. Rubin D. Estimating causal effects from large data sets using propensity scores. Ann Intern Med 1997;127:757–63.

27. Rosenbaum P, Rubin D. The central role of the propensity score in observational studies for causal effects. Biometrika 1983;70:41–55.

28. Drake C, Fisher L. Prognostic models and the propensity score. International J Epidemiol 1995;24:183–87.

29. Blackstone E. Comparing apples and oranges. J Thorac Cardiovasc Surg 2002;123:8–15.

30. Bangert-Drowns RL. Misunderstanding metaanalysis. Evaluation and the Health Professions 1995;18:304–14.

31. Glass GV. Primary, secondary, and metaanalysis research. Educational Researcher 1976;5(10):3–8.

32. Birkmeyer JD. Outcomes research and surgeons. Surgery 1998;124:477–83.

33. Freiman J, Chalmers T, Smith H, Kuebler R. The importance of beta, the type II error and sample size in the design and interpretation of the randomized control trial. N Engl J Med 1978;299:690–94.

34. Hall JA, Rosenthal R. Interpreting and evaluating metaanalysis. Evaluation and the Health Professions 1995;18:393–407.

35. Vatz JB. Metaanalysis: Apples, oranges, or fruitless. Physician Exec 1991;17:40–42.

36. Rouse DJ, Owen J. Decision analysis. Clin Obstet and Gynecol 1998;41:282–95.

37. Pauker S, Kassirer J. Medical progress: Decision analysis. N Engl J Med 1987;316:250–58.

38. Chee NK, Bateman TM. Cost-effectiveness of stress echocardiography and nuclear perfusion imaging. Prog Cardiovasc Dis 2000;43:197–214.

39. Hillman BJ. Outcomes research and cost-effectiveness analysis for diagnostic imaging. Radiology 1994;193:307–10.

40. Udvarhelyi IS, Colditz GA, Rai A, Epstein AM. Cost-effectiveness and cost-benefit analyses in the medical literature: Are the methods being used correctly? Ann Intern Med 1992;116:238–44.

41. Mushlin AI. Challenges and opportunities in economic evaluations of diagnostic tests and procedures. Acad Radiol 1999;6:S128–S131.

42. Cross design synthesis: A new strategy for studying medical outcomes? Lancet 1992;340:944–46.

43. Bossuyt PM, Lijmer JG. Traditional health outcomes in evaluation of diagnostic tests. Acad Radiol 1999;6:S77–S80.

44. Verrilli D, Welch G. The impact of diagnostic testing on therapeutic interventions. JAMA 1996;275:1189–91.

45. Reigleman R, Hirsch R. Introduction to testing a test. In: Studying a study and testing a test: How to read the health science literature. 3rd ed. Boston: Little Brown, 1996:141–44.

46. Yerushalmy J. Statistical problems in assessing methods of medical diagnosis, with special reference to X-Ray techniques. Pub Health Rep 1947:62;1432–49.

47. Fletcher RH. Interpretation of diagnostic tests. Indian J Pediatr 2000:67;49–53.

48. Binder M, Dreiseitl S. The interpretation of test results. J Cutan Med Surg 2000:4;19–25.

49. Henderson R. Assessing test accuracy and its clinical consequences: A primer for receiver operating characteristic curve analysis. Ann Clin Biochem 1993:30;521–39.

50. Fletcher RH, Fletcher SW, Wagner EG. Diagnosis. In: Clinical epidemiology: The essentials, 3rd ed. Baltimore: Williams and Wilkins, 1996:43–74.

51. Einstein A, Bodian C, Gil J. The relationship among performance measures in the selection of diagnostic tests. Arch Pathol Lab Med 1997:121;110–17.

52. Radack KL, Rouan G, Hedges J. The likelihood ratio: An improved measure of reporting and evaluating diagnostic test results. Arch Pathol Lab Med 1986:110;689–93.

53. Hlatky MA, Mark DB, Harrell FE, Lee KL, Califf RM, Pryor DB. Rethinking sensitivity and specificity. Am J Cardiol 1987;59;1195–98.

54. Brenner H, Gefeller O. Variation of sensitivity, specificity, likelihood ratios and predictive values with disease prevalence. Stat Med 1997:16;981–91.

55. Diamond GA. Reverend Bayes' silent majority: An alternative factor affecting sensitivity and specificity of exercise electrocardiography. Am J Cardiol 1986:57;1175–80.

56. Cecil M, Kosinski A, Jones M, et al. The importance of workup (verification) bias correction in assessing the accuracy of SPECT thallium-201 testing for the diagnosis of coronary artery disease. J Clin Epidemiol 49 1996;7:735–42.

57. Miller T, Hodge D, Christian T, Milavetz J, Bailey K, Gibbons R. Effects of adjustment for referral bias on the sensitivity and specificity of single photon emission computed tomography for the diagnosis of coronary artery disease. Am J Med 2002;112:290–97.

58. Altman DG, Bland JM. Diagnostic tests 2: Predictive values. BMJ 1994:309;102.

59. Sonis J. How to use and interpret interval likelihood ratios. Fam Med 1999:31;432–37.

60. Barnard GA, Bayes T. Studies in the history of probability and statistics: IX. Thomas Bayes' essay towards solving a problem in the doctrine of chances. Biometrika 1958;45:293–315.

61. Patterson RE, Horowitz SF. Importance of epidemiology and biostatistics in deciding clinical strategies for using diagnostic tests: A simplified approach using examples from coronary artery disease. J Am Coll Cardiol 1989;13:1653–65.

62. Sackett DL. A primer on the precision and accuracy of the clinical examination. JAMA 1992:267;2638–44.

63. Jaeschke R, Guyatt G, Sackett D. Users' guides to the medical literature: III How to use an article about a diagnostic test: (B) What are the results and will they help me in caring for my patients? JAMA 1994:271;703–07.

64. Visser CA, Kan G, David GK, Lie KI, Durrer D. Two-dimensional echocardiography in the diagnosis of left ventricular thrombus: A prospective study of 67 patients with anatomic validation. Chest 1983;83:228–32.

65. Zweig MH, Campbell G. Receiver-Operating characteristic (ROC) plots: A fundamental evaluation tool in clinical medicine. Clin Chem 1993;39;561–57.

66. Altman DG, Bland JM. Diagnostic tests 3: Receiver operating characteristic plots. BJM 1994;309;188.

67. Greiner M, Pfeiffer D, Smith RD. Principles and practical application of the receiver-operating characteristic analysis for diagnostic tests. Prev Vet Med 2000;45;23–41.

68. Fryback D, Thornbury J. The efficacy of diagnostic imaging. Med Decis Making 1991;11;88–94.

69. Jaeschke R, Gordon G, Sackett D. Users' guides to the medical literature: III How to use an article about a diagnostic test: (A) Are the results of the study valid? JAMA 1994:271;389–91.

## QUESTIONS

1. Which of the following statements have contributed to the increased emphasis on outcomes research?
   A. Need for cost-containment
   B. Unexplained variability in practice patterns
   C. Inappropriate use of medical services
   D. Need for greater accountability
   E. All of the above

2. Which of the following statements are true?
   A. The primary focus of outcomes research is efficacy.
   B. Outcomes research primarily focuses on effectiveness rather than efficacy.

C. Efficacy addresses the question of whether an intervention can work in routine clinical practice.
D. Effectiveness is the usefulness of the medical intervention tested in a randomized control trial.
E. All of the above

**3.** Which of the following data sources can be used in outcomes research?
A. Results from randomized control trials
B. Results from quasiexperimental designs
C. Observational data from large databases
D. Results from effectiveness trials
E. All of the above

**4.** Which of the following statements is true concerning the randomized control trial?
A. The randomization process attempts to control for known and unknown confounding variables.
B. Randomization can reduce conscious and unconscious biases.
C. Randomized control trials are able to assess efficacy of the treatment intervention.
D. One goal of the randomized control trial is to reduce both variability and bias.
E. All of the above

**5.** Effectiveness trials differ in methodology from the randomized control trial. Which of the following statements is true regarding effectiveness trials?
A. Effectiveness trials may not have a random assignment of treatments.
B. Effectiveness trials are significantly less restrictive than randomized control trials.
C. Effectiveness trials are often retrospective and population based.
D. Effectiveness trials may include a broad mix of investigators and occur in office or community hospital settings.
E. All of the above

**6.** Which of the following statements concerning performance measures of diagnostic imaging tests is true?
A. Sensitivity is a measure of how good a test is at not detecting disease in diseased patients.
B. Specificity is a measure of how good a test is at detecting disease in patients who are disease free.
C. Tests that seek to exclude or rule out disease require high specificities.
D. Tests that seek to confirm or rule in a target disorder require a high specificity.

## Chapter 10

# Assessment of Global Ventricular Function

*Nhung T. Lam and Solomon Aronson*

Left ventricular systolic function is a powerful predictor of clinical outcome for a wide range of cardiovascular diseases including ischemic cardiac disease, cardiomyopathy, and valvular heart disease. Data from the CASS registry indicate that left ventricular (LV) function determined by ejection fraction is more important for predicting survival than the number of diseased vessels. Echocardiography provides both a quantitative and qualitative measure of systolic function by estimating global and regional ventricular function and by measuring ventricular volumes and ejection fraction.

## EXAMINATION OF THE LEFT VENTRICLE

Echocardiography, a two-dimensional imaging technique, is used to study a three-dimensional object, the left ventricle, in real time by manipulating the transesophageal echocardiographic (TEE) probe to produce multiple imaging planes. To reproduce and compare measurements, standardized views have been developed based on internal and external references of the ventricle. The imaging planes used to describe and quantitate global left ventricular function include midesophageal four-chamber view (ME 4C) (Fig. 10.1), the midesophageal two-chamber view (ME 2C) (Fig. 10.2), midesophageal long-axis view (ME LAX) (Fig. 10.3), transgastric short-axis view (TG SAX) (Fig. 10.4), and transgastric long-axis view (TG LAX) (Fig. 10.5). During a TEE examination for global ventricular assessment, artifactual shortening of the LV long axis should be avoided or the myocardium at the mid- to apical segments will appear falsely thickened. A foreshortened left ventricle in the four-chamber view may represent a more proximal segment of the anterior wall rather than the true LV apex. The four- and two-chamber views are used to measure mitral inflow velocity, and LV volume and area as surrogates for LV preload.

To obtain the four-chamber view, the TEE probe is inserted into the midesophagus approximately 20 cm, the omniplane is rotated to 10–20 degrees, and the probe is slightly retroflexed. From the four-chamber view, the long axis of the left ventricle is centered in the middle of the sector and the image plane is slowly rotated toward 90 degrees to obtain the two-chamber view. Again, slight angulation and manipulation of the probe is necessary to obtain the two-chamber view, which includes the full length of the left ventricle and avoids foreshortening. The orthogonal axis of the two-chamber view may be used to calculate left ventricular volumes and ejection fraction. The omniplane is rotated towards 120 degrees from the two-chamber view to obtain the long-axis view. This view may be used to study the aortic valve apparatus, the left ventricle, and the LV outflow tract.

From the midesophageal level, the probe is advanced into the stomach to obtain the transgastric midpapillary short-axis view. With the omniplane at 0 degrees, the tip is anteflexed to bring the short axis into view. The short-axis midpapillary plane is preferred intraoperatively because it

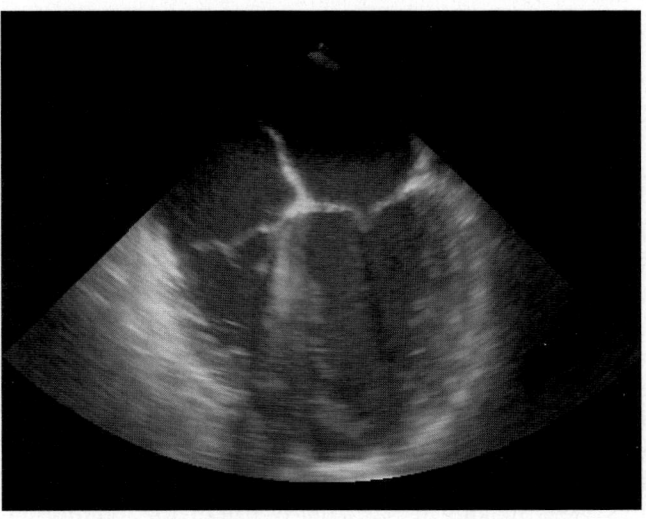

**FIGURE 10.1.** The midesophageal four-chamber view.

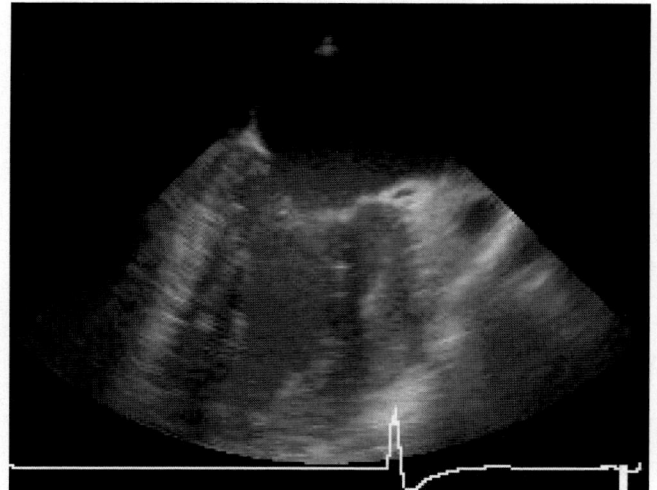

**FIGURE 10.2.** The midesophageal two-chamber view.

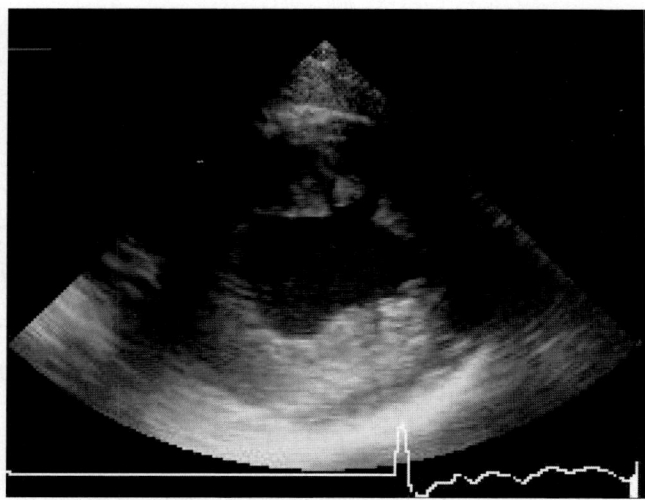

**FIGURE 10.4.** The transgastric short-axis view.

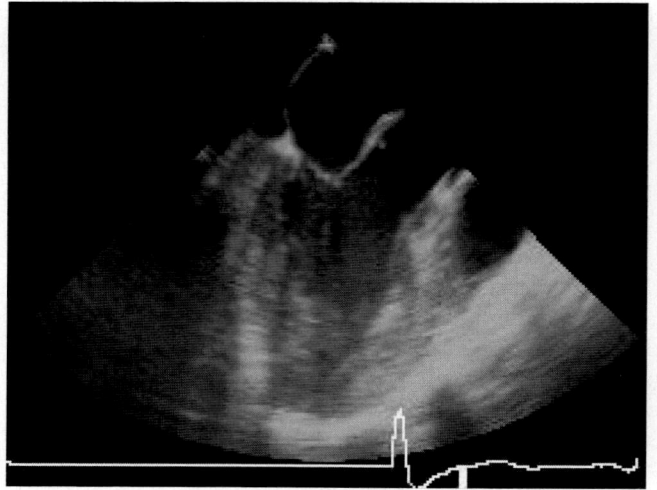

**FIGURE 10.3.** The midesophageal long-axis view.

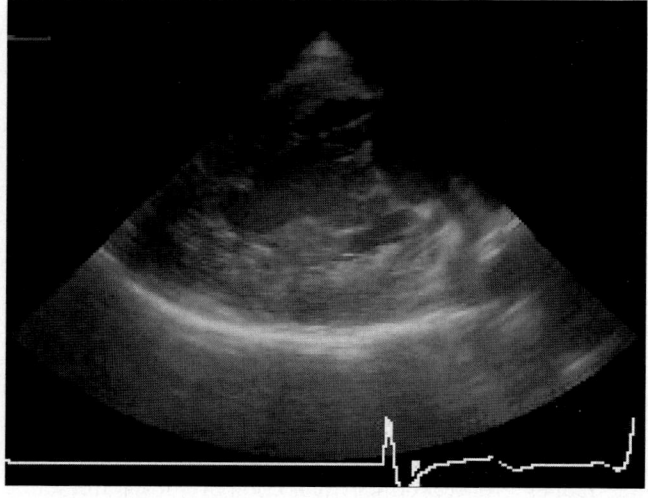

**FIGURE 10.5.** The transgastric long-axis view.

provides information regarding volume, contractility, ventricular dimensions, and thickness. The short axis of the left ventricle can be imaged at many levels; however, only two imaging planes are consistently reproducible from good internal references: the transgastric midpapillary short-axis view through the body of the papillary muscles and the transgastric basal short-axis view through the mitral valve. Intraoperatively, the transgastric midpapillary view reveals changes in volume status that are reflected in the end-diastolic cavity size. Change in fractional area and fractional shortening, surrogates of ejection fraction, can be calculated with this view. Distributions of the three coronary arteries are represented in this view, making it particularly useful for monitoring new regional wall motion abnormalities.

To obtain the two-chamber view of the left ventricle, start at the midesophageal four-chamber view, center the left ventricle in the middle of the imaging, and rotate the omniplane out to 90 degrees. In this view, the inferior wall is at the top of the sector and the anterior wall is at the bottom, directly opposite the inferior wall.

## NORMAL ANATOMY OF THE LEFT VENTRICLE

The left ventricle is a thick-walled, bullet-shaped chamber with average left ventricular wall thickness of 10.9 ± 2.0 mm and an average mass of 92 ± 16 gm/m². In cross section, the left ventricle has a nearly circular configuration that increases in area from base to apex. It is obliquely positioned in the chest with its apex pointing left, slightly anteriorly and inferiorly. It shares a triangular-shaped interventricular septum with the right ventricle in the anteromedial portion. The remainder of the LV wall, called the free wall, is not in contact with any other chamber.

## PHASES OF VENTRICULAR SYSTOLE

In the cardiac cycle, systole starts with mitral valve closure and ends with aortic valve closure. On an electrocardiogram, onset of systole is identified at the peak of the QRS complex and end of systole after repolarization at the end of the T wave. Systole also can be determined by events in the left ventricle (Fig. 10.6). Mitral valve closure marks the beginning of systole and is followed by an isovolumic contraction period. During this period, ventricular pressure rises rapidly while volume stays constant. As ventricular pressure exceeds aortic pressure, the aortic valve opens. The ejection phase follows, marked by acceleration and deceleration. During the first half of the ejection phase when LV pressure exceeds aortic pressure,

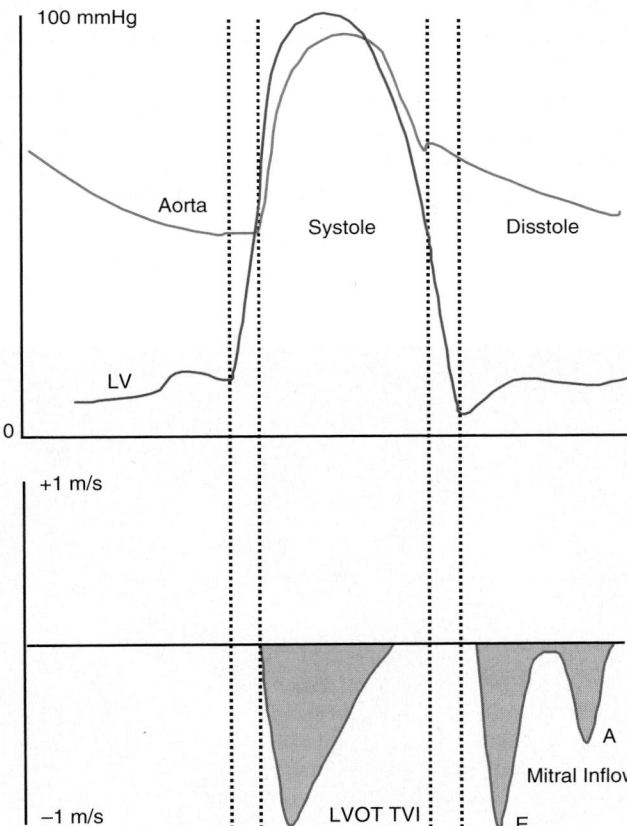

**FIGURE 10.6.** The ventricular cycle and the corresponding Doppler flow velocity profiles in the LV outflow tract and the mitral inflow tract.

blood rushes from the left ventricle into the aorta. Then in the deceleration phase of systole when aortic pressure exceeds ventricular pressure the forward flow of blood at a progressively slower velocity is reflected by the downward slope of the velocity tracing.

## LEFT VENTRICULAR SYSTOLIC FUNCTION

Ventricular systolic function is described by both load-independent and load-dependent indices of myocardial performance. They vary depending on preload and afterload. Therefore, estimates of contractility require measurement of ventricular ejection performance during different loading conditions. The clinical evaluation of ventricular function often relies on evaluating preload, afterload, cardiac output, ejection fraction, end-systolic volumes, and dimensions. Echocardiographic modalities designed for evaluating contractility independent of load include pressure-area relationships.

## EJECTION PHASE INDICES OF LEFT VENTRICULAR PERFORMANCE

LV global systolic performance is commonly expressed in terms of cardiac output, ejection fraction, and fractional shortening. The rate of ejection can be measured by quantifying the peak and mean velocity of fiber shortening. These indices are very sensitive to changes in preload and afterload.

## CARDIAC OUTPUT

Cardiac output is calculated from the equation CO = SV × HR, where SV is stroke volume and HR is heart rate. Stroke volume is defined as the difference between the end-diastolic and end-systolic volume in the left ventricle. Since volume is a three-dimensional parameter, calculation of stroke volume with two-dimensional echo requires measuring a cross-sectional area and the flow through that area with Doppler flow measurement using the equation below:

$$SV = CSA \times VTI$$

where SV is stroke volume, CSA is the cross-sectional area, and VTI is the velocity time integral.

During systole, the left ventricle ejects a given amount of blood (SV) into the cylindrically shaped aorta, which occupies a set volume in the aorta. Stroke volume is calculated by measuring the area and height of this blood column in the aorta. The cross-sectional area at the base of this column is derived by measuring the diameter (D) of the base of the aorta and applying the formula for the area of a circle: $\pi r^2$ or $\pi(D/2)^2$. The height of the column is obtained with Doppler to measure the flow through the aorta during systole. The area under the Doppler systolic flow velocity curve or the velocity time integral (VTI) represents the height of the cylinder. Thus the volume of the cylinder or stroke volume is the product of the CSA and VTI (Fig. 10.7).

Using this method to derive volume from area and flow measurements, we make several assumptions. First, the area measured for the calculation of stroke volume is constant during the entire period of systole. Second, a small error in diameter measurement quadruples the error in the calculation for the cross-sectional area. Third, flow across the area of interest is assumed to be laminar, such that the recorded flow represents the average flow and distance of flow in that region. In the presence of aortic valve disease, stroke volume measurement in the ascending aorta will be inaccurate because flow distal to the valve is not laminar. Fourth, the Doppler beam angle of incidence is assumed to be parallel to the direction of blood flow in that area. Finally, the area and flow measurements must be made at the same anatomic site.

Several investigators have looked into the optimal site for measurements of the Doppler flow velocity. Muhiudeen and colleagues (2) look at the pulmonary artery as a site for cardiac output measurement. They measured the cross-sectional area and pulsed-wave Doppler signal of the pulmonary artery systolic flow. The result correlated modestly with cardiac output measured by the thermodilution method (r = 0.65). Pulmonary systolic flow detected only intraoperative increases in cardiac output

greater than 15% (sensitivity, 71%; specificity, 82%), not decreases (sensitivity, 54%; specificity, 90%). Darmon and colleagues (3) used the transgastric long-axis view to obtain a spectral envelope with the continuous wave beam placed in the path from the LV outflow tract to the ascending aorta. The angle between the Doppler beam and the aortic valve plane was 7 ± 5 degrees with a range of 0 to 18 degrees. For the cross-sectional area, they used the time-averaged shape of the aortic valve aperture, measured in the upper esophageal view at 30 degrees. They obtained the TEE frame where the aortic valve cusp tips were as close to a straight triangle as possible, thus equating this structure to an equilateral triangle. The length of each side of the aortic valve was measured and the three values were averaged before calculation of the area of the aortic valve orifice in systole.

$$AVA = 0.5 \times \text{Cos } 30° \times S^2$$
$$AVA = 0.433 \times S^2$$

When the triangular model was used to calculate aortic valve area, Doppler-derived cardiac output (DCO) correlated tightly with thermodilution results for cardiac output (TCO) (r = 0.93) (Fig. 10.8).

This same group also substantiated the circular model to describe the aortic valve based on the observation that at maximal valve aperture, near peak systole, the aortic valve orifice appears nearly circular (Fig. 10.9). The aortic valve diameter (D) was measured in the longitudinal view, at the hinge points using the inner leaflet surface to inner leaflet surface method (Fig. 10.10). The aortic valve orifice area was then calculated using the equation:

$$AVA = \pi \times (D/2)^2$$

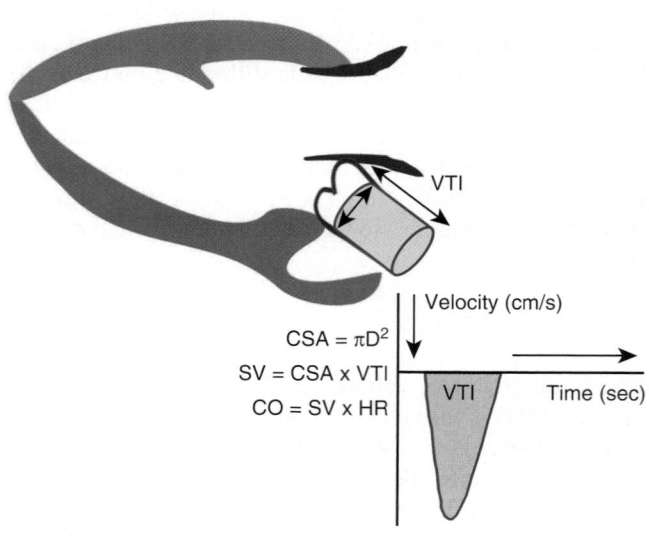

**FIGURE 10.7.** Stroke volume calculation.

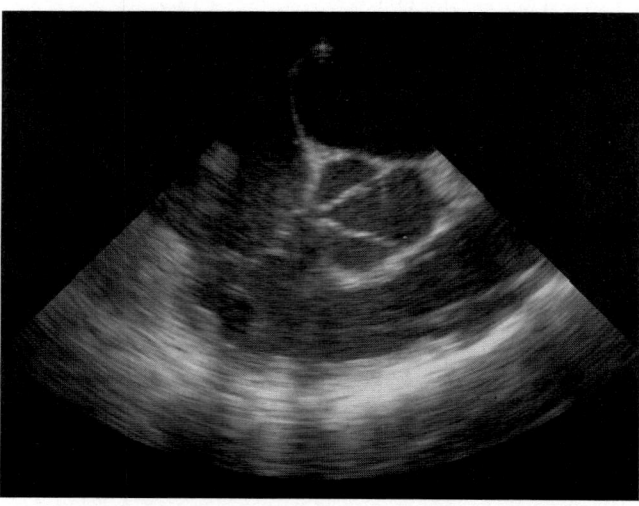

**FIGURE 10.8.** The upper esophageal aortic valve short-axis view demonstrating the aortic valve resembling the shape of an equilateral triangle.

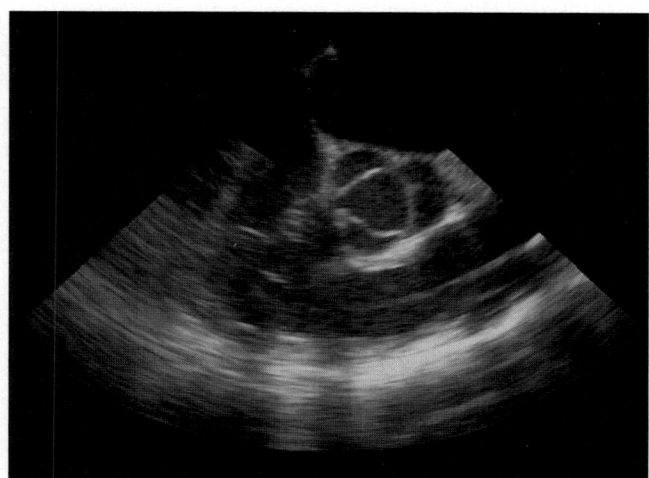

**FIGURE 10.9.** The upper esophageal aortic valve short-axis view demonstrating the aortic valve near peak systole resembling the shape of a circle.

The transgastric long-axis view was used to obtain the Doppler spectral envelope with the continuous wave beam placed in the path from the LV outflow tract to the ascending aorta. CO based on this circular model has a correlation coefficient of 0.88 when compared to the thermodilution method (3).

Perrino and colleagues (4) used the triangular aortic valve method to calculate cardiac output with high reproducibility. In 32 of 33 patients (97%), they were able to image the LV outflow tract in the transgastric long-axis view and calculate cardiac output with a correlation of r = 0.98 for intrasubject changes in cardiac output. Serial changes in cardiac output >1 L/min were tracked correctly in 97% of the cases. The magnitude of change in cardiac output was underestimated by 14% with Doppler-derived cardiac output when compared to the thermodilution method (4). Thus Doppler-derived cardiac output predicted the direction of change with high correlation; in a dynamic setting, it can underestimate the magnitude of the change.

## EJECTION FRACTION

Ejection fraction is calculated by the following formula:

$$EF\% = (EDV - ESV/\, EDV) \times 100\%$$

where EDV, volume at end-diastole; ESV, volume at end systole. The American Society of Echocardiography recommends using the modified Simpson's method to derive the ventricular volumes. (See the section on Preload later in the chapter.) The limitations of the method must be recognized, however. First, endocardial definition is affected by the physics of ultrasound and by anatomic limitations. For example, the lateral wall in the midesophageal four-chamber view is often difficult to visualize and trace because of the anatomic position of the endocardial-ventricular interface in this imaging plane. The border is parallel to the echo beam and therefore appears "blurred" as a result of poor lateral resolution. Signal attenuation by calcium deposits on the mitral annulus can create "drop out" of the echo signal distal to the deposits further complicating endocardial detection of the ventricular walls. The numerous trabeculations in the left ventricle, most notably its apex, may sometimes be falsely identified as the endocardial border. Therefore the endocardium identified by echocardiography is often different than the endocardium identified by angiography, in which the contrast material fills the trabeculations and distinguishes them from the true endocardium. With ultrasound contrast, the true endocardial border is easily revealed.

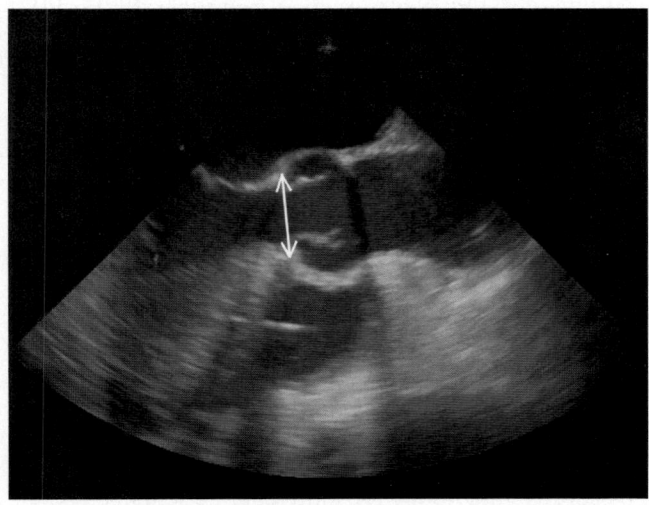

**FIGURE 10.10.** The midesophageal long-axis view demonstrating the aortic valve diameter (D) at the hinge points using the inner leaflet surface to inner leaflet surface method.

## FRACTIONAL AREA CHANGE

Because of the limitations to accurate endocardial detection and the time-consuming nature of calculating volumes, echocardiographers often rely on measuring the fractional area change (FAC) intraoperatively based on the area measured in the transgastric midpapillary view. The equation is as follows:

$$FAC\,\% = \frac{(LVEDA - LVESA)}{LVEDA} \times 100\%$$

where FAC is the fractional area change, LVEDA is the area at end-diastole; LVESA is the area at end-systole.

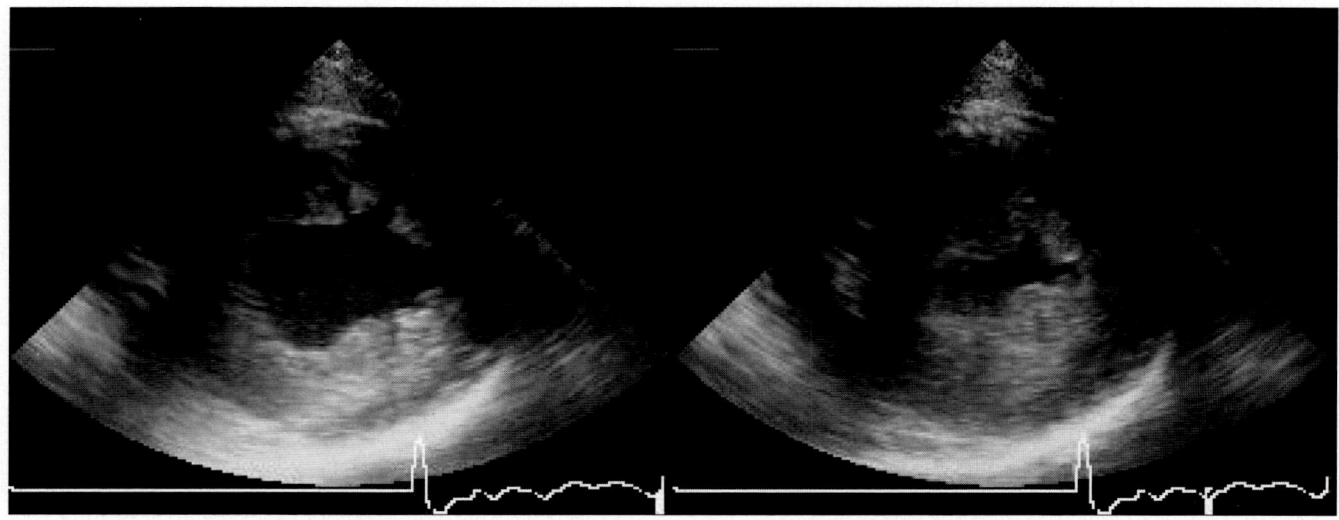

**FIGURE 10.11.** The midpapillary view of the left ventricle at end-diastole **(A)** and end-systole **(B).**

This method measures the percent of change in myocardial dimension as an estimate of LV contractile performance. This index of systolic performance is heavily afterload dependent and slightly preload dependent. Intraoperatively FAC is routinely used as a surrogate for ejection fraction. Several studies with intraoperative TEE using the midpapillary short-axis view to calculate ejection fraction have demonstrated a close correlation between ejection fraction based on fractional area change and radionuclide angiography and scintigraphy (r = 0.96 and r = 0.82, respectively) (Fig. 10.11) (5,6).

## SYSTOLIC INDEX OF CONTRACTILITY (dP/dt)

Although ejection phase indices of LV performance are easy to obtain, their load dependency may confound the accurate assessment of LV systolic function. The maximal rate of pressure increase during the isovolumic phase of ventricular systole $dP/dt_{(max)}$ is sensitive to changes in contractility, insensitive to changes in afterload and wall motion abnormalities, and only mildly affected by changes in preload. Continuous wave Doppler is used to determine the velocity of the mitral regurgitation jet. From that the rate of pressure increase or $dP/dt_{(mean)}$ is determined (7). This method requires that one has a mitral regurgitant jet. Since the method gives the mean dP/dt, the value often underestimates the peak dP/dt. To obtain the dP/dt, the continuous wave velocity profile of the mitral regurgitant jet is optimized. Then the time it takes for the mitral regurgitant velocity to rise from 1 cm/s to 2 cm/s is measured. Using the simplified Bernoulli equation, the velocities are converted into pressures.

$$P = 4V^2 = 4(1)^2 = 4 \text{ mm Hg}$$
$$P = 4V^2 = 4(3)^2 = 36 \text{ mm Hg}$$
$$dP/dt = \frac{4(1)^2 - 4(3)^2}{\Delta t}$$
$$dP/dt = \frac{(36 - 4 \text{ mm Hg} \times 1,000)}{\Delta t}$$

A dP/dt value > 1200 mm Hg/sec or a time of ≤ 27 msec is considered normal and dP/dt value < 1000 mm Hg/sec or a time of ≥ 32 msec is considered abnormal. In one study, dP/dt and −dP/dt indices were determined prospectively in 56 patients with chronic congestive heart failure and low ejection fraction < 50% to predict event-free survival (8).

Unlike ejection phase indices described above, pressure volume relationships describe the contractile state of the myocardium. The slope of the pressure volume loops or the end-systolic elastance is a load-independent indicator of preload-recruitable stroke work and therefore reflects true contractility. Until recently, pressure volume analysis has been difficult to obtain on-line. With the advent of echocardiographic automated border detection, continuous measurement of the LV area as a surrogate for LV volume is possible. Gorcscan and colleagues (9) coupled continuous area measurements obtained with TEE with continuous pressure data measured at the level of the left ventricle in 13 patients undergoing coronary artery bypass grafts. When area was substituted for volume, stroke force from pressure area loops was closely correlated with changes in estimates of stroke work from pressure volume loops for individual patients before bypass (mean correlation r = .99 ± .03) and after bypass (mean correlation r = .96 ± .05). Pressure estimates of end-systolic elastance, maximal elastance, and preload-

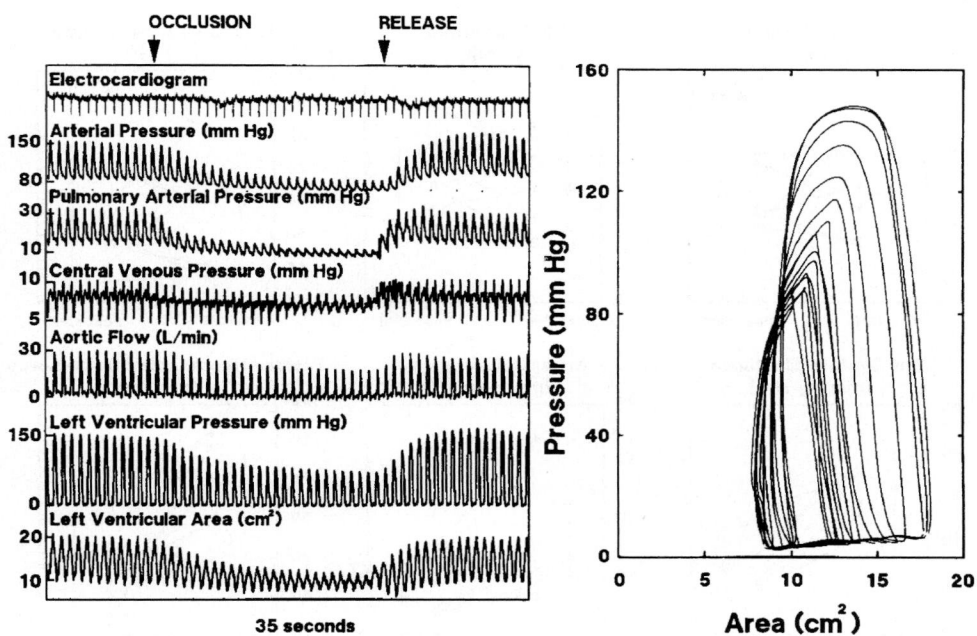

**FIGURE 10.12.** Traces of simultaneous waveform and pressure-area loop data from a patient during an inferior vena caval occlusion maneuver. From: Gorcsan J 3rd, Gasior TA, Mandarino WA, Deneault LG, Hattler BG, Pinsky MR. Assessment of the immediate effects of cardiopulmonary bypass on left ventricular performance by on-line pressure-area relations. Circulation 1994;89(1):180–90.

recruitable stroke force decreased from before to after cardiopulmonary bypass. The load-dependent measures of LV function such as stroke volume, cardiac output, and fractional area change were unchanged after surgery in these patients (Figs. 10.12 through 10.14).

Although contractility independent of different LV loading conditions can be measured using two-dimensional TEE, this method has not been widely adopted because it is cumbersome. Tissue Doppler imaging, a relatively recent addition to the diagnostic imaging modalities available with echocardiography, provides quantitative measurement of global as well as segmental LV function. Tissue Doppler technology is based on the same principles as color flow Doppler mapping.

With advances in Doppler technology, the high velocity and low amplitudes that are characteristic of blood flow can be filtered out to display the high amplitude, low velocity signals that are characteristic of cardiac tissue. Cardiac structures move in a velocity range of 0.06 to 0.24 m/s, approximately ten times slower than myocardial blood flow. Tissue Doppler displays the velocity of the myocardium through the cardiac cycle, with movement towards the transducer depicted as a positive deflection and movement away from the transducer depicted as a

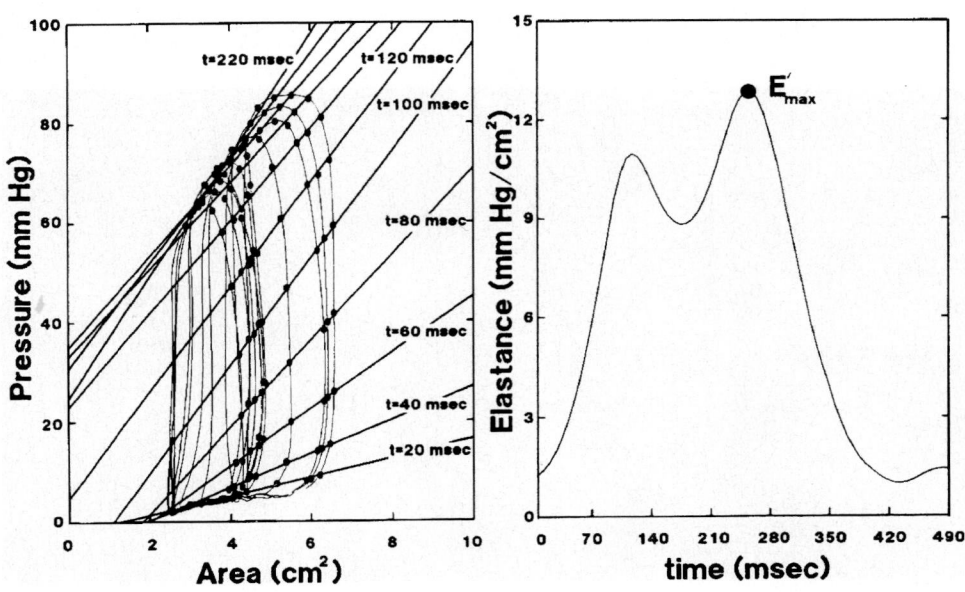

**FIGURE 10.13.** Plots show determination of time-varying elastance from pressure-area loops during inferior vena caval occlusion. **Left panel** shows elastance plots every 20 milliseconds from the onset of systole; **right panel,** corresponding elastance values with maximal elastance (E'max). From Gorcsan J 3rd, Gasior TA, Mandarino WA, Deneault LG, Hattler BG, Pinsky MR. Assessment of the immediate effects of cardiopulmonary bypass on left ventricular performance by on-line pressure-area relations. Circulation 1994; 89(1):180–90.

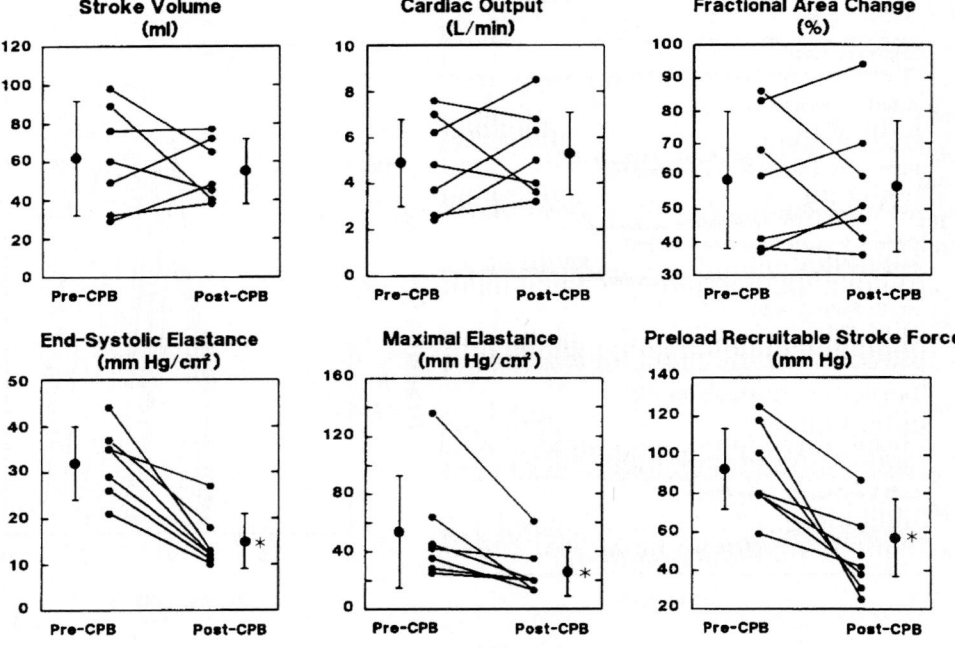

**FIGURE 10.14.** Line plots show results of multiple measures of left ventricular performance before and after cardiopulmonary bypass (CPB) in the same patients with paired data sets. Mean ± SD values are also shown. From Gorcsan J 3rd, Gasior TA, Mandarino WA, Deneault LG, Hattler BG, Pinsky MR. Assessment of the immediate effects of cardiopulmonary bypass on left ventricular performance by on-line pressure-area relations. Circulation 1994;89(1):180–90.

negative deflection. Four distinct velocities are typically seen on the wave form obtained by TEE (Fig. 10.15). The first negative velocity (S1 velocity) is associated with isovolumic contraction. The next negative deflection is the systolic shortening velocity; the peak systolic velocity is $S_2$. These velocities are depicted as negative because as the ventricle contracts there is a net movement towards the apex and away from the transducer. The two velocities in diastole, the E and A velocities, correspond to the Doppler mitral inflow E and A velocities. These are depicted as positive velocities because in diastole the myocardium

moves towards the transducer. The Em is the peak early diastolic myocardial relaxation velocity and Am is the late diastolic velocity associated with atrial contraction.

Myocardial velocity imaging is angle dependent and limited by some of the same variables that limit conventional Doppler echocardiography. The myocardial velocity measured at the site of interest is the sum of all the velocities in that area. In other words, this velocity does not differentiate between the three components that affect the motion of the heart: radial contraction, longitudinal shortening, and rotation. A translational motion of the

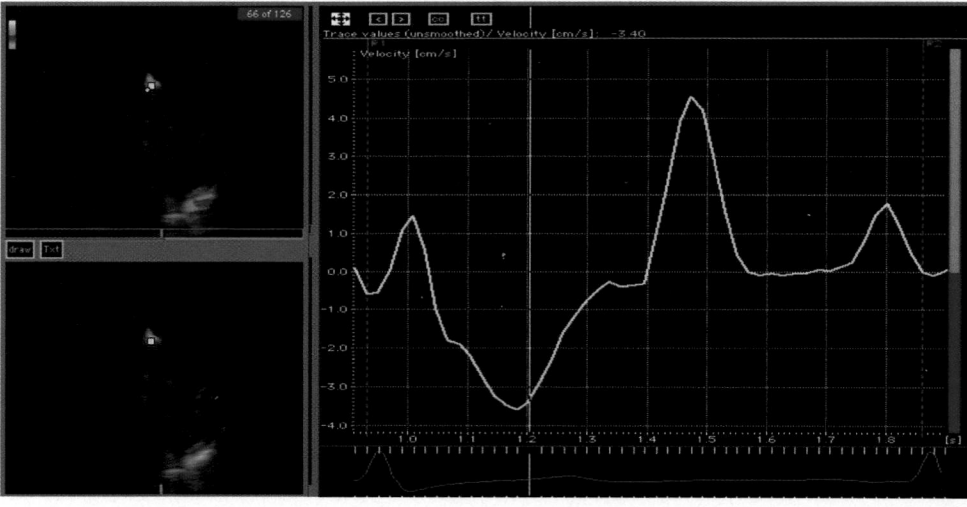

**FIGURE 10.15.** Tissue Doppler velocity tracing with sample site placed at the septal mitral annulus. On the right is the corresponding tissue velocity profile through one cardiac cycle. See text for explanation of the four velocities depicted above.

heart within the thorax can generate a velocity measurable by tissue Doppler imaging. Tissue Doppler imaging does not discriminate between actively contracting myocardium and a "tethered" myocardium. Thus an akinetic segment may demonstrate a velocity if it is being pulled along by an adjacent contracting segment of myocardium. These limitations explain the poor reproducibility of this technique.

Despite these limitations, however, tissue Doppler imaging can be used to measure global ventricular function. The descent of the mitral annulus from the base to the apex is a well described feature of normal left ventricular function. Earlier studies using M-mode and two-dimensional echocardiography have demonstrated the importance of the longitudinal vector of contraction to global LV function. Gulati and colleagues (10) used tissue Doppler M-mode to evaluate the velocity of mitral annular descent. The average peak mitral annular descent velocity correlated linearly with LV ejection fraction (r = 0.86) using radionuclide ventriculograms as the standard of reference. They derived an equation for predicting ejection fraction from average peak mitral annular descent velocity.

$$LVEF = 8.2 \times (\text{average peak mitral annular velocity}) + 3\%$$

When the average peak mitral annular velocity at six sites (septal, lateral, inferior, anterior, posterior, and anteroseptal annulus) was > 5.4 cm/s, the velocity was 88% sensitive and 97% specific for ejection fraction > 50%. A velocity > 5.4 cm/sec at a single annular site predicted an LV ejection fraction > 50% with an 89% sensitivity and 85% specificity. Clinically this has potential value of rapidly estimating global LV function in cases where endocardial border definition is suboptimal for tracing.

Tissue Doppler echocardiography may also be a tool to measure contractility noninvasively. The concept of myocardial strain was introduced in the 1970s to facilitate the understanding of elastic stiffness of myocardial tissue. With tissue Doppler echocardiography, the velocity at two sites along the myocardium can be determined. With strain and strain rate imaging, regional myocardial contractile movement can be measured independent of traction and tethering effects from other regions.

Strain is a dimensionless quantity that represents the percentage change from a resting state to one achieved following the application of a force (stress). The myocardial base descends towards the apex during systole and reverts during diastole (Fig. 10.16). The apex is nearly stationary, moving only a few millimeters in the same direction as the base. As the base moves towards the relatively stationary apex, the tissue velocities decrease from base to apex. Therefore measuring the velocity gradient subtracts its translational component because this motion would affect both sampling points equally.

Strain occurs simultaneously in all three dimensions, longitudinal or meridional, transmural, and circumferential as force is applied to a segment of myocardium. Since myocardial tissue is incompressible and the volume must remain constant, shortening from base to apex must be balanced by thickening. Therefore longitudinal myocardial deformation measured by strain is simultaneously and inversely related to the strain in the other two dimensions.

In general terms, longitudinal strain, $\varepsilon$, means relative deformation, and strain rate (SR) means rate of

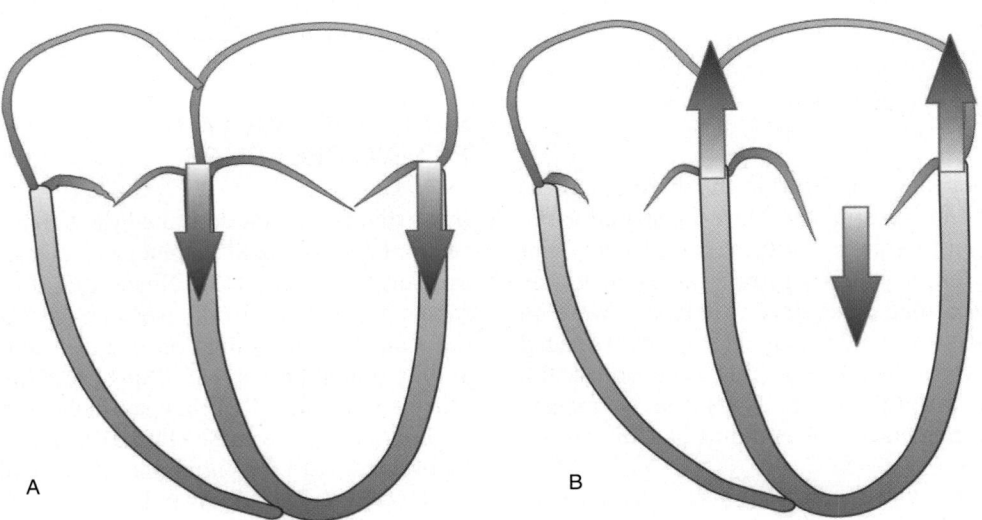

**FIGURE 10.16.** Illustration of systolic shortening mitral annulus moving towards the apex and away from the transducer **(A)**. Diastolic expansion with mitral annulus moving towards the transducer **(B)**.

deformation. If an object has an initial length $L_0$ that after a certain time changes to L, strain is defined as:

$$\varepsilon = \frac{\Delta L}{L_0} = \frac{(L - L_0)}{L_0}$$

The instantaneous change in length (dL) in a small time increment (dt) is related to the velocities ($v_1$ and $v_2$) of the end points of the object:

$$dL = (v_2 - v_1)dt$$

By dividing the equation above by L, we see that the instantaneous change in length per unit length equals the velocity gradient (i.e., strain rate) times the time increment:

$$\frac{dL}{L} = \frac{(v_2 - v_1)dt}{L}$$

Because it is not feasible to track the end points of the object, the velocity gradient SR is estimated from two points with a fixed distance:

$$\frac{dL}{L} \approx \frac{(v_{(r)} - v_{(r+\Delta r)})dt}{\Delta r} = SR\ dt$$

Finally, by integrating this equation from time $t_0$ to t, we arrive at the following relation between strain rate and strain:

$$Log\ \frac{L}{L_0} = \int_{t_0}^{t} SR\ dt$$

where log denotes the natural logarithm and $L_0$ and L denote the object length at times $t_0$ and t, respectively. This gives the equation:

$$\varepsilon = \exp\left(\int_{t_0}^{t} SR\ dt\right) - 1$$

Velocity gradients (strain rates) in the direction of the ultrasonic beam can be estimated from the spatial variation in Doppler shift frequency of the received signal. For calculation of strain, (equation 5) strain rate is integrated throughout each cardiac cycle, starting at peak R wave on the ECG. Because strain rate equals velocity (m/s) divided by distance (m), the units for strain rate is 1/s, and strain, which is the time integral (with units $1/s \times s$), is reported as a fraction or percentage of end-diastolic dimension (11).

Myocardial strain and strain rate imaging is a potentially powerful tool since it allows for quantification of segmental myocardial function that is independent of the tethering effect. A potential application of this technology

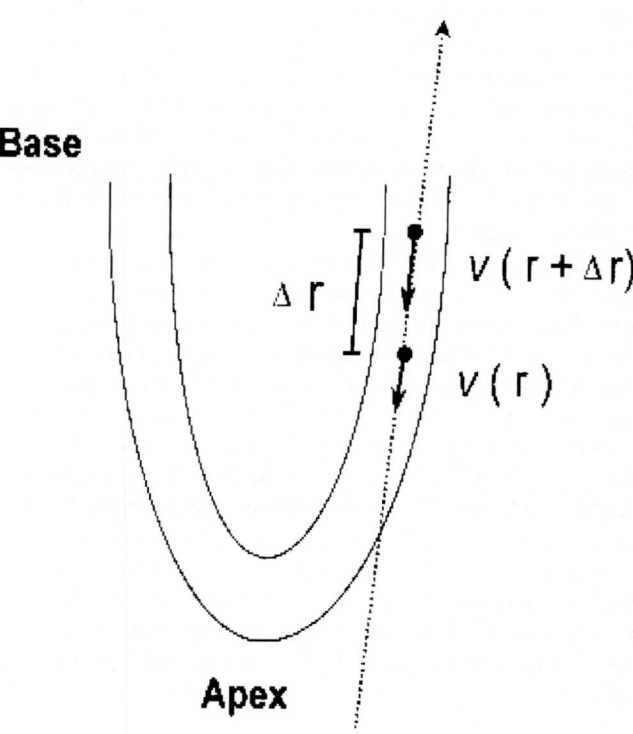

**FIGURE 10.17.** Schematic of how strain rate of tissue segment ($\Delta r$) is estimated from tissue velocity (v). *Dashed line* indicates orientation of ultrasound beam. Distance along beam is denoted r. Strain rate is calculated by subtracting v ($r + \Delta r$) from v (r) over distance ($\Delta r$) between these two points. When velocities are equal, strain rate is zero and there is no compression or expansion. If v ($r + \Delta r$) > (r), strain rate is negative and there is compression. When v (r) exceeds v ($r + \Delta r$), strain rate is positive, indicating expansion. From Urheim. Circulation 2000;102(10): 1158–64.

includes assessment of the contractile reserve of stunned myocardium with or without stress (Figs. 10.17–10.19).

## LEFT VENTRICULAR FILLING PRESSURE

Swan and Ganz first described the clinical use of flow-directed balloon-tipped catheters to measure intracardiac pressures in man (12). Since that introduction, pulmonary artery occlusion pressure has been considered the standard for estimation of mean left atrial pressure and LV filling pressure. LV filling pressure or LV end-diastolic pressure (LVEDP) changes, however, with changes in LV end-diastolic volume (LVEDV), the true indicator of LV preload. With the pulmonary artery catheter, LVEDP is used to estimate a volume index, the LVEDV. The error introduced by this approximation is clinically insignificant in conditions of low LV filling pressures. However, in critically ill patients, the PCWP grossly misrepresents the

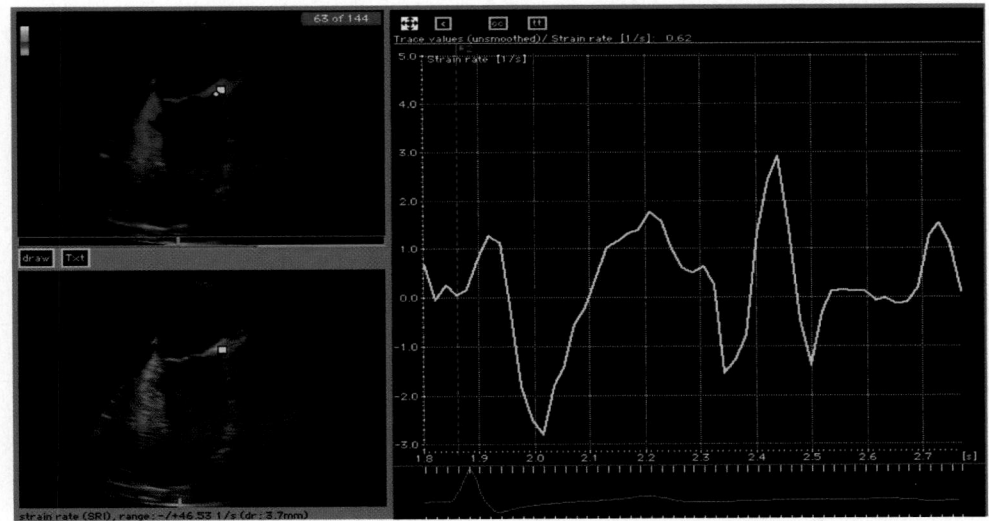

**FIGURE 10.18.** Myocardial strain rate by Doppler (1/s). Of note, strain rate signal has significant noise mainly from random noises in the velocity signal.

LVEDV. Echocardiography, on the other hand, provides an accurate diagnostic tool in any situation for the assessment of LV filling pressure and preload.

## INTERATRIAL SEPTUM

The interatrial septum provides qualitative information regarding the filling pressure of the right and left ventricle. The atrial septum can be examined in the four-chamber view, the bicaval view, or the right ventricular inflow-outflow view. The directional movement of the interatrial septum and its curvature may reflect the pressure relations between the left and right atria. Normally due to higher left-sided pressures, the interatrial septum bulges toward the right atrium. During passive mechanical expiration, right atrial pressure transiently exceeds left atrial pressure, and the atrial septum momentarily bows towards the left atrium. This midsystolic atrial reversal occurs when the corresponding pulmonary artery occlusion pressure (PAOP) is ≤ 15 mm Hg. A rightward midsystolic bowing or absence of the leftward bowing of the interatrial septum indicates PAOP > 15 mm Hg, with a sensitivity of 89%, specificity of 95%, and a positive predictive value of 0.97 (13).

## PULMONARY VEIN FLOW

At the midesophageal level, the TEE transducer is placed behind the left atrium allowing excellent visualization of the left upper pulmonary vein (LUPV) in the two-chamber view. With slight manipulation of the probe, the left lower and right pulmonary veins can easily be identified as well.

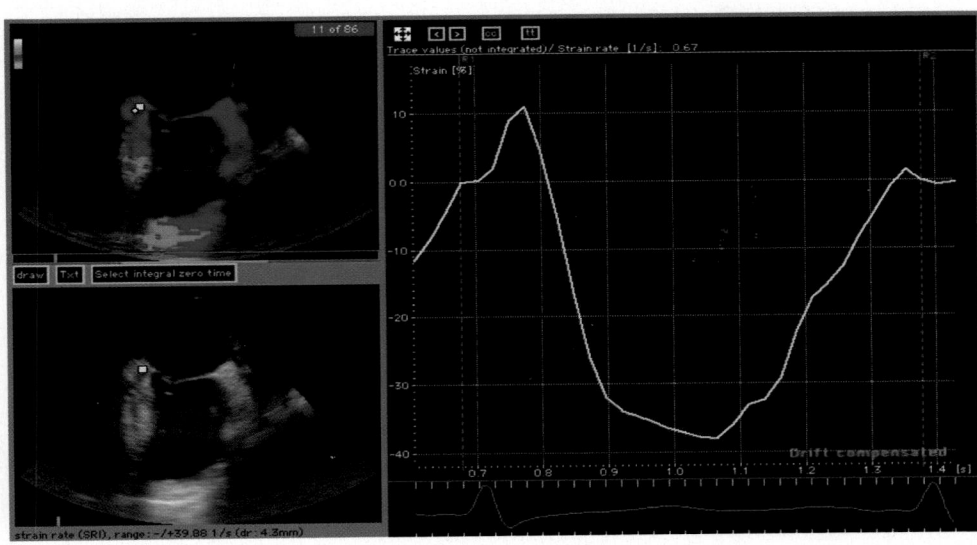

**FIGURE 10.19.** Myocardial strain by Doppler. Negative strain denotes myocardial shortening (compression) while positive strain (expansion) denotes myocardial lengthening. Also during the integration procedure, the random noise is cancelled out and a relatively smooth signal is obtained.

Doppler interrogation of the LUPV in the two-chamber view has several advantages. First, the LUPV can easily be visualized with the aid of color flow Doppler. Second, a long segment of the vein can be visualized enabling proper placement of the pulse wave cursor 1–2 cm into the vein. Lastly, the pulmonary vein visualized here parallels the direction of the Doppler beam thus increasing the accuracy of the Doppler measurements. Orihashi et al. (14) tried to measure pulmonary vein flow by TEE in 15 patients undergoing coronary artery bypass grafting. Using two-dimensional color Doppler TEE, they were able to visualize all four pulmonary veins. They found that the LUPV was most suitable for Doppler flow measurements by TEE. Sampling too close to the left atrium leads to underestimation of atrial reversal velocity. An inadequate signal may be improved by increasing the sample volume size to 3–4 mm. Color flow Doppler may help find the pulmonary vein flow stream as it enters the atrium.

The normal velocity of the pulmonary vein flow is comprised of an antegrade systolic flow (PVs1) produced by the forward flow of blood into the atrium as the left atrial pressure decreases during relaxation (Fig. 10.20). Then, downward movement of the mitral annulus during LV ejection creates a second systolic peak (PVs2) with higher amplitude. In the presence of low left atrial pressure, the biphasic nature of the S wave becomes more prominent because of the temporal dissociation of atrial relaxation and mitral annular motion (15). With TEE, the biphasic systolic wave is commonly seen. The descent of the S wave corresponds with the V wave in the left atrial pressure tracing. The second large flow velocity is the diastolic wave prompted by the antegrade flow of blood from the pulmonary veins into the left ventricle during early diastole. It coincides with the Y descent of the left atrial pressure tracing during early ventricular filling. During this phase, because the left atrium is an open conduit between the pulmonary veins and the left ventricle, the pulmonary veins

▶ **TABLE 10.1.  Determinants of Pulmonary Vein Flow Velocities**

| Velocity | Determinants |
|---|---|
| Early systole (PVs1) | LA relaxation |
| Late systole (PVs2) | RV output, LA compliance, mean LAP |
| Diastole (PVd) | LV relaxation |
| Atrial reversal (PVa) | LA contractility, LV compliance |

reflect abnormalities in the compliance of the left ventricle. The D wave is followed by a retrograde velocity called the A wave, which coincides with atrial contraction during late diastole and represents flow from the atrium into the pulmonary vein during atrial contraction (Table 10.1).

## FACTORS AFFECTING FLOW OF THE PULMONARY VEIN

Sinus tachycardia may cause the systolic and diastolic waves to fuse. The peak systolic to diastolic filling ratio increases with sinus tachycardia because the diastolic filling period is shortened. In patients with atrial fibrillation, systolic forward flow is diminished or absent, and diastolic flow is the main contributor to left atrial filling. Mechanical ventilation may decrease systolic flow during inspiration because of elevated airway pressure and increase diastolic flow at the end of expiration (14). The position of the sample volume in the pulmonary vein affects the flow characteristics as well. The systolic phase decreases as the sample volume is moved closer to the orifice where the pulmonary vein empties into the left atrium. Atrial flow reversal may be detected at a site other than that used to obtain the maximal systolic and diastolic flow velocities. Motion artifact from prominent atrial contraction may make it difficult to detect reversal of atrial contraction because it is a low velocity signal. Sampling from the pulmonary vein in patients with an enlarged left atrium may be difficult because the veins are in the far field of the two-dimensional sector (16).

The shape and size of the pulmonary flow velocity profile provide quantitative and qualitative information about LV preload. Normally, the S wave is equal to or slightly larger than the D wave. The degree of systolic forward flow in the extraparenchymal pulmonary veins is determined by atrial relaxation, LV systolic function (suction effect), mitral regurgitation, and left atrial compliance and pressure. In situations of elevated left atrial pressure (LAP > 15), the S wave is blunted, reflecting that most forward flow into the LA occurs during diastole. Kuecherer and colleagues (17) speculated that the

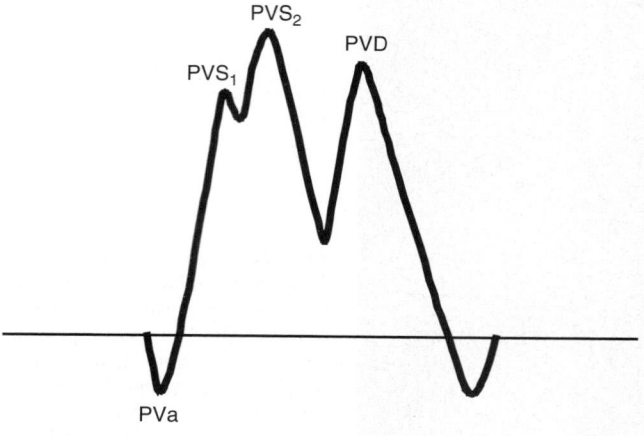

**FIGURE 10.20.** Illustration of the four components of the pulmonary vein Doppler flow velocities. See text for explanation.

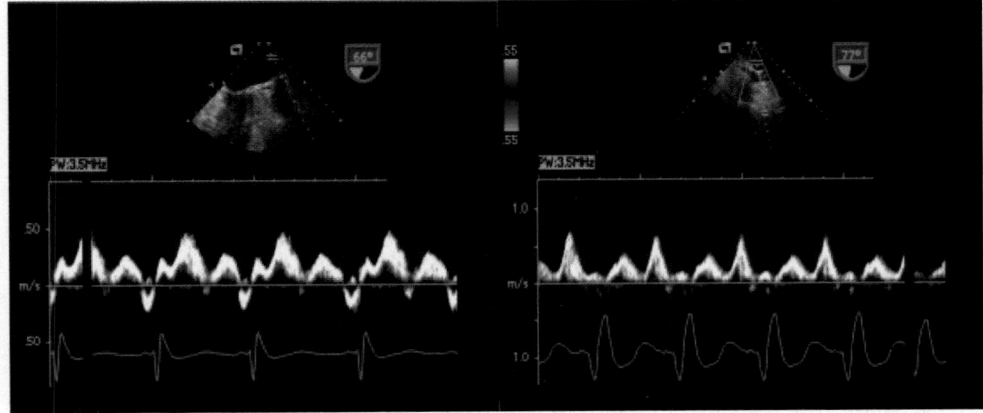

**FIGURE 10.21.** Illustration of low filling pressure (A), where the systolic waveform is greater than the diastolic waveform and the two components of systole, PVs1 and PVs2, are seen clearly. Right, illustration of high left atrial pressure with LAP > 15 mm Hg showing the systolic component blunted and the diastolic waveform greater than the systolic waveform.

decrease in left atrial compliance from increased LAP or left atrial volume or both best explains the shift in pulmonary venous flow. They used TEE Doppler to measure the pulmonary vein inflow velocity in 47 patients during cardiovascular surgery, excluding patients with mitral regurgitation. Fractional area shortening was the index of LV systolic function. They found that the systolic fraction, defined as

$$\text{Systolic Function} = \frac{\text{PV systolic TVI}}{(\text{PV}_{\text{systolic}} \text{ TVI} + \text{PV}_{\text{early diastolic}} \text{ TVI})}$$

correlated strongly with mean pulmonary artery occlusion pressure with (r = −0.88) and LAP measured directly by an intraatrial catheter (r = −0.78). In their study, systolic fraction < 40% usually implied wedge pressure ≥ 20 mm Hg.

Kinnaird et al. (18) reexamined the accuracy of pulmonary venous flow as a predictor of left atrial pressure. Unlike Kuecherer et al. (17), who used both direct LAP and PAOP measurements, Kinnaird used only direct LAP measurements. Measured PAOP consistently overestimated LAP. Kinnaird et al. reported that the deceleration time of the pulmonary vein during early diastole (DT$_D$) was more accurate than pulmonary wedge pressure in predicting LAP in cardiac surgical patients. A close correlation (r = −0.92) was found between LAP and pulmonary vein diastolic deceleration time. A (DT$_D$) of < 175 ms had 100% sensitivity and 94% specificity for LAP > 17 mm Hg. A DT$_D$ > 275ms predicted LAP of ≤ 6 mm Hg with 88% sensitivity and 95% specificity (18).

In summary, systolic flow pattern can be used as an "eyeball index" of LAP during cardiovascular surgery if patients do not have serious mitral regurgitation. The pulmonary vein diastolic deceleration time and the systolic to early diastolic peak velocity ratio are a noninvasive tool for measuring LAP.

Tissue Doppler imaging may also be used in conjunction with conventional Doppler techniques to estimate LV filling pressure. Mitral E wave velocity is directly influenced by LAP and inversely related changes in LV relaxation. Measures of E wave velocity via conventional Doppler correlate poorly with LAP because abnormal relaxation and high filling pressure often coexist in cardiac patients. Nagueh and his colleagues (19) demonstrated that dividing the E wave blood flow velocity by the annulus tissue E velocity (Ea) provides an alternative method to correct the transmitral velocity for the influence of relaxation. They found that the E/Ea correlated well with PCWP (r = 0.87, p < .001) and derived a formula for predicting wedge pressure from the E/Ea ratio.

$$\text{PCWP} = 1.24\,[\text{E/Ea}] + 1.9$$

In patients with sinus tachycardia with fused mitral inflow E and A waves, the E/Ea ratio correlated well with PCWP (r = 0.86, p < .001). As a general guideline, E/Ea >10 predicts a mean PCWP >15 mm Hg with, a 92% sensitivity and 80% specificity.

Kim and Sohn (20) evaluated 200 patients prospectively to compare the ratio of E/Ea to that of invasive left ventricular diastolic pressure measured before atrial contraction (pre-A wave). They found that the E/Ea ratio correlated well with pre-A wave pressure (r = 0.74, p < .001), and the correlation was not dependent on LV systolic function (EF ≥ 50%; r = 0.74 versus EF < 50%; r = 0.70).

The slight discrepancy between the Nagueh and Kim studies may be explained by the following differences. Kim and Sohn used pre-A pressure to represent the LV filling pressure rather than PCWP. Second, the tissue velocity sample volume was placed on the septum in Kim and Sohn's study, whereas Nagueh et al. sampled the lateral mitral annulus. In both studies, an E/Ea ratio of ≥ 9 predicted an elevated left ventricular filling pressure ≥ 12 mm Hg. Kim and Sohn also derived an equation for predicting LV pressure.

$$\text{LV filling pressure} = \text{E/Ea} + 4$$

## PRELOAD

Echocardiography provides several ways to qualitatively and semiqualitatively assess preload as defined by the volume in the ventricle at the end of diastole. Because echocardiography images the heart in a two-dimensional perspective, calculations derived from a single two-dimensional imaging plane provide information regarding area. To derive volume, more than one imaging plane is often necessary. Volumetric calculations must be based on geometric assumptions about the shape of the left ventricle. Geometric models vary: the simple ellipsoid shape, the complex hemi-ellipsoid shape, and the truncated cone ellipsoid shape in which two geometric shapes are used to describe the left ventricle. The accuracy of any model depends on the number of imaging planes used.

TEE is superior to transthoracic echocardiography for detection of the endocardial border. Because of the differences in scanning planes, the validation studies done with TTE cannot be directly applied to TEE. Smith et al. (21) compared LV volumes and ejection fraction derived from transesophageal short-axis and four-chamber images with similar variables obtained from ventriculography. They tested the three commonly used algorithms (Simpson's method, the area length method and the diameter-length method) for predicting volumes using TEE and validated those against ventricular angiography. The modified Simpson's method correlated best with angiography; the area-length method had the next highest correlation. Diastolic and systolic volumes were underestimated with all methods when compared with values assessed with angiography. Measurements of LV length by TEE were smaller for systole and diastole when compared to measurements by ventriculography. The underestimation of ventricular length, possibly because of foreshortening in the four-chamber view, is a major factor contributing to the smaller volumes obtained by TEE.

## CALCULATING VENTRICULAR VOLUMES

The area-length method uses the ellipsoid shape as a model of the left ventricle. Measurement of the LV length is obtained from the midesophageal four-chamber view, and the area calculated from the two-dimensional area is measured in the same long-axis view. In clinical conditions such as dilated cardiomyopathy or LV aneurysms, the ventricle does not resemble the ellipsoid shape; therefore, the equation used to calculate the ventricular volume based on the ellipsoid shape does not apply.

The Simpson's method uses two orthogonal imaging planes to derive volume and makes no geometric assumptions about the ventricle. This method uses the four- and two-chamber view to derive LVEDV, LVESV, and LVEF. The endocardial borders of the selected planes are traced out manually or detected automatically. Then the length of the left ventricle is divided into 20 cylinders of different diameters but equal thickness. This "method of discs" requires that the volumes of the cylinders are calculated and summed to estimate the ventricular volume. Most new models of echocardiography machines calculate the EDV, ESV, and EF automatically after the echocardiographer identifies the four-chamber plane and traces out the endocardium (Fig. 10.22).

When Clements et al. (5) evaluated ventricular area as a surrogate for volume, they used the transgastric midpapillary short-axis view to measure end-systolic area (ESA), end-diastolic area (EDA) and from that calculated fractional area change (FAC). Approximately 87% of the stroke volume is derived from the fiber shortening in the short axis. The level of the midpapillary is ideal for measurement since the papillary muscles provide reproducible internal reference. Clements et al. validated their measurements with simultaneous radionucleotide imaging and found a correlation of r = 0.86 with TEE EDA.

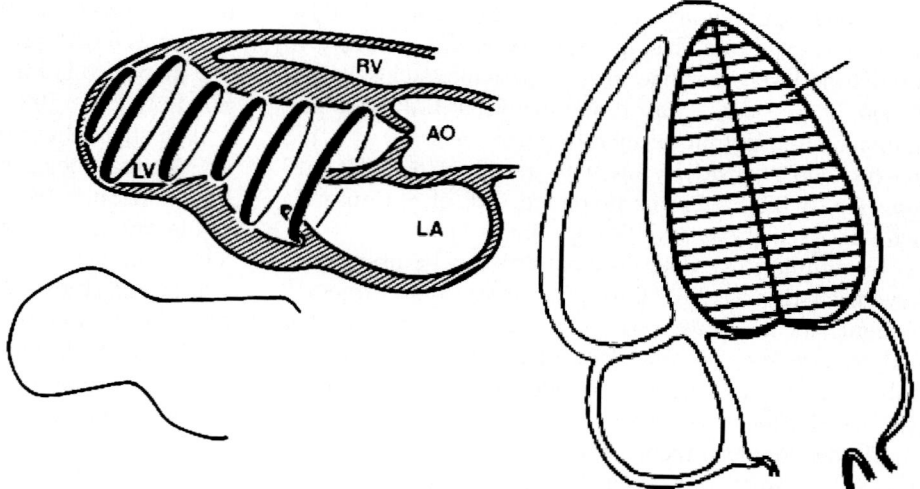

**FIGURE 10.22.** Illustration of the Simpson's method for calculation of LV volumes.

TEE ESA also correlated with radionuclide ESA (r = 0.92) as did the FAC (r = 0.96).

This validation study by Clements et al. supports the use of the LV EDA as a surrogate for preload. In patients with normal or abnormal LV function and graded hypovolemia, acute blood loss caused directional changes in LV EDA. Two-dimensional TEE detected a change in LV EDA with as little as a 2.5% estimated blood volume deficit (approximately 1.75 ml/kg). The mean change in LV EDA was 0.3 cm$^2$/1% estimated blood-volume deficit (22). Reich et al. (23) manipulated blood volumes in pediatric patients following sternal closure after repair of congenital heart lesions and recorded images of the midpapillary short axis during these interventions. Mild reductions in blood volume were identified with high sensitivity (80%–95%) and specificity (80%).

The EDA is measured by acquiring the midpapillary short-axis view and scrolling to the end of diastole as defined by the image frame corresponding to the peak of the QRS complex. Without an ECG for reference, the image on which the LV cavity is largest is selected. Next, with planimetry the borders of the endocardium are traced, using the leading edge to leading edge method and including the papillary muscles in the measurement. After the cavity is traced out, the software package on most machines will automatically give a calculated area and circumference. If the body surface area of the patient is known, the EDA index will be calculated; less than 5.5 cm$^2$/m$^2$ defines hypovolemia.

In summary, two-dimensional TEE can be used to measure LV volumes. Although the absolute volumes calculated underestimate those derived from angiography, detecting change in volume and the direction of change is more important than calculation of absolute volume. The experienced echocardiographer can detect changes in preload by visual inspection of the left ventricle at end-diastole and systole. With decreases in preload, there is a linear decrease in LV EDA and LV ESA. End-systolic cavity obliteration or "kissing ventricle" is a potentially useful "alarm" for hypovolemia. Obliteration can also reflect an increased inotropic state and decreased systemic vascular resistance. Leung and Levine (24) found that although end-systolic cavity obliteration detected by TEE is frequently associated with decreased LV preload, 10% of the time it reflects only an increase in ejection fraction (24). End-systolic cavity obliteration is very sensitive in predicting decreases in ESA (100%), but the specificity for predicting decrease in preload is low (10% to 30%).

## AFTERLOAD

Afterload is the force that acts to resist myocardial shortening during systole. At the level of the arterial system, it is defined in terms of systemic vascular resistance. Alter-

natively, afterload is the stress imposed on the ventricular wall during systole. The use of wall stress to measure myocardial function is based on the principle of equilibrium. The forces acting within the wall must exactly balance the forces acting on the wall. The stress forces acting on the wall are expressed as dynes/cm$^2$. LV wall stress depends on chamber size, myocardial thickness, interventricular pressure, and to some extent configuration. There are three types of ventricular wall stress: circumferential, meridional, and radial (Fig. 10.23). In the ellipsoid model, the forces act on the left ventricle in orthogonal planes. Peak ventricular wall stress occurs during the first third of systole; at the end-systole, ventricular wall stress is about half of the peak value.

Echocardiography can be used to noninvasively measure meridional and circumferential wall stress. Meridional stress acts on the long axis of the left ventricular; the circumferential stress acts on the short-axis of the LV. The shape of the ventricle, which changes throughout the cardiac cycle, affects wall stress. In patients with heart failure, the shape of the left ventricle is spherical. In a spherical model, meridional stress equals circumferential stress. The normal left ventricle resembles the ellipsoid model in which circumferential stress at the end of systole is 2.57 times higher than meridional stress (25). In a dilated failing heart, the left ventricle gradually begins to resemble a sphere, and the meridional and circumferential stress gradually equalize.

Meridional wall stress can be measured with two-dimensional echocardiography using the method that has been validated with angiography (26).

$$\sigma_m \ (dynes/cm^2) = \frac{1.35 \times P \ (LVID)}{4h \ (1 + h/LVID)}$$

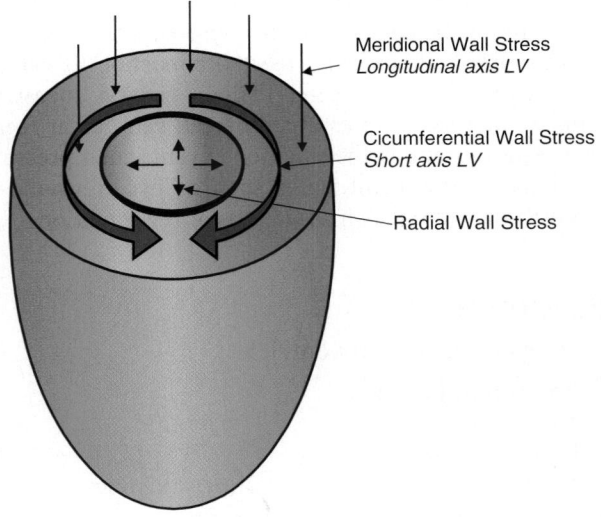

**FIGURE 10.23.** Illustration of the three components of wall stress.

$\sigma_m$, end-systolic meridional wall stress

P, pressure in the LV at the end of systole

LVID, LV internal diameter

h, end-systolic posterior wall thickness

1.35 is the factor to convert the blood pressure from millimeters of mercury to dynes/cm$^2$

Reichek and colleagues (27) used the same equation but substituted systolic blood pressure for LV pressure. When they simultaneously measured pressure using a noninvasive blood pressure cuff and an invasive LV micronometer catheter, they found that the two pressures strongly correlated (r = 0.89). Transthoracic echocardiography using M-mode was used to measure the thickness (h) of the posterior wall. End-systolic stress derived from a noninvasive blood pressure cuff correlated extremely well with stress measured invasively (r = 0.97). The mean value of meridional stress calculated from their study was $64.8 \pm 19.5 \times 10^3$ dynes/cm$^2$.

Meridional wall stress can also be calculated using two-dimensional echocardiography recordings with the formula:

$$\sigma_m(\text{dynes/cm}^2) = 1.33 \times \frac{\text{BP}_{\text{syst}}(\text{A}_m)}{\text{A}_c} \times 10^3$$

$\text{A}_c$

$\text{A}_c$ = Left ventricular cavity area in the short-axis view

$\text{A}_m$ = Myocardial area

$\text{BP}_{\text{syst}}$ = systolic blood pressure

The value for meridional wall stress was slightly higher ($86 \pm 16 \times 10^3$ dynes/cm$^2$) compared to that found with the M-mode (25).

Ventricular wall stress varies throughout the cardiac cycle; end-systolic wall stress indicates afterload. Given the complexity of the calculation this approach has not been widely adopted clinically. Furthermore most of the validation studies were done using TTE. In general, measurements of wall stress to estimate overall ventricular function are most useful in the situation of ventricular pressure or volume predominant states such as hypertension, or with valvular lesions such as stenosis or regurgitation.

### KEY POINTS

TEE exam of the left ventricle

* Four-chamber view
* Two-chamber view
* Long-axis view
* Transgastric midpapillary short-axis view
* Transgastric two-chamber view

Normal anatomy and physiology

* Normal anatomy
* Phases of ventricular systole
* Physiology of left ventricular systolic function

Ejection phases of left ventricular performance

* Cardiac output
* Ejection fraction
* Fractional area change

Isovolumic phases of left ventricular performance

* Doppler-derived dP/dt

Load independent indices of ventricular function

* Pressure area relationships
* Maximal elastance
* Preload recruitable stroke work

Tissue Doppler imaging

* Tissue velocity
* Strain rate imaging
* Strain analysis

Left ventricular filling pressure

* Interatrial septum
* Pulmonary vein flow

Preload

* Area length method
* Modified Simpson's method
* LV EDA

Afterload
End-systolic meridional wall stress

## REFERENCES

1. Gorcsan J, 3rd. Tissue Doppler echocardiography. Current Opinion in Cardiology. 2000;15(5):323–9.
2. Muhiudeen IA, Kuecherer HF, Lee E, Cahalan MK, Schiller NB. Intraoperative estimation of cardiac output by transesophageal pulsed Doppler echocardiography. Anesth 1991; 74(1):9–14.
3. Darmon PL, Hillel Z, Mogtader A, Mindich B, Thys D. Cardiac output by transesophageal echocardiography using continuous-wave Doppler across the aortic valve. Anesth 1994;80(4): 796–805;discussion 25A.
4. Perrino C, Harris S, Luther M. Intraoperative determination of cardiac output using multiplane transesophageal echocardiography. Anesthesia 1998;89:350–7.
5. Clements FM, Harpole DH, Quill T, Jones RH, McCann RL. Estimation of left ventricular volume and ejection fraction by two-dimensional transesophageal echocardiography: comparison of short axis imaging and simultaneous radionuclide angiography. Br J Anaesth 1990;64(3):331–6.
6. Urbanowicz JH, Shaaban MJ, Cohen NH, et al. Comparison of transesophageal echocardiographic and scintigraphic estimates of left ventricular end-diastolic volume index and ejection fraction in patients following coronary artery bypass grafting. Anesth 1990;72(4):607–12.

7. Bargiggia G, et al. A new method for estimating left ventricular dp/dt by continuous wave doppler echocardiography. Validation study at cardiac catheterization. Circulation 1989:80: 1287–92.

8. Kolias TA, Armstrong KD, Armstrong WF. Doppler-derived dP/dt and –dP/dt predict survival in congestive heart failure. J Am Coll Cardiol 2000;36(5):1594–9.

9. Gorcsan J 3rd, Gasior TA, Mandarino WA, Deneault LG, Hattler BG, Pinsky MR. Assessment of the immediate effects of cardiopulmonary bypass on left ventricular performance by on-line pressure-area relations. Circulation 1994;89(1): 180–90.

10. Gulati VK, Katz WE, Follansbee WP, Gorcsan J 3rd. Mitral annular descent velocity by tissue Doppler echocardiography as an index of global left ventricular function. Am J Cardiol 1996;77(11):979–84.

11. Urheim S, Edvardsen T, Torp H, Angelsen B, Smiseth OA. Myocardial strain by Doppler echocardiography. Validation of a new method to quantify regional myocardial function. Circulation 2000;102(10):1158–64.

12. Swan HJ, Ganz W, Forrester J, Marcus H, Diamond G, Chonette D. Catheterization of the heart in man with use of a flow-directed balloon-tipped catheter. N Engl J Med 1970;283 (9):447–51.

13. Kusumoto FM, Muhiudeen IA, Kuecherer HF, Cahalan MK, Schiller NB. Response of the interatrial septum to transatrial pressure gradients and its potential for predicting pulmonary capillary wedge pressure: an intraoperative study using transesophageal echocardiography in patients during mechanical ventilation. J Am Coll Cardiol 1993;21(3):721–8.

14. Orihashi K, Goldiner PL, Oka Y. Intraoperative assessment of pulmonary vein flow. Echocardiography 1990;7(3): 261–71.

15. Nishimura RA, Abel MD, Hatle LK, Tajik AJ. Relation of pulmonary vein to mitral flow velocities by transesophageal Doppler echocardiography. Effect of different loading conditions. Circulation 1990;81(5):1488–97.

16. Klein AL, Tajik AJ. Doppler assessment of pulmonary venous flow in healthy subjects and in patients with heart disease. J Am Soc Echocardiogr 1991;4(4):379–92.

17. Kuecherer HF, Muhiudeen IA, Kusumoto FM, et al. Estimation of mean left atrial pressure from transesophageal pulsed Doppler echocardiography of pulmonary venous flow. Circulation 1990;82(4):1127–39.

18. Kinnaird TD, Thompson CR, Munt BI. The deceleration [correction of declaration] time of pulmonary venous diastolic flow is more accurate than the pulmonary artery occlusion pressure in predicting left atrial pressure. J Am Coll Cardiol 2001;37(8):2025–30.

19. Nagueh SF, Middleton KJ, Kopelen HA, Zoghbi WA, Quinones MA. Doppler tissue imaging: a noninvasive technique for evaluation of left ventricular relaxation and estimation of filling pressures. J Am Coll Cardiol 1997;30(6): 1527–33.

20. Kim Y, Sohn D. Mitral annulus velocity in the estimation of left ventricular filling pressure: prospective study in 200 patients. J Am Soc Echocardiography 2000;13:980–5.

21. Smith M, et al. Value and limitation of transesophageal echocardiography in determination of left ventricular volumes and ejection fraction. JACC 1992;19(6):1213–22.

22. Cheung AT, Savino JS, Weiss SJ, Aukburg SJ, Berlin JA. Echocardiographic and hemodynamic indexes of left ventricular preload in patients with normal and abnormal ventricular function. Anesth 1994;81(2):376–87.

23. Reich DL, Konstadt SN, Nejat M, Abrams HP, Bucek J. Intraoperative transesophageal echocardiography for the detection of cardiac preload changes induced by transfusion and phlebotomy in pediatric patients. Anesth 1993;79(1):10–5.

24. Leung JM, Levine EH. Left ventricular end-systolic cavity obliteration as an estimate of intraoperative hypovolemia. Anesthesiology 1994;81(5):1102–9.

25. Douglas PS, Reichek N, Plappert T, Muhammad A, St John Sutton MG. Comparison of echocardiographic methods for assessment of left ventricular shortening and wall stress. J Am Coll Cardiol 1987;9(4):945–51.

26. Grossman W, Jones D, and Mc Laurin L. Wall stress and patterns of hypertrophy in the human left ventricle. J Clin Invest 1975;56(14).

27. Reichek N, Wilson J, St John Sutton M, Plappert TA, Goldberg S, Hirshfeld JW. Noninvasive determination of left ventricular end-systolic stress: validation of the method and initial application. Circulation 1982;65(1):99–108.

## QUESTIONS

1. All of the following indicate elevated left ventricular filling volumes *except*:
   A. Rightward bowing of the interatrial septum in midsystole.
   B. Blunting of the systolic component of the pulmonary vein flow velocity spectral display.
   C. Pulmonary vein flow systolic fraction < 40%.
   D. E/Ea ratio >10.
   E. Leftward bowing of the interatrial septum in midsystole.

2. Comprehensive exam of left ventricular systolic function include all the following views *except*:
   A. Midesophageal two-chamber view
   B. Midesophageal four-chamber view
   C. Midesophageal long-axis view
   D. Transgastric midpapillary short-axis view
   E. The deep transgastric long-axis view

3. All of the following statements regarding left ventricular wall stress is true *except*:
   A. Meridional wall stress can be calculated using noninvasive BP and myocardial area measured in M-mode.
   B. Meridional wall stress acts on the long axis of the left ventricle.
   C. Circumferential wall stress acts on the long axis of the left ventricle.
   D. In the normal ventricle, circumferential stress at the end of systole is 2.57 times higher than meridional stress.
   E. In the dilated ventricle, circumferential to radial wall stress ratio at the end of systole is 1.

4. Which of the following statements regarding pulmonary vein flow is false?
   A. Tachycardia can cause the systolic and diastolic waveform to fuse.
   B. In patients with atrial fibrillation, diastolic flow is the main contributor to left atrial filling.
   C. With low left atrial pressure, the biphasic nature of the systolic waveform becomes more prominent.
   D. The pulmonary S wave corresponds to the Y descent of the left atrial filling pressure tracing.

5. All of the following statements regarding measurements of stroke volume and cardiac output are true *except*:
   A. Cross-sectional area can be calculated by measuring the LVOT diameter in the midesophageal long-axis view.

B. Cross-sectional area can be calculated by measuring the length of each side of the aortic valve seen in the aortic valve short-axis view.

C. The transgastric long-axis view can be used to obtain the spectral envelope for measuring the velocity time integral used in the stroke volume calculation.

D. The spectral envelope, used to measure the velocity time integral, obtained from the pulmonary artery is equivalent to that from the aorta in the transgastric long-axis view.

# Assessment of Right Ventricular Function

## Gautam Sreeram, Rebecca A. Schroeder, and Jonathan B. Mark

In the past, greater emphasis was placed on descriptive indices of left ventricular function than right ventricular function. In fact, the right ventricle (RV) was often viewed as a simple passive conduit contributing little to overall cardiac performance. More recently, realization of the importance of RV function in maintaining hemodynamic stability has led to a closer examination of the RV.

The asymmetric shape of the RV precludes characterization using simple geometric formulae and complicates assessment of global RV function. Consequently, assessment of RV size and function requires multiple approaches and techniques. Over the past number of years, measurement of RV volume has progressed from simple cross-sectional area planimetry to real-time, three-dimensional echocardiographic renderings of chamber volume (1).

The isovolumic phases of the cardiac cycle are shorter for the RV than for the left ventricle (LV). As a result, while onset of left ventricular contraction normally occurs prior to the onset of right ventricular contraction, RV ejection begins earlier, lasts longer, and has a reduced ejection velocity and a later peak compared with LV ejection. Right ventricular ejection results primarily from inward motion of the RV free wall with smaller contributions from contraction of the RV outflow tract and descent of the base of the heart (2). Right ventricular contraction can be described in terms of movements along major and minor axes, which play an important role in the calculation of some indices of RV function (3).

## STRUCTURE AND FUNCTION OF THE RIGHT VENTRICLE

The RV is an asymmetric, complex chamber, which normally appears crescent shaped in short-axis cross section. The RV medial wall is formed by the ventricular septum that it shares with the LV. The RV free wall may be divided into basal, mid, and apical segments corresponding to the adjacent left ventricular segments in the long-axis,

four-chamber view. Trabeculae carnae or muscle bundles line most of the inner RV chamber (Fig. 11.1).

Right ventricular anatomy may also be described in terms of its inflow and outflow tracts, which reflect the separate embryologic origins of these portions of the RV. The RV inflow tract begins at the tricuspid valve and is located posteroinferiorly, while the anterosuperiorly positioned RV outflow tract leads to the pulmonic valve and pulmonary artery. An encircling muscular ring separates the inflow and outflow portions of the RV and is composed of four distinct muscular bands: the parietal band, crista supraventricularis, septal band, and moderator band (4). Of these, the moderator band is of considerable importance to the echocardiographer. This structure appears as a prominent muscular trabeculation extending from the lower ventricular septum to the RV free wall, and it must not be mistaken for an abnormal intracardiac mass or thrombus.

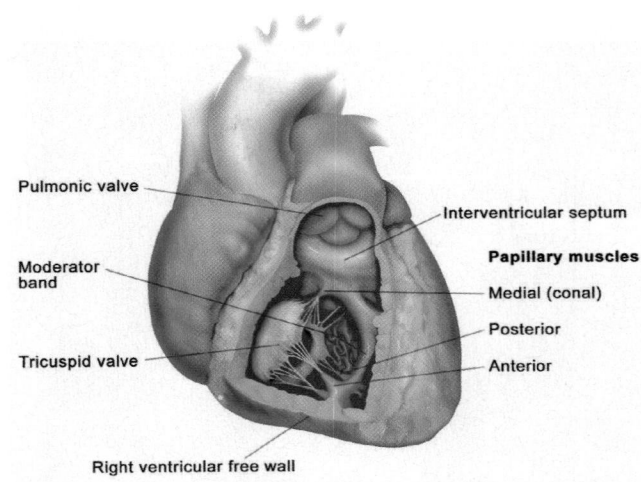

**FIGURE 11.1.** Anatomic drawing of the right ventricle with major structures labeled.

The RV has other distinctive anatomic features that distinguish it from the LV. The inflow RV is heavily trabeculated with the trabeculae carneae, while the outflow RV, or infundibulum, is smoother walled. The papillary muscles that support the tricuspid valve via chordae tendineae are more variable in location and size in the RV compared to the mitral valve support structures. The anterior papillary muscle to the tricuspid valve, which arises from the moderator band, is the only papillary muscle commonly identified during routine transesophageal echocardiography (TEE).

## TRANSESOPHAGEAL ECHOCARDIOGRAPHIC IMAGING OF THE RIGHT VENTRICLE

Because of its unique geometry, multiple images of the RV are required for accurate structural and functional assessment. The most useful TEE scan planes for RV examination include the midesophageal four-chamber view, midesophageal RV inflow-outflow view, transgastric mid short-axis view, and transgastric RV inflow view.

The midesophageal four-chamber view is the single most useful view for assessing overall RV anatomy and global function, and allows evaluation of the apex, mid, and basal segments of this ventricle. In the four-chamber view, the RV appears triangular compared to the elliptical LV and its length extends to only two-thirds of the length of the LV. As a result, the LV, not the RV, normally forms the cardiac apex (Fig. 11.2).

The midesophageal RV inflow-outflow view is sometimes termed the "wrap-around view," because the right atrium (RA), RV, and pulmonary artery (PA) appear to encircle the aortic valve and left atrium, circumscribing a

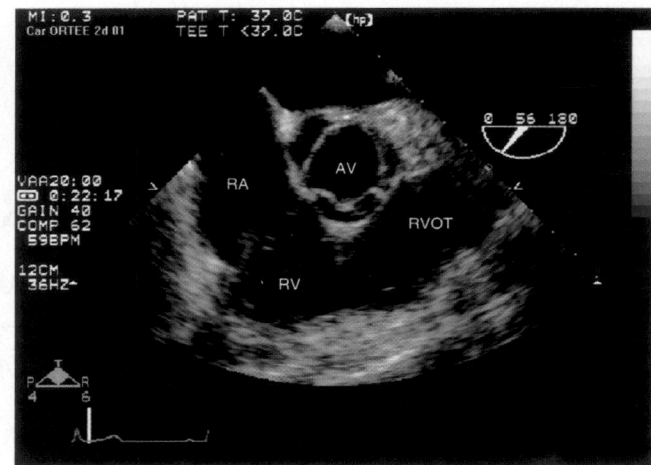

**FIGURE 11.3.** Midesophageal right ventricular inflow-outflow view with right atrium (RA), right ventricle (RV), right-ventricular outflow tract (RVOT), and aortic valve (AV) labeled.

180° to 270° arc (Fig. 11.3). This view is particularly helpful for assessing motion of the RV free wall.

The transgastric mid short-axis view may be obtained in the horizontal scan plane with the TEE probe inserted approximately 35–40 cm from the incisors, with the tip flexed to achieve a true short-axis view. Slight clockwise (rightward) probe rotation will center the RV in the image screen. While this view is used most often to monitor LV function, it also allows assessment of the RV free wall and ventricular septum (Fig. 11.4).

Finally, the transgastric RV inflow view provides a long-axis view of the RV similar to the transgastric two-chamber view of the LV. To acquire this view, begin with the transgastric mid short-axis view of the RV (described above) and advance the multiplane angle to approximately 90° or

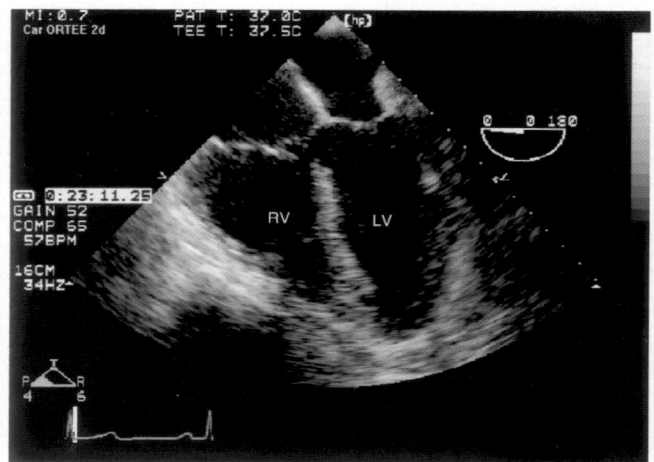

**FIGURE 11.2.** Midesophageal four–chamber view of the right ventricle (RV), left ventricle (LV), right atrium, and left atrium.

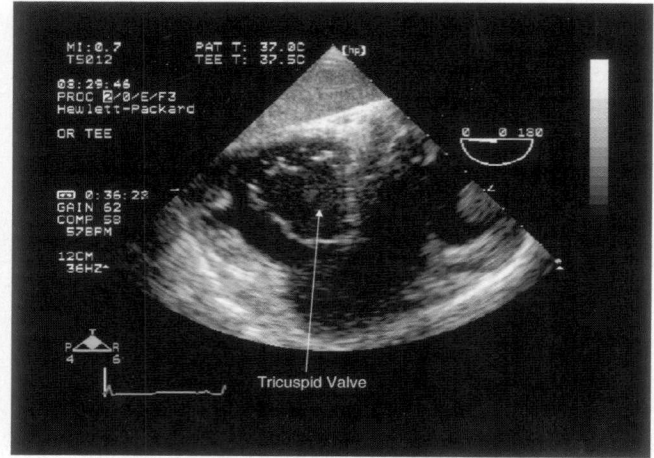

**FIGURE 11.4.** Transgastric mid short-axis view of right ventricle with tricuspid valve seen in cross-section.

until the RA and RV are seen in long axis, with the RV inflow and tricuspid valve centered in the image. Alternatively, one develops the transgastric two-chamber view of the left atrium and ventricle and then rotates the probe clockwise (rightward) until the two right-sided chambers are displayed. Both techniques allow one to obtain the same image of the RV inflow tract and the long axis of the right atrium and ventricle (Fig. 11.5).

Other TEE views may be used to supplement these four standard views in patients who have abnormal RV anatomy and function. The midesophageal long-axis view includes a portion of the RV outflow tract, and often the pulmonic valve can be seen anterior to the aortic valve (Fig. 11.6). The transgastric RV outflow view provides an image with many of the same structures seen in the

midesophageal RV inflow-outflow view, including the RA, RV, PA, and both tricuspid and pulmonic valves (Figs. 11.7a and 11.7b). Not only used for anatomic imaging, this view allows calculation of cardiac output from measurements of the RV outflow tract dimensions and the corresponding blood flow velocity. This view is acquired beginning with the transgastric mid short-axis view, advancing the multiplane angle to approximately 110–140°, and with slight clockwise (rightward) rotation of the TEE probe. Finally, the deep transgastric RV apical view provides an image similar to the deep transgastric long-axis view, but focused instead on the RV, tricuspid valve, and RA (Fig. 11.8). This view is acquired by slight clockwise (rightward) rotation of the probe from the deep transgastric long-axis view.

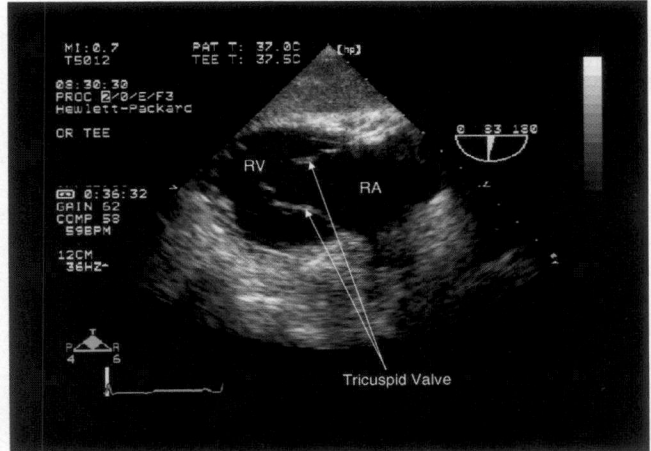

**FIGURE 11.5.** Transgastric RV inflow view with tricuspid valve leaflets clearly seen in open position.

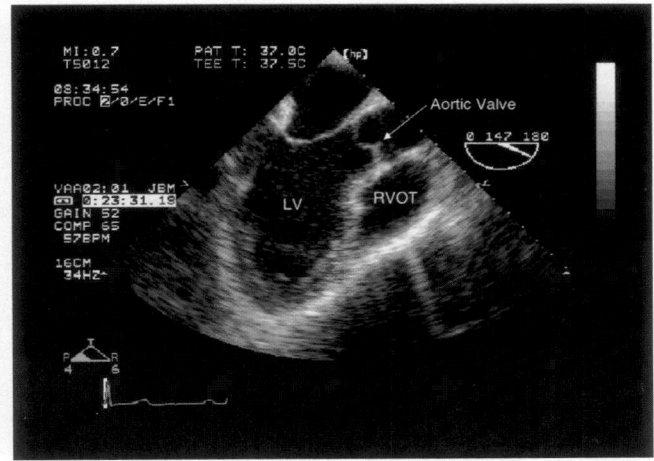

**FIGURE 11.6.** Midesophageal long-axis view of the left ventricle (LV), with the right ventricular outflow tract (RVOT) visible to the right side.

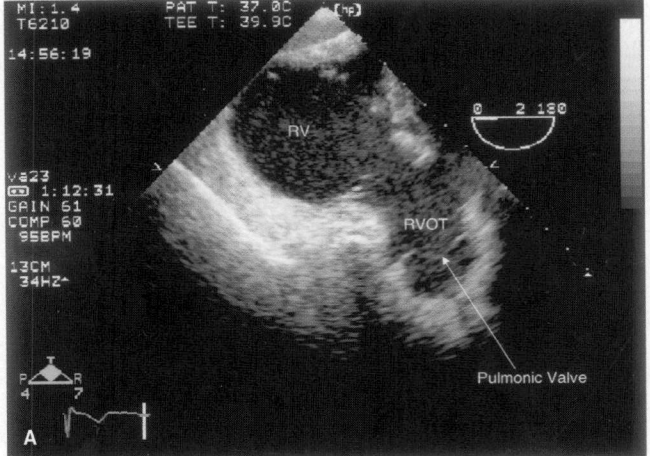

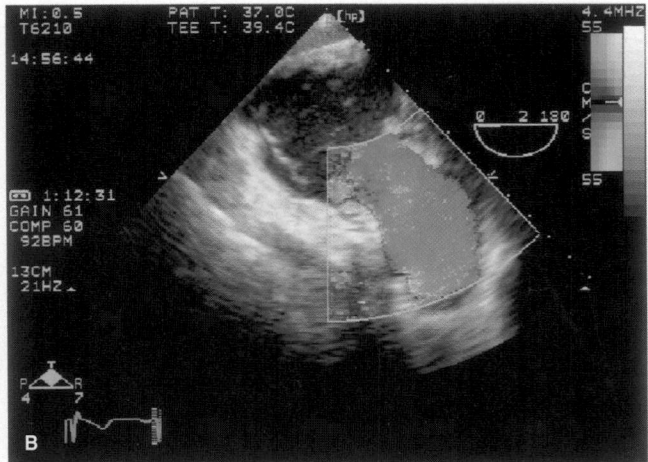

**FIGURE 11.7.** Transgastric right ventricular outflow view with the pulmonic valve visible in the far field, without **(A)** and with **(B)** color-flow Doppler.

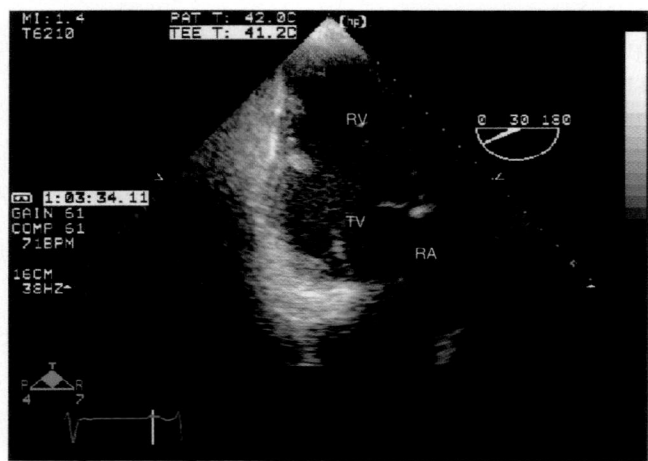

**FIGURE 11.8.** Deep transgastric view of the right ventricle (RV) with the tricuspid valve and right atrium (RA) visible.

## RIGHT VENTRICULAR GLOBAL SYSTOLIC FUNCTION—QUANTITATIVE ECHOCARDIOGRAPHIC ASSESSMENT

Assessment of global right ventricular function includes measurements of RV volume and ejection fraction. Because of the irregular shape of the RV, acquisition of multiple images may be necessary to fully define chamber size and shape. A number of quantitative techniques have been described to measure RV volume and function. First, maximal short-axis and mid short-axis measurements of RV chamber size can be made in a single-plane with normal measurements being 3.5+/−0.2 cm and 2.8+/−0.2 cm, respectively (Fig. 11.9) (3). Second, application of the multiplane method or modified Simpson's rule can be used to determine RV volume (5). Third, in-

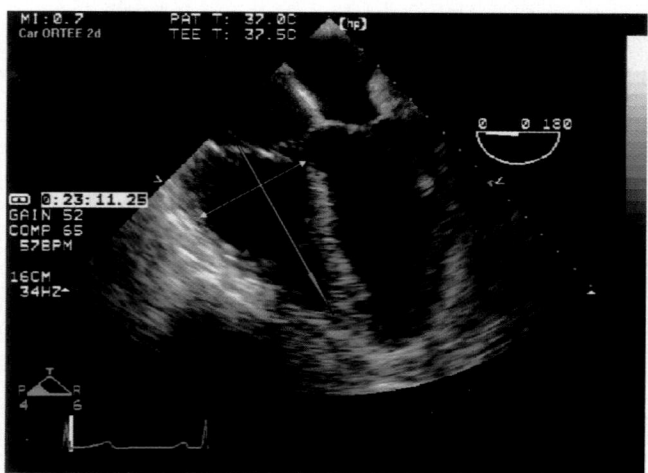

**FIGURE 11.9.** Measurement of RV chamber size: maximal short-axis (*yellow*) and mid short-axis (*blue*) distances measured perpendicular to the long axis of the right ventricle (*green*).

vestigators have estimated RV volume from summation of smaller geometric volumes using models of an ellipsoid, a prism, and a pyramid (6–8). Fourth, right ventricular end-diastolic and end-systolic measurements can be measured by planimetry, and a fractional area change (FAC) ejection fraction calculated where FAC = [(end-diastolic area − end-systolic area)/end-diastolic area] × 100 (9). Fifth, echocardiographic automated border detection allows measurements of the right ventricular cavity area, and the derived end-systolic pressure area and volume relations may be used to assess RV function (10). Finally, three-dimensional echocardiography is being used to determine if more accurate, repeatable estimates of cardiac size can be obtained when compared to conventional two-dimensional imaging (1,11). Given the complexity and potential inaccuracies in all of these methods, quantitative assessment of RV volume is rarely performed in clinical TEE practice.

Because many of the echocardiographic methods described above are cumbersome to use in the operating room, other means of quantifying RV function have been investigated. One method focuses on the unique anatomy of the RV and its pattern of systolic motion. During ventricular systole, long-axis shortening is created by motion of both atrioventricular valve annulae toward the cardiac apex. Because the septal attachment of the tricuspid annulus is relatively fixed, the majority of tricuspid annular motion occurs in its lateral aspect. This gives the motion of the tricuspid annulus a hinge-like appearance, moving more laterally than medially. This motion contrasts with that of the mitral annulus, which has a more symmetrical or piston-like appearance during systole. Tricuspid annular plane systolic excursion (TAPSE) describes this long-axis systolic excursion of the lateral aspect of the tricuspid annulus, and it has been validated as a useful additional measure of global RV systolic function (Figs. 11.10a and 11.10b). Measurement of TAPSE can be expressed as an absolute value (cm or mm) or as a maximal major-axis shortening fraction. Normal TAPSE is 20–25 mm toward the cardiac apex, which is slightly greater than normal mitral annular plane systolic excursion (12). Compared with radionuclide right ventricular ejection fraction as the reference method for assessing global RV function, TAPSE has been found to correlate more closely (r = 0.92) than percent change in RV area during systole (r = 0.81) (13, 14).

## RIGHT VENTRICULAR HYPERTROPHY AND DILATATION

Global evaluation of RV function should include an assessment of the presence or absence of hypertrophy and/or dilatation. Right ventricular hypertrophy results from pressure overload of the ventricle, and common causes include pulmonic valve stenosis and pulmonary hypertension from mitral stenosis or other causes. Right ventricular free wall

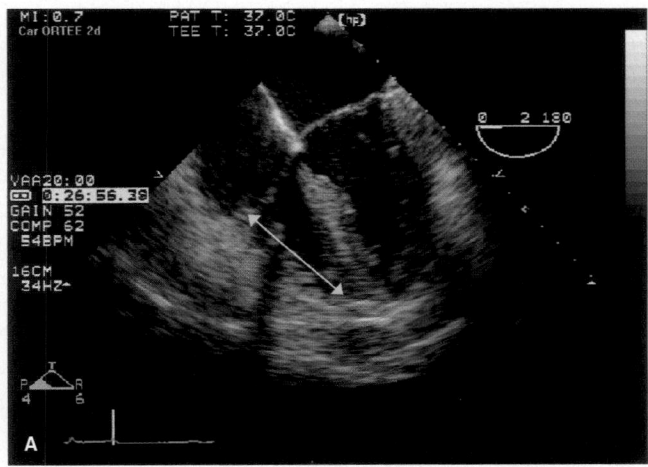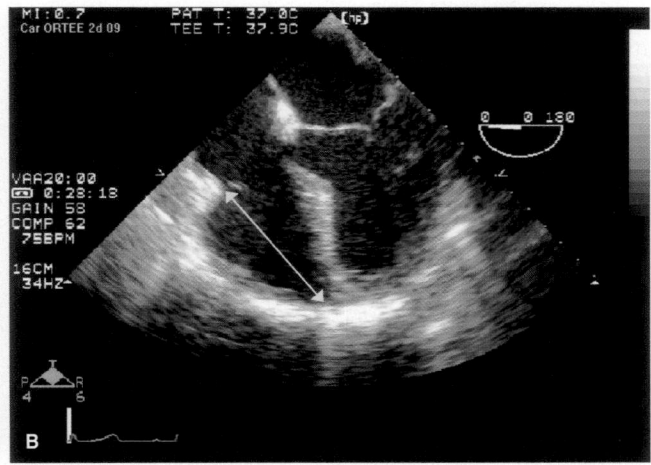

**FIGURE 11.10.** Measurement of tricuspid annular plane systolic excursion (TAPSE), measured during systole **(A)** and diastole **(B)**.

thickness is measured to determine the presence of hypertrophy. Normal RV free wall thickness is less than half that of the LV and measures < 5 mm at end diastole (2), and RV hypertrophy is present when the thickness exceeds 5 mm (15). The diagnosis of mild RV hypertrophy is difficult and confounded by the trabeculations that give the endocardial surface of the chamber an uneven appearance. In patients with chronic cor pulmonale, RV wall thickness may exceed 10 mm when severe pulmonary hypertension raises pulmonary artery pressures to systemic levels (Fig. 11.11). Another clue to the presence of significant RV hypertrophy is the intracavitary trabecular pattern, which becomes more prominent, particularly at the apex. In addition to secondary hypertrophy that results from increased RV systolic pressures, increased RV free wall thickness may be caused less commonly by primary myocardial diseases, such as amyloidosis and endocardial fibroelastosis (16).

Right ventricular dilatation occurs with RV volume overload and often develops in patients with chronic pressure overload. An important clue to the presence of RV dilatation may be found through examination of the cardiac apex. Normally, the RV length extends to only two-thirds the length of the LV. Therefore, in the midesophageal four-chamber view, the cardiac apex is formed by the LV. When the RV rather than the LV forms the cardiac apex, the RV is dilated.

The degree of RV enlargement is usually categorized semiquantitatively by comparing the end-diastolic areas of the RV and LV in the midesophageal four-chamber view. With mild RV dilatation, RV end diastolic area is approximately 60%–100% of the LV area. With moderate dilatation, RV area equals LV area, and with severe RV dilatation, the RV cross-sectional area exceeds that of the LV (Fig. 11.12). A final clue to the presence of RV enlargement

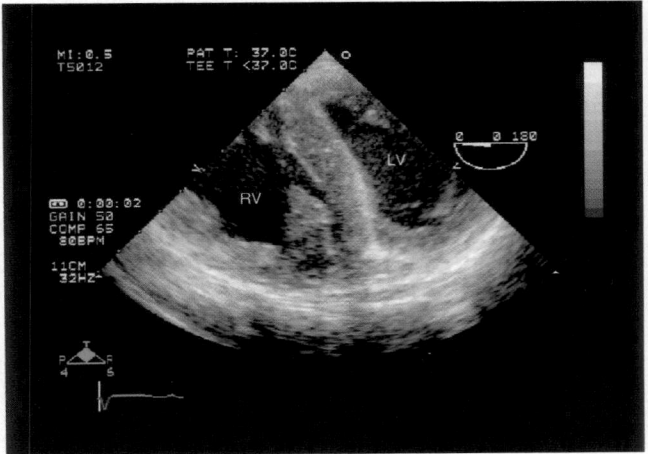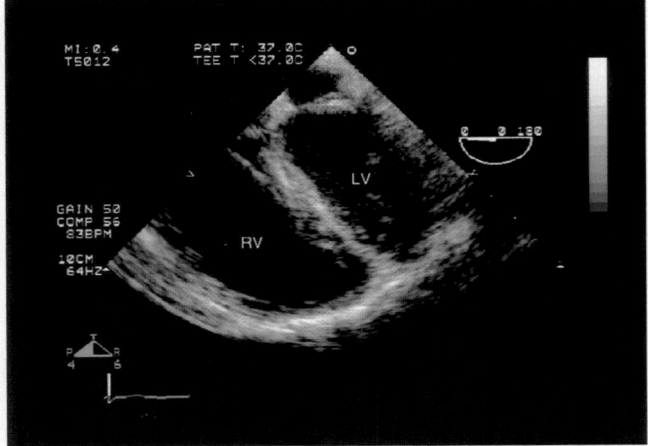

**FIGURE 11.11.** Severe hypertrophy of the right ventricle (RV) with bowing of the interventricular septum into the left ventricle (LV).

**FIGURE 11.12.** Dilation of the right ventricle (RV). Note that the right ventricle fills the apex of the heart displacing the left ventricle (LV).

is gleaned from its shape, because as this chamber dilates, its shape changes from triangular to circular (2,15).

## RIGHT VENTRICULAR SYSTOLIC FUNCTION—QUALITATIVE AND REGIONAL ASSESSMENT

Qualitative assessment of global RV function includes visual assessment of RV end-diastolic and end-systolic areas. Right ventricular free wall excursion and the extent of systolic obliteration of the RV cavity are used as an estimate of RV ejection fraction. Owing to the difficulties in quantitative grading of global RV systolic function, most clinical assessment focuses on these qualitative assessments of chamber size, wall thickness, and systolic function.

One other factor that should be considered during qualitative assessment of RV systolic function is the effect of afterload on RV performance. Because the thin-walled RV is a volume-pumping chamber, its ejection fraction is extremely sensitive to acute increases in PA pressure. In contrast, the thick-walled LV is a pressure-pumping chamber, and its ejection fraction, while influenced by the systemic arterial pressure, is generally preserved despite marked increases in systemic arterial pressure. These hemodynamic factors must be considered for proper interpretation of RV systolic function.

Regional RV function can be impaired when global function remains preserved. This is seen most often in patients with occlusion of the right coronary artery, which provides perfusion to most of the RV except for a small portion of the anterior free wall that may be supplied by the conus branch of the left anterior descending artery (17). The RV is particularly susceptible to injury during cardiac surgery for several reasons. Cardioplegia delivery is often inadequate for RV protection, particularly when retrograde cardioplegia is employed (18), and the anteriorly located RV is more subject to ambient warming from surgical lights. Furthermore, the anterior, nondependent location of the right coronary artery ostium and the proximal anastomotic site of a right coronary artery saphenous vein bypass graft make these favored sites for coronary air or atheromatous embolization.

Compared to assessment of regional LV function, TEE assessment of regional RV function is more difficult, owing both to the relative complexity of RV anatomy and the marked systolic load dependence of RV ejection. Mild degrees of RV hypocontractility are rarely reported, and RV infarction or ischemia is diagnosed only when a portion of the RV free wall is akinetic or dyskinetic (19). Significant RV infarction is typically accompanied by LV inferior wall myocardial infarction, owing to the common right coronary artery blood supply shared by these two portions of the heart (20). Ancillary signs of RV infarction include RA enlargement, RV dilatation, tricuspid regurgi-

tation, and paradoxical ventricular septal motion (21,22). If a patent foramen ovale is present, increases in RA pressure accompanying RV infarction may lead to hypoxemia from right-to-left shunting.

## RIGHT VENTRICULAR OVERLOAD AND THE VENTRICULAR SEPTUM

Examination of the ventricular septum may help distinguish RV volume overload from RV pressure overload. Septal motion is determined primarily by the pattern of myocardial depolarization, the state of musculature contraction, and the pressure gradient between RV and LV. Normally, the LV contains the center of cardiac mass and LV pressures exceed RV pressures throughout the cardiac cycle. Consequently, the ventricular septum functions primarily as part of the LV and maintains a convex curvature toward the RV during systole and diastole. As the RV hypertrophies, the center of myocardial mass moves toward the RV and the ventricular septum flattens. When RV mass exceeds LV mass, paradoxical septal motion appears, with a leftward septal shift that is maximal at end systole and early diastole, corresponding to the time of peak systolic afterloading of the RV (15,23,24). Additional signs of RV pressure overload may include RV dilatation, tricuspid regurgitation from annular dilatation, and RV hypocontractility.

With RV volume overload, diastolic septal distortion and flattening are maximal at end diastole, corresponding to the time of maximal diastolic RV filling (23). During systole, the end-diastolic septal flattening reverses, and there is paradoxical septal motion towards the RV cavity. The abnormal ventricular septal motion caused by RV volume overload should not be confused with the transient abnormality of septal motion that occurs during ventricular pacing. Owing to delayed activation of the LV during RV pacing, a characteristic septal "bounce" may be observed, which reflects the early systolic RV depolarization (25).

## RIGHT VENTRICULAR FUNCTION—HEMODYNAMIC AND DOPPLER ASSESSMENT

Spectral Doppler measurements of right-sided flow patterns can provide important clues to systolic RV function. Measurements of Doppler cardiac output from the RVOT have provided good correlation with thermodilution cardiac output in patients without significant tricuspid valve regurgitation (26). The view of the RVOT required for placement of the pulsed wave sample volume is made by first obtaining the left ventricular mid papillary short-axis view and then rotating the transducer to 110°–140° to obtain a view of the right heart structures.

Hepatic vein flow patterns provide another useful window on right heart filling pressures and global RV systolic function, analogous to the use of pulmonary vein flow patterns to assess LV function. Normal hepatic venous flow patterns have either three or four phasic components (Fig. 11.13). The decline in right atrial pressure during systole results in an initial forward flow toward the RA. This pressure change results from atrial relaxation and apical movement of the tricuspid valve during RV systole and corresponds to the x descent in atrial pressure. A fall in atrial pressure during diastole from early ventricular filling also results in forward caval flow and corresponds to the y descent in atrial pressure. Two small retrograde waves may be seen, one of which results from the end-diastolic atrial contraction. The other small retrograde wave is seen less often, and it appears at end systole, prior to the y descent in RA pressure that drives the forward diastolic hepatic vein flow wave. Impaired RV systolic function is accompanied by a change in the pattern of hepatic vein flow, including blunting of the systolic inflow peak and augmentation of the diastolic inflow peak (27). Alterations in hepatic vein flow patterns following bypass suggest the typically poorer myocardial protection provided for the RV than for the LV (27). In addition, tricuspid regurgitation, which often accompanies systolic RV dysfunction, can obliterate the hepatic vein systolic inflow peak and cause reversed or retrograde systolic flow. (See Chapter 16, Assessment of Tricuspid and Pulmonic Valves.)

In patients with tricuspid regurgitation, continuous wave Doppler can be used to estimate RV systolic pressure, another useful index of right heart function. Measurement of the peak velocity of the tricuspid regurgitant jet allows calculation of the pressure gradient between the RV and RA, which when added to RA pressure, provides

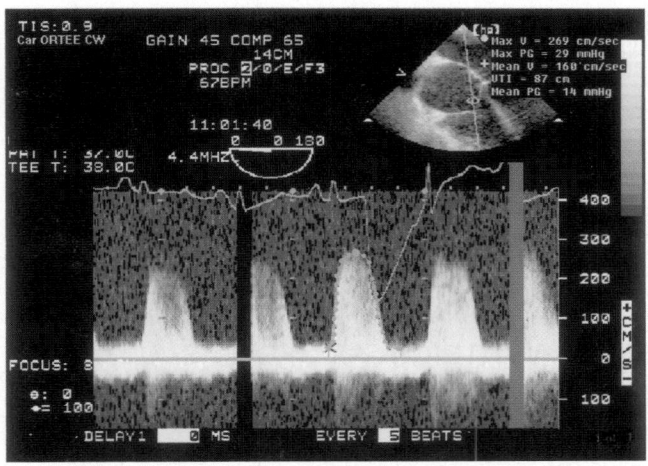

**FIGURE 11.14.** Spectral Doppler analysis of the tricuspid regurgitant jet shows a right ventricular systolic pressure gradient calculation of 29 mm Hg.

an estimate for RV systolic pressure (Fig. 11.14). In the absence of obstruction to RV outflow, this calculated RV systolic pressure provides a good estimate of PA systolic pressure. Because the vast majority of patients with pulmonary hypertension have some degree of tricuspid regurgitation even in the absence of clinical signs, this measurement has widespread application. However, when making this calculation, considerable care must be undertaken to align the ultrasound beam with the regurgitant jet to avoid underestimation of the pressure gradient.

Similarly, PA diastolic pressure can be estimated by using spectral Doppler to measure the end-diastolic velocity of the pulmonic regurgitation jet, which reflects the gradient between the PA and RV at end diastole. This pressure gradient is added to RA pressure to calculate PA diastolic pressure.

Other hemodynamic clues to right heart function can be gleaned from an examination of the inferior vena cava. In spontaneously breathing patients, the inferior vena cava normally changes in size during the respiratory cycle. For example, in a patient with a normal caval diameter (15–25 mm), a decrease in size of at least 50% with inspiration or during an intentional "sniff" indicates that the RA pressure is approximately equal to normal intrathoracic pressures (5–10 mm Hg) (15).

## RIGHT VENTRICULAR DIASTOLIC FUNCTION

Measurements used to assess RV diastolic filling are similar to those used for LV diastolic filling. Velocity inflow patterns across the tricuspid valve to assess E and A velocities can be examined. As with the LV, impaired relaxation of the RV results in a decreased E wave and tall A

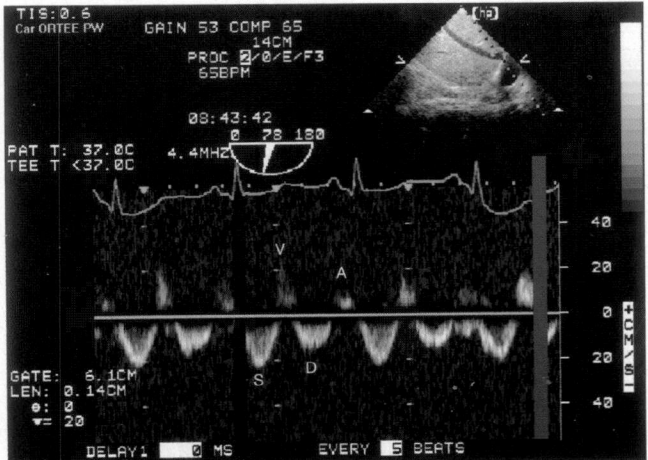

**FIGURE 11.13.** Normal hepatic venous flow patterns with the waves labeled: S, systolic; D, diastolic; V, ventricular; A, atrial.

wave, while restrictive RV physiology results in a tall E wave and small A wave. Because the tricuspid annulus is larger than the mitral annulus and the duration of tricuspid inflow is longer than the time for mitral inflow, the maximal velocities of RV (tricuspid) inflow are lower than the corresponding values for LV inflow (28). Normal values for tricuspid inflow velocities measured by chest wall echocardiography are 0.41 +/− 0.08 m/sec, E wave peak velocity and 0.33 +/− 0.08 m/sec, A wave peak velocity (29).

## RIGHT VENTRICULAR DYSPLASIA

Right ventricular dysplasia is an idiopathic cardiomyopathy in which adipose or collagenous tissue replaces right ventricular myocardium. The right ventricular wall may be of normal thickness or thinned. Reported symptoms and signs include heart murmurs, congestive heart failure, recurrent ventricular tachycardia, and sudden death, particularly in young individuals with a familial predisposition to the disease (30). Echocardiographic features may include isolated or predominant right ventricular dilatation and wall motion abnormalities (hypokinesis or akinesis). When left ventricular involvement is present, a reduced LV ejection fraction will be seen.

### KEY POINTS

- Evaluation of RV function is complicated by the unique anatomy of the RV.
- Techniques to assess RV function may include planimetry of RV chamber sizes, calculation of TAPSE, examination of pulmonary artery flow, assessment of wall motion abnormalities, and calculation of pulmonary artery pressures.
- Examination of ventricular septal motion is useful in distinguishing RV volume overload from RV pressure overload. In RV volume overload, maximal septal distortion occurs at end diastole, while RV pressure overload produces maximal septal distortion at end systole and early diastole, corresponding to the time of peak systolic loading of the RV.
- Signs of RV infarction include akinesis or dyskinesis of the RV, RA enlargement, RV dilatation, tricuspid regurgitation, and paradoxical ventricular septal motion.

## REFERENCES

1. Ota T, Fleishman CE, Strubb M, et al. Real-time, three-dimensional echocardiography: feasibility of dynamic right ventricular volume measurement with saline contrast. Am Heart J 1999;137:958–66.
2. Jiang L, Wiegers SE, Weyman AE. Right ventricle. In: Weyman AE, ed. Principles and practices of echocardiography. Philadelphia: Lea and Febiger, 1994:901–21.
3. Bommer W, Weinert L, Neumann A, et al. Determination of right atrial and right ventricular size by two-dimensional echocardiography. Circulation 1979;60:91–100.
4. Netter FH. The Ciba Collection of Medical Illustrations, Vol. 5, Heart. Ciba Pharmaceutical Co. 1978, p. 9.
5. Pandis IP, Ren J, Kotler MN, et al. Two-dimensional echocardiographic estimation of right ventricular ejection fraction in patients with coronary artery disease. J Am Coll Cardiol 1986;57:811–5.
6. Graham TP, Jarmakani JM, Atwood GF, Canent RV. Right ventricular volume determinations in children. Circulation 1973;47:144–53.
7. Benchimol A, Desser KB, Hastreiter AR. Right ventricular volume in congenital heart disease. Am J Cardiol 1975;36:67–75.
8. Ferlinz J, Gorlin R, Cohn PF, Herman MV. Right ventricular performance in patients with coronary artery disease. Circulation 1975;52:608–15.
9. Davila-Roman VG, Waggoner AD, Hopkins WE, Barzilai B. Right ventricular dysfunction in low output syndrome after cardiac operations: assessment by transesophageal echocardiography. Ann Thorac Surg 1995;60:1081–6.
10. Oe M, Gorcsan J, Mandarino WA, et al. Automated echocardiographic measures of right ventricular area as an index of volume and end-systolic pressure-area relations to assess right ventricular function. Circulation 1995;92:1026–33.
11. Vogel M, White PA, Redington AN. In vitro validation of right ventricular volume measurement by three-dimensional echocardiography. Br Heart J 1995;74:460–3.
12. Hammerstrom E, Wranne B, Pinto FJ, et al. Tricuspid annular motion. J Am Soc Echocardiography 1991;14:131–9.
13. Kaul S, Tei C, Hopkins JM, Shah PM. Assessment of right ventricular function using two-dimensional echocardiography. Am Heart J 1984;107:526–31.
14. Mishra M, Swaminathan M, Malhotra R, Mishra A, Trehan N. Evaluation of right ventricular function during CABG: transesophageal echocardiographic assessment of hepatic venous flow versus conventional right ventricular performance indices. Echocardiography 1998;15:51–8.
15. Otto CM. Echocardiographic evaluation of left and right ventricular systolic function. In: Otto CM, ed. Textbook of clinical echocardiography. Philadelphia: W.B. Saunders Company, 2000:100–31.
16. Child JS, Krivokapich J, Abbasi AS. Increased right ventricular wall thickness on echocardiography in amyloid infiltrative cardiomyopathy. Am J Cardiol 1979;44:1391–5.
17. Wilson BC, Cohn JN. Right ventricular infarction: clinical and pathophysiologic considerations. Ann Intern Med 1988;33:295–309.
18. Christakis GT, Fremes SE, Weisel RD, et al. Right ventricular dysfunction following cold potassium cardioplegia. J Thorac Cardiovasc Surg 1985;90:243–51.
19. D'Arcy B, Nanda NC. Two-dimensional echocardiographic features of right ventricular infarction. Circulation 1982;65:1967–73.
20. Oh JK, Seward JB, Tajik AJ. The Echo Manual (1st ed). Boston: Little, Brown and Company, 1994:82–3.
21. Sharkey SW, Shelley W, Carlyle PF, Rysavy J, Cohn JN. M-mode and two-dimensional echocardiographic analysis of the septum in experimental right ventricular infarction: correlation with hemodynamic alterations. Am Heart J 1985;110:1210–8.
22. Judgutt BI, Sussex BA, Sivaram CA, Rossall RE. Right ventricular infarction: two-dimensional echocardiographic evaluation. Am Heart J 1984;107:505–15.
23. Louie EK, Rich S, Levitsky S, Brundage BH. Doppler echocardiographic demonstration of the differential effects of right ventricular pressure and volume overload on left ventricular geometry and filling. J Am Coll Cardiol 1992;19:84–90.

24. Jardin F, Dubourg O, Bourdarias J-P. Echocardiographic pattern of acute cor pulmonale. Chest 1997;111:209–17.
25. Little WC, Reeves RC, Arciniegas J, Katholi RE, Rogers EW. Mechanism of abnormal interventricular septal motion during delayed left ventricular activation. Circulation 1982;65:1486–91.
26. Maslow A, Comunale ME, Haering JM, Watkins J. Pulsed wave Doppler measurement of cardiac output from the right ventricular outflow tract. Anesth Analg 1996;83:466–71.
27. Nomura T, Lebowitz L, Koide Y, et al. Evaluation of hepatic venous flow using transesophageal echocardiography in coronary artery bypass surgery: an index of right ventricular function. J Cardiothorac Vasc Anesth 1995;9:9–17.
28. Feigenbaum H. Echocardiography (4th ed). Philadelphia: Lea and Febiger, 1986: 157–66.
29. Sidebotham D, Merry A, Legget M. Practical perioperative echocardiography. Philadelphia: Butterworth-Heinemann, 2003: 250.
30. Kullo IJ, Edwards WD, Seward JB. Right ventricular dysplasia: the Mayo Clinic experience. Mayo Clin Proc 1995;70:541–8.

## QUESTIONS

1. In patients with right ventricular volume overload, ventricular septal displacement toward the left ventricle is maximal at which point in the cardiac cycle?
   A. End-diastole
   B. End-systole
   C. Mid-diastole
   D. Mid-systole
   E. Early-diastole

2. Which of the following structures is located in the right ventricle?
   A. Chiari network
   B. Crista terminalis
   C. Eustachian valve
   D. Moderator band
   E. Thebesian valve

3. Which of the following transesophageal echocardiographic scan planes allows visualization of the right ventricular outflow tract?
   A. Bicaval view
   B. Deep transgastric right ventricular apical view
   C. Midesophageal four-chamber view
   D. Midesophageal long-axis view
   E. Transgastric mid short-axis view

4. Which of the following diagnoses is most likely in a patient whose transesophageal echocardiogram shows a 5 mm tricuspid annular plane systolic excursion?
   A. Patent foramen ovale
   B. Pulmonic regurgitation
   C. Right ventricular hypertrophy
   D. Right ventricular infarction
   E. Tricuspid regurgitation

5. Which of the following echocardiographic signs would be expected in a patient with right ventricular dilatation?
   A. Cardiac apex formed by both the right and left ventricles
   B. Exaggerated hepatic vein antegrade systolic inflow wave
   C. Prominent apical muscular trabeculations
   D. Right ventricular cross-sectional area equal to 50% of the left ventricular cross-sectional area
   E. Tricuspid valve leaflet prolapse

# Assessment of Regional Ventricular Function

## *Lori B. Heller and Solomon Aronson*

Assessment of global and regional ventricular function has become the cornerstone for evaluating patients with ischemic heart disease. The dynamic assessment of regional ventricular function is based on echocardiographic derived indices of muscle contraction and relaxation, which are obtained from analysis of moving objects. Echocardiography is therefore an inherently qualitative technique. When using transesophageal echocardiography (TEE) to evaluate regional ventricular function one is really attempting to make inferences about a three-dimensional structure from two-dimensional images. Therefore, multiple images must be acquired from multiple planes and assumptions (explicitly or implicitly) must be made about the shape of the ventricle and the coronary artery distribution within the ventricle.

## SEGMENTAL MODEL OF THE LEFT VENTRICLE

Dividing the LV into segments allows more accurate description of the location of the regional wall motion abnormalities (RWMA) detected with echocardiography and is necessary for their correlation with coronary artery anatomy. Models developed during the era of single plane TEE are based on the transgastric midpapillary short-axis view of the LV and divide the midpapillary image of the LV into four equal segments: septal, anterior, lateral, and inferior. Although simple, there is no true correlation with coronary artery anatomy and the base and the apex are not taken into account. The Society of Cardiovascular Anesthesiology and American Society of Echocardiography has recommended a 16-segment model for regional LV assessment, dividing the basal and mid levels into six segments and the apex into four (Fig. 12.1). An advantage of using this segmental model is a common standard and terminology in discussions about regional function of the LV.

Regional function assessment of the LV can be accomplished quickly and easily in most patients using multi-plane TEE by obtaining five standard views of the LV, three from the midesophageal window and two from the transgastric window (Fig. 12.1).

The first step in obtaining the midesophageal views of the LV is to position the transducer posterior to the left atrium (LA) at the mid level of the mitral valve. The imaging plane is then oriented to simultaneously pass through the center of the mitral annulus and the apex of the LV. In many patients, the esophagus is lateral to this point and the tip of the probe must be flexed to the right to position the transducer directly posterior to the center of the mitral annulus. The LV is usually oriented with its apex somewhat more inferior to the base and the tip of the probe must next be retroflexed to direct the imaging plane through the apex. Getting the proper amount of retroflexion is best done by rotating to multiplane angle 90 degrees and then retroflexing until the apex of the LV is pointing straight down in the image display. The depth should be adjusted to include the entire LV (usually 16 cm). Rotating to multiplane angle 0 degrees should keep the center of the mitral annulus and LV apex in view. The midesophageal four-chamber view is now obtained by rotating the multiplane angle forward from 0 degrees until the aortic valve is no longer in view and the diameter of the tricuspid annulus is maximized, usually between 10 and 30 degrees. The midesophageal four-chamber view shows all three segments (basal, mid, and apical) in each of the septal and lateral walls (Figs. 12.2 and 12.3). The midesophageal two-chamber view can next be obtained by rotating the multiplane angle forward until the right atrium (RA) and the right ventricle (RV) disappear, usually between 90 and 110 degrees. The midesophageal two-chamber view of the LV shows the three segments in each of the anterior and inferior walls (Figs. 12.4 and 12.5). Finally, the midesophageal long-axis view is developed by rotating the multiplane angle forward until the LV outflow tract, aortic valve, and the proximal ascending aorta come into view, usually between 120 and 160 degrees (Figs. 12.6 and 12.7). This view shows the basal and midanteroseptal seg-

*(text continues on page 160)*

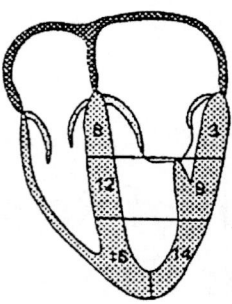
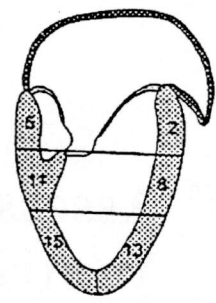

a. four chamber view　　b. two chamber view

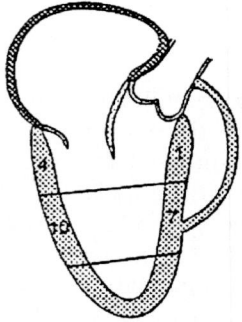
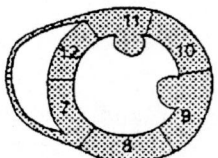

d. mid short axis view

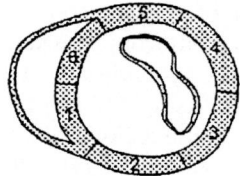

c. long axis view

e. basal short axis view

| Basal Segments | Mid Segments | Apical Segments |
|---|---|---|
| 1= Basal Anteroseptal | 7= Mid Anteroseptal | 13= Apical Anterior |
| 2= Basal Anterior | 8= Mid Anterior | 14= Apical Lateral |
| 3= Basal Lateral | 9= Mid Lateral | 15= Apical Inferior |
| 4= Basal Posterior | 10= Mid Posterior | 16= Apical Septal |
| 5= Basal Inferior | 11= Mid Inferior | |
| 6= Basal Septal | 12= Mid Septal | |

**FIGURE 12.1.** Sixteen-segment model for regional left ventricular assessment. The basal and mid levels are each divided into six segments and the apex into four.

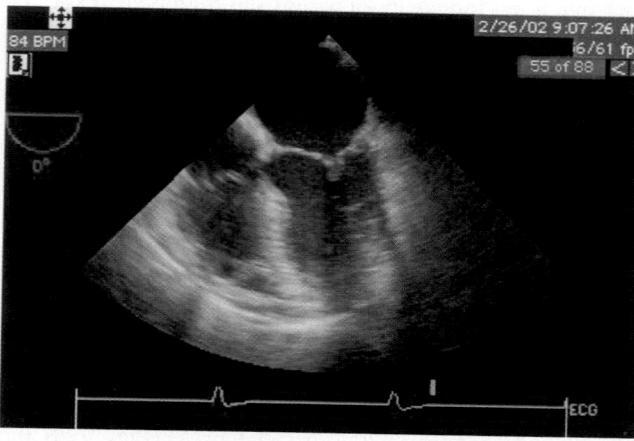

**FIGURE 12.2.** Four-chamber view (obtained at 0–10 degrees) showing the basal, mid, and apical portions of the septal and lateral walls (left and right, respectively).

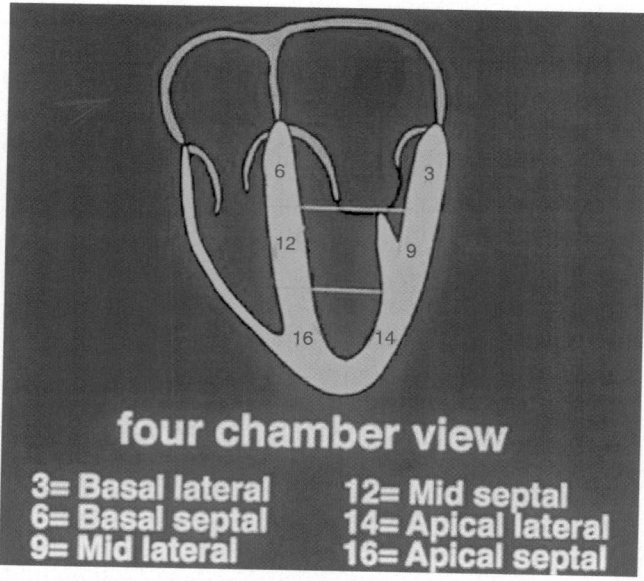

four chamber view

3= Basal lateral　　12= Mid septal
6= Basal septal　　14= Apical lateral
9= Mid lateral　　16= Apical septal

**FIGURE 12.3.** Septal and lateral left ventricular walls according to the 16-segment model.

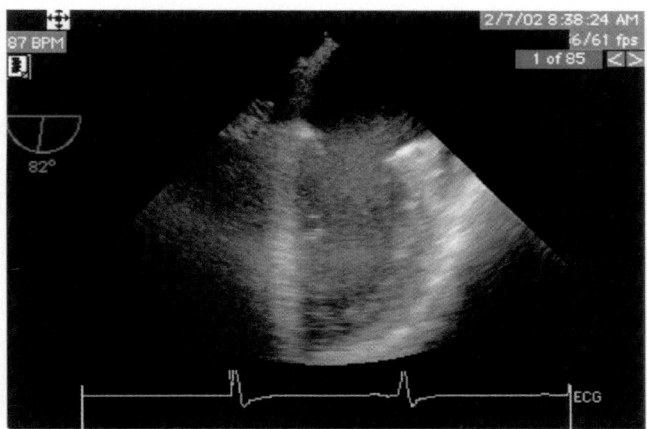

**FIGURE 12.4.** Two-chamber view (obtained at 90–110 degrees) showing the basal, mid, and apical portions of the inferior and anterior walls (left and right, respectively).

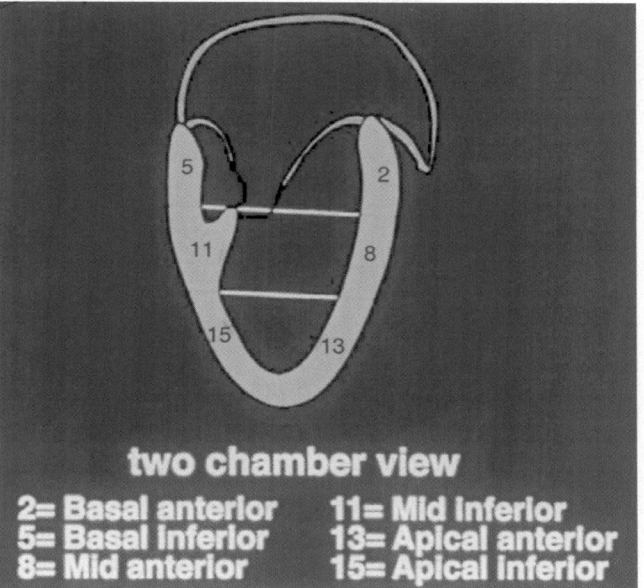

**FIGURE 12.5.** Inferior and anterior left ventricular walls according to the 16-segment model.

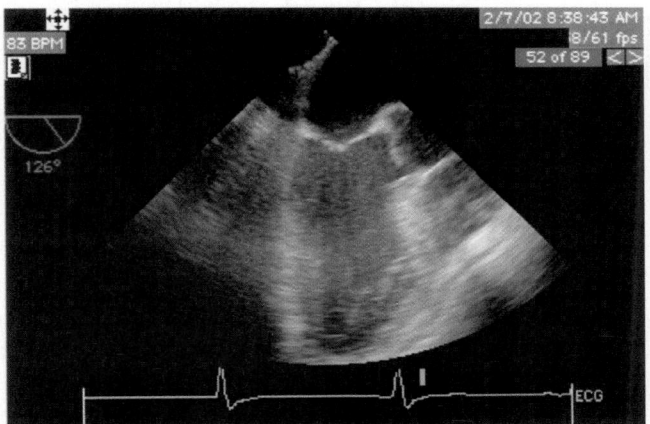

**FIGURE 12.6.** Long-axis view of the left ventricle (obtained at 120–160 degrees) showing the basal, mid, and apical portions of the posterior and anteroseptal walls (left and right, respectively).

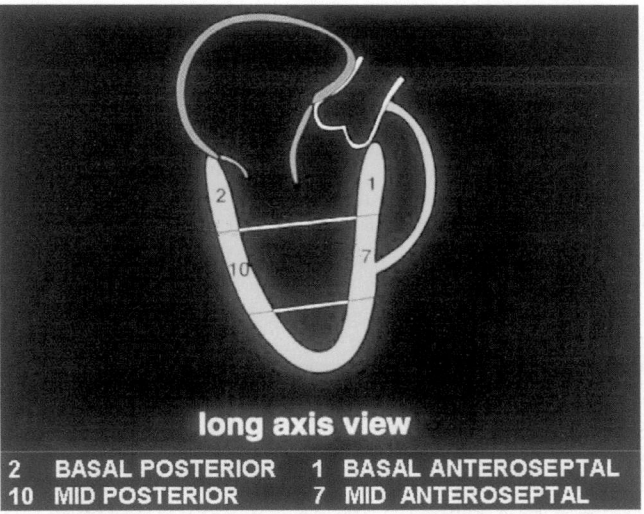

**FIGURE 12.7.** Long-axis view diagram.

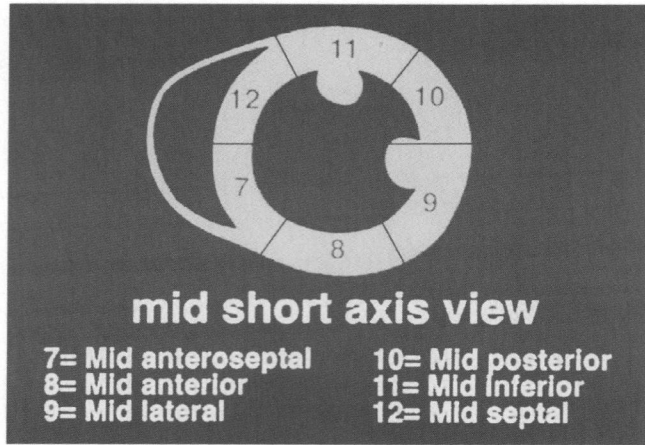

**mid short axis view**

| | |
|---|---|
| 7= Mid anteroseptal | 10= Mid posterior |
| 8= Mid anterior | 11= Mid inferior |
| 9= Mid lateral | 12= Mid septal |

*FIGURE 12.8.* Posterior and anteroseptal walls of the left ventricle according to the 16- segment model.

ments, as well as the basal and midposterior segments. Therefore, with the imaging plane properly oriented through the center of the mitral annulus and the LV apex, one can examine the entire LV without moving the probe and simply rotating the multiplane angle from 0 to 180 degrees.

The transgastric views of the LV are acquired by advancing the probe into the stomach and anteflexing the tip until the heart comes into view. At multiplane angle 0 degrees a short axis of the LV should appear and the probe is then turned to the right or left as needed to center the LV in the display. The depth should be adjusted to include the entire LV, usually 12 cm (Figs. 12.8 and 12.9). There are three levels of transgastric views: basal, where the mitral valve is seen; mid, at the level of the papillary

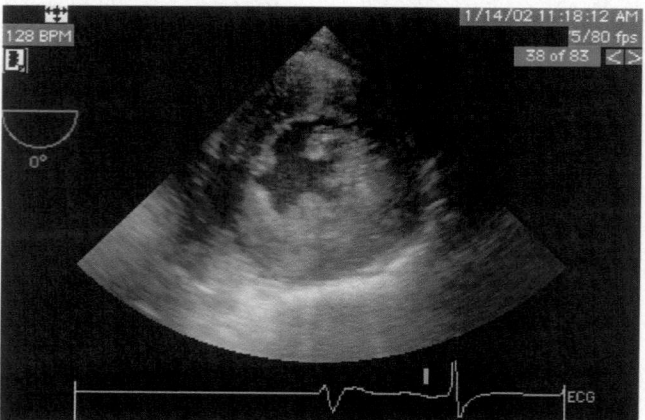

*FIGURE 12.9.* Transgastric short-axis view of the mid portion of the left ventricle. This view is useful for its demonstration of LV preload, as well as for showing portions of the LV supplied by all three of the main coronary arteries.

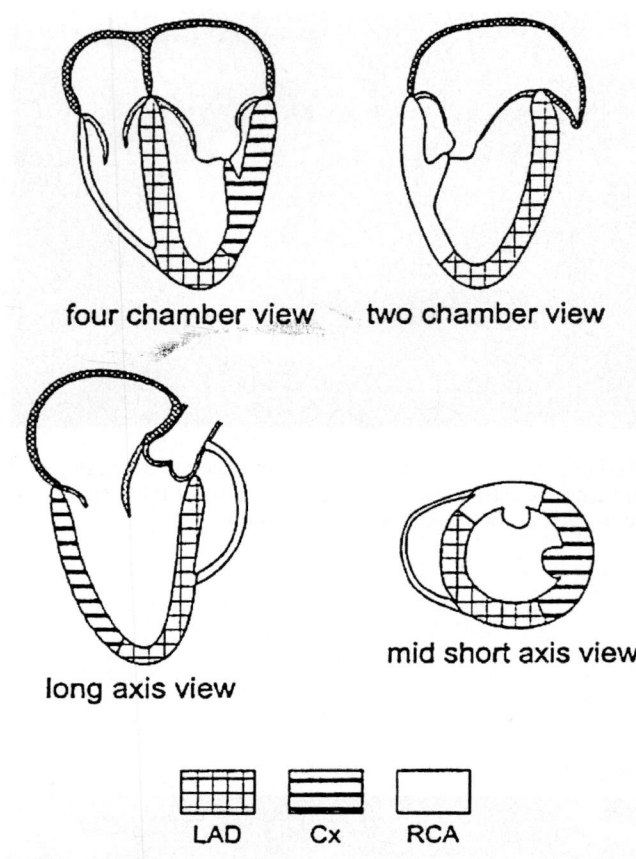

**four chamber view    two chamber view**

**long axis view          mid short axis view**

LAD        Cx        RCA

*FIGURE 12.10.* Short-axis view of the left ventricle according to the 16-segment model.

muscles; and apical. These transverse short-axis views have the advantage of simultaneously showing portions of the LV supplied by the right, circumflex, and the left anterior descending coronary arteries (Figs. 12.10 and 12.11). The midpapillary level, which reveals the approximate center of the left ventricular cavity, is used to determine information regarding the cardiac function and volume status of the patient. Withdrawing the probe from the midpapillary view until the mitral apparatus develops the basal transgastric short-axis view (Fig. 12.11). In some patients, advancing the probe from the mid position develops the apical transgastric short-axis view, but in many the probe moves away from the heart and the image is lost.

The transgastric two-chamber view is developed from the basal transgastric short-axis view by rotating the multiplane angle forward until the apex and the mitral annulus come into view, usually close to 90 degrees (Figs. 12.12 and 12.15). The probe should be turned to the left or right as needed to open up the LV chamber, maximizing its size in the image. This view usually shows the basal and mid segments of the inferior walls, but not the apex.

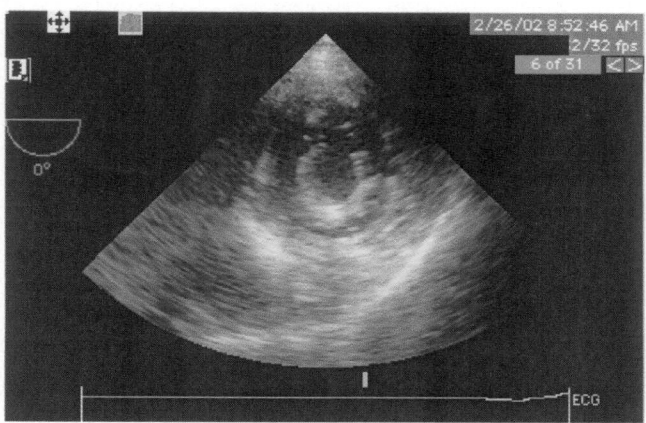

**FIGURE 12.11.** Basal transgastric short-axis view. This view is obtained by withdrawing the probe from the midpapillary short-axis view until the mitral valve comes into view. When looking at this image, the anterior mitral valve leaflet is to the left (toward the RV) and the posterior to the right (toward the lateral wall) of the LV chamber.

When assessing wall motion, it is important to recognize two artifacts of imaging that can occur with any real-time tomographic imaging technique, such as echocardiography: *foreshortening* and *pseudothickening*. Foreshortening occurs when the imaging plane is not correctly aligned along the axis of the chamber being examined, creating an image that is shorter than the true length. With TEE this most commonly occurs at the apex of the LV (Fig. 12.14). Pseudothickening occurs when the heart moves from side to side through the imaging plane, creating the illusion of a change in wall thickness (Fig. 12.15). In order to accurately assess wall motion and thickness, the imaging plane must be perpendicular to the region of the LV being examined.

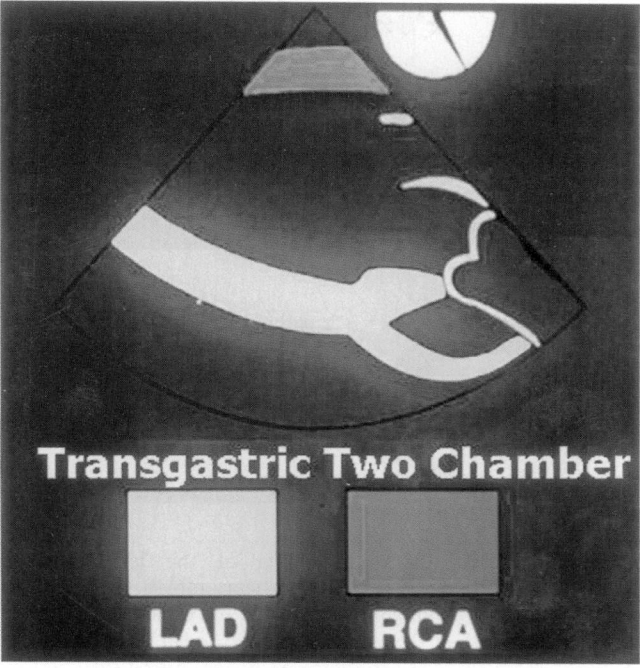

**FIGURE 12.13.** Transgastric two-chamber view illustrating the coronary blood flow pattern.

In current clinical practice, analysis of LV segmental function is based on a qualitative visual assessment of the motion and/or thickening of a segment during systole. Regional wall motion is characterized by observing the movement of the endocardium during systole. As the myocardial oxygen supply-to-demand balance worsens, graded regional wall motion abnormalities progress from mild hypokinesia to severe hypokinesia, akinesia, and finally dyskinesia (1,2). The following qualitative grading

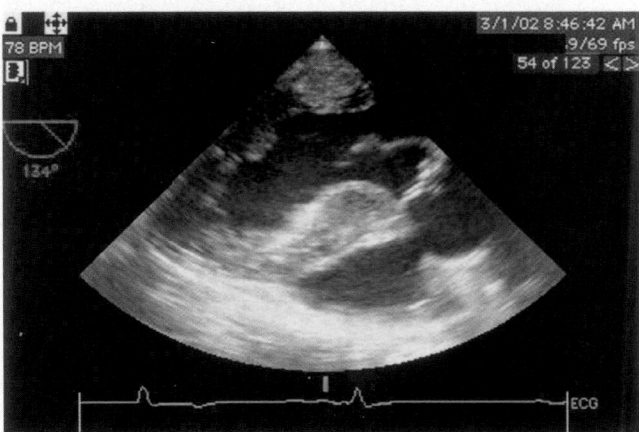

**FIGURE 12.12.** Transgastric two-chamber view. This view is developed by rotating the probe to 85–110 degrees from the basal transgastric short-axis view. This inferior wall is closest to the probe. Opposite from that is the anterior wall.

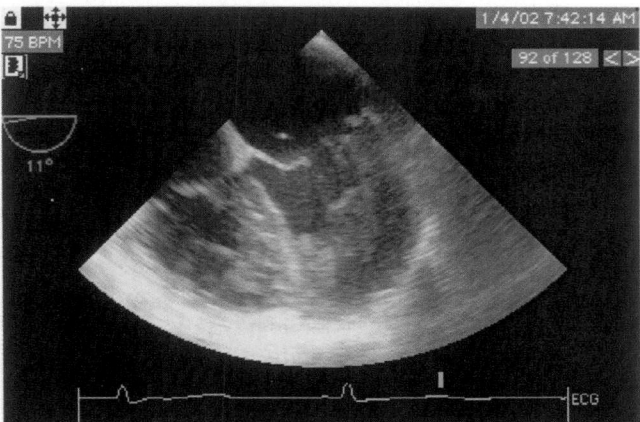

**FIGURE 12.14.** Four-chamber view demonstrating foreshortening of the LV apex. Foreshortening occurs when the imaging plane is not correctly aligned along the axis of the chamber being examined.

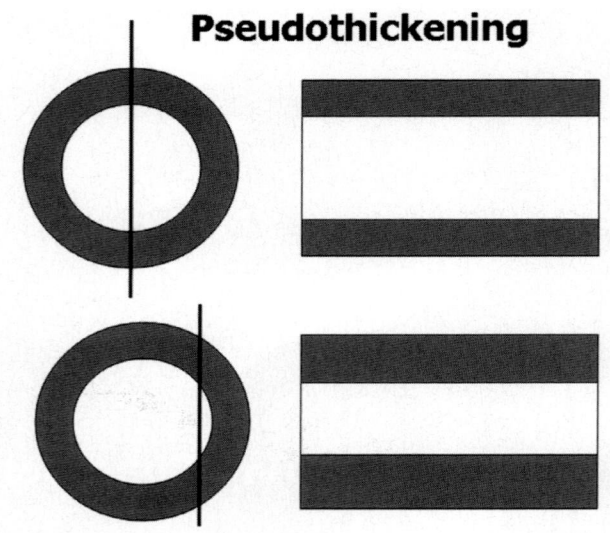

**FIGURE 12.15.** Pseudothickening of the left ventricle. Pseudothickening occurs when the heart moves from side to side through the imaging plane, creating the illusion of a change in wall thickness.

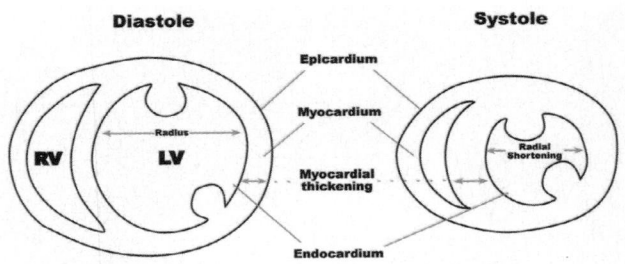

**FIGURE 12.16.** Illustration of LV radial shortening and LV thickening.

scale for wall motion has been used extensively in the intraoperative echocardiography literature and is recommended: 1 = normal, or the endocardium moves toward the center of the LV cavity during systole greater than 30%; 2 = mildly hypokinetic, or the endocardium moves toward the center of the LV cavity < 30%, but greater than 10% during systole; 3 = severely hypokinetic, or the endocardium moves toward the center of the LV cavity but < 10% during systole; 4 = akinetic, or he endocardium does not move or thicken; and 5 = dyskinetic, or the endocardium moves away from the center of the LV cavity during systole (Fig. 12.16 and 12.17). All 16 segments are examined by obtaining five cross-sectional views of the LV, three through the midesophageal window and two through the transgastric window.

## REGIONAL VENTRICULAR FUNCTION AND ISCHEMIA DETECTION

Although new onset of RWMA is the most common way of detecting myocardial ischemia using echocardiography, there are many other important echocardiographic features that are seen in ischemic heart disease. These include abnormal relaxation or diastolic dysfunction, mitral insufficiency with normal mitral valve anatomy, dilation of the ventricle, thin-walled myocardium, and papillary muscle dysfunction. The usefulness of echocardiography for ischemia detection should be based on all findings and not just limited to detection of RWMA. Nev-

ertheless, the relationship of RWMA to ischemia has been compared to changes that occur with surface electrocardiography (ECG), pulmonary capillary wedge pressure (PCWP), and the onset of chest pain. As early as 1935 it was recognized by Tennet and Wiggers that acute myocardial ischemia results in abnormal inward motion and thickening of the affected myocardial region (2). Since then wall motion abnormalities have been shown to occur within seconds of inadequate blood flow or oxygen supply (3). These abnormal contraction patterns typically occur at the same time as regional lactate production (4,5).

The precise sequence of regional functional changes that occurs in the myocardium after interruption of flow has been studied in models of acute ischemia, including percutaneous transluminal coronary angioplasty (6–8). Ischemia of the heart produces a number of changes in mechanical and electrical activity. When ischemia starts, one of the first changes that occurs is abnormal relax-

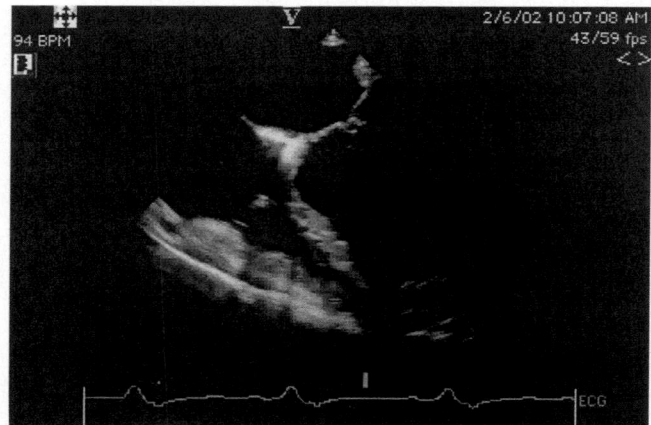

**FIGURE 12.17.** In this four-chamber, midesophageal view the lateral wall thickens and moves towards the center of the ventricle. The apical-septal wall remains still or akinetic, while the basal-septal wall is dyskinetic, moving out towards the right ventricle.

ation of the segment involved. This is followed by a decrease in the systolic function as evidenced by a decrease in wall thickening and decrease in inward motion of the ventricular walls. As the ischemia progresses, the myocardial segment involved will progress from decreased motion (hypokinetic) to the total absence of motion (akinesis). In its most severe form, the segment involved not only fails to contract but cannot withstand the increase in pressure in the ventricle and moves away from the segments that are contracting (dyskinetic). Systolic function is estimated qualitatively and is reflected echocardiographically by regional wall thickening and wall motion during systole. Systolic wall thickening can be calculated from the equation: PSWT = SWT − DWT/SWT × 100, where PSWT = percentage systolic wall thickening, SWT = end systolic wall thickness, and DWT = end diastolic wall thickness.

When evaluating regional wall changes, one must be aware of other factors that influence the movement of the heart as seen on echocardiography. In addition to the inward movement of the walls during systole, the heart is affected by translational and rotational movements. Respiration tends to displace the heart and is an example of translational movement. Translational movement also occurs with the cardiac cycle, for example, displacement of the apex during systole. In the long-axis views, the apex may become foreshortened due to its superior and medial movement. With foreshortening, what appears to be the tip of the heart or apex is really an oblique cut at a higher level and if this is not properly identified, RWMA of the apex can be completely missed. During contraction, the heart tends to rotate along its vertical axis. A way of differentiating rotational movement from regional wall motion is to establish an imaginary point of reference in the center of the ventricle, and observe the movement of the walls towards this central point. Rotational movement will be identified as displacement in a circular fashion in relation to this point instead of displacement towards it.

Clinical studies have indicated that abnormal changes in segmental wall motion occur earlier and are a more sensitive indicator of myocardial ischemia than the abnormal changes detected with an electrocardiogram (4,9–12) or pulmonary artery catheter (13–15). In one study (12), 30 patients undergoing PTCA were simultaneously monitored with twelve-lead electrocardiograms and echocardiography. All the patients had isolated obstructive lesions in their left anterior descending coronary arteries, stable angina, normal baseline electrocardiograms, normal baseline myocardial function with no prior history of infarction and no angiographic evidence of collateralization. In the study, all patients developed segmental wall motion abnormalities (SWMA) approximately 10 seconds after coronary artery occlusion and 27 of the 30

developed repolarization changes in their ECG at approximately 22 seconds.

Smith et al. (11) evaluated 50 patients at high risk for myocardial ischemia during peripheral vascular or cardiac surgery with transesophageal echocardiography (TEE), multilead ECG, and a twelve-lead electrocardiogram. In their study, six patients had repolarization changes diagnostic of ischemia while 24 had new evidence of SWMA. SWMA occurred minutes before ECG changes in three of these six patients and no ST-segment change occurred before or without new SWMA. Three patients who sustained intraoperative myocardial infarctions (MI) developed SWMA in the corresponding area of myocardium, which persisted until the end of surgery, but only one of these three had ischemic ST-segment changes intraoperatively.

The value of pulmonary capillary wedge pressure (PCWP) monitoring for ischemia has also been compared to changes in regional LV function assessed with transesophageal echocardiography. In one study, PCWP, twelve-lead ECG, and left ventricular wall motion were evaluated in 98 patients before coronary artery bypass grafting at predetermined intervals (13). Myocardial ischemia was diagnosed by TEE in 14 patients, and in 10 of the 14 patients ischemia was also detected by repolarization changes on the ECG, while an increase of at least 3 mm Hg in PCWP (an indicator for ischemia) was sensitive only 33% of the time with a positive predictive value of only 16%. Overall, most studies indicate that the sensitivity of wall motion analysis for the detection of myocardial ischemia is generally superior to electrocardiography or pulmonary capillary wedge pressure monitoring.

Although transesophageal echocardiography appears to have many advantages over traditional intraoperative monitors of myocardial ischemia, there remain potential limitations as well. There are various pitfalls that can be encountered in the analysis of wall motion (16). The septum in particular must be given special consideration with respect to wall motion and wall thickness assessment (16–18). The septum is composed of two parts, the lower muscular portion and the basal membranous portion. The basal septum does not exhibit the same degree of contraction as the lower muscular part. At the most superior basal portion, the septum is attached to the aortic outflow track. Its movement at this level is normally paradoxical during ventricular systole. The septum is also a unique region of the left ventricle, because it is a region of the right ventricle as well, and is, therefore, influenced by forces from both ventricles. In addition, sternotomy, pericardiotomy, and cardiopulmonary bypass (CPB) have been suggested to alter the translational and rotational motion of the heart within the chest that may cause changes in ventricular septal motion (18). Consequently, the exact imaging plane for wall motion assessment is critical. The short-axis view of the left ventricle at the level of the midpapillary muscles is used to ensure constant internal landmarks as reference (anterolateral and posteromedial papillary muscles) and to ensure monitoring of the muscular septal region. It must be recognized that although myocardial blood flow from the coronary arteries is best represented at the short-axis, midpapillary muscle level, there may be other myocardial regions that are underperfused and not adequately represented in one echocardiographic imaging plane (19). One solution to this problem is to frequently reposition the probe to view other cross sections of the heart. Another potential problem of wall motion assessment is evaluation of the discoordinated contraction that occurs due to bundle branch block or ventricular pacing. In this situation, the system used to assess SWMA must compensate for global motion of the heart (usually done with a floating frame of reference) and evaluate not only regional endocardial wall motion but myocardial thickening as well.

## REGIONAL VENTRICULAR FUNCTION AND NONISCHEMIA CONDITIONS

Not all SWMA are indicative of myocardial ischemia or infarction (Table 12.1). Clearly, under normal conditions, all hearts 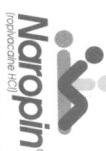 tent mann that most traction p tributable tion to thi artery occlusion. In these models, it is established that myocardial function becomes abnormal in the center of an ischemic zone but it is also true that the myocardial regions adjacent to the ischemic zone become dysfunctional as well. Several studies have reported that the total area of dysfunctional myocardium commonly exceeds the area of ischemic or infarcted myocardium (21,22). The impairment of function in nonischemic tissue has been thought to be caused by a tethering effect. Tethering or the attachment of noncontracting tissue that mechanically impairs contraction in adjacent tissue, which is normally perfused, probably accounts for the consistent overestimation of infarct size by echocardiography when compared to postmortem studies (23). Another limitation of SWMA analysis during surgery is that it does not differentiate stunned or hibernating myocardium from acute ischemia (24), nor does it differentiate the cause of ischemia between increased oxygen demand and decreased oxygen supply. Finally, it should be noted that areas of previous ischemia or scarring may become unmasked by changes in afterload and appear as new SWMA (25).

▶ **TABLE 12.1.** Differential Diagnosis for Regional Wall Motion Abnormalities

| Ischemia |
| --- |
| Infarction |
| Hibernation |
| Stunning |
| Bundle Branch Block |
| Artifact |
| Pacemaker |

Data regarding the significance of intraoperative detection of SWMA suggest that transient abnormalities unaccompanied by hemodynamic or electrocardiographic evidence of ischemia may not represent clinically significant myocardial ischemia and are usually not associated with postoperative morbidity (26). The significance of the severity of SWMA has been studied (3,7). Hypokinetic myocardial segments appear to be associated with minimal perfusion defects compared to significant perfusion defects that accompany akinetic or dyskinetic segments. Hence hypokinesia may be a less predictive marker for postoperative morbidity than akinesis or dyskinesis. Persistent severe SWMA on the other hand are clearly associated with myocardial ischemia and postoperative morbidity (11,27–29).

Intraoperative detection of new or worsened and persistent SWMA during peripheral vascular surgery has been reported to be associated with postoperative cardiac morbidity by several investigators. The occurrence of new segmental wall motion changes during vascular surgery appears to be common (26–29), however, most of the time, transient and clinically insignificant. New segmental wall motion abnormalities that are recognized to persist until the conclusion of surgery on the other hand imply perioperative acute myocardial infarction (11,26–29). Intraoperative wall motion abnormalities, therefore, may be spurious, reversible with or without treatment, or irreversible. The former may be associated with clinically insignificant short periods of ischemia, while the latter is associated with significant ischemia or infarction.

During coronary artery bypass grafting, TEE has helped predict the results of surgery. Following coronary artery bypass grafting to previously dysfunctional segments, immediate improvement of regional myocardial function (which is sustained) has been demonstrated (30, 31). In addition, pre-bypass compensatory hypercontractile segments have been reported to revert toward normal immediately following successful coronary bypass grafting (32). Persistent SWMA following CABG appear to be related to adverse clinical outcomes, while lack of evidence of SWMA following CABG has been shown to be associated with a postoperative course without cardiac morbidity (14).

## ASSESSMENT OF MYOCARDIAL VIABILITY

The perioperative diagnosis of viability after an acute ischemic insult (stunned myocardium) (24) has traditionally been based on clinical signs of an "incomplete" myocardial infarction such as a small creatine phosphokinase leak or non-Q-wave electrocardiographic changes. In patients with chronic coronary artery disease (CAD) who harbor hibernating myocardium (33), evidence of preserved wall thickness (with resting echocardiography) within a hypocontractile region has been a clue to viability. Positron emission tomography (PET) scanning, the gold standard for such assessment, utilizes regional markers of glucose metabolism to demonstrate viability and functional recovery, whereas radionuclear-imaging techniques are predicated on cellular membrane function for perfusion data. Neither PET scanning nor radionuclide imaging techniques however, are practical for intraoperative assessment of viability.

Reversible postoperative ventricular contractile dysfunction that is unrelated to a continuing source of ischemia (i.e., myocardial stunning) has been reported to occur in up to 10% of segments following CABG surgery (34). Identifying ventricular dysfunction caused by inadequate flow remains critical for determining long-term prognosis and perioperative management strategies (Fig. 12.3) (24,35–37). Improvement in regional function after an acute myocardial infarction or ischemic event has been reported to occur up to three weeks after the initial compromising episode, despite adequate restoration of coronary blood flow (24,34). Contractile reserve (the augmented contractile function of a dysynergenic segment) has been demonstrated with dobutamine stress echocardiography (38).

## DOBUTAMINE STRESS ECHOCARDIOGRAPHY (Dse)

Preoperative left ventricular systolic function is among the most powerful predictors of perioperative morbidity and mortality (39) and regional wall motion abnormalities contribute prominently to left ventricular dysfunction (35,40). In patients with coronary artery disease, dysfunctional myocardium at rest may represent either infarcted or viable myocardium (24,33,41). Resting two-dimensional echocardiography, a commonly used imaging modality to detect regional ventricular dysfunction, cannot differentiate acutely dysfunctional but viable myocardium (e.g., stunned myocardium) from chronic but reversibly dysfunctional myocardium (hibernating myocardium) from irreversibly damaged myocardium (infarcted myocardium), because it does not account for coronary blood flow reserve. Because regional left ventricular dysfunction is often reversible and exists in terri-

tories of viable myocardium (30,35,42), provocative testing is necessary to diagnose ischemic and viable segments. Stress echocardiography has emerged as a safe, cost-effective, and sensitive method for the detection of CAD and has been used for risk stratification during the perioperative period (43–45).

Common pharmacologic regimens used during stress echo are dobutamine, dobutamine with atropine, dipyridamole, and adenosine. These techniques have been demonstrated to be safe, with sensitivity and specificity rivaling thallium-201 exercise scintigraphy (46). Of these agents, dobutamine is the most extensively studied. Dobutamine is a racemic mixture of enantiomers with $\alpha 1$, $\beta 1$, and $\beta 2$ effects and a half-life of about 2 minutes (47). The $\alpha 1$ and $\beta 1$ effects are responsible for inotropism independent of endogenous norepinephrine stores (47). The response of regional left ventricular function to dobutamine is useful to characterize myocardial reserve capacity. In the therapeutic dose range (5–20 μg/kg/min) cardiac output is augmented by an increase in ventricular contractility, heart rate, and stroke volume, and a $\beta 2$-mediated decrease in systemic vascular resistance. Contractility increases at higher doses (20–40 μg/kg/min).

Normal resting wall motion and the development of hyperdynamic function with increasing doses of dobutamine are hallmarks of normally perfused myocardium (48–50). The development of new wall motion abnormalities or the worsening of baseline systolic dysfunction with escalating doses of dobutamine indicates myocardial ischemia. Contractile reserve, on the other hand, is consistent with viability and characterized by baseline wall motion abnormalities that improve with low-dose dobutamine (48,49, 51). When such a low-dose augmentation of function is followed by progressive systolic dysfunction with higher doses (biphasic response), the accuracy of predicting postoperative cardiac morbidity or changes in regional function after revascularization is enhanced even further (51). Regional segments that remain akinetic or dyskinetic despite dobutamine infusion are nonviable and likely reflect scar. We often use intraoperative infusion of low-dose dobutamine (prerevascularization) to augment baseline coronary blood flow and assess the changes in regional myocardial function reserve. These changes in function provide a standard to predict regional myocardial flow-function following revascularization (52).

In the left ventricular short-axis view, the left main coronary artery territory typically extends from the anterior septum to the posterolateral wall. The anterior septum and anterior wall typically are perfused by the left anterior descending territory while the lateral and posterior walls are subtended by the circumflex artery territory. The right coronary territory usually includes the inferior wall and posterior septum (Fig. 12.10). Most patients (85%) are right coronary dominant. Dominance is defined by the origin of the blood supply to the inferior surface of the left ventricle. If the circumflex supplies the posterior descending artery, then the system is called left dominant. A codominant system exists if the right coronary artery supplies the posterior descending vessel but provides no further posterolateral branches to the left ventricle.

Dobutamine stress echocardiography has a high sensitivity (82%–85%) and specificity (86%–88%) when compared to angiography in patients with recent myocardial infarction (47,52). A recent review (41) reported that dobutamine echocardiography is slightly more specific than thallium scintigraphy at predicting recovery of regional function after an ischemic event, however sensitivity is slightly less. A possible explanation is that a higher level of myocyte-functional integrity is necessary for demonstration of contractile reserve by dobutamine echo than for evidence of intact membrane function necessary for thallium uptake.

Stress echocardiography has been shown to be an efficient method for risk satisfaction in patients undergoing major vascular surgery (53), and has been used to distinguish hibernating myocardium from nonviable myocardium before coronary revascularization by identifying patients with severe left ventricular dysfunction who had improved regional wall thickening with dobutamine infusion (54).

The application of stress echocardiography intraoperatively allows for online identification of myocardial salvage and viability during coronary revascularization surgery. The ability to intraoperatively differentiate ischemia or infarction of the myocardium from stunning or hibernation of the myocardium can help define the need for revision of the surgical plan or other therapeutic options during coronary bypass surgery, allowing more efficient utilization of resources (such as return to bypass, utilization of a mechanical assist device, or administration of vasoactive drugs).

Barilla et al. (55) reported that patients with viable myocardium treated medically had less recovery of left ventricular systolic function than those who were revascularized. Voci et al. (56) have also shown that microvascular revascularization improves functional outcome. Also of note has been the poor outcome (48% average event rate over 12- to 36-month follow-up periods) seen in patients with viable myocardium when these regions were not revascularized (57,58). The high rate of cardiac events was significantly lower (11%–16%) in patients with viable segments that were revascularized.

## TECHNIQUES TO IMPROVE IMAGE AND ENDOCARDIAL BORDER DETECTION

In order to properly assess regional wall motion and left ventricular function, recognition of the endocardial bor-

der is essential. Automated border detection modalities are based on technology that utilizes machine-derived detection of the tissue-blood interface. Because the difference in amplitude between the integrated backscatter from the myocardium and the blood is so substantial, the machine is able to recognize this border. Analysis of this edge throughout the cardiac cycle can provide information regarding the area, volume, and regional wall motion of the left ventricle (59–62). While this technique eliminates reliance on visual inspection of the endocardial border, most systems are still limited by the quality of the acquired image. An increased echodensity or an artifact in the ventricular cavity can affect the accuracy of this method. Intravenous administration of a contrast agent also enhances endocardial definition. Contrast agents opacify the LV cavity, which allows the border between the blood and the myocardium to be visually identified. In a study by Kornbluth et al., contrast echocardiography was shown to be superior to tissue harmonics in detecting endocardial borders (63).

## KEY POINTS

- *Foreshortening* is a type of imaging artifact that occurs when the transducer beam is not precisely aligned along the long axis of the chamber being imaged. The result is a chamber that appears shorter than its true length and myocardium that is thicker than its true width.
- *Pseudothickening* is another type of imaging artifact and is related to translational movement of the heart and creates the illusion of increased wall thickness.
- The LV is divided into 16 segments, according to guidelines established by the ASE and the SCA. The basal and mid levels of the ventricle are each divided into six segments and the apex is divided into four.
- LV segmental function is graded on a semiquantitative scale of 1 to 5. The numbers correspond to how well the endocardium moves in toward the center of the LV cavity during systole. One represents normal function, or that the endocardium moves in greater than 30%; 2 = mildly hypokinetic, or the endocardium moves < 30%, but > 10%; 3 = severely hypokinetic, or the endocardium moves < 10%; 4 = akinetic, or the endocardium does not move in at all; and 5 = dyskinetic, or the endocardium moves away from the center of the LV cavity during systole.
- There are two principle components to LV regional function: endocardial movement in towards the center of the chamber during systole

and systolic myocardial thickening. A dilated LV cavity, ischemic mitral regurgitation, and LV thrombus offer other indirect clues for ischemia.

- The basal septum is membranous, not muscular, and, therefore, does not exhibit the same degree of contraction as the remaining myocardium.
- While the midpapillary short-axis view of the left ventricle provides a relatively good indicator of overall coronary perfusion and regional wall motion, it must be recognized that not all of the segments are identified in this view. Therefore, one may still have a considerable ischemic area despite normal endocardial motion in this single image.
- New segmental wall motion abnormalities that persist throughout surgery imply perioperative acute myocardial infarction.
- Low-dose dobutamine stress echocardiography can aid in determining areas of limited coronary perfusion and can differentiate between viable and nonviable myocardium.

## REFERENCES

1. Pandian NG, Kerber RE. Two-dimensional echocardiography in experimental coronary stenosis. I. Sensitivity and specificity in detecting transient myocardial dyskinesis: Comparison with sonomicrometers. Circulation 1982;66:597–602.
2. Tennant R, Wiggers CJ. The effect of coronary occlusion on myocardial infarction. Am J Physiol 1935;112:351–61.
3. Vatner SF. Correlation between acute reductions in myocardial blood flow and function in conscious dogs. Circ Res 1980;47:201–7.
4. Waters DD, Luz PD, Wyatt HL, Swan HJ, Forrester JS. Early changes in regional and global left ventricular function induced by graded reductions in regional coronary perfusion. Am J Cardiol 1977;39:537–43.
5. Hauser AM, Gangadharan V, Ramos RG, Gordon S, Timmis GC. Sequence of mechanical, electrocardiographic and clinical effects of repeated coronary artery occlusion in human beings: echocardiographic observations during coronary angioplasty. J Am Coll Cardiol 1985;5:193–7.
6. Massie BM, Botvinick EH, Brundage BH, Greenberg B, Shames D, Gelberg H. Relationship to regional myocardial perfusion to segmental wall motion: a physiological basis for understanding the presence of reversibility of asynergy. Circulation 1978;58:1154–63.
7. Alam M, Khaja F, Brymer J, Marzelli M, Goldstein S. Echocardiographic evaluation of left ventricular function during coronary angioplasty. Am J Cardiol 1986;57:20–5.
8. Labovitz AJ, Lewen MK, Kern M, et al. Evaluation of left ventricular systolic and diastolic dysfunction during transient myocardial ischemia produced by angioplasty. J Am Coll Cardiol 1988;10:748–55.
9. Battler A, Froelicher VF, Gallagher KT, Kemper WS, Ross J. Dissociation between regional myocardial dysfunction and ECG changes during ischemia in the conscious dog. Circulation 1980;62:735–44.
10. Tomoike H, Franklin D, Ross J Jr. Detection of myocardial ischemia by regional dysfunction during and after rapid pacing in conscious dogs. Circulation 1978;58(1):48–56.
11. Smith JS, Cahalan MK, Benefiel DJ, et al. Intraoperative detection of myocardial ischemia in high-risk patients: electrocardiography versus two-dimensional transesophageal echocardiography. Circulation 1985;72:1015–21.
12. Wohlgelernter D, Jaffe CC, Cabin HS, Yeatman LA Jr, Cleman M. Silent ischemia during coronary occlusion produced by balloon inflation: Relation to regional myocardial dysfunction. J Am Coll Cardiol 1987;10:491–8.
13. van Daele ME, Sutherland GR, Mitchell MM, et al. Do changes in pulmonary capillary wedge pressure adequately reflect myocardial ischemia during anesthesia? A correlative preoperative hemodynamic, electrocardiographic, and transesophageal echocardiographic study. Circulation 1990;81:865–71.
14. Leung JM, O'Kelley B, Browner WS, Tubau J, Hollenberg M, Mangano DT. Prognostic importance of postbypass regional wall-motion abnormalities in patients undergoing coronary artery bypass graft surgery. Anesthesiology 1989;71:16–25.
15. Leung JM, O'Kelley BF, Mangano DT. Relationship of regional wall motion abnormalities to hemodynamic indices of myocardial oxygen supply and demand on patients undergoing CABG surgery. Anesthesiology 1990;73:802–14.
16. Clements FM, de Bruijn NP. Perioperative evaluation of regional wall motion by transesophageal two-dimensional echocardiography. Anesth Analg 1987;66:249–61.
17. Rosenthal A, Kawasuji M, Takemura H, Sawa S, Iwa T. Transesophageal echocardiography monitoring during coronary artery bypass surgery. Jpn Circ J 1991;55:109–16.
18. Lehmann KG, Forrester AL, McKenzie WB, et al. Onset of altered interventricular septal motion during cardiac surgery. Circulation 1990;82:1325–34.
19. Chung F, Seyone C, Rakowski H. Transesophageal echocardiography may fail to diagnose perioperative myocardial infarction. Can J Anaesth 1991;38:98–101.
20. Pandian NG, Skorton DJ, Collins SM, Falsetti HL, Burke ER, Kerber RE. Heterogeneity of left ventricular segmental wall motion thickening and excursion in 2–dimensional echocardiograms of normal human subjects. Am J Cardiol 1983;51:1667–73.
21. Lieberman AN, Weiss JL, Jugdutt BI, et al. Two-dimensional echocardiography and infarct size: relationship of regional wall motion and thickening to the extent of myocardial infarction in the dog. Circulation 1981;63:739–46.
22. Lima JA, Becker LC, Melin JA, et al. Impaired thickening of non-ischemic myocardium during acute regional ischemia in the dog. Circulation 1985;71:1048–59.
23. Force T, Kemper A, Perkins L, Gilfoil M, Cohen C, Parisi AF. Overestimation of infarct size by quantitative two-dimensional echocardiography: the role of tethering and of analytic procedures. Circulation 1986;73:1360–8.
24. Braunwald E, Kloner RA. The stunned myocardium: prolonged, postischemic ventricular dysfunction. Circulation 1982;66:1146–9.
25. Buffington CW, Coyle RJ. Altered load dependence of postischemic myocardium. Anesthesiology 1991;75:464–74.
26. London MJ, Tubau JF, Wong MG, et al. The "natural history" of segmental wall motion abnormalities in patients undergoing noncardiac surgery. Anesthesiology 1990;73:644–55.
27. Roizen MF, Beaupre PN, Alpert RA, et al. Monitoring with two-dimensional transesophageal echocardiography. Comparison of myocardial function in patients undergoing supraceliac, suprarenal-infraceliac, or infrarenal aortic occlusion. J Vasc Surg 1984;2:300–5.
28. Smith JS, Roizen MF, Cahalan MK, et al. Does anesthetic technique make a difference? Augmentation of systolic blood pressure during carotid endarterectomy: Effects of phenylephrine versus light anesthesia and of isoflurane versus halothane on the incidence of myocardial ischemia. Anesthesiology 1988;69:846–53.
29. Gewertz BL, Kremser PC, Zarins CK, et al. Transesophageal echocardiographic monitoring of myocardial ischemia during vascular surgery. J Vasc Surg 1987;5:607–13.

30. Topol EJ, Weiss JL, Guzman PA, et al. Immediate improvement of dysfunctional myocardial segments after coronary revascularization: detection by intraoperative transesophageal echocardiography. J Am Coll Cardiol 1984;4(6): 1123–34.

31. Koolen JJ, Visser CA, van Wezel HB, et al. Influence of coronary artery bypass surgery on regional left ventricular wall motion: An intraoperative two-dimensional transesophageal echocardiographic study. J Cardiovasc Anes 1978;1:276–83.

32. Voci P, Billotta F, Aronson S, et al. Changes in myocardial segmental wall motion, systolic wall thickening, and ejection fraction immediately following CABG: An echocardiographic analysis comparing dysfunctional and normal myocardium. J Am Soc Echocardiogr 1991;4:289.

33. Rahimtoola SH. The hibernating myocardium. Am Heart J 1989;117(1):211–21.

34. Bolli R. Myocardial 'stunning' in man. Circulation 1992; 86(6):1671–91.

35. van den Berg EK Jr, Popma JJ, Dehmer GJ, et al. Reversible segmental left ventricular dysfunction after coronary angioplasty. Circulation 1990;81(4):1210–16.

36. Marwick TH, Mehta R, Arheart K, Lauer MS. Use of exercise echocardiography for prognosis evaluation of patients with known or suspected coronary artery disease. J Am Coll Cardiol 1997;30:83–90.

37. Cigarroa CG, de Filippi CR, Brickner ME, Alvarez LG. Dobutamine stress echocardiography identifies hibernating myocardium and predicts recovery of left ventricular function after coronary revascularization. Circulation 1993;88(2): 430–6.

38. Nagueh SF, Vaduganathan P, Ali N, et al. Identification of hibernating myocardium: comparative accuracy of myocardial contrast echocardiography, rest-redistribution thallium-201 tomography and dobutamine echocardiography. J Am Coll Cardiol 1997;29(5):985–93.

39. Alderman EL, Fisher LD, Litwin P, et al. Results of coronary artery surgery in patient with poor ventricular function. Circulation 1983;68(4):785–95.

40. Passamani E, Davis KB, Gillespie MJ, Killip T. A randomized trial of coronary artery bypass surgery. Survival of patients with a low ejection fraction. N Engl J Med 1985;312(26): 1665–71.

41. Lualdi JC, Douglas PS. Echocardiography for the assessment of myocardial viability. J Am Soc Echocard 1997;10:772–80.

42. Brundage BH, Massie BM, Botvinick EH. Improved regional ventricular function after surgical revascularization. J Am Coll Cardiol 1984;3(4):902–8.

43. Davila-Roman VG, Waggoner AD, Sicard GA, Geltman EM, Schechtman KB, Perez JE. Dobutamine stress echocardiography predicts surgical outcome in patients with an aortic aneurysm and peripheral vascular disease. J Am Coll Cardiol 1993;21:957–63.

44. Langan EM 3rd, Youkey JR, Franklin DP, Elmore JR, Costello JM, Nassef LA. Dobutamine stress echocardiography for cardiac risk assessment before aortic surgery. J Vasc Surg 1993;18:905–11.

45. Poldermans D, Fioretti PM, Foster T, et al. Dobutamine-atropine stress echocardiography for assessment of perioperative and late cardiac risk in patients undergoing major vascular surgery. Eur J Vasc Surg 1994;8:286–93.

46. Takeuchi M, Araki M, Nakashima Y, Kuroiwa A. Comparison of dobutamine stress echocardiography and stress thallium-201 single-photon emission computed tomography for detecting coronary artery disease. J Am Soc Echocardiogr 1993;6:593–602.

47. Madu EC, Ahmar W, Arthur J, Fraker TD Jr. Clinical utility of digital dobutamine stress echocardiography in the noninvasive evaluation of coronary artery disease. Arch Intern Med 1994;154:1065–72.

48. Smart SC, Sawada S, Ryan T, et al. Low-dose dobutamine echocardiography detects reversible dysfunction after thrombolytic therapy of acute myocardial infarction. Circulation 1993;88:405–15.

49. Afridi I, Kleiman NS, Raizner AE, Zoghbi WA. Dobutamine echocardiography in myocardial hibernation: optimal dose and accuracy in predicting recovery of ventricular function after coronary angioplasty. Circulation 1995;91(3):663–70.

50. Marcovitz PA, Armstrong WF. Dobutamine stress echocardiography: diagnostic utility. Herz 1991;16(5):372–8.

51. Senior R, Lahiri A. Enhanced detection of myocardial ischemia by stress dobutamine echocardiography utilizing the "biphasic" response of wall thickening during low and high dose dobutamine infusion. J Am Coll Cardiol 1995;26:26–32.

52. Berthe C, Pierard LA, Hiernaux M, et al. Predicting the extent and location of coronary artery disease in acute myocardial infarction by echocardiography during dobutamine infusion. Am J Cardiol 1986;58:1167–72.

53. Boersma E. Predictors of cardiac events after major vascular surgery: role of clinical characteristics, dobutamine echocardiography, and beta-blocker therapy. JAMA 2001;285(14): 1865-73.

54. Kiat H, Berman DS, Maddahi J, et al. Late reversibility of tomographic myocardial thallium-201 defects: an acute marker of myocardial viability. Circulation 1988;76:1456–63.

55. Barilla F, Gheorghiade M, Alam M, Khaja F, Goldstein S. Low-dose dobutamine in patients with acute myocardial infarction identifies viable but not contractile myocardium and predicts the magnitude of improvement in wall motion abnormalities in response to coronary revascularization. Am Heart J 1991;122(6): 1522–31.

56. Voci P, Bilotta F, Caretta Q, Mercanti C, Marino B. Low dose dobutamine echocardiography predicts the early response of dysfunctional myocardial segments to coronary artery bypass grafting. Am Heart J 1995;129:521–6.

57. Di Carli MF, Davidson M, Little R, et al. Value of metabolic imaging with positron emission tomography for evaluating prognosis in patients with coronary artery disease and left ventricular dysfunction. Am J Cardiol 1994;73(8):527–33.

58. Lee KS, Marwick TH, Cook SA, et al. Prognosis of patients with left ventricular dysfunction, with and without viable myocardium after myocardial infarction. Relative efficacy of medical therapy and revascularization. Circulation 1994; 90(6):2687–94.

59. Gorcsan J, 3rd, Lazar JM, Schulman DS, Follansbee WP. Comparison of left ventricular function by echocardiographic automated border detection and by radionuclide ejection fraction. Am J Cardiol 1993; 72(11):810–5.

60. Gorcsan J, 3rd, Morita S, Mandarino WA, et al. Two-dimensional echocardiographic automated border detection accurately reflects changes in left ventricular volume. J Am Soc Echocardiogr 1993;6(5): 482–9.

61. Perrino AC, Jr., Luther MA, O'Connor TZ, Cohen IS. Automated echocardiographic analysis. Examination of serial intraoperative measurements. Anesthesiology 1995;83(2): 285–92.

62. Pinto FJ, Siegel LC, Chezbraun A, Schnittger I. On-line estimation of cardiac output with a new automated border detection system using transesophageal echocardiography: a preliminary comparison with thermodilution. J Cardiothorac Vasc Anesth 1994; 8(6):625–30.

63. Kornbluth M, Liang DH, Brown P, Gessford E, Schnittger I. Contrast echocardiography is superior to tissue harmonics for assessment of left ventricular function in mechanically ventilated patients. Am Heart J 2000;140(2):291–6.

## QUESTIONS

**1.** Normal regional wall motion is based on which two of the following factors?
A. Systolic wall thickening
B. Apical displacement of the LV cavity in systole
C. Epicardial wall motion

D. Endocardial wall motion
E. It is only dependent on one of the above factors

**2.** In order to grade regional wall motion, it is essential to view the myocardium in its entirety, including the epicardium.
A. True
B. False

**3.** Foreshortening can result in:
A. False appearance of a dyskinetic segment
B. Enlargement of the ventricular cavity
C. The appearance of a VSD

D. Myocardial thickening in a scarred, infarcted segment
E. A missed pericardial effusion

**4.** Newly hypokinetic myocardial segments:
A. Indicate hibernating myocardium
B. Are equally indicative of postoperative morbidity as akinesis or dyskinesis
C. Unaccompanied by hemodynamic or EKG evidence of ischemia are usually not associated with postoperative morbidity
D. Signify the need for immediate afterload reduction and beta-blockade

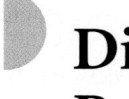

# Diastolic Dysfunction in the Perioperative Setting

Gardar Sigurdsson, Aleksandr Rovner, James D. Thomas, and Robert M. Savage

Congestive heart failure is one of the most common diagnoses made in patients admitted to the hospital in the United States (1,2), and the mortality and morbidity of heart failure incurs high medical costs (3,4). Symptoms of heart failure can be due to systolic dysfunction, diastolic dysfunction, or both. Systolic dysfunction is characterized by decreased forward flow or decreased ejection fraction. Diastolic dysfunction is characterized by elevated left ventricular end diastolic pressure. Both systolic and diastolic dysfunctions can produce the symptoms of fatigue and pulmonary congestion (5–9). Diastolic dysfunction is present in virtually all patients with systolic dysfunction; however, diastolic dysfunction can present without systolic dysfunction. This is called *isolated diastolic dysfunction*. Up to one-third of patients admitted with heart failure symptoms will have isolated diastolic dysfunction (10–12). Because virtually all patients with systolic dysfunction will have diastolic dysfunction, one can state that close to all patients with symptomatic heart failure have diastolic dysfunction. This is why patient care should not exclusively concentrate on systolic dysfunction and the role of diastolic dysfunction has found increasing importance.

Until recently heart failure research has focused on systolic dysfunction, because measuring systolic function by ejection fraction is a simple and reproducible method with prognostic and therapeutic implications. Assessment of diastolic dysfunction is not as widespread due to perceived difficulty in assessing diastolic function (13). The importance of diastolic function is evident in its role as an independent prognostic factor for mortality. The severity of diastolic dysfunction has been shown to predict mortality in patients with or without systolic dysfunction in multiple studies (14–21).

Diastolic dysfunction in general practice is most commonly associated with advanced age, hypertension, and ischemic heart disease. Diastolic dysfunction is also found in idiopathic-dilated cardiomyopathy and cardiomyopathy due to restrictive disease (such as amyloidosis or glycogen storage disease), constriction (such as post-thoracotomy or radiation), or hypertrophy (such as hypertrophic obstructive cardiomyopathy). In the perioperative setting diastolic dysfunction could be due to ischemia, reperfusion injury, hypothermia, cardioplegia, or pericardial effusion.

The assessment of diastolic function can be done by several different methods, including invasive left-ventricular pressure-tip catheter, echocardiographic imaging, magnetic resonance imaging, and nuclear imaging. Bedside clinical assessment of congestive heart failure by studying a patient's history and clinical exam cannot differentiate between systolic and diastolic heart failure (22). The measurement of the left-ventricular filling pressures in the cardiac catheterization laboratory provides an absolute number that is reproducible and can be followed in time. However, it is an invasive procedure and a cumbersome method to use in everyday clinical assessment. In the past two decades, two-dimensional echocardiography has emerged as a reliable and commonly used method to assess left-ventricular diastolic function. With the help of Doppler, it became possible, albeit indirectly, to record left ventricular filling patterns. With innovations in computer software and advances in mechanical technology of Doppler echocardiography, it is possible now to diagnose diastolic dysfunction and follow it in a longitudinal fashion. This method is noninvasive and it has good reliability and reproducibility. Other methods of evaluating diastolic dysfunction have not gained common use but show some promise.

## PATHOPHYSIOLOGY OF DIASTOLIC FUNCTION

### Definition of Diastole

The complexity of diastolic function arises from the multiple factors with different properties that contribute to its physiology. This is in stark contrast to systolic function where the major contribution comes from the left-ventricular myocardial contractility. These factors affecting diastolic function or left-ventricular filling include interactions between left-ventricular relaxation and regional left-ventricular pressure gradients that contribute to the suction effect, pericardial constraint, intraventricular interaction, passive properties of the myocardium, and left atrial contraction—all of these interactions combined contribute and determine how and at what pressure the ventricle fills during the diastolic period (22–26). The physiologic definition of diastole is the phase of the cardiac cycle that starts with the closure of the aortic valve and ends with the closure of the mitral valve (27). The hemodynamics of diastole consists of four phases: isovolumic relaxation, early filling, diastasis, and late filling (Fig. 13.1).

During isovolumic relaxation the left ventricular pressure progressively decreases in an energy-requiring process. The systemic ejection of blood stops when the left ventricular pressure decreases below the pressure in the aorta and the aortic valve closes. When the left ventricular pressure falls below that of the left atrium, the mitral valve opens and the early filling phase of diastole begins.

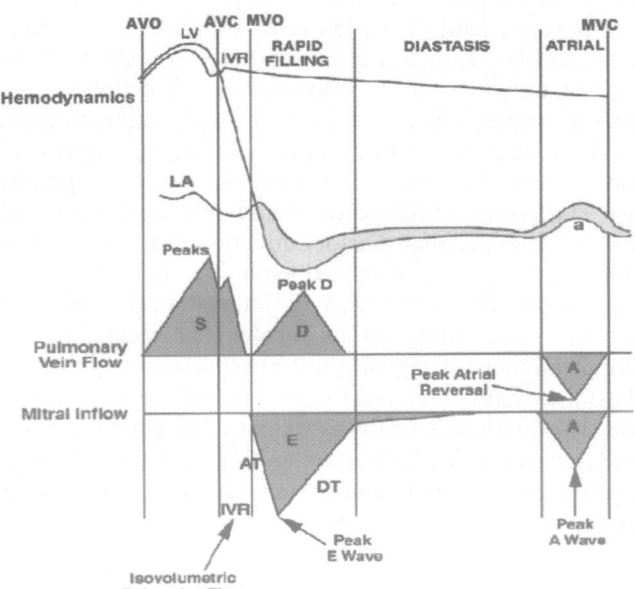

**FIGURE 13.1.** The hemodynamics of diastole consists of four phases: isovolumic relaxation (IVR), early filling (rapid filling), diastasis, and late filling (atrial). The schematic represents the hemodynamic pressure tracings in the aorta, left ventricle (LV), and left atrium (LA); pulsed Doppler tracings of flow in pulmonary veins; and pulsed Doppler tracing of mitral inflow measured at mitral valve tips by transesophageal echocardiographic approach. AVO, Aortic Valve Opening; AVC, Aortic Valve Closure; MVO, Mitral Valve Opening; MVC, Mitral Valve Closure.

When the mitral valve opens, we enter the early filling phase where blood enters the left ventricle down the pressure gradient that develops as the ventricle continues to relax. This small pressure gradient from the base to apex allows the ventricle to fill at low left atrial pressure and can be measured by high fidelity catheters or Doppler echocardiography.

There are several other interactions that produce the forces necessary to accommodate the early filling phase: the rate of decrease in LV pressure, the rate of LV relaxation, the rate of increase of LV pressure from the blood stored in the LA, passive viscoelastic properties of the myocardium, and the potential energy that is stored in the LV at end-systole (28). Also of consequence is the contribution of the filling and geometrical position of the right ventricle as well as the pericardium, which provides a structural constraint to the diastolic filling of the left ventricle (29). When equilibrium between pressure gradients in the LV and LA is reached, the blood flow is usually absent and diastasis begins.

During diastasis the ventricular volume is essentially unchanged. There are no significant pressure gradients between the atrium and the ventricle. The length of diastasis is inversely related to heart rate: As the heart rate increases, the diastasis time decreases.

The left atrial contraction contributes to left ventricular filling during the late filling phase. In a normal adult this constitutes between 15% and 30% of the blood volume (30). As the diastolic period shortens (i.e., during exercise) the atrial contraction moves closer in time to the early filling phase. In normal hearts this phase contributes relatively little to the overall filling of the LV. Clinically, when the ventricle is diseased and the earlier filling becomes impaired, the atrial contribution plays an important role; patients decompensate when atrial fibrillation ensues and the atrial "kick" is lost. Heart failure is another good example: As the LV diastolic function worsens, the LA tries to aid in LV filling. Eventually the LV end-diastolic pressures rise high enough that LA cannot overcome this added "afterload," it dilates and becomes simply a passive conduit between the pulmonary veins and LV (31).

## Active Properties of the Left Ventricle

Relaxation of the left ventricle is an active process that occurs during isovolumic relaxation and the early filling phase. This results in a negative gradient within the left ventricle that facilitates left ventricular filling (32). The active dilatation of the left ventricle is an energy-dependent process requiring adenosine triphosphate (ATP) to allow dissociation of actin from myosin (33). Intracellular calcium also plays an important role. An increase in intracellular calcium is needed to facilitate contraction of the myocyte. A decrease of intracellular calcium is needed to facilitate relaxation (34). Elevated intracellular calcium or deficiency of ATP can lead to diastolic dysfunction.

## PASSIVE PROPERTIES OF THE LEFT VENTRICLE

To appreciate the complexity of the hemodynamic interactions of the diastole, we need to address the intrinsic properties of the cardiac myocytes and the connective tissue matrix that supply the structural support to the contractile elements. These so-called passive properties of the left ventricle include stress and strain at the level of the myocardium and stiffness and compliance at the level of the ventricle.

*Stress* is a force that is applied to the unit of a cross-sectional area. *Strain* is the change in the dimension that is produced by the application of stress. Biological systems exhibit a curvilinear relationship between the applied stress and strain that is produced. The slope of that curve is referred to as *elastic stiffness*. The heart also has viscous elements that contribute to the passive properties. The relationship between strain and viscoelasticity depends on the rate at which stress is applied. Rapid application of stress produces a larger change in strain; the relaxation then follows a different curve in a hysteresis relationship (26,35). The clinical importance of these properties remains unclear.

The change in pressure as it relates to the change in volume (dP/dV) is referred to as *ventricular stiffness*. The inverse of ventricular stiffness is *ventricular compliance* (dV/dP). By measuring the end-diastolic pressure at different end-diastolic volumes, one can construct a pressure-volume loop of the cardiac cycle. There are two important points to consider. In states that produce high end-diastolic pressures (such as severely dilated ventricles), the pressure-volume relationship becomes mathematically complex (27). Also, it is implied that the stiffness can change by either changing the end-diastolic volume or by moving to an entirely new pressure-volume loop (Fig. 13.2) (24,26).

## RELAXATION AS MEASURED BY INDICES DERIVED FROM LEFT VENTRICULAR PRESSURE DATA

As we have described above, the diastolic period consists of several phases with different hemodynamic properties; these can be directly measured from left ventricular pressure data. Because these measurements are relatively simple, a variety of indices of diastolic function based on these pressure measurements was introduced. In the following section, we will discuss three of these indices: isovolumic relaxation time, peak –dP/dt, and the time constant of relaxation.

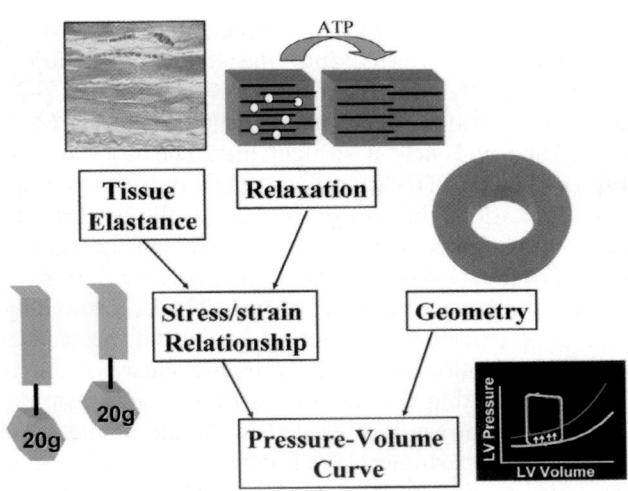

**FIGURE 13.2.** Diastolic function is determined by how the combination of the passive properties of tissue elastance and active ATP require relaxation of the myocytes, influence the ventricles stress/strain relationship, and, together with left ventricular geometry, determine how the ventricle responds to increased volume with increased pressure.

The time that lasts between the closure of the aortic valve and opening of the mitral valve is defined as *isovolumic relaxation time* (IVRT); the volume of left ventricle during this phase is constant (Fig. 13.1). This time can be obtained invasively in the catheterization lab or by using echocardiography. As the disease process progresses, the ventricular relaxation slows and the IVRT will increase (36,37). However, this index has several significant limitations. Aortic or mitral valvular insufficiencies can prolong the IVRT regardless of presence or absence of the disease. Because closure of the aortic valve largely depends on the systemic diastolic pressure, changes in afterload will affect the IVRT, and because opening of the mitral valve depends on left atrial pressure, changes in preload will affect the IVRT as well.

As the left ventricle relaxes the intraventricular pressure declines at a certain rate. The peak negative rate of this pressure drop (–dP/dt) can be measured by taking the first derivative of the left ventricular pressure tracing. With disease processes that affect diastolic function, the peak –dP/dt will be less negative. This index depends on systemic pressure and preload (38,39). Invasive techniques with high fidelity pressure transducers must be used to obtain the peak –dP/dt. One should also realize that the peak –dP/dt is taken at one point in time and does not represent the rate of pressure decline throughout the relaxation of the ventricle during diastole.

Another index of diastolic function that is based on the left ventricular pressure decline is the *time constant of relaxation* (tau). Usually the portion of the LV pressure decline curve that is used is between the peak –dP/dt and an arbitrarily set constant of 5 mm Hg above the end-diastolic pressure. Because the rate of the ventricular pressure drop approaches an exponential decay function, it can be inserted into the following equation: $P_t = P_0 * e^{tau*t}$ as described by Weiss and colleges (40). Taking a logarithm of both sides and then plotting Ln $P_t$ versus time will yield a straight line. The slope of this graph will be tau. The limitations of this index are similar to the limitations that constrain −dP/dt: the need for invasive measurements and the dependents on the loading conditions (39,41–43). Several mathematical variations of this method have evolved with time (27). Unfortunately, there is no current mathematical model that provides a perfect description of the LV pressure decay. There is clear evidence that the rate of the LV pressure drop depends on the forces that existed in systole of the same beat (44). Complex interplay of nonuniformity of the myocardium passive properties (43), cardiac myocyte involvement (biochemical and mechanical), events that happened with previous heartbeats—including torsional and translational motion (23), and other factors make modeling difficult.

## ECHOCARDIOGRAPHIC ASSESSMENT OF DIASTOLIC DYSFUNCTION

With this background describing the factors determining the active, passive, and hemodynamic properties of the LV in the diastole, we will now describe the more conventional methods of two-dimensional Doppler patterns through the mitral valve (Fig. 13.3) and pulmonary veins (Fig. 13.4) that are used to determine the LV inflow and gauge diastolic function. Additionally we will also describe two newer methods; tissue Doppler imaging (Fig. 13.5) and color M-mode (Fig. 13.6). These new methods have gained increasing popularity and appear to be less sensitive to preload than mitral inflow and pulmonary venous flow.

## MITRAL INFLOW PATTERNS

Figure 13.1 demonstrates the normal velocity curve profile obtained when a pulse Doppler is placed at the mitral

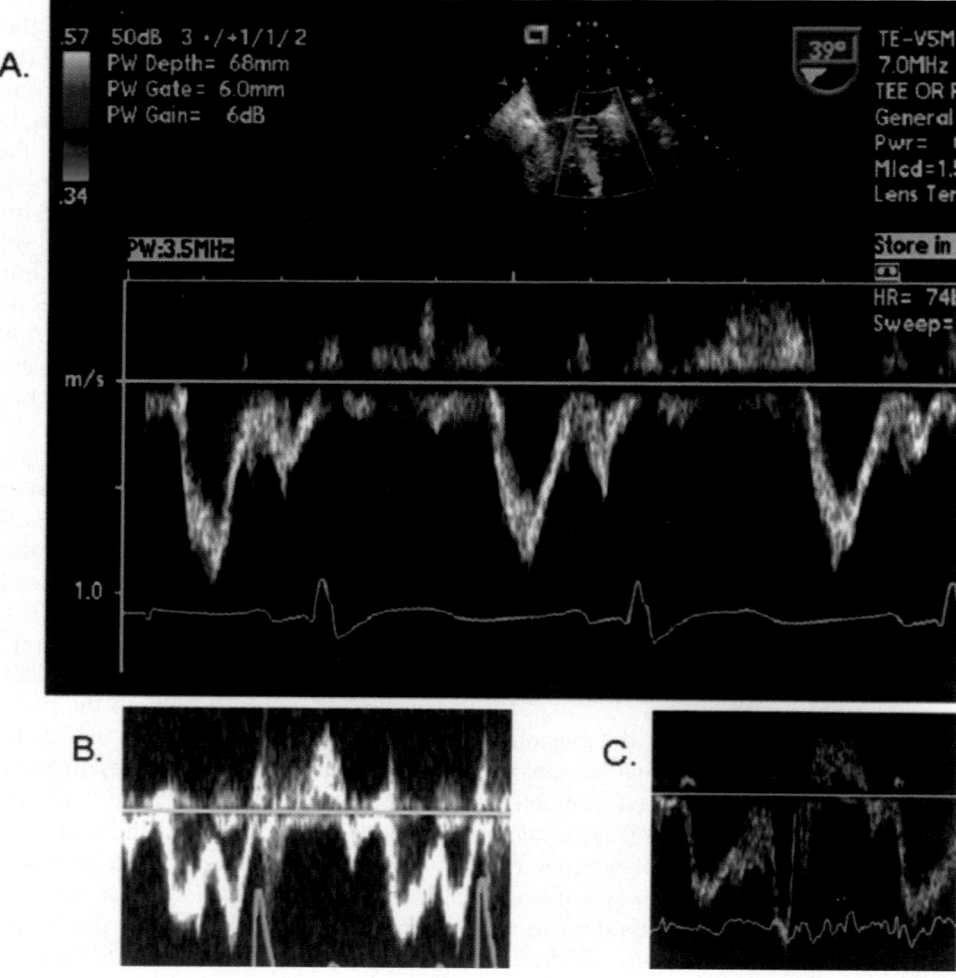

**FIGURE 13.3. A:** Mitral inflow is measured by pulsed Doppler at the level of mitral valve tips. The pattern is stage III diastolic dysfunction (restrictive). **B:** Normal pattern or pseudonormal pattern **C:** Stage I pattern of diastolic dysfunction (abnormal relaxation).

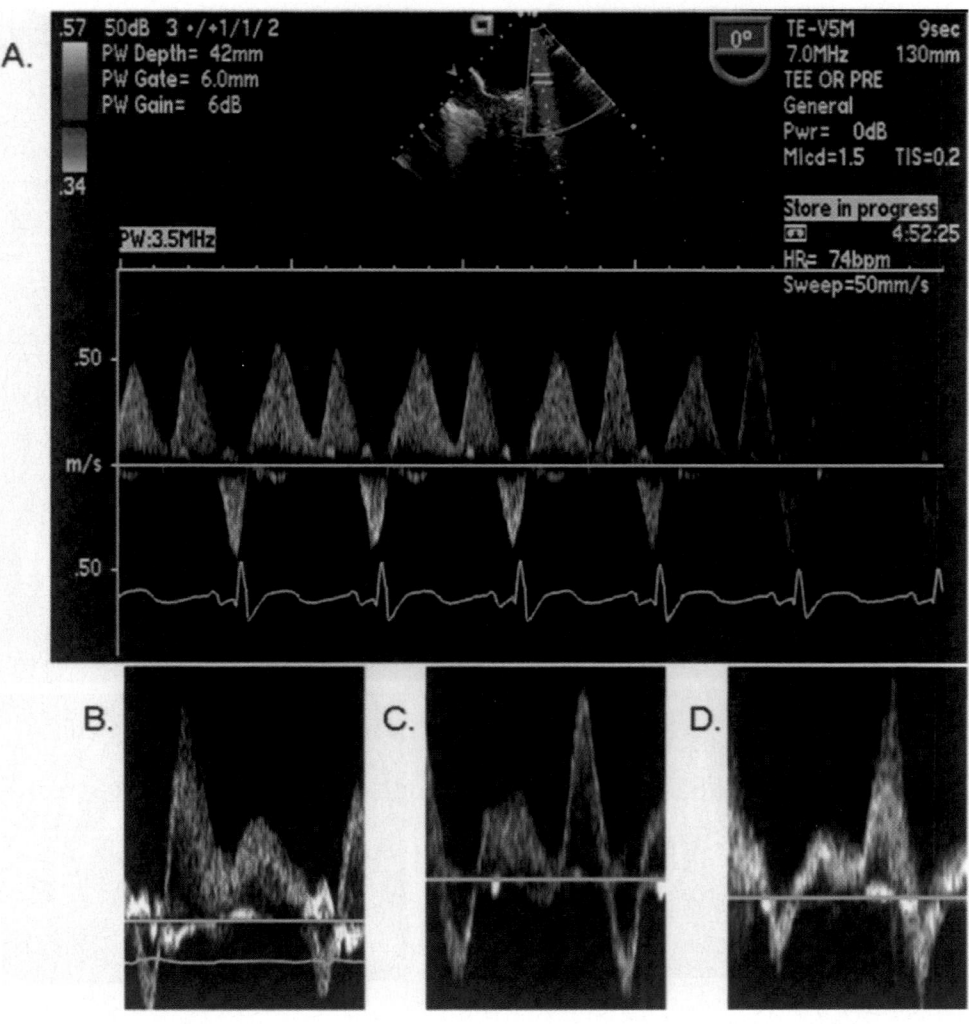

**FIGURE 13.4.** Pulmonary venous flow measured by pulsed Doppler at the orifice of the pulmonary vein. **A:** Normal pattern but large A reversal suggesting high pressure. **B:** Stage I (abnormal relaxation). **C:** Blunting of the S wave and large A reversal suggesting stage II (pseudonormal pattern). **D:** Blunting of S and large D wave suggesting stage III diastolic dysfunction (restrictive).

valve tips during transesophageal echocardiography. The following simple measurements are standard in evaluating diastolic function. The time between the end of the aortic flow (aortic valve closure) and beginning of the mitral inflow (mitral valve opening) represents the IVRT, the E velocity represents the early filling phase, and diastasis is next followed by the A wave that represents the atrial contraction of late filling. Increased age is related to a decrease in E velocity and an increase in A velocity; please see Table 13.1 for further details (45,46). As discussed above, mitral valve inflow velocities are highly dependent on the individual's age, loading conditions, and heart rate. Diastolic function can be staged by mitral inflow into: stage I (delayed relaxation), stage II (pseudonormal), and stage III (restrictive). Note that stage II can only be diagnosed by adding a preload changing maneuver, such as Valsalva or leg raise, or by adding another measure of diastolic function, such as pulmonary venous flow, tissue Doppler imaging, or propagation velocity.

## Stage I: Delayed Relaxation Pattern

Diastolic function is very sensitive to cardiac homeostasis and often becomes abnormal prior to systemic manifestations of the disease. LV relaxation becomes abnormal with diseases such as hypertension and ischemia, and in subjects with increased age. This state introduces specific and reproducible changes in the velocity profile that is obtained at the mitral valve inflow. Because LV relaxation is impaired, the rate of the pressure drop between the LA and LV is slowed, producing a decrease in initial hydrodynamic force that is responsible for the blood entering the LV and manifests with the decrease of the peak E velocity. Although the initial forces are decreased with relaxation, the overall filling will be prolonged continuing into late diastole, producing an increase in the deceleration time. In order to produce a constant stroke volume, during the late filling stage the atrial contraction force will increase to compensate, producing an increase in the peak A velocity.

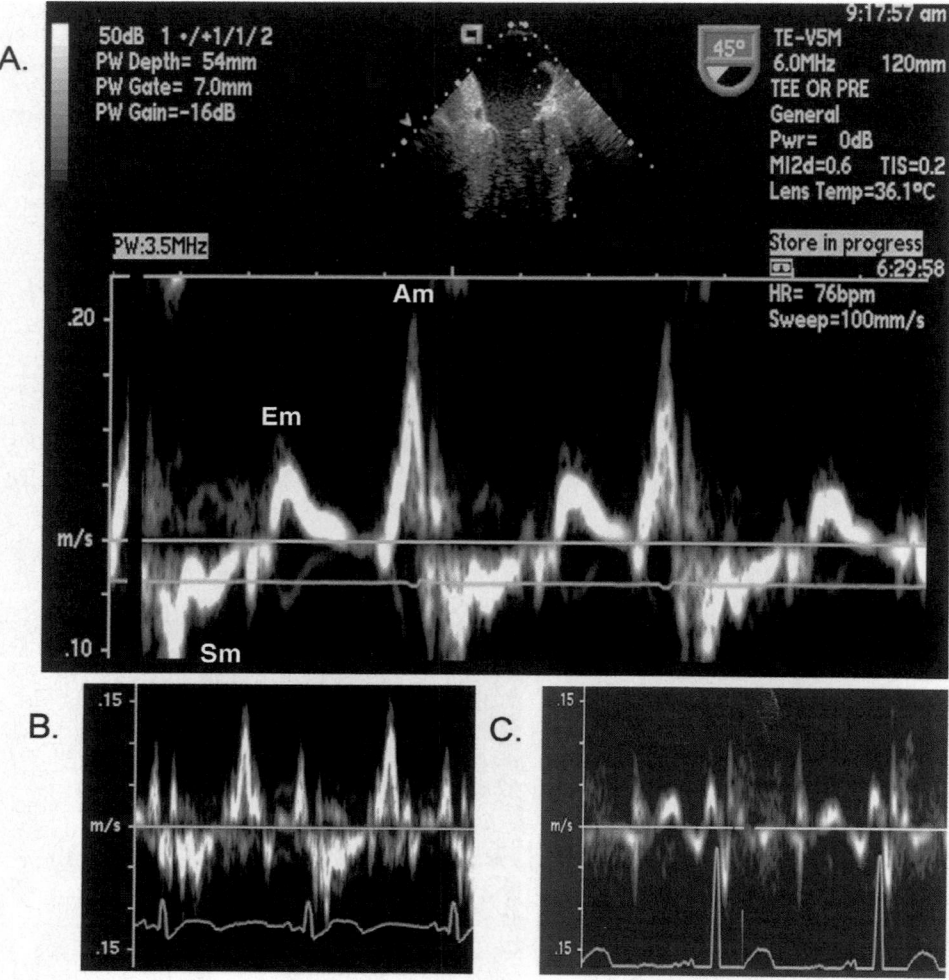

**FIGURE 13.5.** Tissue Doppler imaging with pulsed Doppler sampling at the level of the lateral mitral valve annulus. **A:** Stage I (abnormal relaxation). **B:** Normal with Em velocity above 10 cm/s. **C:** Stage II (pseudonormal) or stage III (restrictive) pattern with Em velocity below 8 cm/s.

To summarize, as the relaxation function of LV becomes less vigorous, the peak E velocity decreases, the peak A velocity increases, the E/A ratio becomes less than one, and the deceleration time increases. These changes define delayed relaxation or stage I of diastolic dysfunction (Fig. 13.7).

## Stage II: Pseudonormal Pattern

As the disease process progresses, the compensatory forces attempt to bring the LV filling to the baseline level. One way to achieve this is to increase the filling pressure or preload by increasing the operating LA pressure. At the same time as the filling pressures increase, the LV compliance decreases further secondary to the progression of the disease. A point is reached when the end-diastolic pressure is just right to increase the peak E velocity; this will produce the inflow velocity profile resembling normal function (47) as demonstrated in Fig. 13.7. This

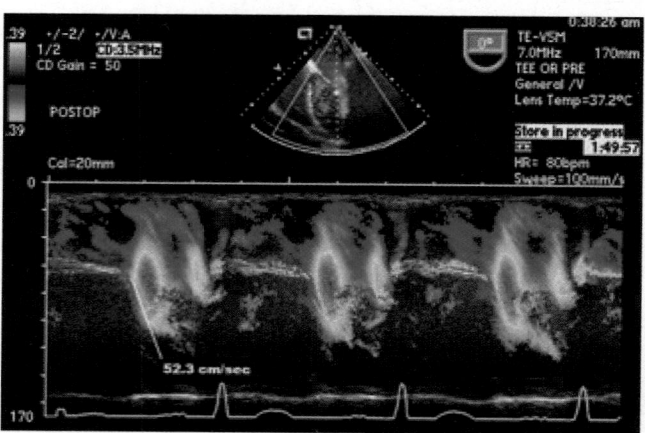

**FIGURE 13.6.** Color M-mode is done by aligning the cursor into the mitral inflow tract with lowering of the Nyquist limit (here at 0.39 m/sec) and adjusting the sweep speed to 100 mm/sec. Velocity flow propagation is measured by assessing the slope of aliasing velocities from the mitral valve and at least 4 cm into the left ventricle. Here it is measured at 52.3 cm/sec, which is normal for a subject older than 50 years.

▶ TABLE 13.1. Normal Values with Different Age and Different Stages of DD

|  | Normal (age 21–49) | Normal (age > 50) | Stage I (delayed relaxation) | Stage II (pseudonormal filling) | Stage III (restrictive filling) |
|---|---|---|---|---|---|
| E/A | > 1 | > 1 | < 1 | 1–2 | > 2 |
| DT (ms) | < 220 | < 220 | > 220 | 150–200 | < 150 |
| IVRT (ms) | < 100 | < 100 | > 100 | 60–100 | < 60 |
| S/D | < 1 | ≥ 1 | ≥ 1 | < 1 | < 1 |
| AR (cm/s) | < 35 | < 35 | < 35 | ≥ 35 | ≥ 25 |
| Em (cm/s) | > 10 | > 8 | < 8 | < 8 | < 8 |
| Vp (cm/s) | > 55 | > 45 | < 45 | < 45 | < 45 |

Unless atrial mechanical failure is present. AR, pulmonary venous peak atrial contraction reversed velocity; DT, early left ventricular filling deceleration time; E/A, early-to-atrial left ventricular filling ratio; Em, peak early diastolic myocardial velocity; IVRT, isovolumic relaxation time; S/D, systolic-to-diastolic pulmonary venous flow ratio; Vp, color M-mode flow propagation velocity.

From Garcia MJ, Thomas JD, Klein AL. New Doppler Echocardiographic applications for the study of diastolic function. JACC 1998;32:865–75, with permission.

pattern of diastolic dysfunction is called pseudonormal or stage II. This presents a major problem in the clinical setting if the diastolic function is assessed only by using mitral valve inflow pattern (48).

To differentiate stage II (pseudonormal pattern) from a normal diastolic function one can employ maneuvers, such as Valsalva, which would decrease preload. When the preload is lowered, the mitral inflow pattern reverts to the delayed relaxation (stage I) pattern with decrease peak E velocity and high peak A velocity (49). In contrast, when diastolic function is normal, the Valsalva procedure will produce a fall in both E and A waves. There are newer echocardiographic techniques, tissue Doppler imaging and color M-mode, which can reliably differentiate the pseudonormal state (50). Pulmonary venous pat-

tern can also be somewhat helpful. We will discuss these methods further later in the text.

## Stage III: Restrictive Pattern

The continuum of the disease process results in increased LV stiffness, worsening the operating LV wall compliance. Eventually, the filling pressures must overcome a very stiff LV to provide a high enough stroke volume. At this point patients have exercise intolerance and symptoms at rest. The mitral valve inflow pattern reflects the increase in filling pressures and poor LV compliance: the peak E velocity is very high and is reached very quickly. Because the LV is stiff, the early filling phase is short and the deceleration time is less than 150 ms. The LA has failed at this stage and provides only a conduit for the blood to pass from the pulmonary veins into the LV. The late filling phase has a small peak A velocity because the LA cannot overcome the LV stiffness. This is termed a restrictive pattern or stage III of diastolic dysfunction.

Stage III (restrictive pattern) has a poor prognosis and high mortality irrespective of the status of the systolic function (16,19,51). There is evidence to suggest that aggressive measures with ACE inhibitors and diuresis may help reverse the restrictive pattern to pseudonormal or delayed relaxation. However, in a subset of patients, the disease process has progressed too far and even with treatment the mitral inflow remains restrictive. This is considered by some investigators to be stage four or irreversible restriction (22). The prognosis for these patients is extremely poor.

## PULMONARY VENOUS FLOW

Another approach that uses pulsed two-dimensional Doppler technique is the interrogation of flow from the pulmonary veins. A normal velocity pattern is represented in Fig. 13.1. Hemodynamically, the pulmonary vein

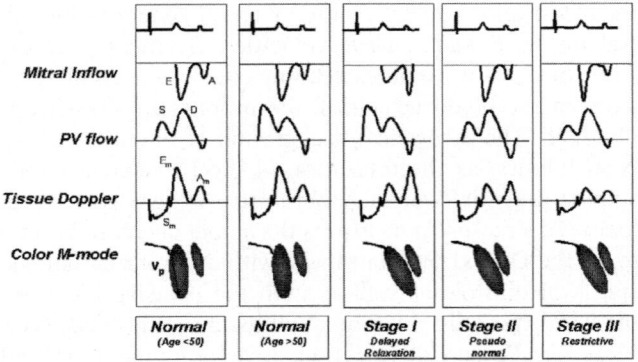

**Patterns of diastolic dysfunction measured by transesophageal echocardiography**

FIGURE 13.7. Diagram using transesophageal echocardiography showing changes in the mitral inflow, PV (pulmonary venous) flow, tissue Doppler, and color M-mode with age and different stages of diastolic dysfunction.

velocity pattern depends more on the compliance and the afterload of the LA rather than on the pressures that are generated by the right ventricle (52,53). The forward flow is comprised from the systolic and diastolic parts. The systolic part sometimes has a biphasic pattern, termed $S_1$ and $S_2$ (54). It follows the atrial contraction and it is thought that the $S_1$ component is directly related to atrial relaxation. The relationship of the $S_2$ component is increased by vigorous downward annular movement due to systole, but decreased by mitral regurgitation. The diastolic part is termed D and physiologically produced by the gradient between the LA and the pulmonary veins during the early filling phase. In general the sum of $S_1$ and $S_2$ flow usually are greater than D. In normal subjects there is a small reversal of flow from the LA into the pulmonary veins with atrial contraction (55). The technical difficulties in obtaining the pulmonary vein flow from the transthoracic approach prompted investigators to evaluate the transesophageal echocardiogram as a tool for this task. Because the transducer location is proximal to the origin of the flow and is parallel to the flow, the pulmonary vein data obtained using the transesophageal technique is more reliable and has better reproducibility (56).

With different loading conditions, the pattern of the pulmonary vein velocity profile changes (57). Nishimura and colleagues found that the mitral inflow peak E velocity and the deceleration time correlate well with the diastolic peak of the pulmonary vein velocity. They also demonstrated a relationship between the mitral inflow and pulmonary vein velocity at different states of LV preload and afterload (58). Combining the information obtained from the conventional two-dimensional pulsed Doppler data from the mitral inflow with that of the pulmonary vein velocities may help to better appreciate the true state of the end-diastolic LV pressure. This may also help to differentiate stage II (pseudonormal pattern) by mitral inflow. The pulmonary vein velocity will reveal blunted S and higher D velocities, although this pattern is also seen in normal young adults (age < 40 years).

## TISSUE DOPPLER IMAGING

Tissue Doppler imaging (TDI) is a technique that involves measurement of the myocardial velocities. It is an extension of the standard two-dimensional Doppler technique. Tissue Doppler imaging can detect the early diastolic motion of the mitral annulus due to LV relaxation (46,59). As shown in Fig. 13.5, the prominent systolic deflection is obtained as well as the Em and Am waves of diastolic motion. Investigators found that placing the sample volume at the mitral annulus for TDI interrogation has good reproducibility (59). Several studies correlated the peak of the early Em velocity of TDI with tau (60,61). There is data to suggest that TDI has less preload dependence

than transmitral pulsed Doppler (61), although in normal hearts this advantage is less clear (62). The Em/Am ratio from TDI behaves similarly to the Em/Am ratio obtained from the mitral inflow using standard two-dimensional pulsed Doppler: it decreases with ischemia and it changes with age (63,64), but unlike transmitral flow it does not pseudonormalize.

Investigators have shown that TDI can be used in several clinical venues. It can differentiate the stages of diastolic function as demonstrated in Fig. 13.7. Another clinical use for TDI is in separating constrictive versus restrictive states. In constriction there are normal Em values, but in restriction they are lowered (50,65–67). Recently, Ommen and colleagues demonstrated a good correlation between catheter-determined LV end-diastolic pressure and the noninvasive estimation using TDI (68).

To summarize, TDI has the potential of becoming the next generation tool to analyze diastolic function. At this time, it is a well-defined adjunct to the prior methods of evaluating diastolic function. TDI can be measured by using presets in place on the echo machine but when not present the pulsed Doppler analysis has to be adjusted towards detecting low velocities, with lowered Doppler gain settings and the filter set towards 100 Hz or lower. Sample volume length also needs to be increased to at least 6 mm compared to 4 mm for pulmonary veins and 2 mm for mitral inflow. The measurements are done in the apical four-chamber views with Doppler focus set at lateral or septal mitral valve annulus.

## COLOR M-MODE DOPPLER: PROPAGATION VELOCITY

Recently, investigators began to use propagation velocity (Vp) obtained from color M-mode Doppler to evaluate LV relaxation (69). Using color kinesis one can describe the flow of blood in the LV by utilizing M-mode. Color M-mode Doppler provides spatiotemporal information on the blood velocities within the LV and it generates the mitral inflow E and A wave velocities. By measuring the slope of the E wave at the leading edge of the color spectrum of the blood velocities, the propagation velocity is obtained. The theoretical background of the utility of Vp is as follows: as the relaxation of the LV decreases, the suction potential worsens; therefore, the peak early E velocities decrease. Vp measures the actual decrease in time to fill the LV and correlates well with different pathologic stages of diastole as well as with the invasive measurements of diastolic function such as tau and –dP/dt (70). Moreover, Vp is relatively insensitive to preload as shown by Garcia and colleagues (71). There is a clear change in Vp as diastolic function worsens, eliminating the ambiguity of the pseudonormalization state of the transmitral inflow pattern.

Garcia and colleagues demonstrated that one could obtain the pulmonary wedge pressure noninvasively using the peak E velocity from the mitral inflow and the Vp data from the color M-mode Doppler (72). Knowing that Vp is inversely proportional to tau and that the peak E velocity is directly proportional to left atrial pressure and has a negative relationship with tau, substituting and rearranging one gets the following: PCPW α E/Vp. This was tested against invasive hemodynamic monitoring in patients admitted to an ICU with good correlation and confirmed in normals (62). Nishihara et al. measured left ventricular pressure in patients with hypertrophic cardiomyopathy and found significant correlation between tau and Vp, but conventional measures of diastolic dysfunction could not be correlated with tau in these patients (73).

Thus, one can utilize the information from the Vp of the color M-mode Doppler together with the conventional pulsed Doppler techniques to differentiate the stages of diastolic dysfunction and to estimate LV filling pressures.

Color M-mode can be performed on all newer echo machines. When the mitral inflow is measured, the sampling cursor has to cover at least 4 cm of the LV below the mitral valve tips. The color-coded Nyquist limit lowered to produce aliasing and helps to better delineate the slope measurements. The measurement of propagating velocity is then done by analyzing the Doppler slope by using the first aliasing velocity measured from the mitral valve (Fig. 13.6).

## FUTURE METHODS OF MEASURING DIASTOLIC FUNCTION

Strain imaging is a recently developed modality that might be useful in analyzing diastolic function (74,75). By changing the filter settings to detect low velocities and high amplitudes, this technique can analyze myocardial velocity changes in the direction of the echo beam. Strain rate (SR) can be analyzed from this data as the difference in velocity between two points divided by the length between these two points (SR = dV/dL, unit sec$^{-1}$) and as such represents the velocity gradient in the direction of the echo beam. Strain (S) can be calculated from SR as it changes over time (S = dSR/dt, no unit), which is a dimensionless index that could be better defined as the proportional changes in the length of a myocardial segment or S = (L0 − L1)/L0, where L0 is initial length and L1 is the compressed length. SR and S imaging of the left ventricle in apical views only measure longitudinal changes in direction of the echo beam; therefore, its measures are relatively independent of translation or rotation (76). Strain imaging can give information on both systolic and diastolic changes, and it has been analyzed in patients with hypertrophic cardiomyopathy (77) and patients with coronary artery disease (78). SR changes with age, loca-

tion of measurement (apex vs. base), and site within each segment (epicardium vs. endocardium) (79).

More recently our laboratory came up with a noninvasive method to determine the intraventricular pressure gradients during diastole by utilizing the velocity data obtained from color M-mode Doppler. While Vp provides important information about the LV filling pattern, it utilizes only one part of data provided by the color M-mode Doppler image. Utilizing full spatiotemporal distribution of the velocities it is possible to calculate noninvasively the transmitral and intraventricular pressure gradients (IVPG) during diastole (83). The presence of the pressure gradient between the LV outflow tract and the aorta during systole is a known entity. Recently diastolic pressure differences have been identified within the left ventricle. Ling and colleagues described the "suction" effect that develops secondary to a pressure drop between the left ventricular base and apex, which aids in the blood flow from the left atrium into the ventricle in a canine model (32). A change in the regional ventricular pressure gradients with positive and negative inotropic agents was subsequently described (80,81). Loss of this suction effect that contributes to the early filling phase was observed when experimental ischemia was produced (82). Ability to measure these gradients and apply them clinically will provide new insights into diastolic function. Until now, the determination of this regional pressure difference was cumbersome, requiring invasive high fidelity pressure monitoring and was not useful in every day clinical practice. With the advent of ultrasound technology, we can use the color M-mode velocity information to determine the diastolic IVPG.

The following is a mathematical representation for the derivation of the pressure gradient measurement from the color M-mode velocity data. The flow of blood in three dimensions across the mitral valve is represented by a differential form of the Navier-Stokes equation for incompressible fluid:

$$-\vec{V} * \left( \frac{P}{\rho} + g \cdot z \right) + \left( \frac{\eta}{\rho} \right) * \vec{V}^2 * \nu = \frac{\partial \nu}{\partial t} + (\nu \cdot \vec{V})\nu$$

The terms in the equation above are as follows: $\vec{V}$, a three-dimensional velocity vector; P, local pressure; ρ, blood density; g, gravitational constant; z, local height; and η, blood viscosity. Because blood viscosity plays an important role only when the unsteady boundary is significant—when a severe obstruction is present and the flow is turbulent—we can disregard the η/ρ term. Also, the hydrostatic g · z term is very small. If we assume the flow to be in a single dimension and then solve the equation for the pressure, it becomes the Euler's equation:

$$\frac{\partial P}{\partial s} = -\rho \left( \frac{\partial \nu}{\partial t} + \nu \frac{\partial \nu}{\partial s} \right)$$

Note that the Euler's equation represents the balance between the pressure force and the combination of acceleration forces and the inertial component of the blood flow. Integrating the Euler's equation with the mitral valve inflow from the left atrium to the left ventricle yields the equation below, which is a simplified form of the unsteady state Bernoulli equation for fluids:

$$\Delta P = \frac{1}{2}\rho(v_{LV}^2[t] - v_{LA}^2[t]) + \rho\int_{LA}^{LV}\frac{\partial v[s,t]}{\partial t}ds$$

Thus the pressure difference is the combination of the convective and inertial forces of the blood flow. Using the spatiotemporal velocity information from the color M-modes we are able to solve the equation for the transmitral pressure gradients as well as the intraventricular pressure gradients. A custom-written computer algorithm takes the raw velocity data and dealiases it as well as provides smoothing. Subsequently, it converts the color pixels into true velocities using the Nyquist limit and then calculates the IVPG (83). A group of investigators from Spain used a similar approach with a different smoothing algorithm to calculate the IVPG (84).

The work done at the Cleveland Clinic validated this noninvasive approach in an animal model as well as in a variety of patient groups with different cardiac pathologies. Greenberg and colleagues validated their noninvasive methodology for estimation of the IVPG in dogs with and without inotropic stimulation (85). Firstenberg demonstrated improvement in the IVPG in patients with coronary disease undergoing coronary revascularization (86). This data was also validated against invasive pressure measurement (87). Similar work was done on patients with hypertrophic obstructive cardiomyopathy; we showed that the IVPG improves with alcohol septal ablation. We validated the noninvasive measurement of the IVPG during myectomies and demonstrated that pressure gradients improve acutely in this patient population (87). There are data to suggest that IVPG change with exercise is the single best predictor of peak oxygen consumption.

IVPG measurement is less dependent on preload and heart rate. The ability to provide noninvasive measurement of the pressure gradients will place this index in permanent clinical use when the process becomes more automated. One must understand the limitations of the noninvasive approach: Blood flow through the mitral valve does not follow a uniform straight line and the unsteady state Bernoulli equation that we used is still in a simplified form. However, we have validated this measurement in several patient groups with good results. IVPG will be a good clinical adjunct to the existing tools used in evaluation of diastolic function.

## LIMITATIONS OF ECHOCARDIOGRAPHIC EVALUATION OF DIASTOLIC FUNCTION

There are many reasons why echocardiography became so popular for evaluating diastolic function. The technique is noninvasive, it is reproducible, and patients can be followed in time. However, there are many drawbacks that keep pulsed Doppler from becoming the gold standard in evaluating diastolic function. Both the transmitral and pulmonary vein velocity profiles are highly dependent on the hemodynamic and physiologic states. Preload dependence has been clearly demonstrated in the velocity profiles of the mitral inflow (88,89). As diastolic function worsens, the relationship between the LV relaxation and mitral velocities starts to follow a parabolic function confounded by preload changes (Fig. 13.8). As the relaxation worsens the peak E velocity is reduced, the peak A velocity is increased, and the DT is slowed. When the filling pressures rise, the peak E velocity increases, the peak A velocity decreases, and the DT normalizes (90).

Age produces dramatic alterations in transmitral and pulmonary vein velocity profiles. There are several factors responsible for these changes (91). As people age, the ventricular mass and wall thickness increases. This leads to increase in stress and stiffness, thus changing the mitral inflow pattern to decrease the peak E velocity and to increase the peak A velocity. As the heart ages there are intrinsic changes in the myocardial fibers and in the supportive collagen scaffold, possibly contributing to the changes in diastolic measurements. Another contributing factor is the increase in both systolic and diastolic blood pressures (92).

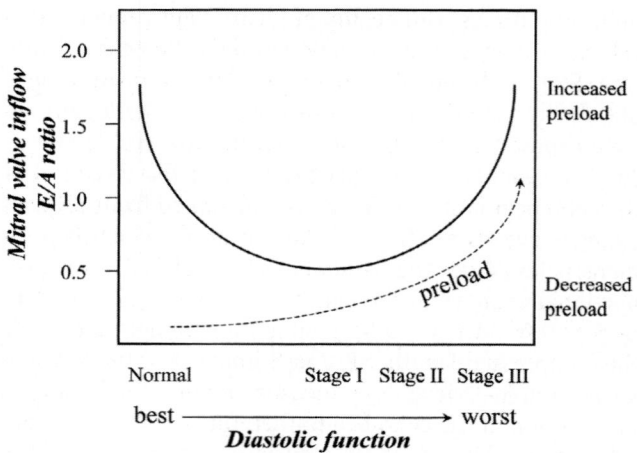

**FIGURE 13.8.** The relationship between preload and patterns of mitral valve inflow, E/A ratio. As preload increases, the E/A ratio increases to the pattern of stage III diastolic dysfunction.

Passive changes in heart rate produce a different change in the transmitral velocity profile compared to increase in heart rate due to exercise. Increased heart rate causes fusion of E and A wave of the mitral inflow.

Mitral valve disease and atrial tachyarrhythmias will significantly affect both mitral inflow and pulmonary venous flow, but in atrial fibrillation it has been suggested that stage III diastolic dysfunction is present if mitral inflow E wave DT is less than 130 ms.

Myocardial infarction can significantly lower TDI values if the infarction is located in areas where the sample volume is placed (base of lateral wall or septum). Aortic valve regurgitation will cause contamination in Vp values irrespective of diastolic dysfunction; therefore, color M-mode has little value in patients where the aortic regurgitant jet intersects the mitral inflow stream (93) (Table 13.2).

## CLINICAL APPLICATION OF MEASURING DIASTOLIC DYSFUNCTION IN THE PERIOPERATIVE SETTING

In the outpatient setting diastolic dysfunction can be readily diagnosed by transthoracic echocardiography but the clinical management is not as well characterized. In stark contrast to evidence-based therapy for systolic heart failure, there is currently no large prospective study on daily therapy of symptomatic diastolic dysfunction. The most obvious treatment for symptomatic diastolic dysfunction has consisted of diuretic therapy (94). Medications, such as angiotensin-converting enzyme inhibitors, angiotensin-receptor inhibitors, and beta-adrenergic inhibitors, have been found beneficial in small substudies and retrospective analysis (95). Treatment with calcium channel blockers is both beneficial (96) and detrimental (97). Multiple prospective trials with Doppler-determined inclusion criteria are underway to determine which of the above-mentioned medications could be beneficial in diastolic dysfunction (95).

In the perioperative setting the diagnosis of diastolic dysfunction is more commonly done with transesophageal echocardiography and its detection can have significant implications towards clinical course and response to surgical and medical management. Diastolic dysfunction has been observed in 30% to 70% of patients planned for cardiac surgery, and in geriatric patients (age > 65) planned for noncardiac surgery the prevalence has been as high as 61% (98). In the perioperative setting patient blood pressure and cardiac output are heavily influenced by volume status. In the setting of normal diastolic function, major volume expansion would be needed to cause elevated left ventricular diastolic pressure or pulmonary venous congestion and the volume expansion will initially lead to improved cardiac performance (99). In the patient with diastolic dysfunction, less volume expansion is needed to cause elevated left ventricular diastolic pressure and pulmonary congestion. By understanding the interplay between different stages of diastolic dysfunction and preload (Fig. 13.8) one can better determine how to manage the patient's volume status. Assessment of diastolic dysfunction could be very helpful in the perioperative setting where its primary role could be to predict how a patient would respond to increasing or decreasing preload. Lattik et al. found exactly this in a pilot study on 14 patients awaiting coronary bypass surgery where the velocity time integral of the E wave/ velocity time integral A wave (VTI E/A) ratio could predict how changes in preload affected cardiac output (100). He then further studied 36 patients undergoing coronary bypass surgery and challenged them with a rapid infusion of a colloid. Again the VTI E/A ratio predicted cardiac output where those with a low ratio (pattern of impaired relaxation) had the greatest likelihood of improvement in cardiac output, as opposed to those with a high VTI E/A ratio (pattern of restriction) where they did not improve cardiac output.

This prediction by diastolic patterns was superior to measurement of pulmonary artery wedge pressure. Multiple studies have shown that pulmonary wedge capillary pressure cannot accurately predict response to a volume

▶ **TABLE 13.2. Comparison of the Most Commonly Used Methods for Assessing Diastolic Dysfunction**

|  | *Where Measured* | *Method* | *Preload Dependence* | *Pitfalls* |
|---|---|---|---|---|
| Mitral Inflow | Tip of mitral valve leaflets | Pulsed Doppler | +++ | Mitral valve disease, atrial arrhythmias |
| Pulmonary Venous Flow | Ostium of pulmonary vein | Pulsed Doppler | +++ | Mitral valve disease, atrial arrhythmias |
| Tissue Doppler | Lateral or medial mitral valve annulus | Pulsed Doppler | + | Myocardial scarring |
| Color M-mode | Left ventricular inflow | Color M-mode | + | Aortic valve regurgitation |

challenge (101,102) and large randomized controlled trials have not been able to prove its role in the perioperative setting (103). Another echocardiography study on perioperative patients found that preexisting diastolic dysfunction could predict difficulty in weaning from cardiopulmonary bypass and increased need for inotropic support (104). Additionally we know that anesthetic agents, such as halothane, desflurane, or isoflurane, can cause diastolic dysfunction (105), and this effect could possibly be reversed with $CaCl_2$ (106) suggesting that these anesthetic agents cause diastolic dysfunction through calcium metabolism. Other medications used specifically in the perioperative setting, such as ketamine or bupivacaine, can cause diastolic dysfunction but not propofol or fentanyl (107–109). Therefore identifying patients with diastolic dysfunction prior to surgery could risk stratify patients and help in determining what medications would suit them best.

In general, analyzing diastolic dysfunction in the perioperative setting could have significant implications on clinical decision making and could result in better patient care and improved clinical outcomes. Large trials comparing outcomes when decisions are made from use of pulmonary artery catheter versus use of Doppler measured diastolic function are needed.

## CONCLUSION

In the past three decades our views on diastolic function have changed with better understanding of the important role it plays in the paradigm of heart failure. The accuracy of determining diastolic dysfunction by echocardiography is confounded by coexisting valvular disease or arrhythmias, acquiring an adequate acoustic window, gaining correct positioning of the Doppler cursor, and using optimal machine settings. Understanding the nature of diastolic dysfunction and mastering its diagnosis could lead to substantial improvement in perioperative patient care, whereas the sensitivity to preload found in some of the measures of diastolic dysfunction could prove helpful in managing patient fluid status. Newer methods of measuring diastolic dysfunction have additive value to older methods, and using more than one method for each patient will improve the accuracy of diagnosing diastolic dysfunction.

### KEY POINTS

- Diastolic dysfunction can be found in virtually all patients with systolic dysfunction.
- Diastolic dysfunction is characterized by elevated diastolic left ventricular pressure.
- More than one method is needed to accurately stage diastolic function.
- Staging of diastolic function can assist in management of perioperative patients.
- Preload dependent changes in mitral inflow can assist in gauging patient volume status.

## REFERENCES

1. Adams KF Jr. New epidemiologic perspectives concerning mild-to-moderate heart failure. Am J Med 2001;110 Suppl 7A:6S-13S.
2. Wexler DJ, Chen J, Smith GL, et al. Predictors of costs of caring for elderly patients discharged with heart failure. Am Heart J 2001;142(2):350–7.
3. Linne AB, Liedholm H, Jendteg S, Israelsson B. Health care costs of heart failure: results from a randomized study of patient education. Eur J Heart Fail 2000;2(3):291–7.
4. Mortality from congestive heart failure—United States, 1980–1990. MMWR Morb Mortal Wkly Rep 1994;43(5):77–81.
5. MacFadyen RJ, MacLeod CM, Shiels P, Russell Smith W, MacDonald TM. Isolated diastolic heart failure as a cause of breathlessness in the community: the Arbroath study. Eur J Heart Fail 2001;3(2):243–8.
6. Gandhi SK, Powers JC, Nomeir AM, et al. The pathogenesis of acute pulmonary edema associated with hypertension. N Engl J Med 2001;344(1):17–22.
7. Little WC, Kitzman DW, Cheng CP. Diastolic dysfunction as a cause of exercise intolerance. Heart Fail Rev 2000;5(4):301–6.
8. Gaasch WH, Levine HJ, Quinones MA, Alexander JK. Left ventricular compliance: mechanisms and clinical implications. Am J Cardiol 1976;38(5):645–53.
9. Packer M. Abnormalities of diastolic function as a potential cause of exercise intolerance in chronic heart failure. Circulation 1990;81(2 Suppl):III78–86.
10. Kitzman DW. Heart failure with normal systolic function. Clin Geriatr Med 2000;16(3):489–512.
11. Stainback RF. Congestive heart failure arising from diastolic dysfunction in the presence of normal left-ventricular systolic function. Tex Heart Inst J 1999;26(1):34–41.
12. Vasan RS, Benjamin EJ, Levy D. Congestive heart failure with normal left ventricular systolic function. Clinical approaches to the diagnosis and treatment of diastolic heart failure. Arch Intern Med 1996;156(2):146–57.
13. Sanderson JE. Diastolic heart failure: fact or fiction? Heart. 2003;89:1281–2.
14. Redfield MM, Jacobsen SJ, Burnett JC Jr, Mahoney DW, Bailey KR, Rodeheffer RJ. Burden of systolic and diastolic ventricular dysfunction in the community: appreciating the scope of the heart failure epidemic. JAMA. 2003;289: 194–202.
15. Hansen A, Haass M, Zugck C, et al. Prognostic value of Doppler echocardiographic mitral inflow patterns: implications for risk stratification in patients with chronic congestive heart failure. J Am Coll Cardiol 2001;37(4):1049–55.
16. Pinamonti B, Zecchin M, Di Lenarda A, Gregori D, Sinagra G, Camerini F. Persistence of restrictive left ventricular filling pattern in dilated cardiomyopathy: an ominous prognostic sign. J Am Coll Cardiol 1997;29(3):604–12.
17. Giannuzzi P, Temporelli PL, Bosimini E, et al. Independent and incremental prognostic value of Doppler-derived mitral deceleration time of early filling in both symptomatic and asymptomatic patients with left ventricular dysfunction. J Am Coll Cardiol 1996;28(2):383–90.
18. Werner GS, Schaefer C, Dirks R, Figulla HR, Kreuzer H. Prognostic value of Doppler echocardiographic assessment

of left ventricular filling in idiopathic dilated cardiomyopa-thy. Am J Cardiol 1994;73(11):792–8.

19. Xie GY, Berk MR, Smith MD, Gurley JC, DeMaria AN. Prognostic value of Doppler transmitral flow patterns in patients with congestive heart failure. J Am Coll Cardiol 1994;24(1):132–9.

20. Yu HCM, Sanderson JE. Different prognostic significance of right and left ventricular diastolic dysfunction in heart failure. Clin Cardiol 1999;5:117–26.

21. Poulsen SH, Jensen SE, Gotzsche O, Egstrup K. Evaluation and prognostic significance of left ventricular diastolic function assessed by Doppler echocardiography in the early phase of a first acute myocardial infarction. Eur Heart J 1997;18(12):1882–9.

22. Nishimura RA. Evaluation of diastolic filling of the left ventricle in health and disease: Doppler echocardiography is the clinician's Rosetta stone. JACC 1997;30(1):8–18.

23. Courtois M, Ludbrook PA, Kovacs SJ. Unsolved problems in diastole. Cardiol Clin 2000;18(3):653–67

24. Gilbert JC, Determinants of left ventricular filling and the diastolic pressure-volume relationship. Circ Res 1989;64:827.

25. Thomas JD. Doppler echocardiography and diastolic function. In Gaasch WH, LeWinter MH, eds. Heart failure and left ventricular diastolic dysfunction. Philadelphia: Lea & Febiger, 1993:192–218.

26. Thomas JD. Echocardiographic Doppler evaluation of left ventricular diastolic function: physics and physiology. Circulation 1991;84:977–90.

27. Choong CY. Left ventricle V: diastolic function—its principles and evaluation. In Weyman AE (ed). Principles and practice of echocardiography. Philadelphia: Lea & Febiger, 1994:721–80.

28. Yellin EL, Nickolic SD. Diastolic suction and the dynamics of left ventricular filling. In Gaasch WH, Lewinter MM, eds. Left ventricular diastolic dysfunction and heart failure. Philadelphia: Lea & Febiger, 1994:89–102.

29. Spadaro J, Bing OH, Gaasch WH, Weintraub RM. Pericardial modulation of right and left ventricular diastolic interaction. Circ Res 1981;48(2):233–8.

30. Arora RR, Machac J, Goldman ME, Butler RN, Gorlin R, Horowitz SF. Atrial kinetics and left ventricular diastolic filling in the healthy elderly. J Am Coll Cardiol 1987;9(6):1255–60.

31. Kono T, Sabbah HN, Rosman H, Alam M, Stein PD, Goldstein S. Left atrial contribution to ventricular filling during the course of evolving heart failure. Circulation 1992;86(4):1317–22.

32. Ling D, Rankin JS, Edwards C, McHale PA, Anderson RW. Regional diastolic mechanics of the LV in the conscious dog. Am J Phys 1979;236 (Heart Circ Physiol 5):H323–H330.

33. Swynghedauw B, Delcayre C, Cheav SL, Callens-el Amrani F. Biological basis of diastolic dysfunction of the hypertensive heart. Eur Heart J. 1992;13[Suppl D]:2–8.

34. Morgan JP, Erny RE, Allen PD, et al. Abnormal intracellular calcium handling, a major cause of systolic and diastolic dysfunction in ventricular myocardium from patients with heart failure. Circulation 1990;81[2 Suppl]:III21–III32.

35. Yellin EL, Meisner JS. Physiology of diastolic function and transmitral pressure-flow relations. Cardiol Clin 2000;18(3):411–33.

36. Ng KS, Gibson DG. Impairment of diastolic function by shortened filling period in severe left ventricular disease. Br Heart J 1989;62(4):246–52.

37. D'Angelo R, Shah N, Rubler S. Diastolic time intervals in ischemic and hypertensive heart disease: a comparison of isovolumic relaxation time and rapid filling time with systolic time intervals. Chest 1975;68(1):56–61.

38. Perlini S, Meyer TE, Foex P. Effects of preload, afterload and inotropy on dynamics of ischemic segmental wall motion. J Am Coll Cardiol 1997;29(4):846–55.

39. Chen C, Rodriguez L, Levine RA, Weyman AE, Thomas JD. Noninvasive measurement of the time constant of left ventricular relaxation using the continuous-wave Doppler velocity profile of mitral regurgitation. Circulation 1992;86(1):272–8.

40. Weiss JL, Frederiksen JW, Weisfeldt ML. Hemodynamic determinants of the time-course of fall in canine left ventricular pressure. J Clin Invest 1976;58(3):751–60.

41. Thomas JD, Flachskampf FA, Chen C, et al. Isovolumic relaxation time varies predictably with its time constant and aortic and left atrial pressures: implications for the noninvasive evaluation of ventricular relaxation. Am Heart J 1992;124(5):1305–13.

42. Schafer S, Fiedler VB, Thamer V. Afterload dependent prolongation of left ventricular relaxation: importance of asynchrony. Cardiovasc Res 1992;26(6):631–7.

43. Gaasch WH, Blaustein AS, Andrias CW, Donahue RP, Avitall B. Myocardial relaxation. II. Hemodynamic determinants of rate of left ventricular isovolumic pressure decline. Am J Physiol 1980;239(1):H1–6.

44. Ariel Y, Gaasch WH, Bogen DK, McMahon TA. Load-dependent relaxation with late systolic volume steps: servo-pump studies in the intact canine heart. Circulation 1987;75(6):1287–94.

45. Garcia MJ, Thomas JD, Klein AL. New Doppler Echocardiographic applications for the study of diastolic function. JACC 1998;32:865–75.

46. Cohen GI, Pietrolungo JF, Thomas JD, Klein AL. A practical guide to assessment of ventricular diastolic function using doppler echocardiography. JACC 1996;27(7):1753–820.

47. Hurrell DG, Nishimura RA, Ilstrup DM, Appleton CP. Utility of preload alteration in assessment of left ventricular filling pressure by Doppler echocardiography: a simultaneous catheterization and Doppler echocardiographic study. J Am Coll Cardiol 1997;30(2):459–67.

48. Elesber AA, Redfield MM. Approach to patients with heart failure and normal ejection fraction. Mayo Clin Proc 2001;76(10):1047–52.

49. Wijbenga AA, Mosterd A, Kasprzak JD, et al. Potentials and limitations of the Valsalva maneuver as a method of differentiating between normal and pseudonormal left ventricular filling patterns. Am J Cardiol 1999;84(1):76–81.

50. Farias CA, Rodriguez L, Garcia MJ, Sun JP, Klein AL, Thomas JD. Assessment of diastolic function by tissue Doppler echocardiography: comparison with standard transmitral and pulmonary venous flow. J Am Soc Echocardiogr 1999;12(8):609–17.

51. Moller JE, Sondergaard E, Poulsen SH, Egstrup K. Pseudonormal and restrictive filling patterns predict left ventricular dilation and cardiac death after a first myocardial infarction: a serial color M-mode Doppler echocardiographic study. J Am Coll Cardiol 2000;36(6):1841–6.

52. Hellevik LR, Segers P, Stergiopulos N, et al. Mechanism of pulmonary venous pressure and flow waves. Heart Vessels 1999;14(2):67–71.

53. Keren G, Bier A, Sherez J, Miura D, Keefe D, LeJemtel T. Atrial contraction is an important determinant of pulmonary venous flow. J Am Coll Cardiol 1986;7(3):693–5.

54. de Marchi SF, Bodenmuller M, Lai DL, Seiler C. Pulmonary venous flow velocity patterns in 404 individuals without cardiovascular disease. Heart 2001;85(1):23–9.

55. Masuyama T, Lee JM, Tamai M, Tanouchi J, Kitabatake A, Kamada T. Pulmonary venous flow velocity pattern as assessed with transthoracic pulsed Doppler echocardiography in subjects without cardiac disease. Am J Cardiol 1991;67(16):1396–404.

56. Castello R, Pearson AC, Lenzen P, Labovitz AJ. Evaluation of pulmonary venous flow by transesophageal echocardiography in subjects with a normal heart: comparison with transthoracic echocardiography. J Am Coll Cardiol 1991;18(1):65–71 .

57. Smiseth OA, Lodemel K, Riddervold F, Blaha M. Changes in pulmonary vein flow pattern during volume loading. Cardiovasc Res 1993;27(3):411–5.

58. Nishimura RA, Abel MD, Hatle LK, Tajik AJ. Relation of pulmonary vein to mitral flow velocities by transesophageal

Doppler echocardiography. Effect of different loading conditions. Circulation 1990;81(5):1488–97.

59. Garcia MJ, Thomas JD. Tissue Doppler to Assess Diastolic Left Ventricular Function. Echocardiography 1999;16(5): 501–8.

60. Oki T, Tabata T, Yamada H, et al. Clinical application of pulsed Doppler tissue imaging for assessing abnormal left ventricular relaxation. Am J Cardiol 1997;79(7):921–8.

61. Sohn DW, Chai IH, Lee DJ, et al. Assessment of mitral annulus velocity by Doppler tissue imaging in the evaluation of left ventricular diastolic function. J Am Coll Cardiol 1997; 30(2):474–80.

62. Firstenberg MS, Vandervoort PM, Greenberg NL, et al. Noninvasive estimation of transmitral pressure drop across the normal mitral valve in humans: importance of convective and inertial forces during left ventricular filling. J Am Coll Cardiol. 2000;36:1942–9.

63. Garcia-Fernandez MA, Azevedo J, Moreno M, et al. Regional diastolic function in ischemic heart disease using pulsed wave Doppler tissue imaging. Eur Heart J 1999;20(7): 496–505.

64. Yamada H, Oki T, Mishiro Y, et al. Effect of aging on diastolic left ventricular myocardial velocities measured by pulsed tissue Doppler imaging in healthy subjects. J Am Soc Echocardiogr 1999;12(7):574–81.

65. Garcia MJ, Rodriguez L, Ares M, Griffin BP, Thomas JD, Klein AL. Differentiation of constrictive pericarditis from restrictive cardiomyopathy: assessment of left ventricular diastolic velocities in longitudinal axis by Doppler tissue imaging. J Am Coll Cardiol. 1996;27:108–14.

66. Bruch C, Schmermund A, Bartel T, Schaar J, Erbel R. Tissue Doppler imaging: a new technique for assessment of pseudonormalization of the mitral inflow pattern. Echocardiography 2000;17(6 Pt 1):539–46.

67. Rajagopalan N, Garcia MJ, Rodriguez L, et al. Comparison of new Doppler echocardiographic methods to differentiate constrictive pericardial heart disease and restrictive cardiomyopathy. Am J Cardiol 2001;87(1):86–94.

68. Ommen SR, Nishimura RA, Appleton CP, et al. Clinical utility of Doppler echocardiography and tissue Doppler imaging in the estimation of left ventricular filling pressures: A comparative simultaneous Doppler-catheterization study. Circulation 2000;102(15):1788–94.

69. Thomas JD, Garcia MJ, Greenberg NL. Application of color Doppler M-mode echocardiography in the assessment of ventricular diastolic function: potential for quantitative analysis. Heart Vessels 1997;Suppl12:135–7.

70. Takatsuji H, Mikami T, Urasawa K, et al. A new approach for evaluation of left ventricular diastolic function: spatial and temporal analysis of left ventricular filling flow propagation by color M-mode Doppler echocardiography. J Am Coll Cardiol 1996;27(2):365–71.

71. Garcia MJ, Smedira NG, Greenberg NL, et al. Color M-mode Doppler flow propagation velocity is a preload insensitive index of left ventricular relaxation: animal and human validation. J Am Coll Cardiol 2000;35(1):201–8.

72. Garcia MJ, Ares MA, Asher C, Rodriguez L, Vandervoort P, Thomas JD. An index of early left ventricular filling that combined with pulsed Doppler peak E velocity may estimate capillary wedge pressure. J Am Coll Cardiol 1997;29(2):448–54.

73. Nishihara K, Mikami T, Takatsuji H, et al. Usefulness of early diastolic flow propagation velocity measured by color M-mode Doppler technique for the assessment of left ventricular diastolic function in patients with hypertrophic cardiomyopathy. J Am Soc Echocardiogr. 2000;13:801–8.

74. Hatle LK, Sutherland GR. Regional myocardial function—a new approach. Eur Heart J 2000;21:1337–57.

75. Urheim S, Edvardsen T, Torp H, et al. Myocardial strain by Doppler echocardiography. Validation of a new method to quantify regional myocardial function. Circulation 2000;102: 1158–64.

76. Castro PL, Greenberg NL, Drinko J, Garcia MJ, Thomas JD. Potential pitfalls of strain rate imaging: angle dependency. Biomed Sci Instrum. 2000;36:197–202.

77. Yang H, Sun JP, Lever HM, et al. Use of strain imaging in detecting segmental dysfunction in patients with hypertrophic cardiomyopathy. J Am Soc Echocardiogr. 2003;16:233–9.

78. Stoylen A, Heimdal A, Bjornstad K, et al. Strain rate imaging by ultrasonography in the diagnosis of coronary artery disease. J Am Soc Echocardiogr 2000;13:1053–64.

79. Sun JP, Popovic ZB, Greenberg NL, et al. Noninvasive quantification of regional myocardial function using Doppler-derived velocity, displacement, strain rate, and strain in healthy volunteers: effects of aging. J Am Soc Echocardiogr 2004; 17:132–8.

80. Falsetti HL, Verani MS, Chen CJ, Cramer JA. Regional pressure differences in the left ventricle. Cathet Cardiovasc Diagn 1980;6(2):123–34.

81. Courtois M, Kovacs SJ Jr, Ludbrook PA. Transmitral pressure-flow velocity relation. Importance of regional pressure gradients in the left ventricle during diastole. Circulation 1988;78(3):661–71.

82. Courtois M, Kovacs SJ, Ludbrook PA. Physiological early diastolic intraventricular pressure gradient is lost during acute myocardial ischemia. Circulation 1990;81(5):1688–96.

83. Greenberg NL, Vandervoort PM, Thomas JD. Instantaneous diastolic transmitral pressure differences from color Doppler M mode echocardiography. Am J Physiol 1996;271(4 Pt 2): H1267–76.

84. Bermejo J, Antoranz JC, Yotti R, Moreno M, Garcia-Fernandez MA. Spatio-temporal mapping of intracardiac pressure gradients. A solution to Euler's equation from digital postprocessing of color Doppler M-mode echocardiograms. Ultrasound Med Biol 2001;27(5):621–30.

85. Greenberg NL, Vandervoort PM, Firstenberg MS, Garcia MJ, Thomas JD. Estimation of diastolic intraventricular pressure gradients by Doppler M-mode echocardiography. Am J Physiol Heart Circ Physiol 2001;280(6):H2507–15.

86. Firstenberg MS, Smedira NG, Greenberg NL, et al. Relationship between early diastolic intraventricular pressure gradients, an index of elastic recoil, and improvements in systolic and diastolic function. Circulation 2001;104(12 Suppl 1): I330–5.

87. Rovner A, Smith R, Greenberg NL, et al. Improvement in diastolic intraventricular pressure gradients in patients with HOCM after ethanol septal reduction. Am J Physiol Heart Circ Physiol. 2003;285(6):H2492–9.

88. Fraites TJ Jr, Saeki A, Kass DA. Effect of altering filling pattern on diastolic pressure-volume curve. Circulation 1997; 96(12):4408–14.

89. Keren G, Milner M, Lindsay J Jr, Goldstein S. Load dependence of left atrial and left ventricular filling dynamics by transthoracic and transesophageal Doppler echocardiography. Am J Card Imaging 1996;10(2):108–16.

90. Appleton CP, Hatle LK, Popp RL. Relation of transmitral flow velocity patterns to left ventricular diastolic function: new insights from a combined hemodynamic and Doppler echocardiographic study. J Am Coll Cardiol 1988;12(2): 426–40.

91. Genovesi-Ebert A, Marabotti C, Palombo C, Giaconi S, Ghione S. Left ventricular filling: relationship with arterial blood pressure, left ventricular mass, age, heart rate and body build. J Hypertens 1991;9(4):345–53.

92. Rittoo D, Monaghan M, Sadiq T, Nichols A, Richardson PJ. Echocardiographic and Doppler evaluation of left ventricular hypertrophy and diastolic function in black and white hypertensive patients. J Hum Hypertens 1990;4(2):113–5.

93. Onbasili OA, Tekten T, Ceyhan C, Ercan E, Mutlu B. A new echocardiographic method for the assessment of the severity of aortic regurgitation: color M-mode flow propagation velocity. J Am Soc Echocardiogr. 2002;15:1453–60.

94. Angeja BG, Grossman W. Evaluation and management of diastolic heart failure. Circulation. 2003;107:659–63.

95. Banerjee P, Banerjee T, Khand A, et al. Diastolic heart failure: neglected or misdiagnosed? J Am Coll Cardiol. 2002;39: 138–141.

96. Setaro J, Zaret BL, Schueman DS, et al. Usefulness of verapamil for congestive heart failure associated with abnormal

left ventricular diastolic performance. Am J Cardiol 1990;66: 981–86.

97. Nishimura RA, Schwartz RS, Holmes DR Jr, Tajik AJ. Failure of calcium channel blockers to improve ventricular relaxation in humans. J Am Coll Cardiol. 1993;21(1):182–8.

98. Phillip B, Pastor D, Bellows W, Leung JM. The prevalence of preoperative diastolic filling abnormalities in geriatric surgical patients. Anesth Analg 2003;97:1214–21.

99. Nozaki J, Kitahata H, Tanaka K, Kawahito S, Oshita S. The effects of acute normovolemic hemodilution on left ventricular systolic and diastolic function in the absence or presence of beta-adrenergic blockade in dogs. Anesth Analg 2002;94: 1120–6.

100. Lattik R, Couture P, Denault AY, et al. Mitral Doppler indices are superior to two-dimensional echocardiographic and hemodynamic variables in predicting responsiveness of cardiac output to a rapid intravenous infusion of colloid. Anesth Analg 2002;94:1092–9.

101. Douglas PS, Edmunds LH, Sutton MS, Geer R, Harken AH, Reichek N. Unreliability of hemodynamic indexes of left ventricular size during cardiac surgery. Ann Thorac Surg. 1987;44:31–4.

102. Swenson JD, Harkin C, Pace NL, Astle K, Bailey P. Transesophageal echocardiography: an objective tool in defining maximum ventricular response to intravenous fluid therapy. Anesth Analg. 1996;83:1149–53.

103. Sandham JD, Hull RD, Brant RF, et al. Canadian Critical Care Clinical Trials Group. A randomized, controlled trial of the use of pulmonary-artery catheters in high risk surgical patients. N Engl J Med 2003;348:5–14.

104. Bernard F, Denault A, Babin D, et al. Diastolic dysfunction is predictive of difficult weaning from cardiopulmonary bypass. Anesth Analg 2001;92:291–8.

105. Pagel PS, Kampine JP, Schmeling WT, Warltier DC. Alteration of left ventricular diastolic function by desflurane, isoflurane, and halothane in the chronically instrumented dog with autonomic nervous system blockade. Anesthesiology. 1991;74:1103–14.

106. Pagel PS, Kampine JP, Schmeling WT, Warltier DC. Reversal of volatile anesthetic-induced depression of myocardial contractility by extracellular calcium also enhances left ventricular diastolic function. Anesthesiology. 1993;78:141–54.

107. Pagel PS, Schmeling WT, Kampine JP, Warltier DC. Alteration of canine left ventricular diastolic function by intravenous anesthetics in vivo. Ketamine and propofol. Anesthesiology. 1992;76:419–25.

108. Hirabayashi Y, Igarashi T, Saitoh K, Fukuda H, Suzuki H, Shimizu R. Comparison of the effects of amrinone, milrinone and olprinone in reversing bupivacaine-induced cardiovascular depression. Acta Anaesthesiol Scand 2000;44: 1128–33.

109. Phillips AS, McMurray TJ, Mirakhur RK, Gibson FM, Elliott P. Propofol-fentanyl anaesthesia in cardiac surgery: a comparison in patients with good and impaired ventricular function. Anaesthesia. 1993;48:661–3.

## QUESTIONS

1. In addition to mitral inflow which of the following is necessary to detect stage II (pseudonormal) of diastolic dysfunction?
   A. Pulsed wave Doppler of pulmonary venous flow
   B. Doppler tissue imaging of the mitral annulus
   C. Color M-mode of the mitral inflow
   D. Any of the above

2. Which of these two choices has higher prevalence in the general population?
   A. Diastolic dysfunction
   B. Systolic dysfunction

3. Which of the following are consistent with diuresis of a patient with a stage II (pseudonormal) pattern of diastolic dysfunction?
   A. Change from stage II (pseudonormal) to stage IV (fixed restrictive) pattern
   B. Change from stage II to stage III (restrictive) pattern
   C. No change in stage II pattern
   D. Change from stage II (pseudonormal) to stage I (abnormal relaxation) pattern

4. Which of the following distinguishes restrictive from constrictive physiology?
   A. Increased Em velocity
   B. Decreased Em velocity
   C. Increased IVRT (isovolumetric relaxation time)
   D. Increased DT (deceleration time)

5. Which of the following distinguishes constrictive from restrictive physiology?
   A. Increased DT (deceleration time) in constrictive physiology
   B. Increased "E" wave in restrictive physiology
   C. Respiratory variation with constrictive physiology
   D. E to A reversal with restrictive physiology

## Chapter 14

# Assessment of the Mitral Valve

*Colleen Gorman Koch*

The mitral valve is aptly named because of its resemblance to a "mitre," a type of folding cap consisting of two similar parts that rise to a peak (1,2). During the Renaissance Andreas Vesalius suggested the term *mitral* because of the valve's resemblance to a bishop's *mitre* (Fig. 14.1) (3,4). His publication of *De Humani Corporis Fabrica* in 1543 constituted a monumental achievement by presenting anatomy as a scientific discipline, ultimately advancing the knowledge of cardiology (5). The intrigue of mitral anatomy, during an age when studies were done in secret and published at risk to the anatomist, is currently captured by transesophageal echocardiography, which provides a window to real-time structure and function of the heart.

## ANATOMY OF THE MITRAL VALVE

Anatomic components of the mitral valve complex include the left atrial wall, the mitral annulus, the anterior and posterior mitral valve leaflets, the chordal tendons, and the anterolateral and posteromedial papillary muscles, which attach the mitral valve to the left ventricular myocardium (6–8). The mitral annulus, which exhibits sphincteric contraction in systole, serves as a basal attachment for the mitral valve leaflets (8). The anterior mitral leaflet is somewhat triangular and subtends approximately one-third of the circumference of the mitral annulus. It has a longer basal-to-margin length than the posterior mitral leaflet. Part of the annulus of the anterior mitral leaflet has a common attachment to the fibrous skeleton of the heart with the left coronary cusp and half of the noncoronary cusp of the aortic valve. (4). The posterior mitral leaflet is shorter and subtends a greater attachment to the mitral annulus than the anterior mitral leaflet. The posterior mitral leaflet has a "true bundle of fibrous tissue," the annulus, separating the left atrium from the left ventricle (6,9,10). While morphologically different, the surface areas of the anterior and posterior mitral valve leaflets are nearly identical (4,6,8,9) and to-

gether exceed the area of the mitral annulus in a relationship of greater than two to one (4,8). The mitral valve leaflets adjoin at the sides of the valve, forming the anterolateral and posteromedial commissures (4). More than 120 chordal tendons subdivide as they project from each papillary muscle to attach to the free edge and body of both mitral valve leaflets. Subdivisions of the choral tendons can be classified as primary (first order), secondary (second order), and tertiary (third order) chordae (4).

Standard nomenclature adopted by the Society of Cardiovascular Anesthesiologists and the American Society of Echocardiography divides the anterior and posterior leaflets into three segmental regions (11). Indentations along the free margin of the posterior mitral leaflet give it a scalloped appearance, allowing identification of individual scallops P1, P2, and P3 (6). The anterior mitral leaflet is also divided into three segments located opposite the corresponding segments of the posterior mitral leaflet: A1, A2, and A3. The P1 and A1 segments are adjacent to the anterolateral commissure, while the P3 and A3 segments are adjacent to the posteromedial commissure (Fig. 14.2) (11).

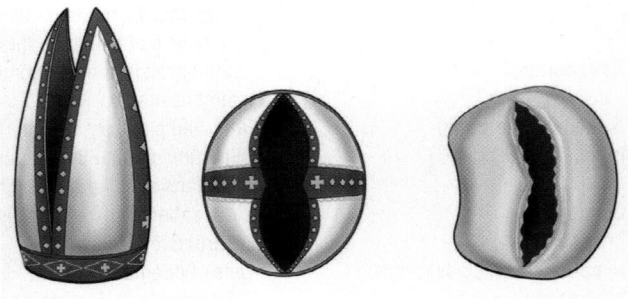

**FIGURE 14.1.** The mitre typically worn by bishops, popes, and cardinals is depicted alongside a cross-sectional image of the mitral valve. Andreas Vesalius, the father of anatomy, noted the striking similarity between the two while performing anatomic dissections in the sixteenth century.

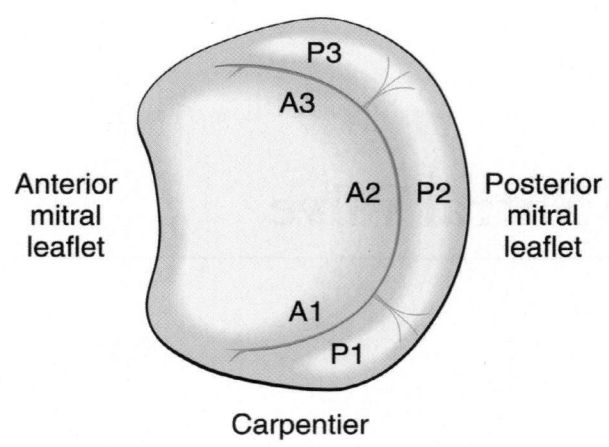

**FIGURE 14.2.** Standard terminology as applied to the mitral valve leaflets is illustrated in this image. The anterior and posterior mitral valve leaflets are each divided into three segmental regions.

## STRUCTURAL INTEGRITY OF THE MITRAL VALVE

### Mitral Regurgitation

The structural integrity of the mitral valve may be compromised by primary valve pathology or secondary disease processes affecting one or more components of the mitral valve apparatus (12). The primary etiology of mitral regurgitation in industrialized countries is from ischemic and degenerative causes (13). Table 14.1 lists a broad range of disease processes that contribute to dysfunction of the mitral valve.

Carpentier and colleagues categorized mitral valve dysfunction based on normal, excessive, or restrictive leaflet motion range (14). Mitral insufficiency with normal leaflet motion occurs in patients with congenital clefts in the leaflet tissue or those with leaflet perforation due to endocarditis. Mitral regurgitation due to excessive leaflet motion can result from chordal rupture leading to segmental leaflet prolapse. Loss of leaflet tissue from rheumatic endocarditis may lead to restricted leaflet motion and subsequent mitral insufficiency (Fig. 14.3) (15).

### Severity Estimation

Echocardiographic grading of mitral regurgitation, as well as determination of ventricular dimensions and function are integral to clinical decision making with regard to the timing for surgical intervention. Application of severity estimation methods is dependent on the technical expertise of the imaging staff, the complexity involved with the measurement technique, associated limitations with the individual method, and time constraints.

Developed methods of estimation can be partitioned into qualitative, semiquantitative, and quantitative techniques. An integration of these techniques in conjunction with clinical features of the patient's presentation will provide an accurate assessment of regurgitant severity and need for surgical intervention.

### Two-Dimensional Echocardiography

Two-dimensional echocardiography provides anatomic details to assist in delineating the underlying etiology of valve dysfunction. A complete transesophageal echocar-

▌ TABLE 14.1. Etiology, Mechanism, and Two-Dimensional Characteristics of Mitral Valve Dysfunction

| Etiology | Mechanism | Two-Dimensional Echocardiographic Appearance |
|---|---|---|
| Rheumatic heart disease | Retractile fibrosis of leaflet tissue and chordal tendons resulting in failure of leaflet coaptation | Thickened leaflet tissue and chordal tendons, restricted leaflet motion, calcium deposition |
| Degenerative | Leaflet prolapse, malalignment of leaflet tissue | Prolapsing/flail leaflet tissue |
| Ischemic (infarction) | Ruptured papillary muscle | Flail leaflet |
| Myocardial disease | Dilatation of annulus, reduced surface area for coaptation | Normal leaflet tissue, increased annular dimensions |
| Congenital | Cleft leaflet, transposed valve | Cleft leaflet, tricuspid valve |
| Endocarditis | Destructive lesions | Perforation, flail leaflets, vegetations |
| Hyperesoinophilic syndrome | Loss of coaptation | Reduced leaflet motion |
| Infiltrative disease | Thickened leaflets impair coaptation | Leaflet thickening |
| Marfan syndrome | Ruptured chordal tendons | Redundant tissue, prolapse, or flail of leaflet tissue |
| Postradiation | Leaflet thickening impairs coaptation | Thickened leaflets, restrictive leaflet motion |
| Carcinoid/ergot alkaloids | Fibrosis of leaflets, failure of coaptation | Leaflet thickening and restriction |

Modified from Rahimtoola S, Enriquez-Sarano M, Schaff H, Frye R. Mitral Valve Disease. In: Fuster V, Alexander R, O'Rourke R, eds. *Hurst's the Heart.* 10th ed. New York: McGraw-Hill 2001, with permission.

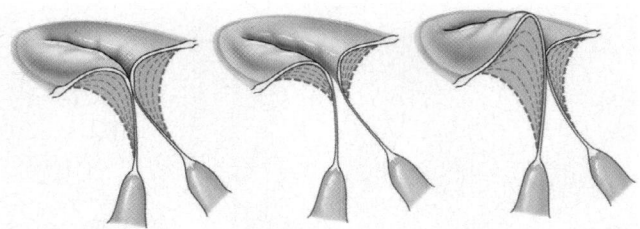

**FIGURE 14.3.** Carpentier's classification of range of mitral leaflet motion is depicted in this illustration as normal, restrictive, and excessive leaflet motion, respectively.

diography (TEE) examination of the mitral valve apparatus and surrounding left ventricular myocardium aid in characterizing valve pathology. Enlargement of the left atrium and increases in the left ventricular systolic and diastolic dimensions are changes detected by two-dimensional echocardiography. Two-dimensional changes suggestive of severe mitral insufficiency include left atrial dimensions of ≥ 5.5 cm and left ventricular diastolic dimensions of ≥ 7 cm (16).

The volume overload imposed on the left ventricle is proportional to the severity of mitral regurgitation present. End-systolic chamber size is considered a sensitive marker for imminent ventricular dysfunction. In particular, it is recommended that asymptomatic and symptomatic patients with severe mitral regurgitation and left ventricular end-systolic diameter of ≥ 4.5 cm undergo corrective surgical intervention (17,18). The impact of volume overload on the left side of the heart is also dependent on the acuity of mitral regurgitation. Initial phases of severe mitral regurgitation result in a dilated left ventricle with hyperdynamic function and an end-systolic cavity volume, which is small, compared to the end diastolic volume. Continued volume overload over time will lead to left ventricular dysfunction. Ideally, with echocardiographic guidance, corrective interventions can be implemented prior to the development of significant and irreversible ventricular dysfunction (18).

## Qualitative Techniques

### Continuous Wave Doppler Signal

Aligning the continuous wave Doppler (CW-Doppler) signal through the mitral regurgitant jet allows visualization of mitral regurgitant signal density and morphology. In general, the signal intensity is reflective of the severity of mitral regurgitation. Mild degrees of mitral regurgitation are detected by CW-Doppler as incomplete envelopes of low CW-Doppler signal intensity, whereas dense complete CW-Doppler signal envelopes of nearly equal intensity to mitral inflow are associated with more severe degrees of mitral regurgitation (Fig. 14.4) (16,19).

### Peak E Wave Velocity

Peak E wave velocity as detected with pulsed wave Doppler of the transmitral flow velocity can be qualitatively related to mitral regurgitation severity. When the degree of mitral regurgitation increases, the added regurgitant volume across the mitral valve will increase the pressure gradient between the left atrium and left ventricle. The increase in pressure gradient, in turn, increases the early mitral inflow velocity (20). Thomas and colleagues investigated the use of peak E wave velocity as an initial screening variable to identify hemodynamically significant mitral regurgitation. Peak E wave velocity was compared to a qualitative echocardiographic evaluation by an expert as well as with regurgitant fraction measurements. An E wave velocity of > 1.2 meters per second (m/s) identified patients with severe mitral regurgitation with a sensitivity of 86%, a specificity of 86%, a positive predictive value of 75%, and a negative predictive value of 92% (20).

## Semiquantitative Techniques

### Spatial Area Mapping

Color flow Doppler is one of the most commonly used semiquantitative methods to estimate the severity of mitral regurgitation (21). Color flow Doppler is based on pulsed wave ultrasound techniques with different signal processing and display formats. Instead of measuring velocities at a single location as with pulsed wave Doppler, color flow Doppler has a number of gates positioned at different depths along many scan lines. Velocity

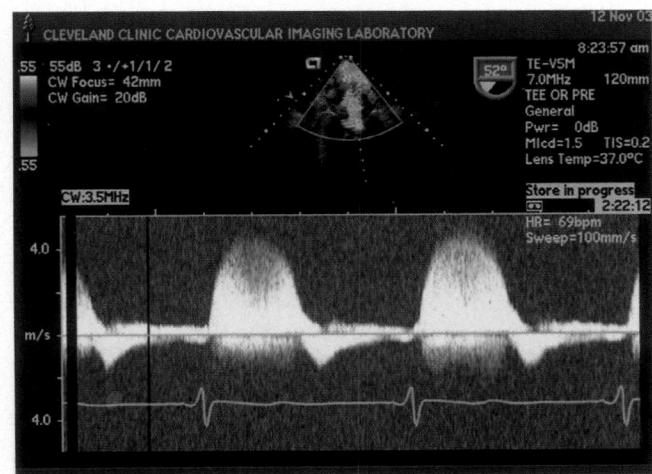

**FIGURE 14.4.** Continuous wave Doppler displays a mitral regurgitant jet as a spectral profile represented above the baseline. This regurgitant signal is of nearly equal intensity to antegrade flow through the mitral valve. This qualitative assessment is consistent with the patient's severe degree of mitral insufficiency.

is encoded into different colors based on the direction of flow to or away from the transducer (22). The extent of the velocity map displayed by color flow Doppler is reflective of the velocity of regurgitant flow rather than absolute regurgitant volume (18). In general, color Doppler can quickly differentiate mild degrees from severe grades of mitral regurgitation (Figs. 14.5 and 14.6).

Color flow Doppler estimates of mitral insufficiency correlate well with the semiquantitative angiographic grades of insufficiency (21). Castello and colleagues compared the correlation between color flow Doppler regurgitant jet area measurements to angiography. A maximal jet area $< 3$ cm$^2$ predicted mild mitral regurgitation with a sensitivity of 96%, a specificity of 100%, and a predictive accuracy of 98%; whereas a maximal regurgitant area of $> 6$ cm$^2$ predicted severe regurgitation with a sensitivity of 91%, specificity of 100%, and predictive accuracy of 98% (23).

Spain and colleagues also reported a good correlation between maximal color flow Doppler jet area and angiographic grades of mitral insufficiency. However, they reported limited correlation between quantitative measurements of mitral regurgitant severity, such as regurgitant volume and regurgitant fraction, with maximal jet area measurements (24).

Rivera and colleagues compared a *visual* assessment method, the color flow Doppler jet area method, and regurgitant fraction measurements for grading the severity of mitral regurgitation. The visual assessment method encompassed integrating information about actual jet dimensions and jet eccentricity as well as chamber geometry to provide an educated assessment of the degree of regurgitation present. They reported that the visual grading method had a better correlation with quantitative

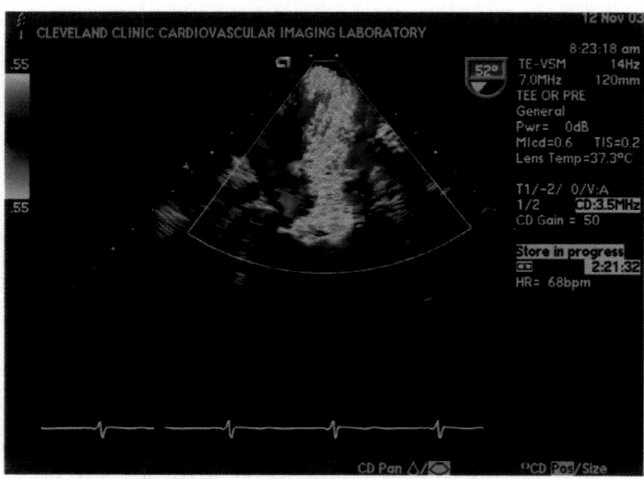

**FIGURE 14.6.** The midesophageal two-chamber view depicts severe mitral insufficiency with color flow imaging. The color flow signal extends to the posterior left atrial wall and displays an area of flow convergence on the left ventricular side of the mitral valve.

measures of regurgitation than jet area measurements (25).

Several technical factors influence the appearance of the color flow signal within the left atrium. Among these are instrumentation settings, such as frame rate, gain settings, and transducer frequency (22). Alterations in color-scale settings impact the effect of entrainment of left atrial blood on the regurgitant jet area. Setting the color scale to the highest possible level will limit the effect of entrainment (26). Maintaining constant technical factors reduces instrumentation errors.

Alterations in intraoperative hemodynamics also influence the jet of mitral regurgitation as detected by color flow Doppler (27,28). Grewal and colleagues (27) reported that slightly more than half of patients with mitral insufficiency improved at least one grade with the induction of general anesthesia. Decreased intravascular volume coupled with a reduction in afterload was thought to contribute to better leaflet coaptation and reduced valvular insufficiency (27).

Compliance and size of the receiving chamber confound the relationship between the size of the regurgitant jet and regurgitant volume (24). Patients with acute, severe mitral regurgitation may display a relatively small jet area secondary to high left atrial pressures due to limited compliance of the left atrium (18).

Eccentric regurgitant jets when imaged by color-flow mapping commonly occupy less overall area compared to jets of similar flow rates directed centrally within the left atrium (29). An eccentric jet has a different observed morphology as compared to free jets secondary to limited expansion due to impingement of the jet along the atrial wall. Consideration of jet morphology in the color flow

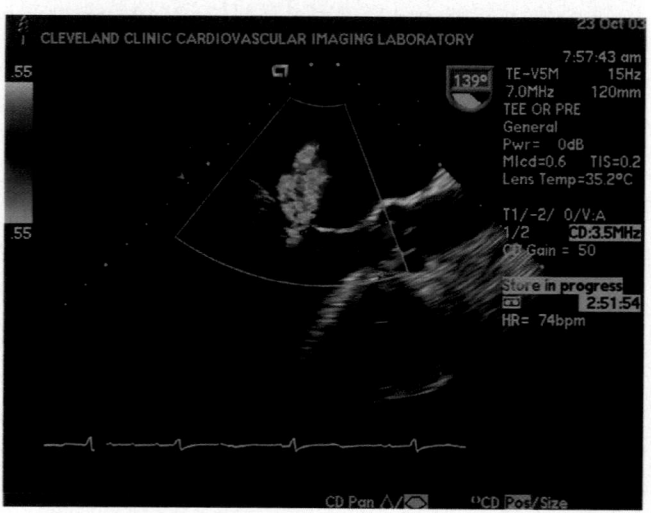

**FIGURE 14.5.** The midesophageal long-axis image of the mitral valve displays a mild grade of mitral insufficiency as represented with color flow Doppler imaging.

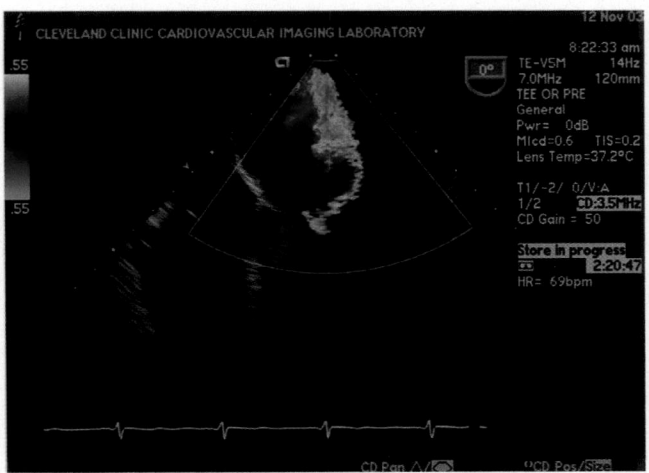

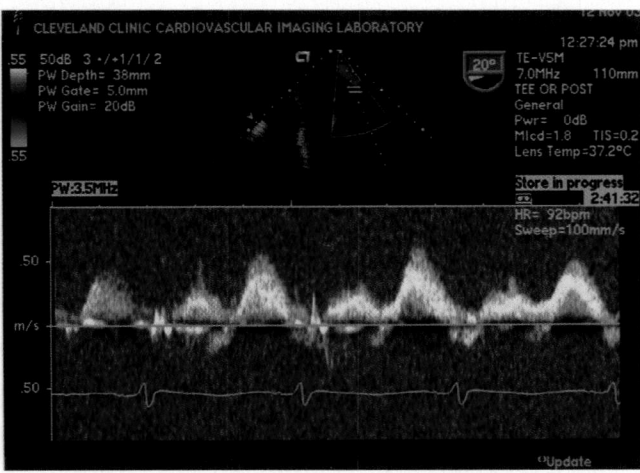

**FIGURE 14.7.** Anterior mitral leaflet prolapse results in an eccentric jet of mitral insufficiency as displayed with color flow imaging from the midesophageal imaging plane. Note the jet of mitral insufficiency is posteriorly directed.

**FIGURE 14.8.** A pulsed wave Doppler sample volume placed within the left upper pulmonary vein reveals a Doppler velocity profile that displays a blunted pulmonary venous waveform pattern.

Doppler assessment is important to avoid underestimating the degree of regurgitation (Fig. 14.7) (29).

### Pulmonary Venous Waveform Patterns

Normal pulmonary venous waveform patterns consist of a biphasic forward systolic waveform occurring during ventricular systole, a forward diastolic velocity waveform that occurs after mitral valve opening, and a retrograde atrial flow reversal waveform that occurs in response to atrial contraction (30). In general, the normal pattern of pulmonary venous flow displays the ratio of systolic waveform to diastolic waveform as greater than or equal to one. Current applications for pulmonary venous waveform patterns include differentiating constrictive pericarditis from constriction, estimation of left ventricular filling pressures, evaluation of left ventricular diastolic dysfunction, and grading the severity of mitral regurgitation (31).

Significant degrees of mitral regurgitation increase left atrial pressure and alter forward flow through the pulmonary veins. Klein and colleagues (32) investigated the relationship between the ratio of peak systolic and peak diastolic flow velocities in the pulmonary veins to varying degrees of mitral regurgitation as measured with TEE color-flow mapping. The ratio of peak systolic and diastolic pulmonary venous waveform velocities were categorized as having a normal pattern where the ratio of peak systolic/diastolic waveform was greater than or equal to one, a blunted pattern where the ratio of peak systolic to peak diastolic waveform was between 0 and < 1 (Fig. 14.8), and reversed systolic waveform represented by a peak systolic velocity value of < 0 (Fig. 14.9). The

sensitivity and specificity for reversed systolic flow detecting 4-plus mitral regurgitation was 93% and 100%, respectively. Blunted systolic flow for detecting 3–plus mitral regurgitation had lower sensitivity and specificity of 61% and 97%, respectively (32).

Pulmonary venous flow patterns may not be a reliable marker of valvular insufficiency for all grades of mitral regurgitation. Pu and colleagues evaluated the relationship between pulmonary venous flow patterns and quantitative indexes of mitral regurgitation in patients with variable degrees of left ventricular function. Quantitative Doppler

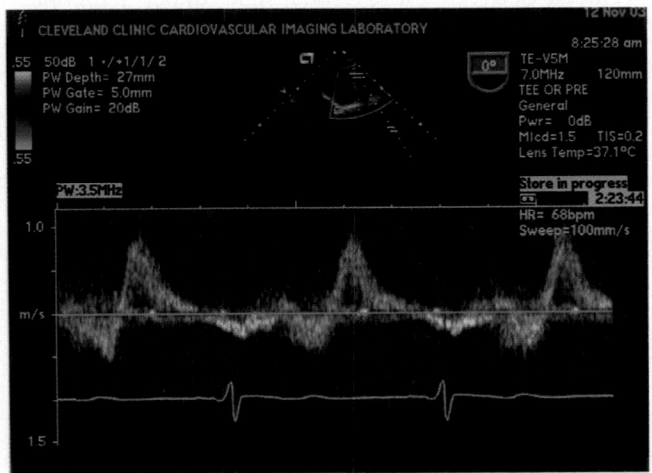

**FIGURE 14.9.** This pulsed wave Doppler profile of the left upper pulmonary vein reveals systolic flow reversal as represented by systolic flow beneath the baseline, which is consistent with severe mitral insufficiency.

measurements included regurgitant orifice area, regurgitant stroke volume, and regurgitant fraction measurements. A normal pulmonary venous waveform pattern had a sensitivity, specificity, and predictive value for detecting a small regurgitant orifice area of less than 0.3 cm$^2$ of 60%, 96%, and 94%, respectively. The reversed pattern was a highly specific marker for detecting a large regurgitant orifice area of greater than 0.3 cm$^2$ with a sensitivity, specificity, and predictive value of 69%, 98%, and 97%, respectively. The blunted pattern was seen in all grades of mitral regurgitation and had low predictive value for grading the severity of mitral regurgitation, particularly in patients with left ventricular dysfunction (33).

Hynes and colleagues reported similar results regarding usefulness of systolic flow reversal as an indicator of severe mitral regurgitation and a normal waveform pattern confirming the absence of significant mitral regurgitation. They reported that the blunted pulmonary venous waveform pattern was more likely associated with left ventricular abnormalities than mitral regurgitation (34).

Pulmonary venous flow patterns are influenced by a number of factors that include changes in myocardial relaxation (35), abnormal left ventricular compliance, systolic and diastolic dysfunction, changes in loading conditions, and left atrial compliance and function (30,31, 36–41). Other cardiac states that alter pulmonary vein flows include arrhythmias, such as atrial fibrillation (31,42).

Klein and colleagues, in a separate investigation, highlighted the importance of sampling both pulmonary veins when grading mitral regurgitation by TEE. They assessed the variability between left and right pulmonary venous flow in the assessment of mitral regurgitation. Discordant pulmonary venous flow as measured by PW Doppler TEE occurred between the left and right upper pulmonary veins at a rate of 37% in those patients with 4-plus mitral insufficiency (43).

Schwerzmann and colleagues reported that combined transmitral E wave velocity and reversed systolic pulmonary venous flow were accurate measures for the determination of moderately severe to severe mitral regurgitation as compared to regurgitant fraction. They reported that reversed systolic pulmonary venous flow with an increased E wave velocity of $> 1$m/s had the sensitivity of 78% and a specificity of 97% for detecting severe mitral regurgitation (100).

## Quantitative Techniques

Among the rationale for the use of quantitative measurements to grade mitral regurgitation are the associated limitations with semiquantitative grading methods. Others have recommended the use of quantifiable methods for patients with greater than mild degrees of mitral regurgitation (45).

### Vena Contracta

The vena contracta is the narrowest part of the regurgitant jet as imaged with color-flow mapping as the jet emerges from the regurgitant orifice. The flow pattern in the region of the vena contracta is organized into a series of parallel flow lines. As flow gradually moves away from the vena contracta it becomes more turbulent and disorganized secondary to entrainment of blood by the regurgitant jet within the left atrium (18).

Hall and colleagues compared the accuracy of the vena contracta width to regurgitant volume and regurgitant orifice area measurements in evaluating the severity of mitral regurgitation. They reported a good correlation between vena contracta measurements and quantitative measures of mitral regurgitation severity. In particular, a vena contracta width of $\geq 0.5$ cm was always associated with a regurgitant volume $> 60$ ml and a regurgitant orifice area $> 0.4$ cm$^2$. A vena contracta width of $\leq 0.3$ cm predicted a regurgitant volume of $< 60$ ml and regurgitant orifice area of $< 0.4$ cm$^2$. They reported a weak correlation between jet area and quantitative measures of mitral regurgitant severity (46).

Grayburn and colleagues reported that the width of the mitral regurgitant jet at its vena contracta was an accurate marker for severe mitral regurgitation. A width of greater than or equal to 6 mm identified angiographically severe mitral regurgitation with a sensitivity and specificity of 95% and 98%, respectively (47).

Limitations of vena contracta measurements include the associated difficulties with localizing the area of the vena contracta and trouble with obtaining good image quality (18). In addition, there are problems regarding axial versus lateral resolution of the ultrasound imaging system (18). This measurement technique is limited by the lateral resolution of color Doppler, which often is unable to distinguish minor variations in the width of the vena contracta (48).

### Regurgitant Orifice Area

The regurgitant orifice area is a reliable quantitative measure of the severity of mitral regurgitation. It can be measured with two-dimensional and pulsed Doppler echocardiography (49) or with the proximal isovelocity surface area (PISA) method (50–52). The PISA method applies the continuity principle to color Doppler mapping in the region of the mitral valve orifice where flow converges toward the mitral regurgitant orifice on the left ventricular side of the mitral valve. As blood flow converges toward the mitral regurgitant orifice it forms a series of isovelocity shells whose surface area is hemispheric in shape (Fig. 14.10) (16,52–57). Color flow Doppler displays a measure of velocity at a specific distance from the regurgitant orifice (Fig. 14.11). By the law of conservation of mass, flow at each layer should be equal to orifice flow because it must all pass through the orifice (53). The

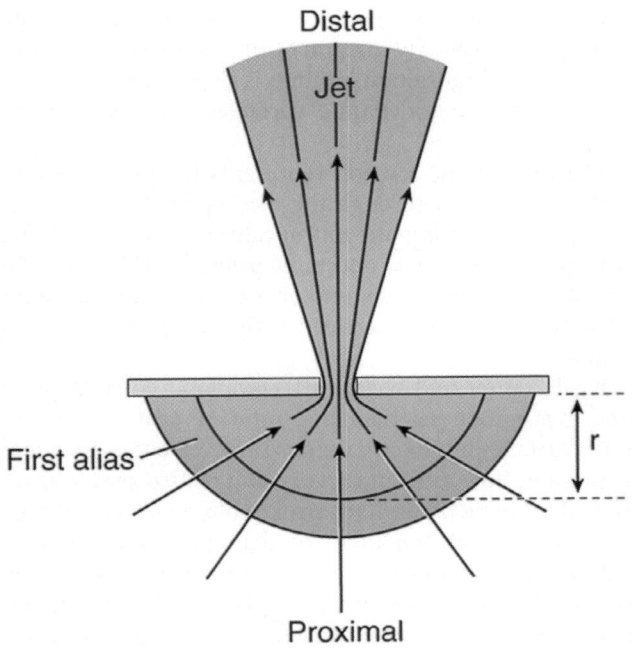

Distal

Jet

First alias — r

Proximal

**FIGURE 14.10.** This illustration of a mitral regurgitant jet depicts the hemispheric shape of the flow convergence region. Where *r* represents the distance from the regurgitant orifice to the first aliasing boundary.

maximal instantaneous flow rate can be calculated as the product of the surface area of the hemisphere and the aliasing velocity ($V_a$)

$$\text{Flow Rate} = 2\,\pi r^2 \times V_a$$

where r is the distance from the regurgitant orifice to the proximal portion of the flow convergence region. Once

the maximal instantaneous flow rate is calculated the regurgitant orifice area (ROA) can be calculated as:

$$\text{ROA} = \text{Flow Rate}/\text{Peak } V_{MR}$$
$$\text{ROA} = 2\,\pi r^2 \times V_a/V_p$$

where $V_{MR}$ is the peak regurgitant velocity of the mitral regurgitant jet. In general, an ROA $\geq 0.4$ cm$^2$ is associated with severe mitral regurgitation (16).

A central assumption with the use of PISA method is that the proximal flow convergence region is hemispheric in shape. When the flow field is constrained, the flow convergence region may become eccentric and assume a nonhemispheric shape (Fig. 14.12). If the flow region is not 180 degrees and hemispheric symmetry of the flow field is assumed, there will be significant overestimation of calculated flow rates. Adjustments are needed to the equation to account for the angle subtended by the constrained flow region (58).

Improperly identifying the regurgitant orifice when making radius measurements will introduce errors in the flow rate and orifice area calculations (52). To circumvent the need to identify the position of the orifice, Sitges and colleagues introduced the concept of *inter-aliasing distance*. The flow rate at any of the multiple flow-convergence zones proximal to the orifice should be equal based on the principle of conservation of mass. With mathematical modeling, a derived radius can be calculated for use in flow convergence calculations that uses the distance between the first and second aliasing boundaries, the inter-aliasing distance (18,59).

To avoid problems with the variability of the regurgitant orifice throughout the cardiac cycle, use of color M-mode of the flow convergence region can provide a

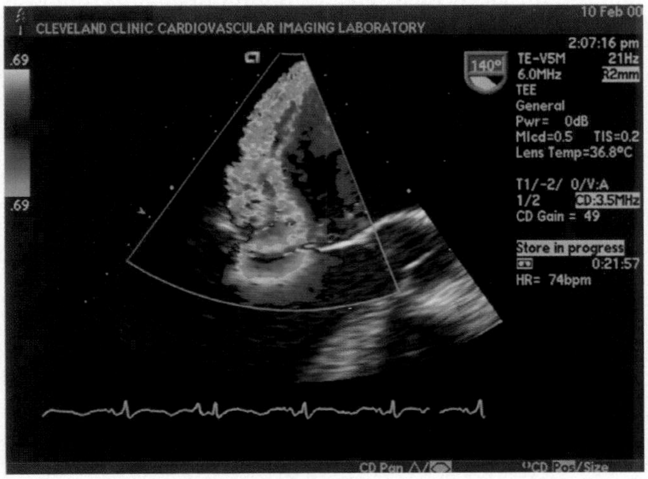

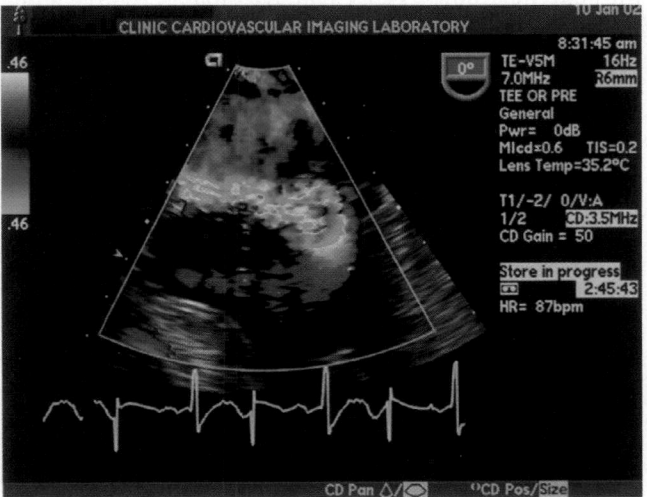

**FIGURE 14.11.** The color Doppler display from the midesophageal long-axis image of the mitral valve depicts a large proximal flow convergence region on the left ventricular side of the mitral valve.

**FIGURE 14.12.** This patient with a partial flail segment of the posterior mitral leaflet displays an eccentric flow convergence region from this midesophageal view.

temporal display of the velocity throughout the cardiac cycle (48).

As real-time, three-dimensional imaging technology improves, imaging the entire geometry of the flow convergence region may reduce errors involved in the quantification of mitral regurgitation with the flow convergence method (60).

Pu and colleagues demonstrated the accuracy of a *simplified* PISA method in the clinical setting (61). Necessary assumptions with the use of the simplified formula include assuming that the pressure difference between the left ventricle and left atrium is 100 mm Hg. Recall that when the peak mitral regurgitant jet velocity is 500 cm/sec, the peak left ventricular to left atrial pressure difference is 100 mm Hg. Furthermore, if the color-aliasing velocity is set at 40 cm/s the formula can be simplified as:

$$ROA = r^2/2$$

where r is the radius of the proximal convergence isovelocity hemisphere.

If the peak jet velocity is greater than 500 cm/sec the regurgitant orifice area will be overestimated; whereas a jet velocity less than 500 cm/sec will underestimate the orifice area. Associated limitations of the conventional PISA method similarly apply to the simplified formula (61).

### Regurgitant Volume and Regurgitant Fraction

Regurgitant volume and regurgitant fraction are quantitative volumetric measurements that assess the amount of regurgitant volume lost from forward stroke volume. They involve measuring the difference between stroke volumes through the regurgitant mitral valve from systemic stroke volume. Measurement of flow volume through the mitral valve will be greater than volume through a competent reference valve (26). Flow across the mitral valve is calculated as the product of the mitral valve area and time velocity integral of mitral inflow,

while flow across the reference valve is the product of the area and time velocity integral of the reference valve (16). The absolute regurgitant volume is dependent on chamber size and hemodynamic variables, such as driving force (18,44).

The regurgitant fraction represents the percentage of stroke volume lost through the incompetent valve and is calculated by dividing the mitral valve regurgitant volume by forward mitral flow and multiplying by 100% (16). In general, a regurgitant volume of > 60 ml and regurgitant fraction of > 55% is associated with severe mitral insufficiency.

Flachskampf and colleagues compared color Doppler area, regurgitant jet diameter, ratio of peak systolic to peak diastolic pulmonary venous flow velocities, maximal regurgitant flow rate, and regurgitant orifice area to invasively determine regurgitant stroke volume. Proximal flow convergence and proximal jet diameter measurements had better discriminatory ability for distinguishing between mild and more severe forms of mitral regurgitation than pulmonary venous waveform patterns and color Doppler jet area. Regurgitant orifice area and maximal regurgitant flow rate had the best correlation with invasively determined regurgitant stroke volume measurements; a regurgitant orifice area of 0.4 cm² had a 100% sensitivity, 93% specificity, 91% positive predictive value, and 100% negative predictive value for detecting angiographic grade 3–4 mitral regurgitation. Proximal jet diameter of 0.65 cm had a 90% sensitivity, 83% specificity, 79% positive predictive value, and a 92% negative predictive value of predicting grade 3–4 mitral regurgitation. Color jet area and pulmonary venous flow velocity profiles did not correlate well with invasive measurements of stroke volume in this investigation (62). Estimation methods for grading mitral regurgitation are summarized in Table 14.2.

Figure 14.13 depicts a summary of the anatomy of the regurgitant jet in relationship to a number of estimation methods. Among the techniques specific aspects of the anatomy of the regurgitant jet are examined: the flow convergence region examines the preregurgitant orifice; the

▶ TABLE 14.2. **Mitral Regurgitation: Severity Estimation**

| Method | Mild | Moderate | Severe |
|---|---|---|---|
| Secondary 2-D changes | Mild LAE | Moderate LAE | Severe LAE |
| Spatial area mapping with color Doppler | < 4.0 cm² | 4.0–8.0 cm² | > 8.0 cm² |
| Pulmonary venous flow profiles | Normal pattern, S waveform ≥ D waveform | Blunted pattern, S waveform < D waveform | Systolic flow reversal, S waveform < 0 |
| Regurgitant volume | 30–40 ml | 40–60 ml | > 60 ml |
| Regurgitant fraction | 10–30% | 30–50% | > 55% |
| Regurgitant orifice area | < 0.2 cm² | 0.3–0.4 cm² | > 0.4 cm² |
| Vena Contracta | ≤ 0.3cm | | ≥ 0.5cm |

*2-D,* two-dimensional; *LAE,* left atrial enlargement; *S,* systolic; D, diastolic; ml, milliliters; cm, centimeters.

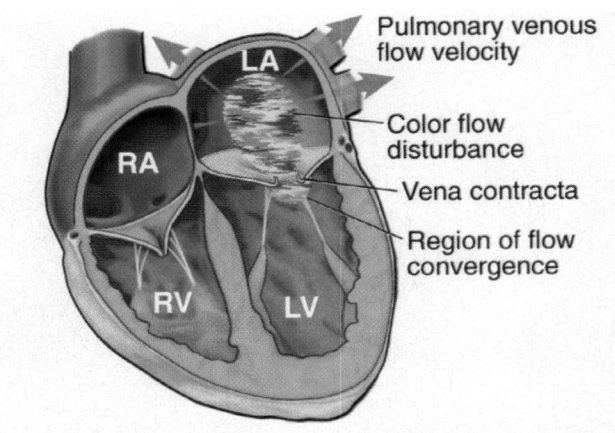

**FIGURE 14.13.** A summary of a number of estimation methods commonly used to determine the severity of mitral insufficiency is displayed in this illustration.

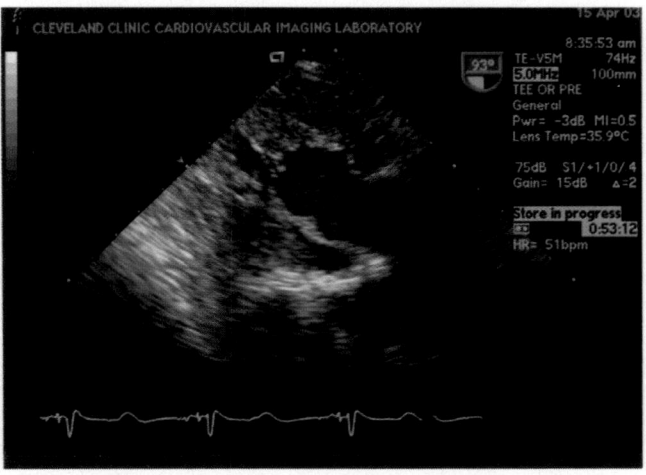

**FIGURE 14.14.** The transgastric long-axis image of the mitral valve and subvalvular apparatus is characteristic of a patient with a parachute mitral valve deformity. The chordal tendons insert into a single papillary muscle.

vena contracta examines the mitral regurgitant orifice; color flow disturbance in the left atrium and alterations in the pulmonary venous waveform patterns involve analysis of the postorifice aspect of the regurgitant jet.

Developments in color-coded display for three-dimensional echocardiography, electron beam-computed tomography, and the use of power-velocity integral at the vena contracta may have broader clinical applications in the future (63–65).

## Mitral Stenosis

Rheumatic carditis caused by a prior episode of rheumatic fever is the leading cause of mitral stenosis in the adult patient (4,66,67). Uncommon etiologies of mitral stenosis include severe mitral annular calcification (68), obstructing lesions such as left atrial tumors (69), and congenital deformities such as a parachute mitral valve or cor triatriatum (4,66,70). Table 14.3 displays mechanisms and characteristic two-dimensional appearances for a number of etiologies of mitral stenosis. Figures 14.14 and

14.15 demonstrate an example of subvalvular obstruction secondary to a parachute mitral valve deformity.

Although the mitral valve is the most commonly affected valve in episodes of acute rheumatic endocarditis, rheumatic heart disease may also involve the pericardium, myocardium, and other heart valves (67,70). Mitral valvulitis results in small vegetations along the mitral leaflet closure line accompanied by valve inflammation (70). Diffuse leaflet thickening results from repeated episodes of carditis interposed with episodes of healing, which results in fibrous tissue formation. In addition, a nonspecific fibrosis and calcium deposition occur as a result of the abnormally deformed valve. There are varying degrees of fibrocalcific fusion of the commissures, contracture and scarring of the leaflet tissue, and fusion and shortening of the chordal tendons.

The rheumatic process advances to varying degrees of mitral stenosis depending upon the number and severity of episodes of rheumatic valvitis. Typically, a time interval

▶ **TABLE 14.3.  Etiology, Mechanism, and Two-Dimensional Appearance of Mitral Stenosis**

| *Etiology* | *Mechanism* | *Two-Dimensional Appearance* |
|---|---|---|
| Rheumatic heart disease | Leaflet and chordal tendon fibrosis and thickening, commissural fusion | Thickened chordal tendons and leaflets, restricted leaflet motion with diastolic doming |
| Left atrial myxoma | Obstruction to inflow | Large mass obstructing mitral inflow |
| Severe mitral annular calcification | Calcium deposition | Calcium deposition from annulus to leaflet tissue |
| Parachute mitral valve deformity | Restricted leaflet opening causing blood to flow through intrachordal spaces | Chordal insertion into single papillary muscle |
| Cor triatriatum | Restriction to mitral inflow due to partition within left atrium | Partition within the left atrium |

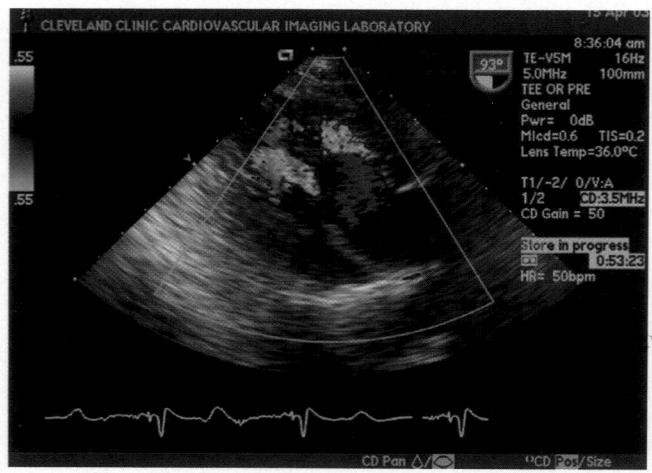

**FIGURE 14.15.** Color flow imaging displays highly turbulent inflow amid the intrachordal spaces from this transgastric long-axis imaging plane in the patient with the parachute mitral valve deformity.

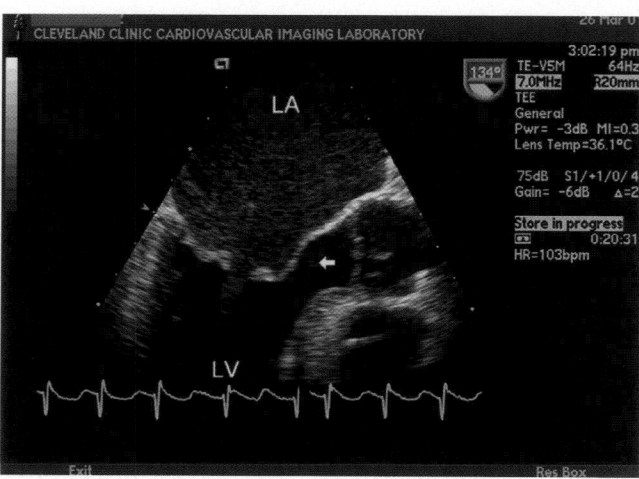

**FIGURE 14.16.** The midesophageal imaging plane depicts the classic diastolic doming or "hockey stick" deformity that characterizes leaflet restriction from the rheumatic mitral disease process.

of several years intervenes between the episode of acute carditis and the appearance of clinically symptomatic mitral stenosis (67). In advanced cases, the mitral valve may become a rigid, funnel-shaped orifice with an almost complete obliteration of the chordal spaces (4,13,66,67,70).

As the mitral valve area becomes progressively reduced, an increase in the transvalvular pressure gradient, left atrial pressure and area occur. The left atrial hypertension can, in turn, result in pulmonary hypertension, right heart dysfunction, and tricuspid insufficiency (4,13,66,67,70).

### Two-Dimensional Echocardiography

The two-dimensional characteristics of rheumatic mitral stenosis follow the pathophysiologic features of rheumatic disease process. There is an enhanced echocardiographic appearance of the mitral valve leaflets due to thickening from variable degrees of tissue fibrosis and calcification. The chordal tendons also appear enhanced on the two-dimensional exam secondary to variable degrees of thickening and contracture (4). The mitral leaflets exhibit restricted leaflet motion. Because the leaflets are anchored at the mitral annulus with fusion of the commissures, the midsection of the leaflets is the only section relatively free to move in diastole. This gives the anterior mitral leaflet an arched appearance, convex toward the left ventricular outflow tract in diastole, resulting in a characteristic diastolic doming or "hockey stick" deformity (Fig. 14.16) (71–73). In advanced degrees of leaflet deformity, the valve can become so severely rigid that there is minimal movement of the valve throughout the cardiac cycle.

Standard chamber dimensions are altered depending on the duration and degree of mitral stenosis. Typically, there is an increase in the left atrial area associated with chronic pressure overload. The presence of left atrial spontaneous echo contrast, an indicator of left atrial blood stasis, may identify patients who are at increased thromboembolic risk (Fig. 14.17) (74,75).

Right ventricular enlargement with dysfunction and tricuspid insufficiency may secondarily result from pulmonary hypertension (72). While left ventricular systolic performance in patients with severe isolated mitral steno-

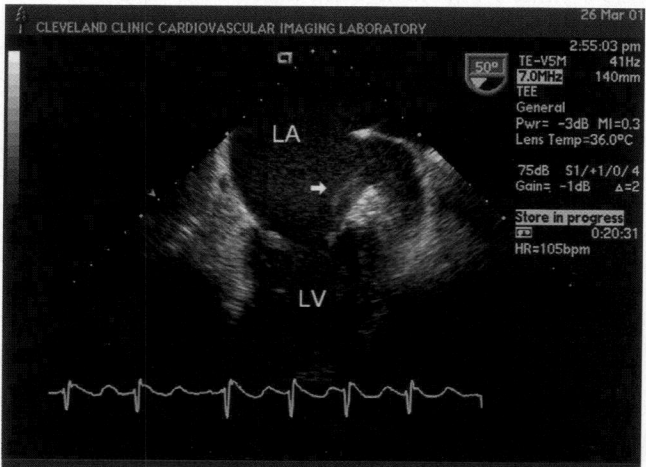

**FIGURE 14.17.** Spontaneous echo contrast or smoke is a hallmark for blood stasis within the chambers of the heart. This transesophageal echocardiographic image depicts the presence of smoke within the left atrial appendage in a patient with severe mitral stenosis. Note there is thrombus formation at the mouth of the left atrial appendage.

sis is similar to that of age-matched controls, there are reductions in diastolic compliance of the left ventricle thought to be a consequence of functional restriction from tethering to a rigid mitral valve apparatus (76).

## Splitability Score

Components of the splitability score as described by Wilkins and colleagues (72) in 1988 are listed in Table 14.4. Wilkins and colleagues examined a number of clinical, hemodynamic, and echocardiographic variables to predict success following percutaneous balloon dilatation of the mitral valve. The echocardiographic variables assessed mitral leaflet mobility, leaflet thickening, subvalvular thickening, and calcification on a scale from 0 to 4. A summation of the component scores resulted in a range of possible scores of 0 to 16, where the highest score represents advanced leaflet deformity. Among the variables, the value for the echocardiographic score was the best predictor of outcome following percutaneous balloon dilatation of the mitral valve. All patients with an echocardiographic score of > 11 had a suboptimal result, whereas all of those patients with a score of < 9 had an optimal result (72). While developed to determine suitability of balloon valvuloplasty, the splitability score serves as a useful intraoperative guide in assessment of the extent of valvular involvement from rheumatic endocarditis.

## Severity Estimation

### Pressure Gradient

The Bernoulli equation describes the relationship between velocity of blood flow and pressure gradient. Because we are unable to directly measure intravascular pressure gradients with Doppler echocardiography, the Bernoulli equation allows us to convert instantaneous velocity of flow across the mitral valve to an instantaneous pressure gradient (77). The Bernoulli equation is:

$$P_1 - P_2 = \frac{1}{2} \rho (V_2{}^2 - V_1{}^2) + \rho_1 \int^2 (DV/DT)\, DS + R(V)$$

| | | |
|---|---|---|
| Convective Acceleration | Flow Acceleration | Viscous Friction |

where $P_1 - P_2$ is the pressure gradient across the valve in millimeters of mercury (mm Hg), P represents the density of blood = $1.06 \times 10^3$ kg/M$^3$, $V_2$ represents the instantaneous velocity of blood distal to the stenotic valve in meters per second (m/s), $V_1$ represents the instantaneous velocity proximal to the stenotic valve (m/s), DV is the velocity vector of the fluid element along its path and DS is the path element. A simplification of the Bernoulli equation allows the pressure drop across a stenotic valve to be calculated from the maximal velocity, $V_2$, as:

$$P_1 - P_2 \text{ (mm Hg)} = 4V^2$$

Modification of the original formula involves eliminating terms that account for viscous losses and flow acceleration. In addition, the proximal velocity term can be ignored if the velocity proximal to the stenosis is significantly less than the velocity distal to the obstruction (26,77–79). The accuracy of the modified Bernoulli equation was demonstrated by Hatle and colleagues in the calculation of the gradient across a stenotic mitral valve (78). Accuracy of the equation has been demonstrated as long as the assumptions have been met: absence of long tubular stenotic lesions (26).

The mean pressure gradient is acquired by tracing the diastolic spectral profile obtained by Doppler interrogation of the inflow velocity across the mitral valve. The

▶ TABLE 14.4. **Echocardiographic Scoring System**

| Grade | Mobility | Subvalvular Thickening | Thickening | Calcification |
|---|---|---|---|---|
| 1 | Highly mobile valve with only leaflet tips restricted | Minimal thickening just below the mitral leaflets | Leaflets near normal in thickness (4–5 mm) | Single area of increased echo brightness |
| 2 | Leaflet mid and base portions have normal mobility | Thickening of chordal structures extending up to 1/3 of chordal length | Midleaflets normal, considerable thickening of margins (5–8 mm) | Scattered areas of brightness confined to leaflet margins |
| 3 | Valve continues to move forward in diastole, mainly from base | Thickening extending to the distal 1/3 of chords | Thickening extending through the entire leaflet (5–8 mm) | Brightness extending into mid-portion of the leaflets |
| 4 | No or minimal forward movement of the leaflets in diastole | Extensive thickening and shortening of all chordal structures extending down to papillary muscles | Considerable thickening of all leaflet tissue (> 8–10 mm) | Extensive brightness throughout much of the leaflet tissue |

Reprinted from Wilkins G, et al. Percutaneous balloon dilatation of the mitral valve: an analysis of echocardiographic variables related to outcome and the mechanism of dilatation. *British Heart Journal* 1988;60:300, with permission.

mean gradient is then determined by averaging instantaneous gradients across the flow period. Current ultrasound software calculates the mean gradient by integrating the area under the diastolic spectral profile curve (26).

Severe mitral regurgitation can result in high transmitral gradients, even with a mildly stenotic valve secondary to the increase in forward flow through the mitral valve in diastole (80). Technical errors involved with measuring pressure gradients with Doppler involve improper alignment of the sampling beam and the flow vector. The calculated pressure gradient will be underestimated if the angle between the flow vector and sampling beam is too large (53,78). Color-flow mapping of mitral inflow displays a turbulent jet extending at the mitral orifice into the left ventricle in diastole. Aligning the sampling beam with inflow depicted by color flow Doppler errors with improper sampling will reduce beam alignment (53). A mean gradient of greater than 10 mm Hg across the mitral valve is considered severe (81).

### Valve Area Calculations

The ultimate goal with each of the methods used to calculate mitral valve area is to provide an echocardiographic-determined valve area as close to the anatomic valve area as possible.

### Planimetry

Planimetry involves the direct measurement of mitral valve area with two-dimensional echocardiography. The valve orifice can be visualized from a transgastric basal short-axis imaging plane, where the image is frozen in early diastole to coincide with maximal valve opening. The orifice margins are directly measured by tracing the internal margins of the mitral valve orifice to provide a valve area measurement in squared centimeters (Fig. 14.18) (82–85). Planimetry has been shown to correlate well with invasively determined valve area calculations (73,82–84).

Limitations with this technique include technical measurement errors, instrumentation factors, and clinical situations where there is poor image quality. Image resolution is critical to obtaining accurate measurements. Calcification of the valve leaflets may result in significant acoustic shadowing that obscures the valve orifice and interferes with the accuracy of the measurement (85). Inadequate imaging plane orientation will result in errors interfering with the ability to identify the true mitral valve orifice. If the plane of the short axis is not at the tip of the mitral valve leaflets, but near the body of the valve leaflet the valve area will be overestimated (Fig. 14.19) (83–86). Scanning the mitral valve orifice superiorly to inferiorly in order to acquire the smallest orifice area will reduce involved with improper imaging plane orientation errors (83,84,86).

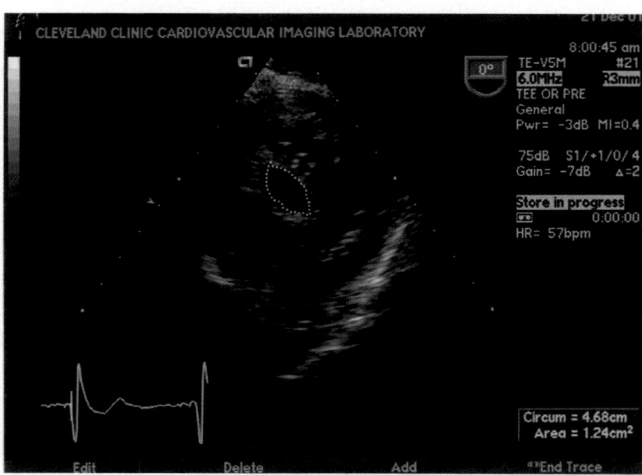

**FIGURE 14.18.** This transgastric short-axis image of the mitral valve depicts the use of planimetry as a method for mitral valve area determination. The mitral valve area is greater than 1.0 cm².

The valve area may be overestimated or underestimated if the gain settings are set too low or too high. If the receiver gain settings are too low, the edges of the valve may be obscured resulting in "echo drop-out" and the valve area will be overestimated (82,86). When the gain settings are set too high there is image saturation and the valve area is underestimated (86). Finally, valve area may be underestimated in patients who have undergone mitral valvuloplasty secondary to the inability to measure the extent of the commissural fractures with planimetry.

### Pressure Half-time

The pressure gradient half-time (PHT) measures the rate of decline in the atrioventricular pressure gradient. It is

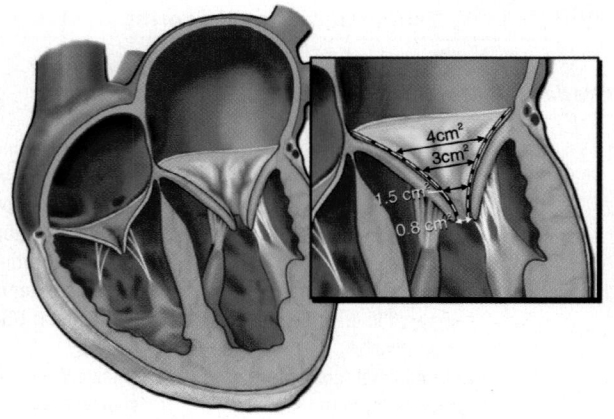

**FIGURE 14.19.** This illustration displays the funnel-shape assumed by the mitral valve orifice in advanced degrees of rheumatic mitral stenosis. If measurements for planimetry are not taken from the appropriate imaging plane, the valve area will be overestimated as demonstrated in this image.

defined as the time required for maximal diastolic pressure difference to decrease by one-half of its initial value. In velocity terms it is equivalent to the time required for the maximum transmitral velocity curve to decrease by a factor of the square root of 2 (87–89). The pressure PHT can be quantitatively related to the severity of mitral stenosis. A normal mitral valve area of 4 cm$^2$ allows the atrioventricular flow to reduce the transmitral pressure difference to negligible values in less than 50 msec after the onset of the diastolic rise in left ventricular pressure (88). As the severity of mitral stenosis increases, there is a proportionately slower rate of pressure decline between the left atrium and left ventricle and the atrioventricular pressure gradient is maintained for a longer period of time (26,85,87–89). A PHT of > 300 m/sec is associated with severe mitral stenosis (88–90).

The rate at which the left atrial and left ventricular pressures equalize is a function of the mitral valve area. The pressure half-time method of determining mitral valve area describes the relative diastolic pressure difference between the left atrium and left ventricle. Increasing PHT occurs with decreasing mitral valve area, independent of the presence of mitral regurgitation (Fig. 14.20) (89).

Hatle and Angelsen (90) originally described the inverse relationship between the PHT measurement and the calculation of mitral valve area. The mathematic relationship between PHT and mitral valve area is described as:

$$MVA\ (cm^2) = 220/PHT\ (msec)$$

where MVA is the mitral valve area in squared centimeters and 220 is an empirically derived constant.

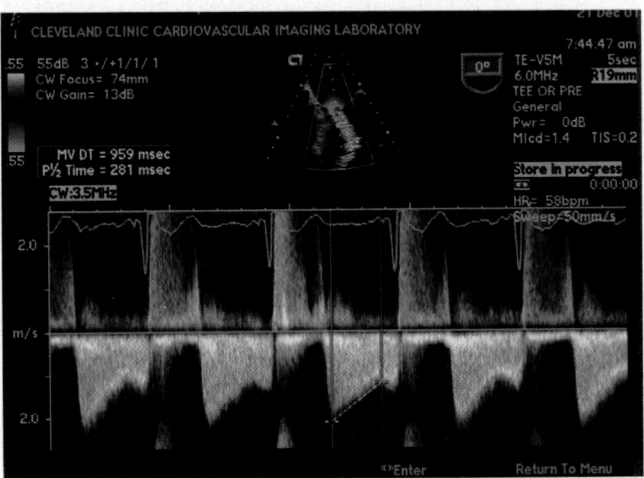

**FIGURE 14.20.** This image displays the Doppler profile of a patient with both mitral stenosis and mitral regurgitation. The Doppler spectral profile beneath the baseline depicts a pressure half-time (PHT) measurement of 281 milliseconds, which is consistent with severe mitral stenosis.

Potential sources of error should be considered when applying the PHT method in specific clinical settings. PHT is influenced by the peak transmitral pressure gradient and left atrial and left ventricular compliances (91). Conditions that alter left atrial or left ventricular compliance, rapid heart rates, or severe aortic insufficiency will impact the measurement accuracy. Moderate-to-severe degrees of aortic insufficiency cause a rapid rise in left ventricular diastolic pressure with a resultant shortening of the PHT and an overestimation in mitral valve area (92–94).

The PHT may be inaccurate for predicting changes in mitral valve area for several days following mitral valvuloplasty. The transient inaccuracies are due to the abrupt changes in left atrial pressure that occur postvalvuloplasty. Following a few days the atrial compliance adapts to the acute decrease in atrial pressure (26). Thomas and colleagues demonstrated inaccuracies of the simple inverse relationship between mitral valve area and pressure half-time in the setting of acute valvotomy. The PHT varied not only with mitral valve area but also with chamber compliance and the peak transmitral gradient. They commented that PHT is determined by more than a simple relationship with mitral valve area, and that changes in these other hemodynamic factors contribute to the breakdown in the inverse relationship after valvotomy (95).

Other clinical conditions that limit the accuracy of the PHT method include atrial septal defects, atrial tachycardias, restrictive cardiomyopathies (87,91,94,95), and abnormal compliance, such as severe left ventricular hypertrophy, ischemia, and severe systemic hypertension (80, 91,94).

### Deceleration Half-time

Deceleration half-time (DHT) is another method to determine mitral valve area by examining the decay of mitral inflow through the stenotic mitral valve. The deceleration time is defined as the time in milliseconds for the peak mitral inflow velocity to reach baseline. As with the PHT method, as the stenosis becomes more severe the decay in the pressure gradient to baseline will be prolonged. The inverse relationship between the DHT and mitral valve area is described as (53):

$$MVA\ (cm^2) = 759/DT\ (msec)$$

where DT is the deceleration time in milliseconds. If the profile of the mitral deceleration time is linear, the PHT is equal to 29% of the deceleration time (16,85).

### Continuity Equation

The continuity equation is based on the law of conservation of mass in hydrodynamics (93). Volumetric flow remains constant through the heart valves in the absence of valvular regurgitation or shunts. Such that flow volume at the mitral valve should equal that at a predetermined reference valve (85,93). The continuity equation is described as:

$$Q \text{ (volumetric flow)} = \text{Area}_1 \times \text{Velocity}_1 = \text{Area}_2 \times \text{Velocity}_2$$

$\text{Area}_1 \times \text{Velocity}_1$ represents volumetric flow in the reference valve. The reference area (Area 1) is a cross-sectional area measurement that assumes the geometric model of a circle: $\pi r^2$. Mean velocities are obtained from the time velocity integrals (TVI) of the spectral profiles generated by Doppler interrogation of the reference valve ($\text{Velocity}_1$) and of the mitral valve ($\text{Velocity}_2$). The equation is rearranged to solve for the mitral stenotic area, $\text{Area}_2$:

$$\text{Area }_2 = \text{Area}_1 \times \text{Velocity}_1 / \text{Velocity}_2$$
$$\text{Stenotic area} = \text{Flow/Velocity across stenosis}$$

The continuity equation provides an accurate measurement of mitral valve area (93). It is particularly useful in clinical situations where the PHT is limited, such as in patients with moderate-to-severe degrees of aortic insufficiency (26,93). The continuity equation is theoretically independent of transvalvular pressure gradient, left ventricular compliance, and changing hemodynamic conditions, such as exercise (91–93). Limitations involve an underestimate of mitral valve area in those patients with concomitant mitral regurgitation secondary to an augmentation of the Doppler measurement of the time velocity integral of the mitral valve (93). In addition, the continuity equation will be inaccurate in circumstances of regurgitation in the reference valve because forward volumetric flows will not be equal (93,96).

### Proximal Isovelocity Surface Area Method

The flow convergence method for calculating mitral valve area applies the use of the basic elements of the continuity equation with the addition of a correction factor to allow for constriction of the flow field by the leaflets. A truly hemispheric shell would occur if the surface of the valve was flat with the leaflets apposed at 180°. The angle subtended by the mitral leaflets creates a funnel-shaped surface; an angle correction factor ($\alpha$/180 degrees) adjusts the hemispheric surface area to avoid introducing errors in the calculation of the volumetric flow rate. The modified formula factors into account the funnel angle formed by the mitral leaflets. Where the instantaneous flow rate (Q) in this region can be calculated as the product of the surface area of a hemisphere ($2\pi r^2$) and the aliasing velocity at the shell (Va):

$$Q = 2\pi r^2 \times \alpha/180° \times Va$$

Flow through this region should equal flow through the restricted orifice based on the continuity principle (54–56). Once the flow rate (Q) is calculated, mitral valve area can be obtained with the use of the continuity equation:

$$\text{MVA (cm}^2) = Q / Vp \text{(cm/s)}$$

where Q = volumetric flow rate and Vp = peak transmitral inflow velocity. The flow convergence method is best applied when there are limitations associated with the continuity equation and the PHT method and in clinical circumstances in which the two-dimensional images are technically poor, thereby limiting the use of planimetry (55). The accuracy of the flow convergence region method in assessing mitral valve area has been validated in a number of studies (56,97). Accurate measurement of mitral valve area can be obtained with this method in the presence of mitral insufficiency (54,98). Calculation of mitral valve area using the flow convergence method can be time-consuming, however its accuracy is not influenced by associated mitral or aortic regurgitation (Fig. 14.21).

### Flow Area

The flow area technique for calculating mitral valve area utilizes color Doppler to image the margins of the mitral inflow. The central laminar core of the color flow jet at the level of the stenotic mitral orifice is imaged in two planes perpendicular to one another, producing major (a) and minor (b) diameter measurements of a presumably

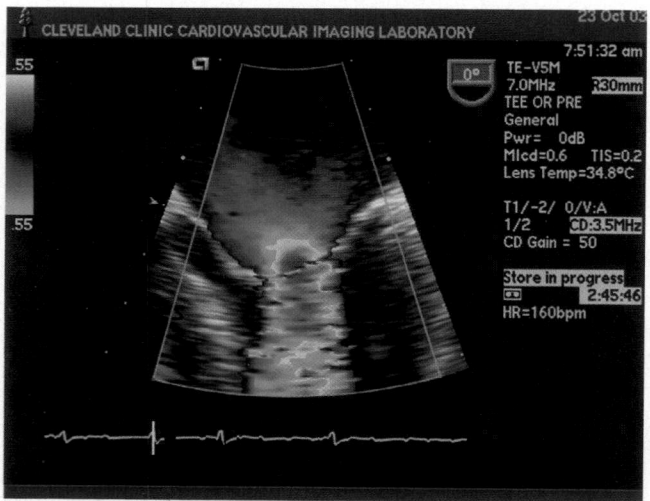

**FIGURE 14.21.** The proximal flow convergence region is detected with color flow Doppler on the left atrial side of the mitral valve in this midesophageal imaging plane. Note the area of the flow convergence region is subtended by the mitral leaflets and is not hemispheric in shape.

▶ **TABLE 14.5.  Techniques for Determining Mitral Valve Area**

| Planimetry | Trace frozen short-axis view in diastole |
|---|---|
| Pressure Half-Time (PHT$_{msec}$) | MVA = 220/PHT |
| Deceleration Time (DT$_{msec}$) | MVA = 759/DT |
| Continuity Equation | MVA = (LVOT$_{area}$) × (LVOT$_{TVI}$) / (MV$_{TVI}$) |
| PISA | MVA = 2πr$^2$ × α/180° × V$_a$/V$_p$ |
| Flow Area | MVA = π/4 × a × b |

*MVA*, mitral valve area in squared centimeters; α, funnel angle; *Va*, aliasing velocity; *Vp*, peak transmitral velocity; *LVOT*, left ventricular outflow tract; T*VI*, time velocity integral; *PISA*, proximal isovelocity surface area.

▶ **TABLE 14.6.  Mitral Stenosis: Severity Estimation**

| Mitral Stenosis Severity Measurement | Mild | Moderate | Severe |
|---|---|---|---|
| Mean gradient (mmHg) | 6 | 6–10 | > 10 |
| PHT (msec) | 100 | 200 | > 300 |
| DHT (msec) | < 500 | 500–700 | > 700 |
| MVA (cm$^2$) | 1.6–2.0 | 1.0–1.5 | < 1.0 |

*PHT*, pressure half-time; *DHT*, deceleration half-time; *MVA*, mitral valve area.

ellipsoid orifice. The valve area is then calculated by applying the equation for the area of an ellipse:

$$(\pi/4) \times (a \times b)$$

This technique is highly dependent on obtaining good image quality (64,86). Faletra and colleagues compared direct measurement of anatomic area to planimetry, PHT, PISA, and the flow area method. The flow area method was reported to be the least reliable of the four methods in this investigation (98).

Techniques for determining mitral valve area are summarized in Table 14.5. Table 14.6 provides grades of severity for mitral stenosis with a number of estimation techniques.

## KEY POINTS

- The mitral valve complex consists of the mitral annulus, anterior and posterior mitral valve leaflets, chordal tendons, and left ventricular myocardium. Structural integrity of the mitral valve requires that all of the elements of the apparatus function appropriately.
- The comprehensive evaluation of a patient with mitral regurgitation includes the integration of qualitative, semiquantitative, and quantitative TEE assessments along with clinical features of the patient's presentation.
- Rheumatic heart disease continues to be the primary etiology of mitral stenosis. Characteristics include variable degrees of leaflet and subvalvular thickening, calcium deposition, and reduction in leaflet mobility.
- The splitability score provides an overall summary score reflecting the degree of leaflet deformity in patients with rheumatic mitral stenosis. Higher scores reflect advanced leaflet deformity.

- The proximal isovelocity surface area method may be applied to quantitatively estimate the degree of mitral regurgitation, as well as the degree of mitral stenosis. A correction factor is applied to estimate valve area for mitral stenosis as the angle subtended by the mitral leaflets creates a funnel-shaped surface.

## REFERENCES

1. The Oxford English dictionary. 2nd ed. Vol. 9, Oxford: Clarendon Press, Oxford University Press, 1989:911.
2. The Catholic encyclopedia. Vol. 15. New York: The Encyclopedia Press, Inc., 1913:405–6.
3. Ross DN. Historical perspective of surgery on the mitral valve. In Duran C, Angell WW, Johnson AD, et al. (eds.): Recent progress in mitral valve disease. London: Butterworth, 1984:5–9.
4. Roberts W, Perloff J. Mitral valve disease: A clinicopathologic survey of the conditions causing the mitral valve to function abnormally. Ann Intern Med 1972;77:939–75.
5. Acierno L. Accurate description by dissection. In: The history of cardiology. New York: The Parthenon Publishing Group, 1994:17–39.
6. Ranganathan N, Lam JH, Wigle ED, et al. Morphology of the human mitral valve: The valve leaflets. Circulation 1970; XLI:459–67.
7. Roberts WC, Perloff JK. Mitral valvular disease: A clinicopathologic survey of the conditions causing the mitral valve to function abnormally. Ann Intern Med 1972;77:939–74.
8. Perloff J, Roberts W. The mitral apparatus. Functional anatomy of mitral regurgitation. Circulation 1972;XLVI:227–39.
9. Edmunds H, Norwood W, Low D. Atlas of Cardiothoracic Surgery. Mitral Valve Reconstruction. 30. Philadelphia: Lea & Febiger, 1990.
10. Ranganathan N, Lam J, Wigle E, Silver M. Morphology of the human mitral valve. II the leaflets. Circulation 1970;XLI:459–67.
11. Shanewise J, Cheung A, Aronson S, et al. ASE/SCA guidelines for performing a comprehensive intraoperative multiplane transesophageal echocardiography examination: Recommendations of the American Society of Echocardiography Council for Intraoperative Echocardiography and Society of Cardiovascular Anesthesiologists Task Force for Certification in Perioperative Transesophageal Echocardiography. J Am Soc Echocardiogr 1999;12:884–98.

12. Gaasch W, O'Rourke R, Cohn L, et al. Mitral valve disease. In Alexander R, Schlant R, Fuster V, eds. Hurst's the heart. 9th ed. New York: McGraw-Hill, 1998:1483.
13. Rahimtoola S, Enriquez-Sarano M, Schaff H, Frye R. Mitral valve disease. In Fuster V, Alexander R, O'Rourke R, eds. Hurst's the heart. 10th ed. New York: McGraw-Hill, 2001:1697–727.
14. Carpentier A, Deloche A, Dauptain J, et al. A new reconstructive operation for correction of mitral and tricuspid insufficiency. J Thorac Cardiovasc Surg 1971;61:1–13.
15. Cosgrove D, Steward W. Mitral valvuloplasty. In Current problems in cardiology. Chicago: Year Book Medical Publishers, Inc., 1989;14:353–416.
16. Oh J, Seward J, Tajik A. Valvular heart disease. In The echo manual. 2nd ed. Philadelphia: Lippincott Williams & Wilkins, 1999:103–32.
17. Bonow R, Carabello B, deLeon A, et al. ACC/AHA guidelines for the management of patients with valvular heart disease: executive summary. A report of the American College of Cardiology/American Heart Association task force on practice guidelines (committee on management of patients with valvular heart disease). Circulation 1998;98:1949–84.
18. Irvine T, Li X, Sahn D, Kenny A. Assessment of mitral regurgitation. Br Heart J 2002;88:11–19.
19. Utsunomiya T, Patel D, Doshi R, et al. Can signal intensity of the continuous wave Doppler regurgitant jet estimate severity of mitral regurgitation? Am Heart J 1992;123:166–71.
20. Thomas L, Foster E, Schiller N. Peak mitral inflow velocity predicts mitral regurgitation severity. J Am Coll Cardiol 1998;31:174–79.
21. Spain MG, Smith MD, Grayburn PA, et al. Quantitative assessment of mitral regurgitation by Doppler color flow imaging: Angiographic and hemodynamic correlations. JACC 1989;13(3):585–90.
22. Edelman SK. Understanding ultrasound physics: Fundamental and exam review. 2nd ed. Bryan, Texas: Tops Printing, Inc. 1997:127–63.
23. Castello R, Lenzen P, Aguirre F, et al. Quantitation of mitral regurgitation by transesophageal echocardiography with Doppler color flow mapping: correlation with cardiac catheterization. J Am Coll Cardiol 1992;19:1516–21.
24. Spain M, Smith M, Grayburn P, et al. Quantitative assessment of mitral regurgitation by Doppler color flow imaging: Angiographic and hemodynamic correlations. J Am Coll Cardiol 1989;13:585–90.
25. Rivera J, Vandervoort P, Morris E, et al. Visual assessment of valvular regurgitation: comparison with quantitative Doppler measurements. J Am Soc Echocardiogr 1994;7:480–87.
26. Quinones M, Otto C, Stoddard M, et al. Recommendations for quantification of Doppler echocardiography: a report from the Doppler quantification task force of the nomenclature and standards committee of the American Society of Echocardiography. J Am Soc Echocardiogr 2002;15:167–80.
27. Grewal K, Malkowski M, Piracha A, et al. Effect of general anesthesia on the severity of mitral regurgitation by transesophageal echocardiography. Am J Cardiol 2000;85:199–203.
28. Konstadt S, Louie E, Shore-Lesserson L, et al. The effects of loading changes on intraoperative Doppler assessment of mitral regurgitation. J Cardiothorac Vasc Anesth 1994;8:19–23.
29. Chen C, Thomas J, Anconina J, et al. Impact of impinging wall jet on color Doppler quantification of mitral regurgitation. Circulation 1991;84:712–20.
30. Oh J, Seward J, Tajik A. Assessment of diastolic function. In: The echo manual. 2nd ed. Philadelphia: Lippincott Williams & Wilkins, 1999:45–57.
31. Tabitha T, Thomas J, Klein A. Pulmonary venous flow by Doppler echocardiography: revisited 12 years later. J Am Coll Cardiol 2003;41:1243–50.
32. Klein A, Borski T, Stewart W, et al. Transesophageal echocardiography of pulmonary venous flow: A marker of mitral regurgitation severity. J Am Coll Cardiol 1991;18:518–26.
33. Pu M, Griffin B, Vandervoort P, et al. The value of assessing pulmonary flow velocity for predicting severity of mitral regurgitation: A quantitative assessment integrating left ventricular function. J Am Soc Echocardiogr 1999;12:736–43.
34. Hynes M, Tam J, Burwash I, et al. Predictive value of pulmonary venous flow patterns in detecting mitral regurgitation and left ventricular abnormalities. Can J Cardiol 1999;15:665–70.
35. Nishimura R, Abel M, Hatle L, et al. Assessment of diastolic function of the heart: background and current applications of Doppler echocardiography. Mayo Clin Proc 1989;64: 181–204.
36. Appleton C, Gonzalez M, Basing M. Relation of left atrial pressure and pulmonary venous flow velocities: importance of baseline mitral and pulmonary venous flow patterns studied in lightly sedated dogs. J Am Soc Echocardiogr 1994; 7:264–75.
37. Klein A, Stewart W, Bartlett J, et al. Effects of mitral regurgitation on pulmonary venous flow and left atrial pressure: An intraoperative transesophageal study. J Am Coll Cardiol 1992;201:345–52.
38. Hofmann T, Keck A, Antigen G, et al. Simultaneous measurement of pulmonary venous flow by intravascular catheter Doppler velocimetry and transesophageal Doppler echocardiography: relation to left atrial pressure and left atrial and left ventricular function. J Am Coll Cardiol 1995;26:239–49.
39. Rossvoll O, Hatle L. Pulmonary venous flow velocities recorded by transthoracic Doppler ultrasound: relation to left ventricular diastolic pressure. J Am Coll Cardiol 1993; 21:1687–97.
40. Pasierski T, Alton M, Person A. Transesophageal echocardiography characterization of pulmonary vein flow not due to atrial contraction or mitral regurgitation. Am J Cardiol 1991;68:415–18.
41. Nishimura R, Abel M, Hatle L, et al. Relation of pulmonary vein to mitral flow velocities by transesophageal Doppler echocardiography: Effect of different loading conditions. Circulation 1990;81:1488–97.
42. Keren G, Sonneblick E, LeJemtel T. Mitral annulus motion: relation to pulmonary venous and transmitral flow in normal subjects and in patients with dilated cardiomyopathy. Circulation 1988;78:621–29.
43. Klein A, Bailey A, Cohen G, et al. Importance of sampling both pulmonary veins in grading mitral regurgitation by transesophageal echocardiography. J Am Soc Echocardiogr 1993;6:115–23.
44. Tribouilloy C, Enriquez-Sarano M, Capps M, et al. Contrasting effect of similar effective regurgitant orifice area in mitral and tricuspid regurgitation: A quantitative Doppler echocardiographic study. J Am Soc Echocardiogr 2002;15:958–65.
45. Enriquez-Sarano M, Tribouilloy C. Quantitation of mitral regurgitation: rationale, approach, and interpretation in clinical practice. Br Heart J 2002;88:1–3.
46. Hall S, Brickner E, Willett D, et al. Assessment of mitral regurgitation severity by Doppler color flow mapping of the vena contracta. Circulation 1997;95:636–42.
47. Grayburn P, Fehske W, Omran H, et al. Multiplane transesophageal echocardiographic assessment of mitral regurgitation by Doppler color flow mapping of the vena contracta. Am J Cardiol 1994;74:912–17.
48. Thomas J. Doppler echocardiographic assessment of valvular regurgitation. Br Heart J. 2002;88:651–57.
49. Enriquez-Sarano E, Bailey K, Seward J, et al. Quantitative Doppler assessment of valvular regurgitation. Circulation 1993;87:841–48.
50. Bargiggia G, Tronconi L, Sahn D, et al. A new method for quantification of mitral regurgitation based on color flow Doppler imaging of flow convergence proximal to the regurgitant orifice. Circulation 1991;84:1481–89.
51. Vandervoort P, Rivera J, Mele D, et al. Application of color Doppler flow mapping to calculate effective regurgitant orifice area: an in vitro study and initial clinical observations. Circulation 1993;88:1150–56.
52. Vandervoort P, Rivera M, Mele D, et al. Application of color Doppler flow mapping to calculate effective regurgitant ori-

fice area: an in vitro study and initial clinical observations. Circulation 1993;88:1150–56.

53. Weyman AE. Left ventricular inflow tract I: The mitral valve, principles and practice of echocardiography. 2nd ed. Malvern, PA: Lea & Febiger, 1994:391–497.

54. Rodriguez L, Thomas JD, Monterroso V, et al. Validation of the proximal flow convergence method: calculation of orifice area in patients with mitral stenosis. Circulation 1993;88: 1157–65.

55. Deng Y, Matsumoto M, Wang X, et al. Estimation of mitral valve area in patients with mitral stenosis by the flow convergence region method: Selection of aliasing velocity. J Am Coll Cardiol 1994;24:683–89.

56. Rifkin R, Harper K, Tighe D. Comparison of proximal isovelocity surface area method with pressure half-time and planimetry in evaluation of mitral stenosis. J Am Coll Cardiol 1995;26:458–65.

57. Vandervoort PM, Rivera M, Mele D, et al. Application of color Doppler flow mapping to calculate effective regurgitant orifice area: An in vitro study and initial clinical observations. Circulation 1993;88:1150–56.

58. Pu M, Vandervoort P, Greenberg N, et al. Impact of wall constraint on velocity distribution in proximal flow convergence zone. Implications for color Doppler quantification of mitral regurgitation. J Am Coll Cardiol 27:1996:706–13.

59. Sitges M, Jones M, Shiota T, et al. Inter-aliasing distance of the flow convergence surface for determining mitral regurgitant volume: a validation study in a chronic animal model. J Am Coll Cardiol 2001;38:1195–1202.

60. Sitges M, Jones M, Shiota T, et al. Real-time three-dimensional color Doppler evaluation of the flow convergence zone for quantification of mitral regurgitation: Validation experimental animal study and initial clinical experience. J Am Soc Echocardiogr 2003;16:38–45.

61. Pu M, Prior D, Fan X, et al. Calculation of mitral regurgitant orifice area with use of a simplified proximal convergence method: initial clinical application. J Am Soc Echocardiogr 2001;14:180–85.

62. Flachskampf F, Frieske R, Engelhard B, et al. Comparison of transesophageal Doppler methods with angiography for evaluation of the severity of mitral regurgitation. J Am Soc Echocardiogr 1998;11:882–92.

63. Buck T, Mucci R, Guerrero L, et al. The power-velocity integral at the vena contracta: A new method for direct quantification of regurgitant volume flow. Circulation 2000;102: 1053–61.

64. Lembcke A, Wiese T, Enzweiler C, et al. Quantification of mitral valve regurgitation by left ventricular volume and flow measurements using electron beam computed tomography: comparison with magnetic resonance imaging. J Comput Assist Tomogr 2003;27:385–91.

65. Sugeng L, Spencer K, Mor-Avi V, et al. Dynamic three-dimensional color flow Doppler: an improved technique for the assessment of mitral regurgitation. Echocardiography 2003;20: 265–73.

66. Olson L, Subramanian R, Ackermann D, et al. Surgical pathology of the mitral valve: A study of 712 cases spanning 21 years. Mayo Clint Proc 1987;62:22–34.

67. Selzer A, Cohn K. Natural history of mitral stenosis: A review. Circulation 1972;45:878–90.

68. Osterberger L, Goldstein S, Khaja F, et al. Functional mitral stenosis in patients with massive mitral annular calcification. Circulation 1981;64:472–76.

69. Nassar W, Davis R, Dillon J, et al. Atrial myxoma. Am Heart J 1972;83:694–704.

70. Oh J, Seward J, Tajik A. Cardiac diseases due to systemic illness, medication, or infection. In: The echo manual. 2nd ed. Philadelphia: Lippincott Williams & Wilkins, 1999:169–79.

71. Otto C. Valvular stenosis: diagnosis, quantitation, and clinical approach, textbook of clinical echocardiography, 2nd ed. Philadelphia: WB Saunders, 2000:229–64.

72. Wilkins G, Weyman A, Abascal V, et al. Percutaneous balloon dilatation of the mitral valve: An analysis of echocardio-

graphic variables related to outcome and the mechanism of dilatation. Br Heart J 1988;60:299–308.

73. Nichol PM, Gilbert BW, Kisslo JA. Two-dimensional echocardiographic assessment of mitral stenosis. Circulation 1977; 55:120–28.

74. Daniel W, Nellessen U, Schroder E, et al. Left atrial spontaneous echo contrast in mitral valve disease: An indicator for an increased thromboembolic risk. J Am Coll Cardiol 1988;11:1204–11.

75. Chen YT, Kan MN, Chen JS, et al. Contributing factors to the formation of left atrial spontaneous echo contrast in mitral valvular disease. J Ultrasound Med 1990;9:151–55.

76. Liu CP, Ting CT, Yang TM, et al. Reduced left ventricular compliance in human mitral stenosis: Role of reversible internal constraint. Circulation 1992;85:1447–56.

77. Feigenbaum H. Hemodynamic information derived from echocardiography. In Echocardiography. 5th ed. Philadelphia: Lea & Febiger, 1994:181–215.

78. Hatle L, Brubakk A, Tromsdal et al. Noninvasive assessment of pressure drop in mitral stenosis by Doppler ultrasound. Br Heart J 1978;40:131–40.

79. Oh J, Seward J, Tajik A. Hemodynamic assessment. In: The echo manual. 2nd ed. Philadelphia: Lippincott Williams & Wilkins, 1999:59–71.

80. Bruce CJ, Nishimura RA. Clinical assessment and management of mitral stenosis, valvular heart disease. In Zoghbi WA, ed. Cardiology Clinics. Philadelphia: WB Saunders Co., 1998: 375–403.

81. Oh J, Seward JB, Tajik A. Valvular heart disease. In: The echo manual. 2nd ed. Philadelphia: Lippincott Williams & Wilkins, 1999:103–32.

82. Otto C. Valvular stenosis: diagnosis, quantitation, and clinical approach, Textbook of clinical echocardiography. 2nd ed. Philadelphia: WB Saunders, 2000:229–64.

83. Henry WL, Griffith JM, Michaelis LL, et al. Measurement of mitral orifice area in patients with mitral valve disease by real-time, two-dimensional echocardiography. Circulation 1975;51:827–31.

84. Wann LS, Weyman AE, Feigenbaum H, et al. Determination of mitral valve area by cross-sectional echocardiography. Ann Intern Med 1978;88:337–41.

85. Bruce C, Nishimura R. Newer advances in the diagnosis and treatment of mitral stenosis. In O'Rourke R, ed. Current problems in cardiology. St. Louis: Mosby Inc., 1998:March: 127–84.

86. Martin RP, Rakowski H, Kleiman JH, et al. Reliability and reproducibility of two-dimensional echocardiographic measurement of the stenotic mitral valve orifice area. Am J Cardiol 1979;43:560–68.

87. Oh J, Seward JB, Tajik A. Valvular heart disease. In: The echo manual. 2nd ed. Philadelphia: Lippincott Williams & Wilkins, 1999:103–32.

88. Libanoff AJ, Rodbard S. Atrioventricular pressure half-time: Measure of mitral valve orifice area. Circulation 1968;38: 144–50.

89. Hatle L, Angelsen B, Tromsdal A. Noninvasive assessment of atrioventricular pressure half-time by Doppler ultrasound. Circulation 1979;60:1096–104.

90. Hatle L, Angelsen B. Pulsed and continuous wave Doppler in diagnosis and assessment of various heart lesions, Doppler ultrasound in cardiology: physical principles and clinical applications. Philadelphia: Lea & Febiger, 1982:76–89.

91. Wranne B, Msee PA, Loyd D. Analysis of different methods of assessing the stenotic mitral valve area with emphasis on the pressure gradient half-time concept. Am J Cardiol 1990;66: 614–20.

92. Braverman AC, Thomas JD, Lee R. Doppler echocardiographic estimation of mitral valve area during changing hemodynamic conditions. Am J Cardiol 1991;68:1485–90.

93. Nakatani S, Masuyama T, Kodama K, et al. Value and limitations of Doppler echocardiography in the quantification of stenotic mitral valve area: Comparison of the pressure half-time and the continuity equation methods. Circulation 1988;77:78–85.

94. Thomas JD, Weyman AE. Doppler mitral pressure half-time: A clinical tool in search of theoretical justification. J Am Coll Cardiol 1987;10:923–29.

95. Thomas JD, Wilkins G, Choong CYP, et al. Inaccuracy of mitral pressure half-time immediately after percutaneous mitral valvotomy: Dependence on transmitral gradient and left atrial and ventricular compliance. Circulation 1988;78:980–93.

96. Karp K, Teien D, Eriksson P. Doppler echocardiographic assessment on the valve area in patients with atrioventricular valve stenosis by application of the continuity equation . J Intern Med 1989;225:261–66.

97. Degertekin M, Basaran Y, Gencbay M, et al. Validation of flow convergence region method in assessing mitral valve area in the course of transthoracic and transesophageal echocardiographic studies. Am Heart J 1998;135:207–14.

98. Faletra F, Pezzano A, Fusco R, et al. Measurement of mitral valve area in mitral stenosis: Four echocardiographic methods compared with direct measurement of anatomic orifices. J Am Coll Cardiol 1996;28:1190–97.

99. Pu M, Thomas J, Vandervoort P, Stewart W, et al. Comparison of quantitative and semiquantitative methods for assessing mitral regurgitation by TEE. Am J Cardiol 2001;87:66–70.

100. Schwerzmann M, Wustmann K, Zimmerli M, et al. Accurate determination of mitral regurgitation by assessing its influence on the combined diastolic mitral and pulmonary venous flow: just 'looking twice'. Eur J Echocardiogr 2001;2:277–84.

## QUESTIONS

1. Standard nomenclature adopted by the Society of Cardiovascular Anesthesiologists and the American Society of Echocardiography applied to the anatomic description of the mitral valve includes:
   A. Division of the anterior and posterior mitral leaflets into two segmental regions labeled A1 and A2 and P1 and P2.
   B. Division of the anterior mitral leaflet into three segmental regions labeled A1, A2, and A3 and the posterior mitral leaflet into three regions labeled P1, P2, and P3.
   C. Division of the anterior mitral leaflet into two segments A1, A2, and the posterior mitral leaflet into three segments labeled P1, P2, and P3.
   D. Division of the leaflet segments by the distribution of the chordal tendons to the individual scallops of the leaflets.

2. Which of the following is most consistent with severe grades of mitral insufficiency:
   A. A continuous Doppler signal that is an incomplete envelope of low signal intensity
   B. A peak E wave velocity of less than 1.2 m per second
   C. A maximal jet area as detected with color Doppler of less than 3.0 cm$^2$
   D. A reversed systolic pulmonary venous waveform as detected with pulsed wave Doppler

3. Results from the which of the quantitative methods are most consistent with severe mitral insufficiency:
   A. A vena contracta width of greater than or equal to 0.5 cm
   B. A regurgitant orifice area of 0.2 cm$^2$
   C. A regurgitant volume of 30 mm
   D. A regurgitant fraction measurement of 10%

4. Severe mitral stenosis is best reflected by which of the following measurements:
   A. A mean pressure gradient of 6 mm Hg
   B. A pressure half-time of 300 msec
   C. A deceleration time of less than 500 msec
   D. A mitral valve area of 2.0 cm$^2$

5. All of the following clinical situations will limit the accuracy of the pressure half-time method except:
   A. Conditions that alter the left atrial or left ventricular compliances
   B. Rapid heart rates
   C. Severe aortic insufficiency
   D. Severe degrees of mitral stenosis

Chapter 15

# Assessment of the Aortic Valve

*Christopher A. Troianos*

Transesophageal echocardiography (TEE) is used intraoperatively to evaluate aortic valve anatomy, function, and hemodynamics. The application of Doppler echocardiography (pulsed wave, continuous wave, and color) with two-dimensional imaging allows for the complete evaluation of stenotic and regurgitant lesions. Qualitative and quantitative assessment permits informed decisions regarding surgical intervention, the type of intervention (repair versus replacement), correction of inadequate surgical repair, and reoperation for complications. Prebypass TEE evaluation also identifies myocardial and valvular abnormalities associated with aortic valvular lesions, and determines the size of valve to be implanted. There are several reasons why valve sizing is important. The size of the valve is always a consideration in deciding whether a valve with only moderate stenosis should be replaced. Patients with small annular diameters may not derive a significant benefit from aortic valve replacement. Preoperative valve sizing is also important when valves of limited availability are to be implanted, i.e., homografts (1). For patients undergoing aortic valve replacement for aortic stenosis, intraoperative TEE has been shown to alter the surgical plan in 13% (2).

Intraoperative TEE among patients with known aortic valve disease undergoing valve replacement is used to confirm the preoperative diagnosis and determine the etiology of valve dysfunction. High-resolution images, owing to the close proximity of the valve and the esophagus, permit accurate diagnosis of the mechanism of valve dys-

function, a key aspect for determining the feasibility of repair versus replacement. The vast majority of aortic valves suitable for repair have regurgitant lesions rather than stenotic lesions. Valve repair for patients with aortic dissection involves resuspension of the cusps and is easily performed and highly successful in the absence of additional leaflet pathology. Valve repair techniques and pathology suitable for repair are discussed later in this book.

Postoperatively, TEE is used to evaluate the success of repair or function of the prosthetic valve. The degree of residual aortic insufficiency is an important aspect of valve repair evaluation. It determines the need for further surgery and possible valve replacement. Aortic valve replacement is associated with fewer regurgitant jets and smaller than the number of jets and jet area associated with mitral valve replacement, but the percentage decrease in regurgitant jet area after protamine administration is similar (3). Patients undergoing the Ross procedure for autograft replacement of their aortic valves also require evaluation of the prosthetic pulmonic valves.

TEE evaluation of left ventricular function is important postoperatively because of the inherent low ventricular compliance present among patients with left ventricular hypertrophy due to long-standing aortic stenosis or chronic hypertension. Left ventricular volume is more accurately determined by two-dimensional echocardiographic assessment of LV cross-sectional area than by filling pressures measured with a pulmonary artery catheter.

▶ TABLE 15.1. Limitations to Determination of Aortic Valve Area by Planimetry

| Limitation | Etiology | Consequence |
|---|---|---|
| Inadequate short-axis view | Leaflet edges not in same plane | Over- or underestimation of area |
| | Severe annular calcification | Shadowing of leaflet edges |
| Heavy calcification | Calcific degeneration of valve | Shadowing of anterior aspect of valve |
| Pinhole aortic stenosis | Advanced disease | Cannot identify valve orifice |

Characteristically, patients with low LV compliance often require volume infusion despite high filling pressures in the post-bypass period. Accurate determination of optimal volume status requires TEE. Clinical information provided by TEE allows appropriate hemodynamic management of patients with aortic valve disease undergoing aortic valve and nonaortic valve surgery before, during, and after general anesthesia.

A comprehensive perioperative TEE examination performed in patients undergoing nonaortic valve surgery may reveal aortic valve disease in patients in whom the diagnosis was not previously apparent. It is important to identify aortic valvular disease because of the surgical and anesthetic implications associated with both aortic stenosis and regurgitation. The increased population of elderly patients presenting for surgery has increased the prevalence of calcific aortic stenosis. Identification of significant aortic stenosis is important for anesthetic management during noncardiac surgery and for surgical management during nonaortic valve cardiac surgery. Aortic valve replacement after previous coronary artery bypass grafting is associated with higher mortality than combined aortic valve and coronary bypass surgery (4). Therefore, it is important to identify even moderate aortic stenosis during coronary bypass surgery, and to consider combination surgery to avoid the higher mortality associated with reoperation. Certain patients have a rapid progression of aortic stenosis, while others have a slower progression. Patients with rapid progression tend to be elderly men with associated coronary artery disease (5,6), or individuals with a smoking history, hypercholesterolemia, and elevated serum creatinine levels (7).

## APPROACH

High-resolution images of the aortic valve provided by TEE result from the close proximity of the valve to the esophagus. The anatomic plane of the aortic valve is oblique compared with the esophageal axis, which is longitudinal within the body. The right, posterior aspect of the valve is inferior to the left anterior aspect of the valve (Fig. 15.1). The implication for TEE imaging is that the transducer must be flexed anteriorly and to the left from the transverse plane of the patient, to align the imaging plane with the plane of the aortic valve. Alternatively, a multiplane TEE probe is rotated forward to between 30 degrees and 60 degrees with anteflexion to develop the short-axis view of the valve (Fig. 15.2). This view is important for tracing the aortic valve orifice area using planimetry and for identifying the site of aortic insufficiency using color flow Doppler. Rotating the multiplane angle forward to between 110 degrees and 150 degrees (orthogonal to the short-axis view) develops the midesophageal aortic valve long-axis (ME AV LAX) view (Fig.

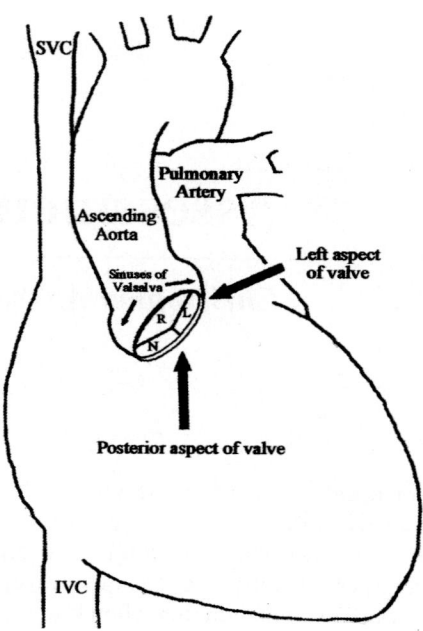

**FIGURE 15.1.** Illustration of the anatomic orientation of the aortic valve and Sinuses of Valsalva within the heart. The aortic valve consists of three cusps: right (R), left (L), and noncoronary (N). The right and posterior aspects of the valve are inferior to the left and anterior aspects of the valve. *SVC*, superior vena cava; *IVC*, inferior vena cava.

15.3). This view provides imaging of the left ventricular outflow tract, aortic valve, and aortic root to differentiate valvular from subvalvular and supravalvular pathology.

Hemodynamic assessment of antegrade and retrograde aortic valve flow requires a parallel orientation of blood flow and the Doppler beam (Fig. 15.4). The midesophageal views used for two-dimensional evaluation are inadequate for this assessment because blood flow is perpendicular to the Doppler beam. Conversely, the two transgastric views are more useful for interrogating flow across the aortic valve, but not as useful for detailed two-dimensional anatomic assessment due to the far field position of the aortic valve in these views. The *deep* transgastric long-axis (deep TG LAX) view is developed from the transgastric mid short-axis view by advancing the probe and flexing the probe to the left until the aortic valve is viewed in the middle or left side of the image in the far field (Fig. 15.5). The transgastric long-axis (TG LAX) view is developed from the transgastric mid short-axis view by rotating the transducer forward from 0 degrees to between 90 and 120 degrees until the aortic valve is viewed on the right side of the image in the far field (Fig. 15.6). Usually one or the other transgastric approach allows sufficient imaging to accomplish aortic valve flow measurement. It is important for the echocardiographer to become familiar with both approaches, because these

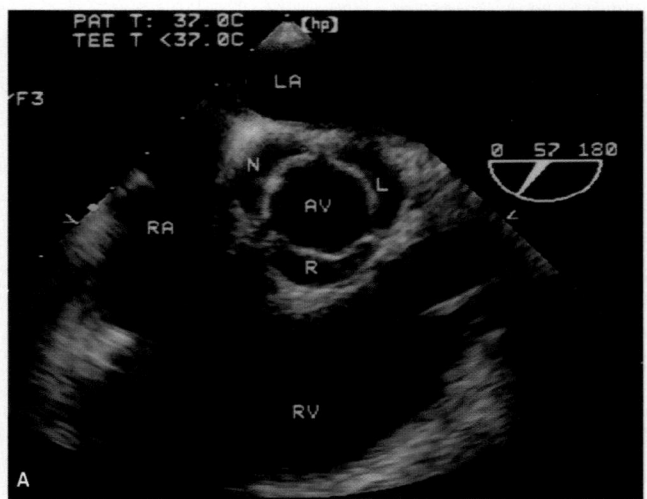 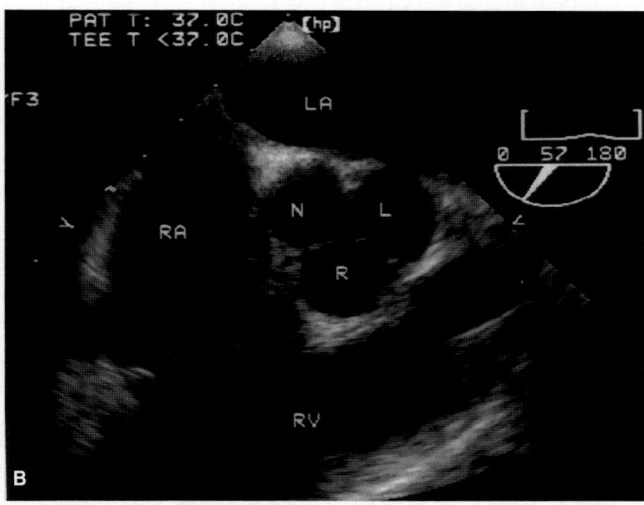

**FIGURE 15.2.** Transesophageal echocardiogram of the midesophageal aortic valve short-axis view during systole **(A)** and diastole **(B)**. A multiplane probe at 57 degrees provided this view in which all three aortic valve cusps are similar in size and appearance, indicating a true short-axis cross section. The aortic valve (AV) is identified by the right (*R*), left (*L*), and noncoronary (*N*) cusps. *LA*, left atrium; *RA*, right atrium; *RV*, right ventricle.

views are often difficult to obtain and require considerable practice and expertise. Stoddard et al. demonstrated 56% feasibility among the first 43 patients studied, as compared to 88% feasibility among the latter 43 patients studied suggesting a significant learning curve in measuring aortic valve blood flow velocity via the transgastric approach (8).

## STRUCTURES

The aortic valve is composed of three cusps that are associated with three bulges or pouch-like dilations in the aortic wall called the Sinuses of Valsalva (Fig. 15.1). Proximal to the aortic valve, the left ventricular outflow tract consists of the inferior surface of the anterior mitral leaflet, the ventricular septum, and the posterior left ventricular free wall. A normal aortic valve appears as two thin lines that open parallel to the aortic walls in the midesophageal aortic valve long-axis (ME AV LAX) view.

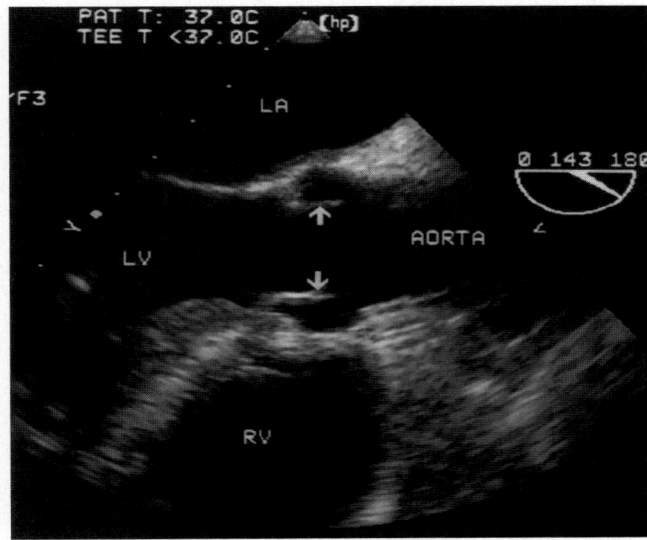

**FIGURE 15.3.** Transesophageal echocardiogram of the midesophageal aortic valve long-axis view during systole. A multiplane probe at 143 degrees provided this view of a normal aortic valve with leaflets (*arrows*) that open parallel to the aortic walls. The proximal ascending aorta is also imaged in this view. *LA*, left atrium; *LV*, left ventricle; *RV*, right ventricle.

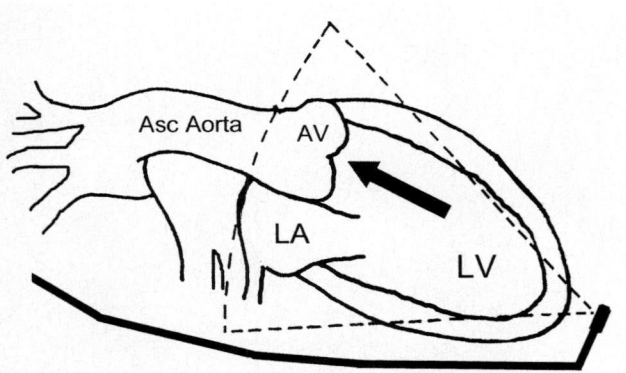

**FIGURE 15.4.** Illustration of the TEE probe position for the deep transgastric view of the aortic valve that allows a parallel orientation of blood flow through the aortic valve (*AV*) and left ventricular outflow tract (*arrow*). *LA*, left atrium; *LV*, left ventricle; *Asc*, ascending. From: Troianos CA. Aortic Valve. In Konstadt SN, Shernan S, & Oka Y, eds. *Clinical Transesophageal Echocardiography: A Problem-Oriented Approach*, 2nd ed., with permission.

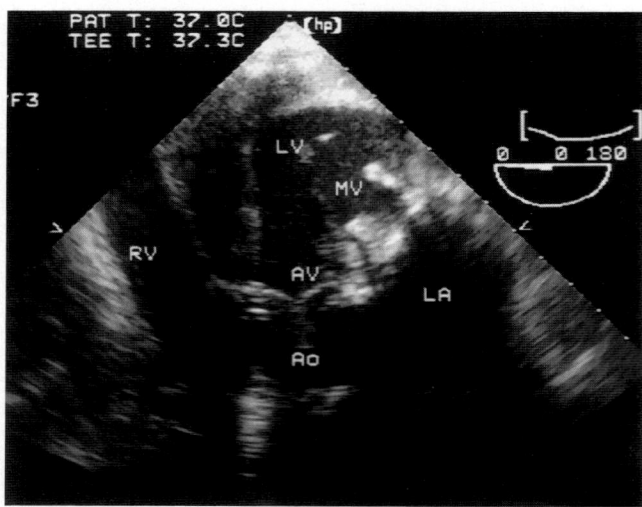

**FIGURE 15.5.** Transesophageal echocardiogram of the deep transgastric view. *AV*, aortic valve; *LA*, left atrium; *LV*, left ventricle; *AO*, ascending aorta; *MV*, mitral valve; *RV*, right ventricle.

The ascending aorta and LVOT are also inspected using this view (Fig. 15.3).

## PATHOLOGY

### Pathophysiology of Aortic Stenosis

The most frequent causes of aortic stenosis are calcific stenosis in the elderly, rheumatic valvulitis, and congenital anomalies (bicuspid, rarely unicuspid) that lead to accelerated leaflet calcification and restriction. The mecha-

nism of stenosis occurs from calcification of the leaflets (calcific, rheumatic, or congenital) or commissural fusion (usually rheumatic). Subaortic stenosis (subaortic membrane or ridge, and asymmetric septal hypertrophy) and supravalvular stenosis (narrowed aortic root) mimic aortic stenosis, but do not represent true valvular stenosis. Many of the echocardiographic techniques used for hemodynamic assessment of the aortic valve, however, can also be used to evaluate the severity of subvalvular and supravalvular pathology. Asymmetric septal hypertrophy or hypertrophic obstructive cardiomyopathy is discussed later in this book.

### Echocardiographic Evaluation of Aortic Stenosis

An important sign of aortic stenosis is leaflet doming during systole (Fig. 15.7). The leaflets are curved toward the midline of the aorta instead of parallel to the aortic wall. Leaflet doming is such an important observation that this finding alone is sufficient for the qualitative diagnosis of aortic stenosis. Coincident with doming is reduced leaflet separation (<15 mm), which is appreciated in both the short- and long-axis views of the aortic valve. The short-axis view of the aortic valve (Fig. 15.8) permits evaluation of leaflet motion and calcification, commissural fusion, and leaflet coaptation. This short-axis view (30 to 60 degrees) is used for measuring the aortic valve orifice area by two-dimensional planimetry, which provides good cor-

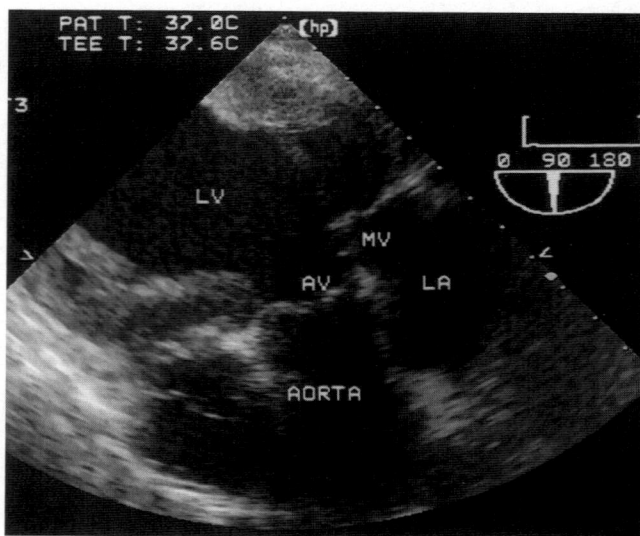

**FIGURE 15.6.** Transesophageal echocardiogram of the transgastric long-axis view. *AV*, aortic valve; *AORTA*, aortic root; *LA*, left atrium; *MV*, mitral valve; *LV*, left ventricle.

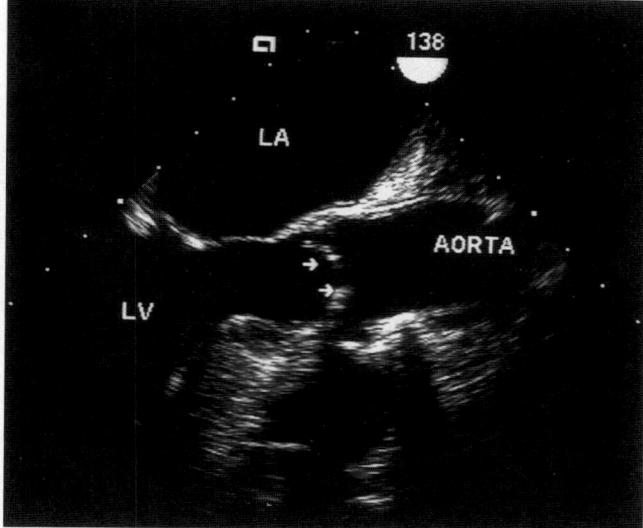

**FIGURE 15.7.** Transesophageal echocardiogram of the midesophageal aortic valve long-axis view during systole in a patient with aortic stenosis. A multiplane probe at 138 degrees provided this view of an aortic valve with doming leaflets (*arrows*). Leaflet doming is a qualitative sign of stenosis. The proximal ascending aorta is also imaged in this view. *LA*, left atrium; *LV*, left ventricle.

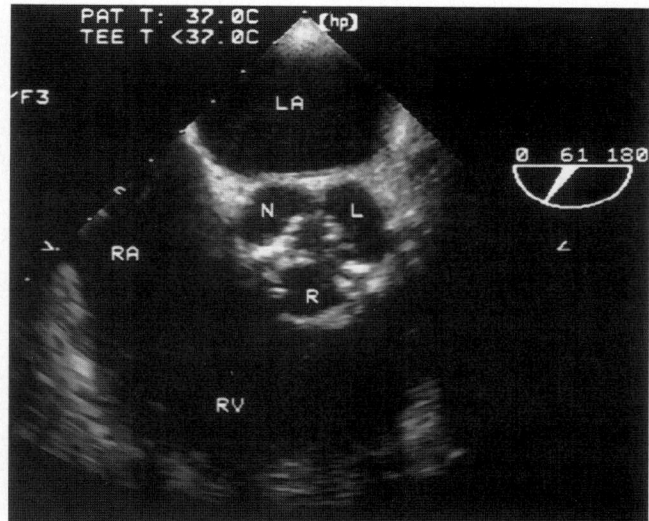

**FIGURE 15.8.** Transesophageal echocardiogram of the midesophageal aortic valve short-axis view during systole in a patient with aortic stenosis. *L, R,* and *N,* left, right, and noncoronary aortic valve cusps, respectively; *LA,* left atrium; *RA,* right atrium; *RV,* right ventricle.

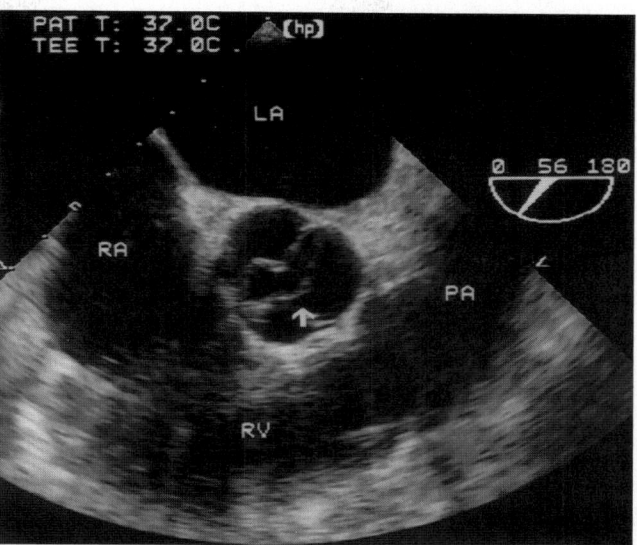

**FIGURE 15.9.** Transesophageal echocardiogram of the midesophageal aortic valve short-axis view in a patient with bicuspid aortic stenosis. *Arrow,* bicuspid aortic valve; *LA,* left atrium; *RA,* right atrium; *RV,* right ventricle; *PA,* pulmonary artery.

relation with other methods used for assessment of aortic stenosis (9). The probe is manipulated to provide the image with the smallest valvular cross-sectional area to ensure that the imaging plane is at the level of the leaflet tips, or smallest orifice. A cross section that is oblique or inferior to the leaflet tips overestimates the orifice size. The valve should appear circular in a true short-axis cross section as all three cusps are viewed simultaneously (9) and appear equal in shape. Multiplane TEE simplifies the location of the actual smallest orifice by imaging the aortic valve, first in long-axis view to identify the smallest orifice at the leaflet tips. The orifice is centered on the image display screen and the transducer position is stabilized within the esophagus as the multiplane angle is rotated backward to the short-axis view. The smallest orifice is traced and the two-dimensional cross-sectional area is displayed. Limitations to this technique are listed in Table 15.1 and include:

1. Inability to obtain an adequate short-axis view
2. Heavy calcification, particularly posterior, that causes shadowing of the valve
3. The presence of "pinhole" aortic stenosis, in which the valve orifice cannot be identified

The short-axis view of the aortic valve identifies congenital abnormalities of the aortic valve, including bicuspid (Fig. 15.9) and unicuspid (Fig. 15.10) valves.

Doppler echocardiography is used to quantitate the severity of aortic stenosis by measuring transvalvular blood velocity. The peak pressure gradient is estimated from the peak velocity measurement using the modified Bernoulli equation:

$$\text{Aortic Valve Gradient} = 4 \times (\text{Aortic Valve Velocity})^2$$

As previously mentioned, the midesophageal views of the aortic valve are not suitable for measuring transaortic velocity because accurate Doppler measurements require a

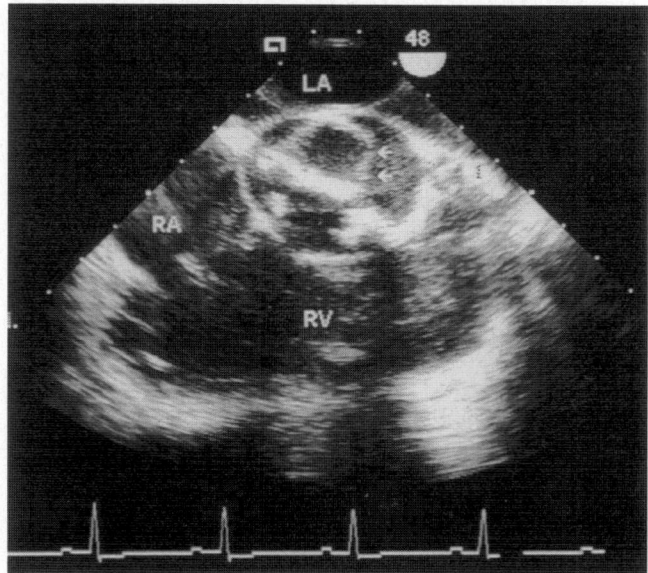

**FIGURE 15.10.** Transesophageal echocardiogram of the midesophageal aortic valve short-axis view in a patient with a unicuspid aortic valve as indicated by the arrows. *LA,* left atrium; *RA,* right atrium; *RV,* right ventricle. From Troianos CA. Perioperative Echocardiography. In: Troianos CA, ed. *Anesthesia for the Cardiac Patient.* St. Louis: Mosby, 2002, with permission.

parallel alignment of the Doppler beam with the blood flow. The deep TG LAX view is developed by advancing the probe beyond the transgastric midpapillary and apical short-axis views, maximally anteflexing the probe and flexing it to the left (Fig. 15.5). This places the probe at the left ventricular apex with the ultrasound beam directed toward the base of the heart (Fig. 15.4). The left atrium appears in the far field, to the right of the aortic valve and aortic root. A parallel alignment with blood flow in the LVOT and through the aortic valve is thus achieved. A parallel alignment of the ultrasound beam and aortic valve flow can also be obtained with the TG LAX view. This view is developed from the transgastric midpapillary short-axis view by rotating the multiplane angle from zero to between 90 and 120 degrees. The left atrium appears on the right side of the screen and the aortic valve is in the far field (Fig. 15.6).

Color flow Doppler and the audible Doppler signal are useful for identifying the location of the narrow high velocity jet (Fig. 15.11). The continuous wave Doppler cursor is placed within the narrow, turbulent jet and the spectral Doppler display is activated. Accurate localization provides a distinctive audible sound and high velocity (> 3 m/sec) spectral Doppler recording that exhibits a fine, feathery appearance and a midsystolic peak (Fig. 15.12). Normal aortic valves have peak velocities of 0.9 to 1.7 m/sec in adults, and peak in early systole. More dominant and dense lower velocities are also evident on the

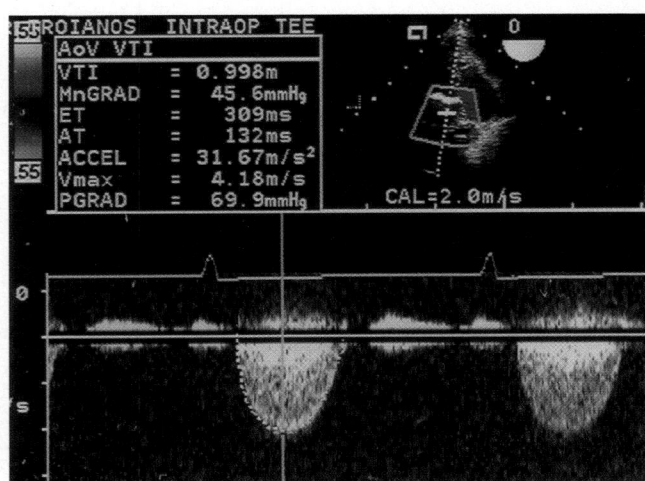

**FIGURE 15.12.** Continuous wave spectral Doppler velocities through a stenotic aortic valve. The fine, feathery appearance of the high (4.18 m/sec) velocities with a midsystolic peak indicates flow through a stenotic aortic valve. The denser lower velocities near the baseline indicate flow through the left ventricular outflow tract.

spectral Doppler display of patients with aortic stenosis and represent the more laminar, lower velocities in the LVOT. Planimetry of the velocity over time spectral Doppler analysis of transaortic blood flow yields the velocity time integral (VTI) and an estimate of mean aortic valve gradient.

A gradient across a stenotic orifice is dynamic because of its dependence on flow. As the flow (or cardiac output) through the valve decreases, the gradient also decreases. Conversely, as flow or the force of contraction increases the gradient also increases. Pressure gradients preoperatively obtained with transthoracic echocardiography utilize the same principles as intraoperative TEE. However, the intraoperative loading conditions, heart rate, and force of contraction may differ markedly from preoperative conditions, yielding disparate gradient data. Doppler-derived gradients also differ from gradients obtained in the cardiac catheterization lab because of the differing techniques employed for gradient determination. A cath lab gradient is usually a peak-to-peak gradient, which represents the difference between the peak left ventricular pressure and the peak aortic pressure. A Doppler gradient, however, is a "peak instantaneous" gradient, which is greater than the peak-to-peak gradient (Fig. 15.13). It is also important to correctly identify the origin of the gradient between the left ventricle and aorta as either valvular, subvalvular, or supravalvular based upon two-dimensional imaging. The shape of the spectral Doppler display differs depending on the etiology of the outflow obstruction. Aortic stenosis produces a rounded pattern with a midsystolic peak (Fig. 15.12), while LVOT obstruction

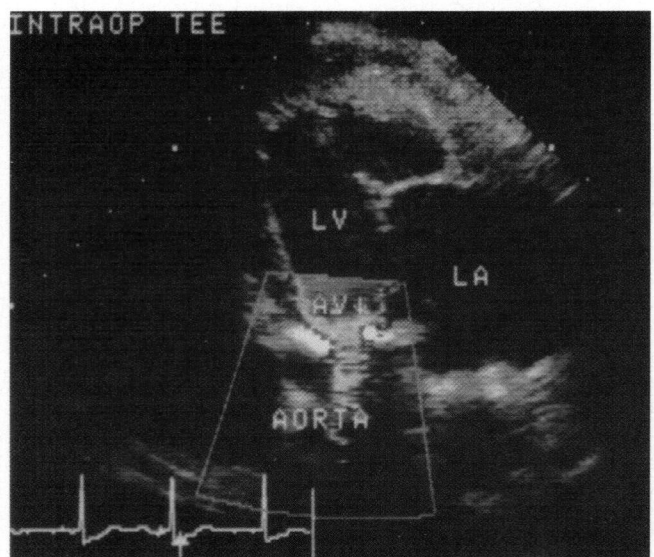

**FIGURE 15.11.** Transesophageal echocardiogram of the deep apical transgastric view with color flow Doppler applied over the stenotic aortic valve. The flow disturbance within the aortic valve (*AV*) identifies the stenotic orifice. *LA*, left atrium; *LV*, left ventricle. From Troianos CA. Perioperative Echocardiography. In: Troianos CA, ed. *Anesthesia for the Cardiac Patient*. St. Louis: Mosby, 2002, with permission.

▶ **TABLE 15.2. Limitations to Assessing the Severity of Aortic Stenosis by Transvalvular Velocity Measurement**

| Etiology of Limitation | Consequence |
|---|---|
| Decreased transvalvular flow | |
|    Severe LV dysfunction | |
|    Severe mitral regurgitation | Decreased pressure gradient |
|    Left to right intracardiac shunt | |
|    Low cardiac output | |
| Increased transvalvular flow | |
|    Hyperdynamic LV function | |
|    Sepsis | Increased pressure gradient |
|    Hyperthyroidism | |

produces a dagger-shaped pattern. Limitations to assessing the severity of stenosis by transvalvular velocity measurement are listed in Table 15.2.

Valve area is considered a more constant and less dynamic assessment of aortic stenosis. Recent evidence indicates that the more pliable valves, such as moderately stenotic or nonrheumatic valves, may open more with increased contractility (10). Nevertheless, determination of aortic valve area with Doppler echocardiography is an important method of valve assessment that is not generally dependent on the state of left ventricular function. The continuity equation is used for calculation of valve area and is based on the assumption that blood flowing through sequential areas of a continuous, intact vascular system must be equal. Blood flowing through the LVOT is thus equated with blood flow through the aortic valve.

$$Aortic\ Valve_{BLOOD\ FLOW} = LVOT_{BLOOD\ FLOW}$$

Substitution of blood flow with the product of velocity (VTI) and cross-sectional area yields:

$$Aortic\ Valve\ Area \times Aortic\ Valve_{VTI} = LVOT_{AREA} \times LVOT_{VTI}$$

Aortic valve area is then calculated as:

$$Aortic\ Valve\ Area = \frac{LVOT_{AREA} \times LVOT_{VTI}}{Aortic\ Valve_{VTI}}$$

$LVOT_{VTI}$ is measured by placing the pulsed wave Doppler sample volume in the LVOT just inferior to the aortic valve (Fig. 15.14) and tracing the spectral Doppler velocity over time. Optimal sampling of LVOT velocity is performed by advancing the sample volume toward the aortic valve until aliasing occurs due to the high velocity stenotic jet, then withdrawing the sample volume into the LVOT until aliasing no longer occurs and the velocity tracing appears laminar. Velocity is thus measured just beneath the aortic valve in the distal LVOT. $LVOT_{AREA}$ is determined using the midesophageal aortic valve long-axis view and measuring the LVOT diameter (d) near the aortic valve annulus (Fig. 15.15) to correspond to the same anatomic location as the pulsed wave Doppler recording of LVOT velocity. $LVOT_{AREA}$ is calculated by assuming that the LVOT is circular and using the formula:

$$AREA = \pi \times (d/2)^2$$

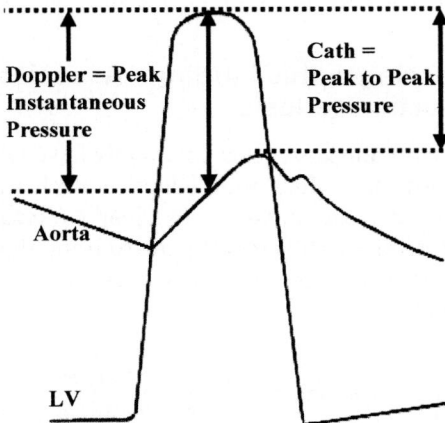

**FIGURE 15.13.** Illustration of the pressure tracings obtained during cardiac catheterization in a patient with aortic stenosis. The pressure gradient obtained with Doppler echocardiography is reflective of the peak instantaneous gradient. The cardiac catheterization gradient is the difference between the peak left ventricular and peak aortic pressures. From Troianos CA. Perioperative echocardiography. In Troianos CA, ed. *Anesthesia for the cardiac patient*. St. Louis: Mosby, 2002, with permission.

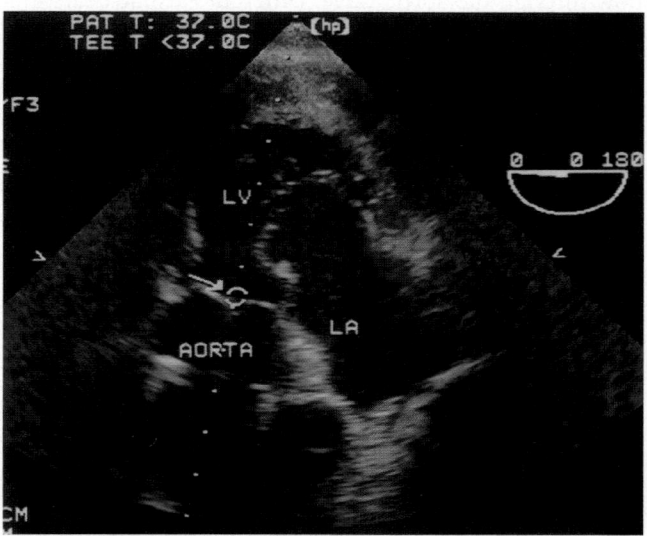

**FIGURE 15.14.** Transesophageal echocardiogram of the deep apical transgastric view with the pulsed wave Doppler sample volume (*arrow*) placed in the LVOT just inferior to the aortic valve. *LA*, left atrium; *LV*, left ventricle.

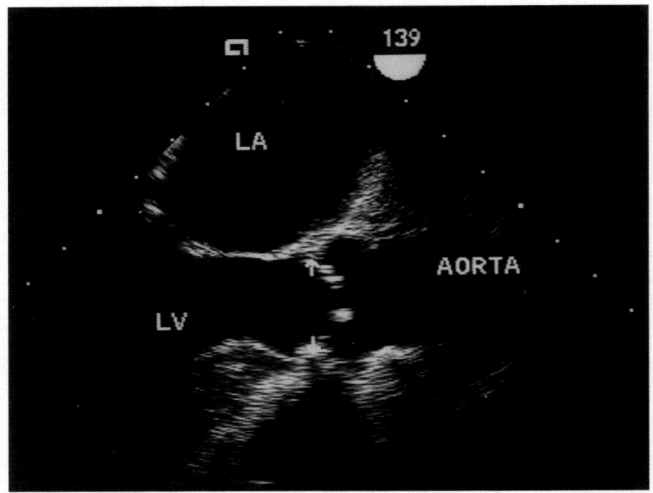

**FIGURE 15.15.** Transesophageal echocardiogram of the midesophageal aortic valve long-axis view during systole, indicating the site of measurement of the left ventricular outflow tract diameter (*arrows*). *LA*, left atrium; *LV*, left ventricle.

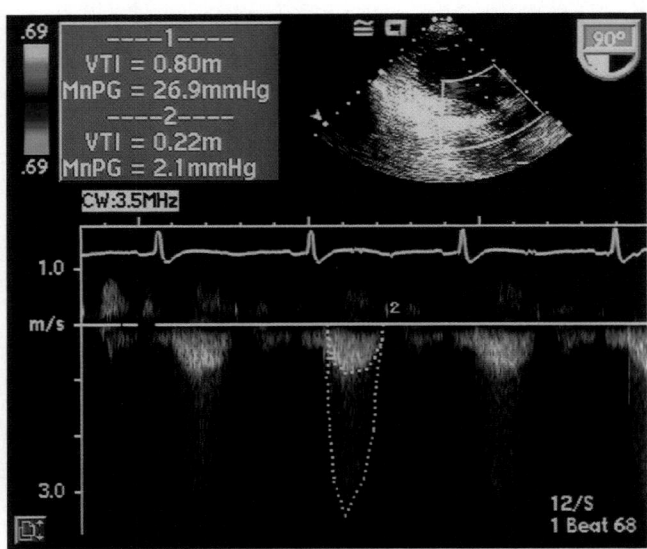

**FIGURE 15.16.** Planimetry of both the aortic valve and left ventricular outflow tract velocities is performed on the same cardiac beat using continuous wave spectral Doppler.

Calculation of LVOT$_{AREA}$ provides the greatest source of error in the continuity equation for valve area calculation. Erroneously foreshortened measurements of LVOT diameter are squared to significantly underestimate the true LVOT$_{AREA}$ and subsequently underestimate actual aortic valve area.

Another source of error with using the continuity equation for determination of aortic valve area is the patient with an irregular cardiac rhythm, such as atrial fibrillation. The equation is based on the conservation of mass, and assumes flow through the LVOT is equal to flow through the aortic valve. Different cardiac beats in a patient with an irregular rhythm have different stroke volumes. It is imperative to measure VTI for both the aortic valve and LVOT using the same cardiac beat. Using the continuous wave spectral Doppler display of aortic valve flow, the aortic valve VTI is traced around the trailing edge of the higher velocity envelope as previously described. However, instead of using pulsed wave Doppler to measure LVOT velocity, the LVOT$_{VTI}$ is traced from the same continuous wave spectral Doppler display as the aortic valve VTI, except that the denser lower velocities within the same cardiac beat are traced (Fig. 15.16). This "double envelope" technique (11) circumvents the problem of different stroke volumes for different beats, but can also be used for patients with a regular rhythm. The author prefers using pulsed wave Doppler for LVOT$_{VTI}$ measurements for patients with a regular rhythm because the continuous wave Doppler beam used to measure aortic valve VTI may not precisely intercept the aortic valve jet and LVOT flow in the same imaging plane or beam intercept angle. An alternative to measuring aortic valve

and LVOT$_{VTI}$ from the same cardiac beat in patients with an irregular rhythm is to measure aortic valve and LVOT$_{VTI}$ of several (seven or more) cardiac beats and take the average VTI for each in calculation of aortic valve area.

The stroke volume affects calculation of aortic valve area—even in patients with a regular sinus rhythm. Use of dobutamine to induce a larger stroke volume yields a slightly larger area that is related to the continuity equation rather than an actual change in valve area (12,13). Limitations to determination of aortic valve area by the continuity equation are summarized in Table 15.3.

## Echocardiographic Findings Associated with Aortic Stenosis

Patients with aortic stenosis commonly have left ventricular hypertrophy, which is an adaptive mechanism in response to chronic pressure overload. Increased wall thickness reduces wall stress by distributing the pressure overload over greater myocardial mass, as indicated by La Place's Law:

$$Wall\ stress = \frac{Pressure \times Volume}{2 \times wall\ thickness}.$$

The major perioperative implication is that estimates of left ventricular filling pressure are not reliable indicators of volume loading because of the associated decreased left ventricular compliance. The second major concern is the development of systolic anterior motion (SAM) of the mitral valve because of the septal hypertro-

▶ **TABLE 15.3.  Limitations to Determination of Aortic Valve Area by the Continuity Equation**

| Limitation | Etiology | Consequence |
|---|---|---|
| Inadequate transgastric view | Patient anatomy | Inability to position Doppler beam parallel to high velocity jet for velocity measurements |
| Inability to identify high velocity jet | Pinhole aortic stenosis | Inability to measure transvalvular flow |
| Inability to measure an accurate LVOT diameter | Anatomic relation between LVOT and esophagus | Error in valve area calculations |

phy after aortic valve replacement for aortic stenosis. Although this condition is well-recognized with asymmetric septal hypertrophy, SAM can also occur in patients with *symmetric* septal hypertrophy after aortic valve replacement. This is usually a manifestation of the abrupt reduction in left ventricular afterload associated with an underfilled left ventricle in patients with septal or concentric hypertrophy. The condition usually resolves with administration of volume, phenylephrine, and discontinuation of inotropic and chronotropic medications.

Patients with aortic stenosis also manifest diastolic dysfunction with long-standing aortic stenosis. Mitral inflow and pulmonary venous flow patterns are examined with deceleration time. Systolic function is preserved until late in the disease progression when left ventricular dilation develops. Systolic dysfunction due to aortic stenosis is usually reversible with valve replacement. Systolic dysfunction due to myocardial infarction may not improve and causes an underestimation of the severity of aortic stenosis by gradient determination.

Many patients with aortic stenosis also have aortic insufficiency (AI). The diastolic regurgitation of blood into the left ventricle increases transaortic blood flow during systole, yielding a higher gradient for a given aortic valve orifice. The presence of AI, however, does not affect continuity equation area calculations because the measurements of systolic flow in the LVOT and the aortic valve both account for the increased systolic flow.

Patients with aortic valve disease may also have mitral valve disease, manifested as mitral stenosis, regurgitation, or both. The presence of mitral stenosis causes an underestimation of the severity of aortic stenosis by gradient determination because of decreased transaortic blood flow.

## Pathophysiology of Aortic Insufficiency

Aortic insufficiency (AI) is caused by either intrinsic disease of the aortic cusps or secondarily from diseases affecting the ascending aorta. Intrinsic valvular problems include rheumatic, calcific, and myxomatous valvular disease; endocarditis, traumatic injury; and congenital

abnormalities. Conditions affecting the ascending aorta that lead to aortic insufficiency include annular dilatation and aortic dissection (secondary to blunt trauma or hypertension), mycotic aneurysm, cystic medial necrosis, Marfan's syndrome, and chronic hypertension. The most common cause of pure aortic insufficiency is no longer postinflammatory, with the decreasing prevalence of rheumatic heart disease among cardiac surgical patients (14). Aortic root dilation is now the most common etiologic factor due to the increased prevalence of degenerative disease, followed by postinflammatory disease and bicuspid valve disease.

## Echocardiographic Evaluation of Aortic Insufficiency

The aortic valve, ascending aorta, and LVOT are inspected using the ME AV LAX view (Fig. 15.3). Normal leaflets are often not visible during diastole, because they are parallel to the Doppler beam when closed. Stenotic leaflets that dome during systole often do not completely coapt during diastole, leading to aortic insufficiency. The diagnosis of leaflet prolapse is made when aortic leaflet tissue is imaged in the LVOT below the annular plane during diastole. An aortic dissection in the aortic root causes disruption of leaflets from the aortic annulus and may also cause leaflet prolapse. Two-dimensional echocardiography is used to determine the etiology of the aortic insufficiency by identifying structural abnormalities of the leaflets or aortic root.

Although two-dimensional echocardiography is not useful for quantifying the severity of AI, there are several associated echocardiographic features. The left ventricle is dilated and more spherical in shape with chronic AI, but not necessarily with acute AI. The mitral valve exhibits premature closure and fluttering of the anterior mitral leaflet during diastole. An eccentric AI jet directed towards the anterior mitral valve leaflet may cause doming of the anterior leaflet with convexity towards the left atrial side of the mitral valve (Fig. 15.17).

Doppler echocardiography is used to quantitate the severity of AI using several techniques that involve color,

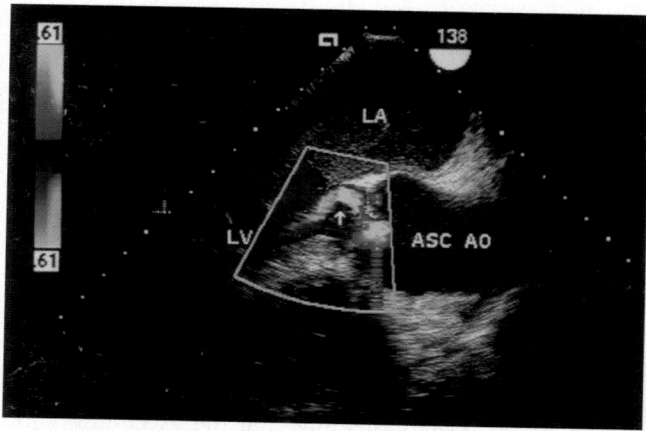

**FIGURE 15.17.** Transesophageal echocardiogram with a color flow Doppler in a patient with eccentric aortic insufficiency. The aortic insufficiency is identified by the color flow disturbance that originates from the aortic valve and directed towards the anterior mitral valve leaflet.

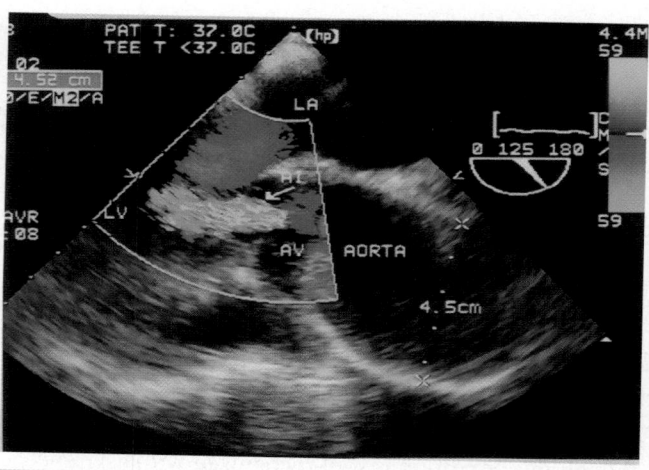

**FIGURE 15.19.** Transesophageal echocardiogram of the midesophageal aortic valve long-axis view with color flow Doppler in a patient with aortic insufficiency (*AI*). *LA*, left atrium; *LV*, left ventricle; *AV*, aortic valve.

pulsed wave, and continuous wave Doppler. These techniques are sensitive and reliable, but all have limitations. Color Doppler applied to ME AV SAX (30 to 50 degrees multiplane angle) is useful for localizing the site of regurgitation (Fig. 15.18). Despite the orthogonal relationship

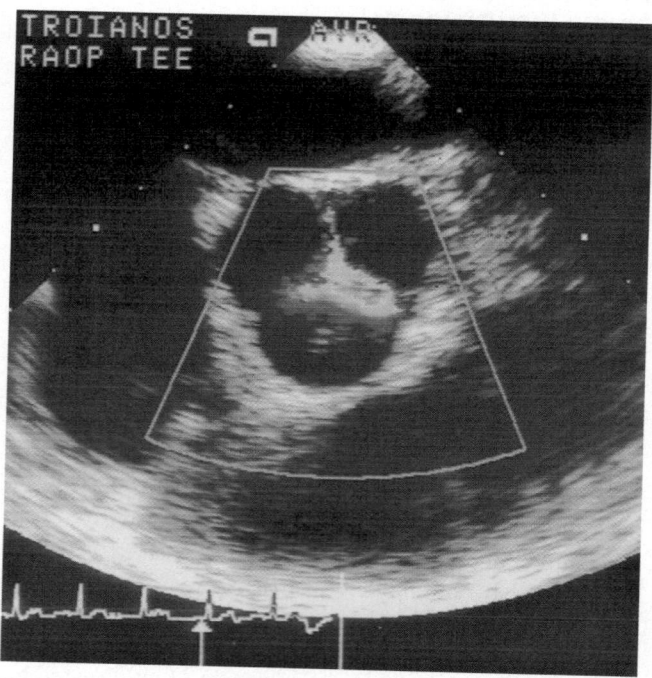

**FIGURE 15.18.** Transesophageal echocardiogram of the midesophageal aortic valve short-axis view with color flow Doppler in a patient with aortic insufficiency. The origin of the aortic insufficiency is predominantly between the right and left coronary cusps. From Troianos CA. Perioperative echocardiography. In Troianos CA, ed. Anesthesia for the cardiac patient. St. Louis: Mosby, 2002, with permission.

between the aortic valve flow and Doppler beam in this short-axis view, the regurgitant orifice is identifiable because the AI jet is usually not completely orthogonal to the Doppler beam, particularly if the jet is eccentric. The ME AV LAX view (120 to 150 degrees multiplane angle) is the most useful for quantitating the severity of AI. Color Doppler reveals a flow disturbance in the left ventricular outflow tract originating from the aortic valve and directed into the left ventricle (Fig. 15.19). A central jet is usually caused by aortic root dilatation, whereas an eccentric jet usually implies a leaflet problem. The width of the jet *at the orifice* compared to the width of the LVOT correlates with angiographic determinants of aortic insufficiency (Table 15.4) (15).

Limitations to use of color flow Doppler echocardiography to estimate the severity of aortic insufficiency are listed in Table 15.5. One such limitation to this technique is that the regurgitant jet orifice and the true LVOT diameter (not foreshortened) may not be in the same imaging plane (16). This limitation is most apparent if "color M-mode" is used to determine the jet/LVOT ratio. Color M-mode refers to the application of M-mode imaging to a color flow Doppler image. M-mode evaluation of the LVOT in the patient with AI is more useful for determina-

▶ **TABLE 15.4. Grading Aortic Insufficiency**

| Severity of Aortic Insufficiency | Jet Width/LVOT Width Ratio (15) | Average Regurgitant Fraction (24) |
|---|---|---|
| 1+ | < 0.25 | 28% |
| 2+ | 0.25 to 0.46 | 33% |
| 3+ | 0.47 to 0.64 | 53% |
| 4+ | > 0.64 | 62% |

▶ **TABLE 15.5. Limitations to Estimating the Severity of Aortic Insufficiency with Color Flow Doppler**

| Limitation | Etiology | Consequence |
|---|---|---|
| Shadowing of LVOT | Prosthetic aortic or mitral valve<br>Mitral annular calcification | Inability to image LVOT or AI jet |
| AI jet is wider in one plane vs. another | Regurgitant orifice asymmetric in its three-dimensional shape | Inaccurate estimate of AI jet width |
| Eccentric jet causing swirling of flow disturbance | Leaflet prolapse | AI jet appears wider than orifice size |

tion of the duration of AI into the diastolic phase rather than the jet/LVOT ratio.

Another limitation to the jet/LVOT ratio method of assessing AI is that the shape of the regurgitant orifice may not be circular or symmetric. An irregularly shaped regurgitant orifice may cause the jet to appear wider in one imaging plane than another (17); hence the importance of examining multiple imaging planes. The AI jet may also be eccentric or converge with the mitral valve inflow, rendering the jet particularly difficult to evaluate in patients with mitral stenosis (18). If color Doppler cannot be applied to the LVOT from the ME AV LAX view because of annular calcification or shadowing of the LVOT from a prosthetic mitral or aortic valve, a *deep* TG LAX or TG LAX view is used. The AI jet in this view appears red or mosaic in color with the jet directed away from the aortic

valve towards the left ventricular cavity (Fig. 15.20). Multiple imaging planes should be utilized to appreciate the three-dimensional character of the jet.

Continuous wave Doppler is also used to determine the severity of AI by measuring the deceleration slope of the regurgitant jet. A deep apical transgastric or transgastric long-axis view aligns the regurgitant jet parallel to the Doppler beam. Color Doppler is useful for identifying the location and direction of the AI jet. The Doppler cursor is placed within the AI color flow Doppler jet and the continuous wave spectral velocity profile is obtained (Fig. 15.21). The velocity of the regurgitant jet declines more rapidly in patients with severe AI because the larger regurgitant orifice allows a more rapid equilibration of the aortic and left ventricular pressures. In other words, if the pressure difference between the aorta and left ventricle approaches zero rapidly, the regurgitant jet velocity also approaches zero more rapidly, creating a steeper slope

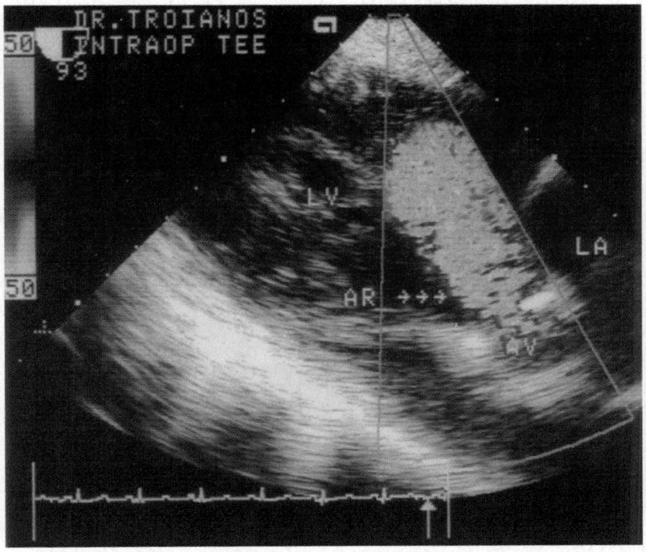

**FIGURE 15.20.** Transesophageal echocardiogram of the transgastric long-axis view with color flow Doppler in a patient with aortic insufficiency (*arrows*). *AV,* aortic valve; *LA,* left atrium; *LV,* left ventricle. From Troianos CA. Perioperative echocardiography. In: Troianos CA, ed. *Anesthesia for the Cardiac Patient.* St. Louis: Mosby, 2002, with permission.

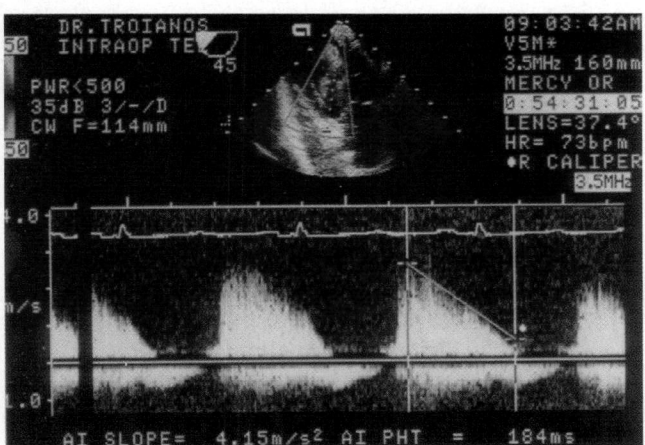

**FIGURE 15.21.** Continuous wave spectral Doppler velocities within the left ventricular outflow tract in a patient with aortic insufficiency. The slope of the velocity deceleration (AI slope = 4.15 m/sec$^2$) indicates the severity of the aortic insufficiency. From Troianos CA. Perioperative echocardiography. In: Troianos CA, ed. *Anesthesia for the Cardiac Patient.* St. Louis: Mosby, 2002, with permission.

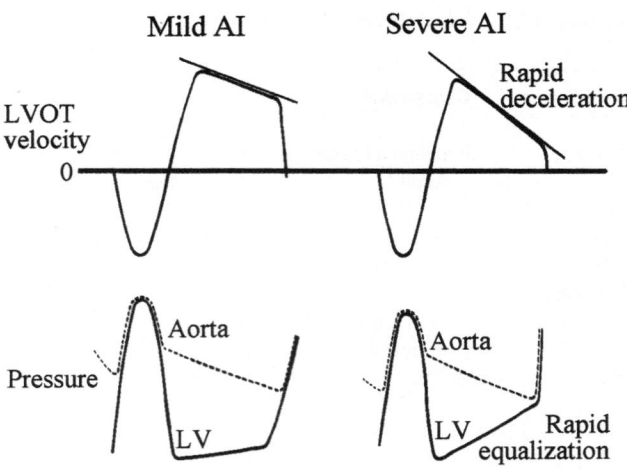

**FIGURE 15.22.** Illustration of the association between the left ventricular outflow tract (LVOT) deceleration slope and the pressure difference between the aorta and left ventricle (LV) during diastole. The deceleration slope is steeper and approaches zero velocity more rapidly with severe aortic insufficiency (AI) as the pressures in the aorta and left ventricle equalize more rapidly. From Troianos CA. Perioperative echocardiography. In: Troianos CA, ed. *Anesthesia for the Cardiac Patient*, St. Louis: Mosby, 2002, with permission and adapted from Feigenbaum H. Echocardiography 1994, 5th ed. Philadelphia: Lea & Febiger, 286, with permission.

(Fig. 15.22). A regurgitant velocity slope greater than 3 m/sec$^2$ is indicative of advanced (3 or 4+) AI (19).

One limitation to this technique is that factors other than regurgitant orifice size influence the deceleration slope (Table 15.6). Systemic vascular resistance and left ventricular compliance affect the rate of deceleration, irrespective of the regurgitant orifice size (20). Decreased systemic vascular resistance (sepsis) and reduced left ventricular compliance (ischemia, cardiomyopathy, acute AI) cause a steeper deceleration slope because aortic and left ventricular pressures equalize more rapidly with these conditions. Another limitation to this technique is that measurement of regurgitant jet velocity is difficult

and unreliable in patients with eccentric jets, because it is difficult to align the Doppler beam with the regurgitant jet.

Pulsed wave Doppler is used to detect retrograde flow in the aorta during diastole. Holodiastolic flow in the abdominal aorta is both sensitive and specific for severe aortic insufficiency. Detection of holodiastolic retrograde flow in the proximal descending thoracic aorta and aortic arch is a sensitive indicator of aortic insufficiency, but is not specific for severe aortic insufficiency. Using the short-axis TEE view of the descending thoracic aorta, the pulsed wave sample volume is placed as distal in the aorta as possible, near the diaphragm. Despite the orthogonal relationship between the aortic flow and Doppler beam in this short-axis view, the flow in the aorta is identifiable because the blood in the aorta tends to swirl as it travels down the aorta. The spectral Doppler display is examined for the duration of diastolic flow. Retrograde flow throughout diastole (holodiastolic) in the distal descending (21) or abdominal aorta (22) (Fig. 15.23) indicates severe aortic insufficiency.

Regurgitant volume and regurgitant fraction can also be used to evaluate the severity of aortic insufficiency. Regurgitant volume is the difference between the systolic flow across the aortic valve and "net forward" cardiac output. In the absence of intracardiac shunts and mitral regurgitation, flow through the pulmonary artery or mitral valve is equivalent to (net) cardiac output. Pulmonary artery blood flow is reliably measured with TEE by measuring the pulmonary artery diameter (d), calculating its area [$\pi(d/2)^2$], and multiplying the area by the pulmonary artery VTI and heart rate (23). Aortic valve systolic flow is the product of aortic valve area and VTI. The aortic regurgitant volume is the difference between aortic valve systolic flow and pulmonary blood flow (cardiac output). Re-

▶ **TABLE 15.6. Limitations to Estimating the Severity of Aortic Insufficiency Using the Deceleration Slope**

| Limitation | Consequence |
|---|---|
| Increased systemic vascular resistance | Steeper slope overestimating AI |
| Decreased left ventricular compliance | Steeper slope overestimating AI |
| Eccentric AI jet | Cannot align Doppler beam with AI jet |

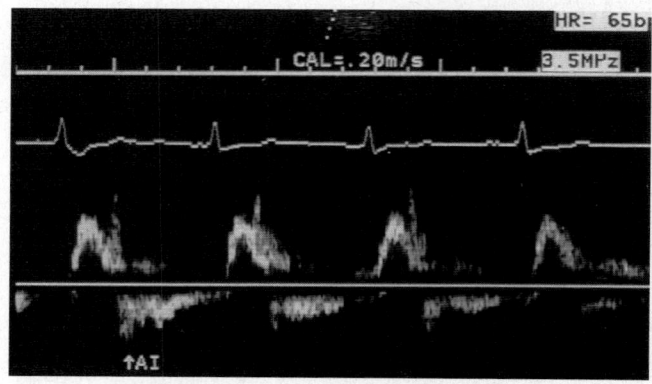

**FIGURE 15.23.** Pulsed wave Doppler spectral velocity of blood flow in the descending thoracic aorta. The retrograde flow throughout diastole (*arrow*) is termed holodiastolic and is associated with severe aortic insufficiency. From Troianos CA. Perioperative echocardiography. In: Troianos CA, ed. *Anesthesia for the Cardiac Patient*. St. Louis: Mosby, 2002, with permission.

gurgitant fraction is expressed as the proportion of aortic valve systolic flow that is regurgitant volume and indicates the severity of AI (Table 15.4) (24).

$$\text{Regurgitant Volume} =$$
$$\text{Aortic Valve Systolic Flow} - \text{Cardiac Output}$$

$$\text{Regurgitant Fraction} = \frac{\text{Regurgitant Volume}}{\text{Aortic Valve Systolic Flow}}$$

The continuity equation could be theoretically used to determine regurgitant orifice size. Diastolic velocities just above (aortic root-VTI) and through the aortic valve (aortic valve-VTI) are determined with Doppler echocardiography and the cross-sectional area of the aortic root is determined with two-dimensional echocardiography (25,26). This technique, however, has not been widely accepted or validated.

$$\text{Aortic Valve Regurgitant Orifice} =$$
$$\frac{\text{Aortic Root}_{AREA} \times \text{Aortic Root Diastolic}_{VTI}}{\text{Aortic Valve Regurgitant Jet}_{VTI}}$$

## Echocardiographic Findings Associated with Aortic Insufficiency

Chronic left ventricular volume overload causes progressive left ventricular dilation over many years, while systolic function is preserved. Ejection fraction is initially normal, while end-diastolic dimensions are increased. In contrast to aortic stenosis, the ventricle remains relatively compliant until systolic dysfunction ensues late in the course of the disease process. Another contrasting feature is that the systolic dysfunction is not reversible. Acute aortic insufficiency is not associated with left ventricular dilation because the adaptive left ventricular dilation has not occurred. This lack of adaptation is associated with a decreased left ventricular compliance and a rapid onset of symptoms. Other echocardiographic findings include premature mitral valve closure and fluttering of the mitral valve leaflets. Depending on the etiology of the AI, aortic root abnormalities may also be present, including aortic dissection or aneurysm.

Aortic insufficiency causes an overestimation of mitral valve area by the pressure half-time method of determining mitral orifice size. The PHT method exploits the relation between mitral inflow deceleration and mitral valve area. Deceleration is based on the equalization of pressure in the left atrium and the left ventricle and is prolonged as mitral orifice size decreases. In the absence of AI, left ventricular volume (and subsequently left pressure) increases via mitral inflow alone. In the presence of AI, left ventricular increases by both mitral inflow and aortic regurgitation, giving the impression that mitral inflow is better than it actually is, underestimating the severity of mitral stenosis.

## KEY POINTS

- The close anatomic proximity between the aortic valve and the esophagus permits accurate diagnosis of the mechanism of aortic valve dysfunction, valve sizing for valve replacement, and identification of associated lesions.
- Complete evaluation of the aortic valve utilizes two-dimensional imaging and pulsed wave, continuous wave, and color Doppler for quantitative evaluation of stenotic and regurgitant lesions.
- Velocity measurement of aortic valve flow provides an estimate of valve gradient using the modified Bernoulli equation. The force of ventricular contraction and transaortic blood flow determine transvalvular velocity in addition to the size of the stenotic orifice. The severity of aortic stenosis is underestimated in patients with severe left ventricular dysfunction. These patients require area determination to assess the severity of aortic stenosis.
- There is often a discrepancy between Doppler and cardiac catheterization derived gradient measurements due to differences in technique and measurements. Doppler-derived measurements usually exceed catheterization measurements.
- Aortic valve area is determined by planimetry or by using the continuity equation.
- Aortic insufficiency is caused by conditions affecting the aortic cusps or secondarily from diseases affecting the ascending aorta.
- Two-dimensional echocardiography is useful for identifying the etiology of aortic insufficiency and associated lesions, but not for assessing the severity of regurgitation.
- Color, pulsed wave, and continuous wave Doppler are used to quantify the severity of regurgitation, but each technique has limitations.

## REFERENCES

1. Oh CC, Click RL, Orszulak TA, et al. Role of intraoperative transesophageal echocardiography in determining aortic annulus diameter in homograft insertion. J Am Soc Echocardiogr 1998;11:638–42.
2. Nowrangi SK, Connolly HM, Freeman WK, Click RL. Impact of intraoperative transesophageal echocardiography among patients undergoing aortic valve replacement for aortic stenosis. J Am Soc Echocardiogr 2001;14:863–6.
3. Morehead AJ, Firstenberg MS, Shiota T, et al. Intraoperative echocardiographic detection of regurgitant jets after valve replacement. Ann Thorac Surg 2000;69:135–9.
4. Odell JA, Mullany CJ, Schaff HV, et al. Aortic valve replacement after previous coronary artery bypass grafting. Ann Thorac Surg 1996;62:1424–30.

5. Peter M, Hoffmann A, Parker C, et al. Progression of aortic stenosis. Chest 1993;103:1715–9.

6. Bahler RC, Desser DR, Finkelhor RS, et al. Factors leading to progression of valvular aortic stenosis. Am J Cardiol 1999; 84:1044–8.

7. Palta S, Pai AM, Gill KS, et al. New insights into the progression of aortic stenosis: implications for secondary prevention. Circulation 2000;101:2497–502.

8. Stoddard MF, Hammons RT, Longaker RA. Doppler transesophageal echocardiographic determination of aortic valve area in adults with aortic stenosis. Am Heart J 1996;132: 337–42.

9. Hoffmann R, Flachskampf FA, Hanrath P. Planimetry of orifice area in aortic stenosis using multiplane transesophageal echocardiography. J Am Coll Cardiol 1993;22:529–34.

10. Shively BK, Charlton GA, Crawford MH, et al. Flow dependence of valve area in aortic stenosis: Relation to valve morphology. J Am Coll Cardiol 1998;31:654–60.

11. Maslow AD, Mashikian J, Haering JM, et al. Transesophageal echocardiographic evaluation of native aortic valve area: Utility of the double-envelope technique. J Cardiothorac Vasc Anesth 2001;15:293–9.

12. Rask LP, Karp KH, Eriksson NP. Flow dependence of the aortic valve area in patients with aortic stenosis: assessment by application of the continuity equation. J Am Soc Echocardiogr 1996;9:295–9.

13. Lin SS, Roger VL, Pascoe R, et al. Dobutamine stress Doppler hemodynamics in patients with aortic stenosis: feasibility, safety, and surgical correlations. Am Heart J 1998; 136:1010–6.

14. Cosgrove DM, Rosenkranz ER, Hendren WG, et al. Valvuloplasty for aortic insufficiency. J Thorac Cardiovasc Surg 1991;102:571–7.

15. Perry GJ, Helmke F, Nanda NC, et al. Evaluation of aortic insufficiency by Doppler color flow mapping. J Am Coll Cardiol 1987;9:952–9.

16. Reynolds T, Abate J, Tenney A, et al. The JH/LVOH method in the quantification of aortic regurgitation: How the cardiac sonographer may avoid an important potential pitfall. J Am Soc Echo 1991;4:105–8.

17. Taylor AL, Eichhorn EJ, Brickner ME, et al. Aortic valve morphology: An important in vitro determinant of proximal regurgitant jet width by Doppler color flow mapping. J Am Coll Cardiol 1990;16:405–12.

18. Masuyama T, Kitabatake A, Kodama K, et al. Semiquantitative evaluation of aortic regurgitation by Doppler echocardiography: Effects of associated mitral stenosis. Am Heart J 1989;117:133–9.

19. Grayburn PA, Handshoe R, Smith MD, et al. Quantitative assessment of the hemodynamic consequences of aortic regurgitation by means of continuous wave Doppler recordings. J Am Coll Cardiol 1987;10:135–41.

20. Griffin BP, Flachskampf FA, Siu S, et al. The effects of regurgitant orifice size, chamber compliance, and systemic vascular resistance on aortic regurgitant velocity slope and pressure half-time. Am Heart J 1991;122:1049–56.

21. Sutton DC, Kluger R, Ahmed SU, et al. Flow reversal in the descending aorta: a guide to intraoperative assessment of aortic regurgitation with transesophageal echocardiography. J Thorac Cardiovasc Surg 1994;108:576–82.

22. Takenaka K, Sakamoto T, Dabestani A, et al. Pulsed Doppler echocardiographic detection of regurgitant blood flow in the ascending, descending and abdominal aorta of patients with aortic regurgitation. J Cardiol 1987;17:301–9.

23. Savino JS, Troianos CA, Aukburg S, et al. Measurement of pulmonary blood flow with transesophageal two-dimensional and Doppler echocardiography. Anesthesiology 1991; 75:445–51.

24. Kitabatake A, Ito H, Inoue M, et al. A new approach to noninvasive evaluation of aortic regurgitant fraction by two-dimensional Doppler echocardiography. Circulation 1985;72: 523–9.

25. Reimold SC, Ganz P, Bittl JA, et al. Effective aortic regurgitant orifice area: Description of a method based on the conservation of mass. J Am Coll Cardiol 1991;18:761–8.

26. Yeung AC, Plappert T, St. John Sutton MG. Calculation of aortic regurgitation orifice area by Doppler echocardiography: An application of the continuity equation. Br Heart J 1992;68:236–40.

## QUESTIONS

1. An 80-year-old patient with a 15% left ventricular ejection fraction presents for coronary artery bypass grafting and possible aortic valve replacement. Preoperative cardiac catheterization revealed a left ventricular to aorta gradient of 20 mm Hg. What is the best way to determine the severity of aortic stenosis in this patient?
   A. Determine aortic valve area using the continuity equation.
   B. Determine mean aortic valve gradient using the modified Bernoulli equation.
   C. Measure maximal aortic valve cusp separation via the aortic valve long-axis view.
   D. Measure peak transaortic valve velocity using continuous-wave Doppler via the deep transgastric view.

2. A patient with aortic stenosis was found to have a 30 mm Hg aortic valve gradient via cardiac catheterization, but a 50 mm Hg gradient using continuous wave Doppler echocardiography via the deep transgastric view. What is the most likely explanation for this discrepancy?
   A. Doppler beam-aortic valve flow angle greater than 20 degrees
   B. Peak-to-peak cardiac catheter pressure gradient determination versus peak instantaneous pressure gradient determination via echo
   C. "Pin-hole" aortic stenosis
   D. Severe aortic regurgitation associated with aortic stenosis

3. The etiology of aortic insufficiency is best determined with
   A. color flow Doppler echocardiography.
   B. continuous wave Doppler echocardiography.
   C. pulsed wave Doppler echocardiography.
   D. two-dimensional echocardiography.

4. Which of the following would cause an aortic valve regurgitant velocity deceleration slope of 5 m/sec?
   A. Increased left ventricular compliance
   B. Mild aortic insufficiency
   C. Phenylephrine administration to a patient with a competent aortic valve
   D. Severe aortic insufficiency

# Assessment of the Tricuspid and Pulmonic Valves

*Rebecca A. Schroeder, Jonathan B. Mark, and Katherine A. Grichnik*

Evaluation of the right-sided cardiac valves with transesophageal echocardiography (TEE) is easily accomplished with two-dimensional imaging through several standard windows as well as color flow Doppler (CFD) and spectral Doppler analysis. The primary function of these valves is to regulate blood flow from the periphery to the pulmonary vascular bed and to maximize the efficiency of the right ventricle (RV). Although the valves are well seen with transthoracic echocardiographic (TTE) techniques, detailed TEE assessment can add additional information and is invaluable in situations unsuitable for TTE.

## STRUCTURE AND FUNCTION OF THE TRICUSPID VALVE

The tricuspid valve (TV) has several important characteristics that differentiate it from the other cardiac valves. It has three thin membranous leaflets that are not sup-

ported by a substantial fibrous annulus and are much less distinct, separated more by indentations in a continuous sheet of tissue rather than true commissures. The TV consists of large anterior and septal leaflets and a smaller posterior leaflet, each attached to papillary muscles by way of chordae tendinae and affixed to the annulus and a portion of the RV free wall (Fig. 16.1). The area of the TV, 7–9 cm², is significantly greater than that of any other valve (1).

The TV apparatus, while similar to that of the mitral valve, is more complex and variable. The anterior papillary muscle is the largest and arises from a linear band of cardiac muscle that runs perpendicular to the papillary muscle known as the moderator band. It attaches to the ventricular septum near the apex of the right ventricle and may be mistaken for an intracardiac mass (Fig. 16.2). The posterior papillary muscle is frequently small and at times even absent. A diminutive septal papillary muscle is also present (Fig. 16.1). An alternative nomenclature describes two papillary muscles: a right anterior muscle and a posterior muscle that may have multiple heads. The tricuspid

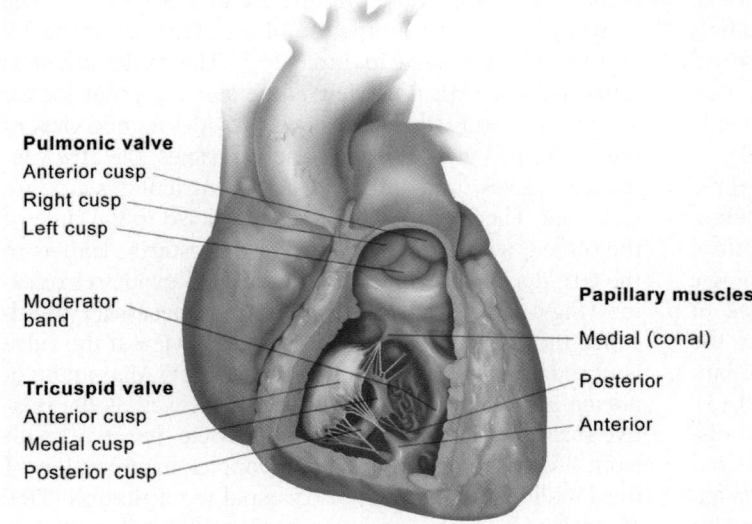

Pulmonic valve
Anterior cusp
Right cusp
Left cusp

Moderator band

Tricuspid valve
Anterior cusp
Medial cusp
Posterior cusp

Papillary muscles
Medial (conal)
Posterior
Anterior

**FIGURE 16.1.** Anatomic drawing of right ventricle with valves labeled, anterior view. (Reprinted with permission from Konstadt SN, Shernan S, Oka Y, eds. *Clinical Transesophageal Echocardiography: A Problem Oriented Approach*, 2nd ed. Philadelphia: Lippincott Williams & Wilkins.)

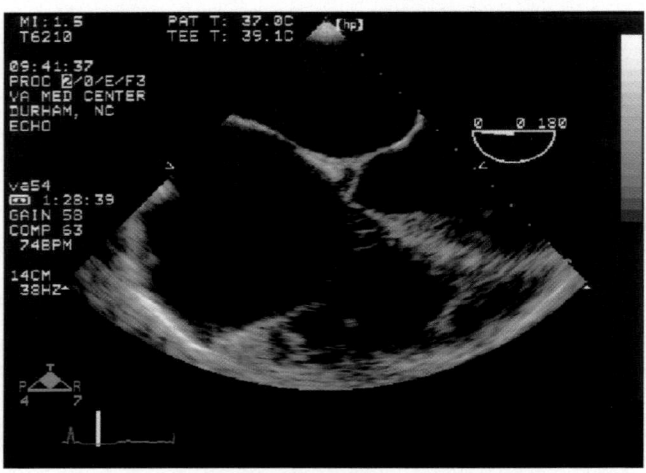

**FIGURE 16.2.** TEE of modified midesophageal four-chamber view showing moderator traversing the right ventricle near the apex. Note right atrial enlargement.

annulus lies in a slightly more apical position than the mitral annulus, with its inferior margin near the entrances of the inferior vena cava and coronary sinus into the right atrium. The contribution of tricuspid annular motion to RV function is quite important. Downward or apical movement of the annulus significantly augments RV stroke volume, even more than the analogous movement of the mitral annulus. With loss of annular motion, systolic shortening of the RV free wall decreases substantially, significantly diminishing effective right heart function (2).

## STRUCTURE AND FUNCTION OF THE PULMONIC VALVE

The pulmonic valve (PV) is most similar in structure and function to the aortic valve (AV). Due to its position on the right side, a lower pressure system, the pulmonic leaflets are somewhat thinner. The three PV leaflets are termed anterior, left, and right. The latter two are situated posterior to the anterior leaflet and may be more correctly termed the right posterior and left posterior (Fig. 16.1).

The valvular apparatus of the PV consists of the three cusps, their associated sinuses of Valsalva, and a sinotubular junction, similar to that of the AV. This structural similarity is a consequence of their common embryologic origin. Both semilunar valves develop from ridges of subendocardial tissue that form at the orifices of the aorta and the pulmonary trunk after partition of the bulbus cordis and the truncus arteriosus has occurred (3). The annulus of the PV is much more ill-defined and distensible than that of the AV because the pulmonary root attaches directly to RV muscle rather than to a fibrous annular ring. The geometric relationships between the valve annulus and sinotubular junction are similar on the right and left sides of the heart, resulting in a pulmonic sinotubular junction that is 10% to 15% smaller than the PV annulus diameter (4). The pulmonic valve area is similar to that of the AV, approximately 2 cm²/m². The anterior and right posterior PV leaflets and their associated sinuses of Valsalva are slightly larger than the left posterior (5). Other features common to both the PV and the AV are the *nodulus Arantii* (small fibrous nodules in the free margin of the cusp) and the *lunula* (thin half-moon-shaped areas along the free edge of each cusp that can have perforations not considered clinically important) (6).

## TRANSESOPHAGEAL ECHOCARDIOGRAPHIC EVALUATION OF THE TRICUSPID AND PULMONIC VALVES

### Two-Dimensional and Color Flow Doppler

A complete evaluation of the right-sided valves includes standard two-dimensional (2-D) views, CFD, and spectral Doppler examination of the right-sided chambers, the TV, the PV, and their supporting structures, the vena cavae, the hepatic veins, and the proximal main pulmonary artery (PA). TEE may prove less effective in visualizing the TV and PV compared to the MV and AV due to the anterior location of the right-sided valves. Examination of the TV may be especially difficult in the presence of a calcified or prosthetic mitral annulus, or thickened atrial septum. Furthermore, visualization of all three leaflets of the PV is difficult with either TTE or TEE.

The Society of Cardiovascular Anesthesiologists, in collaborative effort with the American Society of Echocardiography (SCA/ASE), has recently published TEE practice guidelines detailing standard imaging planes useful for evaluating the TV and the PV (7). The relevant views for examination of the right heart, the TV and the PV are listed in Table 16.1. The midesophageal four-chamber (ME 4-C) view is the starting point for assessing the right-sided valves and provides a good view of the TV. In this view, the atria and ventricles, the atrioventricular valves, and the atrial and ventricular septa are well seen. The TV septal leaflet is displayed to the right of the screen, with either the anterior or posterior leaflets to the left, depending on the degree of TEE probe retroflexion (Figs. 16.3A and 16.3B). It may be necessary to advance the probe slightly to optimize this view if the valve is obscured by a calcified or prosthetic AV. Anatomic abnormalities of the TV are easily seen, as well as the relative sizes of the right atrium and ventricle that may result from TV pathology. Color flow Doppler examination of the TV allows assessment of tricuspid regurgitation (TR). The valve should be interrogated throughout its superior-

▶ TABLE 16.1.   Suggested Views for Imaging Tricuspid and Pulmonic Valves

| View | Transducer Position (degrees) | Right-Sided Structures Imaged |
|---|---|---|
| Midesophageal four-chamber | 0–10 | RA, RV, TV, IAS, IVS |
| Midesophageal RV inflow-outflow | 60–90 | TV, RV, RVOT, PV |
| Midesophageal bicaval | 100–120 | RA, IAS, SVC, IVC |
| Modified midesophageal bicaval | 120–140 | RA, IAS, SVC, IVC, TV |
| Midesophageal aortic valve short axis | 30–60 | PV, main PA |
| Upper-esophageal aortic arch short axis | 90 | PA, PV, aortic arch |
| Transgastric TV short axis | 0–20 | TV (anterior, posterior, and septal leaflets) |
| Transgastric RV inflow (long axis) | 100–120 | RV, RA, TV, chordae, papillary muscles |
| Transgastric hepatic | 90–120 | Hepatic veins |
| Transgastric RV outflow | 70–90 | RVOT, PV |
| Deep transgastric RV outflow | 0 | RVOT, PV |

PA, pulmonary artery; PV, pulmonic valve; RA, right atrium; RV, right ventricle; TV, tricuspid valve; IAS, interatrial septum; IVS, interventricular septum; RVOT, right ventricular outflow tract; SVC, superior vena cava; IVC, inferior vena cava

to-inferior aspect and across its transverse dimension (0, 30, and 60 degrees) to completely map the TR jet and determine the severity of regurgitation. Spectral Doppler examination of the valve may be attempted in this imaging plane, but the angle of interception between the direction of flow and the ultrasound beam may preclude an accurate result. The PV is not visualized in the ME 4-C view.

At the same midesophageal level, advancement of the transducer multiplane angle to between 60 and 90 degrees will display the midesophageal RV inflow-outflow view. In this view, the posterior leaflet of the TV will appear to the left side of the screen display and the anterior leaflet to the right. In the far right field, the PV is visible, separating the proximal PA and right ventricular outflow

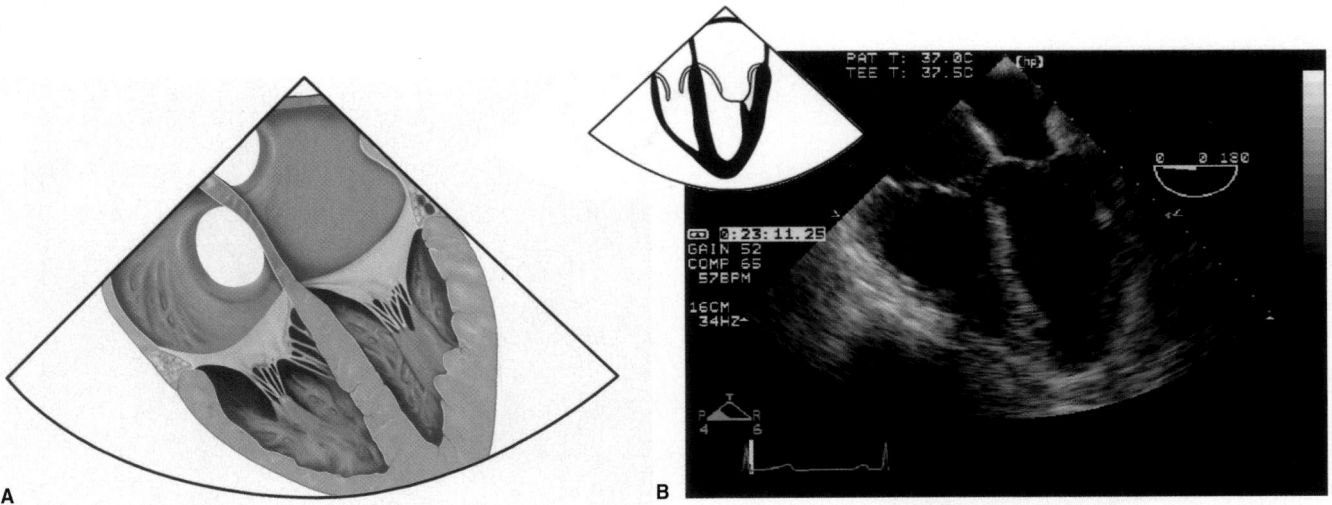

**FIGURE 16.3. A:** Anatomic drawing of the midesophageal four-chamber view. (Reprinted with permission from Konstadt SN, Shernan S, Oka Y, eds. *Clinical Transesophageal Echocardiography: A Problem Oriented Approach,* 2nd ed. Philadelphia: Lippincott Williams & Wilkins.) **B:** TEE of midesophageal four-chamber view with corresponding icon.

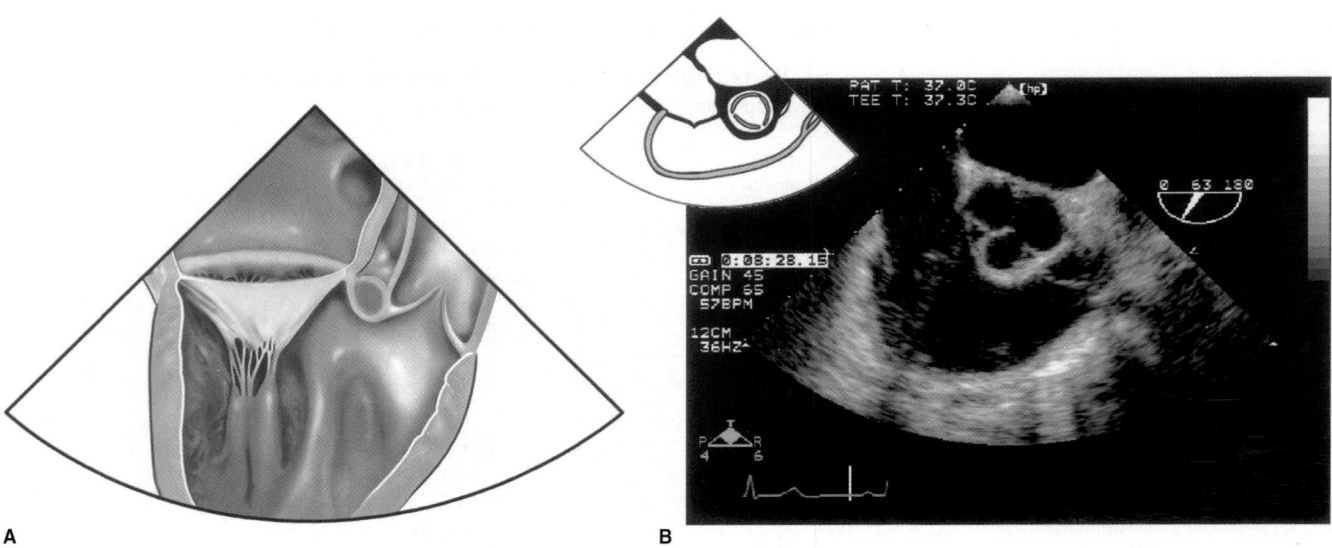

**FIGURE 16.4. A:** Anatomic drawing of right ventricular inflow-outflow view. (Reprinted with permission from Konstadt SN, Shernan S, Oka Y, eds. *Clinical Transesophageal Echocardiography: A Problem Oriented Approach,* 2nd ed. Philadelphia: Lippincott Williams & Wilkins, Figure 10.3.) **B:** TEE of right ventricular inflow-outflow view with corresponding icon.

tract (RVOT) (Figs. 16.4A and 16.4B). Rotation of the probe to the left (counterclockwise) may improve the image of the proximal main PA allowing evaluation of its first few centimeters for abnormalities. Of note, although the PV leaflets may not be clearly imaged in this view, CFD may still be used to detect pulmonic regurgitation (PR).

A third imaging plane for examining RV inflow can be acquired beginning with the midesophageal bicaval view (110–140 degrees of transducer rotation) (Figs. 16.5A and 16.5B) and applying slight counterclockwise probe rota-tion. The Eustachian valve is often well seen on the left side of the display. In this modified bicaval view, the basal RV and portions of the TV appear in the left far field and allow evaluation of TV inflow and regurgitation (Figs. 16.6A and 16.6B). In addition, the direction of blood flow and the ultrasound beam vector are closely aligned in this view, thereby allowing accurate spectral Doppler assessment of transvalvular flow. Pulsed wave Doppler (PW) analysis of TR peak jet velocity allows estimation of RV and PA systolic pressures (Fig. 16.6C). Also, the severity of

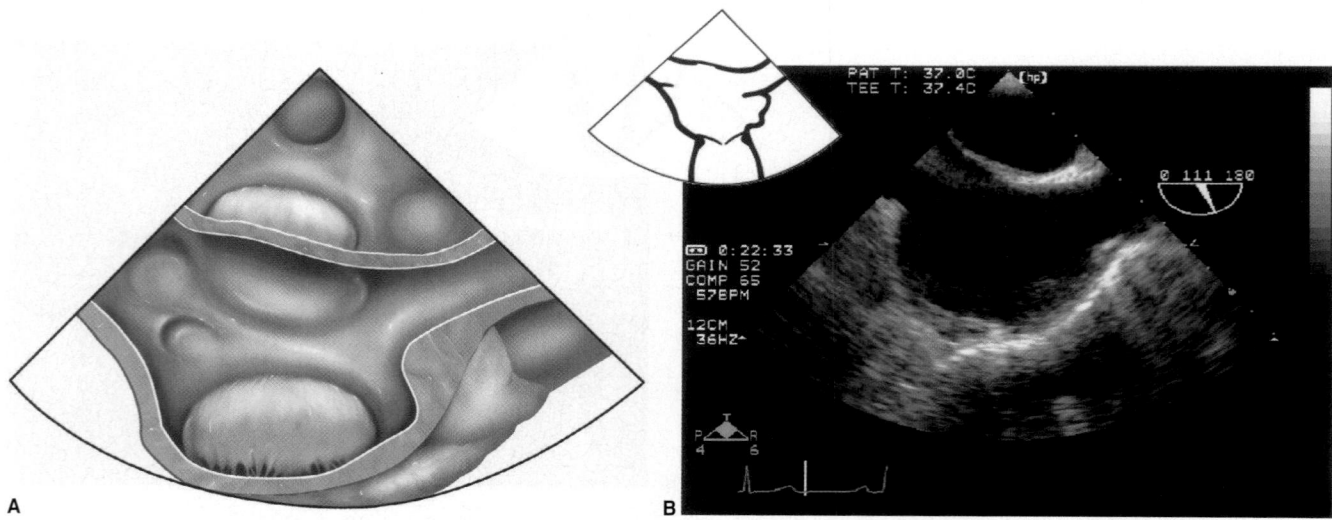

**FIGURE 16.5. A:** Anatomic drawing of bicaval view. (Reprinted with permission from Konstadt SN, Shernan S, Oka Y, eds. *Clinical Transesophageal Echocardiography: A Problem Oriented Approach,* 2nd ed. Philadelphia: Lippincott Williams & Wilkins.) **B:** TEE of bicaval view with corresponding icon.

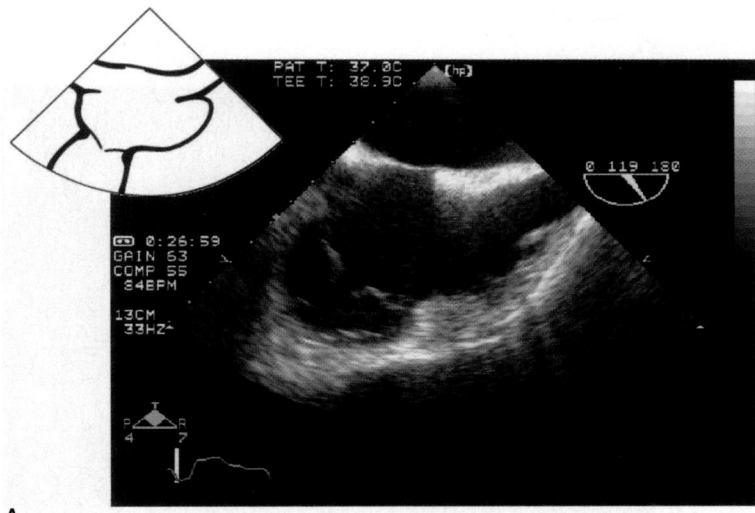

**FIGURE 16.6. A:** TEE of modified bicaval view with corresponding icon. **B:** Color Doppler of the tricuspid valve from the modified bicaval view. **C:** Spectral Doppler interrogation of the tricuspid valve.

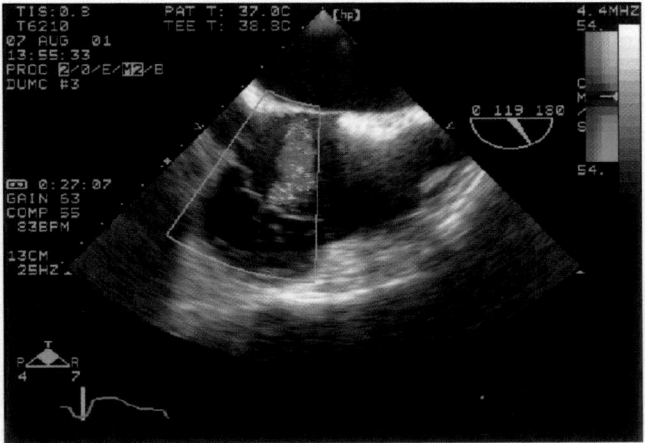

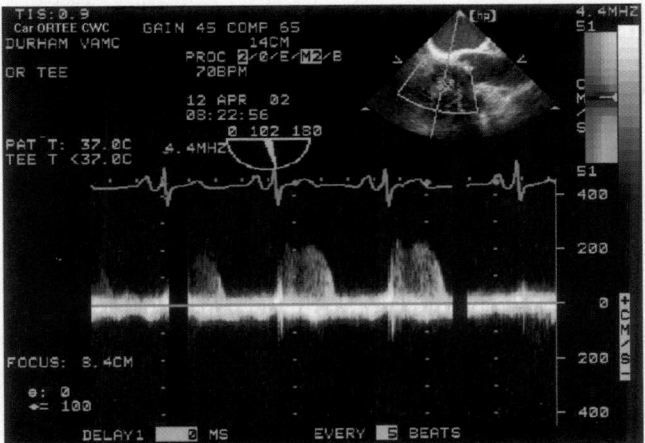

TV stenosis may be assessed using continuous wave (CW) Doppler techniques.

Imaging of the PV may be augmented with the midesophageal short-axis view of the AV (ME AV SAX). This view is developed at 30–60 degrees of transducer rotation, with the display showing the PV and the main PA to the right of the AV (Fig. 16.7A). In this scan plane, the right posterior pulmonic leaflet appears posteromedial and the anterior pulmonic leaflet appears more lateral on the display (Fig. 16.7B) (8). This is another excellent view in which to inspect the proximal pulmonary artery for pathology.

Also useful for PV imaging is the upper esophageal (UE) aortic arch short-axis view (Fig. 16.8A). In this window, the PA and the PV appear on the left side of the screen, well aligned in long axis with the ultrasound beam vector (Fig. 16.8B). Hence, it is one of the best views for assessing the severity of pulmonic stenosis (PS) and PR. Turning the probe slightly to the left (counterclockwise) and retroflexing may improve the view of the PV. This view provides the best longitudinal assessment of the main PA.

Transgastric (TG) views of the TV are useful, although slightly more difficult to obtain. A short axis of the RV is obtained by visualizing the short axis of the left ventricle and rotating the probe to the right (clockwise). By anteflexing the probe and withdrawing slightly, the three leaflets of the TV come into view, in a manner somewhat analogous to that of the short axis of the leaflets of the mitral valve (Fig. 16.9). The anterior leaflet appears in the left far field, the posterior in the near left, and the septal to the right of the display. The TG RV inflow view is also developed from the TG midpapillary, short-axis view of the left ventricle by turning the probe slightly rightward (clockwise), centering the RV on the display, and advancing the multiplane angle to between 100 and 120 degrees

*(text continues on page 225)*

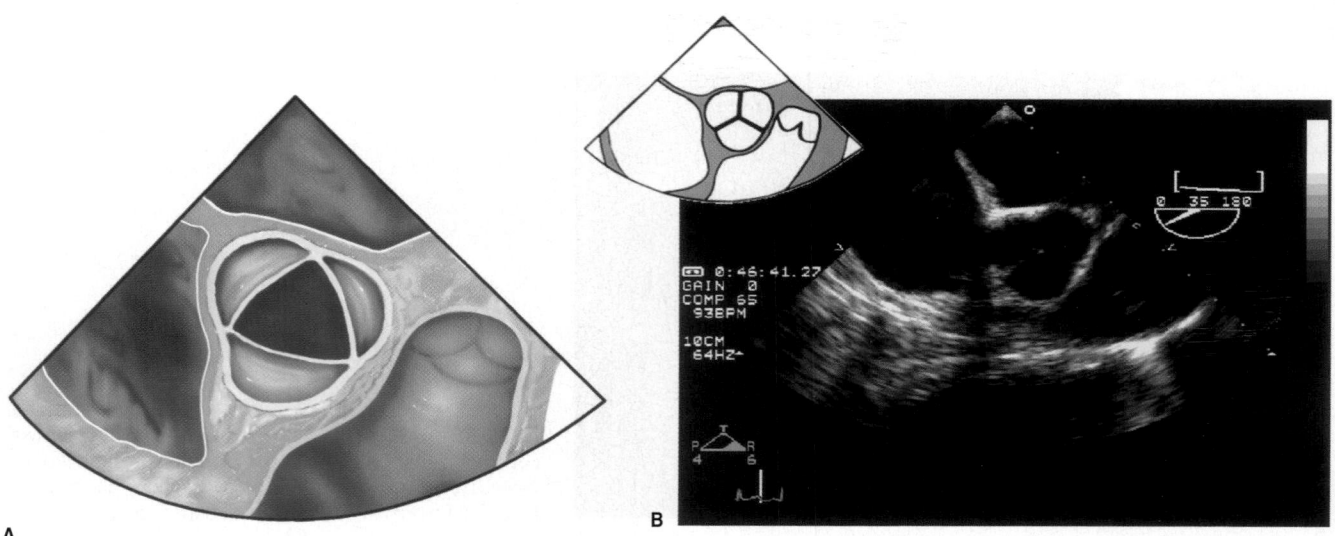

**FIGURE 16.7. A:** Anatomic drawing of midesophageal aortic valve short-axis view with right ventricular outflow tract seen. (Reprinted with permission from Konstadt SN, Shernan S, Oka Y, eds. *Clinical Transesophageal Echocardiography: A Problem Oriented Approach,* 2nd ed. Philadelphia: Lippincott Williams & Wilkins.) **B:** TEE of midesophageal aortic valve short axis with corresponding icon.

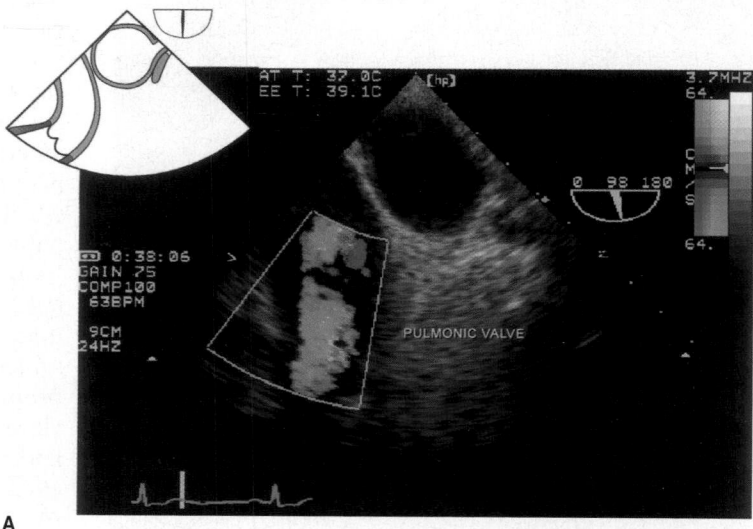

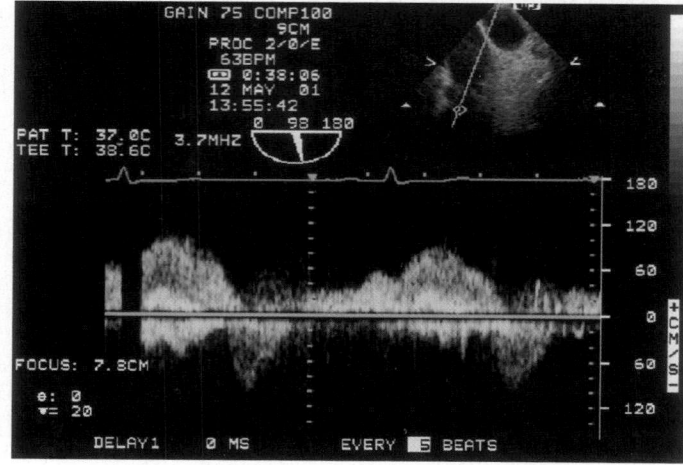

**FIGURE 16.8. A:** TEE of upper esophageal aortic arch short-axis view with color Doppler flow across the pulmonic valve. **B:** TEE of upper esophageal aortic arch short-axis view with spectral Doppler across the pulmonic valve demonstrating forward systolic flow and retrograde flow during diastole. (Reprinted with permission from Konstadt SN, Shernan S, Oka Y, eds. *Clinical Transesophageal Echocardiography: A Problem Oriented Approach,* 2nd ed. Philadelphia: Lippincott Williams & Wilkins.)

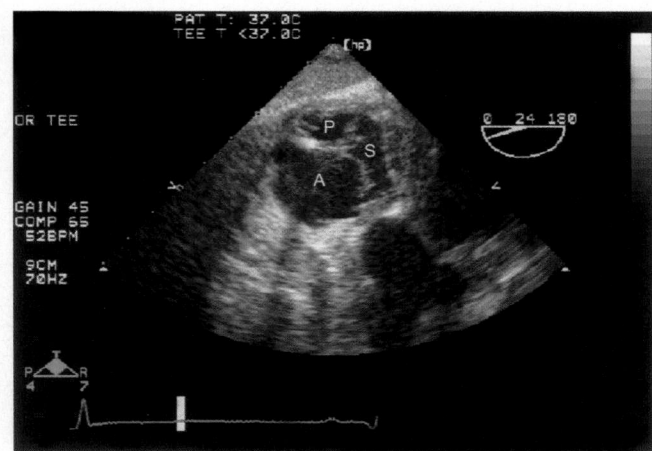

**FIGURE 16.9.** TEE of tricuspid valve short axis with leaflets labeled. (Reprinted with permission from Konstadt SN, Shernan S, Oka Y, eds. *Clinical Transesophageal Echocardiography: A Problem Oriented Approach,* 2nd ed. Philadelphia: Lippincott Williams & Wilkins.)

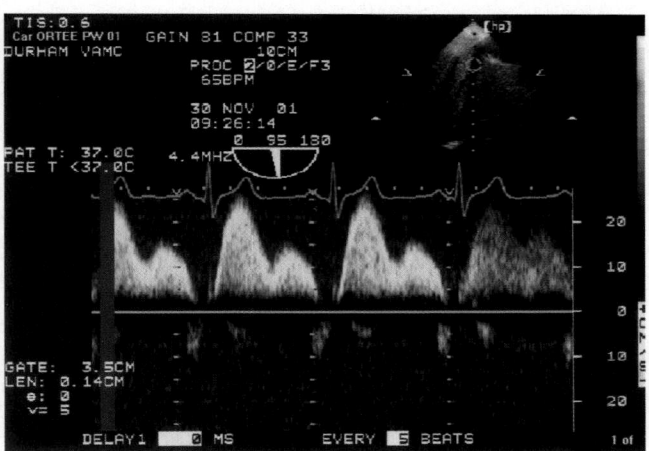

**FIGURE 16.11.** TEE of normal hepatic venous flow.

(Fig. 16.10). This scan plane provides the best view of the TV supporting structures, including the chordae tendinae and papillary muscles. The RV appears on the left, and the RA on the right of the display screen. From this scan plane, the TEE probe can be rotated further rightward (clockwise) to image the hepatic veins, most easily identified with CFD. Pulsed wave Doppler can then be used to evaluate hepatic flow patterns (Fig. 16.11). The PV and the RVOT can also be imaged from this probe location. From the TG RV inflow view at between 100 and 120 degrees, reducing the multiplane angle slowly toward zero and anteflexing brings the RVOT and the PV into view somewhere between 60 and 90 degrees (TG RV outflow view) (Fig. 16.12A) (7). At times, the aortic valve may appear just to the right of the PV, demonstrating the inti-

mate relationship between the two semilunar valves (Fig. 16.12B).

Finally, further advancing the TEE probe to the deep transgastric position at zero degrees, rightward (clockwise) probe rotation and anteflexion will reveal another view of the RVOT and the PV (Figs. 16.13A and B). It is important to evaluate the proximal main PA whenever visible, as abnormalities may reflect PV pathology, or be the cause of it.

An additional view, not technically part of TV and PV imaging, is a view of the short axis of the aorta and superior vena cava with the distal portion of the main PA seen to the right of the screen, and the proximal right PA appearing at the top of the screen in long axis. This view is developed from the aortic valve short-axis view by slow withdrawal of the TEE probe until these structures come into view. Often, a pulmonary artery catheter can be seen in both the SVC and the right main PA in this view. The left PA is usually obscured by the bronchial structures.

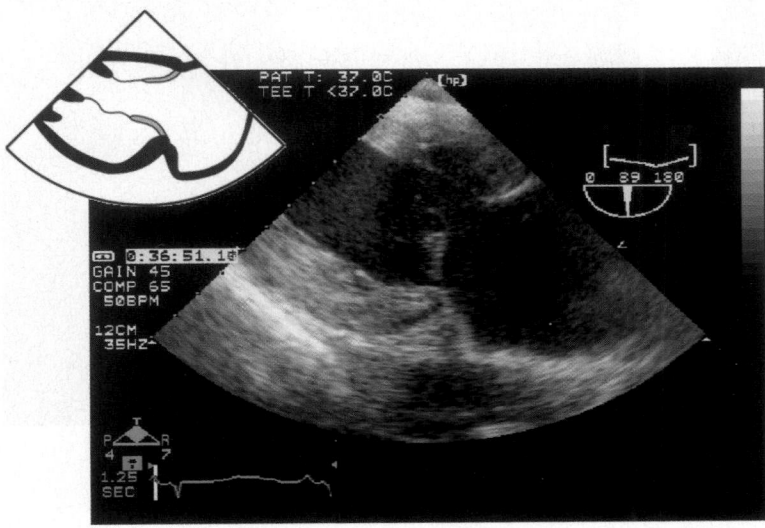

**FIGURE 16.10.** TEE of transgastric right ventricle view with corresponding icon.

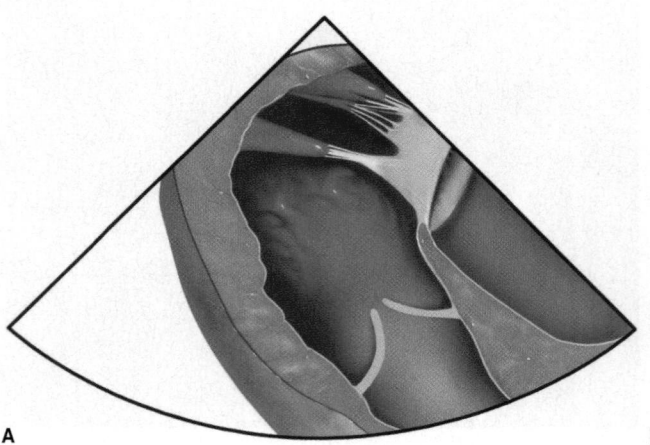
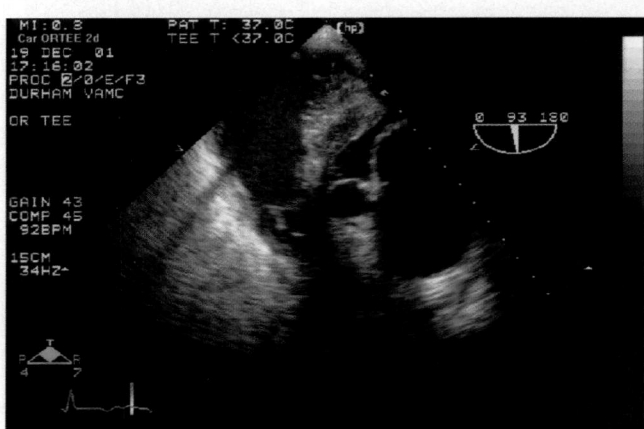

**FIGURE 16.12. A:** Anatomic drawing of transgastric right ventricular outflow view with pulmonic valve prominent. (Reprinted with permission from Konstadt SN, Shernan S, Oka Y, eds. *Clinical Transesophageal Echocardiography: A Problem Oriented Approach,* 2nd ed. Philadelphia: Lippincott Williams & Wilkins.) **B:** TEE of transgastric right ventricular outflow tract on the left and left ventricular outflow tract on the right. The aortic and pulmonic valves are clearly seen.

Any of the echocardiographic imaging artifacts may confound evaluation of the TV and the PV. Especially pertinent to imaging of the right-sided structures, however, are pacing wires and intracardiac catheters that may cause acoustic shadowing or be misinterpreted as intracardiac masses, clots, or vegetations (Fig. 16.14) (9).

## Spectral Doppler

Evaluation of flow through the TV and the PV is performed using spectral Doppler techniques. Analysis of tricuspid flow is optimally performed using the modified bicaval view, the ME RV inflow-outflow view, or the ME 4-C

view, depending on which view provides the most parallel alignment of flow with the ultrasound beam. The sample volume should be placed between the leaflet tips during diastole to assess diastolic filling patterns. Analogous to transmitral flow, characteristic early (E) wave and A (atrial) wave Doppler peaks correspond respectively to early ventricular filling and late diastolic filling from atrial contraction. From these recordings, E velocity, A velocity, E/A velocity ratio, and E-wave deceleration time may be measured or calculated. Typical pathologic patterns of diastolic dysfunction include impaired relaxation (E < A) and restriction (E ≫ A) of RV filling. It is important to note that tricuspid inflow patterns have lower ab-

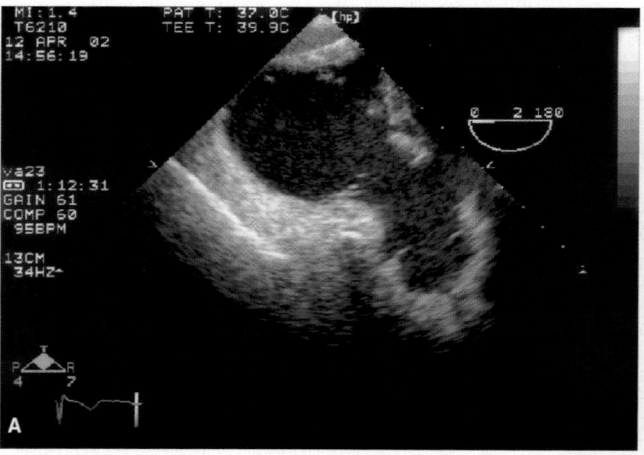
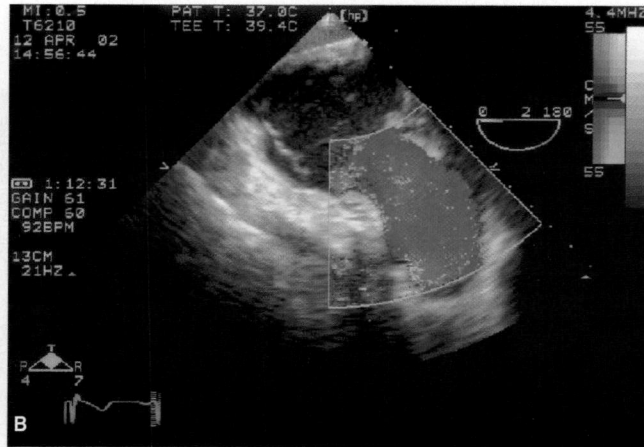

**FIGURE 16.13. A:** TEE of deep transgastric right ventricular outflow tract. **B:** TEE of deep transgastric right ventricular outflow view with color flow Doppler demonstrating transpulmonic flow.

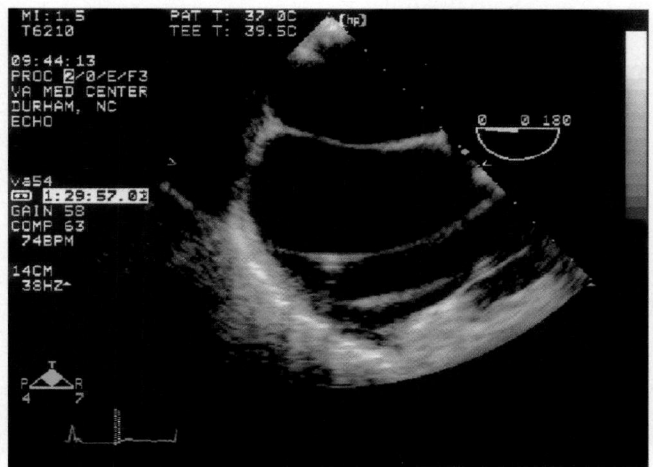

**FIGURE 16.14.** TEE focused on right atrium to demonstrate the pulmonary artery catheter echographic characteristics.

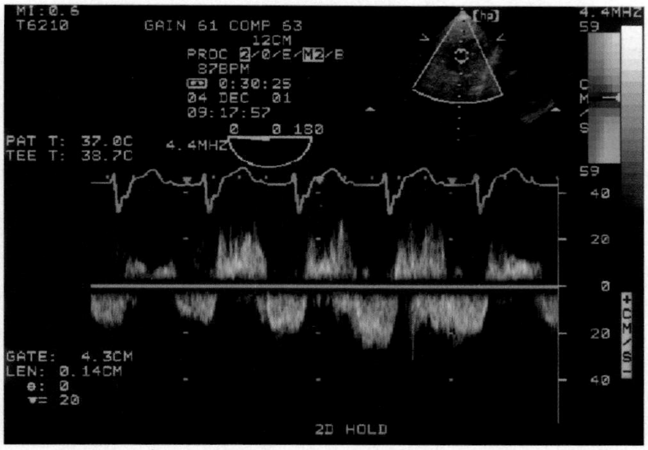

**FIGURE 16.15.** Spectral Doppler of hepatic venous flow in a patient with severe tricuspid regurgitation.

solute velocities than the corresponding mitral inflow velocities owing to the lower pressures generated by the RV and the larger cross-sectional area of the TV.

Useful information concerning TV and RV function may often be obtained by analysis of hepatic venous flow patterns. Normal venous flow in the hepatic veins is similar to pulmonary venous flow, with antegrade systolic (S) and diastolic (D) waves, and a retrograde atrial (A) wave resulting from atrial contraction (Fig. 16.11). At times, an additional small retrograde wave appears at end systole and is termed a *V-wave*. This additional retrograde wave likely results from tricuspid annular motion at end systole. When right atrial pressure is increased, the S-wave and the S/D ratio decrease while the A-wave increases. Severe TR eliminates the normal antegrade S-wave, and produces a reversed flow signal during systole (Fig. 16.15). In patients with atrial fibrillation no A-wave is seen in the hepatic venous or TV inflow patterns.

Spectral Doppler assessment of the TV may provide a great deal of pertinent hemodynamic information. As mentioned earlier, PA systolic pressure (PAS) may be estimated by measuring the peak velocity of the TR jet, using the simplified Bernoulli equation to estimate the transvalvular gradient and adding an estimate of RA pressure (Fig. 16.6C) (Table 16.2). In turn, RA pressure can be estimated by measuring respiratory variation in the size of the inferior vena cava in spontaneously breathing patients. If the diameter decreases by 50% or more during inspiration (sniffing), RA pressure is less than 10 mm Hg.

For accurate results, quantitative spectral Doppler measurements must be made carefully, assuring that the ultrasound beam is parallel to the flow vector. Misinterpretation may result from unintentional contamination of the Doppler signal from high velocity jets of mitral regurgitation or aortic stenosis that are difficult to differen-

tiate. The TR jet may be distinguished by identifying the low velocity antegrade diastolic flow signal that results from flow through the TV. Contrast enhancement of the TR jet with agitated saline injection may also help make the signal envelope more visible.

Spectral Doppler assessment of PV flow usually follows CFD qualitative assessment of PR and PS and is best accomplished in the UE aortic arch short axis or one of the two transgastric views of the RVOT and the PV (Figs. 16.8B, 16.12B, and 16.13A). Color flow Doppler is helpful to define the direction of flow and assist in alignment of the Doppler beam for PW and CW techniques. Because flow through the PV is roughly perpendicular to that through the AV, the two are rarely confused. Normal blood flow through the PV is directed in an

▶ **TABLE 16.2. Formulas Useful for Assessing the Tricuspid Valve, Pulmonic Valve, and Pulmonary Artery Blood Flow**

RVSP or PASP = 4 $V^2$ + CVP
  V = peak velocity of the tricuspid regurgitant jet

PADP = 4$V^2$ + RVDP or CVP
  V = late end-diastolic velocity of the pulmonary regurgitant jet

PAMP = 4$V^2$
  V = early peak velocity of the pulmonary regurgitant jet

SV = Area × VTI
  PV area × VTI$_{PV}$
  0.785 × (PV diameter)$^2$ × VTI$_{PV}$

*RV,* right ventricle; *RA,* right atrium; *PA,* pulmonary artery; *V,* velocity; *RVSP,* right ventricle systolic pressure; *PASP,* pulmonary artery systolic pressure; *CVP,* central venous pressure; *PADP,* pulmonary artery diastolic pressure; *RVDP,* right ventricle diastolic pressure; *SV,* stroke volume; *PAMP,* pulmonary artery mean pressure; *VTI,* velocity time integral; *PV,* pulmonic valve.

anterior-to-posterior and slightly right-to-left direction with respect to the patient. Peak flows through the PV range between 0.5 m/s and 1.0 m/s, with an average of 0.75 m/s (10). Pulmonic stenosis is diagnosed when the peak gradient between the RV and the PA reaches 25 mm Hg, which corresponds to a peak velocity of 2.5 m/s. Doppler flow patterns of regurgitant flow may also be used to estimate PA pressures. The early peak gradient derived from the PR jet can provide an approximate mean PA pressure (MPAP), and the late minimal gradient yields an estimate of PA diastolic pressure (PAD). Pulsed wave Doppler can be used to assess RV stroke volume as well as in calculation of regurgitant and shunt fractions (Table 16.2) (11).

## Tricuspid Regurgitation

Mild TR is extremely common in the normal population. It has an overall incidence of 65%, but may be seen in up to 93% of patients over 70 years of age (12). This "physiologic" TR, however, should have a high velocity, turbulent jet that appears small with CFD imaging. The most common causes of clinically significant TR are annular dilation and altered RV anatomy that result from pulmonary hypertension (PHTN), constrictive pericarditis, pulmonic stenosis, or RV ischemia or infarction. Moderate or severe TR may also develop in patients with rheumatic disease, endocarditis, carcinoid heart disease, tumors, endomyocardial fibrosis, or mechanical valve damage resulting from trauma or iatrogenic injury from cardiac catheters (Fig. 16.16) (13–15).

Assessing severity of TR and deciding whether it is physiologic or pathologic may be difficult. Normal TR jet velocity is 2.0–2.5 m/sec (16). Higher velocities may indicate PHTN or PS, both of which will increase the pressure gradient between the RA and the RV. Lower TR jet velocities accompany more severe degrees of regurgitation, and

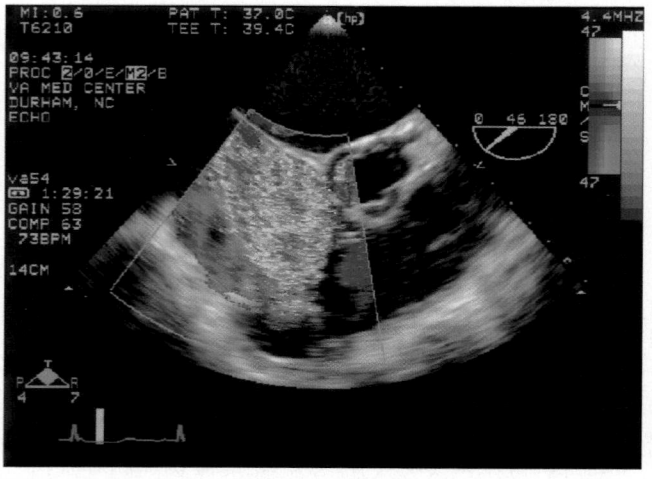

*FIGURE 16.16.* TEE showing severe tricuspid regurgitation.

▶ **TABLE 16.3.** **Tricuspid Regurgitation Classification Schemes**

| | RA Area (%) | TR Jet Area (cm²) | Length of TR Jet (cm) |
|---|---|---|---|
| Trace | | < 2 | < 1.5 |
| Mild | ≤ 20 | 2–4 | 1.5–3.0 |
| Moderate | 21–33 | 4–10 | 3.0–4.5 |
| Severe | ≥ 33 | > 10 | > 4.5 |

*TR, tricuspid regurgitation; RA, right atrium.*

a laminar regurgitant flow pattern indicates unrestricted, severe TR. There are several alternative methods used to evaluate TR, and these should be considered complementary. On 2-D examination, findings of RV volume overload suggest severe TR unless another etiology is identified. These signs include RV and RA enlargement, flattening of the ventricular septum, dilation of the tricuspid annulus, SVC, IVC, or hepatic veins, and leftward displacement of the atrial septum. The proximal isovelocity surface area (PISA) method of determining the size of the regurgitant orifice may be useful in quantifying the degree of TR, although this is rarely done (17). In addition, PWD analysis of the hepatic veins may show reversed flow during systole (Fig. 16.15). As always, clinical correlation is extremely important because chronic valvular disease can increase RA compliance and obviate many of these findings.

Several CFD grading systems for TR have been reported in the literature (Table 16.3). The first focuses on the longitudinal extension of the jet into the RA and the other two focus on estimation of the CFD regurgitant jet area. All three systems classify TR into three or four grades that roughly correspond to trace or trivial, mild, moderate, and severe regurgitation (18–20). Although these results correlate well with angiographic data, it is important to remember that all of these methods are semiquantitative at best, and subject to technical and physiologic factors that affect jet length and area.

## Pulmonic Regurgitation

Color flow Doppler analysis is used to map the extent of the PR jet into the RVOT. Trace and mild degrees of PR, of minimal clinical significance, are diagnosed when the PR jet is less than one centimeter in length and only appears in late diastole (Fig. 16.17). Pathologic PR is defined as a pandiastolic jet of greater dimension. However, PR is considered clinically significant only when the jet extends more than two centimeters into the RVOT or reaches within one centimeter of the TV, regurgitant flow is holodiastolic, and PWD velocity is greater than 1.5 m/sec (21,22). Most PR jets are central, although a prolapsed or restricted pulmonic leaflet may result in an eccentric signal. The appearance of turbulent flow alone to identify

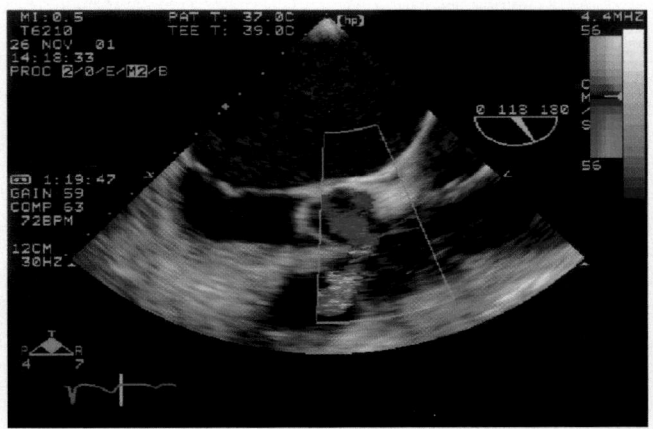

**FIGURE 16.17.** TEE of aortic valve short-axis view demonstrating moderate pulmonic valve insufficiency.

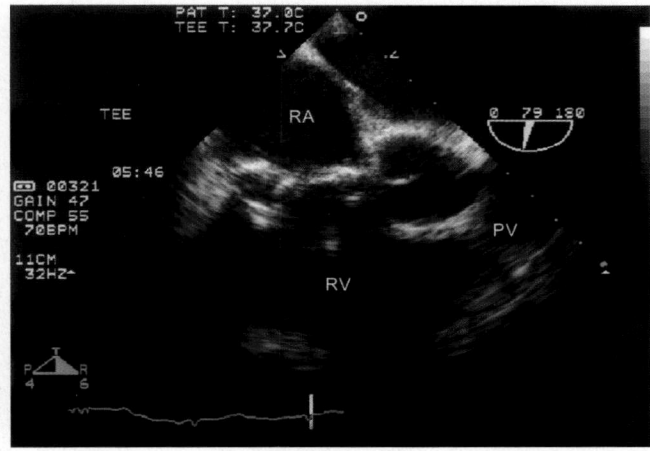

**FIGURE 16.18.** TEE demonstrating severe tricuspid stenosis.

the jet as pathologic is unreliable, owing to the small pressure gradient between the PA and the RV. Furthermore, PR jet velocity may vary greatly with respiration. Hence, accurate and meaningful measurements of flow velocity must include averaging over several cardiac cycles. In the setting of tachycardia, color M-mode of the RVOT may be useful (23).

## Tricuspid Stenosis

Tricuspid stenosis (TS) is most commonly of rheumatic etiology, and in these cases, the mitral valve is invariably involved. Other causes of tricuspid stenosis (TS) include congenital anomalies, endocarditis, methysergide toxicity, carcinoid heart disease, and endomyocardial fibrosis. Characteristic findings on 2-D examination include doming of the leaflets during diastole, thickening of the leaflets—especially at their tips, restricted leaflet motion, and commissural fusion (Fig. 16.18). Doppler evaluation of TV inflow will show increased peak velocities (E waves > 1.5 m/sec) (24,25). Of note, when TS results from carcinoid syndrome, the leaflets appear more fixed and retracted and do not display the typical doming seen in rheumatic TS.

## Pulmonic Stenosis

Similarly to TS, pulmonic stenosis (PS) is characterized by leaflet doming due to commissural fusion, leaflet thickening, and restricted systolic motion. Other relevant echocardiographic findings that may confirm the clinical significance of stenosis include poststenotic dilatation of the main PA and its primary branches. Interestingly, the left PA will often be more dilated than the right (21,25). Hypertrophy of the RV, flattening of the ventricular septum producing a characteristic D-shaped left ventricle,

RA enlargement, and moderate-to-severe TR all suggest RV pressure overload. In this setting, a search for coexisting congenital anomalies is important.

The peak pressure gradient across the PV indicates PS severity. Gradients less than 25–30 mm Hg are considered mild. Twenty-five to approximately 50–65 mm Hg reflects moderate stenosis; greater than this level is considered severe (21). Other descriptions in the literature have defined severe PS as a transvalvular pressure gradient that exceeds 80 mm Hg or a RV systolic pressure of greater than 100 mm Hg (5). Indications for intervention, such as balloon valvuloplasty, surgical repair or valve replacement, are determined by symptoms, including exertional dyspnea, angina, and syncope, or objective evidence of severe PS by echocardiography or catheterization. Stenotic lesions should be easily visible with CFD mapping of the PV and proximal PA. They will appear as highly turbulent lesions with marked aliasing of the color signal.

## CONGENITAL DISEASES OF THE TRICUSPID AND PULMONIC VALVES

### Ebstein's Anomaly

Ebstein's anomaly of the TV is an isolated congenital malformation in which the leaflets are displaced downward toward the RV apex with the posterior, septal, and a portion of the anterior leaflets originating from the RV wall rather than the tricuspid annulus (Fig. 16.19A). Frequently, the chordae tendinae are missing altogether and the leaflets are significantly redundant. The valve itself is usually incompetent with an orifice area much smaller than normal. The portion of the RV remaining above the valve is thin and severely hypokinetic and often termed "atrialized" (Fig. 16.19B) (6,17). Clinical presentation is highly variable

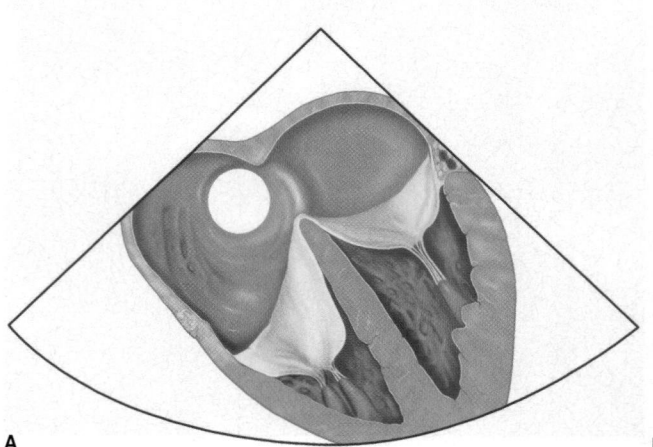
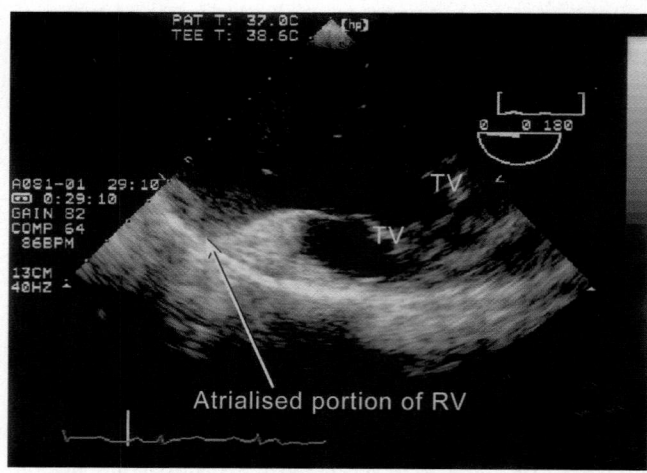

**FIGURE 16.19.** **A:** Anatomic drawing of valvular abnormalities in Ebstein's anomaly. **B:** TEE of patient with Ebstein's Anomaly showing apical displacement of the tricuspid valve leaflet and the thin, "atrialized" portion of the affected right ventricular wall. (Reprinted with permission from Konstadt SN, Shernan S, Oka Y, eds. *Clinical Transesophageal Echocardiography: A Problem Oriented Approach,* 2nd ed. Philadelphia: Lippincott Williams & Wilkins.)

and dependent on the degree of apical displacement of the valve and distortion of RV anatomy and function. Generally, greater degrees of valvular displacement and smaller portions of residual normal RV cavity result in more severe symptoms and a worse prognosis. If accompanied by an atrial septal defect (ASD), these patients may present with cyanosis as very young children (3).

## Tricuspid Atresia

In rare cases, tricuspid atresia may present in a young adult. In this condition, there is no normal flow through the tricuspid annulus, and the only egress from the RA is via the foramen ovale or an ASD. Pulmonary flow only occurs through a patent ductus arteriosus (PDA) or a ventricular septal defect (VSD) and is highly dependent on the size of these connections. Most patients present in the first months of life with cyanosis, but if the sizes of these left-to-right shunts are optimal, they may remain clinically stable for many years. In such cases, they will present with congestive failure of the left ventricle due to long standing volume overload (3).

## Congenital Anomalies of the Pulmonic Valve

In the adult population, isolated RVOT obstruction is usually part of a complex congenital anomaly and is rare. The obstruction may be above, below, or at the level of the PV, with the most common abnormality being valvular PS. Supravalvular stenosis may involve narrowing of the PA, especially near the bifurcation of the main PA into its primary branches. This often coexists with other con-

genital abnormalities, such as an ASD, a VSD, or a PDA. Subvalvular stenosis may involve infundibular or subinfundibular hypertrophy that may accompany PS and is often paired with a VSD. More unusual causes of RVOT obstruction include a right sinus of Valsalva aneurysm that encroaches on the RVOT, postoperative mediastinal hematomas, primary sarcomas, pericardial cysts, and iatrogenic obstruction following repair of complex cardiac abnormalities (8,26). Complete RVOT obstruction presenting in the neonate, such as critical PS or pulmonary atresia, cannot occur as an isolated lesion (27). These patients require a shunt or other corrective procedure to palliate or repair the condition.

Congenital PS usually presents in newborns although it may remain undiagnosed into adulthood. Valvular PS accounts for 10%–12% of all congenital heart disease in the United States (5). Other causes of valvular PS include commissural fusion, leaflet dysplasia, congenital bicuspid valve, rubella embryopathy, rheumatic heart disease, and senile calcification. TEE is particularly useful for monitoring these patients during balloon valvuloplasty (28). Laminar flow on CFD and a reduced peak gradient by CWD are evidence of a successful procedure.

## ACQUIRED DISEASES OF THE TRICUSPID AND PULMONIC VALVES

### Endocarditis

Echocardiography is the diagnostic test of choice for detecting vegetations and perivalvular abscesses. Furthermore, TEE is often preferable to TTE due to the low negative predictive value of the latter (29,30). Vegetations vary in appearance from flat, small sessile lesions involving a single leaflet to large bulky, friable, echodense, or oscillating masses that may obstruct flow through the valve, especially the TV (Fig. 16.20). The most common organisms are *Staphylococcus aureus* and *Pseudomonas aeruginosa*. Tricuspid endocarditis is less common than mitral or AV endocarditis, except amongst intravenous drug abusers (29,31,32). When using TEE to evaluate endocarditis, it is especially important to evaluate the chordae tendinae and other supporting structures. This is due to the fact that these may be involved in the infectious/inflammatory process (29,31,32). Even more rare than tricuspid disease is isolated endocarditis of the PV. The PV is the least commonly involved valve in cases of multivalvular endocarditis, and usually occurs in patients with other predisposing factors, including a structurally abnormal PV, immunosuppression and intravenous drug abuse (33,34). Indwelling intravascular catheters or wires are another risk factor for right-sided endocarditis (35,36). Complications of tricuspid and pulmonic endocarditis include septic pulmonary emboli or infarcts and RV failure.

## Carcinoid Heart Disease

Carcinoid heart disease occurs almost exclusively in patients with primary carcinoid tumors that do not drain into the portal circulation, such as ovarian tumors, or in patients with hepatic metastases of their primary gastrointestinal carcinoid tumors. Vasoactive amines, such as serotonin and bradykinin, are chronically secreted and lead to fibrosis of the "downstream" endocardial surfaces of the right heart valves, including the ventricular surface of the TV and the pulmonary arterial surface of the PV. Right-sided cardiac valve involvement occurs in 50% of patients with carcinoid tumors and can be rapidly progressive (37). Of note, TEE has been used to monitor somatostatin analog therapy in patients with carcinoid heart disease (38). Cardiac surgical intervention is indicated only for severe valvular disease because carcinoid is a slow-growing tumor and carcinoid-related death more commonly results from cardiac failure than primary tumor growth.

Echocardiographically, carcinoid heart disease produces short, thickened valvular leaflets that eventually become immobile retracted cusps that often remain fixed in the open position and result in severe TR (Fig. 16.21). As mentioned above, the typical doming seen in rheumatic valvular stenosis differs from this pattern of tricuspid disease. Interestingly, the PV may develop PS with or without PR. Acute palliation of PS in advanced disease has resulted in a hypercontractile RV with residual subvalvular dynamic RVOT obstruction, parenthetically called the "suicide RV" (39).

## Rheumatic Disease

The right heart valves can be affected by rheumatic heart disease in several ways. Rheumatic mitral stenosis and/or regurgitation may produce pulmonary hypertension, resulting in RV enlargement, tricuspid annular dilatation, and functional TR. Acute rheumatic carditis is characterized by myocardial and valve leaflet edema and leukocyte infiltration with eventual erosion of the leaflet tips. Ultimately, bead-like vegetations develop along the line of valve coaptation. Capillaries invade the vegetations during the healing phase, and fibrous nodules develop, frequently involving scarring and fusion of the chordae tendinae. The free edges of the cusps become shortened at the site of healed vegetations, and chordal contracture and commissural fusion develop. Tricuspid regurgitation rather than TS usually results. Despite the volume overload of the RV, it maintains its normal size in most cases

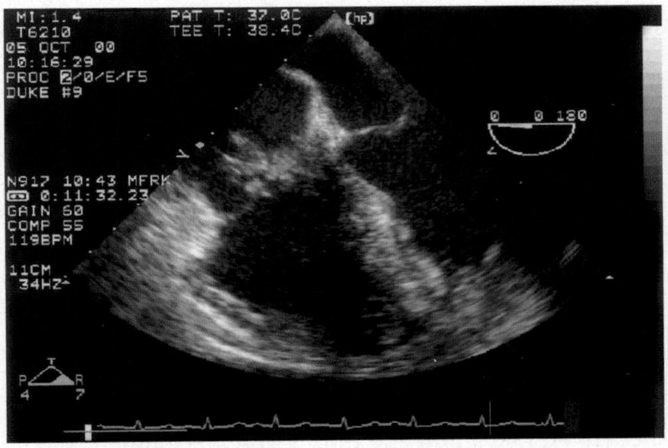

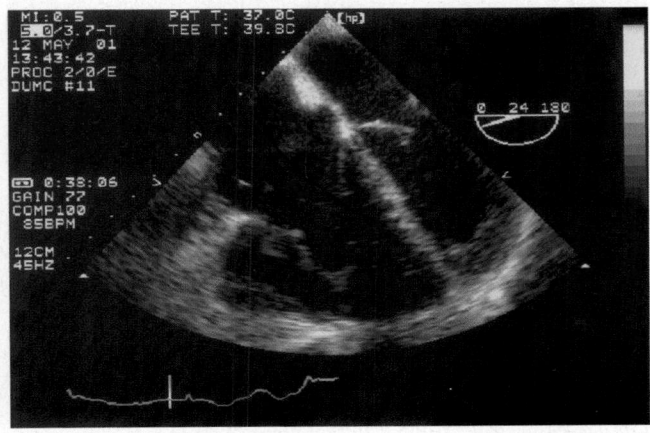

**FIGURE 16.20.** TEE of tricuspid valve vegetation in a patient with endocarditis.

**FIGURE 16.21.** TEE of tricuspid valve in a patient with carcinoid heart disease.

(17). There have been a few case reports of PV involvement, including one involving all four cardiac valves, but these are relatively rare (40).

## Other Pathologic Conditions

Functional regurgitation of the TV is probably the most common form of TV dysfunction. It results from annular dilatation, most frequently caused by chronic RV ischemia, cardiomyopathy, or volume overload (13–15). Similarly, PHTN of any etiology can cause abnormalities of TV or PV structure and function. Enlargement of the annular ring causes relative displacement of the valve supporting structures, leading to faulty coaptation of the leaflet tips and central regurgitation. Multiple regurgitant jets are commonly seen. M-mode echocardiography may be useful in differentiating severe PHTN from valvular PR with PS as causes for right-sided valvular dysfunction or RV failure. Early systolic closure of the PV and an absent A wave occur with severe PHTN but not with valvular PS (41). Also, PWD measurements across the PV may show rapid early PA systolic flow acceleration and midsystolic slowing.

Tricuspid valve prolapse (TVP) is relatively rare and is remarkable if found in isolation. Prolapse of both atrioventricular valves usually coexists and is most commonly seen in patients with floppy valve syndromes, such as Ehlers-Danlos syndrome, Marfan's syndrome, Ebstein's anomaly, or septum secundum ASD. The anterior and septal leaflets are most commonly involved and the resulting regurgitant jet is often eccentric. Diagnosis of TVP is made by identifying displacement of valve leaflet tissue

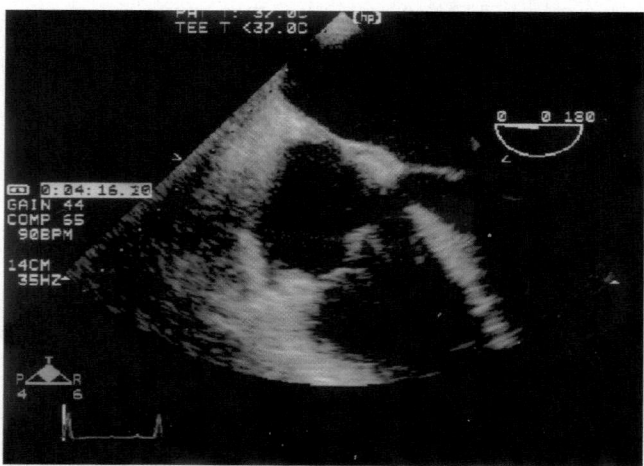

**FIGURE 16.22.** TEE showing tricuspid valve prolapse. (Reprinted with permission from Konstadt SN, Shernan S, Oka Y, eds. *Clinical Transesophageal Echocardiography: A Problem Oriented Approach,* 2nd ed. Philadelphia: Lippincott Williams & Wilkins.)

beyond the annular plane into the right atrium (Fig. 16.22) (17).

Heart disease associated with systemic lupus erythematosus (SLE) is characterized by myocarditis, pericarditis, and endocarditis and may involve the TV. Valvular leaflets may become thickened and stenotic after multiple episodes of lupus endocarditis. Lesions are small, berry-shaped excrescences that appear on both the atrial and ventricular sides of the leaflets as well as on the chordae tendinea, papillary muscles, and the mural endocardium. Characteristic vegetations located on both sides of the TV differentiate SLE disease from rheumatic disease in which the lesions only appear on the atrial side of the TV (42).

Papillary fibroelastomas are rare benign cardiac tumors that usually involve the AV, although they may occasionally appear on the PV or the TV. These masses appear as small, mobile, echodense masses attached to the valve leaflets and may be difficult to differentiate from clot or endocarditis. In general, however, these tumors do not cause TR or PR (43,44).

Twenty percent of all cardiac myxomas occur in the right heart with three-quarters of these originating from the RA. These can affect the TV by prolapsing into the TV annulus and causing dynamic RV inflow obstruction (24). Renal cell carcinomas may encroach upon the RA and TV and cause obstructive symptoms. Traumatic disruption of the TV causing acute TR, while uncommon, may result from deceleration injuries and produce endothelial tears, hemorrhage into valvular cusps, or rupture of the papillary muscles (45). Either the TV or the PV may be injured iatrogenically during catheterization procedures, although routine PA catheter placement has not been shown to cause significant right-sided valvular dysfunction (46).

## The Ross Procedure

In certain cases, the PV may be used to replace another valve, most often the AV, in a procedure known as the PV autograft or the Ross procedure. The PV has been used to replace the mitral valve as well, although this is much more uncommon (47,48). Prior to the surgical procedure, TEE is used to meticulously rule out any congenital abnormality of the PV. The diameter of the PV annulus should be 10%–15% larger than the diameter of its adjacent sinotubular junction, as measured by TEE. Similar measurements are made of the AV. The sizes of the donor and the recipient site should be within 2 mm of each other to avoid distortion of either the transplanted valve annulus or the recipient site sinotubular junction. Size mismatch may result in autograft valvular incompetence. In a recent series of 81 patients undergoing this procedure, David et al. reported the range of AV annulus diameters to be 19–35 mm and the PV annulus diameters to be 19–27 mm (4). In cases with size discrepancies, the aortic annulus diameter can be reduced by plication of the annulus and annuloplasty to achieve geometric parity (49). After the harvested PV has been placed in the aortic position, a PV cadaveric homograft is implanted. TEE measurements are also used for appropriate sizing of this graft. Postoperatively, suture lines of the PV homograft are visible with TEE, but there are few other visible echocardiographic changes. However, PR or even PS may develop postoperatively, necessitating balloon valvuloplasty, PA stenting, or even PV replacement with a bioprosthetic or mechanical valve (50).

Of note, there is also a variation of the Ross procedure, known as the "semilunar valve switch" in which the native AV is repaired and reimplanted into the pulmonic position rather than using a cadaveric homograft for the PV. However, in one report, neopulmonic valvular stenosis was present in 54% of patients undergoing this procedure (51).

## KEY POINTS

- Clinically significant TR is most commonly secondary to left-sided pathology or pulmonary hypertension.
- The best views in which to evaluate the TV are the midesophageal four-chamber view, the RV inflow-outflow view, the midesophageal modified bicaval view, and the transgastric RV inflow view.
- Most useful views for evaluation of the PV are the midesophageal RV inflow-outflow view, the transgastric RV inflow view, and the upper esophageal aortic arch short-axis view.
- Differentiation of physiologic from pathologic TR involves examination of hepatic venous flow patterns, peak TR jet velocity, relative right ventricular and atrial size, and pattern on color flow Doppler analysis.
- The TV apparatus is distinguished by its poorly defined annulus, its large anterior and small septal and posterior leaflets, and its corresponding large anterior, small septal, and posterior papillary muscles.
- The PV apparatus differs from the AV structure by its ill-defined annulus and slightly smaller size.
- Estimations of PA systolic pressure are best made from the midesophageal modified bicaval view. By this approach, the direction of TR flow is best aligned with the direction of the ultrasound beam.
- In the Ross procedure, the PV is transplanted to the AV position and replaced with a homograft.

- The ascending main pulmonary artery can be well visualized in multiple views, allowing anatomic assessment of this structure. The right main pulmonary artery can also be visualized and assessed for pathology, as well as positioning of a pulmonary artery catheter.

## REFERENCES

1. Hauck A, Freeman D, Ackermann D, et al. Surgical pathology of the tricuspid valve: a study of 363 cases spanning 25 years. Mayo Clin Proc 1988;63:851–63.
2. Isaaz K, Munoz L, Lee E, et al. Quantitation by Doppler echo of the motion of the cardiac base in normal man. [Abstract] Circulation 1989;80(suppl II):169.
3. Gersony WM, Pruitt A, Riemenschneider TA. The cardiovascular system. In: Behrman RE, Vaughan III VC, Nelson WE, eds. Nelson textbook of pediatrics. 13th ed. Philadelphia: W.B. Saunders Company, 1987;943–1032.
4. David TE, Omran A, Webb G, Rakowski H, Armstrong S, Sun A. Geometric mismatch of the aortic and pulmonary root causes aortic insufficiency after the Ross Procedure. J Thorac Cardiovasc Surg 1996;112:1231–9.
5. Brickner ME, Hillis LD, Lange RA. Congenital heart disease in adults: First of two parts. N Engl J Med 2000;342:256–63.
6. Netter FH. Heart. 1st ed. Summitt, NH: CIBA-GEIGY Corporation, 1981:6–10.
7. Shanewise JS, Cheung AT, Aronson S, et al. ASE/SCA guidelines for performing a comprehensive intraoperative multiplane transesophageal examination: recommendations of the American Society of Echocardiography Council for Intraoperative Echocardiography and the Society of Cardiovascular Anesthesiologists Task Force for Certification in Perioperative Transesophageal Echocardiography. Anesth Analg 1999; 89:870–84.
8. Shively BK. Transesophageal echocardiographic (TEE) evaluation of the aortic valve, left ventricular outflow tract, and pulmonic valve. Cardiol Clin 2000;18(4):711–29.
9. Song MH, Usui M, Usui A, Watanabe T, Ueda Y. Giant vegetation mimicking cardiac tumor in tricuspid valve endocarditis after catheter ablation. Jpn J Thorac Cardiovasc Surg 2001; 49(4):255–7.
10. "Doppler flow imaging." In: Feigenbaum H, ed. Echocardiography, 5th ed. Philadelphia: Lippincott, Williams & Wilkins, 1993:101–5.
11. Maslow A, Comunale ME, Haering JM, Watkins J. Pulsed wave Doppler measurement of cardiac output from the right ventricular outflow tract. Anesth Analg 1996;83(3):466–71.
12. Klein AL, Burstow DJ, Tajik AJ, et al. Age-related prevalence of valvular regurgitation in normal subjects: a comprehensive color flow examination of 118 volunteers. J Am Soc Echocardiogr 1990;3:54–63.
13. Braunwald E. Valvular heart disease. In: Braunwald E, Zipes DP, Licina MG, eds. A textbook of cardiovascular medicine. 6th ed. Philadelphia: W.B. Saunders Company, 2001: 1643–722.
14. Cohen SR, Sell JE, McIntosh CL, Clark RE. Tricuspid regurgitation in patients with acquired, chronic, pure mitral regurgitation. I. Prevalence, diagnosis, and comparison of preoperative clinical and hemodynamic features in patients with and without tricuspid regurgitation. J Thorac Cardiovasc Surg 1987;94(4):481–7.
15. Morrison DA, Ovitt T, Hammermeister KE. Functional tricuspid regurgitation and right ventricular dysfunction in pulmonary hypertension. Am J Cardiol 1988;62(1):108–12.
16. "Cardiac diseases due to systemic illness." In: Oh JK, Seward JB, Tajik AJ, eds. The echo manual. 1st ed. Boston: Little, Brown and Company, 1994:169–79.

17. Zaroff JG, Picard MH. Transesophageal echocardiographic (TEE) evaluation of the mitral and tricuspid valves. Cardiol Clin 2000;18(4):731–50.

18. Miyatake K, Okamoto M, Kinoshita N, et al. Evaluation of tricuspid regurgitation by pulsed Doppler and two dimensional echocardiography. Circ 1982;66:777–84.

19. Rivera JM, Vandervoort PM, Morris E, et al. Visual assessment of valvular regurgitation: comparison with quantitative Doppler measurements. J Am Soc Echocardiogr 1994;7:480–7.

20. Nagueh SF. Assessment of valvular regurgitation with Doppler echocardiography. Cardiol Clin 1998;16:405–19.

21. Kerut EK, McIlwain EF, Plotkin GD. Handbook of echo-Doppler interpretation. 1st ed. Armonk, NY: Futura Publishing Company, 1996:123–37.

22. Reynolds T, ed. The echocardiographer's pocket reference. 2nd ed. Phoenix: Arizona Heart Institute, 2000:410–11.

23. Frasco PE, deBruijn NP. Valvular heart disease. In Estafanous EF, Barash PG, Reeves JG, eds. Cardiac anesthesia: principles and clinical practice. 2nd ed. Philadelphia: Lippincott, Williams and Wilkins, 2001;557–84.

24. Otto CM. Echocardiographic evaluation of ventricular diastolic filling and function. In: Textbook of clinical echocardiography. 2nd ed. Philadelphia: W.B. Saunders Company, 2000;329–59.

25. Rumbak MJ, Scott M, Walsh FW. Left hilar mass in a 62–year-old man: severe pulmonary valve stenosis with a poststenotic aneurysm. South Med J 1996;89(8):824–5.

26. Liau CS, Chu IT, Ho FM. Unruptured congenital aneurysm of the sinus of Valsalva presenting with pulmonic stenosis. Cath Cardiovasc Interv 1999;46:210–3.

27. Vargas-Barron J, Espinol-Zavaleta N, Rijlaarsdam M, Keirns C. Tetralogy of Fallot with absent pulmonic valve and total anomalous pulmonary venous connection. J Am Soc Echocardiogr 1999;12:160–3.

28. Tumbarello R, Bini RM, Sanna A. Omniplane transesophageal echocardiography: an improvement in the monitoring of percutaneous pulmonary valvulolasty. G Ital Cardiol 1997;27:168–72.

29. Ryan EW, Bolger AF. Transesophageal echocardiography (TEE) in the evaluation of infective endocarditis. Cardiol Clin 2000;18(4):773–87.

30. Birmingham GD, Rahko PS, Ballantyne F 3rd. Improved detection of infective endocarditis with transesophageal echocardiography. Am Heart J 1992;123(3):774–81.

31. San Roman JA, Vilacosta I, Zamorano JL, Almeria C, Sanchez-Harguindey L. Transesophageal echocardiography in right-sided endocarditis. J Am Coll Cardiol 1993;21(5):1226–30.

32. Clifford CP, Eykyn SJ, Oakley CM. Staphylococcal tricuspid valve endocarditis in patients with structurally normal hearts and no evidence of narcotic abuse. QJM 1994;87(12):755–7.

33. Schaefer A, Meyer GP, Waldow A, Weiss T, Hausmann D, Drexler H. Images in cardiovascular medicine: pulmonic valve endocarditis. Circulation 2001;103:E53–E54.

34. Akram M, Khan IA. Isolated pulmonic valve endocarditis caused by group B streptococcus-a case report and literature review. Angiology 2001;52:211–5.

35. Kamaraju S, Nelson K, Williams DN, Ayenew W, Modi KS. Staphylococcus lugdunnsis pulmonary valve endocarditis in a patient on chronic hemodialysis. Am J Neph 1999;19:605–8.

36. Hearn CJ, Smedira NG. Pulmonic valve endocarditis after orthotopic liver transplantation. Liver Transpl Surg 1999;5:456–7.

37. Moyssakis IE, Rallidis LS, Guida GF, et al. Incidence and evolution of carcinoid syndrome in the heart. J Heart Valve Dis 1997;6:625–30.

38. Denney WD, Kemp WE, Anthony LB, Oates JA, Byrd BF. Echocardiographic and biochemical evaluation of the development and progression of carcinoid heart disease. J Am Coll Cardiol 1998;32:1017–22.

39. Congenital heart disease. (Accessed September 8, 2004, at http://www.rchc,rush.edu/congenital_heart_disease.htm.)

40. Kumar N, Rasheed K, Gallo R, Al-Halees Z, Duran CM. Rheumatic involvement of all four heart valves—preoperative echocardiographic diagnosis and successful surgical management. Eur J Cardiothorac Surg 1995;9(12):713–4.

41. Echocardiography-pulmonic stenosis. (Accessed September 8, 2004, at http://www.umdnj.edu/~shindler/ps.html.)

42. Roldan CA, Shively BK, Crawford MH. An echocardiographic study of valvular heart disease associated systemic lupus erythematosus. N Engl J Med 1996;335(19):1424–30.

43. Saad RS, Galvis CO, Bshara W, Liddicoat J, Dabbs DJ. Pulmonary valve papillary fibroelastoma. Arch Path Lab Med 2001;125:933–4.

44. Wolfe JT 3rd, Finck SJ, Safford RE, Persellin ST. Tricuspid valve papillary fibroelastoma: echocardiographic characterization. Ann Thorac Surg 1991;51(1):116–8.

45. Leszek P, Zielinski T, Rozanski J, Klisiewicz A, Korewicki J. Traumatic tricuspid valve insufficiency: a case report. J Heart Valve Dis 2001;10(4):545–7.

46. Sherman SV, Wall MH, Kennedy DJ, et al. Do pulmonary artery catheters cause or increase tricuspid or pulmonic regurgitation? Anesth Analg 2001;92:1117–22.

47. Kouchoukos NT, Davila-Roman VG, Spray TL, Murphy SF, Perrillo JB. Replacement of the aortic root with a pulmonary autograft in children and young adults with aortic-valve disease. N Engl J Med 1994;330:1–6.

48. Kabbani SS, Ross DN, Jamil H, Hannoud A, et al. Mitral valve replacement with a pulmonary autograft: initial experience. J Heart Valve Dis 1999;8:359–67.

49. Azari DM, DiNardo JA. The role of transesophageal echocardiography during the Ross Procedure. J Cardio thorac Vasc Anesth 1995;9:558–61.

50. Hokken RB, Bogers AJ, Taams MA, et al. Does the pulmonary autograft in the aortic position in adults increase in diameter? An echographic study. J Thorac Cardiovasc Surg 1997;113:667–74.

51. Roughneen PT, DeLeon SY, Eidem BW, et al. Semilunar valve switch procedure: autotransplantation of the native aortic valve to the pulmonary position in the Ross procedure. Ann Thorac Surg 1999;67:745–50.

## QUESTIONS

Pick the false statement in each of the numbered items below.

**1.** The pulmonic valve
   A. is well seen in the deep transgastric RV outflow view.
   B. is embryologically derived from the same structure as the aortic valve.
   C. is replaced with a mechanical valve as part of the Ross procedure.
   D. may have *nodulus arantii*.

**2.** Tricuspid regurgitation
   A. is always pathologic.
   B. may be used to assess intracardiac pressures.
   C. is graded by color flow jet extension into the right atrium.
   D. is graded by reversal of hepatic venous flow.
   E. is unrelated to the velocity of the regurgitant jet.

**3.** Carcinoid heart disease
   A. is characterized by right-sided cardiac valvular lesions.

B. may be monitored by TEE for regression of disease with medical therapy.

C. is an uncommon cause of death in patients with carcinoid syndrome.

D. results in fixed immobile valves characterized by regurgitation and stenosis.

E. tends to occur on the ventricular surface of the TV and the arterial surface of the PV.

4. Stenotic right-sided cardiac valves
   A. are characterized by leaflet doming for all disease processes.

B. may be assessed by the velocity of the regurgitant jet.

C. are commonly associated with rheumatic heart disease.

D. are suggested by right atrial enlargement.

E. may involve commissural leaflet fusion.

## Chapter 17

# Assessment of the Thoracic Aorta

*Steven Konstadt*

This chapter will cover three main topics. First, it will describe the echocardiographic approach to the examination of the aorta. The anatomic proximity of the esophagus and aorta makes it possible for an echocardiographer to interrogate nearly the entire thoracic aorta with the exception of the distal ascending and proximal arch portions. Then it will define the normal anatomy of the aorta, and finally it will discuss the pathologic conditions of the thoracic aorta.

The three pathologic conditions to be addressed are aortic dissection, aortic aneurysm, and aortic atherosclerosis. Acute dissection of the ascending aorta is a true medical emergency, often necessitating immediate surgical repair. The key to instituting appropriate therapy in acute dissection of the ascending aorta, therefore, is an accurate and rapid diagnosis and anatomical assessment of the aorta. Aortic aneurysm is the most common diagnosis of patients having elective surgery of the aorta. Though there is no universally accepted definition of an aneurysm, it is well accepted that aneurysms are dangerous and need to be treated. Neurologic dysfunction after cardiopulmonary bypass remains a major source of the morbidity and mortality associated with cardiac surgical procedures. Because atheroembolic phenomena are a predominant cause of adverse neurological outcomes in this patient population, atheromatous disease of the thoracic aorta is a significant risk factor for neurologic injury after cardiopulmonary bypass. Echocardiography may help to identify the patients at risk, and may provide risk reduction strategies.

## ECHOCARDIOGRAPHIC APPROACH (TEE VIEWS, EPIAORTIC SCANNING)

In the pre- and postoperative periods, the thoracic aorta can be interrogated by transesophageal echocardiography. Additionally, in some patients, transthoracic images may be obtainable. In the intraoperative period after ster-

notomy, the thoracic aorta can be interrogated by both transesophageal and epiaortic techniques.

Transthoracic images of the ascending aorta may be obtained from the sternal notch by directing the probe towards the aortic valve using a standard transthoracic probe (Fig. 17.1). One limitation of this approach is the footprint of the probe and the size of the sternal notch window. Another problem with this approach is the relatively poor image quality compared to the other echocardiographic imaging options.

The Society of Cardiovascular Anesthesiologists and the American Society of Echocardiography have defined six views to interrogate the thoracic aorta by transesophageal echocardiography. However, it must be realized that these views are not single images to obtain, but rather *six imaging planes* to be used to evaluate the aorta. In most of the views, the probe must be manipulated to obtain multiple images in that orientation. The six imaging planes are

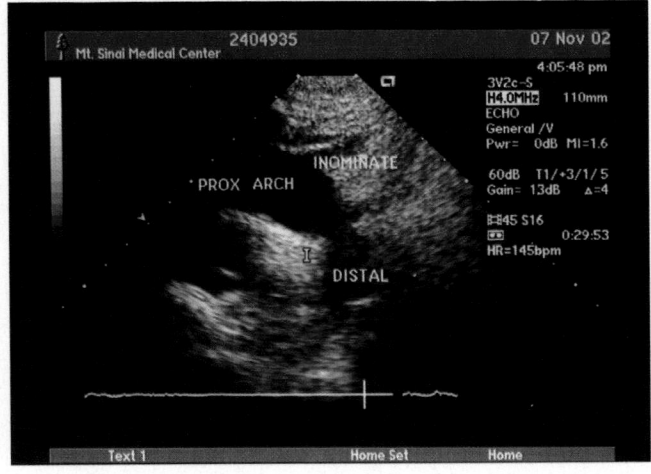

**FIGURE 17.1.** Transthoracic long-axis image of the ascending aorta.

1. Midesophageal (ME) ascending aorta SAX (short axis)
2. ME ascending aorta LAX (long axis)
3. Upper esophageal (UE) aorta arch
4. UE aorta arch LAX
5. Descending aorta SAX
6. Descending aorta LAX

The ME ascending aorta SAX view is obtained in the 0-degree imaging plane with the probe at approximately 25 cm from the lips (Fig. 17.2). Frequently, anteflexion of the tip is needed to improve probe contact and therefore image quality. Though this view is called a midesophageal view, it is obtained closer to the lips than the "ME" views of the mitral valve, and therefore could be considered a UE view. In this view, a cross section of the ascending view of the aorta is obtained. This view is useful for qualitatively assessing the aortic anatomy and measuring the overall diameter of the aorta and the wall thickness. It is also useful for the assessment of the superior vena cava and the detection of pericardial fluid. Visualization of the main pulmonary artery and right pulmonary artery allows verification of proper pulmonary artery catheter placement.

The ME ascending LAX view is obtained by rotating the imaging plane to between 90 and 110 degrees (Fig. 17.3). This view is useful for defining the wall thickness and tissue characteristics, aortic contour, aortic dimensions, and blood flow patterns in the ascending aorta. With respect to wall dimensions, this view is very useful to determine the relative diameter of the ascending aorta along its course. Unfortunately, because of the interposition of the airway between the esophagus and aorta only about 80% of the ascending aorta is visualized and in some patients more than 40% of the ascending aorta is not seen (1). In this view, though flow is not completely parallel with the Doppler beam, it is still possible to inter-

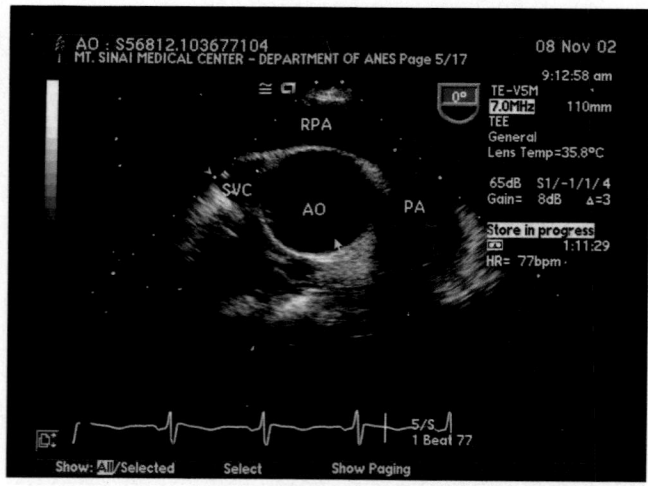

**FIGURE 17.2.** Midesophageal (ME) ascending short-axis view (SAX). *RPA,* right pulmonary artery; *SVC,* superior vena cava; *PA,* pulmonary artery; *AO,* ascending aorta.

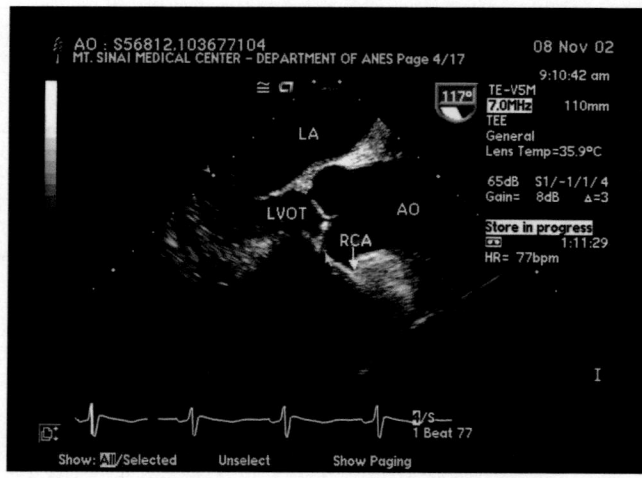

**FIGURE 17.3.** ME ascending aorta long-axis view (LAX). *LA,* left atrium; *LVOT,* left ventricular outflow tract; *RCA,* right coronary artery; *AO,* aorta.

rogate ascending flow. Aortic flow patterns are very important to differentiate abnormal pathology from imaging artifacts.

After imaging the ascending aorta, it is usually easiest to image the descending aorta. The descending aorta is located by starting in the ME four-chamber view and rotating the shaft of the echo probe 180 degrees. Once the descending aorta is visualized, adjust the depth setting to center the aorta in the image. At this point, it is also important to set the probe at the highest imaging frequency to obtain the best resolution. Insert the probe to the level of the diaphragm where the image of the descending aorta disappears. Then slowly withdraw the probe while keeping the image centered with slight rotational adjustments. The entire descending aorta can be interrogated in this fashion. These short-axis views are useful to define the wall thickness and tissue characteristics, aortic dimensions, and aortic flow patterns (Fig. 17.4). It is also possible to detect left-sided pleural effusions and atelectasis in these views. The aorta should imaged in the same fashion in the 90-degree imaging plane to obtain long-axis views of the descending aorta (Fig. 17.5). The long-axis views are most useful for defining the presence of branch vessels and the spatial relationship of the short-axis findings. Flow patterns are also very useful in these images.

The aortic arch is most easily located at the end of the interrogation of the descending aorta as the probe is being withdrawn. At the arch in the 0-degree imaging plane, the short-axis view of the aorta will transition to a long-axis view—the UE aortic arch LAX view (Fig. 17.6). To optimize visualization of the arch, it is often necessary to rotate the shaft of the probe in a clockwise direction. It may also be helpful to manipulate the degree of flexion in

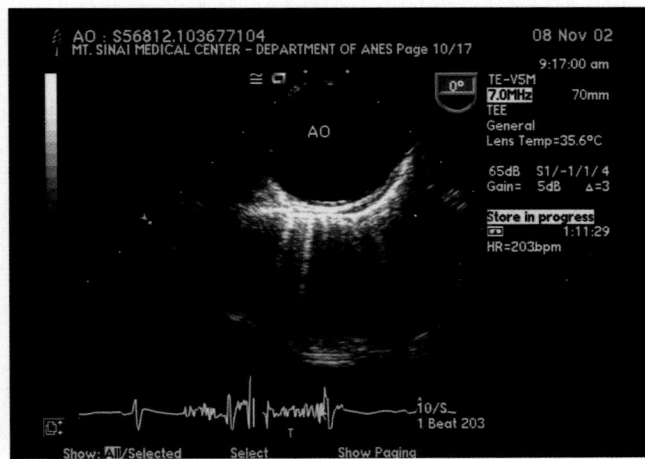

**FIGURE 17.4.** Descending aorta SAX.

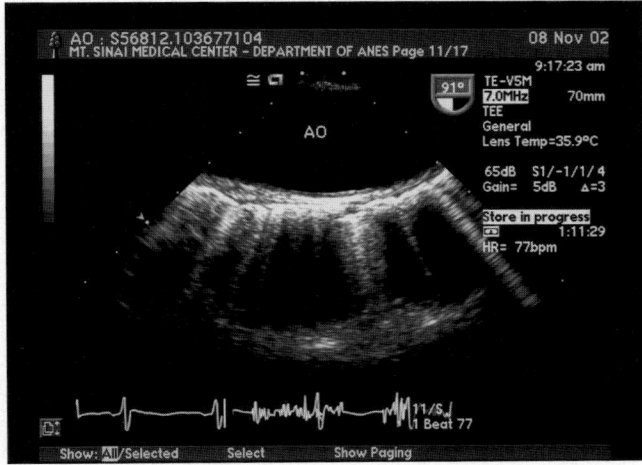

**FIGURE 17.5.** Descending aorta LAX.

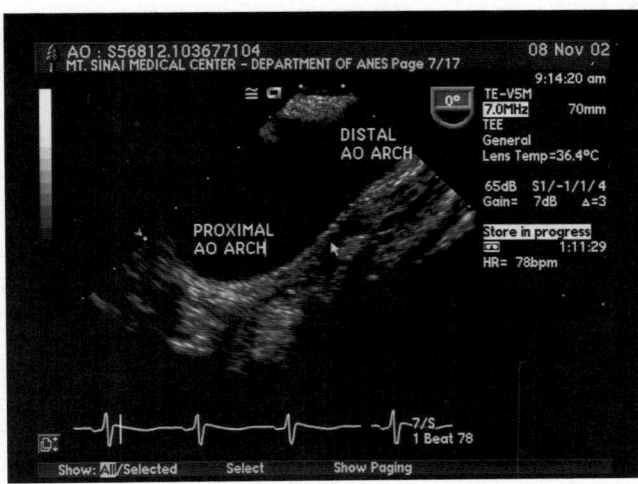

**FIGURE 17.6.** Upper esophageal (UE) LAX.

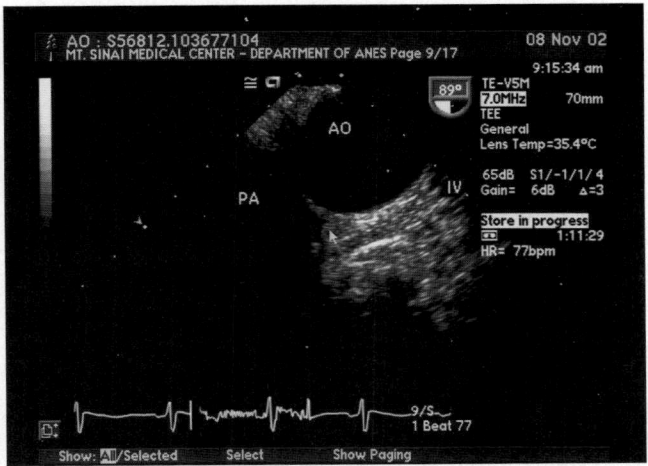

**FIGURE 17.7.** UE aorta arch SAX. *AO,* aorta; *PA,* pulmonary artery; *IV,* innominate vein.

the tip. The LAX view is useful for defining the aortic dimensions, wall contour, and branch vessels. The innominate vein is often seen in this view. After the visualization in the long axis is complete, to obtain the short-axis views of the arch, it is necessary to rotate the imaging plane to 90 degrees (Fig. 17.7). Starting at distal arch, multiple short-axis views of the arch and branch vessels can be obtained by clockwise rotation of the shaft of the probe. At the proximal portion of the arch the main pulmonary artery and left pulmonary may be visualized. In both the LAX and SAX views it is important to consider the wall thickness and tissue characteristics, aortic dimensions, and blood flow patterns. Even using all of these views, it is still not possible to image the entire thoracic aorta. In addition to the blind spot in the distal ascending aorta created by the airway, there are limited LAX and SAX scan planes of the ascending aorta. Additionally, the aorta is subject to many types of artifacts. To overcome these problems during surgical procedures with a sternotomy, it is possible to image the entire ascending aorta by epiaortic echocardiography. Epiaortic scanning can be performed with either sector or linear probes. The sector probes have a smaller footprint and are easier to move within the chest, but have poorer lateral resolution. On the other hand, linear probes have a larger footprint but offer better lateral resolution. In rare circumstances, it may be desirable to place a probe under the arch and this can be accomplished with a transesophageal probe. All of these probes must be sterilely wrapped. Other than the theoretical possibility of introducing contamination and the necessary 5 to 10 minutes for the examination, there are no known complications of epiaortic scanning. However, there are several important imaging considerations.

First, the depth and zoom settings should be optimized to maximize the aortic size. Second, it is necessary to cre-

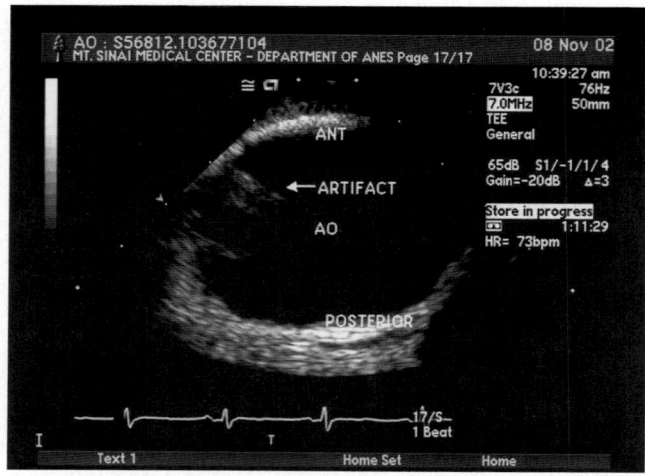

**FIGURE 17.8.** Epiaortic SAX view. *ANT,* anterior; *AO,* aorta. Note the hazy density on the left side of the image. This is a typical artifact seen in the aorta.

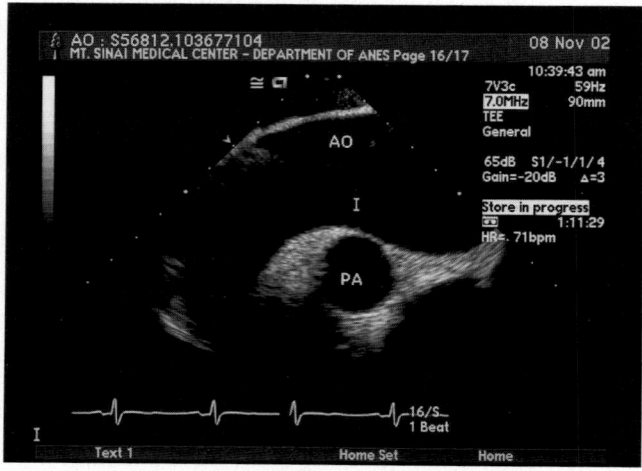

**FIGURE 17.9.** Epiaortic LAX. *AO,* aorta; *PA,* pulmonary artery.

ate a standoff from the aorta to the probe to visualize the anterior wall of the aorta. This can be accomplished with gel or water. The aorta is best interrogated in both the long- and short-axis imaging planes (Figs. 17.8 and 17.9).

## STRUCTURES (NORMAL ANATOMY)

The aorta is the largest artery of the body with a normal diameter of up to 3.5 cm. It contains a considerable amount of elastic tissue and smooth muscle in its wall to prevent disruption. The aortic wall is composed of three layers: intima, media, and adventitia. The intimal surface is a thinly lined layer with a confluent monolayer of flattened endothelial cells resting on a thin basal lamina. The endothelium regulates vasomotor tone, plays an intimate role in the coagulation cascade, and mediates inflammatory and immunologic responses. The media consists of smooth muscle cells enmeshed in a matrix of connective tissue components (collagen, elastin, and occasional fibroblasts) arranged in a laminated and intertwined fashion in a spiral pattern (2). This layer accounts for up to 80% of the aortic wall thickness and provides mechanical and structural support to the aorta along with vascular tone (3).

The adventitia is a looser layer of tissue containing collagen, lymphatics, and the vasa vasorum. It is responsible for providing nutrients to the aortic wall.

The aorta begins at the aortic valve and is divided into four parts:

1. Ascending aorta
2. Transverse aortic arch
3. Descending thoracic aorta
4. Abdominal aorta

The ascending aorta arises from the left ventricle posterior to the right ventricular infundibulum and the pulmonary valve. It courses superiorly and slightly rightward. The proximal portion of the aorta is comprised of the sinuses of Valsalva. These three sinuses bulge outward to allow full excursion of the aortic leaflets during ventricular systole and to accommodate the retrograde flow during diastole. The middle third of the ascending aorta is to the right of the main pulmonary artery, anterior to the right pulmonary artery, and anteromedial to the superior vena cava. The distal third of the ascending aorta courses superiorly, and runs posteriorly and leftward at the level of the aortic arch. This part of the aorta lies anterior to the trachea and the right mainstem bronchus, superior to the pulmonary artery, and posterior to the innominate vein.

The aortic arch gives rise to three branches from its superior aspect:

1. The innominate (brachiocephalic) artery
2. The left common carotid artery
3. The left subclavian artery.

All three branches course posterosuperiorly. The innominate and the left common carotid arteries are in close proximity to the anterior aspect of the trachea, while the left subclavian artery lies to the left of the trachea. The descending thoracic aorta begins distal to the left subclavian artery at the level of the ligamentum arteriosum. This area is referred to as the aortic isthmus. At the distal portion of the aortic arch and the beginning of the descending thoracic aorta, the aorta courses caudally and lies in close proximity to the esophagus in the left thoracic cavity. As the aorta descends in the thoracic cavity, it curves to course posteriorly to the esophagus. Finally, at the level of the distal portion of the descending thoracic aorta, the aorta will lie directly posterior to the esophagus.

## PATHOLOGY

This section will focus on three main diseases of the aorta: atherosclerosis, aortic aneurysm, and aortic dissection. One of the important considerations in the evaluation of aortic pathology is the differentiation of pathology from imaging artifact. So this section will also illustrate some of the common imaging artifacts encountered in the interrogation of the aorta.

## Atherosclerosis

Neurologic injury after procedures with cardiopulmonary bypass (CPB) continues to be a major problem and occurs in 1%–10% of the patients (4). Because there is very little one can do to treat this injury, prevention is the only real option. It is unclear which factor or factors are primarily responsible for this neurological injury after CPB; however, cerebral embolization and cerebral hypoperfusion continue to be the major focus of study. The watershed zones of infarction in the brain are areas thought to be at high risk for ischemic injury from decreases in perfusion pressure due to their position at the border of two distinct territories of perfusion. Because these areas rely on small arteriolar connections, they are subject to malperfusion based on decreased perfusion pressure, but they are also susceptible to embolic events based on their small caliber and their location as branches of major arteries. Retinal microvascular lesions, as well as pathologic subcapillary arteriolar dilatations in the brain have been demonstrated after CPB.

Prior investigations that focused on cerebral hypoperfusion, nonpulsatility, and air embolization as the major etiologic factors for stroke have been supplanted by studies of atheroemboli, which are now believed to be responsible for a majority of cerebral embolic events during open or closed cardiac procedures (5–9). Valvular surgery and open cardiac procedures were once thought to be higher risk procedures for micro- and macroembolization because of the entrainment of air into cardiac chambers and the potential for embolization of calcific and thrombotic debris (10). Atherosclerosis of the ascending thoracic aorta and aortic arch is now recognized as one, if not the major predictor of postoperative stroke after cardiac surgery (11). Additional evidence for the role of aortic atherosclerosis was provided by an autopsy study (n = 221) by Blauth et al. (12). The study found that atheroemboli were more common after coronary revascularization than after valvular procedures, p = 0.008. Peripheral vascular disease and ascending aortic atherosclerosis were significant independent risk factors for atheroemboli. A direct correlation between age and ascending aortic atherosclerosis was found, as well as a high correlation between ascending aortic atherosclerosis and atheroembolic events. Of the 98 patients who did not have atherosclerosis of the ascending aorta only 2 had autopsy evidence of embolic phenomena. Forty-six of the 123 patients with atherosclerosis of the ascending aorta had autopsy evidence of embolic events.

When aortic instrumentation is planned, the presence of ascending, transverse, and descending aortic atheromatous disease is a harbinger of potential cerebral embolization. Using echocardiographic techniques, aortic atherosclerosis can and should be diagnosed prior to anticipated instrumentation. Ascending aortic plaque is often soft, friable, and not able to be palpated by the cardiac surgeon. A number of investigations have shown that palpation underestimates the incidence of aortic plaque when compared with diagnosis via echocardiographic techniques (13,14). Its presence may only be recognized after it is seen oozing from an aortotomy site. After aortotomy, the embolization of atherosclerotic debris may have already occurred with resultant adverse sequelae. Thus, the preoperative identification of aortic plaque, made possible by improved echocardiographic technologies, has become an area of intense interest and research.

### Risk Factors

In order to accurately assess clinical risk for the development of stroke (stroke having an incidence of only 1%), sufficient numbers of patients must be studied in order to attain statistical power. For this reason, many of the studies that have identified risk factors have been necropsy studies, retrospective chart review, or prospective multicenter studies. Additionally, different criteria for diagnosis and assessment make comparison of studies quite difficult.

TEE evidence of thoracic aortic atherosclerosis has been shown to be a good predictor of the presence of ascending aortic atherosclerosis as seen by epicardial echocardiography, and may thus be a useful screen for patients at risk for cerebral embolization (Fig. 17.10) (15). Further, a negative TEE exam for atherosclerosis is helpful to exclude the possibility of ascending atherosclerosis by epicardial examination. Descending aortic atherosclerosis is a risk factor for embolic complications during aortic surgery (16). Its presence alone may also pose a risk to patients undergoing CPB procedures because these patients undergo extracorporeal perfusion with potential femoral cannulation and femoral instrumentation (17,18).

Severe atherosclerotic disease of the thoracic aorta is prevalent in elderly patients (19) and is probably an underestimated source of cerebral emboli during cardiac surgery (20). The presence of aortic knob calcification on radiographic films correlates well with atherosclerotic disease detected by echocardiographic means and should be considered a specific marker for atherosclerotic disease (21,22).

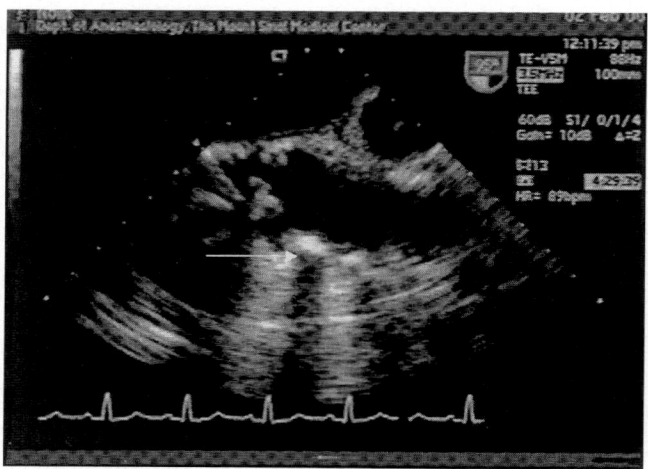

**FIGURE 17.10.** TEE atherosclerosis. ME LAX ascending aortic view with severe plaque at the sinotubular junction indicated by the arrow. Note the shadowing below the calcified plaque.

Davila-Roman et al. (23) relied heavily upon epiaortic ultrasonography (EPI) to detect aortic atherosclerosis in high-risk patients (Fig. 17.11). An analysis of preoperative variables that are known to correlate with atherosclerosis revealed that age and diabetes were the only significant independent predictors of severe atherosclerosis diagnosed by EPI of the ascending aorta.

These investigators divide the ascending aorta into three equal segments between the aortic root and the innominate artery. Mild atherosclerosis was defined as intimal thickening (< 3 mm) involving only one segment of the ascending aorta, moderate atherosclerosis was defined as intimal thickening (> 3 mm) in one or two segments, and severe atherosclerosis was defined as marked

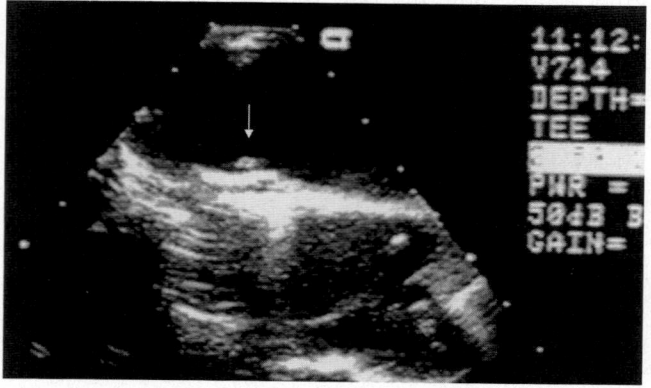

**FIGURE 17.11.** Epiaortic atherosclerosis. Long-axis view of the distal ascending aorta. Note the plaque on the anterior wall of the aorta that was detectable by palpation. Also note the pedunculated mobile plaque indicated by the arrow that was not detected by palpation.

intimal thickening (> 3 mm) in all three segments or circumferentially around the aorta. As expected, palpation of the ascending aorta significantly underestimated the severity and incidence of severe atherosclerosis. An analysis of preoperative variables that are known to correlate with atherosclerosis revealed that age and diabetes were the only significant independent predictors of severe atherosclerosis of the ascending aorta (by epiaortic ultrasonography). Based on the results of epiaortic ultrasonography, these investigators devised an algorithm that allowed revision of the planned surgical procedure to avoid areas of moderate or severe atherosclerosis. In a descriptive uncontrolled study, the algorithm was as follows. In patients with moderate aortic disease, potential alterations in the surgical procedure included femoral artery cannulation, change in the site for the aortic cross-clamp, avoidance of aortic cross-clamp using fibrillatory arrest, alteration of site of vein graft anastomoses, relocation of the cardioplegia needle, and the avoidance of antegrade cardioplegia by using retrograde cardioplegia. In patients with severe atherosclerotic disease, techniques included femoral artery cannulation with or without graft replacement of the ascending aorta using hypothermic circulatory arrest. Although permanent neurologic deficits occurred in 1% of the patients overall, no permanent neurologic deficits were present in the patients with severe atherosclerotic disease who had aggressive modifications of the surgical technique. Patients with moderate or severe atherosclerotic disease, who had only minor modifications of the surgical procedure, still had a 6.3% stroke rate (24). There were no strokes in the patients with severe carotid occlusive disease who underwent concomitant carotid endarterectomy and cardiac surgical procedures.

Using historical controls, other authors have reported similar success when employing measures to avoid instrumentation of the atherosclerotic ascending aorta based on the results of palpation (25) and/or ultrasonography (26–29). Various strategies have been employed to prevent potential atheroembolism from the ascending aorta; however, studies in larger numbers of patients or randomized trials are necessary to determine if the incidence of stroke can truly be reduced.

More recently, investigators have divided perioperative strokes into early and late events. This is done because they believe that different etiologic factors may play a role. Though there is disagreement in the literature as to whether early or late strokes are more common, one interesting finding is the relationship of late stroke and intimal lesions at the cannulation and clamp sites detected by epiaortic scanning postdecannulation. New lesions were found in 3.4% of the studied patients, and 30% of these patients developed a stroke (30). This study suggests that epiaortic scanning may be indicated postbypass to evaluate the sites of surgical manipulation.

## Implications

Cerebral dysfunction after cardiac surgery remains a major source of morbidity despite advances in surgical, medical, and perfusion techniques. Though the etiology of stroke and neuropsychologic dysfunction is multifactorial, evidence has been presented that supports that a large component of cerebral dysfunction is a result of embolism of atherosclerotic debris from the thoracic aorta. Transesophageal echocardiography is a sensitive and relatively noninvasive method for detecting atherosclerotic plaque in the thoracic aorta. If TEE monitoring is available, patients at high risk for atherosclerotic disease of the ascending aorta can be identified both by historical data and echocardiographic imaging. Once identified as high risk, epiaortic ultrasonography should be performed to further delineate the sites of severe atherosclerosis so that surgical modifications can be made.

## Aortic Aneurysm

There is no universally accepted definition of an aneurysm. Generally, an aneurysm is a localized dilation of an artery. An aortic aneurysm may be described as a permanent dilation that is at least 1.5 times the diameter of the expected normal value (31). Aneurysms can be further described according to their location, morphology, and etiology. Location is commonly used to classify aortic aneurysms for both clinical significance and surgical approach. Typically, the aneurysm can be localized to the sinuses of Valsalva (aortoannuloectasia), ascending arch, descending arch, and abdominal portions of the aorta. This type of classification may be misleading, because other portions of the aorta may also be involved. Approximately 6% of thoracic aortic aneurysms affect the distal aorta and arch, while 11% involve the thoracoabdominal aorta (32). Sixty-five percent of all aortic aneurysms occur in the abdominal aorta.

The morphology of an aneurysm is either fusiform or saccular. Fusiform aneurysms are sausage-like in shape; they are dilated symmetrically throughout the *full circumference* of the aorta (Fig. 17.12). Saccular aneurysms involve an outpouching of a *portion of the circumference* of the aortic wall. Aneurysms may also be classified morphologically as either true or false (pseudoaneurysm). True aneurysms involve all layers of the aortic wall. A pseudoaneurysm is a contained rupture that extends through all layers of the aortic wall. The integrity of the vasculature is maintained by surrounding tissues and the chronic inflammatory reaction to extravasated blood (33).

### Clinical Manifestations

Most patients with thoracic aortic aneurysms are asymptomatic at time of presentation and the aneurysms are

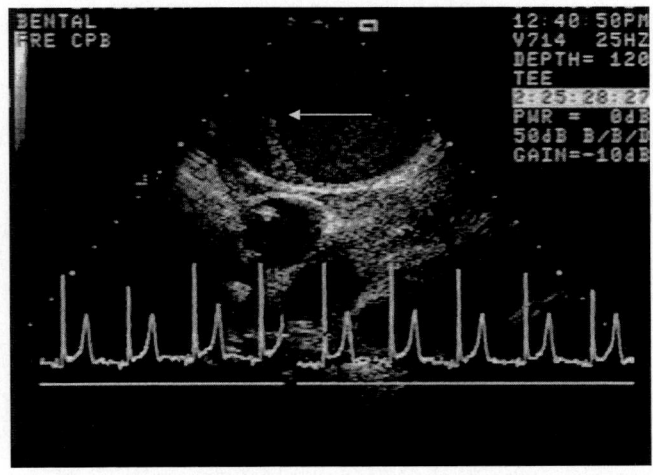

**FIGURE 17.12.** Ascending aortic aneurysm. This is an epiaortic scan of an ascending aortic aneurysm measuring nearly 6 cm in diameter (see cm markers on the side of the image). Also note that the arrow points to an intimal dissection flap that was missed on both preoperative CT and TEE. Though aneurysmal aortas are more likely to dissect, they are also more likely to have missed dissections than smaller aortas.

only detected while the patient is being investigated for other diseases. Signs and symptoms of thoracic aneurysms are usually secondary to enlargement of the aneurysm with impingement upon adjacent structures. Aneurysms of the ascending aorta frequently present with symptoms of congestive heart failure from aortic regurgitation. Rarely they can present with symptoms of compression of the coronary arteries, trachea, or superior vena cava. Descending thoracic aortic aneurysms can frequently present with symptoms of cough or hemoptysis from compression and/or erosion of the left main stem bronchus and pulmonary parenchyma. Because the left recurrent laryngeal nerve wraps around the ligamentum arteriosum, hoarseness may result if it is stretched and damaged. The physical examination is usually unremarkable in patients with thoracic aortic aneurysms; the only signs of an aneurysm may be an audible murmur or signs of superior vena caval compression.

### Diagnosis

Chest radiography may detect large thoracic aortic aneurysms as widening of the mediastinal silhouette, enlargement of the aortic knob, and tracheal deviation. Smaller aneurysms may be missed by conventional x-ray examinations, making this modality notoriously poor in the diagnosis of aortic disease; furthermore, masses in adjacent regions and interference from the cardiac silhouette may obscure the diagnosis of aortic disease (34). Although angiography remains the "gold standard" and remains important to delineate pathology involving the coronary arteries and the heart, computerized tomography and magnetic resonance imaging are quickly replacing angiography as the most useful tools for imaging the thoracic aorta. These modalities are also useful for evaluating the involvement of structures adjacent to the aneurysm. Transesophageal echocardiography is quickly becoming an alternative when a rapid diagnosis is necessary, especially in the management of suspected aortic dissection.

In addition to defining the size and extent of the aortic aneurysm, TEE can provide additional important information. For example, clots can form in a dilated aorta due to the relatively low blood velocity. It is important to identify this for the surgeon to prevent embolization. TEE can also identify chronic and acute dissection in these susceptible aortas. Other important uses of TEE in the evaluation of aortic aneurysm are as follows:

1. Timing of surgery based on valve morphology
2. Decision of valve sparing versus valve replacement surgery
3. Determination of which part of the aortic pathology to repair first depends on the severity of aortic insufficiency (AI)
4. AI as an indicator of acute dissection
5. Efficacy of open and endovascular repair

Thus intraoperative TEE plays an important role in the evaluation and treatment of aortic aneurysm.

## Aortic Dissection

### Pathophysiology

Blood accumulation in the medial layer is the characteristic feature of aortic dissection. The dissection of the medial layer may either be localized or split longitudinally. The plane of dissection usually courses along the greater curvature of the ascending aorta and the arch of the aorta, while in the descending aorta it is mainly located lateral to the true lumen but may also spiral along its longitudinal axis. The dissection usually does not occupy more than half of the circumference of the aorta. Most often, the dissection starts at a tear (rent) in the intimal layer that allows blood to flow between the intimal and medial/adventitial layers. The dissection usually propagates distally from the intimal tear but proximal propagation can also occur. One or more secondary (reentry or exit) tears may also be present distally. Also, a dissection can occur without any evidence of an intimal tear. It is proposed that this type of aortic dissection is due to medial layer weakness and hemorrhage of vessels in the vasa vasorum.

### Incidence

The incidence of aortic dissection is about 5 per million population per year. Predisposing factors include arterial hypertension, age, connective tissue disorders (Marfan's syndrome), congenital lesions (bicuspid aortic valve and coarctation of the aorta), iatrogenic causes (cardiac catheterization, intraaortic balloon counterpulsation, and aortic cannulation site), trauma, and pregnancy. The disease predominantly affects men (3:1 male:female ratio), with an average age of onset from the fifth to the seventh decades of life.

### Classification

Aortic dissections may be described by either the DeBakey or Stanford (Daily) classification systems. In the DeBakey types I and II, the dissections originate in the ascending aorta, while type III dissections begin in the descending aorta. The DeBakey type I dissection extends from the ascending aorta and arch to the descending aorta, while type II dissections are limited to the ascending aorta. The Stanford system simplified the classification into two groups: type A or type B. Type A describes those dissections that involve the ascending aorta, regardless of the origin of the tear or the extent of dissection (DeBakey types I and II are both included). Type B dissections involve only the descending aorta. Many clinicians have adopted the use of the simplified Stanford classification because it delineates two distinct risk groups and therapeutic approaches. Stanford type A accounts for between 50% and 85% of cases of aortic dissection, and is associated with a mortality of 90%–95% without surgical intervention. The acute mortality rate of a Stanford type B dissection is about 40% and, accordingly, the therapeutic approach is more conservative.

### Diagnosis

Because urgent surgical repair has such a pivotal role in the treatment of type A aortic dissection, it is imperative that a rapid diagnosis be made in any case where the index of suspicion is high. TEE has overcome some of the major disadvantages of the other diagnostic modalities. It is a minimally invasive procedure that has a proven safety record (35). An examination can be performed within about fifteen to twenty minutes and a diagnosis can usually be obtained at the same time. The test is easily performed at the bedside in critically ill patients. The close anatomic relationship of the esophagus to the aorta and the heart allows TEE to provide excellent high-quality images without significant interference from the overlying structures (lungs and chest wall). With the introduction of biplane and multiplane TEE probes, a more complete definition of the distal ascending aorta and aortic arch are possible. TEE is performed in real time allowing for its unique ability to give functional and hemodynamic information. This enables the evaluation of the aortic valve for regurgitation, the pericardial space for tamponade, and the left ventricle for evidence of dysfunction. Flow in both the true and false lumina can be analyzed with Doppler color flow imaging (DCFI) and pulsed (PW) or continuous (CW) wave Doppler allowing for an alternative technique to identify intimal tears when not directly visualized by two-dimensional imaging (Fig. 17.13). The coronary arteries can be observed for possible involvement in the dissection process.

Nonetheless, TEE has some limitations. There is still the risk (albeit small) for the probe to cause damage in the regions of the oropharynx, esophagus, or stomach. Hypotension and/or hypertension can occur rapidly secondary to complications from the aortic dissection (i.e., tamponade) or from stimulation of the oropharynx by the TEE probe, respectively; therefore, continuous intraarterial pressure monitoring is usually indicated. Additionally, because of the risk of aspiration of gastric contents in this patient population, endotracheal intubation should be considered.

### Comparison of Diagnostic Modalities

Several studies have compared the use of aortography, CT, MRI, and TEE for diagnosing acute aortic dissection. In 1989, Erbel et al. compared monoplane TEE to CT and aortography and found that TEE can provide an accurate diagnosis in a relatively short time. Of the 164 patients studied with suspected acute aortic dissections, only one false negative and two false positives occurred with

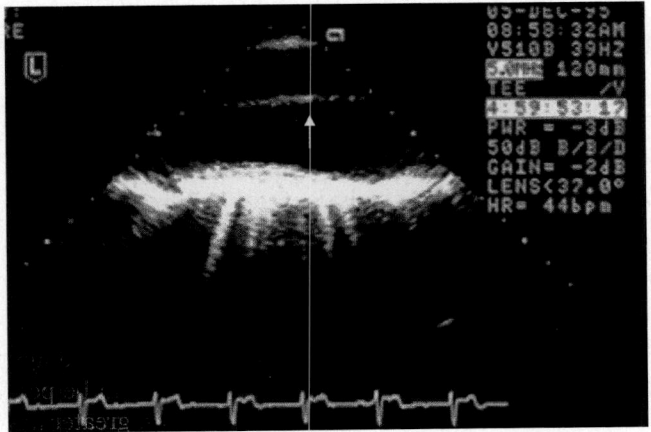

**FIGURE 17.13.** Descending aortic dissection. LAX view of a type B dissection. The arrow is in the false lumen pointing toward the intimal flap. The lack of symmetry of the two lumina suggests this is not an artifact. This could be confirmed by differential color flow patterns across the two sides of the flap.

TEE, for a sensitivity of 99%, a specificity of 98%, and positive and negative predictive values of 98% and 99%, respectively. CT scan had a slightly higher specificity (100%) but a lower sensitivity (83%) and negative predictive value (86%) than TEE. Angiography did not fare as well for sensitivity, specificity, and positive or negative predictive values compared to TEE. The authors state that reverberations in the region of the ascending aorta were the main cause for the two false positive exams by TEE (36).

Two years later, Ballal et al., reported on the value of TEE for diagnosing acute aortic dissections when aortography, surgery, and/or autopsy were used to confirm their findings. Once more, TEE was shown to be a highly accurate diagnostic test having a sensitivity, specificity, and positive and negative predicative values of 97%, 100%, 100%, and 96%, respectively (37). In a study by Nienaber and associates published in 1992, monoplane TEE was compared to MRI for the diagnosis of acute aortic dissection. The sensitivity for TEE and MRI was 100%, but MRI had a higher specificity than TEE (100% vs. 68%, respectively). Transthoracic echocardiography (TTE) did not perform as well when compared to either of these modalities. The lower specificity (higher incidence of false positives) of TEE compared to MRI was again attributable to reverberations in the ascending aorta or extensive plaque formations in this region as well (38). In 1993, Nienaber et al. reported on their expanded experience of 110 patients and confirmed the excellent sensitivity of TEE (98%) irrespective of the location of the dissection (39). As in their previous study, TEE had a lower specificity than MRI (77% vs. 100%, respectively; six false positive findings for TEE) contradicting the high specificity found by the studies of Erbel et al. and Ballal et al. In a study by Simon et al., it was reconfirmed that TEE was an excellent test for identifying aortic dissections (sensitivity and specificity, 100%) (40). It can be seen from that study, however, that the ability of TEE to correctly ascertain the type (location) of dissection caused a decrease in specificity for type A dissections (86%, one false positive) and a decrease in sensitivity for type B dissections (88%). Therefore, it appears that the level of accuracy of TEE depends on the location of the dissection within the aorta. Regardless, recent studies have reiterated that TEE is an accurate test for diagnosing acute aortic dissections and support its use as the first test to be performed in the acute setting because TEE:

1. Is minimally invasive
2. Requires no contrast
3. Allows for real-time analysis of the cardiovascular system
4. Can be performed at the bedside in critically ill patients
5. Can be performed in a short period of time (41,42)

Despite the many advocates of using TEE as the first diagnostic test, it appears that MRI, when practical, is a more sensitive and specific test for locating the exact location and extent of an aortic dissection. If the previous studies were repeated with multiplane probes and more experienced echocardiographers, it is likely that the apparent advantages might disappear.

### Limitations

A common denominator in these earlier studies was the decreased specificity of TEE in diagnosing dissections accurately in the ascending aorta and its inferior ability to detect type B dissections compared to MRI. It is generally agreed that the former problem was mainly due to artifacts generated in the ascending aorta. Appelbe et al. describe an in vitro model that could predict a curvilinear artifact emulated by reverberations in the ascending aorta at predictable distances from the transducer. The distance between the transducer to the left atrial wall that abuts the aorta was equal to the distance from this portion of the left atrial wall and the artifact. In their retrospective analysis of in vivo TEE examinations, it was demonstrated that this artifact was primarily limited to those patients whose aortic diameter exceeded the distance of the left atrium. In these cases, the reverberation artifact appeared to lie within the lumen of the aorta, mimicking an intimal flap (43). As for TEE's decreased ability to detect dissections of the descending abdominal aorta, this appears to be secondary to the anatomical divergence of the aorta from the esophagus in the abdomen.

It is also important to note that many of these studies were limited because the authors mainly used monoplane (transverse) TEE probes that offer only limited views of the ascending aorta. Biplane or multiplane probes can provide additional tomographic images of the ascending aorta, which may have improved the specificity of the earlier studies. Despite these additional views, however, visualization of the distal ascending aorta to the midtransverse aortic arch is somewhat limited because of the interposition of the trachea and the right mainstem bronchus between the esophagus and the aorta (44). TTE in the suprasternal window may afford visualization of this region when TEE fails. Nevertheless, in subsequent studies, TEE has continued to compare favorably to MRI and appears to perform better than CT, TTE, and angiography in its ability to rapidly diagnose acute aortic dissection.

### Secondary Diagnoses

In addition to revealing the presence and extent of an aortic dissection, special features of the TEE can be used to diagnose and define several important aspects of the dissection. TEE is one of the best methods for accurately identifying the structural and functional status (using DCFI and CW Doppler) of the aortic valve, which has im-

portant surgical implications. TEE is also valuable for assessing the degree of involvement and integrity of the coronary arteries in aortic dissection. TEE visualizes approximately 70%–88% and 25%–50% of the left and right coronary artery ostia, respectively. Of the seven patients with proven involvement of the coronary ostium in the study by Ballal et al., six were correctly diagnosed by TEE (9). There are situations, however, where coronary angiography is required to define the need for coronary artery bypass grafting (CABG) or coronary angioplasty (e.g., ascending aortic dissection with an acute MI). Aortography should be considered if cardiac catheterization is planned. Flow patterns of the true and false lumina and the location of intimal tears can be further assessed using DCFI and PW Doppler. This can lead to identification of patients at risk for malperfusion. The diagnosis of a left pleural or pericardial effusion or even blood clots in the pericardium can be obtained more rapidly with TEE compared with CT or MRI. TEE can also give real-time analysis of cardiac function, which is very critical for medical, surgical, and anesthetic management. Rare complications of aortic dissections have also been reported that were diagnosed by TEE and missed by other modalities. An example is aortic intussusception, where the intimal flap partially or totally separates from the aorta and migrates distally causing obstruction of blood flow to extremities or major organs (45).

From the data presented above and from expert consensus, it can be concluded that both TEE and MRI are highly accurate and should be considered among the first diagnostic studies to be performed for the initial evaluation of suspected aortic dissections. CT scanning and aortography also have a solid place in the armamentarium of diagnostic modalities. Each diagnostic test offers distinct advantages and disadvantages. In order to justify the use of any one of these tests, each case must be evaluated on an individual basis, and individual practitioners' and institutional preferences should also be considered. Irrespective of this, it seems logical to include TEE in nearly 100% of cases. The exam can be performed rapidly, is portable, and can be safely done in hemodynamically unstable patients at their bedside. Furthermore, a diagnosis is generally obtained within minutes of the examination. If there is a type A dissection and the primary physicians are satisfied with the information obtained by TEE, then the patient can be operated upon without further delay. If the TEE shows a type B dissection, then medical therapy can be instituted. Additional diagnostic tests can be performed at a later time in order to assess, with greater accuracy, the extent of the dissection. If the TEE is equivocal, then another diagnostic test can be obtained. Therefore, the advantages and limitations of TEE and other modalities (i.e., CT, MRI, aortography) must be considered in the diagnostic evaluation of the patient with suspected aortic dissection.

## KEY POINTS

- Aortic diseases are life threatening.
- Careful evaluation with multiple views, multiple imaging approaches, and Doppler.
- Consider the pathophysiologic implications.
- Understand the surgical plan and react accordingly.
- Understand limitations and artifacts.

## REFERENCES

1. Konstadt SN, Reich DL, Quintana C, et al. The ascending aorta: how much does transesophageal echocardiograpy see? Anesth Analg 1994;78:240–4.
2. Davies MG, Hagen PO. Physiology of the arterial system, including the effects of nitric oxide. In Sabiston DC, Lyerly HK, eds. Textbook of surgery: the biological basis of modern surgical practice, 15th ed. Philadelphia: W.B. Saunders Company, 1997:1620.
3. Orihashi K, Sisto DA. Aorta. In Oka Y, Goldiner PL, eds. Transesophageal echocardiography. Philadelphia: JB Lippincott, 1992:189–225.
4. Shaw PS, Bates B, Cartlidge NEF, et al. Neurologic and neuropsychological morbidity following major surgery: Comparison of coronary artery bypass and peripheral vascular surgery. Stroke 1987;18:700–7.
5. Mills SA. Risk factors for cerebral injury and cardiac surgery. Ann Thorac Surg 1995;59:1296–99.
6. Yao FS, Barbut D, Hager DN, Trifiletti RR, Gold JP. Detection of aortic emboli by transesophageal echocardiography during coronary artery bypass surgery. J Cardiothorac Vasc Anesth 1996;10:314–17.
7. Barbut D, Gold JP. Aortic atheromatosis and risks of cerebral embolization. J Cardiothorac Vasc Anesth 1996;10:24–29.
8. Lynn GM, Stefanko K, Reed JF III, Gee W, Nicholas G. Risk factors for stroke after coronary artery bypass. J Thorac Cardiovasc Surg 1992;104:1518–23.
9. Breuer AC, Furlan AJ, Hanson MR, et al. Central nervous system complications of coronary artery bypass graft surgery: prospective analysis of 421 patients. Stroke 1983;14:682–87.
10. Nussmeier NA. Adverse neurologic events: risks of intracardiac versus extracardiac surgery. J Cardiothorac Vasc Anesth 1996;10:31–37.
11. Bull DA, Neumayer LA, Hunter GC, et al. Risk factors for stroke in patients undergoing coronary artery bypass grafting. Cardiovasc Surg 1993;1:182–85.
12. Blauth CI, Cosgrove DM, Webb BW, et al. Atheroembolism from the ascending aorta. An emerging problem in cardiac surgery. J Thorac Cardiovasc Surg 1992;103:1104–12.
13. Marschall K, Kanchuger M, Kessler K, et al. Superiority of transesophageal echocardiography in detecting aortic arch atheromatous disease: identification of patients at increased risk of stroke during cardiac surgery. J Cardiothorac Vasc Anesth 1994;8:5–13.
14. Duda AM, Letwin LB, Sutter FP, Goldman SM. Does routine use of aortic ultrasonography decrease the stroke rate in coronary artery bypass surgery? J Vasc Surg 1995;21:98–109.
15. Konstadt SN, Reich DL, Kahn R, Viggiani RF. Transesophageal echocardiography can be used to screen for ascending aortic atherosclerosis. Anesth Analg 1995;81:225–8.
16. Kassirer JP. Atheroembolic renal disease. N Engl J Med 1969; 280:812–8.
17. Karalis DG, Chandrasekaran K, Victor MF, et al. Recognition and embolic potential of intra-aortic atherosclerotic debris. J Am Coll Cardiol 1991;17:73–8.
18. Hartman GS, Yao FS, Bruefach M 3, et al. Severity of aortic atheromatous disease diagnosed by transesophageal echocardiography predicts stroke and other outcomes associated with coronary artery surgery: a prospective study. Anesth Analg 1996;83:701–8.
19. Mitchell MM, Frankville DD, Weinger MB, Dittrich HC. Detection of thoracic aortic atheroma with transesophageal echocardiography in patients without symptoms of embolism. Am Heart J 1991;122:1768–71.
20. Simons AJ, Carlson R, Hare CL, et al. The use of transesophageal echocardiography in detecting aortic atherosclerosis in patients with embolic disease. Am Heart J 1992; 123:224–6.
21. Witteman JCM, Kannel WB, Wolf PA, et al. Aortic calcified plaques and cardiovascular disease (The Framingham Study). Am J Cardiol 1990;66:1060–4.
22. Toyoda K, Yasaka M, Nagata S, Yamaguchi T. Aortogenic embolic stroke: A transesophageal echocardiographic approach. Stroke 1992;23:1056–61.
23. Davila-Roman VG, Barzilai B, Wareing TH, et al. Intraoperative ultrasonographic evaluation of the ascending aorta in 100 consecutive patients undergoing cardiac surgery. Circulation 1991;84:III47–III53.
24. Wareing TH, Davila-Roman VG, Daily BB, et al. Strategy for the reduction of stroke incidence in cardiac surgical patients. Ann Thorac Surg 1993;55:1400–8.
25. Bar-El Y, Goor DA. Clamping of the atherosclerotic ascending aorta during coronary artery bypass operations. J Thorac Cardiovasc Surg 1992;104:469–74.
26. Ribakove GH, Katz ES, Galloway AC, et al. Surgical implications of transesophageal echocardiography to grade the atheromatous aortic arch. Ann Thorac Surg 1992;53:758–63.
27. Hosoda Y, Watanabe M, Hirooka Y, et al. Significance of atherosclerotic changes of the ascending aorta during coronary bypass surgery with intraoperative detection by echography. J Cardiovasc Surg 1991;32:301–6.
28. Swanson SJ, Cohn LH. Excision of focal aortic arch atheroma using deep hypothermic circulatory arrest. Ann Thorac Surg 1995;60:457–8.
29. Ohteki H, Itoh T, Natsuaki M, et al. Intraoperative ultrasonic imaging of the ascending aorta in ischemic heart disease. Ann Thorac Surg 1990;5:539–42.
30. Ura M, Sakata R, Nakayama Y, et al. Ultrasonic demonstration of manipulation-related aortic injuries after cardiac surgery. JACC 2000;35:1303–10.
31. Johnston KW, Rutherford RB, Tilson MD, Shah DM, Hollier L, Stanley JC. Suggested standards for reporting on arterial aneurysms. Subcommittee on Reporting Standards for Arterial Aneurysms, Ad Hoc Committee on Reporting Standards, Society for Vascular Surgery and North American Chapter, International Society for Cardiovascular Surgery. J Vasc Surg 1991;13:452–58.
32. Dapunt OE, Galla JD, Sadeghi AM, Lansman SL, Mezrow CK, de Asla RA, Quintana C, Wallenstein S, Ergin AM, Griepp RB. The natural history of thoracic aortic aneurysms. J Thorac Cardiovasc Surg 1994;107;1323–32.
33. Isselbacher EM, Eagle KA, Desanctis RW. Diseases of the aorta. In Braunwald E ed. Heart disease, 5th ed. Philadelphia: W.B. Saunders Company, 1997:1546.
34. Chen JT. Plain radiographic evaluation of the aorta. J Thorac Imaging 1990;5;1–17.
35. Daniel WG, Erbel R, Kasper W, et al. Safety of transesophageal echocardiography: A multicenter survey of 10,419 examinations. Circulation 1991;83:817–21.
36. Erbel R, Daniel W, Visser C, et al. Echocardiography in diagnosis of aortic dissection. Lancet 1989;1:457–69.
37. Ballal RS, Nanda NC, Gatewood R, et al. Usefulness of transesophageal echocardiography in assessment of aortic dissection. Circ 1991;84:1903–14.
38. Nienaber CA, Spielmann RP, von Kodolitsch Y, et al. Diagnosis of thoracic aortic dissection: Magnetic resonance imaging versus transesophageal echocardiography. Circ 1992;85:434–47.
39. Nienaber CA, von Kodolitsch Y, Nicolas V, et al. The diagnosis of thoracic aortic dissection by noninvasive imaging procedures. N Engl J Med 1993;1:328.

40. Simon P, Owen AN, Havel M, et al. Transesophageal echocardiography in the emergency surgical management of patients with aortic dissection. J Thor Card Surg 1992;103:1113–18.
41. Chirillo F, Cavallini C, Longhini C, et al. Comparative diagnostic value of transesophageal echocardiography and retrograde aortography in the evaluation of thoracic aortic dissection. Am J Cardiol 1994;74:590–95.
42. Laissy JP, Blanc F, Soyer P, et al. Thoracic aortic dissection: Diagnosis with transesophageal echocardiography versus MR imaging. Radiology 1995;194:331–36.
43. Appelbe AF, Walker PG, Yeoh JK, et al. Clinical significance and origin artifacts in transesophageal echocardiography of the thoracic aorta. J Am Coll Cardiol 1993;21:754–60.
44. Konstadt SN, Reich DL, Quintana C, et al. The ascending aorta: How much does the transesophageal echocardiography see? Anesth Analg 1994;78:240–44.
45. Hudak AM, Konstadt SN. Aortic intussusception: A rare complication of aortic dissection. Anesth 1995;82:1292–94.

## QUESTIONS

1. What portion of the thoracic aorta is not well visualized by TEE?
   A. Proximal descending aorta
   B. Proximal ascending aorta
   C. Distal ascending aorta
   D. Midaortic arch
   E. Distal aortic arch

2. Type A aortic dissections may least likely result in all of the following *except*
   A. Aortic regurgitation
   B. Mitral regurgitation
   C. Pericardial effusion
   D. Coronary ischemia
   E. Pleural effusion

3. The normal diameter of the ascending aorta is
   A. < 3.5 cm
   B. 3.5–4.5 cm
   C. 4.5–5.5 cm
   D. 1.5–2.5 cm
   E. None of the above

4. The best view to evaluate the cannulation site is
   A. Midesophageal long-axis view
   B. Upper esophageal long-axis view
   C. Upper esophageal short-axis view
   D. Epiaortic short-axis view
   E. Midesophageal short-axis view

## Chapter 18

# Assessment of Prosthetic Valves

*Michelle Capdeville and Michael G. Licina*

The first clinical artificial heart valve was introduced more than 45 years ago. Mechanical and biological prostheses developed in parallel. In 1953, Huffnagel treated aortic regurgitation by placing a caged ball valve in the descending thoracic aorta (1). In 1956, Murray implanted a cadaveric aortic valve in a similar fashion (2). With the subsequent development of cardiopulmonary bypass techniques, intracardiac valve replacement became possible, with Starr and Edwards performing the first successful valve replacement using a caged ball prosthesis in 1960 (3).

## TYPES OF PROSTHETIC VALVES

Currently available prosthetic heart valves can be divided into two broad categories: mechanical and bioprosthetic. Multiple sizes are available for each valve type (Table 18.1). With prolonged implantation of a prosthetic valve, regardless of type, one can expect to see some degree of malfunction or failure, making this a form of palliative treatment (4,5).

## Mechanical Valves

The term "profile" is frequently used when describing prosthetic valves and refers to the height from the base of the prosthesis to the top of the struts.

### High Profile Valves

#### Ball-Cage Valves

Ball-cage valves were the earliest mechanical valves used. The Starr-Edwards valve is the only ball-cage valve currently in use in the United States. Other modifications of this valve have included the Smeloff-Sutter valve and the Magovern-Cromie sutureless valve.

#### Starr-Edwards Valve

The Starr-Edwards prosthesis is the most well known caged ball valve, having the longest history and most extensive follow-up. It was designed in 1960 and consists of a metal cage and a round silastic ball (poppet or occluder) with a circular sewing ring. Over the years this valve has undergone constant modification to eliminate problems, such as thrombogenicity, noise, and hemolysis (Fig. 18.1) (6).

▶ TABLE 18.1. Prosthetic Valve Types

| ADVANTAGES | DISADVANTAGES |
|---|---|
| **Mechanical Valves:**<br>Durability<br>Low profile (bileaflet and tilting disc models)<br>Low incidence of structural failures | **Mechanical Valves:**<br>Higher incidence of thromboembolism<br>Anticoagulant-related hemorrhage<br>Hemolysis<br>Higher incidence of perivalvular leak |
| **Bioprosthetic Valves:**<br>Reduced incidence of thromboembolism<br>Lower incidence of perivalvular leak<br>Fewer bleeding complications | **Bioprosthetic Valves:**<br>Tissue degeneration (worse in younger patients)<br>More flow obstruction with smaller sizes (especially stented valves)<br>Poor long-term durability |

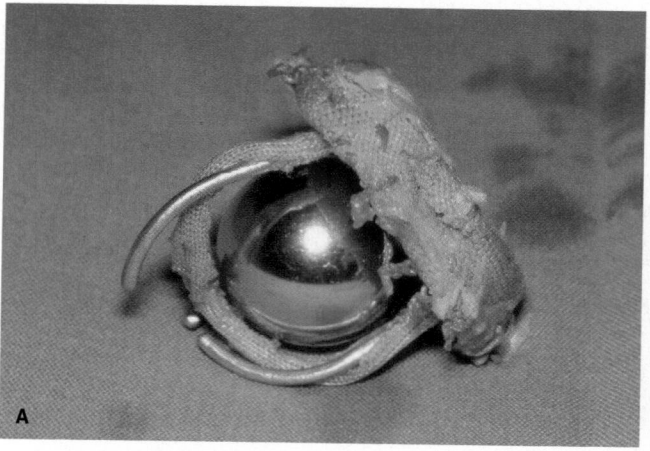

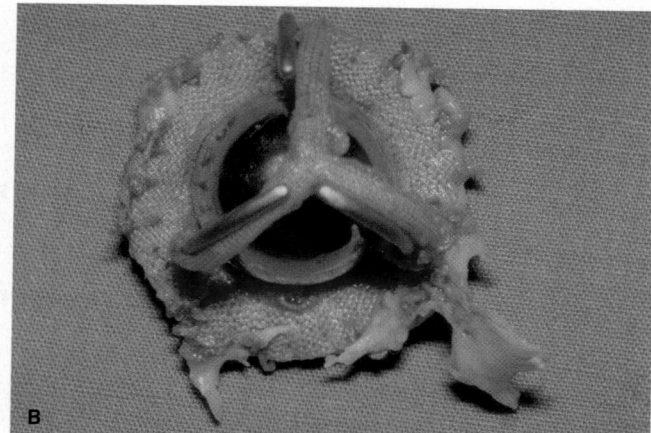

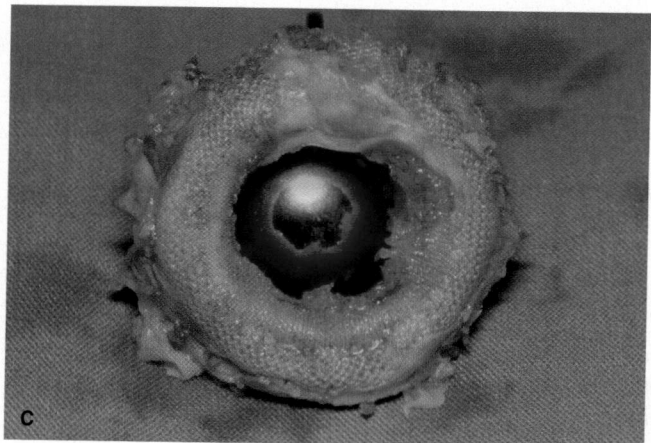

**FIGURE 18.1. A–C:** Various views of an excised Starr-Edwards valve with surgically bent strut.

When blood flows across the valve, the ball moves to the apex of the cage; the ball moves to the base of the cage to close the valve and prevent regurgitation. The motion of the ball, with its continually changing points of contact, is thought to reduce the risk of thrombus formation. These valves have a high profile with the potential for left ventricular outflow tract obstruction in the mitral position. They also have a relatively small orifice and can cause some degree of hemolysis, though the latter is relatively insignificant in the absence of a perivalvular leak. Axisymmetrical and turbulent flow occurs because of the central obstruction by the ball and flow around its edges (flow downstream remains evenly distributed and converges). Stagnation can occur behind the ball, predisposing to thromboembolism. These valves have a very small regurgitant volume.

The Starr-Edwards valve has three orifices: a primary orifice at the annulus; a secondary orifice at the angle made by the ball in the open position and the annular opening; and a tertiary orifice between the ball perimeter and the ventricular or aortic walls. Therefore, a large primary orifice can result in a small tertiary orifice because of the larger size ball. This is because the ball must be larger than the valve opening in order for it to occlude the

orifice completely. Consequently, in the mitral position, a relatively large ball lying in the middle of the ventricle partially obstructs blood flow. Compared to other mechanical valves, the inlet orifice diameter compared to the overall valve diameter is less favorable. Effective orifice size may not reflect the actual (larger) measured orifice because the former is affected by the shape of the valve orifice (Fig. 18.2).

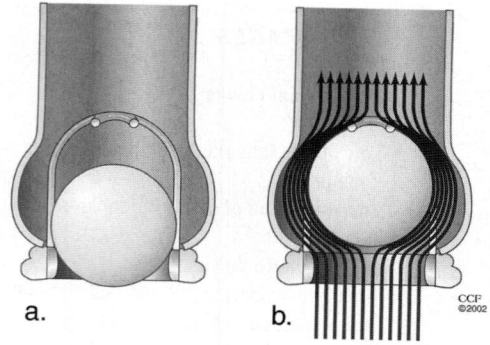

**FIGURE 18.2. A:** Ball-cage valve in a closed position. **B:** Complex flow around a ball-cage valve. This illustrates how the effective orifice area is affected by a high profile valve.

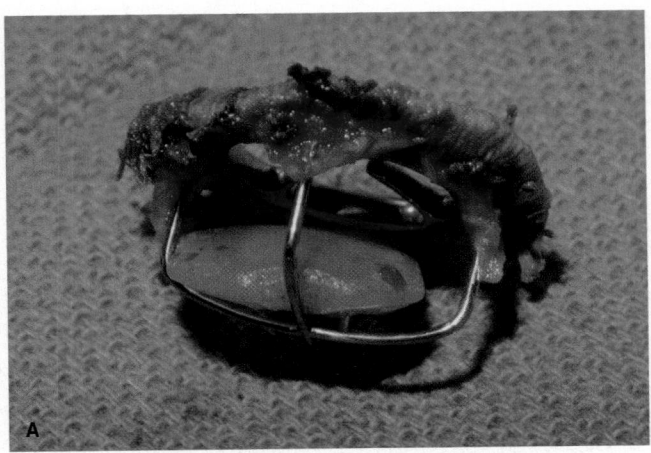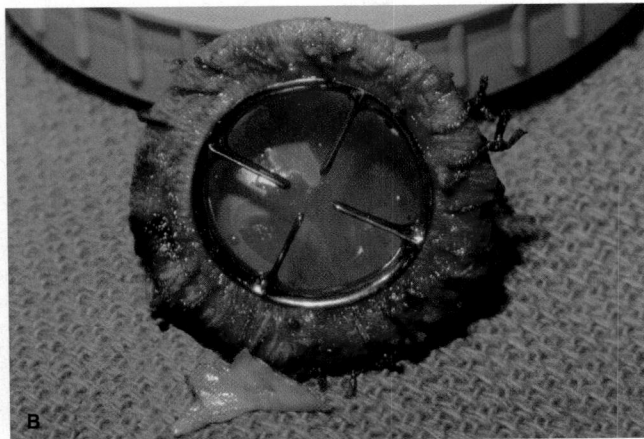

**FIGURE 18.3. A – B:** Various views of a surgically excised Kay-Suzuki valve (disc-cage).

### Caged Disc Valves

Caged disc valves include the Cooley-Cutter, the Beall, the Cross-Jones, the Harken, the Starr-Edwards (6500 series), the Kay–Suzuki, and the Kay-Shiley. Although these valves have all been discontinued, some are still functional more than 20 years after implantation (Fig. 18.3).

### Low Profile Valves

The introduction of low profile valves reduced the "mass to orifice ratio," thereby improving hemodynamics. Most low profile mechanical valves are made of pyrolitic carbon to reduce thrombogenicity and improve durability.

### Tilting Disc Valves

Tilting disc valves were introduced in 1967 with the goal of achieving a low profile and reducing bulk within the left ventricular cavity. They have an intermediate range of valve obstruction. The circular disc of the valve is attached to the sewing ring by way of an eccentric strut/hinge mechanism. Back pressure on the larger portion of the disc causes the valve to close. The opening angle of the disc is important, because the gradient will increase when the angle is less than 60 degrees from the sewing ring. The opening angle is typically 60–70 degrees. To ensure proper valve closure, this angle must be less than 90 degrees. If the opening angle is too great, the regurgitant volume will increase. A certain amount of valvular insufficiency is felt to be beneficial as it reduces the problem of periprosthetic flow stagnation, which could lead to thrombosis. In the open position, there is an area of stagnation behind the valve because the opening angle is less than 90 degrees. Flow across tilting disc valves is complex. These valves have a major orifice (70% of flow) and a minor orifice. The orientation of the orifice is important because it affects flow dynamics. As blood flow opens the disc, it is directed laterally through each orifice (Figs. 18.4 and 18.5) (7–10).

### Bjork-Shiley Valve

The Bjork-Shiley valve was originally manufactured in 1969. It was removed from the United States market because of problems with strut fractures due to weld fractures and disc embolization. It consists of a free-floating disc, which is suspended in a stellite cage with a major inflow and minor outflow C-shaped struts.

The Bjork-Shiley Monostrut valve was subsequently developed and eliminated the two-armed welded outflow strut entirely; instead it has a single thick arm, which is part of the housing in a single piece. It is still sold in Europe.

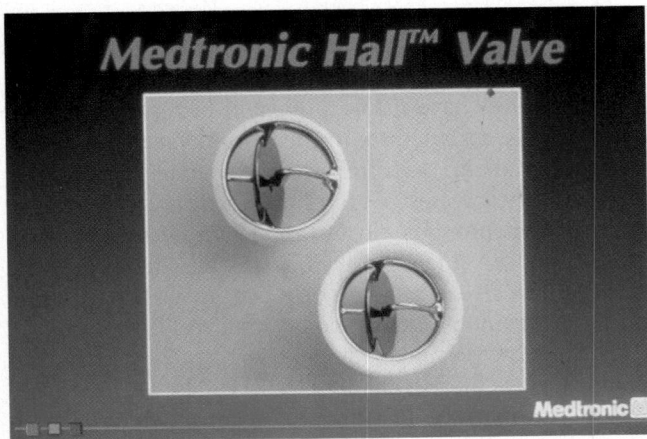

**FIGURE 18.4.** An example of Medtronic's single-disc valve.

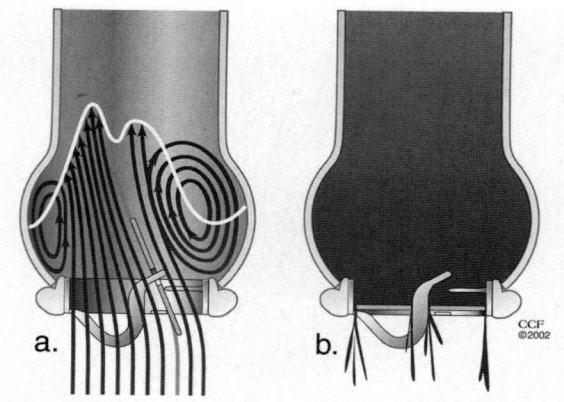

FIGURE 18.5. **A:** Complex flow pattern around a single-disc valve with a major and minor orifice flow pattern represented. **B:** Closed single-disc valve shows the characteristic regurgitant (washing) jets.

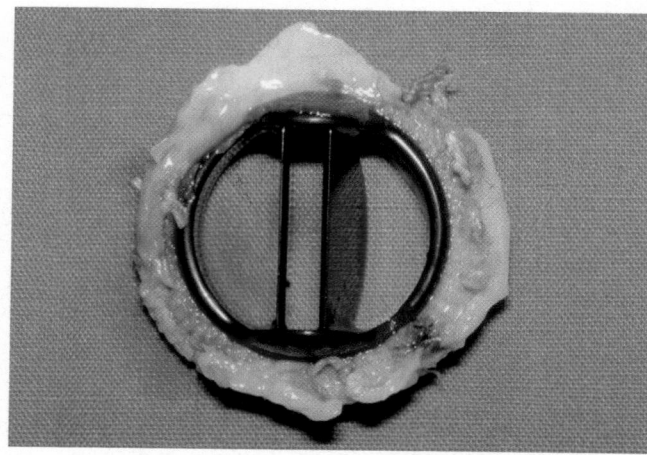

FIGURE 18.6. A surgically excised St. Jude valve with the leaflets in the open position.

### Medtronic Hall Valve

The Medtronic Hall valve, previously known as the Hall-Kaster valve, was developed in 1975. It is the most commonly implanted single-disc valve in the United States. It consists of a disc, housing, struts, and ring. The disc moves up and down on the S-shaped guide strut. It is still in use (Fig. 18.4).

### OmniScience Valve

The OmniScience valve is a descendant of the Lillehei-Kaster disc valve. It was manufactured in 1978. It has a curved pivoting disc, a one-piece cage, and a sewing ring.

### Wada Cutter Valve

The Wada Cutter valve is a single-disc valve with two metal struts at the sides of the valve housing to hold the disc in place. It was manufactured in 1967, and subsequently discontinued in 1972.

### Bileaflet Valves

Bileaflet valves have the advantage of being less obstructive (flow is across three orifices) and have the lowest pressure gradients, especially with the smaller sizes. They also have the greatest regurgitant fraction (10%), due in part to asynchronous closure of the leaflets and a long closing arc. Advantages of the bileaflet prostheses over the tilting disc valves include a reduced area of stagnation, and a larger unobstructed and symmetrical flow area.

Bileaflet valves make up approximately 90% of the mechanical valve market share in the U.S. The St. Jude valve is the prototype "gold standard" against which all mechanical prostheses are compared (Figs. 18.6–18.8).

### St. Jude Valve

The St. Jude valve was manufactured in 1977. It has two semicircular leaflets attached to a sewing ring by a midline hinge mechanism. The leaflets pivot open (no rotation) during valve opening. When the valve opens there are two large lateral semicircular openings and a smaller central rectangular opening. The leaflets open to 85 degrees from horizontal and the angle of closure is at 30 to 35 degrees to the orifice plane (varies with valve size). Because of the large opening angle, the effective valve orifice closely approximates the area of the sewing ring. This wide angle of excursion, however, allows for significant backflow across the valve (approximately 10% regurgitant volume) (11).

### Carbomedics Valve

The Carbomedics valve was introduced in 1986. It is structurally different from the St. Jude valve but has the

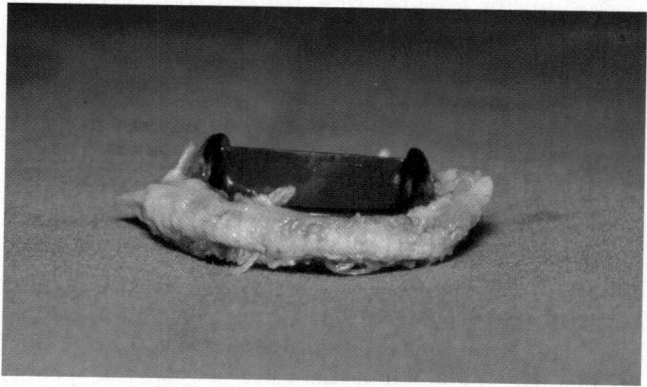

FIGURE 18.7. Surgically excised St. Jude valve revealing its low profile nature.

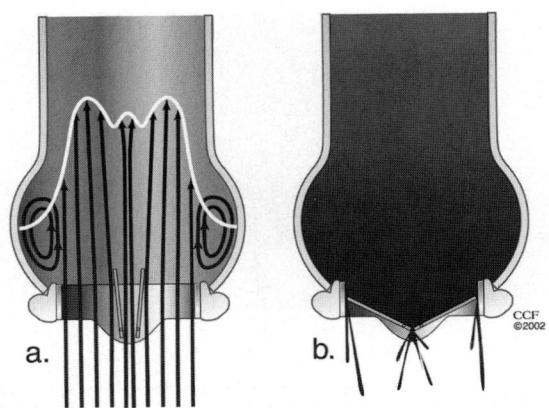

**FIGURE 18.8. A:** A bileaflet valve in the open position revealing the near laminar flow pattern. **B:** A bileaflet valve in the closed position showing the characteristic regurgitant (washing) jets.

same echocardiographic characteristics. Pressure gradients across this prosthesis are similar to the St. Jude valve.

### Other Bileaflet Valves

Other manufactured bileaflet mechanical prostheses include the Edwards Duromedics valve (withdrawn due to disc fractures), the Medtronic Parallel valve (withdrawn due to a high incidence of thromboembolism), and the On-X valve, which was manufactured in 1996.

## Bioprosthetic Valves

The first use of intracardiac tissue valves occurred in 1962 when Heimbecker et al. implanted a stentless cadaveric aortic valve in the mitral position (12), and Ross implanted the same in the aortic position (13,14). The low availability of these cadaveric valves led to the subsequent use of heterografts in 1965 by Binet et al. (15). Limited durability was improved by the use of glutaraldehyde preservation as described by Carpentier et al. in 1969 (16); ease of implantation was facilitated by mounting these valves on a stent as described by Reis et al. in 1971 (17).

Tissue valves are distinguished by their tissue composition. They are typically made of animal (heterograft, xenograft) or human tissue (homograft), and the tissue can be of valvular or nonvalvular origin. Today's bioprosthetic valves are made of biologic material and include homograft valves, porcine aortic valves, and bovine pericardial tissue valves. These valves are well suited for patients at risk for hemorrhage, women who plan to bear children, and those who will not reliably follow a strict anticoagulation regimen. Unfortunately, the bioprostheses have a limited durability. This is generally due to progressive collagen disruption and calcification, leading to stenosis and eventual leaflet disruption.

Mitral bioprostheses have a higher failure rate than aortic bioprostheses. This is believed to be related to mechanical closure stress, bending of the struts by left ventricular contraction, and atrial fibrillation. A greater back pressure between the left ventricle and atrium in systole compared to the aorta and left ventricle in diastole has also been implicated.

Smaller sized valves have a greater obstruction to flow. Flow characteristics are improved in the larger sized valves when compared to mechanical prostheses, and there is less shear stress to blood elements. Valve orientation during insertion is unimportant because the orifice is central. Care must be taken, however, to ensure that the struts do not impinge on the left ventricular outflow tract for mitral prostheses.

### Mitral Homograft Valves

Homografts are cryopreserved human cadaveric valves either stented or unstented. They are harvested shortly after death (when the endothelium is still viable). Stented mitral homografts have not proven very successful, with a high incidence of failure within 5 years due to leaflet thickening, calcification, and the development of valvular insufficiency.

Mitral homografts are more difficult to implant, and the patient's valve size must be known beforehand. Early attempts at homograft mitral valve replacement yielded a high failure rate because of technical problems, including inadequate sizing of the graft and early dehiscence of the papillary muscle anastomosis. Good results have recently been reported in Europe (18–22).

### Aortic Homograft Valves

Aortic homografts are cryopreserved human cadaveric aortic valves. Typically, a mini root replacement is done with reimplantation of the coronary ostia. This is an attractive alternative for younger patients and patients with endocarditis. Another advantage of these valves is a notable resistance to infection. Earlier methods of chemical preservation led to early valve failure (24). Antibiotic sterilization and cryopreservation have resulted in significant improvements in long-term valve performance (25). Size limits the availability of this type of valve because the patient's annulus must match that of the homograft.

The Ross procedure is a double valve procedure in which the patient's pulmonic valve is placed in the aortic position as an autograft, and the pulmonic valve is then replaced with an aortic homograft (26). The right and left coronary ostia must be reimplanted (some surgeons use an inclusion technique where the pulmonic valve is inserted into the aortic root without removing the coronary ostia). A major concern with this procedure is the risk of injury to the first septal perforator (near the base of the pulmonic valve), which can lead to high septal infarction and death. The procedure is well suited to younger, growing patients because the autograft can continue to grow with the cardiovascular tree (Fig. 18.9) (23).

### Stented Porcine Valves

The stented porcine bioprostheses in current use are the Carpentier-Edwards and Hancock valves. These valves consist of a stented preserved porcine aortic valve attached to a sewing ring. Prior to mounting, the valve leaflets are treated with glutaraldehyde, which reduces their antigenicity. These leaflets are stiffer than those on a homograft, because the tissue is nonviable. As a result of this stiffness, incomplete valve opening occurs at low flow rates.

The greatest disadvantage of these valves is their lack of long-term durability. Patient age greatly affects the rate of degeneration, with the highest failure rates occurring in patients under 20 years of age. This is thought to be due to a more active immune reaction to the foreign tissue. Valve failure is generally due to stenosis (cusp calcification), leaflet thickening, leaflet fracturing, or insufficiency (torn leaflets).

Porcine valve degeneration usually occurs gradually, but can also have an acute onset. The valve surface tends to undergo endothelial denudation with basement membrane exposure, leading to the deposition of fibrin, platelet aggregates, activated leukocytes, and small focal calcium deposits. The fixation process also makes the collagen more brittle. Approximately 10% of these valves have some degree of central regurgitation. With mitral annular calcification, the sewing ring may be distorted, leading to regurgitation (Fig. 18.10) (27–35).

### Hancock Porcine Valve

The Hancock valve, a treated stented porcine aortic valve, was the first commercially successful bioprosthetic valve.

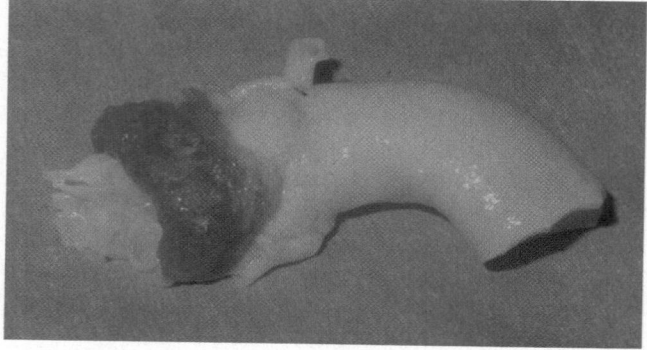

**FIGURE 18.9.** Aortic valve homograft. Please note a portion of the left ventricular outflow tract muscle with the anterior mitral valve leaflet attached along with a section of the ascending aorta.

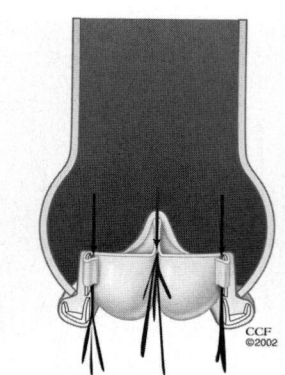

**FIGURE 18.10.** A cross-sectional view of a stented bioprosthetic valve showing the characteristic regurgitant (washing) jets.

It was manufactured in 1970 and is still widely used. It comes in two models, which look alike on echocardiographic exam.

### Carpentier-Edwards Porcine Valve

The Carpentier-Edwards treated aortic porcine valve has been on the market since 1976, and is the most frequently implanted biological valve. The frame is flexible and the sewing ring is saddle-shaped.

### Bovine Pericardial Valves

Pericardial valves make up approximately 40% of the U.S. tissue valve market and 16% of all valves implanted in the U.S. Their first clinical use was in 1971. Bovine pericardial valves are similar to porcine valves; however, the three leaflets are made from bovine pericardium. The advantages over porcine valves include unlimited size and easy modification of valve design.

The most common causes of pericardial valve failure were abrasion of the leaflets by the support frame and leaflet calcification leading to valvular incompetence. Cusp tears tended to occur along the free edges of the cusp and at the leaflet crease. The cloth covering of the stents was believed to cause abrasion of the pericardial commissures and cusps. Cusp perforations were also caused by long suture ends. Calcification of pericardial valves tended to occur in the line of flexion parallel to the annulus (porcine valves tend to become calcified at the commissures) (Fig. 18.11) (36,37).

### Ionescu-Shiley Valve

The Ionescu-Shiley valve is the prototype and was first manufactured in 1976. Premature failure typically occurred after 6 to 8 years. Some of the failures were due to tears occurring along the suture line of the valve leaflets to the stent posts. This valve is no longer commercially available.

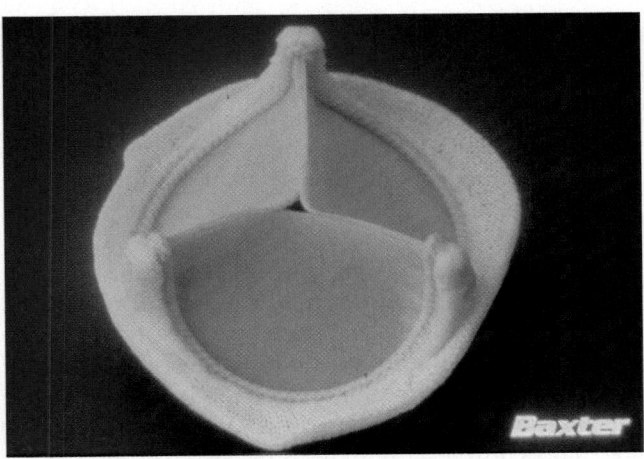

*FIGURE 18.11.* The Baxter pericardial valve.

### Carpentier-Edwards Perimount Valve

The Carpentier-Edwards Perimount pericardial bioprosthesis was introduced clinically in 1981 and approved for commercial use in the U.S. in 1991. It is the only pericardial valve that is commercially available in the United States. Its design is similar to the CE porcine valve, with thicker leaflets. It is made for use in the aortic position and recently for the mitral position. The valve shows a similar durability profile to the porcine valve.

### Stentless Porcine Valves

The Medtronic Freestyle stentless aortic xenograft and the St. Jude Medical Toronto stentless porcine valve (SPV) are the two stentless aortic valves currently available on the U.S. market. The Prima valve is another stentless valve undergoing clinical trials, but it is not yet commercially available.

Because mechanical and stented aortic prostheses are relatively stenotic, the stentless valves were developed in an effort to provide a larger effective orifice area. Benefits of these stentless valves include regression of left ventricular hypertrophy, a factor that has been linked to survival (38–41). Both valves are derived from the porcine aortic root and lack any sewing ring or supporting struts. They have a single layer of polyester covering around the outer base of the valve (Fig. 18.12).

### ECHOCARDIOGRAPHIC EVALUATION OF PROSTHETIC HEART VALVES

Because of the large number of prostheses, a wide range of sizes, and a wide variety of pathologic findings, the echocardiographer must have a good understanding of the appearance and function of the commonly implanted prosthetic heart valves.

A complete examination should include evaluation of:

- Function of the prosthesis
- Chamber size
- Presence of intracardiac densities (e.g., thrombus, vegetations, pannus formation)
- Ventricular function
- Valvular lesions
- Hemodynamic measurements (gradients, effective orifice area)
- Regurgitant jets (normal vs. pathologic)

The 2D and color flow Doppler examination of prosthetic valves can be challenging because of:

- Dense reverberations
- Dense sewing ring
- Sound beam attenuation by prosthesis (flow masking) (43–45)

### NORMAL IMAGING

Prosthetic heart valves have characteristic echo appearances. They produce a certain degree of acoustic shadowing and characteristic reverberations. Acoustic shadowing occurs because of the highly reflective material in prosthetic valves and usually occurs on the opposite side of the prosthesis. Reverberations need to be distinguished from vegetations or thrombus.

The elongated appearance of parts of the prosthesis on the echo exam is due to the differential speed of sound through the dense prosthesis versus through the tissue. The valve's occluding mechanism determines the pattern of flow and shadowing/artifact. The sewing ring should be examined closely for stability (i.e., no rocking motion),

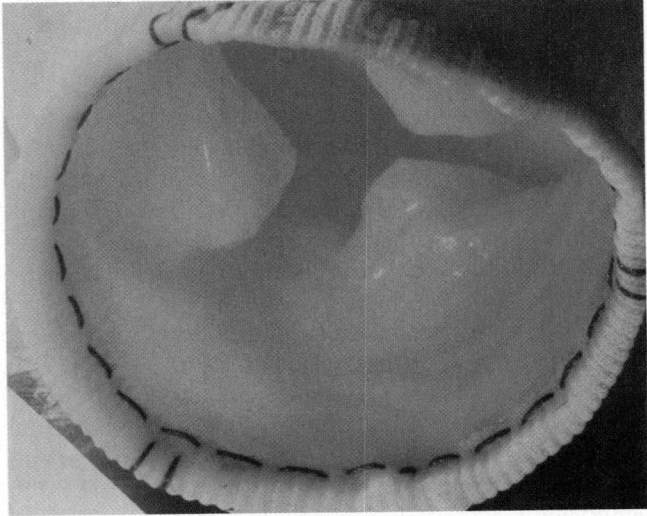

*FIGURE 18.12.* The Medtronic Freestyle stentless aortic valve.

and disc/leaflet/poppet motion should be thoroughly evaluated. All valves should be scanned from multiple views and planes.

Baseline function should be determined after valve replacement prior to hospital discharge (immediate post-cardiopulmonary bypass results may be different from findings prior to hospital discharge). This allows monitoring of valve function over time. The type and size of valve should be documented, as well as previously measured gradients and duration of implantation (46,47).

## HEMODYNAMIC MEASUREMENTS

Normal Doppler hemodynamic measurements for the prosthetic mitral valve include:

- Early peak velocity (E wave) of mitral inflow
- Mean gradient
- End-diastolic gradient
- Pressure half-time
- Estimated valve orifice area
- Tricuspid regurgitation velocity (to estimate PA pressure)

Normal Doppler hemodynamic measurements for the prosthetic aortic valve include:

- Peak and mean gradients
- Dimensionless ratio

### Valve Gradients by CW Doppler

Each valve type and size has its own hemodynamic characteristics. Even though peak and mean valvular gradients are only grossly correlated to the size of the prosthesis, such measurements are important in practice. They can reflect increased stroke work and can be abnormally elevated because of pathologic stenosis/obstruction, a high cardiac output state, increased stroke volume (e.g., regurgitation), or a mismatch between prosthesis size and body size. With the exception of the Starr-Edwards valve, the diameter of the valve is generally the size of the sewing ring. The point to remember is that transvalvular gradients obtained by Doppler are very flow-dependent. With increasing prosthetic valve size there is a notable decrease in peak velocity and mean gradient for all valve types (48,49).

There is a very good correlation between simultaneous Doppler mean and catheter gradients using the simplified Bernoulli equation (50). In a simultaneous Doppler/catheter study, left atrial pressure (LAP) by transseptal puncture correlated well with the mean Doppler gradient; however, pulmonary capillary wedge pressure (PCWP) significantly overestimated the mean gradient in several cases.

Normal prosthetic gradients depend on the size and type of the prosthesis, valve location, and ventricular function. For all measurements, an average of several beats should be taken (especially when there is an irregular cardiac rhythm). Furthermore, measurement of exercise hemodynamics can uncover mild dysfunction, and may augment the differences noted between different prostheses (51,52).

The phenomenon of "pressure recovery" must be considered because it can become a source of error. The point of highest velocity and lowest pressure occurs at the narrowest point in a prosthetic valve or at the vena contracta downstream (minimum jet cross section). Velocity decreases and pressure increases ("pressure recovery") as one moves further from the prosthesis because of re-expansion of flow downstream. The pressure gradient will therefore depend on where the pressure is sampled. "Pressure recovery" is more significant in prosthetic than native valves (especially aortic prostheses). Valve design and size will influence the extent of pressure recovery. As a result, Doppler-derived gradients can be misleading (53). For example, peak velocities should be measured using CW Doppler across a lateral orifice for bileaflet valves. If velocity is measured across a central orifice it may lead to an overestimation of the degree of stenosis.

### Effective Orifice Area

Effective orifice area (EOA) is superior to transvalvular gradients as a measure of prosthetic valve function and performance. All valve prostheses are mildly stenotic and the EOA is always less than the anatomic area. The prosthesis EOA gives a more flow-independent measure of resistance, as with stenotic native valves. Gradients, on the other hand, are more dependent on flow, diastolic filling time, heart rate, valve size, and valve type. Unfortunately, measurement of EOA for mitral prostheses has been imprecise (54–65). For native mitral valves, it is generally measured using the pressure half-time method as described by Hatle (55):

$$EOA = 220/T_{1/2}$$

The pressure half-time method, however, has not been validated for prosthetic valves (mechanical or bioprosthetic), and has been shown in some studies to overestimate the true EOA of mitral bioprostheses (56,66). Pressure half-time probably cannot detect early prosthetic obstruction; however, it can differentiate a high peak velocity secondary to stenosis from that due to a high stroke volume. Increased flow velocity across a prosthetic valve does not always indicate obstruction. For example, a high output state or severe prosthetic regurgitation can cause an increase in velocity. With a mitral prosthesis, the pressure half-time is useful in distinguishing whether an increased gradient (i.e., velocity) is secondary to increased flow or obstruction. Obstruction of an aortic prosthesis will lead to an increased velocity unless the cardiac output is decreased.

Data provided by the manufacturer about pressure and flow suggests that the EOA increases with increasing pressure and flow, and that there is not a unique area for each prosthesis. The explanation for this finding is that bioprosthetic leaflet inertia occurs at low flow. Dumesnil suggests that the overestimation of EOA by pressure half-time seen in most patients with bioprostheses is due to opening inertia of the prosthesis early in diastole, leading to a higher initial gradient and steeper deceleration slope when the valve opens (56). Bileaflet mechanical prostheses, on the other hand, open fully at low flows, with minimal variation in orifice area between valves. Therefore, EOA and measured manufacturer's area should be similar.

For patients with no aortic or mitral regurgitation, and an aortic or mitral prosthesis, the continuity equation can be used:

$$EOA = \frac{(LVOT\ area) \times (LVOT\ TVI)}{(Prosthesis\ TVI)}$$

The continuity equation is the preferred method with prostheses provided there is no significant aortic insufficiency (AI) or mitral regurgitation (MR). Areas calculated with the continuity equation correlate well with areas derived from an in vitro hydraulic model, while those calculated using the pressure half-time method do not (64). Note that TVI must be used in the equation (not velocity) for mitral prostheses, and LVOT area is calculated from the external diameter of the sewing ring for aortic prosthesis calculations. The LVOT diameter is generally within 1 to 2 mm of the external sewing ring diameter (68,69). The simplified continuity equation has been validated for aortic prostheses using velocity in the formula (68,70), however, the software on newer instruments allows for TVI to be easily measured.

An alternate continuity equation method (71) has also been described and can be used in the presence of aortic or mitral regurgitation for mitral or tricuspid prosthesis EOA. The external sewing ring diameter is used to approximate LA diameter near the sewing ring; pulse wave (PW) Doppler is used to measure LA TVI with the sample volume just above the sewing ring; CW Doppler is used to measure MVR TVI:

$$EOA = \frac{(Sewing\ ring\ D)^2 \times (0.785) \times LA\ TVI}{MVR\ TVI}$$

This latter method compares favorably with the standard continuity equation method, but neither compares well with the pressure half-time method.

The PISA (proximal isovelocity surface area) method (72) has also been used to calculate forward flow and estimate the EOA of St. Jude mitral prostheses:

$$Q = \frac{2\Pi r^2\ v_a \cdot v}{v - v_a}$$

and

$$EOA = \frac{Q}{v}$$

where Q, instantaneous flow rate; r, radius from orifice (measured to the level of the prosthetic annulus); $v_a$, aliasing velocity; v, peak transorifice velocity (across lateral orifice of St. Jude prosthesis, measured with CW). $v/(v - v_a)$ is a correction factor for flow underestimation (isotach flattening near orifice secondary to finite size and low transorifice velocity of the prosthesis). The valve orifice is assumed to be at the level of the prosthetic annulus. It is suggested that this method might improve the noninvasive assessment of prosthetic mitral valve obstruction.

The dimensionless ratio, also known as the Doppler velocity index (DVI), velocity ratio (VR), or dimensionless obstructive index (DOI) is the ratio of the velocity or velocity time integral of the LVOT to the aortic prosthesis (68,73).

$$DOI = \frac{v_{LVOT}}{v_{max}}$$

or

$$DOI = \frac{TVI_{LVOT}}{TVI_{prosthesis}}$$

It is useful to help differentiate increased velocity across an aortic prosthesis, which is secondary to obstruction (DOI ≤ 0.25), versus increased velocity due to aortic insufficiency (DOI ≥ 0.3). This ratio remains unchanged unless either the LVOT dimension changes (a less likely occurrence) or the dimension of the prosthetic aortic valve orifice changes.

A double-envelope technique has been described for the evaluation of prosthetic aortic valves. With this method, left ventricular outflow tract velocity and aortic valve velocity are simultaneously obtained from transgastric views using CW Doppler. It was suggested that obtaining subvalvular and valvular peak velocities from the same Doppler trace might reduce the beat-to-beat variability that can occur with nonsimultaneous measurements, and might simplify use of the continuity equation (74).

Three-dimensional (3D) TEE is a newer ultrasonic modality that has been used for quantitative assessment of mechanical prosthetic valve area. Orifice area assess-

▶ **Normal Prosthetic Mean Gradients from the Mayo Clinic Prosthesis Project**

| Mitral Prosthesis | N | Peak Velocity (m/sec) | Mean Gradient (mm Hg) | EOA (cm²) (pressure half-time) | % Valves with Trivial or Mild MR |
|---|---|---|---|---|---|
| Ball-Cage | 161 | 1.8 ± 0.3 | 4.9 ± 1.8 | 2.4 ± 0.7 | 7.5 |
| Bjork-Shiley | 79 | 1.7 ± 0.3 | 4.1 ± 1.6 | 2.6 ± 0.6 | 20.3 |
| Heterograft | 150 | 1.6 ± 0.3 | 4.1 ± 1.5 | 2.3 ± 0.7 | 24.7 |
| St. Jude | 66 | 1.6 ± 0.4 | 4.0 ± 1.8 | 3.0 ± 0.8 | 24.2 |
| Total | 456 | 1.7 ± 0.3 | 4.4 ± 1.7 | 2.5 ± 0.7 | 17.8 |

For all mitral prostheses, as size increases the gradient decreases.

| Aortic Prosthesis | N | Peak Velocity (m/sec) | Mean Gradient (mm Hg) | Dimensionless Obstructive Index |
|---|---|---|---|---|
| Heterograft | 215 | 2.4 ± 0.5 | 13.3 ± 6.1 | 0.42 ± 0.12 |
| Ball-Cage | 158 | 3.2 ± 0.6 | 22.8 ± 8.6 | 0.32 ± 0.09 |
| Bjork-Shiley | 142 | 2.5 ± 0.6 | 13.7 ± 7.0 | 0.40 ± 0.10 |
| St. Jude | 74 | 2.6 ± 0.6 | 15.1 ± 7.3 | 0.39 ± 0.10 |
| Homograft | 33 | 1.9 ± 0.4 | 7.8 ± 2.7 | 0.56 ± 0.12 |
| Medtronic Hall | 24 | 2.6 ± 0.4 | 15.1 ± 5.2 | 0.39 ± 0.08 |
| Total | 646 | 2.6 ± 0.7 | 15.7 ± 8.2 | 0.39 ± 0.12 |

With the exception of the ball-cage prostheses, prosthetic aortic gradients decreased with increasing valve size.

| Tricuspid Prosthesis | N | Peak Velocity (m/sec) | Mean Gradient (mm Hg) | Pressure Half-Time (msec) | % Valves with Trivial or Mild TR |
|---|---|---|---|---|---|
| Heterograft | 43 | 1.3 ± 0.2 | 3.2 ± 1.1 | 145 ± 37 | 20.9 |
| Ball-Cage | 35 | 1.3 ± 0.2 | 3.2 ± 0.8 | 140 ± 48 | 8.6 |
| St. Jude | 7 | 1.2 ± 0.3 | 2.7 ± 1.1 | 108 ± 32 | 28.6 |
| Bjork-Shiley | 1 | 1.3 | 2.2 | 144 | 0 |
| Total | 86 | 1.3 ± 0.2 | 3.1 ± 1.0 | 140 ± 42 (N = 69) | 16.3 |

For tricuspid prostheses, respiratory variation accounted for average differences between maximum and minimum values for peak velocity (0.5 ± 0.2 m/sec), mean gradient (0.3 ± 0.2 mm Hg), and pressure half-time (81.6 ± 36.9 msec) (76–78).

ment by 3D TEE offers the advantage of being independent of flow, heart rate, MR, AI, systolic, and diastolic LV function. Further study is warranted with this newer technology (75).

## Prosthetic Valve Regurgitation

Degree of prosthetic aortic regurgitation is difficult to assess by color flow Doppler. For aortic prostheses, a low pressure half-time (≤ 250 msec), a restrictive mitral inflow pattern, an increased LVOT velocity (> 1.5 m/sec), and diastolic flow reversal in the aorta are suggestive of severe aortic regurgitation. For a mitral prosthesis, a normal pressure half-time (≥ 150 msec), reversal of flow in the pulmonary veins, and an increased peak inflow velocity (≥ 2.5 m/sec) are suggestive of severe mitral regurgitation.

## ECHOCARDIOGRAPHIC CHARACTERISTICS OF SPECIFIC VALVE TYPES

Unless otherwise specified, the descriptions below will focus on prosthetic valves in the mitral position.

### Starr-Edwards Valve

During diastole, blood entering the left ventricle goes around the ball. The ring, tip of the cage, and the leading and trailing edges of the ball give off strong echoes. In systole, the trailing edge of the ball has an artifactual elongated appearance with a large portion extending outside the cage (into the left atrium). The ring can be seen, as can the tip of the cage, the leading edge of the ball within the cage, and the trailing edge of the ball. In diastole, reverberations from the prosthesis are seen in the left ventricle.

The "closing volume" of the prosthesis is the volume displaced by the ball in early systole as the ball moves towards the sewing ring. This is seen as a small central early systolic regurgitant volume in the left atrium. This needs to be distinguished from pathologic regurgitation which is holosystolic. CW gradients should be measured around the periphery of the ball where flow velocities are the highest.

Echocardiography has been used to detect cloth cover tears in the fully covered Starr-Edwards valve (61) (Fig. 18.13). Such tears appeared as elongated echogenic masses attached to the cage and floating downstream, with normal transvalvular gradients (79).

## Disc Valves

### Bjork-Shiley Valve

During systole, when the disc closes, a characteristic rectangular reverberation is seen in the left ventricle. In diastole, there is flow across the major and minor orifices of the valve, with convergence of the two jets into one as they pass the tip of the disc.

In this valve, only peripheral regurgitant jets are seen (only one disc without a central hole). The jets are narrow (< 10 mm) and short (< 30 mm). Knowledge of the specific type of Bjork-Shiley valve is important as "normal" jet sizes differ (Fig. 18.14; see also Fig. 18.5B) (80–83).

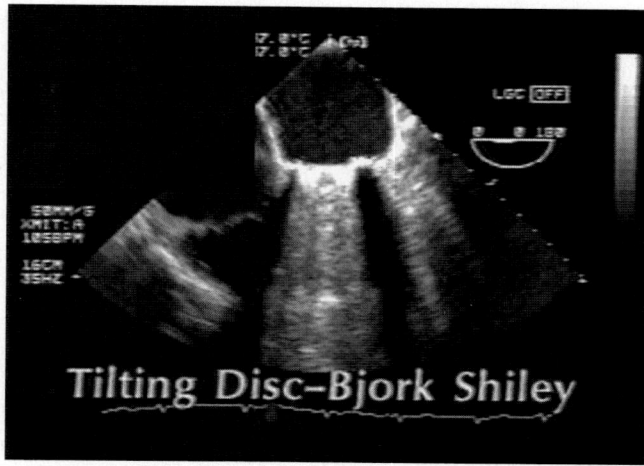

**FIGURE 18.14.** Tilting-disc valve in the mitral position showing reverberation and acoustic shadowing artifacts.

### Medtronic-Hall Valve

The ring, which is located just inside the mitral annulus, causes acoustic shadowing (increased echogenicity adjacent to the annulus). The strut is seen as a strong echo dot with side lobes just above the annulus level between the dot and the ring. The disc is seen as a strong echo line in the left ventricle. Disc reverberations are more prominent in systole.

There are usually two peripheral jets and one central regurgitant jet. The central jet originates at the small gap formed between the strut and central hole of the disc. Peripheral jets occur at the gap between the ring and disc. These "normal" regurgitant jets are usually small and narrow. These washing jets eliminate stagnation on the underside of the valve.

## Bileaflet Valves

### St. Jude Valve

Regurgitant jets in the St. Jude valve occur at the hinge points. There is one central jet and two peripheral jets. The central jet is due to the gap between the disc leaflets. Color flow Doppler mapping of the St. Jude valve shows regurgitant flow at the periphery (between the disc and sewing ring) and centrally (between the leaflets). These jets are three-dimensional, and therefore can appear convergent or divergent, depending on the imaging plane. The CW Doppler beam should be directed through the lateral orifices of the valve. The phenomenon of "pressure recovery" (see above) occurs across St. Jude prostheses and can lead to an overestimation of the true valve gradient when the central orifice is used. This occurs because some of the gradient recorded by Doppler is "recovered" as flow emerges from the valve. Pressure recovery is limited to the central orifice of the valve (85). The gradient

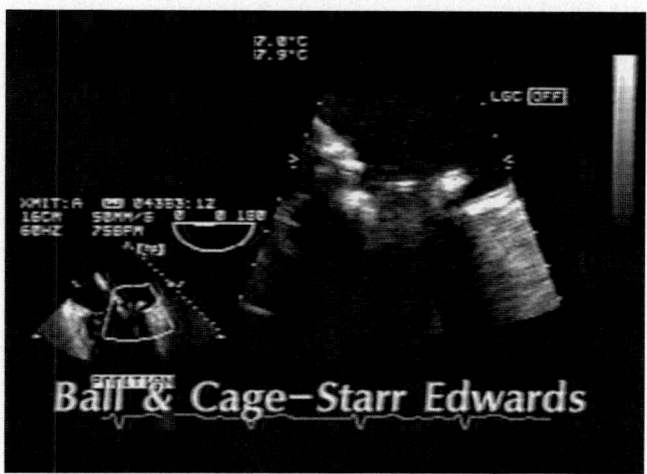

**FIGURE 18.13.** Starr-Edwards valve in the mitral position.

measured across the central orifice can be 40%–50% higher than that measured across the lateral orifices, which are the preferred measurement sites (Figs. 18.15, 18.16, and 18.9) (84,85).

## CarboMedics Valve

Color flow Doppler of the CarboMedics valve normally shows four washing jets, one on either side of each pivot point. One jet is often more prominent than the others. Regurgitant jets are more significant compared to the St. Jude valve (86–88).

## Stented Bioprosthetic Valves

Valve stents are usually oriented towards the septum in a mitral prosthesis. It is important to look for extraneous echoes, leaflet excursion, leaflet thickening, leaflet prolapse/flail, and stability of the sewing ring. It is also important to make sure the stents do not create an obstruction by impinging upon the left ventricular outflow tract. Perimount bovine pericardial valves have prominent washing jets (central where the three leaflets coapt and between the leaflets where they attach to the sewing ring), which may be considered excessive if you are not familiar with the normal color flow of this valve (Figs. 18.11, 18.17, and 18.18) (89–90).

## Stentless Bioprosthetic Valves

Depending on the method of valve implantation, the echocardiographic appearance of stentless aortic bioprostheses will vary. If the valve has been implanted using a subcoronary or root inclusion technique (where the bioprosthesis is within the native aortic root), a space can be

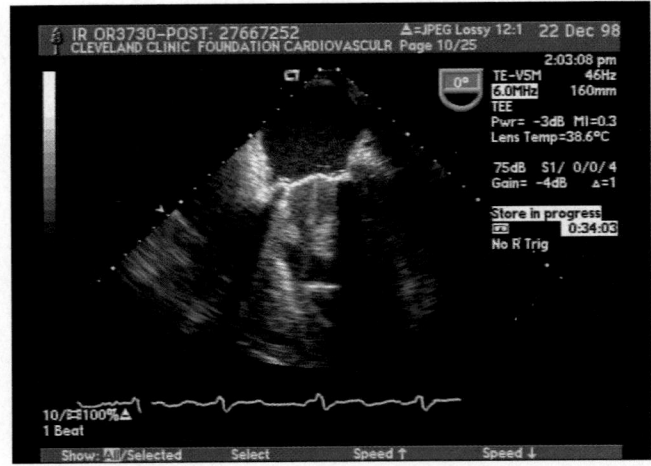

**FIGURE 18.16.** Closed bileaflet valve in the mitral position. Notice the acoustic shadowing and reverberation artifacts.

detected between the native aortic wall and the porcine aortic wall. This is a normal finding, provided there is no detectable color flow within this space. The presence of color flow within this space is suggestive of a dehiscence of the proximal or distal suture line. This space generally disappears within 6 months when the porcine wall becomes fully adherent to the native aortic wall. If the valve has been implanted using the root replacement technique, the coronary ostia are reimplanted. In this case, the echocardiographic appearance is very similar to that of an aortic valve homograft (38,91).

### Aortic Valve Homografts

The unstented homografts placed in the aortic position are nearly identical in appearance and flow characteris-

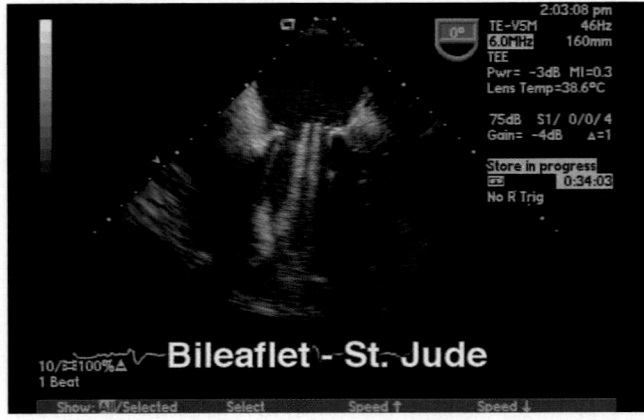

**FIGURE 18.15.** Open bileaflet valve in the mitral position. Notice the acoustic shadowing and reverberation artifacts in the left ventricular cavity.

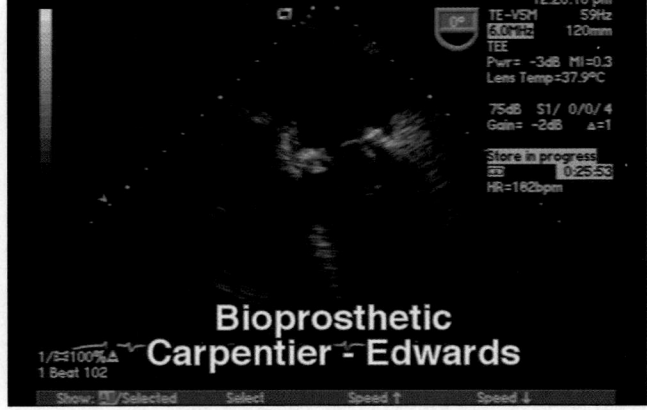

**FIGURE 18.17.** Bioprosthetic Carpentier-Edwards valve in the mitral position. A thin leaflet can be seen along the lateral wall and a strut in the left ventricular cavity.

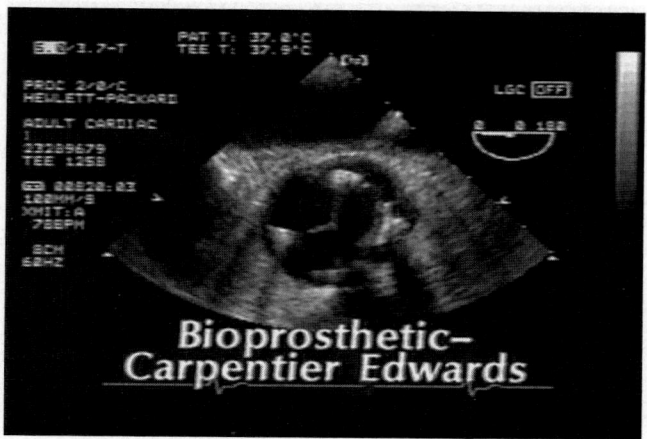

**FIGURE 18.18.** Bioprosthetic Carpentier-Edwards valve in the aortic position. You can see the three cusps, which are closed, and the three struts with the annular ring around the valve.

tics to the native aortic valve. In a normally functioning aortic valve homograft the only distinguishing echocardiographic feature is an increase in echo density around the suture line.

## PROSTHETIC VALVE DYSFUNCTION AND COMPLICATIONS

### Prosthetic Valve Stenosis

Compared to native valves, prosthetic valves are relatively obstructive, with the degree of obstruction being a function of valve type and size. Because there is such a wide range of normal velocities across prosthetic valves, the diagnosis of prosthetic valve stenosis can prove challenging.

Degree of stenosis is generally assessed by measuring: peak velocity, mean velocity, velocity time integral, valve area (pressure half-time), and effective valve orifice area (continuity equation and Gorlin formula) for mitral prostheses. For aortic prostheses, peak and mean velocities, velocity time integral, and dimensionless ratio are measured. Even though Doppler gradients can be indicative of prosthetic valve obstruction, one must keep in mind that transvalvular gradients obtained by Doppler are very flow-dependent. Prosthetic orifice area gives a more flow-independent measure of resistance, as with stenotic native valves.

In order to determine if a prosthetic valve is stenotic, it is best to compare Doppler-derived estimates of gradients or valve areas to the expected value for a valve of particular size and type. When a prosthetic valve has been implanted, a baseline echocardiographic study should be obtained prior to hospital discharge. Gradient values can be used for future follow-up comparison. Measurements and calculations should be made in the same manner,

specifying the method and mathematical formula employed. Trends and deviation from baseline values may be more revealing than absolute numbers. And of course, 2D echo information can provide information on the etiology of prosthetic valvular stenosis (92,93).

Thrombosis and pannus formation are the most common causes of prosthetic valve stenosis in mechanical valves (94,95). Pannus formation is fibroconnective tissue ingrowth from the sewing ring and typically occurs after many years of valve implantation. It can interfere with valve closure and opening by impinging on the hinge mechanism of a mechanical valve. This can lead to flow obstruction (restricted opening) or regurgitation (restricted closure). Its formation is unaffected by routine anticoagulation. Obstruction with normal disc motion has also been demonstrated in a patient with a Bjork-Shiley aortic prosthesis who developed annular pannus ingrowth (96). Stenosis can also be due to an undersized prosthesis or other structural problems, such as the leaflet being stuck in the closed position.

Acute disc or leaflet immobilization has been described in mechanical prostheses (97–102). Restricted occluder motion can be complete, partial, or intermittent. The occluder may be fixed in the open or closed position. If sutures are not cut short enough, or become unraveled, they can get caught in the valve housing and cause sticking. Mitral chordal remnants and even the left ventricular wall can interfere with proper disc/leaflet motion. Left ventricular outflow tract obstruction can occur with retention of the anterior mitral leaflet during mitral valve replacement. With ball-cage valves, one can see ball variance, where the ball swells and becomes partially stuck in the cage.

Identification of thrombus on a prosthetic valve can be difficult, especially if it is nonobstructive. TEE can be used to monitor thrombolysis of thrombosed prosthetic valves (103–106). TEE can help assess thrombus size, location, and aid in treatment decisions, such as thrombolysis, anticoagulation, and surgery.

Opening angle can sometimes be measured. The echocardiographer should have an understanding of normal occluder motion for each type of prosthesis (Figs. 18.19–18.21).

### Prosthetic Valve Regurgitation

Because of the location of the TEE transducer behind the left atrium, prosthetic mitral regurgitation can be well-visualized with color flow Doppler (107–114). TEE is far superior to TTE (115) in the evaluation of prosthetic mitral regurgitation (28% vs. 95% mitral, 29% vs. 44% aortic). Prosthetic aortic regurgitation originating from the posterior side of the prosthesis can be well appreciated by TEE, while anteriorly located aortic insufficiency may be

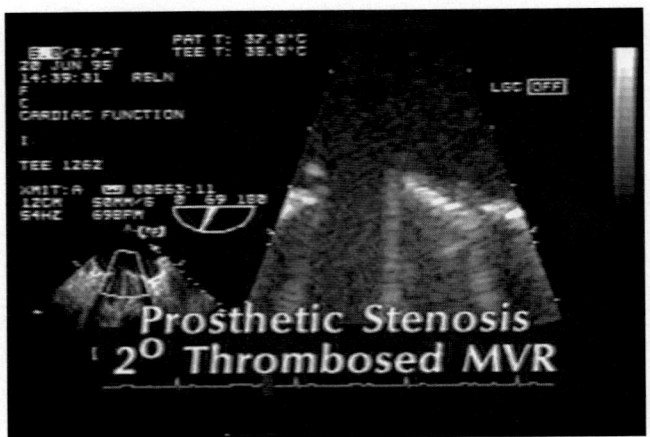

**FIGURE 18.19.** A St. Jude mitral valve with one leaflet in the open position and the other leaflet in the closed position secondary to thrombosis.

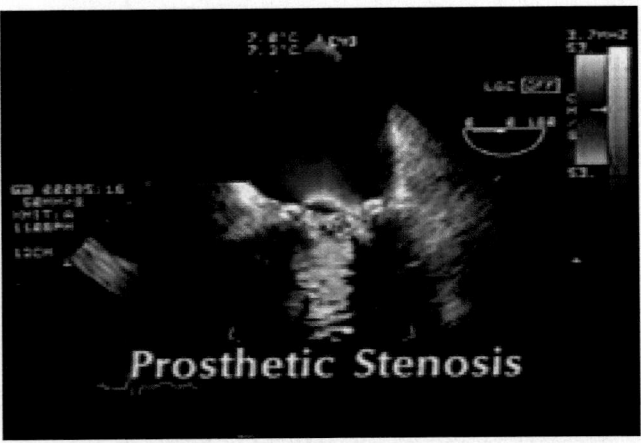

**FIGURE 18.21.** Prosthetic stenosis of a bioprosthetic valve. Note the large PISA on the left atrial side of the valve indicating severe prosthetic stenosis

difficult to visualize, especially if there is shadowing from a mitral prosthetic valve or ring, or dense mitral annular calcification.

An understanding of normal prosthetic regurgitation is necessary. "Normal" regurgitant jets are short, narrow, flame-like, laminar, and of low velocity. This type of regurgitation can be subdivided into two categories based on timing of flow. "Closure backflow" occurs during valve closure, as the prosthetic disc or ball displaces blood into the left atrium for a mitral prosthesis. "Leakage backflow" can be transvalvular or paravalvular, and occurs after valve closure (116). With the exception of the Starr-Edwards caged ball prosthesis, which demonstrates only closure backflow jets, all mechanical prostheses show some degree of closure and leakage backflow due to their

design. Leakage backflow occurs at hinge points, around struts, or between the ring and central occluder (117). Most often these regurgitant jets are of no hemodynamic significance. Pathologic jets tend to show increased color variance, and are longer and broader than normal physiologic jets.

Regurgitation can be quantified by examining volume of color jet in LA, density of CW signal, PISA on ventricular side of regurgitant orifice, and systolic reversal of flow in pulmonary vein(s). Flow convergence should be looked for on the ventricular side of the regurgitant prosthesis (72). This proximal flow acceleration is indicative of significant valvular regurgitation.

Regurgitation can be perivalvular, transvalvular, or a combination of both. Both etiologies can lead to shearing of red blood cells and intravascular hemolysis (see below). It is more commonly seen with mechanical than biological prostheses, and is believed to be due in part to the inflexibility of the mechanical valve annulus. Endocarditis is also an important cause of periprosthetic leaks and should be ruled out.

With valvular regurgitation secondary to prosthetic valve dehiscence, there is a rocking motion of the prosthesis at its site of attachment. A perivalvular leak originates at the junction of the annulus and prosthetic sewing ring. Systolic and diastolic flows should be sought across a suspected periprosthetic defect.

Preservation of the mitral subvalvular apparatus during mitral valve replacement is commonly performed, and has been associated with improved long-term survival and better preservation of left ventricular function (118). Mitral regurgitation secondary to obstruction of a St. Jude mitral prosthesis by entrapment of preserved subvalvular mitral tissue several years after implant has been described (119).

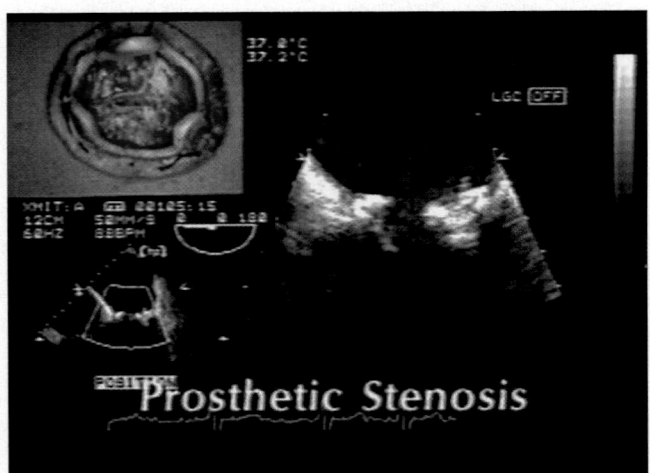

**FIGURE 18.20.** The stenosis of a mitral CE valve. It shows calcification and thickening of the leaflets.

Surgical technique has also been implicated, especially with the use of running, small-sized sutures (leads to suture fracture). Over- and undersizing of the valve can lead to valve dehiscence, as can severe annular calcification, which makes suture placement and proper valve seating difficult. In some instances, the surgeon will bend the prosthetic ring to make it fit.

Disc escape or embolization, most commonly associated with the Bjork-Shiley valve, has been described for several mechanical prostheses and is generally a fatal complication (Figs. 18.22–18.24) (120,121).

With bioprostheses, transvalvular regurgitation is usually due to cusp degeneration. With mechanical valve, transvalvular regurgitation may be caused by a thrombus, which prevents proper mechanical disc motion or proper seating of the valve poppet; it may also be caused by variance in the shape of the mechanical ball or disc.

Immediately after prosthetic valve insertion, perivalvular leaks are frequently seen. Most leaks usually disappear in approximately 2 weeks when the sewing ring has become endothelialized. Some jets decrease in size after insertion with the reversal of heparin with protamine following cardiopulmonary bypass.

## Prosthetic Valve Endocarditis (PVE)

Prosthetic valve endocarditis is a devastating complication of valve replacement. Early detection and treatment rely on accurate diagnosis. TEE is considered the best approach for defining anatomic valve abnormalities, dysfunction, periprosthetic leak, fistulous communications, and abscess formation. The sensitivity of TEE in the detection of PVE is 85%–90% (five times more sensitive than TTE). With TTE, reverberations from the prosthesis

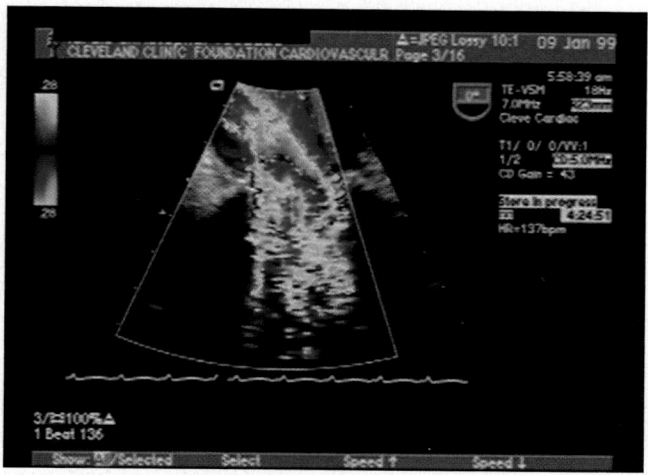

**FIGURE 18.23.** This image shows the regurgitation secondary to loss of the single-disc valve.

make it very difficult to see vegetations. TEE is indicated in all patients suspected of having PVE.

Vegetations are seen as echodense, mobile, "shaggy" appearing structures representing infected material containing bacteria, fibrin, platelets, and white and red blood cells. The rate of PVE is similar between mechanical and biological prostheses. Ring abscesses and septal muscle abscesses are more common in prosthetic valvular than native valvular endocarditis. All parts of the prosthesis must be inspected for vegetations and disruption. The initial infective growth tends to occur on the sewing ring of mechanical valves. Bioprosthetic valves tend to have vegetations on diseased or disrupted leaflets.

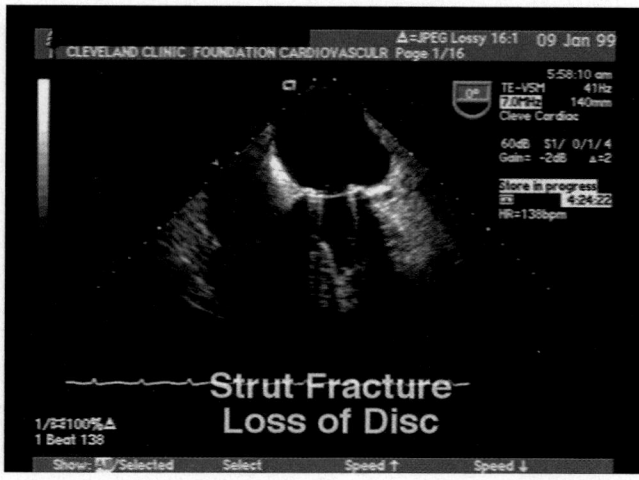

**FIGURE 18.22.** This image shows a single-disc mitral valve in which the disc is absent and the picture shows the annular ring with an echo lucency where the disc should be.

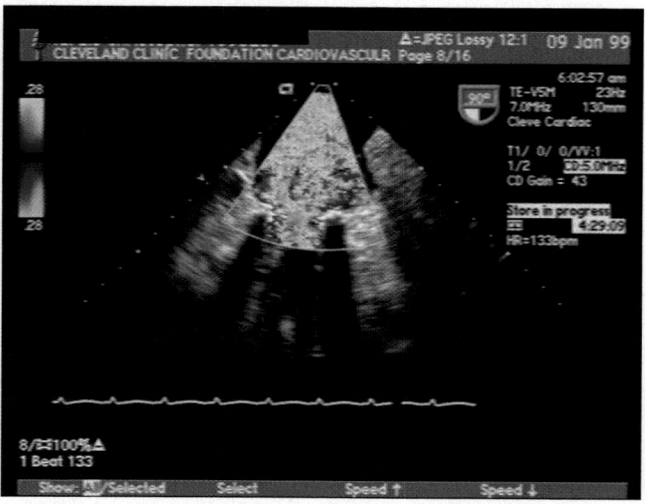

**FIGURE 18.24.** This image shows the regurgitation secondary to loss of the single-disc valve.

Differentiation of thrombus from vegetation (diagnosis based on clinical picture) can be quite difficult, particularly with mechanical valves and small lesions. The entire perivalvular region must be scanned to rule out multicentric abscesses. A torn or disrupted sewing ring cloth can be mistaken for vegetations.

A perivalvular abscess has the appearance of an echolucent or echodense region within the annulus or perivalvular tissue. Early on, a perivalvular abscess may appear homogeneous. Later, necrosis can lead to an echolucent and heterogeneous appearance. Some abscesses may be multicentric; some may form fistulae with other cardiac chambers or vascular spaces (best seen with color flow Doppler). Systolic motion of an abscess cavity is suggestive of communication with a cardiac chamber or great vessel. Color flow Doppler imaging facilitates the diagnosis of such communications (Figs. 18.25–18.28) (122–127).

## Structural Abnormalities

Fibrin strands are often seen on otherwise structurally and functionally normal prostheses. They are more commonly seen on the atrial side of St. Jude mechanical valves and are not clearly associated with endocarditis, thrombosis, or embolization (128,129). Their etiology, incidence, and significance remain unclear, and many still consider them a potential source of embolization (130). In one report, a strand from a degenerated mitral bioprosthetic valve was analyzed and found to consist of a sparsely cellular component with extracellular amorphous of fibrillary areas (predominantly collagen) (131). Valvular strands have also been detected during thrombolytic therapy, suggesting a fibrotic or thrombotic origin.

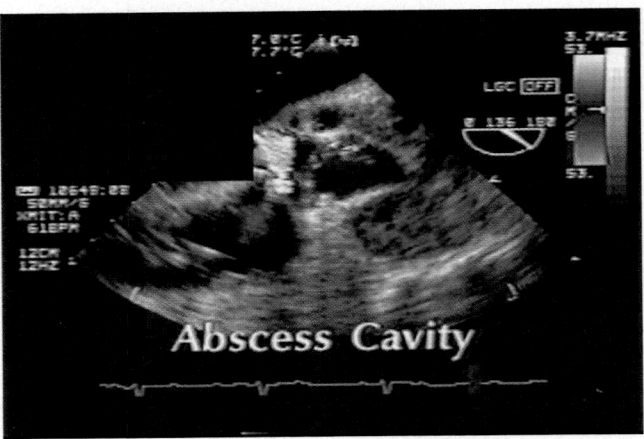

**FIGURE 18.26.** This image shows aortic regurgitation secondary to this abscess of the aortic homograft.

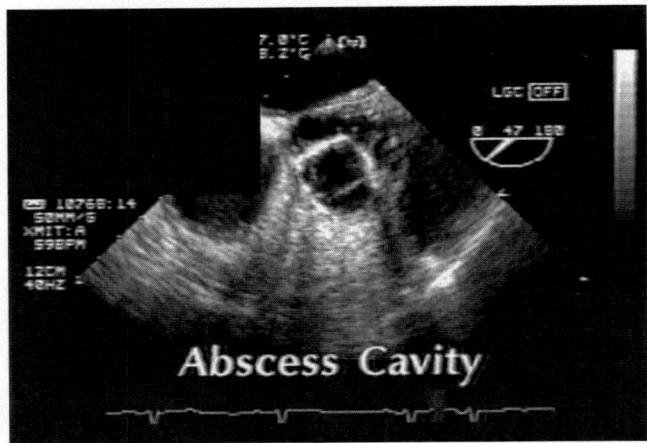

**FIGURE 18.27.** This image shows a cross section of the infected abscessed aortic homograft. Superiorly you may see part of the ring abscessed cavity.

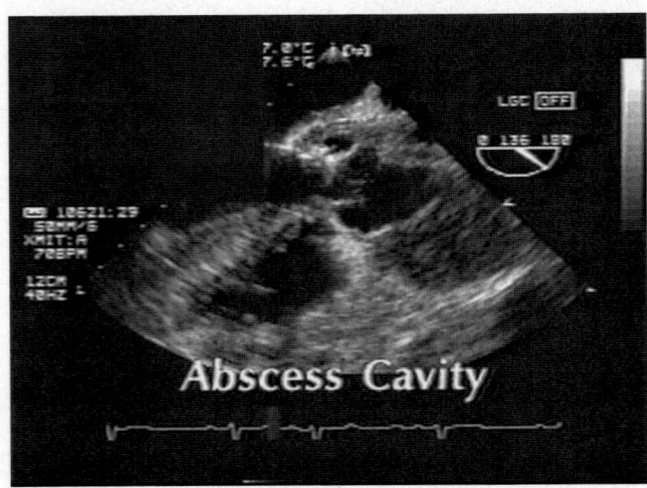

**FIGURE 18.25.** This image shows an abscess cavity with a ring abscess around an aortic homograft.

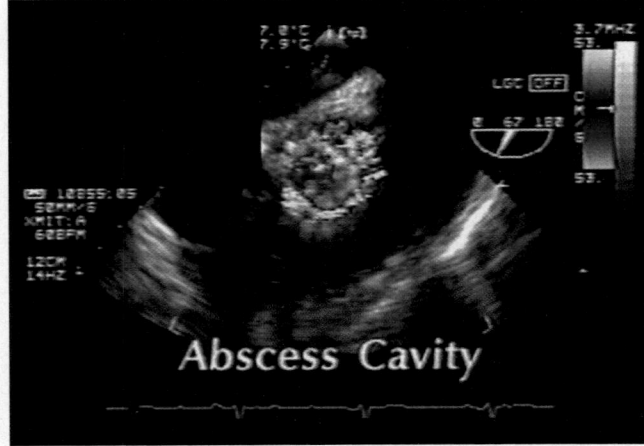

**FIGURE 18.28.** This image shows the cross-sectional view of the infected abscess cavity and aortic homograft and the color shows the ring abscess around this valve.

## ASSOCIATED COMPLICATIONS

### Thromboembolism

Thromboembolism continues to be one of the major drawbacks of mechanical prostheses. It includes systemic emboli, nonhemorrhagic strokes, and transient ischemic attacks. It is believed to be due to a combination of flow stasis at hinge points and the sewing ring, and a lack of endothelialization (132).

A number of factors contribute to this complication including adequacy of anticoagulation, atrial fibrillation, low cardiac output, multiple valve replacement, endocarditis, and previous history of thromboembolism.

### Hemorrhage

Hemorrhage is generally related to anticoagulation.

### Hemolysis

Hemolysis from prosthetic regurgitation is related to high shear stress, which is in turn related to the configuration of the resulting flow disturbance. Regurgitant flow patterns seen in patients with hemolysis secondary to a mitral prosthesis have been shown to be associated with rapid acceleration/deceleration, high peak shear rates, or both. (In vitro shear stresses > 3000 dynes/cm$^2$ can cause red blood cell destruction.) The site of origin of the flow disturbance (central vs. paravalvular) and type of prosthesis are less important than the nature of the flow disturbance produced by the regurgitant lesion and the resulting increased shear stress.

The development of hemolytic anemia with valve prostheses has been attributed to high shear stresses, pressure fluctuations, turbulent flow, the interaction of red blood cells with foreign surfaces, and abnormalities of the red cell membrane. Perivalvular regurgitant jets can denude an endothelialized prosthesis, exposing its foreign surface and increasing the risk of hemolysis. With the early ball-cage valves, the incidence of hemolysis was as high as 6% to 15%. Improved design reduced this frequency. Hemolysis is more significant with malfunctioning prostheses than normal prostheses.

Evidence suggests that acceleration and deceleration may be important causes of hemolysis, the absence of a perivalvular leak does not preclude the development of clinical hemolysis, and hemolysis is not related to the severity of mitral regurgitation. Collision with rapid deceleration was the most common pattern associated with hemolysis. Regurgitation through small single or multiple orifices, and flow fragmentation or collision were associated with more hemolysis than flow through larger single orifices. This was thought to be due to the greater flow acceleration across smaller orifices. Collision with rapid deceleration was found to be the most common mechanism associated with hemolysis (133).

### KEY POINTS

- The echocardiographic evaluation of prosthetic heart valves is complex and requires a thorough knowledge of the different types of valves available, how they function, and their echocardiographic appearance during normal function and dysfunction.
- The echocardiographic examination of all prosthetic valves can be limited by acoustic shadowing and reverberations by the echo-dense areas of the valve.
- TEE and TTE are complementary in the evaluation of all prosthetic heart valves.
- Causes of prosthetic valve dysfunction include: degeneration, thrombosis, dehiscence, obstruction, and infection.
- The Doppler examination of prosthetic valves can be used to assess gradients, keeping in mind that each type of valve has its own degree of obstruction, and that gradients are highly dependent on valve type, size, location, flow, and cardiac function.
- Effective orifice area is a superior measure of prosthetic valve performance compared to transvalvular gradients because it is a flow-independent measurement.
- All prosthetic valves (with perhaps the exception of stentless porcine valves and aortic homografts) are relatively stenotic compared to native valves, and have distinct "normal" regurgitant flow patterns.

## REFERENCES

1. Huffnagel CA, Harvey WP. The surgical correction of aortic insufficiency. Bull Georgetown U Med Cent 1953;6:60.
2. Murray G. Homologous aortic-valve-segment transplants as surgical treatment for aortic and mitral insufficiency. Angiology 1956;7:466.
3. Starr A, Edwards ML. Mitral replacement: clinical experience with a ball valve prosthesis. Ann Surg 1961;154:726–40.
4. Grunkemeier GL, Starr A, Rahimtoola SH. Prosthetic heart valve performance: Long-term follow-up. Curr Probl Cardiol 1992;17:335–406.
5. Whittlesey D, Geha AS. Selection and complications of cardiac valvular prostheses. In Baue AE, Geha AS, Hammond GL, Laks H, Naunheim, eds. Glenn's thoracic and cardiovascular surgery. Appleton and Lange CN: 1991:1719–28.
6. Pluth JR. The Starr-Edwards mitral valve. In Ionescu MI, Cohn LH, eds. Mitral valve disease: diagnosis and treatment. London: Butterworth and Co. (Publishers) Ltd., 1985:217–20.
7. Lepley D Jr, Flemma RJ, Mullen DC. The Bjork-Shiley tilting disc valve in the mitral position. In Ionescu MI, Cohn LH, eds. Mitral valve disease: diagnosis and treatment. London: Butterworth and Co. (Publishers) Ltd., 1985:221–32.

8. Lindblom D, Bjork VO, Semb BKH. Mechanical failure of the Bjork-Shiley valve. Incidence, clinical presentation, and management. J Thorac Cardiovasc Surg 1986;92:894–907.

9. Sugita T, Yasuda R, Watarida S, Onoe M, Tabata R, Mori A. Minor strut fracture of the Bjork-Shiley mitral valve. Nippon Kyobu Geka Zasshi 1990;38:1049–52.

10. Bjork VO, Lindblom D, Henze A. The monostrut strength. Scand J Thorac Cardiovasc Surg 1985;19:13–19.

11. Matloff JM, Chaux A, Czer LSC, DeRobertis MA, Gray RJ. A four year experience with the St. Jude mitral valve prosthesis. In Ionescu MI, Cohn LH, eds. Mitral valve disease: diagnosis and treatment. London: Butterworth and Co. (Publishers) Ltd., 1985:233–4.

12. Heimbecker RO, Baird RJ, Lajox TZ, et al. Homograft replacement of the human mitral valve: a preliminary report. J Can Med Assoc 1962;86:805.

13. Ross DN. Homograft replacement of the aortic valve. Lancet 1962;2:487.

14. Duran CMG, Gunning AJ. A method for placing a total homologous aortic valve in the subcoronary position. Lancet 1962;2:488.

15. Binet JP, Duran CMG, Carpentier A, Langlois J. Heterologous aortic valve transplantation. Lancet 1965;2:1275.

16. Carpentier A, Lemaigre G, Robert L, Carpentier S, Dubost C. Biological factors affecting long term results of valvular heterografts. J Thorac Cardiovasc Surg 1969;58:467–83.

17. Reis RL, Hancock WD, Yarbrough JW, Glancy DL, Morrow AG. The flexible stent: A new concept in the fabrication of tissue heart valve prostheses. J Thorac Cardiovasc Surg 1971;62:683–9.

18. Reardon MJ, Oury JH. Evolving experience with cryopreserved mitral valve allografts. Curr Opin Cardiol 1998;13:85–90.

19. Kumar AS, Kumar DA, Chander H, Saxena A. Experience with homograft mitral valve replacement. J Heart Valve Dis 1998;7:225–8.

20. Acar C. Mitral valve homograft. Adv Card Surg 1997;9:1–13.

21. Vrandecic M, Gontijo B, Fantini F. Homograft replacement of the mitral valve. J Thorac Cardiovasc Surg 1996;112:678–9.

22. Reardon MJ, Oury JH. Evolving experience with cryopreserved mitral allografts. Curr Opin Cardiol 1998;13:85–90.

23. Yacoub M, Rasmi NRH, Sundt TM, et al. Fourteen year experience with homovital homografts for aortic valve replacement. J Thorac Cardiovasc Surg 1995;110:186–94.

24. Cohen DJ, Myerowitz PD, Young WP, et al. The fate of aortic valve homografts 12 to 17 years after implantation. Chest 1988;93:482–4.

25. Kirklin JK, Smith D, Novick W, et al. Long-term function of cryopreserved aortic homografts: A ten year study. J Thorac Cardiovasc Surg 1993;106:154–66.

26. Oury JH. Clinical aspects of the Ross procedure: Indications and contraindications. Semin Thorac Surg 1996;65:496–502.

27. DiSesa VJ, Collins JJ Jr, Cohn LH. Mitral valve replacement with the porcine bioprosthesis. In Ionescu MI, Cohn L, eds. Mitral valve disease: diagnosis and treatment. London: Butterworth and Co. (Publishers) Ltd., 1985:243–52.

28. Jones M, Rodriguez ER, Eidbo EE, Ferrans VJ. Cuspal perforations caused by long suture ends in implanted bioprosthetic valves. J Thorac Cardiovasc Surg 1985;90:557–63.

29. Orszulak TA, Schaff HV, Danielson GK, Pluth JR, Puga FJ, Piehler JM. Results of reoperation for periprosthetic leakage. Ann Thorac Surg 1983;35:584–9.

30. Thiene G, Bortolotti U, Valente M, et al. Mode of failure of the Hancock pericardial valve xenograft. Am J Cardiol 1989;63:129–33.

31. Riddle JM, Magilligan DJ, Stein PD. Surface morphology of degenerated porcine bioprosthetic valves four to seven years following implantation. J Thorac Cardiovasc Surg 1981;81:279–87.

32. Ishihara T, Ferrans VJ, Boyce SW, Jones M, Roberts WC. Structure and classification of cuspal tears and perforations in porcine bioprosthetic cardiac valves implanted in patients. Am J Cardiol 1981;48:665–78.

33. Thubrikar MJ, Deck JD, Aouad J, Nolan SP. Role of mechanical stress in calcification of aortic bioprosthetic valves. J Thorac Cardiovasc Surg 1983;86:115–25.

34. Magilligan DJ, Lewis JW Jr, Tilley B, Peterson E. The porcine bioprosthetic valve: twelve years later. J Thorac Cardiovasc Surg 1985;89:499–507.

35. Curcio CA, Commerford PJ, Rose AG, Stevens JE, Barnard MS. Calcification of glutaraldehyde-preserved porcine xenografts in young patients. J Thorac Cardiovasc Surg 1981; 81:621–5.

36. Kopf GS, Geha AS, Hellerbrand WE. Fate of left-sided cardiac bioprosthesis valves in children. Arch Surg 1986;121:488–90.

37. Ionescu MI, Silverton NP, Tandon AP. The pericardial xenograft in the mitral position. In Ionescu MI, Cohn LH, eds. Mitral valve disease: diagnosis and treatment. London: Butterworth and Co. (Publishers) Ltd., 1985:243–52.

38. Bach DS. Echocardiographic assessment of stentless aortic bioprosthetic valves. J Am Soc Echocardiogr 2000;13:941–8.

39. Del Rizzo DF, Abdoh A. Clinical and hemodynamic comparison of the Medtronic Freestyle and Toronto SPV stentless valves. J Card Surg 1998;13:398–407.

40. Jin XY, Westaby S, Gibson DG, Pillai R, Taggart DP. Left ventricular remodeling and improvement in Freestyle stentless valve haemodynamics. Eur J Cardiothorac Surg 1997;12:63–9.

41. Pibarot P, Dumesnil JG, Leblanc MH, Cartier P, Metras J. Changes in left ventricular mass and function after aortic valve replacement: A comparison between stentless and stented bioprosthetic valves. J Am Soc Echocardiogr 1999; 12:981–7.

42. Chen W, Schoen FJ, Levy RJ. Mechanism of efficacy of 2–amino oleic acid for inhibition of calcification of glutaraldehyde-pretreated porcine bioprosthetic heart valves. Circulation 1994;90:323–9.

43. Feigenbaum H. Acquired valvular heart disease: prosthetic valves. In Feigenbaum H, ed. Echocardiography, 5th ed., 1993: 297–314.

44. Oka Y, Kato M, Strom J. Mitral valve. In Oka Y, Goldiner PL, eds. Transesophageal echocardiography. Philadelphia: JB Lippincott Co., 1992:99–151.

45. Clements FM, de Bruijn NP. Interventional echocardiography and the mitral valve. In Clements FM, de Bruijn NP, eds. Transesophageal echocardiography. Little, Brown and Co., 1991:111–31.

46. Renee BA, Brink VD, Visser CA. Comparison of transthoracic and transesophageal color Doppler flow imaging in patients with mechanical prostheses in the mitral valve position. Am J Cardiol 1989;63:1471–4.

47. Khandheria BK, Seward JB, Oh JK, et al. Value and limitations of transesophageal echocardiography in assessment of mitral valve prostheses. Circulation 1991;83:1956–68.

48. Levine RA, Jimoh A, Cape EG, McMillan S, Yoganathan AP, Weyman AE. Pressure recovery distal to a stenosis: Potential cause of gradient "overestimation" by Doppler echocardiography. J Am Coll Cardiol 1989;13:706–15.

49. Reisner SA, Meltzer RS. Normal values of prosthetic valve Doppler echocardiographic parameters: A review. J Am Soc Echocardiogr 1988;1:201–10.

50. Burstow DJ, Nishimura RA, Bailey KR, et al. Continuous wave Doppler echocardiographic measurement of prosthetic valve gradients: A simultaneous Doppler-catheter correlative study. Circulation 1989;80:504–14.

51. Tatineni S, Barner HB, Pearson AC, Halbe D, Woodruff R, Labovitz AJ. Rest and exercise evaluation of St. Jude Medical and Medtronic Hall prostheses: Influence of primary lesion, valvular type, valvular size, and left ventricular function. Circulation 1989;80(3 Pt I):I-16–23.

52. Leavitt JI, Coats MH, Falk RH. Effects of exercise on transmitral gradient and pulmonary artery pressure in patients

with mitral stenosis or a prosthetic mitral valve: A Doppler echocardiographic study. J Am Coll Cardiol 1991;17:1520–6.

53. Bech-Hanssen O, Caidahl K, Wallentin I, Brandberg J, Wranne B, Ask P. Aortic prosthetic valve design and size: Relation to Doppler echocardiographic findings and pressure recovery—An in vitro study. J Am Soc Echocardiogr, 2000; 13:39–50.

54. Cooper DM, Stewart WJ, Schiavone WA, et al. Evaluation of normal prosthetic valve function by Doppler echocardiography. Am Heart J 1987;114:576–82.

55. Hatle L, Angelsen B, Tromsdal A. Noninvasive assessment of atrioventricular pressure half-time by Doppler ultrasound. Circulation 1979;60:1096–104.

56. Dumesnil JG, Honos GN, Lemieux M, Beauchemin J. Validation and applications of mitral prosthetic valvular areas calculated by Doppler echocardiography. Am J Cardiol 1990;65: 1443–8.

57. Henneke KH, Pongratz G, Bachmann K. Limitations of Doppler echocardiography in the assessment of prosthetic valve hemodynamics. J Heart Valve Dis 1995;4:18–25.

58. Nakatani S, Masuyama T, Kodama K, Kitabatake A, Fuji K, Kamada T. Value and limitations of Doppler echocardiography in the quantification of stenotic mitral valve area: Comparison of the pressure half-time and the continuity equation methods. Circulation 1988;77:78–85.

59. Bitar JN, Lechin ME, Salazar G, Zoghbi WA. Doppler echocardiographic assessment with the continuity equation of St. Jude Medical mechanical prostheses in the mitral valve position. Am J Cardiol 1995;76:287–93.

60. Bhatia S, Moten M, Werner M, et al. Frequency of unusually high transvalvular Doppler velocities in patients with normal prosthetic valves. J Am Coll Cardiol 1987;9:238A.

61. Chambers JB, Jackson G, Jewitt DE. Limitations of Doppler ultrasound in the assessment of the function of prosthetic mitral valves. Br Heart J 1990;63:189–94.

62. Loyd D, Ask P, Wranne B. Pressure half-time does not always predict mitral valve area correctly. J Am Soc Echocardiogr 1988;1:313–21.

63. Leung DY, Wong J, Rodriguez L, Pu M, Vandervoort PM, Thomas JD. Application of color Doppler flow mapping to calculate orifice area of St. Jude mitral valve. Circulation 1998;98:1205–11.

64. Mohan JC, Agrawal R, Arora R, Khalilullah M. Improved Doppler assessment of the Bjork-Shiley mitral prosthesis using the continuity equation. Int J Cardiol 1994;43:321–6.

65. Williams GA, Labovitz AJ. Doppler hemodynamic evaluation of prosthetic (Starr-Edwards and Bjork-Shiley) and bioprosthetic (Hancock and Carpentier-Edwards) cardiac valves. Am J Cardiol 1985;56:325–32.

66. Chambers JB, Cochrane T, Black MM, Jackson G. Assessment of the Hatle and Gorlin orifice formulae in mitral bioprostheses using Doppler ultrasound. Eur Heart J 1988;9 (Suppl. 1):209.

67. Chambers J, Deveral P, Jackson G, Sowton E. The Hatle orifice area formula tested in normal bileaflet mechanical mitral prostheses. Int J Cardiol 1992;35:397–404.

68. Rothbart RM, Castriz JL, Harding LV, Russo CD, Teague SM. Determination of aortic valve area by two-dimensional and Doppler echocardiography in patients with normal and stenotic bioprosthetic valves. J Am Coll Cardiol 1990;15: 817–24.

69. Chafizadeh ER, Zoghbi WA. Doppler echocardiographic assessment of the St. Jude Medical prosthetic valve in the aortic position using the continuity equation. Circulation 1991; 83:213–23.

70. Dumesnil JG, Honos GN, Lemieux M, Beauchemin J. Validation and applications of indexed aortic prosthetic valve areas calculated by Doppler echocardiography. J Am Coll Cardiol 1990;16:637–43.

71. Miller FA Jr, Khanderia BK, Freeman WK, Seward JB, Tajik AJ. Mitral prosthesis effective orifice area by a new method using continuity of flow between left atrium and prosthesis. J Am Coll Cardiol 1992;193:214A.

72. Cohen GI, Davison MB, Klein AL, Salcedo EE, Stewart WJ. A comparison of flow convergence with other transthoracic echocardiographic indexes of prosthetic mitral regurgitation. J Am Soc Echocardiogr 1992;5:620–7.

73. Saad RM, Barbetseas J, Ohnos L, Rubio N, Zoghbi WA. Application of the continuity equation and valve resistance to the evaluation of St. Jude Medical prosthetic aortic valve dysfunction. Am J Cardiol 1997;80:1239–42.

74. Maslow AD, Haering JM, Heindel S, Mashikian J, Levine R, Douglas P. An evaluation of prosthetic aortic valves using transesophageal echocardiography: The double-envelope technique. Anesth Analg, 2000;91:509–16.

75. Mannaerts H, Li Y, Kamp O, et al. Quantitative assessment of mechanical prosthetic valve area by 3–dimensional transesophageal echocardiography. J Am Soc Echocardiogr 2001; 14:723–31.

76. Lengyel M, Miller FA Jr, Taylor CL, Larson-Keller JJ, Seward JB, Tajik AJ. Doppler hemodynamic profiles of 456 clinically and echo-normal mitral valve prostheses. Circulation 1990; 82(Suppl 3):III-43(abst).

77. Miller FA, Callahan JA, Taylor CL, Larson-Keller JJ, Seward JB. Normal aortic valve prosthesis hemodynamics: 609 prospective Doppler examinations. Circulation 1989;80(Suppl 2): II-169(abst).

78. Connolly H, Miller FA Jr, Taylor CL, Naessens JM, Seward JB, Tajik AJ. Doppler hemodynamic profiles of 82 clinically and echocardiographically normal tricuspid valve prostheses. Circulation 1993;88:2722–7.

79. Shapira Y, Feinberg MS, Hirsch R, Nili M, Sagie A, Fernberg MS. Echocardiography can detect cloth tears in fully covered Starr-Edwards valves: a long-term clinical and echocardiographic study. Am Heart J 1997;134:665–71.

80. Temesvari A, Mohl W, Kupilik N. Characterization of normal leakage flow of monostrut tilting disc prosthetic mitral valves by multiplane transesophageal echocardiography. J Am Soc Echocardiogr 1997;10:155–8.

81. Lindower PD, Dellsperger KC, Johnson B, Chandran KB, Vandenberg BF. Variability of regurgitation in Bjork-Shiley mitral valves and relationship to disc occluder design: an in vitro two-dimensional color-Doppler flow mapping study. J Heart Valve Dis 1996;5(Suppl 2):S178–83.

82. Holen J, Simonsen S, Froysaker T. An ultrasound Doppler technique for the noninvasive determination of the pressure gradient in the Bjork-Shiley mitral valve. Circulation 1979;9:436–42.

83. Dittrich H, Nicod P, Hoit B, Dalton N, Sahn D. Evaluation of Bjork-Shiley prosthetic valves by real-time two dimensional Doppler echocardiographic flow mapping. Am Heart J 1988; 115:133–8.

84. Panidis IP, Ren JF, Kotler MN, et al. Clinical and echocardiographic evaluation of the St. Jude cardiac valve prostheses: Follow-up of 126 patients. J Am Coll Cardiol 1984;4:454–62.

85. Vandervoort PM, Greenberg NL, Powell KA, Cosgrove DM, Thomas JD. Pressure recovery in bileaflet heart valve prostheses. Localized high velocities and gradients in central and side orifices with implications for Doppler-catheter relation in aortic and mitral position. Circulation 1995;92:3464–72.

86. Chambers J, Cross J, Deverall P, Sowton E. Echocardiographic description of the CarboMedics bileaflet prosthetic heart valve. J Am Coll Cardiol 1993;21:398–405.

87. Soo CS, Ca M, Tay M, Yeoh JK, Sim E, Choo M. Doppler echocardiographic assessment of CarboMedics prosthetic valves in the mitral position. J Am Soc Echocardiogr 1994; 7:159–64.

88. Chakraborty B, Quek S, Pin DZ, Siong CT, Kheng TL. Evaluation of normal hemodynamic profile of CarboMedics prosthetic valves by Doppler echocardiography. Angiology 1997; 48:1055–61.

89. Fawzy ME, Halim M, Ziady G, Mercer E, Phillips R, Andaya W. Hemodynamic evaluation of porcine bioprostheses in the mitral position by Doppler echocardiography. Am J Cardiol 1987;59:643–6.

90. Firstenberg MS, Morehead AJ, Thomas JD, et al. Short-term hemodynamic performance of the mitral Carpentier-Edwards Perimount Pericardial Valve. Ann Thorac Surg 2001;71:S285–88.

91. Baur LHB, Jin XY, Houdas Y, et al. Echocardiographic parameters of the Freestyle bioprosthesis in aortic position: The European experience. J Am Soc Echocardiogr 1999;12:729–35.

92. Lytle BW, Cosgrove DM, Taylor PC, et al. Reoperations for valve surgery: Perioperative mortality and determinants of risk for 1,000 patients, 1958–1984. Ann Thorac Surg 1986;432:632–43.

93. Roberts WC, Sullivan MF. Clinical and necropsy observations early after simultaneous replacement of the mitral and aortic valves. Am J Cardiol 1986;58:1067–84.

94. Barbetseas J, Pistavos C, Lalos S, Psarros T, Toutouzas P. Partial thrombosis of a bileaflet mitral prosthetic valve: Diagnosis by transesophageal echocardiography. J Am Soc Echocardiogr 1993;6:91–3.

95. Dinarevic S, Redington A, Rigby M, Sheppard MN. Left ventricular pannus causing inflow obstruction late after mitral valve replacement for endocardial fibroelastosis. Pediatr Cardiol 1996;17:257–9.

96. Nakatani S, Andoh M, Okita Y, Yamagishi M, Miyatake K. Prosthetic valve obstruction with normal disc motion: Usefulness of transesophageal echocardiography to define cause. J Am Soc Echocardiogr 1999;12:537–9.

97. Van Son JA, Steinseifer U, Reul H, Knott E, Vincent JG, Lacquet LK. Jamming of prosthetic heart valves by suture trapping: Experimental findings. J Thorac Cardiovasc Surg 1989;37:288–93.

98. Waggoner AD, Perez JE, Barzilai B, Rosenbloom M, Eaton MH, Cox JL. Left ventricular outflow obstruction resulting from insertion of mitral prostheses leaving the native leaflets intact: Adverse clinical outcome in seven patients. Am Heart J 1991;122:483–8.

99. Shahid M, Sutherland G, Hatle L. Diagnosis of intermittent obstruction of mechanical mitral valve prostheses by Doppler echocardiography. Am J Cardiol 1995;76:1305–9.

100. Jaggers J, Chetham PM, Kinnard TL, Fullerton DA. Intraoperative prosthetic valve dysfunction: Detection by transesophageal echocardiography. Ann Thorac Surg 1995;59:755–7.

100. Vesely L, Boughner D, Song T. Tissue buckling as a mechanism of bioprosthetic valve failure. Ann Thorac Surg 1988;46:302–8.

101. Pai GP, Ellison RG, Rubin JW, Moore HV, Kamath MV. Disc immobilization of Bjork-Shiley and Medtronic Hall valves during and immediately after valve replacement. Ann Thorac Surg 1987;44:73–6.

102. Young E, Shapiro SM, French WJ, Ginzton LE. Use of transesophageal echocardiography during thrombolysis with tissue plasminogen activator of a thrombosed prosthetic mitral valve. J Am Soc Echocardiogr 1992;5:153–8.

103. Lee TM, Chu SH, Wang LC, Lee YT. Thrombolysis for obstructed CarboMedics mitral valve prosthesis. Ann Thorac Surg 1995;59:509–11.

104. Oliver JM, Gallego P, Gonzalez A, Dominguez FJ, Gamallo C, Mesa JM. Bioprosthetic mitral valve thrombosis: Clinical profile, transesophageal echocardiographic features, and follow-up after anticoagulant therapy. J Am Soc Echocardiogr 1996;9:691–9.

105. Gueret P, Vignon P, Fournier, et al. Transesophageal echocardiography for the diagnosis and management of nonobstructive thrombosis of mechanical mitral valve prosthesis. Circulation 1995;9:103–10.

106. Meloni L, Aru G, Abbruzzese PA, et al. Regurgitant flow of mitral valve prostheses: An intraoperative transesophageal echocardiographic study. J Am Soc Echocardiogr 1994;7:36–46.

107. Chen YT, Kan MN, Chen JS, et al. Detection of prosthetic mitral valve leak: A comparative study using transesophageal echocardiography, transthoracic echocardiography, and auscultation. J Clin Ultrasound 1990;18:557–61.

108. Yoshida K, Yoshikawa J, Akasaka T, Nishigami K, Minagoe S. Value of acceleration flow signals proximal to the leaking orifice in assessing the severity of prosthetic mitral valve regurgitation. J Am Coll Cardiol 1992;19:333–8.

109. Foster GP, Isselbacher EM, Rose GA, Torchiana DF, Akins CW, Picard MH. Accurate localization of mitral regurgitant defects using multiplane transesophageal echocardiography. Ann Thorac Surg 1998;65:1025–31.

110. Lindower PD, Dellsperger KC, Johnson B, Chandran KB, Vandenberg BF. Variability of regurgitation in Bjork-Shiley mitral valves and relationship to disc occluder design: An in vitro two-dimensional color-Doppler flow mapping study. J Heart Valve Dis 1996;5(Suppl 2):S178–83.

111. Hixson CS, Smith MD, Mattson MD, Morris EJ, Lehoff SJ, Salley RK. Comparison of transesophageal color flow Doppler imaging of normal mitral regurgitant jets in St. Jude Medical and Medtronic Hall cardiac prostheses. J Am Soc Echocardiogr 1992;5:57–62.

112. Dhasmana JP, Blackstone EH, Kirklin JW, Kouchoukos NT. Factors associated with periprosthetic leakage following primary mitral valve replacement with special consideration of the suture technique. Ann Thorac Surg 1983;35:170–8.

113. Bedderman C, Borst HG. Comparison of two suture techniques and materials: Relationship to perivalvular leaks after cardiac valve replacement. Cardiovasc Dis (Bull Tex Heart Inst) 1978;5:354.

114. Mohr-Kahaly S, Kupferwasser I, Erbel R, Oelert H, Meyer J. Regurgitant flow in apparently normal valve prostheses: Improved detection and semiquantitative analysis by transesophageal two-dimensional color-coded Doppler echocardiography. J Am Soc Echocardiogr 1990;3:187–95.

115. Dellsperger KC, Wieting DW, Baehr DA, Bard RJ, Brugger JP, Harrison EC. Regurgitation of prosthetic heart valves: Dependence on heart rate and cardiac output. Am J Cardiol 1983;51:321–8.

116. Flachskampf FA, Guerrero JL, O'Shea JP, Weyman AE, Thomas JD. Patterns of normal transvalvular regurgitation in mechanical valve prostheses. J Am Coll Cardiol 1991;18:1493–8.

117. Popovic Z, Barac I, Jovic M, Panic G, Miric M, Bojic M. Ventricular performance following valve replacement for chronic mitral regurgitation: Importance of chordal preservation. J Cardiovasc Surg 1999;40:183–90.

118. Agostini F, Click RL, Mulvagh SL, Abel MD, Dearani JA. Entrapment of subvalvular mitral tissue causing intermittent failure of a St. Jude mitral prosthesis. J Am Soc Echocardiogr 2000;13:1121–3.

119. van der Graaf Y, de Waard F, van Herwerden LA, Defauw J. Risk of strut fracture of Bjork-Shiley valves. Lancet 1992;339:257–61.

120. Novaro GM, Robbins MA, Firstenberg MS, Prior DL, Stewart WJ, Rodriguez LL. Disc embolization of a Bjork-Shiley convexo-concave mitral valve: A cause of sudden cardiovascular collapse and mesenteric ischemia. J Am Soc Echocardiogr 2000;13:417–20.

121. Blumberg EA, Karalis DA, Chandrasekaran K, et al. Endocarditis-associated paravalvular abscesses. Do clinical parameters predict the presence of abscess? Chest 1995;107:898–903.

122. Parker FB Jr, Greiner-Hayes C, Tomar RH, Markowitz AH, Bove EL, Marvasti MA. Bacteremia following prosthetic valve replacement. Ann Surg 1983;197:147–51.

123. Rutledge R, Kim J, Applebaum RE. Actuarial analysis of the risk of prosthetic valve endocarditis in 1,598 patients with mechanical and bioprosthetic valves. Arch Surg 1985;120:469–72.

124. Lytle BW. Surgical treatment of prosthetic valve endocarditis. Semin Thorac Cardiovasc Surg 1995;7:13–19.

125. Mugge A, Daniel WG, Frank G, Lichtlen PR. Echocardiography in infective endocarditis: Reassessment of prognostic implications of vegetation size determined by transthoracic and transesophageal approach. J Am Coll Cardiol 1989;14:631–8.

126. Shively BK, Gurule FT, Rolden CA, Leggett JH, Schiller NB. Diagnostic value of transesophageal compared with transthoracic echocardiography in infective endocarditis. J Am Coll Cardiol 1991;18:391–7.

127. Stoddard MF, Dawkins PR, Longaker RA. Mobile strands are frequently attached to the St. Jude Medical mitral valve prosthesis as assessed by two-dimensional transesophageal echocardiography. Am Heart J 1992;124:671–4.

128. Narins CR, Eichelberger JP. The development of valvular strands during thrombolytic therapy detected by transesophageal echocardiography. J Am Soc Echocardiogr 1996; 9:888–90.

129. Isada LR, Torelli JN, Stewart WJ, Klein AL. Detection of fibrous strands on prosthetic mitral valves by transesophageal echocardiography: Another potential embolic source. J Am Soc Echocardiogr 1994;7:641–5.

130. Ionescu AA, Newman GR, Butchart EG, Fraser AG. Morphologic analysis of a strand recovered from a prosthetic mitral valve: No evidence of fibrin. J Am Soc Echocardiogr 1999;641–51.

131. Cohn LH. Thromboembolism after mitral valve replacement. Recent progress. In Duran CMG, Angell W, Johnson A, et al, eds. Mitral Valve Disease. London: Butterworth, 1984:330–9.

132. Garcia MJ, Vandervoort P, Stewart WJ, et al. Mechanisms of hemolysis with mitral prosthetic regurgitation: Study using transesophageal echocardiography and fluid dynamic simulation. J Am Coll Cardiol 1996;27:399–406.

## QUESTIONS

1. Low profile mechanical valves
   A. Have an increased mass-to-orifice ratio
   B. Are bileaflet valves, such as the St. Jude and Carbomedics valves, which are less obstructive than tilting-disc valves
   C. Are not MRI compatible
   D. Are less durable than porcine bioprostheses

2. Stentless porcine valves, such as the Medtronic Freestyle and St. Jude SPV valves, are characterized by
   A. A smaller effective orifice area than stented porcine bioprostheses
   B. A sewing ring with supporting struts
   C. Earlier regression of left ventricular hypertrophy
   D. Uniform echocardiographic appearance regardless of implantation technique

3. A prosthetic perivalvular leak
   A. Originates within the sewing ring
   B. Demonstrates diastolic but not systolic color flow across the defect
   C. Is always caused by endocarditis
   D. Is seen as a rocking motion of the prosthesis at its site of attachment

4. Transvalvular gradients obtained by Doppler are
   A. Flow-dependent
   B. Flow-independent
   C. Unrelated to ventricular function
   D. Unaffected by valvular regurgitation

5. The sensitivity of TEE in the detection of prosthetic valve endocarditis is:
   A. 25%–40%
   B. 40%–50%
   C. 60%–75%
   D. 85%–90%

## Chapter 19

# Assessment of Cardiac Masses

*Kirk Spencer*

The identification of intracardiac masses is an important use of echocardiography. TEE provides an unparalleled window into the heart. TEE allows improved definition of mass size, shape, and mobility compared to the transthoracic window (1–9). The higher frequency and proximity of TEE probes provide superior evaluation of the tissue characterization of a mass, which can be useful in differential formulation. In addition, clarification of mass location, attachment, extent, and myocardial involvement are easily accomplished with TEE (5,7,10–12). The benefit of TEE is particularly strong for the evaluation of masses in the LAA, RA, and aorta or in those patients with technically limited transthoracic images (1,7,9). Three-dimensional reconstruction from the TEE window allows dynamic presentation of views simulating intraoperative visualization of cardiac masses (13,14).

Cardiac surgery for intracardiac masses is an indication for intraoperative TEE that has been recognized (15). Although patients may have had preoperative TTE and even TEE exams, a complete intraoperative evaluation is paramount for confirmation of the mass prior to surgical exploration (15–17). Likewise, rapid and accurate interpretation after the discovery of an unsuspected cardiac mass in the operating room is essential (18–20). Once a cardiac mass is confirmed, intraoperative TEE is useful for guiding the surgical approach for removal (10, 21–23). In addition, placement of surgical cannula in the presence of cardiac masses, whether in the IVC, SVC, or aorta, may be guided using TEE (17,24). Intraoperative TEE to assess the hemodynamic effects of a cardiac mass can prove invaluable. Lastly, intraoperative TEE allows assessment of the surgical intervention. Intraoperative TEE permits evaluation for residual mass as well as sequelae of mass removal on valvular and myocardial function prior to leaving the operating room (15).

The value of intraoperative TEE during surgery for cardiac masses was highlighted in a recent series (17). In this study, 9 in 75 patients had their surgical course altered by intraoperative transesophageal echocardiogra-

phy. Six patients had the operative procedure altered due to the detection of additional pathology. This included one patient with a right atrial myxoma in whom an unknown LA myxoma was detected. One subject with an RA mass had alteration of the caval cannulation site. One intraoperative TEE failed to confirm a LA thrombus and surgery was cancelled. Three patients went back on cardiac bypass for valve repair after mass removal based on information provided by the intraoperative TEE.

## APPROACH/STRUCTURES

Equally important as complete knowledge of pathologic masses within the heart is an understanding of the normal structures, anatomic variants, and artifacts encountered during a transesophageal examination that may be confused with pathologic findings. Detailed knowledge of these normal findings prevents undo concern or delay in the operative setting to pursue further evaluation or solicit opinions regarding a structure, which is, in fact, a normal variant. Correct interpretation of normal intracardiac masses may in fact prevent surgical evaluation or inappropriate medical therapy for these structures. Patients referred for surgical removal of intracardiac masses have been spared operation by a thorough and knowledgeable intraoperative transesophageal echocardiographic examination. Though some of the structures detailed in the paragraphs below may seem, to an experienced transesophageal echocardiographer, as unlikely to be mistaken for a pathologic finding, all of these structures have been confused with pathology at one time or another (3,8).

## IVC/SVC/RIGHT ATRIUM

The right atrium and vena cava can be imaged in a midesophageal bicaval view, which displays a long axis of the vena cava as it enters the right atrial cavity. In this view, the eustachian valve is noted at the juncture of the inferior vena cava and right atrium. This structure projects into the right atrial cavity and can be mistaken for an intracardiac mass. There is wide variation in eustachian valves among patients and although typically thin and mobile, eustachian valves may be thick and rigid. It is the typical location of the eustachian valve that allows it to be discerned from a pathologic structure.

One might also see a Chiari network in the RA. This structure consists of a meshwork of fibers originating about the margin of the eustachian and thebesian valves and attaches in the area of the crista terminalis. This network represents the vestigial remains of the right valvulae venosae and septum spurium that fail to resorb into the wall of the RA (25). Echocardiographically, this structure appears as a thin mobile filamentous echodensity within the RA cavity (Fig. 19.1) (26,27). The anatomic variation in Chiari networks is quite wide because many patients have no visible Chiari network and others have prominent ones. Distinction of this structure from an intracardiac mass is made by its typical echocardiographic appearance and by noting, that although the body is mobile, this structure is tethered at its margins. These remnants are seldom clinically important, but have been reported as sources of entrapment for emboli and right heart catheters (28,29).

Within the body of the right atrium itself, several structures are noteworthy for potential confusion with pathologic masses. The right atrial wall is trabeculated with pectinate muscles that must be noted as normal variants. Pectinate muscles are discerned by their perpendicular alignment from the right atrial wall and their regular spacing from one another. When the SVC is viewed in long axis, there is a prominent ridge at the juncture of the SVC and the right atrium, the crista terminalis. There

is somewhat wide anatomic variation in this ridge and it may appear quite prominent in some patients. Its location adjacent to the right atrial appendage can sometimes be confused with a right atrial appendage thrombus.

When there is a loculated pericardial effusion behind the right atrium, the right atrial wall may appear to be an intracardiac linear density. This abnormality can be readily discerned with the injection of agitated saline, which delineates the right atrial cavity. The tricuspid annulus may accumulate fat and be prominent. Particularly if imaged off-axis, this may appear to represent an intracardiac mass between the RA and RV. This can readily be discerned by imaging in multiple planes and noting smooth continuity with the rest of the cardiac structures (Fig. 19.2).

Two normal anatomic variants of the interatrial septum can also be confused with intracardiac masses, the first of which is lipomatous hypertrophy. Pathologically, lipomatous hypertrophy represents a benign proliferation in which mature adipocytes infiltrate the interatrial septum. This fatty involvement is more prominent at the cephalad and caudal ends sparing the fossa ovalis, giving the interatrial septum a dumb-bell shaped appearance (Fig. 19.3). Fatty infiltration of the interatrial septum is denoted not only by its typical pattern of involvement, but also by the hyperrefractile nature of the fatty deposits that may cast a prominent acoustic shadow. Although this disorder represents a spectrum of interatrial septal thickening, diagnostic thickness criteria of 1.5–2.0 cm have been proposed (30–33). At the other end of the spectrum, lipomatous hypertrophy can reach massive proportions and infiltrations several centimeters in diameter have been reported (34,35).

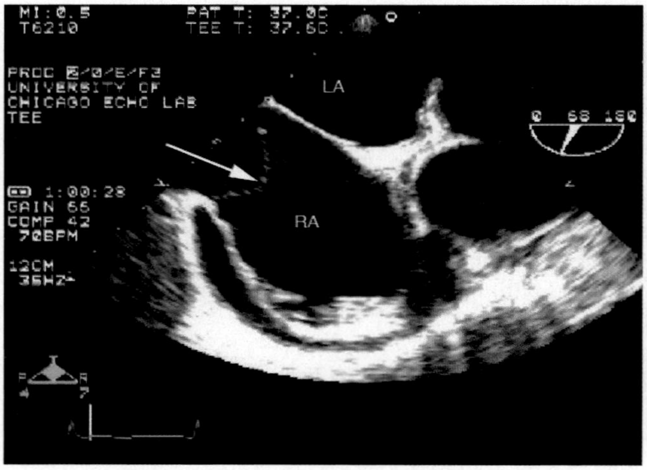

**FIGURE 19.1.** This linear right atrial mass (*RA*) is a Chiari network, which is a normal variant. *LA*, left atrium.

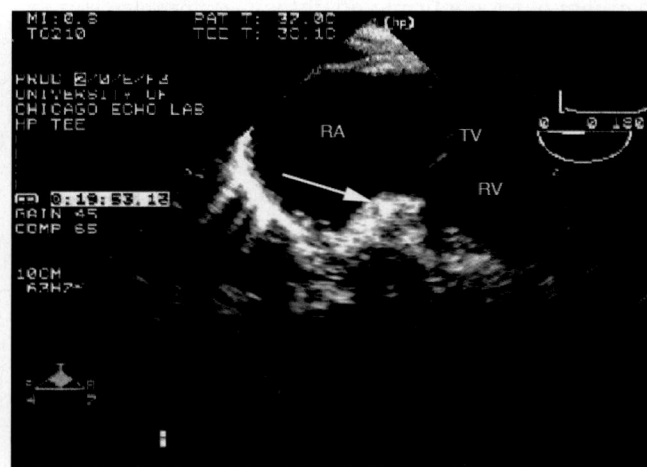

**FIGURE 19.2.** A view of the right atrium (*RA*), tricuspid valve (*TV*), and right ventricle (*RV*) showing a prominent tricuspid annulus (*arrow*), which can be confused with an intracardiac mass.

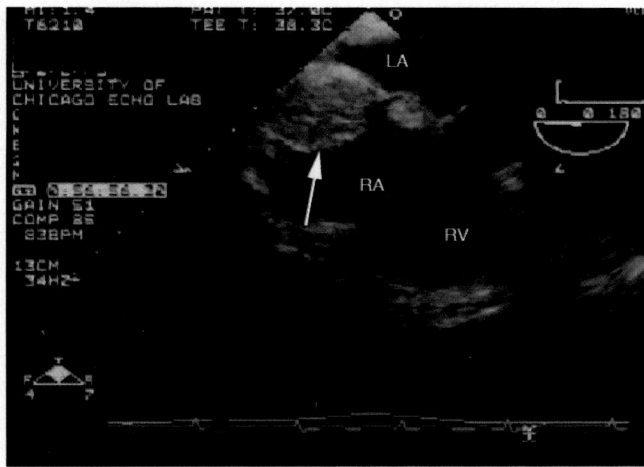

**FIGURE 19.3.** Interatrial septum with lipomatous hypertrophy (*arrow*). Note the sparing of the fossa ovalis. *RA,* right atrium; *LA,* left atrium; *RV,* right ventricle.

An interatrial septal aneurysm, which has a prevalence of between 2% and 10%, is another anatomic variant that can mimic an intracardiac mass (36–38). The definitions of redundant septum and aneurysmal septum are somewhat arbitrary. Published criteria define an interatrial septal, aneurysm as a redundancy of at least 1.5 cm of the septum, with a displacement past the midline of at least 1 cm (36,39). In some patients the redundancy of the interatrial septum is prominent with excursions of several centimeters into the left or right atrium depending on interatrial pressures (Fig. 19.4). When imaging off-axis, the aneurysmal portion of the septum may protrude into and out of plane giving the appearance of a mobile interatrial mass. This may present during intraoperative trans-

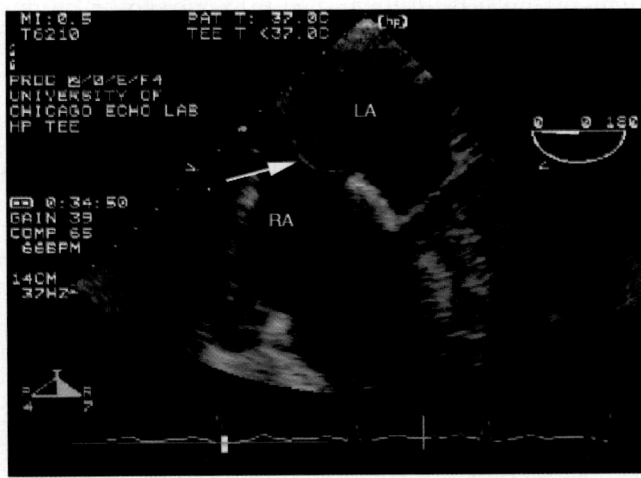

**FIGURE 19.4.** Midesophageal four-chamber view demonstrating an interatrial septal aneurysm (*arrow*). *RA,* right atrium; *LA,* left atrium.

esophageal echocardiography as an unexpected mass, despite a preoperative transthoracic echocardiogram, because of TEE's superior rate of detection for this lesion (37,39).

## RIGHT VENTRICLE/ PULMONARY ARTERY

There are several normal structures within the right ventricle and right ventricular outflow track that can be confused with pathologic intracardiac masses. Within the right ventricular chamber itself, the primary structures to beware of are the ventricular trabeculations. The right ventricle is a heavily trabeculated chamber and in the setting of right ventricular pressure overload, these trabeculations may become quite prominent. Even in the normal right ventricle, there is a prominent muscular band, the moderator band, which is a normal finding. Catheters within the right ventricle must of course be discerned from intracardiac masses. Although this would seem straightforward, because catheters are curvilinear structures being interrogated with a flat imaging plane, only small portions of the catheter may be visualized at any one time. This may give the appearance of small mobile intracardiac echodensities. In addition, because catheters are echodense, they are prone to forming reverberation and side lobe artifacts, which must not be mistaken for pathologic structures.

Within the pulmonary artery itself, the primary consideration is not confusing ultrasound clutter for an intraluminal mass. The main pulmonary artery is typically imaged in the midesophageal RV inflow-outflow view. This puts the pulmonary artery in the far field where, because of ultrasound beam spreading, there is often prominent clutter. With adjustment of the ultrasound imaging controls, such as gain and focus, as well as manipulating the probe itself this clutter artifact can usually be "cleaned up." Clutter artifact is also prominent in near field. When the right pulmonary artery is being imaged from the midesophageal ascending aortic short-axis view, there is often prominent clutter within the right pulmonary artery. Again, attention to focus and gain can minimize this artifact and avoid the false interpretation of a right pulmonary artery thrombus.

## PULMONARY VEINS/LEFT ATRIUM/LEFT ATRIAL APPENDAGE

A normal structure that can be confused with an intracardiac mass in the LA is the fold of tissue between the left upper pulmonary vein and the LA proper. This ridge has anatomic variation and at times can be prominent. In addition, though this ridge is typically linear, the end of the ridge may appear somewhat bulbous giving it a "Q-tip" appearance. This can be confused with an LA or LAA thrombus. Another structure that can lead to the erroneous diagnosis of an LAA mass is the transverse sinus. When there is fluid in this pericardial reflection it may appear to be continuous with the LAA cavity. The LAA wall may then appear to be a linear mass. In addition, this structure often has echodense fibrinous material in it that can be confused with an LAA thrombus.

The left atrial appendage is a structure that commonly has features suggesting an intracardiac mass. The left atrial appendage has pectinate muscles that may simulate left atrial appendage thrombus. Pectinate muscles typically have a tissue characterization more similar to muscle than thrombus. In addition, the pectinate muscles typically emanate perpendicular from the left atrial appendage wall and appear multiple in a somewhat regularly spaced pattern. A multiplane approach to the evaluation of left atrial appendage is essential. The LAA often has multiple lobes (40) and the tissue separating these infoldings may be confused with thrombus.

Another phenomenon, although not truly a normal anatomic finding but nevertheless doesn't represent an intracardiac mass, is left atrial spontaneous echo contrast or "smoke." Spontaneous echo contrast in the left atrial chamber is noted by its echodense swirling pattern and may be confused with left atrial thrombus. Within the left atrial appendage, particularly in situations of low appendage flow such as atrial fibrillation, dense spontaneous echo contrast can be very difficult to discern from intraappendage thrombus (Fig. 19.5). Confirming the presence of a thrombus in multiple planes can be helpful to prevent misinterpretations.

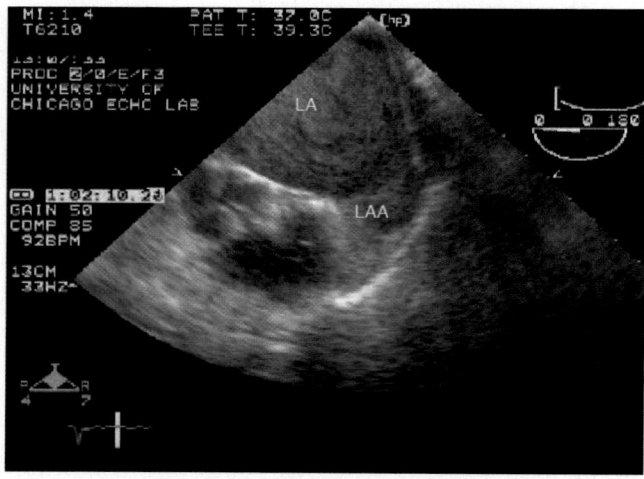

**FIGURE 19.5.** Spontaneous echo contrast in a patient with severe mitral stenosis. Though the left atrial appendage (*LAA*) appears to have a thrombus, this actually represents dense spontaneous echo contrast. *LA,* left atrium.

## LEFT VENTRICLE

Several normal structures within the left ventricular cavity, when imaged along tangential planes, can lead to the false diagnosis of an intracardiac mass. The LV papillary muscles are usually easily discerned from pathologic masses by their location and attachments to the submitral apparatus, as well as having a tissue characterization that is similar to that of the myocardium. When imaging from a midesophageal four-chamber view, the base of the interventricular septum may appear prominent, suggesting an intramyocardial mass. However, far more commonly is the presence of sigmoid septum. This is a normal variant of aging in which remodeling of the left ventricular cavity projects the basilar interventricular septum into the left ventricular outflow tract.

The left ventricular cavity can also have thin linear structures, which cross the chamber particularly near the left ventricular apex. These false chords are common normal anatomic variants. Lastly, the left ventricular apex is often foreshortened and difficult to completely image from a midesophageal four-chamber view. This foreshortening can give the appearance that the apex is filled in and thus lead to the erroneous conclusion of an apical thrombus. When evaluating the left ventricular apex from the transesophageal approach, care must be taken to retroflex the probe to fully elongate the left ventricular cavity. Additional imaging from the transgastric long-axis and reverse four-chamber views may be helpful.

## AORTA

False positive masses in the thoracic aorta are primarily ultrasound artifacts. As the aorta is in the near field when imaging from the esophagus, near field clutter is common and must be distinguished from intraaortic thrombus or atheroma. This is done by noting that the aorta can be moved independent of the clutter and that the clutter often extends outside the borders of the aorta. Linear artifacts can be noted in the descending or ascending aorta. If not appreciated as artifacts these can lead to erroneous conclusions that have significant clinical implications. The mechanism of these artifacts has been elucidated and distinction from true pathology is often possible (41).

## PATHOLOGY

Most pathologic cardiac masses represent thrombus, infection, or tumor. A transesophageal echocardiographic examination cannot definitively diagnose an intracardiac mass, as this requires histologic confirmation. However, a reasonably secure diagnosis can usually be made by incorporating the echocardiographic location and appearance of the mass with available clinical data. In addition, there may be associated echocardiographic findings that substantially alter the differential diagnostic choices for an intracardiac mass.

Cardiac involvement by malignancy may be primary (origin within the heart) or secondary/metastatic (origin distant from heart). Metastatic neoplasms are far more common than are primary tumors by a 20–30:1 ratio (42–44). Of metastatic involvement of the heart, the most common tumors are lung, breast, and lymphoma/leukemia followed by esophageal and uterine (42–44). Cardiac involvement may occur from direct invasion or metastatic spread from distant disease. Certain tumors, such as melanoma, have a predilection for metastasizing to the heart. Although most secondary involvement of the heart by malignancy is pericardial (~75%), it is the myocardial and intracardiac involvement this chapter focuses on, because these present as cardiac masses.

Intraoperative TEE evaluation of metastatic disease of the heart is not simply an imaging exercise. Patients with metastatic tumor of the heart who have made it to the operating room may be there for attempt at surgical cure. In this case, careful TEE evaluation of tumor extent and myocardial infiltration is crucial. If intraoperative and preoperative tumor staging differ, the surgical approach may be aborted or altered (45). In addition, patients may be undergoing palliative surgery to relieve the hemodynamic effects of tumor involvement (for example, intracardiac obstruction). Intraoperative evaluation of hemodynamic improvement after tumor resection is vital to operative success.

Primary cardiac tumors are less commonly found with an incidence of 0.1%–0.3% in autopsies series (42,44,46). Most (75%–80%) are benign; more than one-half of these are myxomas. Less common cardiac tumors include rhabdomyoma, fibroma, and hemangioma. Primary malignant cardiac tumors are almost exclusively types of sarcoma (> 95%) (47–49). Of sarcomas, the angiosarcoma and rhabdomyosarcoma are the most common (50). Those tumors suitable for primary resection can be evaluated with intraoperative TEE to guide surgical therapy.

Cardiac involvement by tumors may be asymptomatic or cause significant morbidity, such as pericardial tamponade, arrhythmias, or congestive heart failure. The lack of malignant potential does not always indicate a "benign" clinical course because nonmalignant intracavitary tumors may produce obstruction to blood flow or partially dislodge, causing embolization.

## IVC/SVC/RIGHT ATRIUM

The most common intracardiac mass in the vena cava and right atrium is a thrombus. Right atrial thrombi oc-

cur in several settings. Thrombi from the deep venous system may embolize and become entrapped in the right atrium (51). This clinical scenario likely happens far more frequently than detected as most thromboemboli rapidly pass through the right atrium. Thromboemboli originally from peripheral veins appear as mobile serpiginous irregular masses in the right atrium that do not have a point of attachment to the right atrial wall. These thrombi may become entrapped in the foramen ovale, which is a mechanism for paradoxical embolization (1,52).

Another cause of right atrial thrombus is in situ formation, which occurs in conditions with low atrial blood flow, such as right atrial dilatation in cardiomyopathic states and atrial fibrillation. In situ thrombi typically are homogenous echodensities adherent to the right atrial wall with a broad base of attachment. Although right atrial thrombi have been reported along the interatrial septum, this is unusual. Right atrial thrombi commonly have mobile irregularities extending from their surface. These projections may be large enough to prolapse into the RV cavity during diastole (Fig. 19.6).

Right atrial thrombi associated with atrial fibrillation typically form on the right atrial free wall or within the right atrial appendage (Fig. 19.7). In patients with atrial fibrillation, approximately 15% of cardiac thrombi are located within the right atrial appendage. Right atrial appendage thrombi are best visualized in a midesophageal bicaval view. Careful movement of the probe into and out of the esophagus is required to interrogate the entire body of the right atrial appendage.

A special case of in situ right atrial thrombus formation is that associated with intracardiac catheters. Superior vena caval catheters, particularly hemodialysis

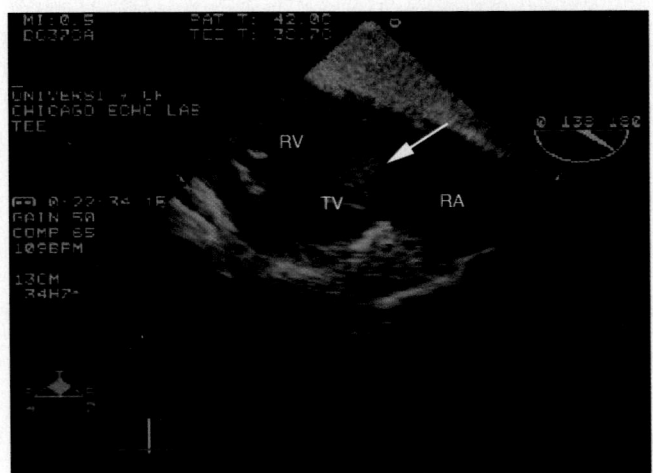

**FIGURE 19.6.** Transgastric long-axis view of the tricuspid valve (*TV*), showing a large right atrial thrombus (*arrow*) prolapsing through the tricuspid valve. *RA*, right atrium; *RV*, right ventricle.

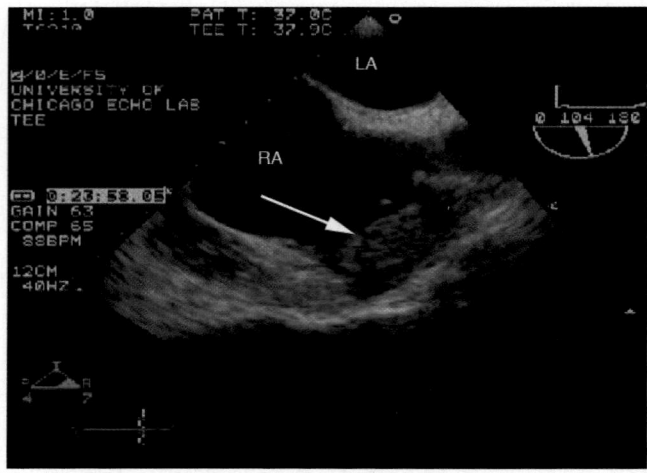

**FIGURE 19.7.** Large thrombus in the right atrial appendage (*arrow*). *RA*, right atrium; *LA*, left atrium.

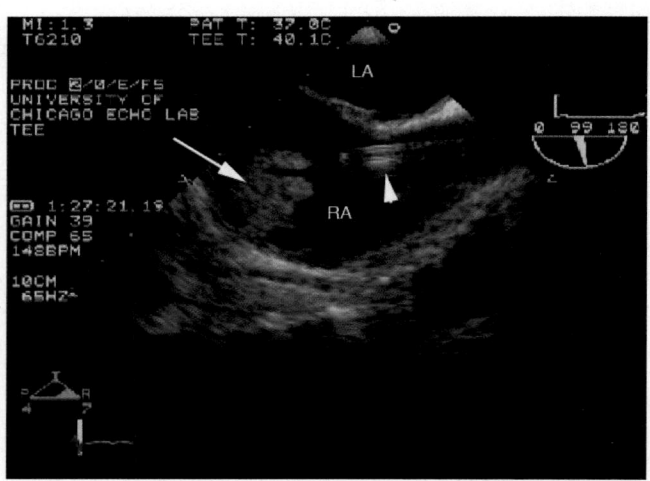

**FIGURE 19.9.** Bicaval view of the right atrium (*RA*) with a catheter (*arrowhead*) in the superior vena cava protruding into the right atrial cavity. There is a large thrombus (*arrow*) in the right atrium formed around the catheter.

catheters that are stiff and have higher flows, may lead to endocardial damage that serves as a nidus for mural thrombus formation. Given the orientation of the vena cava and right atrium, superior vena caval catheter-associated thrombi most commonly form near the inferior vena cava—right atrial junction, often on or near the eustachian valve (Fig. 19.8). Right atrial thrombi in this location and others, associated with patients with chronic renal failure, typically are more inhomogeneous and partially calcified.

Lastly, right atrial thrombi may form around a foreign body, such as catheter or electrode (Fig. 19.9). Small mo-

bile echodensities are commonly associated with functioning catheters in asymptomatic patients. More substantial thrombi may form around catheters and become quite large (Fig. 19.10). A catheter-associated thrombus may involve and extend into the superior vena cava leading to partial obstruction (Fig. 19.11). Differentiation of atrial thrombus from other right atrial masses is done by noting the typical location of thrombi and the presence of associated thrombogenic conditions. Additionally, thrombi may appear laminated and partially calcified.

Right atrial masses may also represent primary cardiac tumors. Of these, the most common is a myxoma.

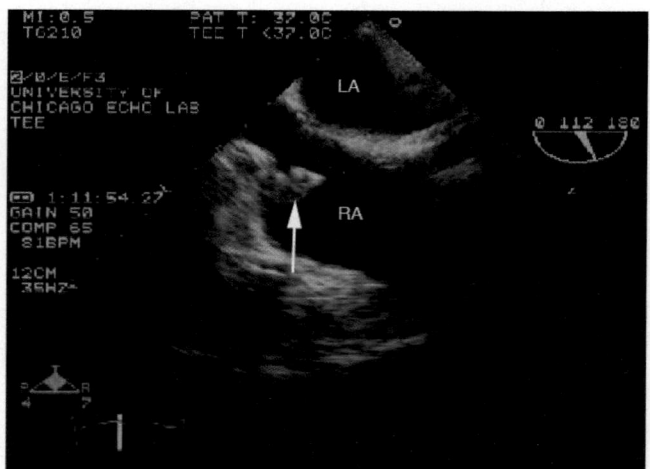

**FIGURE 19.8.** Bicaval view of the right atrium (*RA*) demonstrating a mural thrombus (*arrow*) at the junction of the inferior vena cava. The location of this thrombus is typical for patients with dialysis catheters in the superior vena cava, which causes endothelial injury of the right atrial wall.

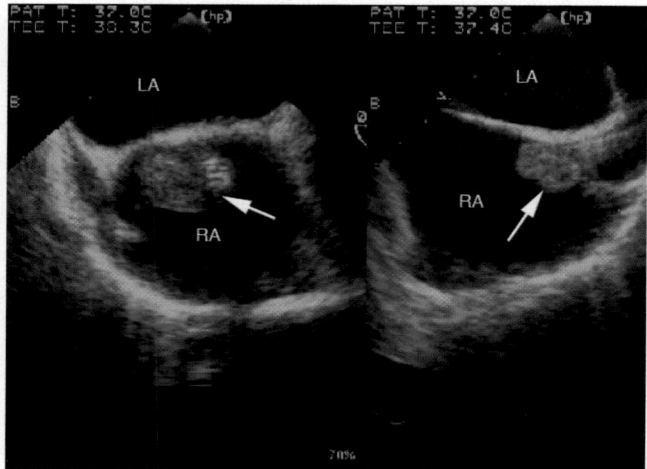

**FIGURE 19.10.** **Right panel:** Bicaval view, there is a catheter in the superior vena cava with thrombus (*arrow*) attached to the end of it. **Left panel:** Short axis of the right atrium demonstrating the catheter with extensive thrombus. *RA*, right atrium; *LA*, left atrium.

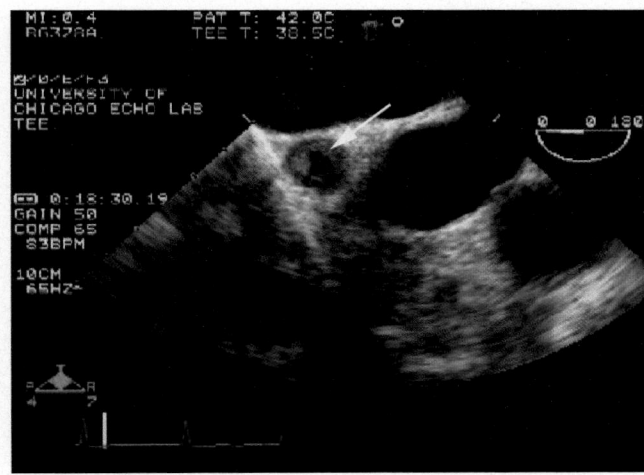

**FIGURE 19.11.** Short axis of the superior vena cava demonstrating thrombus (*arrow*).

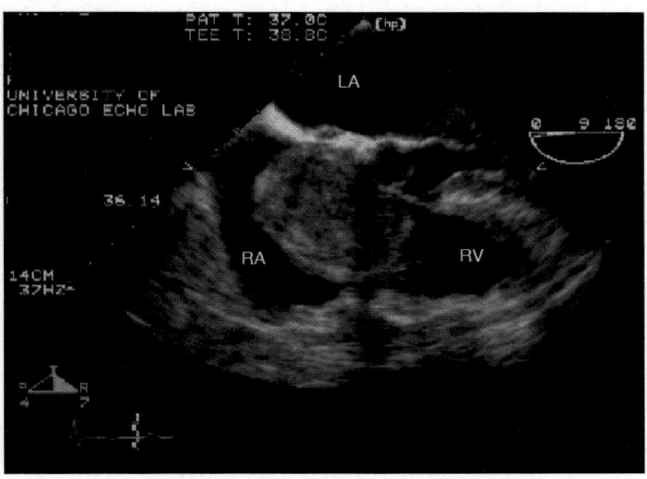

**FIGURE 19.13.** Large right atrial myxoma prolapsing into the tricuspid valve. Transesophageal evaluation of the hemodynamic effects of this mass would be essential. *RA*, right atrium; *LA*, left atrium; *RV*, right ventricle.

These typically have well-defined borders and somewhat inhomogeneous tissue characterization (Fig. 19.12). Right atrial myxomas represent 20%–25% of all cardiac myxomas (42,53,54). Like left atrial tumors, right atrial myxomas are usually mobile and if large enough, may obstruct the tricuspid orifice in diastole (Fig. 19.13). Right atrial myxomas can be imaged from the midesophageal four-chamber and bicaval view as well as the transgastric RV inflow view. Complete TEE assessment of RA myxomas includes evaluation of tumor attachment, size, and mobility as well as tricuspid valve function (55).

Other primary benign tumors of the heart involve the right atrium infrequently. Of the primary malignant cardiac tumors, angiosarcoma is the most common (Fig. 19.14) (56). This tumor originates in the right atrium in 80% of cases and presents as a large mural mass that frequently extends into the pericardium and vena cava (47–49,56,57).

Right atrial masses may also represent secondary involvement of the right atrium by malignancy. This may happen through intravascular extension or extracardiac invasion of the right atrium (Fig. 19.15). Tumor extension along the inferior vena cava into the right atrium is a common form of secondary cardiac involvement in certain malignancies, such as renal cell carcinoma, Wilms' tumor, hepatoma, and uterine leiomyomatosis (10,58–63).

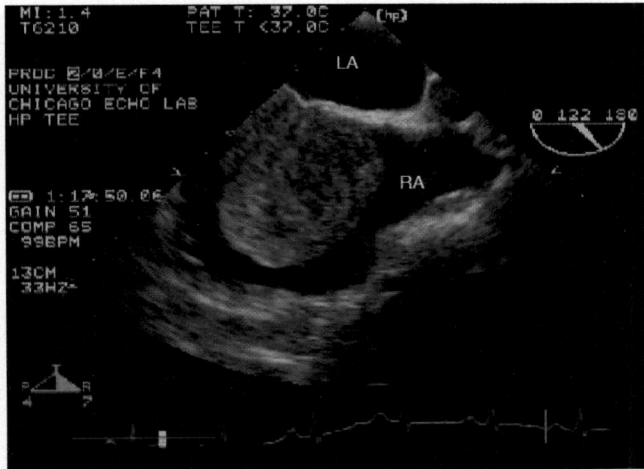

**FIGURE 19.12.** Large right atrial myxoma. The characteristic shape and attachment of this mass to the interatrial septum in the area of the fossa ovalis makes a myxoma very high on the differential. *RA*, right atrium; *LA*, left atrium.

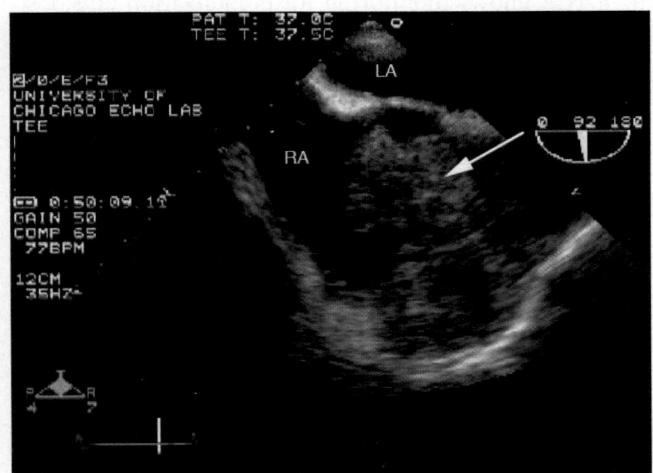

**FIGURE 19.14.** Although the location of this mass (*arrow*) in the right atrial appendage protruding into the right atrial cavity would suggest thrombus, this in fact, was pathologically shown to be an angiosarcoma. *RA*, right atrium; *LA*, left atrium.

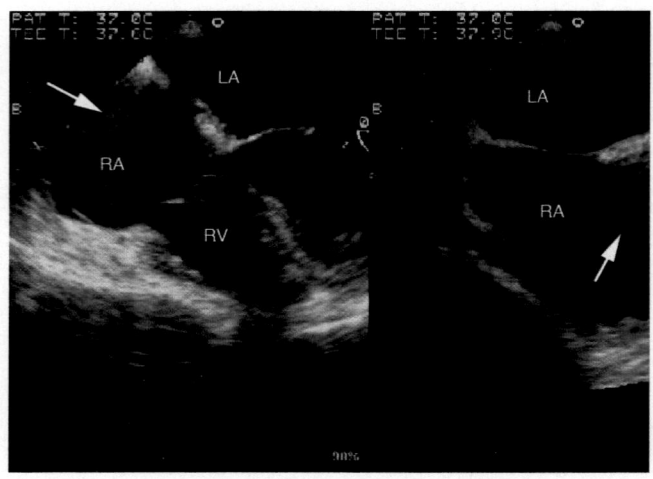

**FIGURE 19.15.** Two views of the right atrium demonstrating a lymphoma (*arrow*) that had infiltrated the right atrium. *RA*, right atrium; *LA*, left atrium; *RV*, right ventricle.

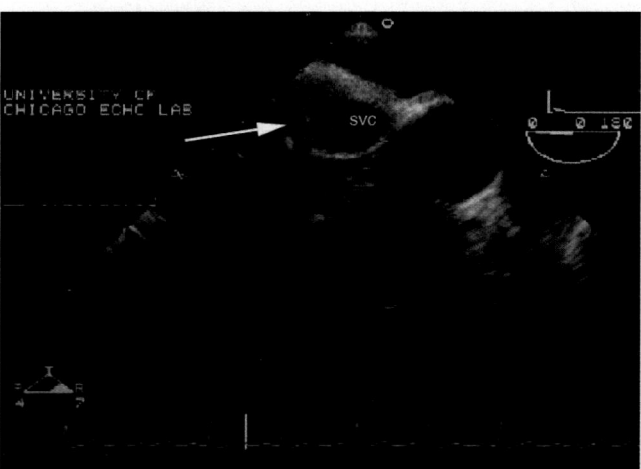

**FIGURE 19.16.** Short axis of the superior vena cava (*SVC*) demonstrating an intraluminal mass that most commonly would represent thrombus. However, this mass also appears to be external to the superior vena cava (*arrow*) and the definition of the superior vena cava wall has been obscured. This represents external infiltration of the superior vena cava by a mediastinal lymphoma.

These tumors appear as elongated mobile masses protruding into the right atrial cavity from the inferior vena cava. These tumors may become quite large, occupying most of the right atrial cavity causing tricuspid valve obstruction (69). Mobile tumor components may prolapse across the tricuspid valve into the right ventricular cavity.

Intraoperative TEE may be useful during resection of these RA tumors. Using the midesophageal bicaval view, the distal IVC, and RA chamber are well visualized. By advancing the probe in this view, more proximal aspects of the IVC may be visualized. The intraoperative exam should define the cephalic extent of tumor, extent of caval occlusion, and mobility of tumor, all of which help plan surgical strategy (61–63,65). During resection, intraoperative TEE allows monitoring for embolization and positioning of cannula and occlusion balloons (10,45,50, 66–70). Once resection is complete, intraoperative TEE is essential to look for residual tumor and IVC patency.

Direct invasion of the right atrium and great venous vessels is also possible. Most typically this occurs from breast, lung, and esophageal cancers. Invasion of the right atrium or vena cava from extracardiac tumors is noted echocardiographically by careful inspection of the wall. Finding continuity between an intraatrial and an extracardiac mass, which are similar in tissue characterization, is highly suggestive of tumor invasion (Fig. 19.16).

## RIGHT VENTRICLE/ PULMONARY ARTERY

The right ventricle and pulmonary artery are relatively uncommon sights for intracardiac masses. Although in situ right ventricular thrombi occur, this is less common

than the other cardiac chambers. Identification of thrombus can be challenging in the heavily trabeculated RV. Thrombi are most likely to form in situations of low flow states or in the presence of RV regional wall motion abnormalities. RV thrombi are most likely to be located in the apex and have ultrasound characteristics distinctly different from the myocardium (Fig. 19.17). The RV apex should be viewed from both the midesophageal four-chamber and transgastric RV inflow views to confirm the presence of a RV thrombus.

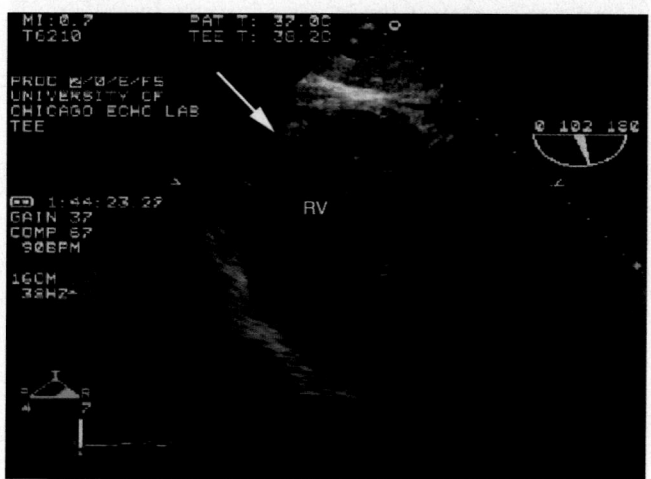

**FIGURE 19.17.** Transgastric long axis of the tricuspid valve (*TV*) showing a large apical right ventricular (*RV*) thrombus (*arrow*).

Thrombi in the pulmonary artery are exclusively the result of emboli from the deep venous system and can be visualized using TEE (71–74). Evaluation of the pulmonary artery and pulmonary branches is critical in hemodynamically unstable patients as the specificity of a pulmonary artery thrombus detected with transesophageal echocardiography is excellent (Fig. 19.18) (72,75–77). In addition, intraoperative TEE to detect residual emboli during pulmonary embolectomy is beneficial. Intraoperative TEE may document residual thrombus in up to 30% of embolectomy procedures (15). The main PA can be visualized using the midesophageal RV inflow-outflow and ascending aortic short-axis views. The proximal LPA and initial 4 to 6 cm of the RPA can be visualized from the midesophageal ascending aortic short- and long-axis views.

Benign and malignant primary tumors of the right ventricle are uncommon but nearly all types, including myxoma, rhabdomyoma, fibroma, and rhabdomyosarcoma, have been noted (47–49,78). Like other cardiac chambers, direct invasion of the right ventricle from extracardiac tumor can result in myocardial replacement and intracardiac extension of tumor. Right ventricular masses may also be the result of right atrial masses that prolapse through the tricuspid valve into the right ventricular chamber.

Although involvement of the pulmonary artery by lung carcinoma is not uncommon, this typically involves external compression rather than presenting as an intracardiac mass (79). Inspection of the PA for hemodynamically significant compression using intraoperative TEE in lung cancer patients is pertinent. Tumor may also involve the PA via embolization. Intracardiac RA tumors may partially dislodge spontaneously or during surgical manipulation (70). These tumor emboli may become entrapped in the proximal pulmonary arterial tree and be visualized using TEE as heterogeneous, irregular intraluminal masses (69,80).

## PULMONARY VEINS LEFT ATRIUM/LEFT ATRIAL APPENDAGE

The majority of intracardiac masses in the LA are cardiac thrombi. Although, LA thrombi can be located in any portion of this chamber (Figs. 19.19 and 19.20), the vast majority are located in the LAA. Complete visualization of the LAA requires careful multiplane interrogation, as they are often complex multilobed structures (81). Left atrial thrombi have a tissue characterization that differs from the surrounding cardiac structures (Fig. 19.21). LA clots often appear laminated and have irregular or lobulated borders. Although the base of attachment to the LA wall is broad, LA thrombi may be mobile or have mobile projections. Rarely, thrombi may detach from the LA wall after they have become so large they cannot escape the LA cavity and become free-floating (82).

In addition to echocardiographic appearance and location, the clinical setting influences differentiation of thrombus from other LA masses. In patients with risk factors for atrial stasis, such as atrial fibrillation, mitral stenosis, or LV dysfunction, thrombus must be high on the differential list of a LA mass. This is especially true when there is TEE evidence of atrial stasis, such as spontaneous echo contrast. Using intraoperative TEE in patients with atrial fibrillation, one may expect to find a thrombus in 5%–15% of cases (83,84). Although initially

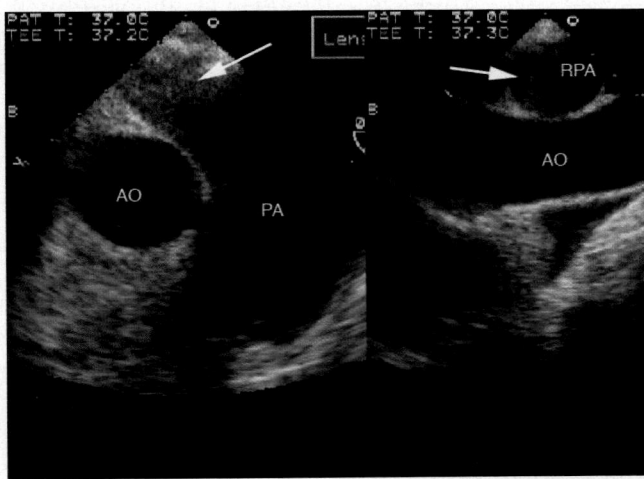

**FIGURE 19.18.** The first panel shows the short axis of the ascending thoracic aorta (*Ao*) with pulmonary artery (*PA*) bifurcation. The right pulmonary artery (*RPA*) has an intraluminal mass consistent with thrombus (*arrow*). The second panel shows the ascending aorta in long axis with a cross section of the right pulmonary artery demonstrating thrombus.

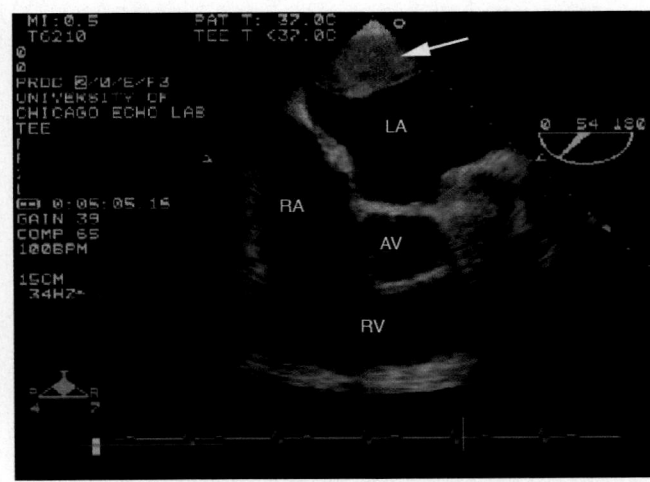

**FIGURE 19.19.** Short-axis view of the aortic valve (*AV*). A large mural thrombus (*arrow*) can be noted in the left atrial chamber (*LA*). *RA,* right atrium; *RV,* right ventricle.

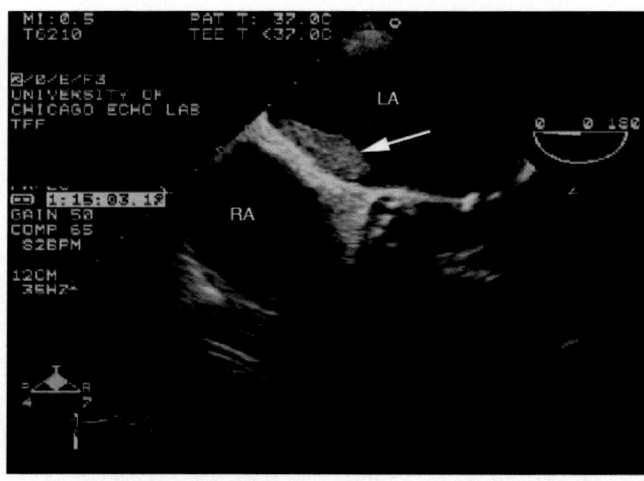

**FIGURE 19.20.** Atypical left atrial thrombus (*arrow*) located on the interatrial septum. Because of the location of this mass, it would be difficult to distinguish from a myxoma with certainty. *RA,* right atrium; *LA,* left atrium.

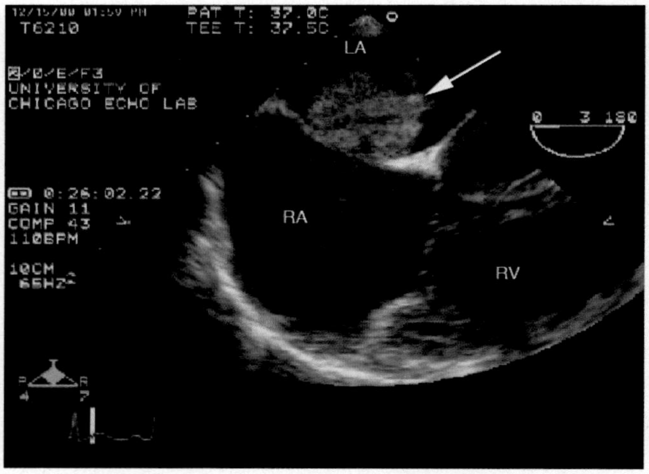

**FIGURE 19.22.** Left atrial myxoma (*arrow*) attached to the interatrial septum. Note the projections from the main body of the myxoma. *RA,* right atrium; *LA,* left atrium; *RV,* right ventricle.

thought to be uncommon in atrial flutter, LA thrombi are also present in that disorder (85). Transesophageal echocardiography is both highly sensitive and specific for thrombus detection in the left atrium and left atrial appendage (86–88).

The most common primary cardiac tumor is an atrial myxoma, which occurs 75%–80% of the time in the left atrium (42,53,54,89). Left atrial myxomas characteristically appear as rounded or oval structures. Although they may appear fairly smooth, close inspection often reveals multiple villous projections (Fig. 19.22). Most LA myxomas (~90%) arise from the interatrial septum, though they may arise from nearly any location in the atrium, including the appendage (Fig. 19.23) (90). Myxomas are

typically attached to the atrial septum via a stalk that arises from or near the fossa ovalis. The presence of a stalk is not essential for the diagnosis because up to 10% of myxomas may be sessile (91). Pedunculated myxomas with long stalks may be quite mobile and move toward the mitral valve during diastole and back into the left atrial chamber in systole. A very large myxoma can, in fact, occupy most of the LA volume and interfere with left ventricular inflow.

Atrial myxomas are typically distinguished from other left atrial masses by their characteristic shape and appearance, as well as their site of origin. However, final diagnosis requires histologic confirmation. Intraoperatively the TEE operator must confirm the presence of a myx-

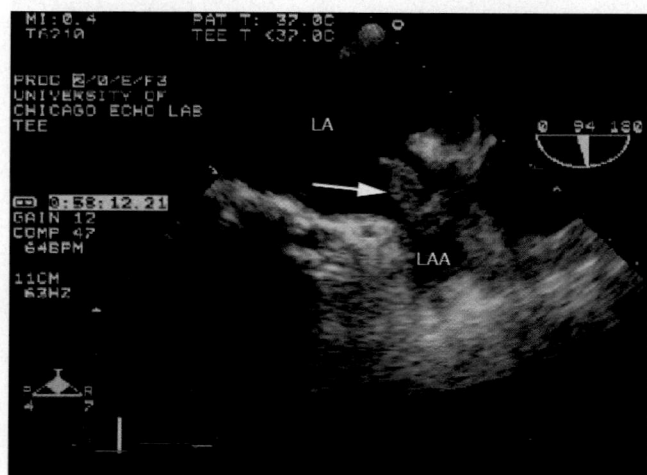

**FIGURE 19.21.** Large mobile left atrial appendage (*LAA*) thrombus (*arrow*).

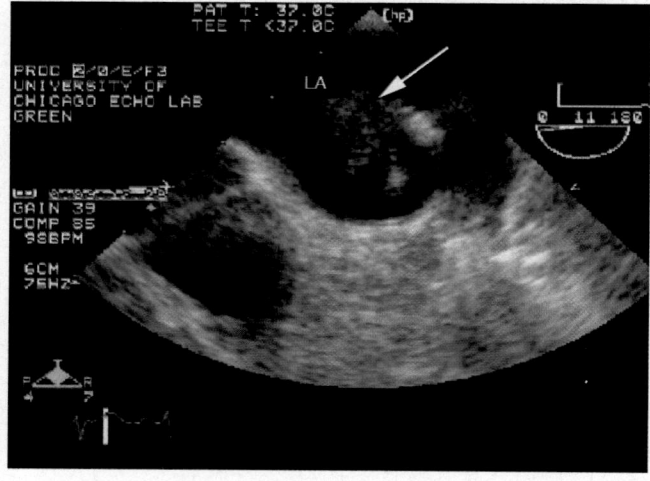

**FIGURE 19.23.** Atypical left atrial myxoma attached near the mouth of the left atrial appendage. *LA,* left atrium.

oma and identify the extent of involvement of the interatrial septum. Careful inspection of the remaining atrium and contralateral atrium is essential as these tumors may occasionally be multiple or biatrial. Intraoperative TEE is also used to look for mitral valve dysfunction (both obstruction and regurgitation) resulting from the myxoma. Evaluation of the integrity of the mitral valve and interatrial septum after resection prior to leaving the operating room is also important. Recently, 3-D TEE has allowed superior visualization of the size and attachment, as well as mitral involvement of LA myxomas (13,14).

Other primary cardiac tumors (benign or malignant), such as rhabdomyosarcoma, are unusual within the left atrium, but have been reported on occasion (92). Secondary involvement of the left atrium by cardiac tumors occurs in two manners. The first is invasion of the left atrium from extracardiac extension of a tumor, most commonly from breast, lung, or esophageal cancer (Fig. 19.24). Lung carcinomas may also invade the left atrium hematogenously through one of the pulmonary veins (93,94). A homogeneous mass filling a pulmonary vein and entering the left atrium should be highly suspicious for bronchogenic carcinoma.

## LEFT VENTRICLE

There are many masses that can be found within the left ventricular cavity; however, the most common are thrombi. Thrombi occur primarily in one of two situations, either global left ventricular systolic dysfunction or regional akinesis/dyskinesis of the ventricular apex. Less commonly, thrombi may be seen in inferobasilar aneurysms. Apical LV thrombi appear as masses with increased echogenicity and clearly delineated borders adja

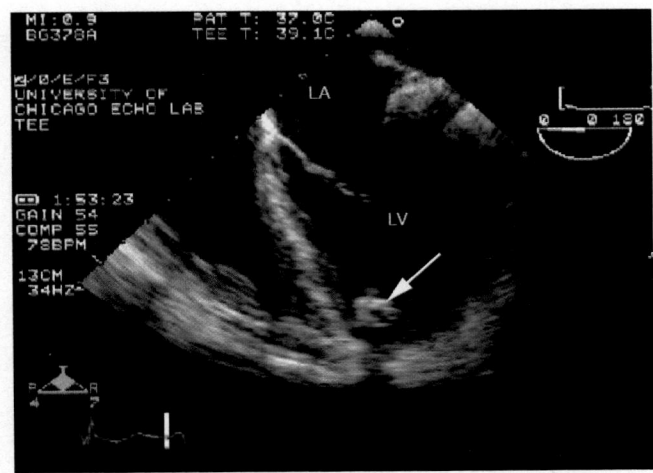

**FIGURE 19.25.** Midesophageal four-chamber view demonstrating a left ventricular (*LV*) apical partially calcified thrombus (*arrow*). *LA*, left atrium.

cent to but distinct from the endocardium (Figs. 19.25 and 19.26). The acoustic quality of thrombi are distinctly different from the surrounding myocardium. Thrombi should be visualized in both systole and diastole as well as in more than one view to ensure differentiation from artifact and tangential cuts through the LV apex. Although large pedunculated thrombi are easy to visualize, small thrombi and mural thrombi may be difficult to demonstrate from the transesophageal approach.

Complete visualization of the left ventricular apex from the midesophageal two- and four-chamber views requires significant retroflexion such that maintaining contact may be difficult. Despite this, several studies have shown the superiority of TEE over TTE for visualization

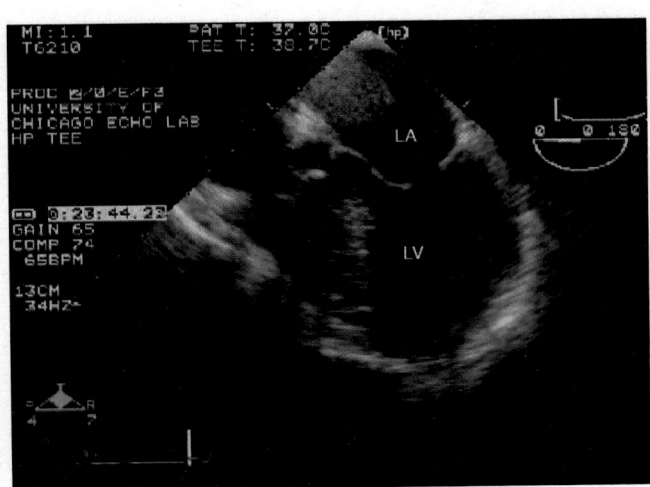

**FIGURE 19.24.** Infiltration into the left atrium (*LA*) of a lung carcinoma (*arrow*). *LV*, left ventricle.

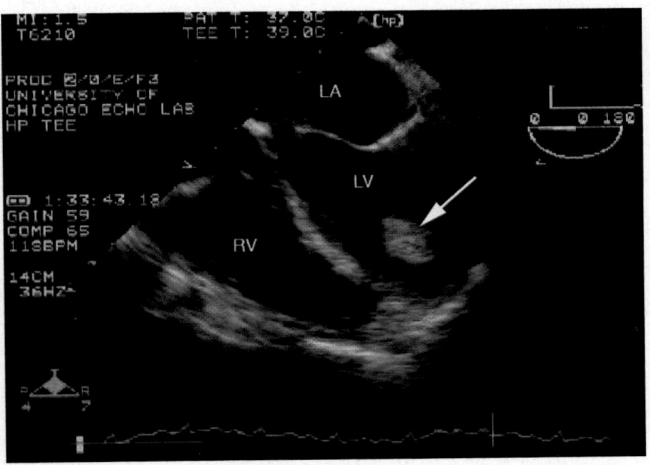

**FIGURE 19.26.** Midesophageal four-chamber view demonstrating a large left ventricular (*LV*) thrombus (*arrow*). *LA*, left atrium; *RV*, right ventricle.

of apical thrombus (7,95), although others have not (1). Intraoperative assessment of the LV for thrombus may be particularly helpful in patients with TTE exams that are equivocal for apical thrombus. In this group, TEE confirms clot in more than 50% (95). Use of the transgastric two-chamber and the deep transgastric long-axis views may be useful to visualize the LV apex. Intraoperative identification of an apical clot may allow alteration of the surgical procedure to minimize LV manipulation or even remove the clot. Because apical thrombi may be dislodged or fragmented during bypass surgery, careful inspection of the LV apex in susceptible patients prior to removal of the cross-clamp may prevent intraoperative embolization (19).

There are several primary tumors that involve the left ventricle. Unlike atrial tumors, primary tumors of the LV tend to be intramural. Rhabdomyomas are the most common primary cardiac tumors in pediatric patients and are often multiple (42,47–49). These are primarily ventricular tumors with nearly equal frequency in the right and left ventricles. Rhabdomyomas typically are more echodense than the myocardium and may be intramural or intracavitary. Fibromas are the second most common tumors in the left ventricle and most frequently are intramural, involving the interventricular septum or anterior free wall. These tumors range in size from 3 to 10 cm and central calcification is common (96,97). Left ventricular myxomas are uncommon (98) as are fibroelastomas. Malignant primary tumors of the heart, the majority of which are sarcomas, are more commonly right-sided but can occur in the left ventricle (47–49).

Secondary involvement of the left ventricle by malignancies may occur by direct invasion of an extracardiac mass. Myocardial involvement can be diagnosed by noting a change in the tissue characterization of a segment of myocardium and akinesis of the myocardium that has been infiltrated (99). If this occurs adjacent to a homogeneous extracardiac mass, tumor infiltration should be suspected. Tumor infiltration can progress rapidly and extensive myocardial replacement by tumor can occur, leading to severe heart failure and arrhythmias (100–102).

## AORTA

The most common aortic mass is an atheroma. Atheromas occur with greatest frequency in the descending aorta and aortic arch and least commonly in the ascending aorta. Aortic atheromatous disease represents a spectrum of abnormality. Early atheromatous disease is defined by intimal thickening or minor plaque formation. Higher grade atheromas protrude into the aortic lumen. These plaques are heterogeneous and frequently have calcification. Atheromas typically involve a portion of the circumferential extent of the aorta, though in severe cases

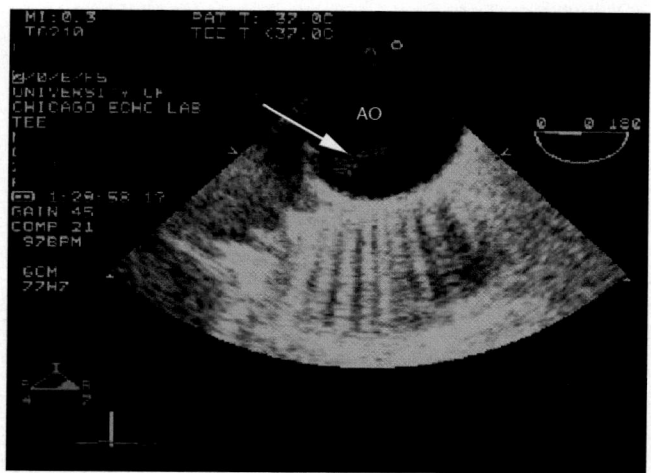

**FIGURE 19.27.** Short axis of the descending thoracic aorta (*Ao*) showing a large protruding mobile atheroma (*arrow*).

the aorta can be involved in its entire circumference. Large atheroma may have highly mobile protruding components that likely represent thrombus (Fig. 19.27). More extensive thrombus may be seen in aneurysmal segments of the thoracic aorta (Fig. 19.28).

Aortic plaques more than 4 to 5 mm in thickness or with mobile components are markers for significant embolic risk during cardiac surgery (103–107). Identification of the extent and location of atheroma on intraoperative TEE prior to aortic manipulation may help reduce perioperative stroke risk (15). Preliminary data using ultrasound-guided selection of the site for aortic cannulation and cross-clamping revealed the potential to reduce the risk of perioperative stroke due to embolization of atherosclerotic debris (108,109). This is discussed more in the chapter on assessment of aortic disease.

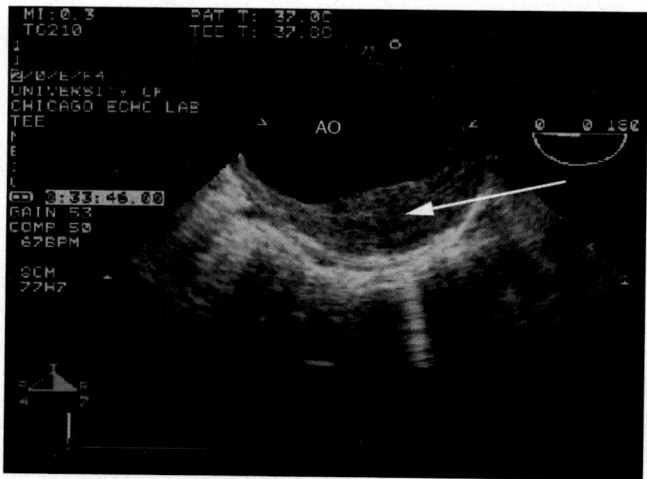

**FIGURE 19.28.** Dilated segment of the descending thoracic aorta (*Ao*) with extensive thrombus (*arrow*).

Primary tumors of the aorta are rare. Secondary involvement of the aorta by tumor, although uncommon, has been reported. Primary lung malignancies often extend to invade local structures that may include the thoracic aorta. TEE has been used to help stage periaortic invasion of lung cancer in patients with a suspicion of aortic involvement by CT scanning (110). Aortic involvement by lung carcinoma may be confused with aortic pathology, such as intramural hematoma (111).

## KEY POINTS

- TEE allows improved definition of cardiac mass size, shape, mobility, tissue characterization, location, attachment, and extent of myocardial involvement compared to the transthoracic window.
- Intraoperative TEE can be invaluable in guiding the surgical approach for removal of an intracardiac mass, assessing the hemodynamic effects of a cardiac mass, and evaluating for residual mass and sequelae of mass removal on valvular and myocardial function.
- Knowledge of the normal structures, anatomic variants, and artifacts that can be confused with pathologic masses during a transesophageal examination is essential.
- Most pathologic cardiac masses represent thrombus, infection, or tumor.
- A reasonably secure diagnosis of a cardiac mass can usually be made by incorporating the location and appearance of the mass with associated echocardiographic findings and clinical data.
- Cardiac involvement by malignancy is most commonly due to secondary or metastatic disease.
- Primary cardiac tumors are uncommon and most (75%–80%) are benign. Of these more than one-half are myxomas.
- The lack of malignant potential does not always indicate a "benign" clinical course because nonmalignant intracavitary tumors may produce obstruction of blood flow or partially dislodge, causing embolization.

## REFERENCES

1. Mugge A, Daniel WG, Haverich A, Lichtlen PR. Diagnosis of noninfective cardiac mass lesions by two-dimensional echocardiography. Comparison of the transthoracic and transesophageal approaches. Circulation 1991;83:70–8.
2. Obeid AI, Marvasti M, Parker F, Rosenberg J. Comparison of trans-thoracic and transesophageal echocardiography in diagnosis of left atrial-myxoma. Am J Cardiol 1989;63:1006–8.
3. Alam M, Sun I. Transesophageal echocardiographic evaluation of left atrial mass lesions. J Am Soc Echocardiogr 1991;4:323–30.
4. Leibowitz G, Keller NM, Daniel WG, et al. Transesophageal versus transthoracic echocardiography in the evaluation of right atrial tumors. Am Heart J 1995;130:1224–7.
5. DeVille JB, Corley D, Jin BS, de Castro CM, Hall RJ, Wilansky S. Assessment of intracardiac masses by transesophageal echocardiography. Tex Heart Inst J 1995;22:134–7.
6. Shyu KG, Chen JJ, Cheng JJ, Hwang JJ, Kuan P, Lien WP. Comparison of transthoracic and transesophageal echocardiography in the diagnosis of intracardiac tumors in adults. J Clin Ultrasound 1994;22:381-9.
7. Reeder GS, Khandheria BK, Seward JB, Tajik AJ. Transesophageal echocardiography and cardiac masses. [See comments.] Mayo Clin Proc 1991;66:1101–9.
8. Alam M, Sun I, Smith S. Transesophageal echocardiographic evaluation of right atrial mass lesions. J Am Soc Echocardiogr 1991;4:331–7.
9. Alam M, Rosman HS, Grullon C. Transesophageal echocardiography in evaluation of atrial masses. Angiology 1995;46:123–28.
10. Koide Y, Mizoguchi T, Ishii K, Okumura F. Intraoperative management for removal of tumor thrombus in the inferior vena cava or the right atrium with multiplane transesophageal echocardiography. J Cardiovasc Surg 1998;39:641–7.
11. Aru GM, Falchi S, Cardu G, Meloni L, Lixi G, Martelli V. The role of transesophageal echocardiography in the monitoring of cardiac mass removal: a review of 17 cases. J Card Surg 1993;8:554–7.
12. Milano A, Dan M, Bortolotti U. Left atrial myxoma: excision guided by transesophageal cross-sectional echocardiography. Int J Cardiol 1990;27:125–7.
13. Borges AC, Witt C, Bartel T, Muller S, Konertz W, Baumann G. Preoperative two- and three-dimensional transesophageal echocardiographic assessment of heart tumors. Ann Thorac Surg 1996;61:1163–167.
14. Borges AC, Bartel T, Mueller S, Bohm J, Baumann G. Assessment of myxoma with dynamic three-dimensional echocadiography: A helpful new approach for the surgical management. Am J Noninvasive Cardiol 1994; 8:313–16.
15. Task Force on Perioperative Transesophageal Echocardiography. Practice guidelines for perioperative transesophageal echocardiography. A report by the American Society of Anesthesiologists and the Society of Cardiovascular Anesthesiologists Task Force on Transesophageal Echocardiography. Anesthesiology 1996;84:986–1006.
16. Ofori CS, Sharma BN, Moore LC, Warshafsky G, Bennett R, Gradman AH. Disappearing cardiac masses—the importance of intraoperative transesophageal echocardiography. J Heart Valve Dis 1994;3:688–9.
17. Dujardin KS, Click RL, Oh JK. The role of intraoperative transesophageal echocardiography in patients undergoing cardiac mass removal. J Am Soc Echocardiogr 2000;13:1080–3.
18. Brooker RF, Butterworth JF, Klopfenstein HS. Intraoperative diagnosis of left atrial-myxoma. Anesth Analg 1995;80:183–84.
19. Maslow A, Lowenstein E, Steriti J, Leckie R, Cohn W, Haering M. Left ventricular thrombi: Intraoperative detection by transesophageal echocardiography and recognition of a source of post CABG embolic stroke: a case series. Anesthesiology 1998;89:1257–62.
20. Leslie D, Hall TS, Goldstein S, Shindler D. Mural left atrial thrombus: a hidden danger accompanying cardiac surgery. J Card Surg 1998;39:649–50.
21. Schuetz WH, Welz A, Heymer B. A symptomatic papillary fibroelastoma of the left-ventricle removed with the aid of transesophageal echocardiography. Thorac Cardiovasc Surg 1993;41:258–60.
22. Kawahito S, Kitahata H, Tanaka K, et al. Intraoperative management of a pediatric patient undergoing cardiac tumor

resection with the aid of transesophageal and epicardial echocardiography. Anesth Analg 1999;88:1048–50.

23. Mora F, Mindich BP, Guarino T, Goldman ME. Improved surgical approach to cardiac tumors with intraoperative two-dimensional echocardiography. Chest 1987;91:142–4.

24. Rousou JA, Tighe DA, Rifkin RD, et al. Echocardiography allows safer venous cannulation during excision of large right atrial masses. Ann Thorac Surg 1998;65:403–6.

25. Ralston L, Wasdahl W. Chiari's network. A J Med 1958; 810–13.

26. Zema MJ, Temkin ML, Caccavano M. Echocardiographic appearance of the Chiari network. J Clin Ultrasound 1985;13: 671–4.

27. Werner JA, Cheitlin MD, Gross BW, Speck SM, Ivey TD. Echocardiographic appearance of the Chiari network: differentiation from right-heart pathology. Circulation 1981;63: 1104–9.

28. Goedde TA, Conetta D, Rumisek JD. Chiari network entrapment of thromboemboli: congenital inferior vena cava filter. Ann Thorac Surg 1990;49:317–8.

29. Goldschlager A, Goldschlager N, Brewster H, Kaplan J. Catheter entrapment in a Chiari network involving an atrial septal defect. Chest 1972;62:345–6.

30. Burke AP, Litovsky S, Virmani R. Lipomatous hypertrophy of the atrial septum presenting as a right atrial mass. Am J Surg Pathol 1996;20:678–85.

31. Ghods M, Lighty G, Ren J, Constantinescu D, Garden J, Elia E. Lipomatous hypertrophy of the atrial septum. Echocardiography 1994;4:21–26.

32. Pochis WT, Saeian K, Sagar KB. Usefulness of transesophageal echocardiography in diagnosing lipomatous hypertrophy of the atrial septum with comparison to transthoracic echocardiography. Am J Cardiol 1992;70:396–8.

33. Fyke FE, 3rd, Tajik AJ, Edwards WD, Seward JB. Diagnosis of lipomatous hypertrophy of the atrial septum by two-dimensional echocardiography. J Am Coll Cardiol 1983;1: 1352–7.

34. Saric M, Applebaum R, Culliford A, Huang J, Scholes J, Kronzon I. Massive atrial septal lipomatous hypertrophy. Echocardiography 1999;16:833–34.

35. Shirani J, Roberts WC. Clinical, electrocardiographic and morphologic features of massive fatty deposits ("lipomatous hypertrophy") in the atrial septum. J Am Coll Cardiol 1993;22:226–38.

36. Olivares-Reyes A, Chan S, Lazar EJ, Bandlamudi K, Narla V, Ong K. Atrial septal aneurysm: a new classification in two hundred five adults. J Am Soc Echocardiogr 1997;10:644–56.

37. Schneider B, Hofmann T, Meinertz T, Hanrath P. Diagnostic value of transesophageal echocardiography in atrial septal aneurysm. International Journal of Cardiac Imaging 1992; 8:143–52.

38. Pearson AC, Nagelhout D, Castello R, Gomez CR, Labovitz AJ. Atrial septal aneurysm and stroke: a transesophageal echocardiographic study. J Am Coll Cardiol 1991;18:1223–9.

39. Mugge A, Daniel WG, Angermann C, et al. Atrial septal aneurysm in adult patients. A multicenter study using transthoracic and transesophageal echocardiography. [See comments.] Circulation 1995;91:2785–92.

40. Veinot JP, Harrity PJ, Gentile F, et al. Anatomy of the normal left atrial appendage: a quantitative study of age-related changes in 500 autopsy hearts: implications for echocardiographic examination. Circulation 1997;96:3112–5.

41. Vignon P, Spencer KT, Rambaud G, et al. Differential transesophageal echocardiographic diagnosis between linear artifacts and intraluminal flap of aortic dissection or disruption. Chest 2001;119:1778–90.

42. Roberts WC. Primary and secondary neoplasms of the heart. Am J Cardiol 1997;80:671–82.

43. Abraham KP, Reddy V, Gattuso P. Neoplasms metastatic to the heart: review of 3314 consecutive autopsies. Am J Cardiovasc Pathol 1990;3:195–8.

44. Lam KY, Dickens P, Chan AC. Tumors of the heart. A 20-year experience with a review of 12,485 consecutive autopsies. Arch Pathol Lab Med 1993;117:1027–31.

45. Sigman DB, Hasnain JU, Del Pizzo JJ, Sklar GN. Real-time transesophageal echocardiography for intraoperative surveillance of patients with renal cell carcinoma and vena caval extension undergoing radical nephrectomy. J Urol 1999;161: 36–8.

46. Reynen K. Frequency of primary tumors of the heart. Am J Cardiol 1996;77:107.

47. Fenoglio JJ, Jr., McAllister HA J, Ferrans VJ. Cardiac rhabdomyoma: a clinicopathologic and electron microscopic study. Am J Cardiol 1976;38:241–51.

48. Smythe JF, Dyck JD, Smallhorn JF, Freedom RM. Natural history of cardiac rhabdomyoma in infancy and childhood. [see comments]. Am J Cardiol 1990;66:1247–9.

49. Burke AP, Virmani R. Cardiac rhabdomyoma: a clinicopathologic study. Mod Pathol 1991;4:70–4.

50. Goldman JH, Foster E. Transesophageal echocardiographic (TEE) evaluation of intracardiac and pericardial masses. Cardiol Clin 2000;18:849–60.

51. Pasierski TJ, Alton ME, Van Fossen DB, Pearson AC. Right atrial mobile thrombus: improved visualization by transesophageal echocardiography. Am Heart J 1992;123:802–3.

52. Nellessen U, Daniel WG, Matheis G, Oelert H, Depping K, Lichtlen PR. Impending paradoxical embolism from atrial thrombus: correct diagnosis by transesophageal echocardiography and prevention by surgery. J Am Coll Cardiol 1985; 5:1002–4.

53. Burke A, Virmani R. More on cardiac myxomas. [letter; comment]. N Engl J Med 1996;335:1462–63; discussion 1463–4.

54. Markel ML, Waller BF, Armstrong WF. Cardiac myxoma. A review. Medicine 1987;66:114–25.

55. Smith ST, Hautamaki K, Lewis JW, Serwin J, Alam M. Transthoracic and transesophageal echocardiography in the diagnosis and surgical management of right atrial myxoma. Chest 1991;100:575–6.

56. Janigan DT, Husain A, Robinson NA. Cardiac angiosarcomas. A review and a case report. Cancer 1986;57:852–9.

57. Frohwein SC, Karalis DG, McQuillan JM, Ross JJ, Jr., Mintz GS, Chandrasekaran K. Preoperative detection of pericardial angiosarcoma by transesophageal echocardiography. Am Heart J 1991;122:874–5.

58. Kullo IJ, Oh JK, Keeney GL, Khandheria BK, Seward JB. Intracardiac leiomyomatosis-echocardiographic features. Chest 1999;115:587–91.

59. Podolsky LA, Jacobs LE, Ioli A, Kotler MN. TEE in the diagnosis of intravenous leiomyomatosis extending into the right atrium. Am Heart J 1993;125:1462–64.

60. Tierney WM, Ehrlich CE, Bailey JC, King RD, Roth LM, Wann LS. Intravenous leiomyomatosis of the uterus with extension into the heart. Am J Med 1980;69:471–75.

61. Sogani PC, Herr HW, Bains MS, Whitmore WF, Jr. Renal cell carcinoma extending into inferior vena cava. J Urol 1983; 130:660–3.

62. Skinner DG, Pritchett TR, Lieskovsky G, Boyd SD, Stiles QR. Vena caval involvement by renal cell carcinoma. Surgical resection provides meaningful long-term survival. Ann Surg 1989;210:387–92; discussion 392–4.

63. Hatcher PA, Paulson DF, Anderson EE. Accuracy in staging of renal cell carcinoma involving vena cava. Urol 1992;39: 27–30.

64. Basso LV, Gradman M, Finkelstein S, Gonzalezlavin L. Tricuspid-valve obstruction due to intravenous leiomyomatosis. Clin Nucl Med 1984;9:152–55.

65. Treiger BF, Humphrey LS, Peterson CV, et al. Transesophageal echocardiography in renal cell carcinoma: an accurate diagnostic technique for intracaval neoplastic extension. J Urol 1991;145:1138–40.

66. Mizoguchi T, Koide Y, Ohara M, Okumura F. Multiplane transesophageal echocardiographic guidance during resection of renal cell carcinoma extending into the inferior vena cava. Anesth Analg 1995;81:1102–5.

67. Milne B, Cervenko FW, Morales A, Salerno TA. Massive intraoperative pulmonary tumor embolus from renal cell carcinoma. Anesthesiology 1981;54:253–5.

68. Allen G, Klingman R, Ferraris VA, Fisher H, Harte F, Singh A. Transesophageal echocardiography in the surgical management of renal cell carcinoma with intracardiac extension. J Cardiovasc Surg 1991;32:833–6.

69. Katz ES, Rosenzweig BP, Rorman D, Kronzon I. Diagnosis of tumor embolus to the pulmonary artery by transesophageal echocardiography. J Am Soc Echocardiogr 1992;5:439–43.

70. O'Hara JF, Jr., Sprung J, Whalley D, Lewis B, Zanettin G, Klein E. Transesophageal echocardiography in monitoring of intrapulmonary embolism during inferior vena cava tumor resection. J Cardiothorac Vasc Anesth 1999;13:69–71.

71. Nixdorff U, Erbel R, Drexler M, Meyer J. Detection of thromboembolus of the right pulmonary artery by transesophageal two-dimensional echocardiography. Am J Cardiol 1988;61:488–9.

72. Leibowitz D. Role of echocardiography in the diagnosis and treatment of acute pulmonary embolism. J Am Soc Echocardiogr 2001;14:921–26.

73. Rittoo D, Sutherland GR, Samuel L, Flapan AD, Shaw TR. Role of transesophageal echocardiography in diagnosis and management of central pulmonary artery thromboembolism. Am J Cardiol 1993;71:1115–8.

74. Wittlich N, Erbel R, Eichler A, et al. Detection of central pulmonary artery thromboemboli by transesophageal echocardiography in patients with severe pulmonary embolism. J Am Soc Echocardiogr 1992;5:515–24.

75. Pruszczyk P, Torbicki A, Kuch-Wocial A, Szulc M, Pacho R. Diagnostic value of transesophageal echocardiography in suspected haemodynamically significant pulmonary embolism. [See comments.] Heart 2001;85:628–34.

76. Pruszczyk P, Torbicki A, Pacho R, et al. Noninvasive diagnosis of suspected severe pulmonary embolism: transesophageal echocardiography vs spiral CT. [See comments.] Chest 1997;112:722–8.

77. Krivec B, Voga G, Zuran I, et al. Diagnosis and treatment of shock due to massive pulmonary embolism: approach with transesophageal echocardiography and intrapulmonary thrombolysis. [See comments.] Chest 1997;112:1310–6.

78. Fagan LF, Castello R, Barner H, Moran M, Labovitz AJ. Transesophageal echocardiographic diagnosis of recurrent right ventricular myxoma 2 years after excision of right atrial myxoma. Am Heart J 1990;120:1456–8.

79. Waller BF, Fletcher RD, Roberts WC. Carcinoma of the lung causing pulmonary arterial stenosis. Chest 1981;79:589–91.

80. Nagasaka S, Taniguchi S, Kobayashi S, et al. Successful treatment of intraoperative pulmonary tumor embolism from renal cell carcinoma. Heart Vessels 1997;12:199–202.

81. Ernst G, Stollberger C, Abzieher F, et al. Morphology of the left atrial appendage. Anat Rec 1995;242:553–61.

82. Wrisley D, Giambartolomei A, Lee I, Brownlee W. Left atrial ball thrombus: review of clinical and echocardiographic manifestations with suggestions for management. Am Heart J 1991;121:1784–90.

83. Manning WJ, Silverman DI, Gordon SP, Krumholz HM, Douglas PS. Cardioversion from atrial fibrillation without prolonged anticoagulation with use of transesophageal echocardiography to exclude the presence of atrial thrombi. [See comments.] N Engl J Med 1993;328:750–5.

84. Klein AL, Grimm RA, Murray RD, et al. Use of transesophageal echocardiography to guide cardioversion in patients with atrial fibrillation. [See comments.] N Engl J Med 2001;344:1411–20.

85. Wood KA, Eisenberg SJ, Kalman JM, et al. Risk of thromboembolism in chronic atrial flutter. Am J Cardiol 1997;79:1043–7.

86. Manning WJ, Weintraub RM, Waksmonski CA, et al. Accuracy of transesophageal echocardiography for identifying left atrial thrombi—a prospective, intraoperative study. Ann Intern Med 1995;123:817–22.

87. Aschenberg W, Schluter M, Kremer P, Schroder E, Siglow V, Bleifeld W. Transesophageal two-dimensional echocardiography for the detection of left atrial appendage thrombus. J Am Coll Cardiol 1986;7:163–66.

88. Mugge A, Kuhn H, Daniel WG. The role of transesophageal echocardiography in the detection of left atrial thrombi. Echocardiography 1993;10:405–17.

89. Heath D. Pathology of cardiac tumors. Am J Cardiol 1968;21:315–27.

90. Feinglass NG, Reeder GS, Finck SJ, Shine TS, Maniu CV. Myxoma of the left atrial appendage mimicking thrombus during aortic valve replacement. J Am Soc Echocardiogr 1998;11:677–9.

91. St John Sutton MG, Mercier LA, Giuliani ER, Lie JT. Atrial myxomas: a review of clinical experience in 40 patients. Mayo Clin Proc 1980;55:371–6.

92. Awad M, Dunn B, al Halees Z, et al. Intracardiac rhabdomyosarcoma: transesophageal echocardiographic findings and diagnosis. J Am Soc Echocardiogr 1992;5:199–202.

93. Weg IL, Mehra S, Azueta V, Rosner F. Cardiac metastasis from adenocarcinoma of the lung. Echocardiographic-pathologic correlation. Am J Med 1986;80:108–12.

94. Onuigbo WI. Direct extension of cancer between pulmonary veins and the left atrium. Chest 1972;62:444–6.

95. Chen C, Koschyk D, Hamm C, Sievers B, Kupper W, Bleifeld W. Usefulness of transesophageal echocardiography in identifying small left-ventricular apical thrombus. J Am Coll Cardiol 1993;21:208–15.

96. Parmley LF, Salley RK, Williams JP, Head GB. The clinical spectrum of cardiac fibroma with diagnostic and surgical considerations—noninvasive imaging enhances management. Ann Thorac Surg 1988;45:455–65.

97. Takahashi K, Imamura Y, Ochi T, et al. Echocardiographic demonstration of an asymptomatic patient with left-ventricular fibroma. Am J Cardiol 1984;53:981–82.

98. Wrisley D, Rosenberg J, Giambartolomei A, Levy I, Turiello C, Antonini T. Left ventricular myxoma discovered incidentally by echocardiography. Am Heart J 1991;121:1554–5.

99. Lestuzzi C, Biasi S, Nicolosi GL, et al. Secondary neoplastic infiltration of the myocardium diagnosed by two-dimensional echocardiography in seven cases with anatomic confirmation. J Am Coll Cardiol 1987;9:439–45.

100. Lee PJ, Spencer KT. Pseudoaneurysm of the left ventricular free wall caused by tumor. J Am Soc Echocardiogr 1999;12:876–8.

101. Lynch M, Cobbs W, Miller RL, Martin RP. Massive cardiac involvement by malignant lymphoma. Cardiology 1996;87:566–8.

102. Miyazaki T, Yoshida T, Mori H, Yamazaki K, Handa S, Nakamura Y. Intractable heart failure, conduction disturbances and myocardial infarction by massive myocardial invasion of malignant lymphoma. J Am Coll Cardiol 1985;6:937–41.

103. Tunick PA, Kronzon I. Atheromas of the thoracic aorta: clinical and therapeutic update. J Am Coll Cardiol 2000;35:545–54.

104. Heinzlef O, Cohen A, Amarenco P. An update on aortic causes of ischemic stroke. Curr Opin Neurol 1997;10:64–72.

105. Blauth CI, Cosgrove DM, Webb BW, et al. Atheroembolism from the ascending aorta. An emerging problem in cardiac surgery. J Thorac Cardiovasc Surg 1992;103:1104–11; discussion 1111–2.

106. Davila-Roman VG, Barzilai B, Wareing TH, Murphy SF, Schechtman KB, Kouchoukos NT. Atherosclerosis of the ascending aorta. Prevalence and role as an independent predictor of cerebrovascular events in cardiac patients. Stroke 1994;25:2010–16.

107. Katz ES, Tunick PA, Rusinek H, Ribakove G, Spencer FC, Kronzon I. Protruding aortic atheromas predict stroke in elderly patients undergoing cardiopulmonary bypass: experience with intraoperative transesophageal echocardiography. J Am Coll Cardiol 1992;20:70–7.

108. Ribakove GH, Katz ES, Galloway AC, et al. Surgical implications of transesophageal echocardiography to grade the atheromatous aortic arch. Ann Thorac Surg 1992;53:758–61; discussion 762–3.

109. Wareing TH, Davila-Roman VG, Barzilai B, Murphy SF, Kouchoukos NT. Management of the severely atherascle-

rotic ascending aorta during cardiac operations. A strategy for detection and treatment. J Thorac Cardiovasc Surg 1992;103:453–62.

110. Wang KY, Lin CY, Kuo-Tai J, Yuan L, Chang HJ. Use of transesophageal echocardiography for evaluation of resectability of lung cancer. Acta Anaesthesiologica Sinica 1994;32:255–60.

111. Draznin J, Spencer KT. Squamous cell carcinoma masquerading as a thoracic intramural hematoma. Echocardiography 2001;18:175–7.

## QUESTIONS

1. Which of the following statements is false concerning neoplastic masses in the heart?
   A. Metastatic neoplasms are far more common than are primary tumors by a 20–30:1 ratio.
   B. Lung and breast tumors are two of the more common malignant tumors involving the heart.
   C. Melanomas have a predilection for metastasizing to the heart.
   D. Most secondary involvement of the heart by malignancy is myocardial.

2. Which of the following statements regarding primary tumors of the heart is false?
   A. Most primary cardiac tumors are benign.
   B. Cardiac lipomas are the most common benign primary cardiac tumor.
   C. Most primary malignant cardiac tumors are types of sarcoma.
   D. The most common location for a primary malignant tumor of the heart is the right atrium.

3. Which of the following statements regarding cardiac thrombi is true?
   A. Approximately 50% of cardiac thrombi in patients with atrial fibrillation are found in the right atrium.
   B. Detection of any irregularity on the wall of the left atrial appendage is highly suspicious for thrombus because the left atrial appendage is typically smooth walled.
   C. LV apical thrombi should be visualized in both systole and diastole, as well as in more than one view.
   D. Transesophageal echocardiography allows definitive distinction between cardiac thrombi and cardiac tumors.

# Assessment of Congenital Heart Disease in the Adult Patient

## Isobel Russell and Elyse Foster

*This chapter is, in large part, based on an original review that is currently in press: Russell IA, Rouine-Rapp K, Stratmann G, Miller-Hance W. Congenital Heart Disease in the Adult: A Review with Internet-Accessible Transesophageal Echocardiography, Anesthesia and Analgesia.*

Advances in cardiac surgery, anesthesia, intensive care, and diagnosis over the last 50 years have permitted survival of 85% of infants with congenital heart disease (CHD) into adulthood. In fact, for the first time, the number of adults with CHD equals the number of children with the disorder (1). Although accurate statistics are lacking, the number of adults with CHD in the United States has reached a conservative estimate of approximately 800,000, which is increasing at the rate of 5% per year. It was estimated that by the year 2002, the number of adults with simple, moderate, and complex forms of CHD would be approximately 370,000, 300,000, and 120,000, respectively (1). These figures are underestimates because they do not include patients that are diagnosed in adulthood, but are based on the widely varying reported prevalence rates of congenital heart disease. It is estimated that the number of patients with congenital heart disease reaching adulthood is approximately 16,000 per year in the United States alone (1). The recent consensus report (1) suggests that these patients should receive care in regional centers for adult congenital heart disease and the patients should keep their own copies of information on operations, cardiac catheterizations, and other diagnostic tests, such as echocardiograms in the form of a "health passport."

## INDICATIONS

Indications for TEE in adult patients with congenital heart disease should follow established guidelines by the American Society of Anesthesiologists and the Society of Cardiovascular Anesthesiologists (2) and the American College of Cardiology/American Heart Association Task Forces (3). It should be emphasized that a complete diagnosis of the congenital heart lesion should be defined prior to performance of intraoperative TEE. The lesion, coexisting pathology, hemodynamics, cardiac size, and function should be well delineated whether by cardiac catheterization, transthoracic echocardiography, or transesophageal echocardiography (4–6). Intraoperative TEE should not be used as a replacement for an inadequate preoperative evaluation.

Here are summaries from the two reports on the indications for intraoperative TEE for congenital heart disease.

a) "Practice guidelines for perioperative transesophageal echocardiography."

Most cardiac defects requiring repair under cardiopulmonary bypass are a category 1 indication for intraoperative TEE, including pre- and post-cardiopulmonary imaging (category 1 is defined as that being supported by the strongest evidence or expert opinion substantiating that TEE is useful in improving clinical outcomes) (2).

b) "ACC/AHA guidelines for the clinical application of echocardiography."

Monitoring and guidance during cardiothoracic procedures associated with the potential for residual shunts, valvular regurgitation, obstruction or myocardial dysfunction is a class 1 indication (defined as conditions for which there is evidence and/or general agreement that a given procedure or treatment is useful and effective) (3). This was defined under the indications for TEE in pediatric patients with congenital heart disease but is applicable to adolescents and adults with CHD.

## Approach

Image orientation, nomenclature guidelines, and a comprehensive intraoperative echocardiographic examination should follow those suggested by the American Society of Echocardiography (7) and ASE/SCA guidelines (8). Appropriate TEE views for evaluation of congenital heart lesions are described in Table 20.1 and Fig. 20.1. Assessment of the connections of the various cardiac segments, atrial arrangement or situs, venoatrial, atrioventricular, and ventriculoarterial connections should be performed. Septal and valvar structures should then be evaluated, including assessment of flow velocities with Doppler echocardiography. In general, the approach for each lesion is to define the intracardiac anatomy and associated defects, assess the ventricular function, and evaluate any residual lesions (Table 20.2). Comprehensive reference atlases include *Pediatric Echocardiography*, edited by N. Silverman (Williams and Wilkins), *Transesophageal Echocardiography in Congenital Heart Disease*, edited by O. Stumper and G. Sutherland (Little, Brown and Company), and *Congenital Heart Disease in Adults*, edited by J. K. Perloff and J. S. Child (W. B. Saunders).

Congenital heart disease can be classified in several ways: according to the underlying physiology of either shunt; obstructive, regurgitant, and mixed lesions; according to the presence and absence of cyanosis; or according to the level of complexity of the lesion. For purposes of simplicity, this chapter will organize the lesions according to level of complexity, with greater emphasis on the more common lesions.

## SIMPLE LESIONS

### Atrial Septal Defects

Atrial septal defects (ASD) are one of the most common defects in the adult population, accounting for one-fourth

▶ **TABLE 20.1. Congenital Heart Lesions—Appropriate TEE Views for Evaluation of Congenital Heart Lesions**

| *Lesion* | *TEE Plane* |
|---|---|
| Atrial Septal Defects | • ME four-chamber for ostium secundum and primum defects<br>• ME bicaval for interatrial septum for sinus venosus defects and possible anomalous pulmonary veins |
| Ventricular Septal Defects | • ME four-chamber, LAX for perimembranous, inlet and muscular VSDs, chamber sizes, presence of ventricular septal aneurysm<br>• ME AV LAX, deep TG LAX views for evaluation of the aortic valve for insufficiency and herniation<br>• ME RV inflow and outflow for pulmonic valve insufficiency |
| Atrioventricular Septal Defects | • ME four- and two- chamber for the bridging leaflets and their attachments, extent of intracardiac defects, size of septal defects, and extent of AV valve regurgitation |
| Aortic Stenosis (valvular and subvalvular) | • Deep TG LAX for aortic stenosis, insufficiency, and aortic root size<br>• ME AV SAX evaluation of aortic valve morphology<br>• ME four-chamber for LV hypertrophy and function assessment |
| Transposition of the Great Arteries | • ME four-chamber to evaluate AV valve regurgitation and baffle assessment after Senning/Mustard procedures<br>• ME bicaval view additionally for caval junctions and pulmonary veins<br>• TG mid SAX for ventricular function and SWMA<br>• Deep TG LAX for ventriculoarterial connections and anastomas after arterial switch |
| Tetralogy of Fallot | • ME AV LAX and deep TG LAX for definition of aortic override and obstruction of the right ventricular outflow tract and estimation of gradients<br>• ME RV inflow-outflow for RVOT evaluation<br>• ME four-chamber view for position and extension of VSD and other additional VSDs |
| Truncus Arteriosus | • ME four-chamber view for VSD position and extent<br>• ME AV SAX to evaluate truncal valve<br>• ME AV LAX and deep TG LAX for evaluation of truncal insufficiency and determination of truncal anatomy |
| Patent Ductus Arteriosus | • Difficult to visualize by 2D TEE, but ductal flow can be visualized in the ME asc aortic SAX view by presence of abnormal continuous high velocity aliased flow |
| Pulmonic Valve Stenosis | • ME RV inflow-outflow and deep TG LAX view for outflow tract evaluation and gradient estimation<br>• ME asc aortic SAX for evaluation of pulmonic valve and main pulmonary artery |
| Single Ventricles | • ME four-chamber, two-chamber and deep TG LAX for atrioventricular morphology and atrioventricular and ventriculoarterial connections<br>• ME bicaval view for evalution of Glenn anastomosis |

*asc,* ascending; *AV,* aortic valve; *LAX,* longitudinal axis; *ME,* midesophageal; *RV,* right ventricle; *RVOT,* right ventricular outflow tract; *SAX,* short axis; *SWMA,* segmental wall motion abnormality; *TG,* transgastric.

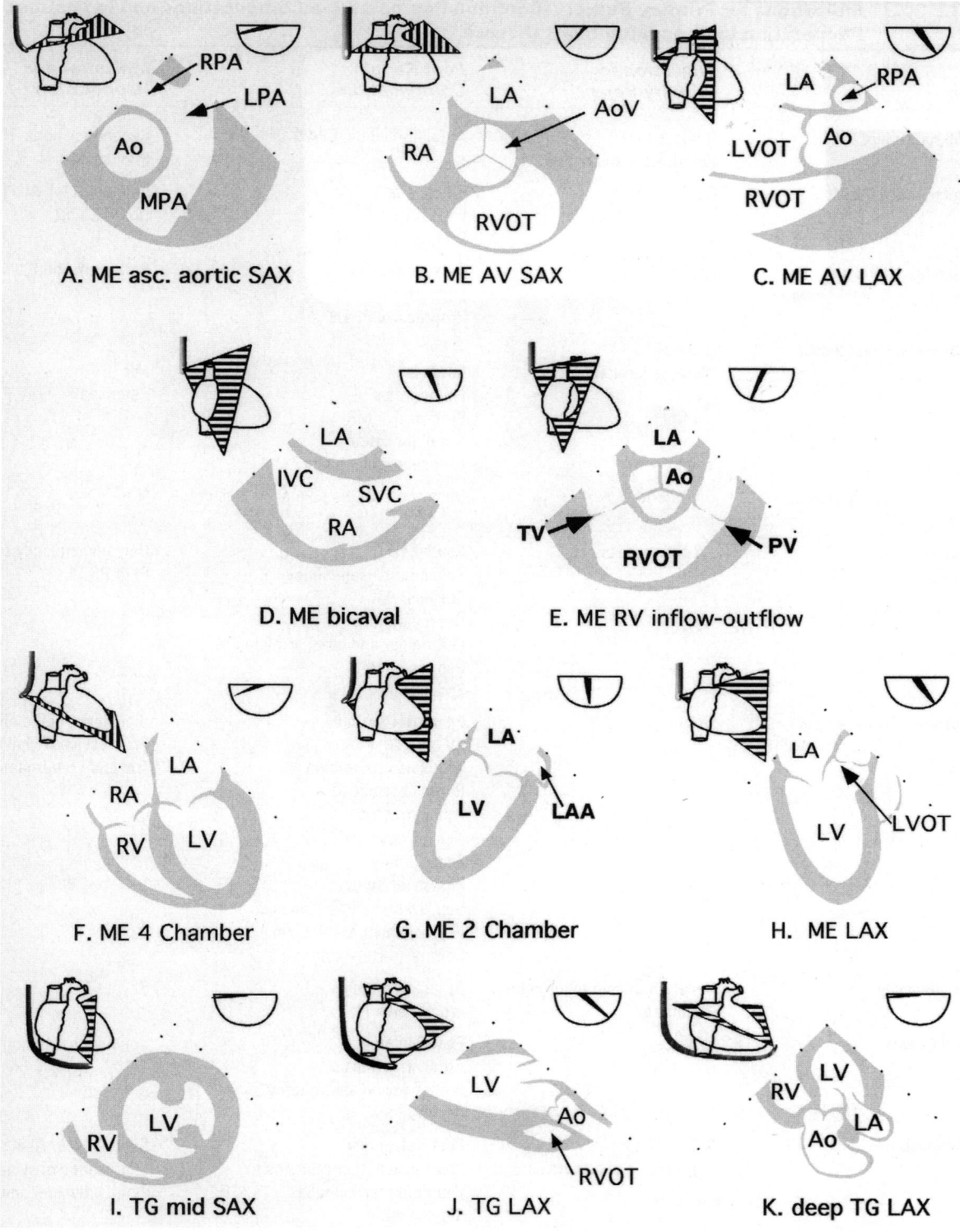

**FIGURE 20.1.** Cross-sectional views depicting imaging planes useful for assessment of congenital heart defects. The appropriate multiplane angle is indicated by the icon on the right adjacent to each view. The imaging plane is indicated by the schematic drawing of the heart on the left. *asc.*, ascending; *Ao*, aorta; *AoV*, aortic valve; *IVC*, inferior vena cava; *LA*, left atrium; *LAA*, left atrial appendage; *LAX*, long axis; *LPA*, left pulmonary artery; *LV*, left ventricle; *LVOT*, left ventricular outflow tract; *ME*, midesophageal; *MPA*, main pulmonary artery; *RA*, right atrium; *RPA*, right pulmonary artery; *RV*, right ventricle; *RVOT*, right ventricular outflow tract; *SAX*, short axis; *SVC*, superior vena cava; *TG*, transgastric; *TV*, tricuspid valve.

▶ **TABLE 20.2.   Indications for Primary Surgery, Common Postoperative Complications and Indications for Reoperation in Congenital Heart Disease**

| Lesion | Indication for Primary Repair | Post-Repair Complications | Indication for Reoperation |
|---|---|---|---|
| Atrial Septal Defect | Qp:Qs ≥ 1.8:1<br>Paradoxical embolization | Atrial fibrillation, CVA* | Secundum: none<br>Primum: MR |
| Ventricular Septal Defect | Qp:Qs ≥ 1.5:1 | Patch leak<br>Endocarditis*<br>Progressive PHTN | Patch leak when<br>Qp:Qs ≥ 1.5:1 |
| Patent Ductus Arteriosus | Qp:Qs > 1.5:1 | Persistent shunt<br>Endoarteritis*<br>Progressive PHTN | Persistent shunt |
| Atrioventricular Canal Defect | Qp:Qs > 1.5:1<br>Mitral regurgitation | Patch leak<br>Endocarditis<br>Progressive MR<br>Atrial fibrillation<br>Atrioventricular block | MR<br>Patch leak |
| Anomalous Pulmonary Venous Drainage | Qp:Qs > 1.5:1 | Obstruction of the pulmonary veins | N/A |
| Tetralogy of Fallot | No previous repair | Patch Leak<br>Pulmonary insufficiency<br>Residual PS<br>Heart block<br>Ventricular and atrial arrhythmias<br>Sudden death<br>Endocarditis | Hemodynamically significant PI or PS |
| Transposition of Great Vessel | N/A | **Postatrial Switch:**<br>RV failure<br>Tricuspid regurgitation<br>Baffle obstruction<br>Atrial arrhythmias<br>Heart block<br>Endocarditis<br>**Postatrial Switch:**<br>Supravalvar aortic stenosis<br>   (neopulmonic stenosis)<br>Coronary artery stenosis | Significant baffle obstruction<br>Progressive RV failure<br>Tricuspid regurgitation |
| Ebstein's Anomaly | Severe tricuspid regurgitation<br>RV failure | Atrial arrhythmias<br>Progressive TR | Severe TR |
| Tricuspid Atresia | N/A | **Post-Fontan**<br>Atrial arrhythmias<br>Protein losing enteropathy<br>Ascites | Conduit obstruction |
| Aortic Stenosis | AVA < 0.8 cm² in<br>   presence of symptoms | **Post-Valvotomy**<br>Progressive AI or restenosis<br>Ventricular arrhythmias<br>Sudden death<br>Endocarditis | Severe AS or AI in the<br>   presence of symptoms<br>   or LV dysfunction |
| Subaortic Stenosis | Gradient > 30 mm Hg or<br>   the development of AI<br>   at a lower gradient | Progressive AI<br>Restenosis<br>Endocarditis | Severe AI or recurrent<br>   stenosis in the presence<br>   of symptoms |

*(continued)*

▶ **TABLE 20.2.   Indications for Primary Surgery, Common Postoperative Complications and Indications for Reoperation in Congenital Heart Disease** (Continued)

| Lesion | Indication for Primary Repair | Post-Repair Complications | Indication for Reoperation |
|---|---|---|---|
| **Pulmonary Stenosis** | Transpulmonary gradient > 50 mm Hg<br>Transpulmonary gradient < 50 mm Hg with RV hypertrophy or symptoms | Restenosis<br>Pulmonic valve insufficiency<br>Endocarditis rare | Severe PS or PI in the presence of symptoms |
| **Coarctation of Aorta** | Upper extremity HTN<br>Transcoarct gradient > 25 mm Hg | Residual HTN<br>Saccular aneurysm<br>Dissecting aneurysm<br>Circle of Willis aneurysm<br>CVA<br>Premature CAD<br>AS/AI<br>Endocarditis or endarteritis | Recurrent coarctation<br>AS/AI (see above)<br>CAD<br>Saccular or dissecting aneurysm |

*Qp:Qs,* pulmonary to systemic flow ratio; *CVA,* cerebrovascular accident; *PHTN,* pulmonary hypertension; *MR,* mitral regurgitation; *PI,* pulmonic valve insufficiency; *PS,* pulmonary stenosis; *AS,* aortic stenosis; *TR,* tricuspid regurgitation, *RV,* right ventricle; *AVA,* aortic valve area; *CAD,* coronary artery disease.
*These complications are most common when repair performed at age > 40; *endocarditis and endarteritis likely only in the presence of persistent shunt.

to one-third of all lesions, occurring more commonly in women (9). There are four types of atrial septal defects:

1. Ostium secundum defect (70%), which occurs in the midseptum region of the fossa ovalis. Varying degrees of mitral valve prolapse and mitral regurgitation can occur, but hemodynamically significant lesions are uncommon.
2. Ostium primum defect (15%–25%), which is also a form of a partial atrioventricular canal defect and consists of an ASD in the lower part of the interatrial septum. Abnormalities of the atrioventricular valve can occur with a "cleft" anterior mitral valve and septal tricuspid valve leaflet with variable degrees of regurgitation.
3. Sinus venosus defect (10%) is usually superior and posterior in relation to the superior vena cava (more frequently) and/or inferior vena cava. These defects are frequently associated with an anomalous drainage of one or more pulmonary veins into the right atrium or superior vena cava (10).
4. Coronary sinus defects (extremely rare) occur between the left atrium and coronary sinus and can be associated with a persistent left superior vena cava.

Imaging with intraoperative TEE is performed following the guidelines in Table 20.1 to confirm the presence, size, and location of the defect; degree of atrioventricular valve regurgitation; ventricular function; and associated anomalies, such as anomalous pulmonary veins (Fig. 20.2). Postoperatively, TEE is used to detect residual

shunts by color Doppler and contrast, assess ventricular function, and assess for pulmonary venous obstruction and valvar regurgitation. To evaluate for residual shunts, we use agitated saline contrast because the microbubbles are readily apparent even when a very small number of microbubbles cross a defect (11). The method used is to vigorously agitate 0.5–1.0 cc of the patient's blood between two syringes with 10 cc of saline (12).

A defect in the interatrial septum allows pulmonary venous return to pass from the left to the right atrium. Because this left-to-right shunt increases the venous return to the right ventricle, the right ventricular stroke volume and pulmonary blood flow are increased compared with the systemic blood flow. Right ventricular volume overload results. Indirect evidence of an atrial septal defect includes right-sided chamber enlargement and appearance of saline contrast in the left heart chambers. Color flow Doppler echocardiography can demonstrate flow across the atrial septum and detect mitral or tricuspid regurgitation.

Primary or patch closure of an atrial septal defect in childhood provides excellent operative results and nearly normal long-term survival in adults (13,14). Additionally, a recent retrospective study suggested improved 10-year survival in patients over the age of 40 years treated surgically (95%) compared with those treated medically (84%) (14). A prospective clinical trial (15) randomized adult patients with secundum atrial septal defects with shunt ratios > 1.7:1 to surgical versus medical management, showing improved survival with surgical closure. However, late repair does not appear to reduce the incidence

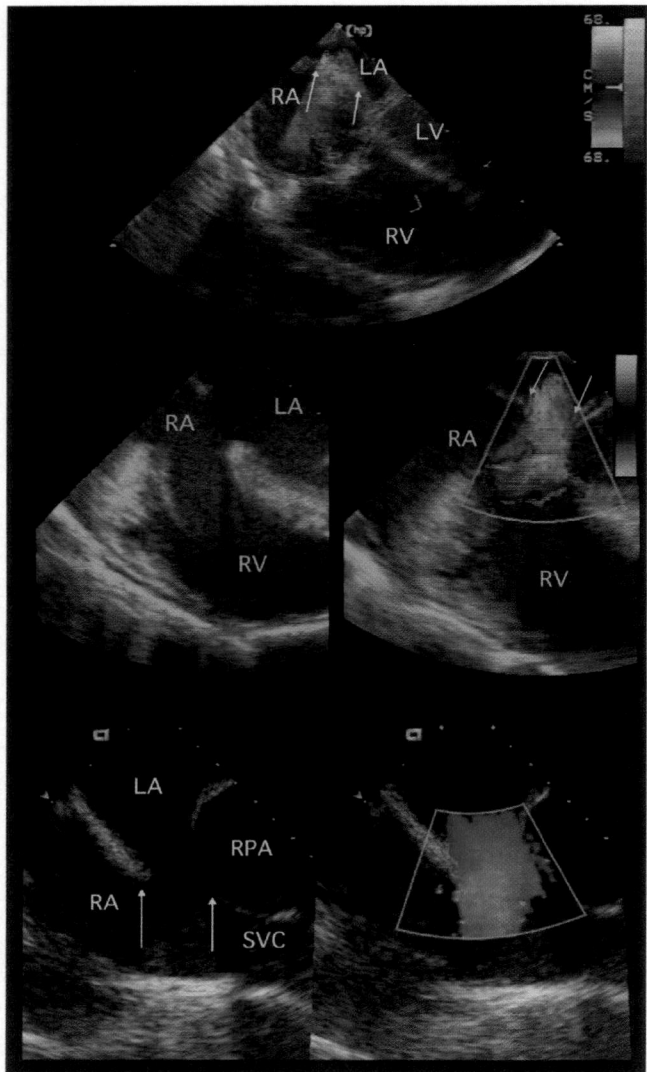

**FIGURE 20.2.** Atrial septal defects. **Top:** Secundum atrial septal defect (midesophageal four-chamber view). **Middle:** Primum atrial septal defect (midesophageal four-chamber view). **Bottom:** Sinus venosus atrial septal defect (midesophageal bicaval view). *Arrows* indicate the defect in the atrial septum. Left-to-right shunting is demonstrated by blue color flow Doppler. *LA,* left atrium; *LV,* left ventricle; *RA,* right atrium; *RV,* right ventricle; *RPA,* right pulmonary artery; *SVC,* superior vena cava.

of arrhythmias, which are generally related to preoperative atrial dilatation or postoperative incisional reentry (16). Operative patch closure is generally recommended if the shunt is large with a pulmonary blood flow-to-systemic blood flow ratio of 1.8:1 or higher and right ventricular enlargement. Percutaneous closure with a variety of devices is becoming increasingly available and can be considered in adults. Patients with smaller shunts have a lower incidence of congestive heart failure, pulmonary hypertension, and arrhythmias but are at risk for para-

doxical embolization. In patients with ostium primum defects, surgical valve repair with or without annuloplasty may reduce the severity of the mitral and tricuspid regurgitation. If severe mitral regurgitation persists, valve re-repair or replacement is necessary.

## Ventricular Septal Defects

Ventricular septal defects are the most common cardiac abnormality in infants and children (9). Patients with unoperated ventricular septal defects are encountered less frequently than those with atrial septal defect, because large defects are usually closed surgically in childhood when there is evidence of congestive heart failure or pulmonary hypertension. In infancy and childhood, defects have a high rate of spontaneous closure (90% of those that close do so by the time the child is 10 years of age).

Ventricular septal defects can be classified by anatomic location into four types:

1. Perimembranous ventricular septal defects (70%) are found in the membranous region of the septum and can extend into the muscular, inlet, or outlet regions.
2. Muscular ventricular septal defects (20%) are located within the trabecular portion of the septum, and can be in the central or apical areas. Multiple defects can occur, either two or three or multiple small ones known as "swiss cheese septum."
3. Doubly committed or subarterial ventricular septal defects (so called "supracristal") (5%) are found just below the aortic and pulmonary valves and may have associated aortic cusp herniation and aortic regurgitation.
4. Inlet ventricular septal defects (5%) occur close to the atrioventricular valves in the posterior and inlet portions of the septum.

TEE is particularly helpful in evaluation of these defects (Table 20.1). If the left-to-right shunt is large, the left atrium and left ventricle are dilated. Right ventricular dimension is normal unless there is pulmonary hypertension. Preoperatively TEE confirms the presence; size; and location of the defect, degree of atrioventricular and aortic valve regurgitation (Fig. 20.3). The peak velocity across the VSD can be used to estimate the right ventricular systolic pressure and pulmonary artery systolic pressure (17). Postoperatively, TEE is used to detect residual shunts by color Doppler and contrast and to assess ventricular function, residual aortic or pulmonic insufficiency, and right ventricular outflow tract obstruction.

The ventricular septal defect permits a left-to-right shunt to occur at the ventricular level and the physiologic consequences are determined by the size of the defect and the relative resistance of the systemic and pulmonary vascular beds. If the ventricular septal defect is small and restrictive, there is a large pressure difference between the left and the right ventricles in systole. If the ventricular

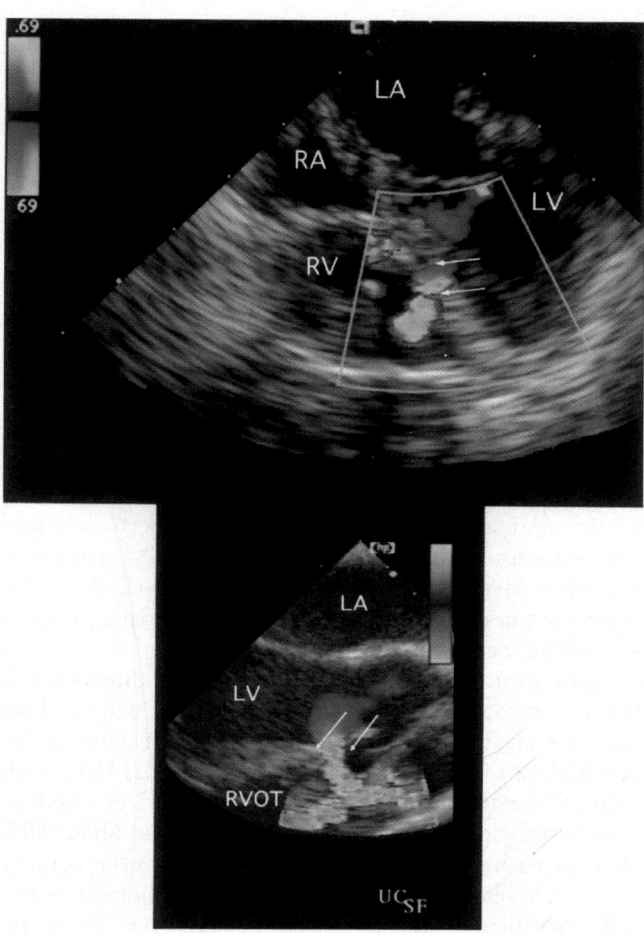

**FIGURE 20.3.** Ventricular septal defects. **Top:** Residual muscular ventricular septal defect (midesophageal four-chamber view) as indicated by the *arrows*, with color flow Doppler demonstrating the left-to-right ventricular shunting. **Bottom:** Subarterial (doubly committed) ventricular septal defect with color flow Doppler demonstrating the left-to-right-ventricular shunting into the right ventricular outflow tract. *LA*, left atrium; *LV*, left ventricle; *RA*, right atrium; *RVOT*, right ventricular outflow tract.

septal defect is large (nonrestrictive), there is no pressure difference between the left and the right ventricles; then, the magnitude of the shunt depends on the ratio of pulmonary vascular resistance to systemic vascular resistance. If the pulmonary vascular resistance is lower than the systemic vascular resistance, the left-to-right shunt can be large. When the increased pulmonary blood flow returns to the left ventricle, left ventricular diastolic volume and stroke volume increase.

By the time the patient has reached adolescence or early adulthood, there is virtually no chance that the ventricular septal defect will close spontaneously (Table 20.2). If the left-to-right shunt is large, congestive heart failure is possible. If a large ventricular septal defect is associated with pulmonary hypertension, the chance of the

development of pulmonary vascular disease is high. In adults diagnosed with ventricular septal defect, the overall 10-year survival after initial presentation is approximately 75%. Functional class greater than 1, cardiomegaly, and elevated pulmonary artery pressure (> 50 mm Hg) are clinical predictors of an adverse prognosis (7).

## Complete AV Septal Defect

In complete AV septal defect, there is failure of the endocardial cushions to close the atrial and ventricular septum, affecting the complete formation of the mitral and tricuspid valves. As a result, patients have a ventricular septal defect, an atrial septal defect, and varying degrees of AV valve regurgitation. With large left-to-right shunts at the atrial and ventricular levels and systemic pressures in the right ventricle because of the ventricular septal defect, pulmonary vascular disease occurs very early. Most adults with uncorrected complete atrioventricular septal defects (AVSD) are cyanotic with Eisenmenger's syndrome, and are not candidates for correction. When the repair has been performed in childhood, residual mitral or tricuspid regurgitation often remains.

TEE is useful for defining the type and extension of the septal defects (Table 20.1) and the morphology of the "bridging leaflets," which span the common orifice. Proposed by Rastelli et al., the attachment of the anterosuperior leaflet defines the various types of AVSDs (a, b, and c) (18). TEE of an AVSD demonstrates complete absence of the crux of the heart, with both low atrial and high ventricular septal defects (Fig. 20.4). In the adult, color flow imaging and Doppler studies usually show regurgitation

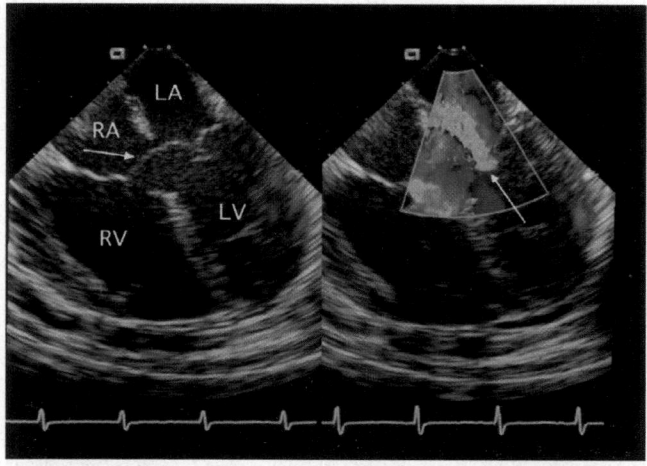

**FIGURE 20.4.** Atrioventricular septal defects. Atrioventricular septal defect (midesophageal four-chamber view) demonstrating the anterior-bridging leaflet (*arrow*) and interatrial and interventricular defects. The right frame demonstrates color flow Doppler of the left-sided atrioventricular valve regurgitation (*arrows*). *LA*, left atrium; *LV*, left ventricle; *RA*, right atrium; *RV*, right ventricle.

of both AV valves and evidence of pulmonary artery hypertension.

The lesions in these patients are usually corrected in infancy. The surgery consists of patch closure of the atrial and ventricular septal defects and repair of the AV valves. The unoperated adult with a complete AV septal defect is rarely a candidate for a complete repair because of the frequent and early development of pulmonary vascular disease, but she or he may be a candidate for heart-lung transplantation or lung transplantation with intracardiac repair (Table 20.2). For the patient who has been corrected in infancy, the most common postoperative sequela is progressive mitral valve regurgitation owing to an inadequate repair.

## Congenital Aortic Stenosis

The pathophysiology of congenital aortic stenosis is similar to that of acquired aortic stenosis. However, in congenital left ventricular outflow tract obstruction, the anatomic level of obstruction can be supravalvular or subvalvular whereas in acquired aortic stenosis, it is almost always valvular. Valvular aortic stenosis is due to a malformed valve that is usually functionally bicuspid, occurring in 2%–3% of the population (Fig. 20.5). Patients with the most severely malformed and stenotic valves may require intervention in childhood. Even with a less-restricted orifice, the disturbed flow through the valve causes progressive thickening and calcification and may eventually result in severe stenosis and varying degrees of valvular insufficiency that become manifest later in life. In supravalvular aortic stenosis, the narrowing is usually above the level of the sinuses of Valsalva. Therefore, the coronary arteries arise from the aorta proximal to the obstruction and are subjected to an elevated systolic pressure equal to that of the left ventricle. The high pressures cause coronary artery dilatation and may accelerate atherosclerosis.

In the most common form of subaortic stenosis, there is a discrete membrane immediately below the aortic valve, resulting in a systolic jet that traumatizes the valve leaflets, leading to aortic regurgitation. There is frequent association of left ventricular outflow tract obstruction with coarctation of the aorta and also mitral valve abnormalities.

TEE is diagnostic in valvular aortic stenosis with direct visualization of the valve leaflets by two-dimensional imaging and measurement of the pressure gradient across the left ventricular outflow tract by Doppler interrogation. Identification of associated lesions, especially aortic coarctation, and left ventricular hypertrophy and function should also be assessed. TEE can also visualize a subaortic membrane or supravalvar stenosis. With discrete membranous subvalvular aortic stenosis, progressive aortic regurgitation can occur.

After aortic valvotomy for severe stenosis during childhood, approximately one-fourth of patients will need repeat surgery for recurrent stenosis or progressive aortic insufficiency in the next 25 years (Table 20.2) (19). With medical treatment, approximately one-third of children with systolic gradients below 50 mm Hg and about 80% of those with gradient 50 to 79 mm Hg will need surgery within 25 years (19). With symptomatic, hemodynamically significant valvular aortic stenosis (i.e., an aortic valve area less than 0.8 cm²) and a flexible noncalcified valve, balloon valvotomy may have therapeutic success similar to that of operative valvotomy—even in young adults. However, when there is calcification or associated aortic insufficiency, valve replacement is required. An alternative is the Ross procedure, which involves placement of a homograft in the pulmonary valve position and the native pulmonary valve in the aortic position. The advantages of this innovative, although technically challenging, approach is that it obviates the need for anticoagulation without using bioprosthetic valves, which have an excessive rate of degeneration, however it is not as advantageous in the adult because growth is not a major issue.

## Coarctation of the Aorta

In the most common form of aortic coarctation, there is narrowing immediately distal to the takeoff of the left subclavian artery or more commonly at the level of the insertion of the ligamentum arteriosus. The constriction may take the form of a shelf or a localized hourglass narrowing of the distal arch proximal to the ligamentum. It is difficult to visualize the actual site of the coarctation in the adult patient with TEE. However, color Doppler studies of the descending aorta may detect flow acceleration

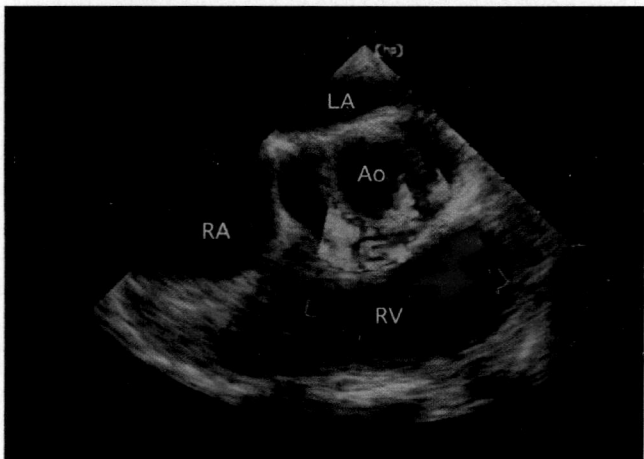

**FIGURE 20.5.** Bicuspid aortic valve. Bicuspid aortic valve (midesophageal aortic valve short-axis view) demonstrating the two cusps, instead of three, during systole. *Ao*, aortic valve; *LA*, left atrium; *RA*, right atrium; *RV*, right ventricle.

or turbulent jets (20). An associated bicuspid aortic valve can also be identified by TEE. Angiography or MRI is usually needed to define the site and extent of narrowing.

Arterial hypertension is usually present proximal to the aortic obstruction (Table 20.2). Repair should be undertaken when the coarctation is severe enough to cause proximal hypertension and the gradient across the coarctation is greater than 25 to 30 mm Hg. Most of these patients will have multiple collateral vessels seen on aortography and atheromatous changes at the site of the coarctation, which can complicate surgery. If the gradient is less than 20 mm Hg and no collaterals are present, repair is not indicated. In some patients, primary balloon dilatation has been used successfully. Aortic aneurysms can occur around the area of the coarctation or elsewhere in the aorta and in the branches of the circle of Willis (so-called berry aneurysms).

## Pulmonic Valvular Stenosis

Although pulmonic valve stenosis is congenital in origin, it may be progressive. The obstruction to outflow puts an afterload burden on the right ventricle, resulting in concentric right ventricular hypertrophy. Severe right ventricular hypertrophy with increased systolic compression may compromise intramural coronary flow. Because of the increased RV myocardial oxygen demand, this situation can lead to subendocardial ischemia.

TEE demonstrates the stenotic doming pulmonary valve and thickening of the free wall of the right ventricle (Fig. 20.6). The orifice can range from a pinhole to several millimeters but is rarely critical in the adult. The pulmonary valve is best seen in the basal horizontal views

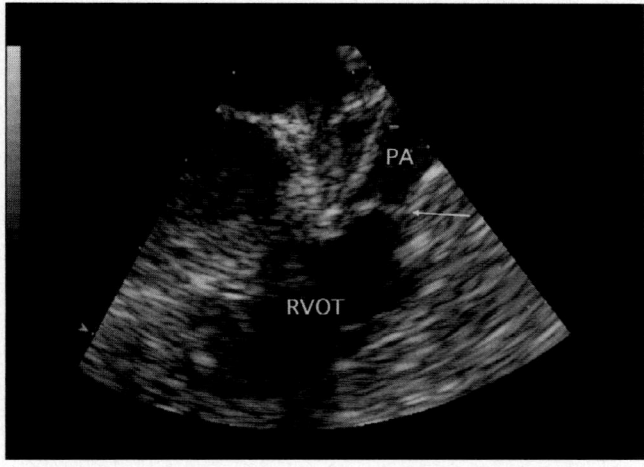

**FIGURE 20.6.** Pulmonic valve stenosis. Pulmonic valve stenosis (midesophageal right ventricular inflow-outflow view) demonstrating the doming stenotic valve (*arrow* points to the pulmonic valve). *PA,* pulmonic artery; *RVOT,* right ventricular outflow tract.

where it is seen in long axis (ME asc aortic SAX and RV inflow-outflow view) (Fig. 20.1, Table 20.1). Accurate measurements of the pressure gradient across the right ventricular outflow tract are possible with Doppler interrogation, usually from the transgastric view.

It is unusual to see an adult with severe valvular pulmonary stenosis. Adult patients with valvular pulmonary stenosis usually do well, but eventually right ventricular failure can occur. Surgical valvotomy has been an extremely successful operation for long-term relief of pulmonary valve obstruction. A recent natural history study of surgically treated severe (gradient ≥ 80 mm Hg) pulmonic stenosis demonstrated an excellent 25-year survival of 95%, equivalent to the normal population (Table 20.2) (21). In the adult, severe pulmonary valve stenosis requiring intervention is defined as a peak systolic gradient in excess of 60 mm Hg, although intervention may be recommended for lesser degrees of stenosis in the presence of symptoms. In patients with severe valvular pulmonary stenosis, percutaneous balloon valvuloplasty is the current treatment of choice and has replaced surgical valvotomy in patients with flexible valves.

## Patent Ductus Arteriosus

The patent ductus arteriosus, which accounts for 10% of cases of congenital heart disease, connects the proximal descending aorta with the pulmonary artery at its bifurcation. The magnitude of the left-to-right shunt depends on the size of the patent ductus and the pulmonary vascular resistance–to–systemic vascular resistance ratio in a manner similar to that of the ventricular septal defect.

On two-dimensional echocardiography, the ductus itself is rarely seen, but visualization of abnormal, continuous, high-velocity "aliased" flow within the main pulmonary artery near the left branch is seen on color flow Doppler imaging (22,23). Pulmonary artery systolic pressures can also be estimated (24).

The marked increase in pulmonary blood flow results in left-sided volume overload with an increase in the size of the left atrium, left ventricle, ascending aorta, and aortic arch. The left ventricular volume overload can result in congestive heart failure. Similar to a large VSD, the high pressure, high flow state can cause severe pulmonary hypertension and Eisenmenger's syndrome as a result of pulmonary vascular disease. In a young or middle-aged person with a small patent ductus arteriosus, percutaneous closure is the treatment of choice today. In the past, closure, by ligation and division of the patent ductus, was performed to prevent the long-term danger of infective endarteritis. Currently, some centers are closing smaller patent ductuses percutaneously using coils or intravascular devices with an approximately 95% success rate at intermediate follow-up; long-term follow-up is not yet available. With a large left-to-right shunt, especially with elevated pulmonary artery pressures, ligation of the patent ductus arteriosus, preferably with division, is indicated at any age.

## Coronary Artery Anomalies

Although coronary artery anomalies are rare, they should be considered a potential cause in young patients (usually in the second or third decades of life) presenting with symptoms suggestive of ischemia, including exertional syncope or chest pain. The most common coronary anomalies seen in adults are anomalous origin of the left circumflex coronary artery from the right sinus of Valsalva, coronary to pulmonary artery fistulas, coronary cameral fistulas (fistulous connection between the coronary artery and the coronary chamber, usually right atrium or right ventricle), and abnormal origin of the left coronary artery from the anterior sinus of Valsalva or the right coronary artery from the left posterior sinus of Valsalva.

## COMPLEX LESIONS

### Tetralogy of Fallot

Tetralogy of Fallot, the most common cyanotic defect after infancy refers to a combination of four lesions consisting of:

1. An interventricular septal defect
2. Infundibular stenosis with or without valvular pulmonic stenosis
3. An aorta overriding the ventricular septal defect
4. Right ventricular hypertrophy, which is a compensatory response to the other lesions

The right ventricular obstruction and large ventricular septal defect result in a high right ventricular pressure that is similar to left ventricular pressure. When the resistance due to the right ventricular outflow obstruction is greater than systemic vascular resistance, there is a right-to-left shunt, arterial desaturation, and if severe, cyanosis. If the right ventricular outflow obstruction is not severe, there may be little or no right-to-left shunt. The shunt may even be left-to-right, and the pulmonary valve and arteries may be normal or large. This lesion is sometimes referred to as "pink" or "acyanotic" tetralogy of Fallot. In tetralogy of Fallot, associated abnormalities include a right-sided aortic arch in about 25% of patients, atrial septal defect in 10% (so-called pentalogy of Fallot) and coronary anomalies in 10%. In adult patients with a perimembranous VSD, there can be acquired hypertrophy of right ventricular muscle bundles, resulting in dynamic outflow obstruction with pathophysiology similar

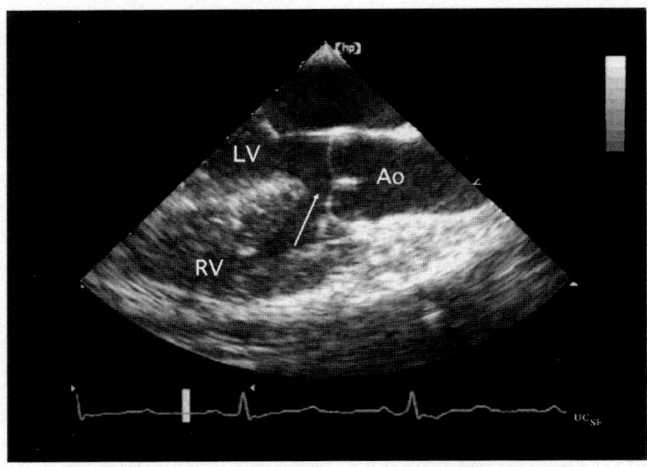

**FIGURE 20.7.** Tetralogy of Fallot. Tetralogy of Fallot (midesophageal long-axis view) showing the aortic override over the ventricular septum. The *arrow* points to the ventricular septal defect. *Ao,* aorta; *LV,* left ventricle; *RV,* right ventricle.

to tetralogy of Fallot. This entity has been termed "double chambered right ventricle."

TEE is particularly useful for definition of the degree of aortic override, which is best seen by the longitudinal plane (Fig. 20.7). In patients with unrepaired tetralogy of Fallot, TEE demonstrates severe right ventricular hypertrophy including the infundibulum usually with a thickened, malformed pulmonary valve. There is a large perimembranous ventricular septal defect in the vicinity of the membranous septum with evidence of right-to-left shunting and a dilated overriding aorta. The gradient across the right ventricular outflow tract can be measured by spectral Doppler. Most patients with tetralogy of Fallot have had palliative operations or corrective surgery by the time they are teenagers. Occasionally, a patient reaches the third decade of life without surgery. Sometimes patients present with only palliative systemic to pulmonary arterial shunts such as Blalock-Taussig shunt (subclavian to pulmonary artery), Potts' shunt (descending aorta to left pulmonary artery), or Waterston's shunts (ascending aorta to right pulmonary artery). Before surgical correction was possible, most patients died in the second decade of life.

Although it is an extremely successful operation, total intracardiac repair for tetralogy of Fallot has several potential significant postoperative residua, including residual right ventricular outflow tract obstruction, pulmonary valve regurgitation, peripheral pulmonary artery stenosis of one or both pulmonary arteries, ventricular septal patch leaks and arrhythmias (Table 20.2). In the early and intermediate follow-up period, important residual right ventricular outflow tract obstruction appears to be the major source of morbidity and mortality. However, in the late follow-up period, pulmonary insufficiency with eventual right ventricular failure owing to volume over-load and ventricular arrhythmias may lead to disability and even death. Survival in postoperative tetralogy of Fallot is about 90% at about 30 years after surgery (25). Thus, most adults with tetralogy of Fallot come to surgery for correction of significant hemodynamic sequelae, especially pulmonary valve repair and less frequently for residual VSD.

## Truncus Arteriosus

In truncus arteriosus, the embryonic truncus fails to divide into an aorta and a pulmonary artery, retaining the single semilunar valve and a VSD. The pulmonary, aortic and coronary arteries thus arise from the single truncal root. Classification is based on the anatomic origin of the pulmonary arteries from the single trunk (26,27). Either the pulmonary trunk arises separately from the common trunk and close to the truncal valve (Type I), or as separate vessels from the truncus (Types II and III).

In the unoperated child, TEE can demonstrate the presence of a single semilunar valve, the size of the VSD and provide evidence of left ventricular volume (Fig. 20.8). If the pulmonary arteries arise without stenosis from the truncus and the VSD is large, pulmonary blood flow will be markedly increased, volume loading the LV, and causing heart failure and pulmonary hypertension. Without surgery as an infant, the patient will not survive to adulthood. If the pulmonary arteries are stenotic at their origin, there will be a systolic ejection murmur and the pulmonary blood flow may be low, normal or only mildly increased. Survival of the unoperated adult is the exception.

The truncus patient is usually managed surgically by closing the VSD and incorporating the semilunar valve on the left side as the aortic valve. A valved conduit is placed from the RV to the pulmonary artery. If the semilunar valve is severely incompetent, valve replacement may be necessary. Depending on the severity of the pulmonary artery stenoses, varying techniques including surgical and balloon catheter techniques are used to relieve the obstruction. Residual obstruction to the pulmonary arteries, truncal valvular regurgitation, and obstruction of the conduit can be late complications, which may bring the adult patient to surgery.

## Transposition of the Great Arteries

These infants are born with the great arteries arising from the wrong ventricle. The aortic valve arises anteriorly from the right ventricle and the pulmonic valve posteriorly from the left ventricle. Without cross-connections, such as a patent foramen ovale, atrial septal defect, ventricular septal defect, or patent ductus arteriosus, this lesion is incompatible with life.

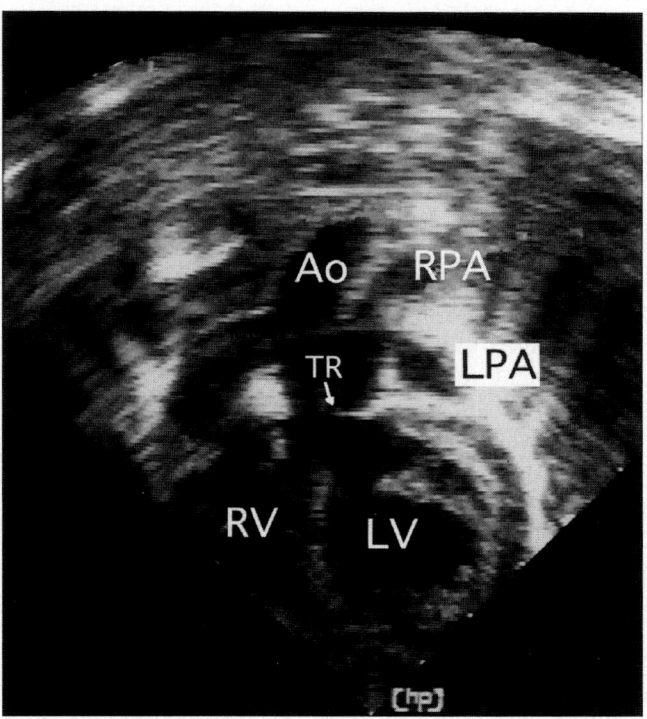

**FIGURE 20.8.** Truncus arteriosus. Truncus arteriosus (deep transgastric long-axis view, with apex of the heart displayed at the bottom) showing the biventricular origin of the large central vessel arising above the ventricular septal defect. The right and left pulmonary arteries (*RPA, LPA*) and the aorta (*Ao*) originate from the large common arterial trunk. *TR,* truncal vessel. (Reproduced with slight modification from: Muhiudeen IA et al. Transesophageal transgastric echocardiography in infants and children. J Am Soc Echocardiogr 1995;8:231, with permission.)

Infants with this condition rarely survive without intervention. With only rare exceptions, adults have had a palliative atrial switch procedure (such as the Mustard or Senning procedures), after which the right ventricle usually continues to serve the systemic circulation. More recently, an arterial switch operation, the Jatene procedure, was developed to reconnect the great arteries to their proper ventricle, reconnect the coronary arteries to the new aortic location, and restore a "normal" circulation (Table 20.2).

TEE evaluation with multiple planes, including contrast injection, should include baffle assessment after the Senning and Mustard procedure to evaluate potential baffle leaks or pulmonary venous obstruction by the intra-atrial baffle (Table 20.1). Evaluation of ventricular function is important because patients with an atrial switch procedure are at risk from failure of the systemic "right" ventricle. Patients with the arterial switch operation (Jatene procedure) can have coronary artery obstruction, atrial or ventricular patch leaks, aortic valvular regurgitation, and supravalvular obstruction at the site of the aortic and pulmonary artery anastomoses. Medical therapy to treat failure of the systemic right ventricle includes afterload reduction with vasodilators, digoxin, and diuretics. Noninvasive and invasive studies may demonstrate the need for further surgical palliative procedures.

## Physiologically Corrected Transposition (L-Transposition)

L-transposition is characterized by malposition of the great vessels and ventricular inversion, with the left ventricle connected to the right atrium and pulmonary artery and the right ventricle connected to the left atrium and aorta. Blood flow is physiologically correct, but an anatomic right ventricle serves as the systemic ventricle. Most previously undiagnosed adults with this lesion usually have no other abnormalities. Corrected transposition is frequently discovered as a result of the physical findings due to accompanying congenital defects, such as VSD and subpulmonic valve stenosis. With no other abnormalities, this lesion may remain undetected until the patient presents with syncope, owing to complete heart block.

Without additional lesions, patients with corrected transposition may live to old age. The development of complete heart block is common and occurs at a rate of approximately 5% per year in adults. In the presence of severe accompanying lesions, surgical correction may be possible. The systemic ventricle, an anatomic right ventricle, may show progressive failure requiring medical treatment. Adult patients with l-TGV rarely come to surgery. Patients previously operated upon for PS may have conduit stenosis or valve failure, and tricuspid regurgitation may result from RV failure. However, tricuspid valve replacement or repair is rarely beneficial.

TEE examination should include identification of ventricular morphology and function and associated lesions, such as VSD and pulmonary outflow tract obstruction.

## Ebstein's Anomaly

In Ebstein's anomaly, the septal and posterior leaflets of the tricuspid valve are dysplastic and displaced from the tricuspid annulus apically into the body of the right ventricle (28–30). Thus, a portion of the right ventricle is above the tricuspid valve (the atrialized right ventricle) and enlarges the true right atrium. The valve may be regurgitant, and if a patent foramen ovale or an atrial septal defect is present (80% of patients), there can be a large right-to-left shunt. These patients are cyanotic, are likely to present in infancy, and may have had palliative procedures with atrial septal defect closure. The presentation in adolescents or adults is more likely related to progressive tricuspid regurgitation and heart failure or arrhythmias than to cyanosis. Nevertheless, some patients with severe displacement of the tricuspid valve can live normal lives with minimal symptoms.

The TEE is diagnostic, with a normal basal attachment of the large redundant anterior leaflet and displaced immobile septal and posterior leaflets, demonstrating the morphology of the abnormal tricuspid valve with a tricuspid regurgitant jet arising apically within the right ventricle (Fig. 20.9). The right atrium and ventricle are enlarged.

Once the patient has survived childhood, the prognosis is favorable, even with severe displacement of the tricuspid valve. If the tricuspid regurgitation is severe, then the ability to increase cardiac output may be diminished and the patient may have progressive limitation of activity with fatigability. Closure of an atrial septal defect and reconstruction of the tricuspid valve with an annuloplasty or even replacement has been done with success. If atrial tachycardia is present with an anomalous atrioventricular conduction pathway (Wolff-Parkinson-White syndrome), radiofrequency ablation of the AV pathway can successfully treat the paroxysmal atrial tachycardia.

## Single Ventricle

A number of CHD lesions are included in the single ventricle category. Hypoplasia of either the RV or LV results in a single functional ventricle. This category includes hypoplastic left heart syndrome, double-inlet left ventricle, and tricuspid atresia.

TEE evaluation should include multiple views to evaluate atrioventricular and ventriculoarterial connections and ventricular size and morphology. Adult patients with a single ventricle lesion may have a modified Blalock

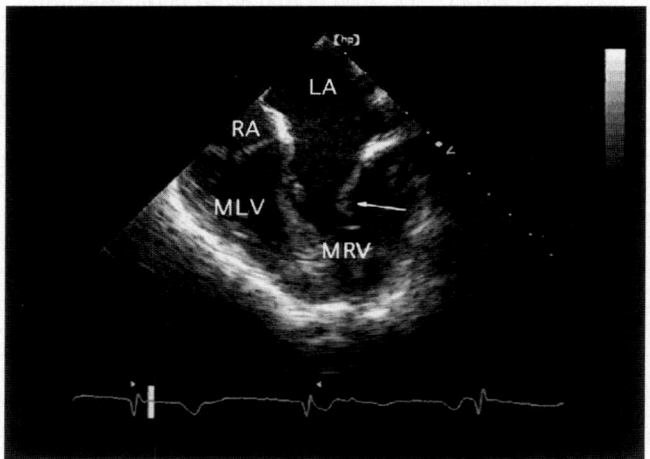

**FIGURE 20.9.** Corrected transposition with Ebstein deformity of the tricuspid valve. Corrected transposition of the great arteries with the morphologic right ventricle (*MRV*) below the left atrium (*LA*) and the morphologic left ventricle (*MLV*) below the right atrium (*RA*). The septal leaflet of the tricuspid valve is inferiorly displaced well below the insertion of the mitral valve (midesophageal four-chamber view). *LA*, left atrium; *RA*, right atrium.

Taussig shunt, a Glenn anastomosis (SVC to PA cavopulmonary connection) (31), or a Fontan connection (total caval to pulmonary connection) (32,33). Visualization of the Glenn anastomosis is not always possible by TEE, but it can sometimes be demonstrated using longitudinal planes.

The Fontan procedure includes a variety of surgical approaches that connect either the right atrium or the vena cavae directly to the pulmonary arteries, bypassing the RV. Pulmonary blood flow is propelled by the systemic venous pressure and negative inspiratory force, reducing the volume overload to the LV. TEE is particularly useful for evaluation of ventricular function and valvar regurgitation. The Glenn or Fontan procedure is usually performed in childhood but occasionally adults are candidates for the procedure. Patients with the Fontan procedure can do well into the third and fourth decades. Successful pregnancies have been reported in these patients. The patients have an elevated systemic venous pressure and can have ascites and peripheral edema for months after surgery. Eventually these resolve, but later complications include chylous pleural effusions, protein losing enteropathy, and eventual ventricular failure. Atrial tachyarrythmias, especially in those patients where the right atrium is part of the connection to the pulmonary artery, can be a difficult problem.

Adult patients with single-ventricle physiology may come to surgery for:

1. Revision of previous Fontan or Glenn procedures
2. Primary Fontan or Glenn procedures
3. Revision of arteriopulmonary shunts
4. Transplantation

## Dextrocardia and Dextroposition

With dextrocardia and situs inversus, the vena cava, atria, ventricles, and great vessels are all reversed and, thus, connected appropriately. Frequently, there are associated congenital heart lesions and the right lung may be hypoplastic.

## CONCLUSIONS

In many medical centers, TEE is now the standard of care for intraoperative assessment of patients with congenital heart disease. In noncardiac surgery, TEE can be used to evaluate ventricular volume, function, underlying pathology, and to assess any residual lesions. TEE clearly has significant perioperative impact in the care of patients with CHD undergoing cardiac surgery, diagnosis can be confirmed, altered, and the surgical plan revised in as many as 5% to 7% of cases.

## KEY POINTS

- Atrial septal defects (ASD) are one of the most common defects in the adult population. There are four types of atrial septal defects: ostium secundum defect (70%), ostium primum defect (15% to 25%), sinus venosus defect (10%), and coronary sinus ASDs (< 2%).
- Ventricular septal defects are the most common cardiac abnormality in infants and children, and have a high rate of spontaneous closure. Primary closure is indicated for a Qp:Qs > 1.8:1 in the absence of Eisenmenger's physiology.
- Atrioventricular septal defects include a ventricular septal defect, an atrial septal defect, and varying degrees of AV valve regurgitation.
- **Congenital Aortic Stenosis.** The anatomic level of obstruction can be supravalvular, valvular, or subvalvular. Aortic stenosis is due to a malformed valve that is usually functionally bicuspid.
- Tetralogy of Fallot, the most common cyanotic defect after infancy, consists of an interventricular septal defect, infundibular stenosis with or without valvular pulmonic stenosis, an aorta overriding the ventricular septal defect, and right ventricular hypertrophy,
- **Transposition of the Great Arteries.** The aortic valve arises from the right ventricle and the pulmonic valve arises from the left ventricle.
- **Physiologically Corrected Transposition (L-Transposition).** Transposition consists of malposition of the great vessels and ventricular inversion, with the left ventricle connected to the right atrium and pulmonary artery and the right ventricle connected to the left atrium and aorta. VSD and PS are the most common associated lesions. Complete heart block is frequent.
- In Ebstein's anomaly the leaflets of the tricuspid valve are dysplastic and displaced from the tricuspid annulus apically into the body of the right ventricle. Interatrial septal defects or PFO are present in 50% of patients.
- A number of CHD lesions comprise what is known as single ventricles, usually resulting in hypoplasia of the RV or LV.

## REFERENCES

1. Care of the adult with congenital heart disease. 32nd Bethesda Conference, Bethesda, Maryland, October 2-3, 2000, 2001. Vol. 37. J Am Coll Card.
2. Thys D, Abel M, Bollen B, et al. Practice guidelines for perioperative transesophageal echocardiography. Anesthesiology 1996;84:986–1006.

3. Cheitlin M, Alpert J, Armstrong W, et al. ACC/AHA guidelines for the clinical application of echocardiography. A report of the American College of Cardiology/American Heart Association Task Force on Practice Guidelines. (Committee on Clinical Application of Echocardiography). Circulation 1997;95: 1686–744.

4. Child JS. Transthoracic and transesophageal echocardiographic imaging: anatomic and hemodynamic assessment. In: Perloff JK, Child JS, eds. Congenital heart disease in adults. Philadelphia: W. B. Saunders, 1998:91–128.

5. Child JS, Marelli AJ. The application of transesophageal echocardiography in the adult with congenital heart disease. In: Maurer G, ed. Transesophageal Echocardiography. New York: McGraw-Hill, 1994:159–88.

6. Kaplan S, Adolph RJ. Pulmonary valve stenosis in adults. Cardiovasc Clin 1979;10:327–39.

7. Schiller NB, Maurer G, Ritter SB, et al. Transesophageal echocardiography. J Am Soc Echocardiogr 1989;2:354–7.

8. Shanewise JS, Cheung AT, Aronson S, et al. ASE/SCA guidelines for performing a comprehensive intraoperative multiplane transesophageal echocardiography examination: recommendations of the American Society of Echocardiography Council for Intraoperative Echocardiography and the Society of Cardiovascular Anesthesiologists Task Force for Certification in Perioperative Transesophageal Echocardiography. Anesth Analg 1999;89:870–84.

9. Brickner ME, Hillis LD, Lange RA. Congenital heart disease in adults. N Engl J Med 2000;342:256–63.

10. Maxted W, Finch A, Nanda NC, Kim KS, Sanyal R. Multiplane transesophageal echocardiographic detection of sinus venosus atrial septal defect. Echocardiography 1995;12:139–45.

11. Van Hare G, Silverman N. Contrast two-dimensional echocardiography in congenital heart disease: Techniques, indications and clinical utility. J Am Coll Cardiol 1989; 13:673–86.

12. Valdes-Cruz LM, Pieroni DR, Roland JM, Shematek JP. Recognition of residual postoperative shunts by contrast echocardiographic techniques. Circulation 1977;55:148–52.

13. Murphy JG, Gersh BJ, McGoon MD, et al. Long-term outcome after surgical repair of isolated atrial septal defect. Follow-up at 27 to 32 years. N Engl J Med 1990;323:1645–50.

14. Konstantinides S, Geibel A, Olschewski M, et al. A comparison of surgical and medical therapy for atrial septal defect in adults. N Engl J Med 1995;333:469–73.

15. Attie F, Rosas M, Granados N, Zabal C, Buendia A, Calderon J. Surgical treatment for secundum atrial septal defects in patients > 40 years old. A randomized clinical trial. J Am Coll Cardiol 2001;38:2035–42.

16. Gatzoulis MA, Freeman MA, Siu SC, Webb GD, Harris L. Atrial arrhythmia after surgical closure of atrial septal defects in adults. N Engl J Med 1999;340:839–46.

17. Silbert DR, Brunson SC, Schiff R, Diamant S. Determination of right ventricular pressure in the presence of a ventricular septal defect using continuous wave Doppler ultrasound. J Am Coll Cardiol 1986;8:379–84.

18. Rastelli G, Kirklin JW, Titus JL. Anatomic observations on complete form of persistent common atrioventricular canal with special reference to atrioventricular valves. Mayo Clin Proc 1966;41:296–308.

19. Keane JF, Driscoll DJ, Gersony WM, et al. Second natural history study of congenital heart defects. Results of treatment of patients with aortic valvar stenosis. Circulation 1993;87:I16–27.

20. Simpson IA, Sahn DJ, Valdes-Cruz LM, Chung KJ, Sherman FS, Swensson RE. Color Doppler flow mapping in patients with coarctation of the aorta: new observations and improved evaluation with color flow diameter and proximal acceleration as predictors of severity. Circulation 1988;77: 736–44.

21. Hayes CJ, Gersony WM, Driscoll DJ, et al. Second natural history study of congenital heart defects. Results of treatment of patients with pulmonary valvar stenosis. Circulation 1993;87:I28–37.

22. Mugge A, Daniel WG, Lichtlen PR. Imaging of patent ductus arteriosus by transesophageal color-coded Doppler echocardiography. J Clin Ultrasound 1991;19:128–9.

23. Takenaka K, Sakamoto T, Shiota T, Amano W, Igarashi T, Sugimoto T. Diagnosis of patent ductus arteriosus in adults by biplane transesophageal color Doppler flow mapping. Am J Cardiol 1991;68:691–3.

24. Marx GR, Allen HD, Goldberg SJ. Doppler echocardiographic estimation of systolic pulmonary artery pressure in patients with aortic-pulmonary shunts. J Am Coll Cardiol 1986;7:880–5.

25. Murphy JG, Gersh BJ, Mair DD, et al. Long-term outcome in patients undergoing surgical repair of tetralogy of Fallot. N Engl J Med 1993;329:593–9.

26. Calder L, Van Praagh R, Van Praagh S, et al. Truncus arteriosus communis: clinical, angiographic, and pathologic findings in 100 patients. Am Heart J 1976;92:23–38.

27. Collett RW, Edwards JE. Persistent truncus arteriosus: a classification according to anatomic types. Surg Clin North Am 1949;29:1245–70.

28. Roberson DA, Silverman NH. Ebstein's anomaly: echocardiographic and clinical features in the fetus and neonate. J Am Coll Cardiol 1989;14:1300–7.

29. Quaegebeur JM, Sreeram N, Fraser AG, et al. Surgery for Ebstein's anomaly: the clinical and echocardiographic evaluation of a new technique. J Am Coll Cardiol 1991;17:722–8.

30. Vargas-Barron J, Rijlaarsdam M, Romero-Cardenas A, et al. Transesophageal echocardiographic study of Ebstein's anomaly. Echocardiography 1995;12:253–61.

31. Trusler GA, Williams WG, Cohen AJ, et al. William Glenn lecture. The cavopulmonary shunt. Evolution of a concept. Circulation 1990;82:IV131-8.

32. Fyfe DA, Ritter SB, Snider AR, et al. Guidelines for transesophageal echocardiography in children. J Am Soc Echocardiogr 1992;5:640–4.

33. Stumper O, Sutherland GR, Geuskens R, Roelandt JR, Bos E, Hess J. Transesophageal echocardiography in evaluation and management after a Fontan procedure. J Am Coll Cardiol 1991;17:1152–60.

## QUESTIONS

1. The most common atrial defect in the adult population is:
   A. Primum atrial septal defect
   B. Secundum atrial septal defect
   C. Sinus venosus atrial septal defect
   D. Coronary sinus atrial septal defect

2. Longitudinal plane imaging is extremely useful for which of the following lesions?
   A. Atrioventricular septal defect
   B. Secundum atrial septal defect
   C. Patent ductus arteriosus
   D. Tetralogy of Fallot

3. After an arterial switch for transposition of the great arteries, all of the following can occur *except*:
   A. Supravalvar aortic stenosis
   B. Left ventricular dysfunction
   C. Protein-losing enteropathy
   D. Coronary artery stenosis

# Decision Making in Critical Care

Chapter 21

# TEE in the Critical Care Setting

*Scott T. Reeves, Kim J. Payne, James Ramsay,*
*Jack Shanewise, Stephen Insler, and William J. Stewart*

## TRAUMA AND CRITICAL CARE

In 2003 a task force cosponsored by the American College of Cardiology, American Heart Association, and American Society of Echocardiography published guidelines for clinical application of echocardiography, including trauma and critical care. The full-text article is available from the Web sites of each organization and the summary is published in the journals of each group (1). As is the case with most such guidelines, they are structured in terms of recommendations according to the level of scientific support, with "Class I" indications defined as "conditions for which there is evidence and/or general agreement that a given procedure or treatment is useful and effective." Other levels of evidence are "Class IIa" where there is some divergence of opinion but the weight of evidence is in favor of utility/efficacy; "Class IIb" where the weight of evidence is less compelling; and "Class III" where the evidence suggests either a lack of utility or even harm. Table 21.1 lists the conditions relevant to critical care and trauma where the 2003 guidelines suggest Class I indications. In addition, Class I or IIa indications for echocardiography exist for many conditions that may coexist or present in the critically ill (e.g., known or suspected native or prosthetic valve endocarditis; chest pain and/or myocardial ischemic syndromes; dyspnea, edema, or cardiomyopathy; pericardial disease; suspected thoracic aortic disease; and pulmonary/pulmonary vascular disease).

TEE provides a particular benefit in the critically injured and the critically ill. Unlike the echocardiography laboratory where adequate images can be obtained from the transthoracic exam in > 90% of patients (2), the percentage of successful, diagnostic TTE exams in the critically ill is approximately 50% (3–8). Several reports of TEE in this population are based entirely on patients in whom TTE could not obtain adequate images (9–13); in all of these reports, the success rate in obtaining an adequate TEE exam was > 90%. Conditions limiting the effectiveness of TTE are listed in Table 21.2. In addition,

there are the "usual" indications for preferential use of TEE (high-resolution imaging of structures nearer to the esophagus than the chest wall) in many critically ill or injured patients. It has been suggested that TTE is not cost-effective in critically ill surgical patients and the usual progression of TTE followed by TEE should be replaced by directly performing a TEE exam in this population (14). Most would not agree with this view because TTE is a noninvasive, rapid test, becoming even more available to clinicians with the recent appearance of handheld transthoracic devices (Figs. 21.1 and 21.2). In critically ill and injured patients these smaller, portable devices suffer the same drawbacks as listed in Table 21.2, and are not currently able to provide the full echocardiography examination, but they are small, simple, and convenient to use and can facilitate an urgent, focused, qualitative assessment in many patients (10). The fact remains, however,

▌ TABLE 21.1. Class I Indications for Echocardiography in the Critically Ill and Critically Injured (1)

**Critically Ill**
1. The hemodynamically unstable patient
2. Suspected aortic dissection (TEE)

**Critically Injured**
1. Serious blunt or penetrating chest trauma (suspected pericardial effusion or tamponade)
2. Mechanically ventilated multiple-trauma or chest trauma patient
3. Suspected preexisting valvular or myocardial disease in the trauma patient
4. The hemodynamically unstable multiple-injury patient without obvious chest trauma but with a mechanism of injury suggesting potential cardiac or aortic injury (deceleration or crush)
5. Widening of the mediastinum, postinjury suspected aortic injury (TEE)
6. Potential catheter, guidewire, pacer electrode, or pericardiocentesis needle injury with or without signs of tamponade.

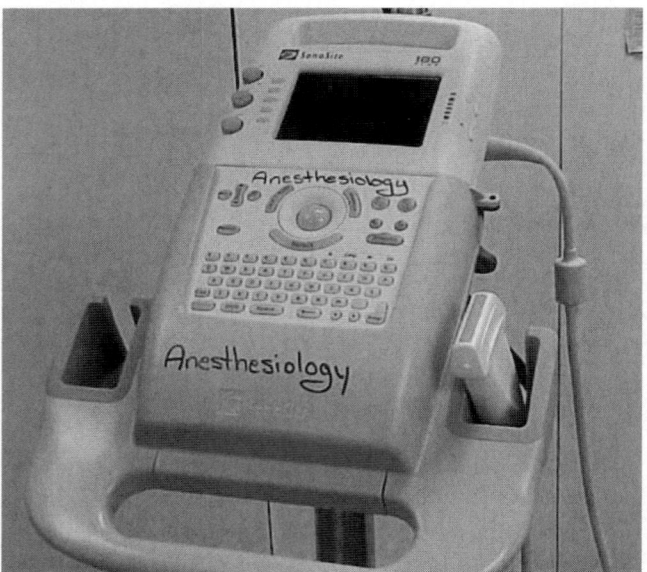

*FIGURE 21.1.* Handheld ultrasound unit made by Sonosite, Inc. (Vascular access probe is shown; a 2 MHz cardiac probe is available.)

that definitive diagnosis for approximately 50% of critically ill or injured patients will require a TEE exam.

In this chapter the use of echocardiography to assess the hemodynamically unstable patient in the intensive care unit (ICU) or emergency room (ER) will be discussed, followed by evaluation of the patient with unexplained hypoxemia (question of intracardiac shunt), and the patient with suspected endocarditis. Finally the assessment of the patient with trauma, and with suspected aortic dissection will be presented. Table 21.3 lists these and other common indications for echocardiography in the ICU.

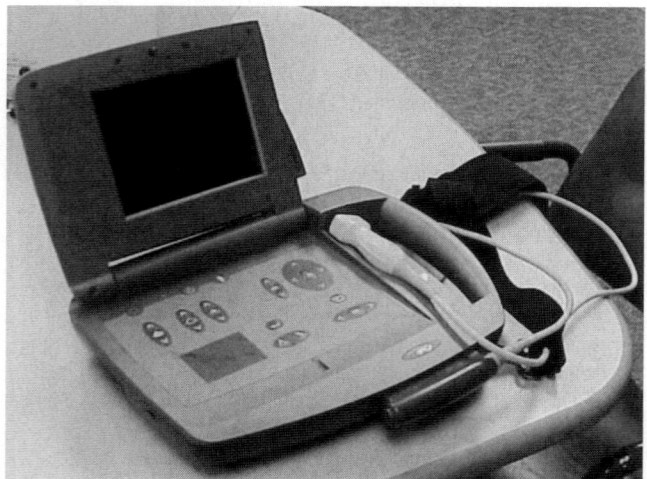

*FIGURE 21.2.* Handheld ultrasound unit made by Philips Inc.

▶ **TABLE 21.2. Conditions Limiting Success of Transthoracic Imaging in the ICU**

Mechanical ventilation
    Especially PEEP > 15 cm $H_2O$
Inaccessible windows
    Surgical dressings and drains
    Chest tubes
    Thoracic or upper abdominal incisions
Pneumothorax, pneumopericardium, or subcutaneous emphysema
Surgery-induced fluid collections or cardiac position changes
Inability to position patient
Inability of patient to cooperate for respiratory maneuvers
Obesity
Severe chronic obstructive pulmonary disease

## The Hemodynamically Unstable Patient

"Hemodynamic instability" usually refers to unexplained hypotension or hypotension not responding appropriately to fluid or vasopressor therapy. This is a common clinical problem in the ER and ICU. Some conditions associated with hypotension and the associated echocardiographic findings are indicated in Table 21.4. Heidenreich et al. studied 60 patients with unexplained hypotension, finding adequate images with TTE in 36%, but in 97% with TEE (4). He reported new diagnoses in 28%, leading to surgery in 20%. Sohn et al. (11) performed 127 examinations over 7 years, and found "severe cardiovascular abnormalities" accounting for unstable hemodynamics in 52%, with 21% undergoing urgent procedures based on the TEE findings. Several other reports suggest significant changes in therapy or surgical intervention following TEE examination in many ICU populations including those with hypotension (5,8,11,12). In addition to imaging specific pathologies that may indicate a need for surgical repair or intervention, assessment of ventricular size

▶ **TABLE 21.3. Common Reasons for Requesting Echocardiography in the ICU and ER**

Hypotension with lack of response to fluid administration
    Assessment of intravascular volume status
    Assessment of myocardial function: left and right
Known or suspected chest trauma
    Suspected aortic dissection
Suspicion of pulmonary embolus (right heart function; look for clot)
Suspicion of new valvular disease (e.g., mitral regurgitation)
Prosthetic valve dysfunction
Suspicion of endocarditis
Suspicion of pericardial disease (e.g., tamponade)
Hypoxemia with suspicion of intracardiac shunt
Chest pain
Complications of myocardial infarction

▶ TABLE 21.4. **Some Common Conditions Associated with Hypotension**

| Condition | Useful Views | TEE Findings |
|---|---|---|
| Hypovolemia | TG SAX of LV | Decreased EDA |
| | TG LAX of LV | Increased FAC |
| | | "Kissing" papillary muscles |
| Vasodilation | TG SAX of LV | Normal EDA |
| | | Increased FAC |
| | ME 4 Ch, 2 Ch, LAX | No severe valvular regurgitation |
| Decreased | TG SAX of LV | Increased EDA, decreased FAC |
| Systolic | TG LAX of LV | Increased ESA, decreased FAC |
| Function | | |
| Pericardial Tamponade | ME 4 ch; TG SAX | Effusion |
| | and LAX of LV | Diastolic collapse of right-sided |
| | | chamber/chambers |
| Aortic Dissection | ME 5 ch and LAX; | Intimal flap |
| | ascending/descending Ao | Two lumens in aorta (no flow in 1) |
| | | Aortic regurgitation |
| | | Pericardial effusion |
| Pulmonary Embolus | ME 4 ch; RV in/out; | Dilated RA and RV |
| | PA views (upper E) | Small LA and LV |
| | | TR/PR jets |
| | | Flow through PFO |
| | | Echogenic density |

Modified from Lobato EB, Urdaneta F. "TEE in the ICU" in *A practical approach to TEE*. Perrino AC, Reeves ST eds. Philadelphia: Lippincott Williams & Wilkins 2003;272–85, with permission.

and contractility in combination with diastolic properties permits differentiation between cardiac and noncardiac causes of hypotension. Not surprisingly, TEE is of particular value after cardiac surgery, when mechanical ventilation, incisional dressings, and chest tubes are always present. Three reports in this population demonstrate how TEE may prompt additional surgery and prevent unnecessary reoperation in the postoperative cardiac patient (15–17). Denault et al. elegantly describe the value of repeat TEE examination after lung transplantation, providing not only diagnostic information, but also the placement of the intraaortic balloon pump, cannulae for extracorporeal membrane oxygenation, and weaning from the latter therapy were all facilitated by use of TEE (18).

## Echocardiography versus the Pulmonary Artery Catheter

Most of the information available from the pulmonary artery catheter (PAC) can also be obtained from echocardiography. The principal drawbacks to the latter are that it requires significant training and expertise that is not widely available in the ER and ICU, and echocardiography usually provides only a single, diagnostic examination. Invasive monitoring skills are more widespread, and the PAC is used to guide or monitor therapy in a way that would be impractical for echocardiography (although the use of handheld devices as referred to above, and in-

creased echocardiography training for ER and ICU physicians may change this). On the other hand, provided an echocardiographer is available, echocardiography can provide diagnostic information faster than the time required to place and obtain information from a PAC (19), and imaging provides a diagnostic capacity not available from the PAC.

A number of investigators have examined the role of echocardiography when a PAC is already present. In the study by Heidenreich referred to above, a PAC was present in 38% of the patients; 63% had changes in therapy after TEE (4). After cardiac surgery, Reichert et al. found a disagreement in diagnosis in 50% of patients when TEE and PAC were compared (15). Costachescu et al. found TEE was associated with a higher interobserver reliability in the assessment of hemodynamic instability after cardiac surgery than hemodynamic monitoring (17). In a medical-surgical population excluding postcardiac surgery patients, Poelaert et al. found 44% of patients who had a PAC in place had therapy changed after TEE, whether the primary illness was cardiac or septic (20). In an attempt to understand this discrepancy, Bouchard et al. compared ventricular performance assessments from the PAC (left ventricular stroke work index, or LVSWI) with fractional area change (FAC) and regional wall motion score index from TEE in 60 patients during and after cardiac surgery (21). They found no correlation between LVSWI and FAC, and postulate that changes in ventricular compliance, loading conditions, and ventricular function alter the pressure-volume relationship of the left ventricle in a manner that leads to discordant interpretations between the two techniques. This is illustrated in Fig. 21.3 with the use of pressure-volume curves. A simple example would be the effect of acute preload reduction, which decreases LVSWI, but increases FAC (ejection fraction). The use of both techniques (PAC and TEE) simultaneously to aid clinical decision making has not been assessed in a prospective manner; however, many investigators have suggested that use of pressure parameters alone (from the PAC) can lead to erroneous conclusions regarding ventricular filling and function.

## Unexplained Hypoxemia: Intracardiac Shunt

In clinical medicine hypoxemia is caused by three disorders:

1. Hypoventilation
2. Impaired gas exchange (most commonly low ventilation–perfusion ratio, or poor ventilation of perfused alveoli; less commonly diffusion impairment)
3. True shunt

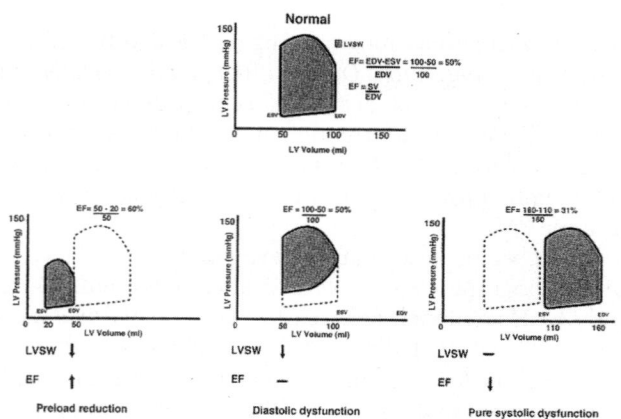

**FIGURE 21.3.** Pressure-volume relationship with left ventricular *(LV)* pressure on the y-axis and LV volume on the x-axis. The stroke volume *(SV)* is end-diastolic volume *(EDV)* minus end-systolic volume *(ESV)*; the ejection fraction *(EF)* is equal to SV divided by EDV. Three scenarios are presented to explain discrepancy between changes in LV stroke work *(LVSW)* and EF. On the left, acute preload reduction was associated with a leftward displacement of the pressure-volume relationship. This results in a reduction of LVSW and an increase in EF. In the middle panel, diastolic dysfunction was associated with an upsloping of the pressure-volume relationship. This results in a reduction in LVSW, but no change in EF. Finally, in the right panel, pure systolic dysfunction was associated with a rightward displacement of the pressure-volume relationship. In this condition, LVSW will be unchanged, but EF will be reduced. Reproduced from Bouchard MJ, et al. Crit Care Med 2004;32: 644-48, with permission.

The latter may be intrapulmonary (e.g., lobar collapse) or intracardiac (e.g., patent foramen ovale or PFO). It is not uncommon for more than one of these disorders to occur simultaneously in the critically ill. When there is true shunt, a decrease in the cardiac output resulting in a decreased mixed venous saturation can further worsen the arterial hypoxemia.

Transesophageal echocardiography is the technique of choice for detection of intracardiac shunt (22). In addition, the TEE exam provides an assessment of overall cardiac function and views of other intrathoracic pathology (pericardial or pleural effusions, collapsed portions of the lung, pulmonary embolus). In those patients with persistent unexplained hypoxemia (i.e., not explained by the chest radiograph), echocardiography should be performed to search for an intracardiac shunt, the most common of which is PFO. While less common, atrial septal defects of all types as well as associated anomalous pulmonary venous drainage can best be detected by TEE (23).

## Patent Foramen Ovale

In utero, blood from the placenta bypasses the lungs by crossing from the right atrium (RA) to left atrium (LA) through the foramen ovale, a fenestration in the septum secundum located in the fossa ovalis. The fossa ovalis is bordered by a section of the septum primum, which acts as a one-way flap valve. At birth when LA pressure exceeds RA pressure the flap valve functionally seals, but may not form a permanent closure. A Mayo clinic adult autopsy study demonstrated a 27% incidence of "probe-patent" foramen ovale (24). In disease states associated with elevations in the RA pressure, this potential channel can open allowing right-to-left shunting. Some examples in the critical care setting include acute pulmonary embolism, right ventricular infarction, and use of high levels of positive end expiratory pressure (PEEP). Less common circumstances include cardiac tamponade and distortion of mediastinal structures that may occur postpneumonectomy. A review of perioperative implications of PFO was recently published (25).

Echocardiographic detection of a PFO and associated intracardiac shunt requires visualization of the atrial septum, color flow mapping, and right-sided injection of echo contrast (contrast echocardiography). Usually the best TEE views of the fossa ovalis are from the midesophageal level; scanning from the horizontal to the vertical plane with the probe rotated to the right will allow a complete assessment, with the best views in the vertical plane (Fig. 21.4). With unenhanced two-dimensional scanning, the size of the fossa ovalis and the mobility of its flap valve can be assessed. The presence of an atrial septal aneurysm, defined as a transient bulging of the fossa ovalis region of the interatrial septum greater than

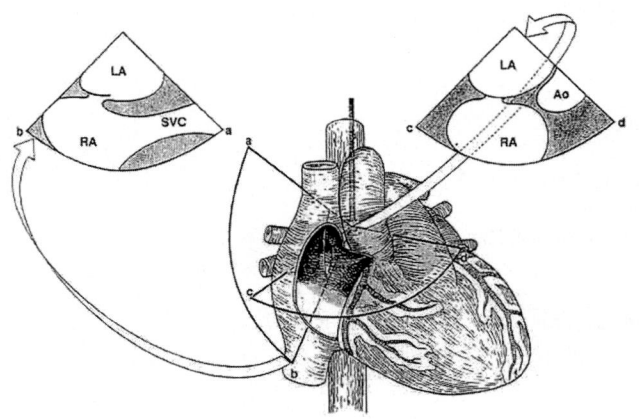

**FIGURE 21.4.** Schematic drawing demonstrating anatomy of interatrial septum as viewed from the right atrial perspective. The potential superiority of the vertical plane *(sector image to the left)* to delineate opening of the PFO *(black shadow in the cranial portion of the fossa ovalis)* is related to its craniocaudal orientation. A horizontal cut *(sector image to the right)* is less likely to intersect the potential separation between the septum primum and septum secundum. The transducer is situated behind the LA. *LA,* left atrium; *RA,* right atrium; *SVC,* superior vena cava; *Ao,* aorta. Reproduced from Chenzbraun A, et al. J Am Soc Echocardiogr 1993;6:417–21, with permission.

15 mm in the absence of chronically elevated atrial pressures, is associated with up to a 90% incidence of PFO (26).

Detection of flow across a PFO requires color flow mapping and contrast echocardiography. Color flow mapping of this region using a low Nyquist limit (30 cm/sec) may detect shunt in either (or both) direction(s). The pressure gradient between the RA and LA can be transiently augmented in an intubated patient by releasing a sustained positive intrathoracic pressure (20 cm water for a few cardiac cycles), or in a spontaneously breathing patient by release of a Valsalva maneuver. The increase in right-sided venous return provoked by this maneuver should cause the interatrial septum to "bulge" to the left, and result in visible flow across the foramen ovale if it is patent. If flow through a PFO is causing hypoxemia, this maneuver should not really be necessary.

## Contrast Echocardiography

The definitive test for presence of a PFO is contrast echocardiography, performed by injecting agitated, microbubble-containing solution rapidly into the RA (27). This test does not require actual imaging of the PFO or flow, both of which may sometimes be difficult—especially with TTE. Approximately 5 ml of saline, 3 ml of the patient's blood, and 0.2 ml–2.0 ml of air are rapidly injected between two 10-ml syringes connected to a stopcock, until the solution is opaque but with no large visible

air bubbles. While imaging both atria (Fig. 21.4), the 10-ml solution is rapidly injected into a venous catheter as close to the RA as possible, resulting in "opacification" (made white with microbubbles) of the RA. A right-to-left shunt is diagnosed if microbubbles appear in the LA within three to five cardiac cycles of RA opacification; late appearance can be due to transpulmonary flow. Crude quantification is possible with a small shunt defined as 3–10 bubbles, a medium shunt 10–20, and a large shunt > 20 bubbles (28). If the right-to-left shunt is causing arterial hypoxemia, the contrast test will be positive.

## Suspected Endocarditis

Infective endocarditis (IE) may present as critical illness (cardiac failure, dysrhythmias, sepsis), and critically ill patients may develop endocarditis due to infection of indwelling devices and the presence of an immunocompromised state. Because critically ill patients often have nonspecific signs and symptoms, and are usually receiving antibiotics that reduce the sensitivity of blood cultures, echocardiography plays a critical role in diagnosis. A recent review suggests that TEE is cost-effective as an initial strategy (as opposed to TTE) when the pretest (pre-echo) probability of endocarditis based on clinical findings and laboratory results is as low as 4% (29).

Strict diagnostic criteria for IE were originally proposed by von Reyn et al. in 1981 (30), then revised by Durack et al. in 1994 (the "Duke" criteria) (31). Diagnosis is made based on either (1) pathologic (surgery or autopsy) findings or (2) clinical plus echocardiographic findings. Table 21.5 outlines the clinical criteria defined by Durack et al. They suggest the presence of 2 major criteria, 1 major and 3 minor, or 5 minor criteria all be considered "definite by clinical criteria." In an evaluation of the Durack criteria in more than 100 patients with IE, Roe et al. found that TEE was critically important, resulting in a diagnostic reclassification in approximately 25% of patients, 90% of which were from "possible" to "definite" IE (32).

The hallmark lesion of IE is the vegetation, defined as a mass adherent to the endocardium consisting of pathologic microorganisms interwoven with platelets, fibrin strands, and blood cells. Vegetations typically occur where normal endocardium has been partially denuded or altered by abnormal flow such as regurgitation, the most common site being the "upstream" side of a regurgitant valve (e.g., the LA side of the mitral valve or LV side of the aortic valve). Vegetations usually occur on valves, but may occur on a chamber wall where the endocardium has been disrupted by abnormal flow, such as a regurgitant jet. Lesions may be relatively slow growing (months) or, in the case of very pathogenic organisms such as *staphylococcus aureus*, rapidly growing to more than a centimeter in size over a few days. A variable amount of

**TABLE 21.5. Criteria for the Diagnosis of Infective Endocarditis (IE)**

Major Criteria
Positive blood culture
    Typical organism for IE from two separate blood cultures*
                OR
    Persistently positive blood culture with organism consistent with IE from
      (i)   Blood cultures drawn more than 12 hours apart, or
      (ii)  All of 3 or a majority of 4 or more separate cultures at least 1 hour apart
Evidence of endocardial involvement
    Positive echocardiogram for IE
      (i)   Oscillating intracardiac mass on valve or supporting structures, or in the path of
            regurgitant jets, or on implanted material, in the absence of an alternative
            anatomic explanation
      (ii)  Abscess
      (iii) New partial dehiscence of prosthetic valve, or
            new valvular regurgitation (change in murmur not sufficient)
Minor Criteria
    Predisposition: predisposing heart condition or intravenous drug use
    Fever ≥ 38° C
    Vascular phenomena: arterial emboli, septic pulmonary infarcts, mycotic aneurysm,
        intracranial hemorrhage, conjunctival hemorrhage, Janeway lesions
    Immunologic phenomena: glomerulonephritis, Osler nodes, Roth spots, rheumatoid factor
    Microbiologic evidence: positive blood culture but not meeting major criteria**
    Echocardiogram: consistent with endocarditis but not meeting major criteria

*Viridans streptococci, Streptococcus bovis, HACEK group (Haemophilus spp., Actinobacillus actino-
  mycetemconitans, Cardiobacterium hominis, Eikenella spp., and Kingella kingae); or community-
  acquired staphylococcus aureus or enterococci, in the absence of a primary focus.
**Excluding single-positive culture for coagulase negative staphylococci and organisms that do not
  cause endocarditis or serologic evidence of active infection with appropriate organism (31).

destruction of the involved region of the heart occurs, usually resulting in new or worsening regurgitation; the infection can become invasive leading to localized abscess and/or fistula formation. The echocardiographic appearance is an echodense mass exhibiting a variable amount of independent motion (Fig. 21.5). Vegetations may vary in size from microscopic (below the resolution of TEE) to several centimeters in size, with fungal vegetations of the tricuspid valve tending to be the largest.

## Vegetation Detection by TTE versus TEE

Similar to the discussion above regarding the assessment of hemodynamic instability in the ICU, at least 6 investigations in the last 15 years have compared TTE with TEE in the diagnosis of IE. These studies have been summarized by Shanewise and Martin (33), demonstrating a sensitivity of TTE of 28%–63% versus 86%–100% with TEE. The *specificity* of the two techniques is similar: once a vegetation is seen with either TTE or TEE it is generally due to IE, however TEE provides a much greater sensitivity and is the technique of choice. The less invasive TTE is likely to be performed first in most cases, however, if negative the TTE should be promptly followed by TEE. Several of the studies also found TEE to be much more sensi-

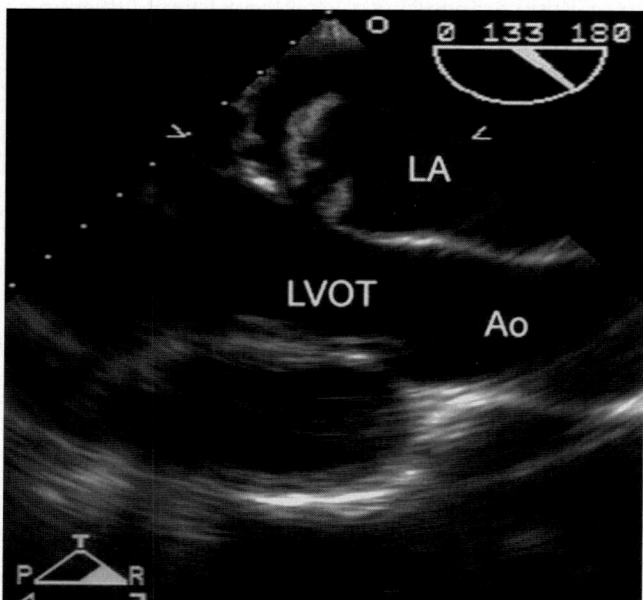

**FIGURE 21.5.** Midesophageal long-axis TEE view showing a large vegetation on the mitral valve with perforation through the anterior leaflet. *LA,* left atrium; *LVOT,* left ventricular outflow tract; *Ao,* ascending aorta.

tive in the detection of associated pathology, such as chordal rupture, valve perforation, and abscess formation. All used single-plane TEE; a recent study by Reynolds et al. in 114 cases of suspected IE confirmed that with the use of modern equipment TTE still detects only 55% of lesions seen with TEE (34).

The echocardiographic exam for IE should be a complete, standard exam including careful, multiplane imaging of all the valves and associated structures, as well as complete Doppler echocardiographic assessment. In some patients (especially those with prosthetic valves), it may be necessary to use TTE and TEE to obtain adequate views. Care must be taken to evaluate the tissues surrounding any valves with suspicious findings, looking for fistulae and abscesses. Echocardiography can also be used to assess prognosis in IE, because vegetation size and mobility are predictive of outcome (greater size and mobility, worse outcome). One study found that vegetations larger than 10 mm were associated with a 47% risk of embolization (35); another found that 25% of mitral vegetations versus 10% of aortic vegetations were associated with embolization (36). In all series, embolization is a major risk factor for adverse outcome. Thus, large mobile vegetations of the mitral valve are likely to be associated with a poor prognosis.

## Trauma

Chest trauma alone accounts for 25% of fatalities from automobile accidents. Due to its noninvasive nature, transthoracic echocardiography (TTE) is initially used as a screening tool for evaluating patients with significant chest trauma. However, as described above there are multiple technical limitations with TTE. Transesophageal echocardiography provides consistently superior resolution of multiple cardiac structures in the setting of trauma, and is especially useful in assessing the thoracic aorta, mitral valve, and posterior structures, such as the left atrial appendage, the intraatrial septum, and the pulmonary veins (37–40).

In a prospective multicenter trial, Garcia-Fernandez has demonstrated the utility of TEE in the assessment of patients with blunt chest trauma and compared TEE findings with those provided by the electrocardiogram and cardiac isoenzyme assays (40). As outlined in Table 21.6, Garcia-Fernandez demonstrated that 56% of patients had pathologic findings on TEE attributed to blunt chest trauma (Fig. 21.6).

## Blunt Cardiac Trauma

### Cardiac Tamponade

The initial clinical manifestations of acute traumatic cardiac tamponade as described in Beck in 1935 still hold true and include hypotension, increased jugular venous

▶ TABLE 21.6. **Transesophageal Echocardiographic Findings in 117 Prospectively Evaluated Patients with Blunt Chest Trauma**

| Location | Percent |
|---|---|
| I. Myocardial | |
|    A. Abnormal regional wall motion | |
|      RV ventricular wall hypokinesis | 24% |
|      LV anterior-septal hypokinesis/akinesis | 11% |
|      LV interior-posterior hypokinesis | 3% |
|    B. RV dilation | 13% |
|    C. Interventricular septal rupture | 1% |
| II. Pericardial | |
|      Pericardial effusion | 11% |
|      Cardiac tamponade | 1% |
| III. Valvular | |
|      MV leaflet disruption | 1% |
|      MV chordal rupture | 1% |
|      TV prolapse | 1% |
| IV. Aorta | |
|      Aortic rupture | 7% |
|      Aortic dissection | 1% |
| V. Normal exam | 44% |

Adapted from Garcia-Fernandez MA, Lopez-Perez JM, Perez-Castellano N, et al. Role of transesophageal echocardiography in the assessment of patients with blunt chest trauma: Correlation of echocardiographic findings with the electrocardiogram and creatine kinase monoclonal antibody measurements. Am Heart J 1998;135:426–81.

distention, and quiet distant heart sounds (41). These signs are very frequent in patients who suffer cardiac trauma or rupture when there is an acute increase in intrapericardial pressure. As fluid accumulates within the pericardial sac, there is a progressive limitation of ventricular diastolic filling, a reduction of stroke volume, and hence, a decreased cardiac output. If the pericardial effusion accumulates over time, one will typically see the classical nontraumatic manifestations of cardiac tamponade, which include pulsus paradoxus, tachycardia, increased jugular venous pressure, and hypotension.

### Pathophysiology

If one were to consider the heart to be in a fixed, enclosed space when tamponade is present, the normal rise and fall of intrathoracic pressures during spontaneous ventilation can have profound effects on atrial and ventricular filling. Specific changes in these filling patterns have been identified in cardiac tamponade in which greater interdependence of the ventricles occurs as a result of the fluid-filled pericardium. When a spontaneously breathing patient with cardiac tamponade inhales, intrathoracic pressure falls resulting in an increase venous return to the right atrium and right ventricle, resulting in a leftward shift of the interventricular septum and decreasing

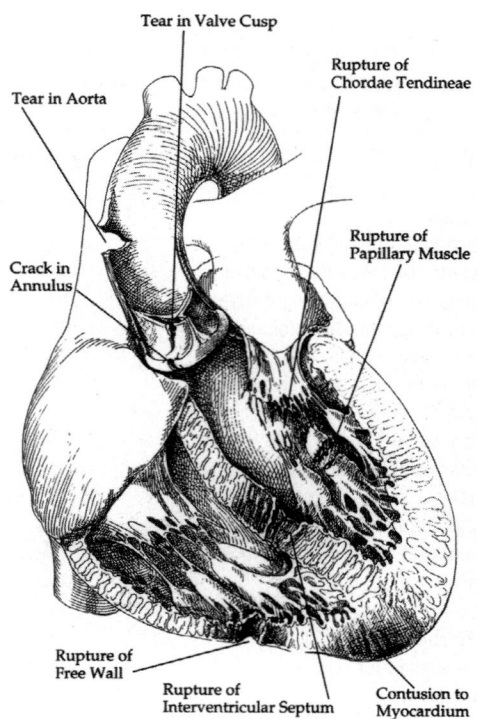

Tear in Valve Cusp

Tear in Aorta

Rupture of
Chordae Tendineae

Crack in
Annulus

Rupture of
Papillary Muscle

Rupture of
Free Wall

Rupture of
Interventricular Septum

Contusion to
Myocardium

**FIGURE 21.6.** Blunt trauma, such as that caused by the impact of the chest against the steering wheel in an automobile accident, may injure various cardiac structures. Myocardial contusion is the most frequent injury, but rupture may occur at several sites, including the interventricular septum, the walls of the cardiac chambers, the papillary muscles, and the chordae tendineae. The sheering forces that accompany abrupt deceleration may also cause tearing of the aorta and the valve cusp and cracking of the annulus. From Dale DC, Federman BD eds. Scientific American Medicine. Web MD Corporation 2001, section 8, page 8, reproduced with permission.

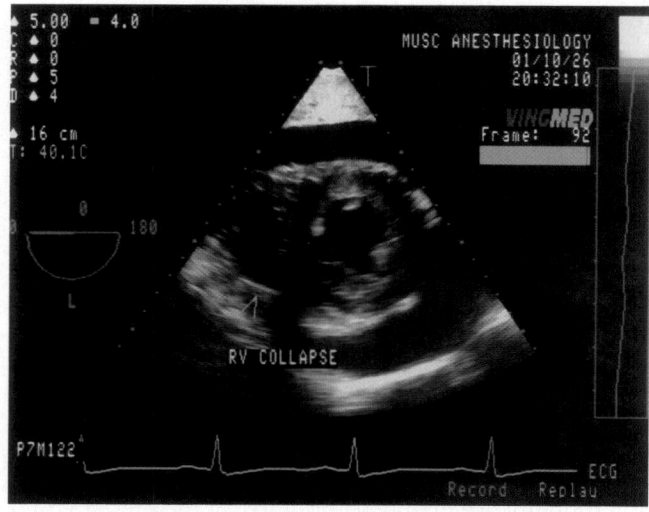

A

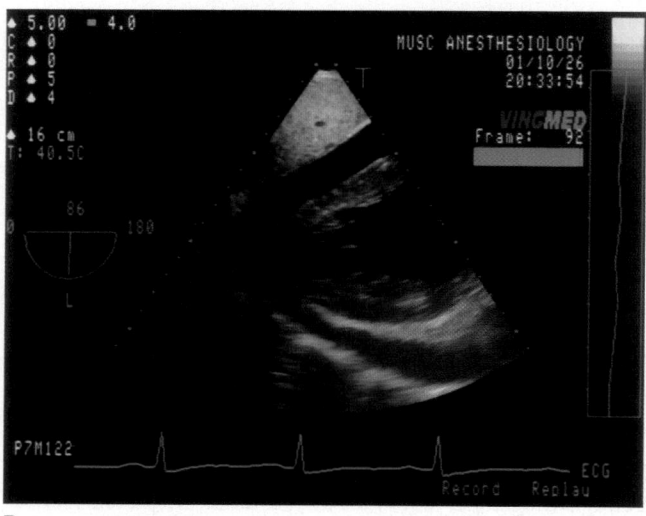

B

**FIGURE 21.7. A:** Transgastric short-axis view demonstrating very large pericardial effusion with right ventricular collapse as demonstrated by the arrow during diastole. **B:** A longitudinal view at approximately 90% of the left ventricle, again demonstrating significant circumferential pericardial effusion.

filling on the left side of the heart. This pathophysiology will lead to the classical Doppler manifestations of a decreased left ventricular filling with inspiration, a delay of mitral valve opening, lengthening of the isovolemic relaxation time, and a decreased mitral E-wave velocity. Conversely on expiration, there is an increased intrathoracic pressure resulting in decreased venous return to the right side of the heart and a reciprocal increased return to the left side of the heart. For the patient undergoing positive pressure ventilation, a reciprocal pattern of tricuspid and mitral filling may occur.

### Echocardiographic Diagnoses

The most sensitive 2-D manifestation of cardiac tamponade is right ventricular collapse during diastole in a patient with a pericardial effusion. Figures 21.7A and 21.7B demonstrate a patient with a large circumferential pericardial effusion of greater than 1 cm. Figure 21.8 shows the right ventricular diastolic collapse in the same pa-

tient. Right atrial invagination can also be seen occurring in late diastole (Fig. 21.9) (42,43). The ability to time right-sided chamber collapse has been simplified by utilizing the freeze frame technology available in echocardiographic systems, allowing the echocardiographer the ability to follow the EKG frame-by-frame to visualize right atrial and ventricular collapse in early diastole. Timing of the chamber collapse can also be made by coordinating it with mitral valve opening.

It is extremely important to realize that cardiac tamponade is a clinical syndrome and requires bedside diagnosis. Echocardiographic manifestations may actually precede clinical manifestations in cardiac tamponade. In

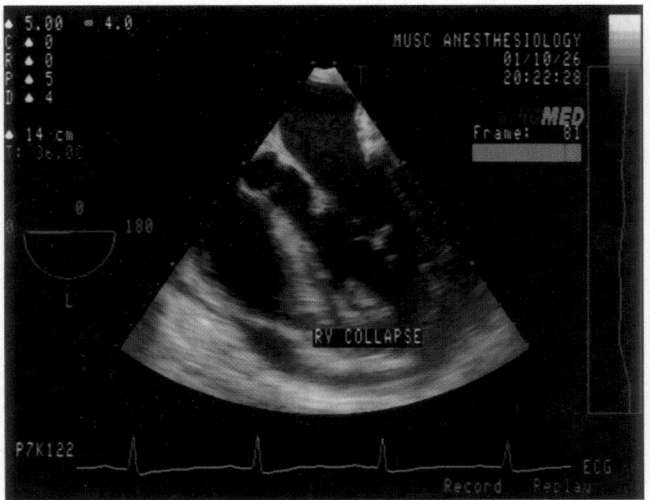

**FIGURE 21.8.** Right ventricular collapse in a five-chamber midesophageal view in early diastole.

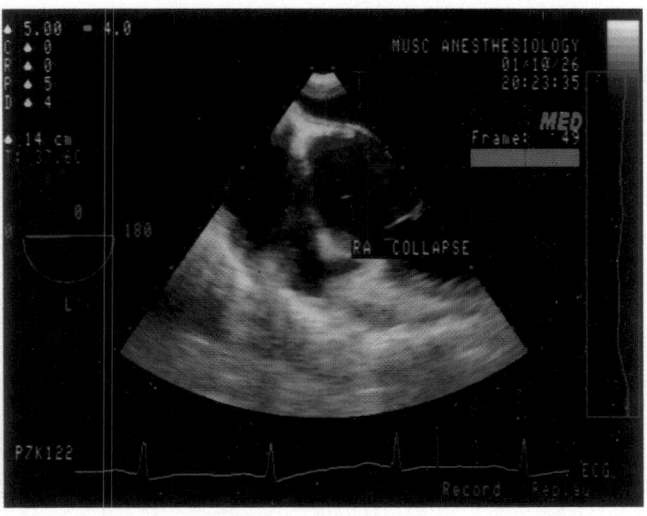

**FIGURE 21.9.** Right atrial collapse in early diastole.

addition, echo manifestations may be completely absent. In a prospective study of 110 patients with moderate or large pericardial effusions, Merce et al. demonstrated that 10% of patients did not have any evidence of right atrial or right ventricular collapse (43). The usual explanation for right ventricular and atrial collapse is that these chambers are low-pressure chambers and, therefore, have thin walls and are easily compressed by the elevated pericardial pressure. If right ventricular pressure is significantly elevated, resulting in right ventricular hypertrophy, right ventricular collapse may not be present (42,43). The authors have also seen the elimination of right ventricular and right atrial collapse with aggressive volume expansion in the trauma patient.

Other 2-D manifestations of tamponade can include left atrial and ventricular collapse. This usually occurs when the left atrial and left ventricular pressures are low. This phenomenon is not uncommon following cardiac surgical procedures where a loculated pericardial effusion or an intrapericardial clot may affect left atrial and left ventricular filling as demonstrated in Figs. 21.10A and 21.10B. Finally, inferior vena cava distention with a lack of inspiratory variation may be present.

### Doppler Echocardiography

As has already been discussed, there is minimal respiratory variation of mitral inflow in the normal patient.

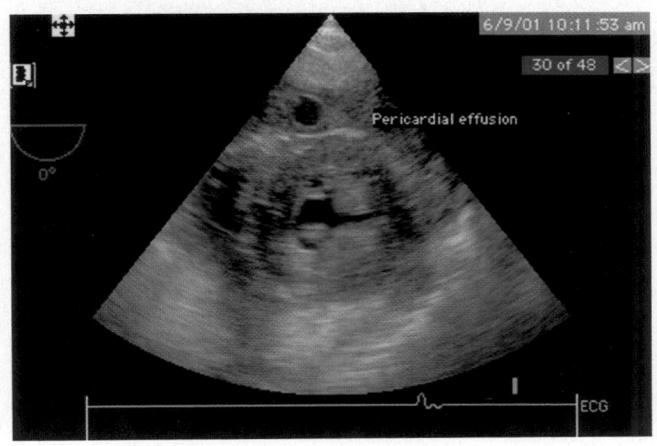

A

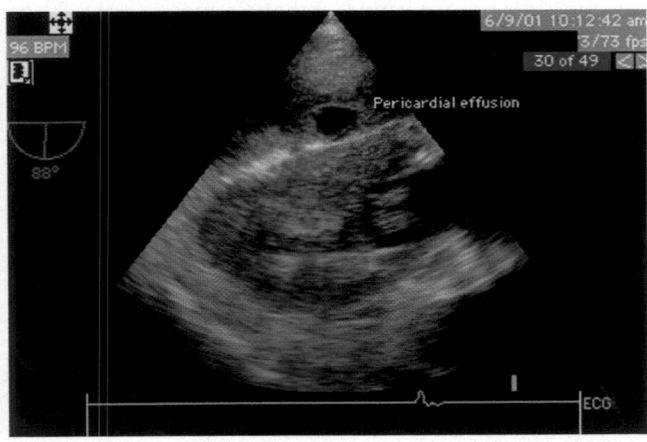

B

**FIGURE 21.10. A:** Short-axis transgastric view demonstrating a loculated posterior pericardial effusion in a patient status postcardiac surgery. The effusion measures a little over 1 cm posteriorly. **B:** The same patient in the transesophageal long-axis view with the loculated posterior pericardial effusion.

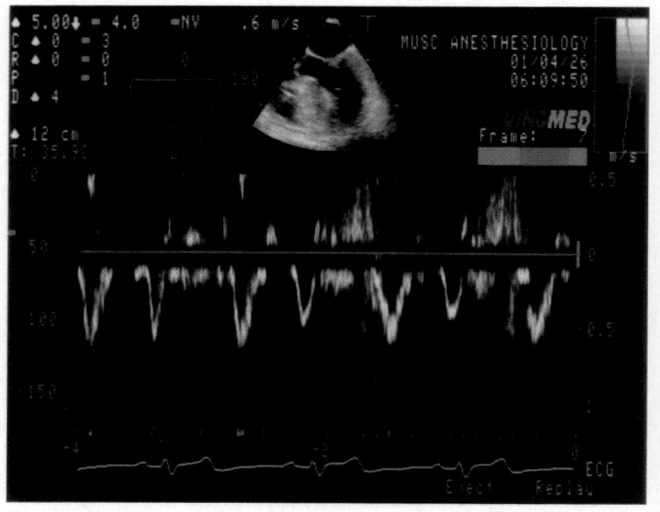
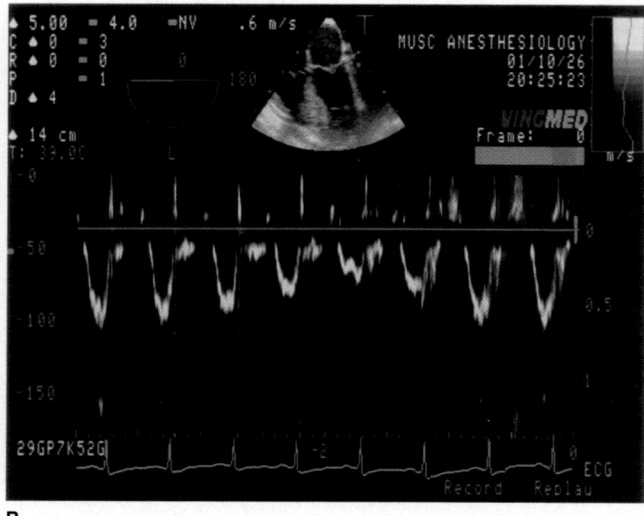

**FIGURE 21.11. A:** Normal mitral in-flow E-wave velocities. **B:** The significant respiratory variation of mitral in-flow E-wave velocities in a patient with cardiac tamponade. Note the significant decrease in the mitral E-wave during inspiration in this spontaneously breathing patient.

However, in the spontaneously breathing patient with cardiac tamponade, inspiration will produce a decrease in left-sided filling and, therefore, will reduce early diastolic velocity through the mitral valve. Figures 21.11A and 21.11B demonstrate a significant drop in the height of the early diastolic E-wave velocity across the mitral valve during inspiration. With the onset of expiration, one will see an increase in the mitral valve E-wave diastolic velocity and a shortening of the isovolemic relaxation time. Doppler of the tricuspid valve reveals an increase in the tricuspid valve E-wave velocity with inspiration and a decrease in the tricuspid valve E-wave velocity with expiration (Fig. 21.12).

Diastolic pulmonary venous forward flow will decrease during inspiration and increase during expiration in a spontaneously breathing patient with cardiac tamponade. During expiration, hepatic venous flow will be reduced in both systole and diastole. In addition, hepatic venous diastolic flow reversal may actually occur with expiration. Table 21.7 summarizes the clinical and echocardiographic manifestations of cardiac tamponade (38,39). These correlations have been demonstrated during spontaneous respiration and may not be equally applicable during positive pressure ventilation.

### Myocardial Contusion and Rupture

Most patients with RV contusions are asymptomatic at presentation. In a prospective study involving 117 patients, Garcia-Fernandez demonstrated that TEE is extremely safe and effective in diagnosing acute cardiac injuries following blunt chest trauma (38). TEE was found to be much more specific and sensitive than EKG

or CK-MB analysis for detection of cardiac damage following blunt chest trauma. Due to its close proximity to the sternum, the anterior right ventricular wall is the most vulnerable to cardiac contusions. In one study, the right ventricle was affected in 32% of patients, the left ventricle in 15%, and both ventricles in 5% of patients who had blunt chest trauma (38). It was also noted, as will be discussed shortly, that the higher pressures on the left side of the heart resulted in a higher incidence of mitral and aortic valve injuries compared to right-sided valves.

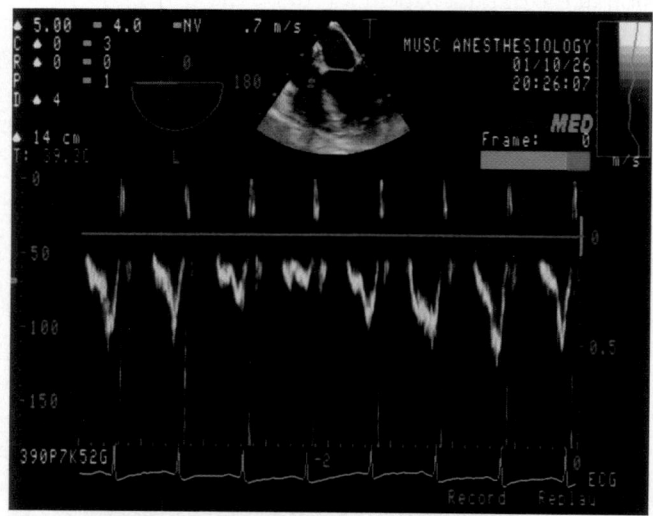

**FIGURE 21.12.** Midesophageal four-chamber view demonstrating a profound decrease in the tricuspid E-wave velocity with the onset of expiration.

▶ **TABLE 21.7. Pericardial Tamponade Clinical and Echocardiographic Manifestations**

| *Clinical* |
| --- |
| Elevated jugular venous pressures |
| Pulsus paradoxus |
| Hypotension |
| Low cardiac output |

| *2-D Echo* |
| --- |
| Swinging heart (electrical alternans) |
| RA collapse late diastole |
| RV collapse early diastole |
| Dilated IVC without inspiratory collapse |
| LA collapse in late diastole and early systole |

| *Doppler (Spontaneous Ventilation)* | |
| --- | --- |
| Respiratory variation in mitral and tricuspid inflow | |
| Inspiration | Increased tricuspid E-wave velocity |
| | Decreased mitral E-wave velocity |
| Expiration | Decreased tricuspid E-wave velocity |
| | Increased mitral E-wave velocity |
| Hepatic flow | |
| Expiration | severely decreased diastolic forward flow or flow reversal |
| | Atrial component flow reversal |

## Echo Manifestations of Myocardial Contusion

Pandian et al., in an acute canine model of blunt chest trauma, demonstrated that echo manifestations of myocardial contusion consist of:

1. Increased ventricular wall echocardiographic brightness
2. An increase in diastolic wall thickness
3. Impaired regional wall systolic function (44)

Most clinicians define cardiac contusions as a presence of wall motion abnormalities in either or both ventricles in the absence of a transmural myocardial infarction on EKG (45). Figure 21.13 demonstrates the dilated right ventricle typically seen following RV contusion. This patient had segmental wall motion abnormalities involving the anterior wall of the right ventricle.

RV contusions are associated with depression of overall RV ejection fraction. Both mean end systolic and diastolic volumes will increase creating an appropriate increase in right ventricular preload in order to maintain cardiac output. Significant reductions of cardiac output of 30% to 40% can occur and may last for several weeks following the incident (46,47).

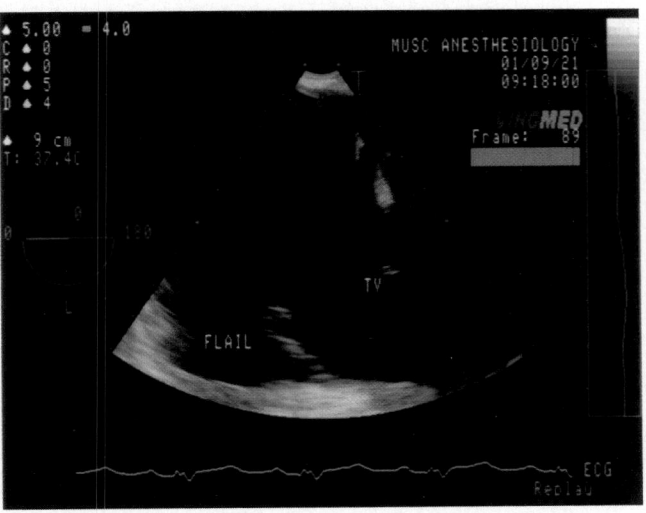

**FIGURE 21.13.** A dilated right ventricle following blunt cardiac trauma. The force of the trauma resulted in a flailed anterior leaflet of the tricuspid valve. The patient also had hypokinesis and thinning of his anterior right ventricular free wall.

## Cardiac Rupture

Both ventricles are prone to rupture if the impact occurs during the brief period of time during late diastole and early systole when the chambers are fully distended and the valves are closed, thus providing no outlet for the release of the increased intracardiac pressure (48). When the left ventricle is involved, the injury usually will be isolated to the apex and the septum, whereas the majority of right ventricular ruptures occur on the anterior apical wall. In contrast to the left ventricle, atrial ruptures occur most often during systole when venous return distends the atrium (37).

## Valve Injury

Blunt chest trauma resulting in significant injury to a normal valve is uncommon. However, valvular injury may occur with the aortic valve most frequently involved, followed by the mitral valve, the tricuspid valve, and finally the pulmonic valve (49). Fortunately, transesophageal echocardiography can help delineate valve pathology if utilized as a screening tool for blunt chest trauma when there is a high index of suspicion for a valve injury. Figures 21.14A–C demonstrate midesophageal aortic valve short-axis and midesophageal five-chamber views of the aortic valve with a laceration of the right coronary cusp due to blunt chest trauma. Aortic valve injury most frequently involves rupture along its base at the cusps' attachment site to the annulus, and less frequently occurs due to a frank tear in a cusp. Devineni has proposed that the sudden transmission of the increased intrathoracic

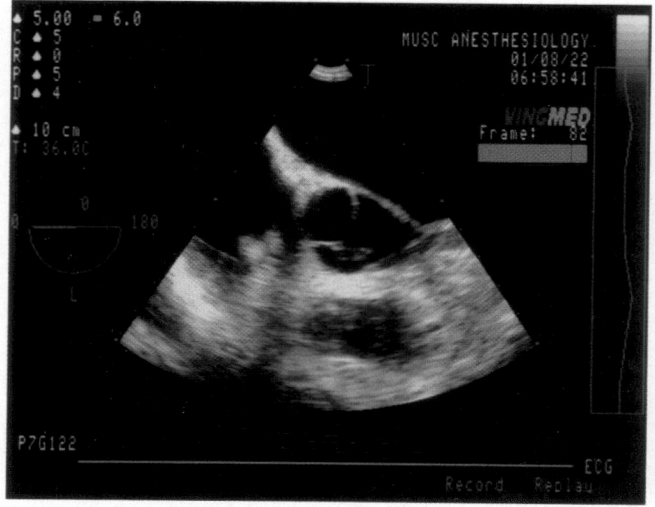

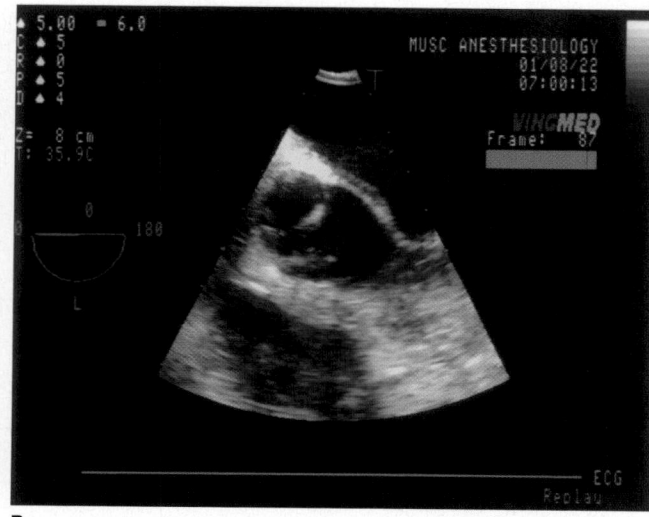

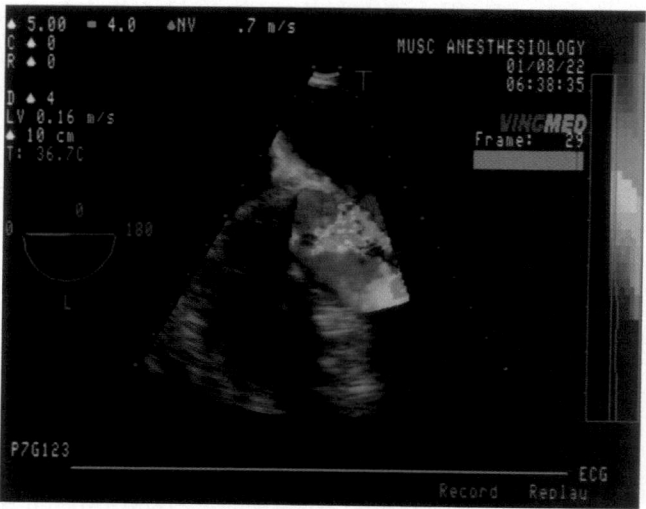

**FIGURE 21.14. A:** A slightly off-axis aortic valve short-axis view with a tear in the right coronary cusp following blunt chest trauma. **B:** Flailing of a segment of the right coronary cusp into the left ventricular outflow track. **C:** An eccentric severe jet of the aortic insufficiency resulting from the torn right coronary cusp.

pressure to the aorta and left ventricle at the time of compressive chest trauma while the aortic and mitral valves are closed results in a blowout type of injury to the aortic valve (49). Acute avulsion of one of the coronary cusps may occur, when the aortic valve is closed in early diastole and the pressure gradient across the aortic valve is maximal.

Mitral valve injury will present as rupture of the chordae tendinae or papillary muscles. Actual leaflet tears will occasionally occur. The mechanism of injury appears to be acute elevations in intraventricular pressure during diastole when the mitral valve is closed and the ventricle is distended. Because the chordae tendinae that are anchoring the anterior leaflet are thicker than those anchoring the posterior leaflet, the posterior leaflet is more often involved in blunt chest trauma (37). Figures 21.15A and 21.15B demonstrate a traumatic rupture of the posterior medial papillary muscle.

Tricuspid valve injury is even less common than aortic or mitral valve injury. Its mechanism is again felt to be secondary to an abrupt elevation in right ventricular pressure during diastole when the tricuspid valve is closed and the ventricle is distended. One might expect an increase incidence secondary to the close proximity of the sternum to the right ventricle, however, this has not been documented in the literature. Figure 21.13 demonstrates an acute RV anterior papillary muscle rupture and a profoundly dilated right ventricle following blunt chest trauma.

## Aortic Dissection

Acute aortic dissection has been shown to have an extremely high mortality of 1% per hour among untreated patients during the first 48 hours. It is therefore imperative that a quick and an accurate diagnosis is made in order to initiate treatment and improve survival. Aortography was

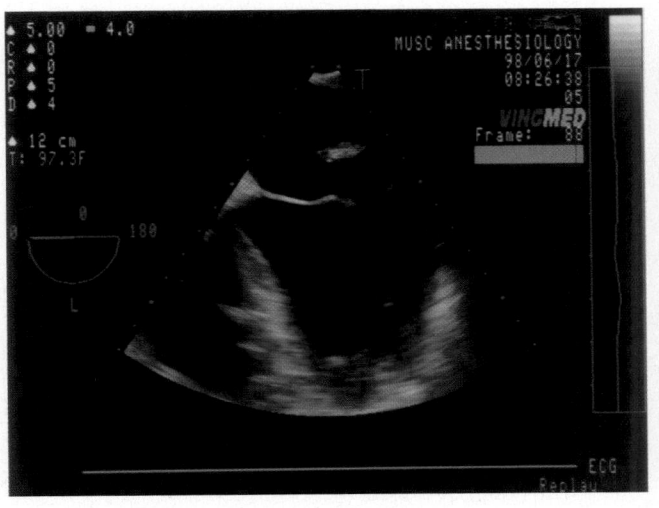

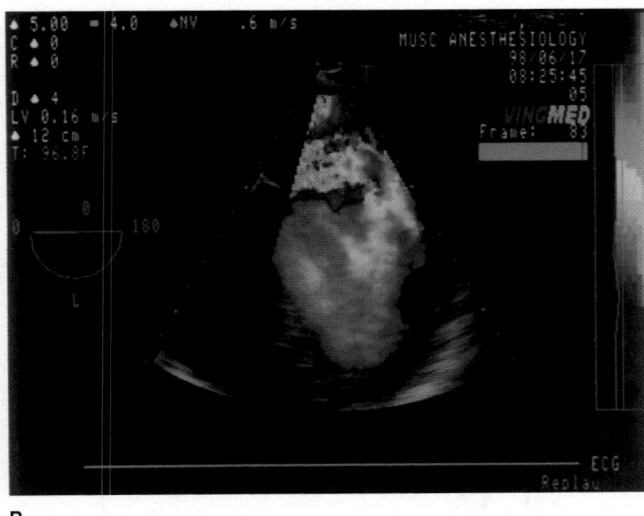

A                                                                    B

**FIGURE 21.15. A:** A flailed, ruptured posterior medial papillary muscle of the mitral valve, resulting in posterior leaflet flailing following blunt cardiac trauma. **B:** Severe eccentric jet of mitral regurgitation resulting from the posterior leaflet flail.

previously considered the gold standard for evaluation of patients with suspected aortic dissection. However, transesophageal echocardiography, due to its wide availability, noninvasiveness, ease of performance at the bedside, and cost, is becoming the diagnostic modality of choice in major trauma centers throughout the United States. Table 21.8 summarizes the diagnostic performance of different modalities in patients suspected of having an aortic dissection.

### Classification Systems

The Debakey classification system was proposed in 1965 (50) and classified dissections as Type I, where the dissec-

tion starts in the ascending aorta and involves variable portions of the descending aorta; Type II, where the dissection is confined only to the ascending aorta; and Type III, where the dissection starts distal to the left subclavian artery and involves either exclusively the descending thoracic aorta (3-A) or extends into the abdominal segment of the descending aorta (3B). In 1970, the Stanford Classification (51) was devised, which separates aortic dissections into Type A where the dissection involves the ascending aorta and Type B where the dissection is confined to the descending thoracic aorta. The two classification systems are compared in Fig. 21.16.

### Review of Transesophageal Echocardiography Image Planes

TEE is ideal for evaluating the thoracic aorta secondary to its close proximity to the esophagus. The relationship of the esophagus and the thoracic aorta changes as one moves from the upper thorax towards the diaphragm. At the distal arch, the aorta lies anterior to the esophagus. It moves posterior to the esophagus by the time one reaches the level of the diaphragm. This changing anatomical relationship makes it difficult to designate anterior and posterior as well as left and right orientation of the descending aorta. One must have a systematic approach when evaluating the thoracic aorta in order to be able to communicate with cardiothoracic surgeons and others. The approach we find most useful is to estimate distances from known anatomical landmarks. In the ascending aorta, the aortic valve is used as a defining landmark, whereas in the descending aorta the distance of the structure from the left subclavian artery is utilized. This

▶ **TABLE 21.8. Diagnostic Performance of Imaging Modalities in the Evaluation of Suspected Dissection**

| Diagnostic Performance | Angio | CT | MRI | TEE |
|---|---|---|---|---|
| Sensitivity | ++ | ++ | +++ | +++ |
| Specificity | +++ | +++ | +++ | ++/+++ |
| Site of intimal tear | ++ | + | +++ | ++ |
| Presence of thrombus | +++ | ++ | +++ | + |
| Presence of aortic insufficiency | +++ | - | + | +++ |
| Pericardial effusion | - | ++ | +++ | +++ |
| Branch vessel involvement | +++ | + | ++ | + |
| Coronary artery involvement | ++ | - | - | ++ |

**Note:** +++, excellent; ++, good; +, fair; - , not detected; *Angio,* angiography; *CT,* computed tomography; *MRI,* magnetic resonance imaging; *TEE,* transesophageal echocardiography.
**Source**: Modified from Cigarro JE, Isselbacher EM, DeSanctis RW, et al. Diagnostic imaging in the evaluation of suspected aortic dissection: old standards and new directions. N Engl J Med 1993;328:35, with permission. Copyright by the Massachusetts Medical Society.

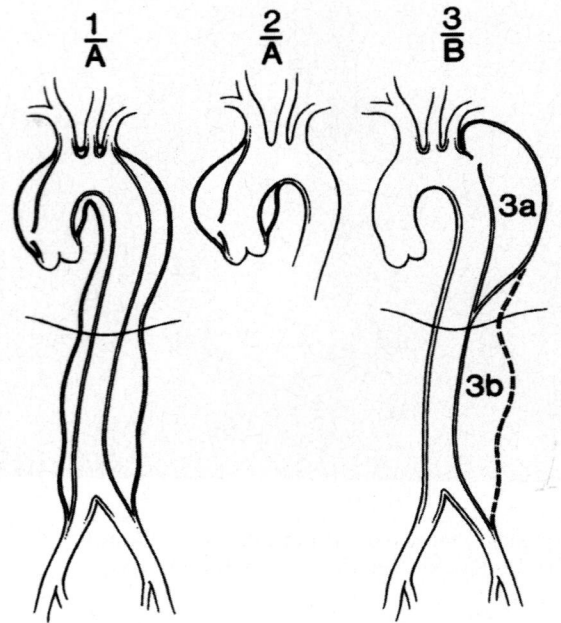

**FIGURE 21.16.** The Stanford (A and B) and Debakey (I, II, III) classification systems for thoracic aorta dissections. From Crawford ES, Crawford JL. *Diseases of the Aorta*, Baltimore: Williams & Wilkins, 1984:174, with permission.

approach is different than what is used in the echocardiography suite where one is concerned with follow-up examinations. In the echocardiography lab, the depth of the lesion from the incisors is most frequently utilized.

There are two areas that must be carefully examined when looking for acute aortic dissections; these include the area just distal to the aortic valve in the region of the sinotubular junction—the propagation site for acute ascending aortic dissections,—and just distal to the left subclavian artery—the propagation site for descending dissections. While one is performing an examination, one must remember that the air-filled trachea is interposed between the esophagus and the distal ascending aorta and proximal aortic arch. This area is not clearly visualized even with multiplane TEE technology. Therefore, a high index of suspicion must be utilized for any abnormality in this area.

### Transesophageal Echocardiography Evaluation for Aortic Dissection

The goals of perioperative TEE for the evaluation of aortic dissection include:

1. Establishment of the diagnosis
2. Localization of primary and secondary entry sites
3. Differentiation of the true from the false lumen
4. Evaluation of the aortic valve for insufficiency
5. Establishing the involvement of coronary arteries
6. Estimation of left ventricular function
7. Ruling out associated conditions, such as pericardial infusions or tamponade

### Establishment of the Diagnosis

Aortic dissection occurs when blood dissects the intima from the media. A majority of examinations are associated with an intimal flap seen as a mobile linear echo within the vascular lumen. It is imperative that this intimal flap is demonstrated in two planes in order to establish the diagnosis. The identification of flow within the true and false lumens on either side of an intimal flap are highly sensitive features of aortic dissection (Figs. 21.17A and 21.17B) (52–55). Additional 2-D findings consistent with aortic dis-

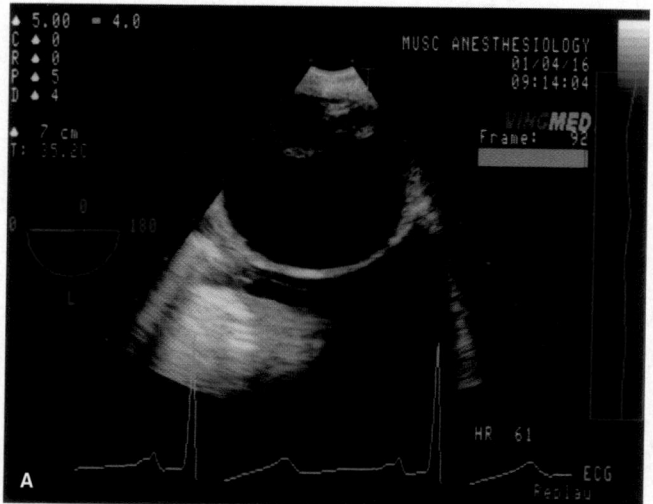

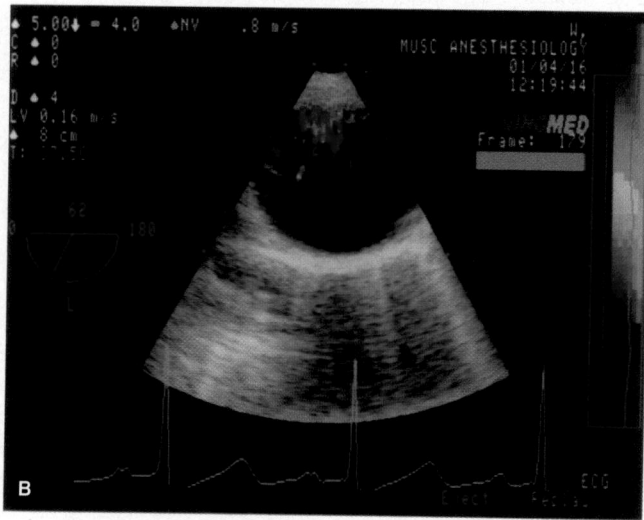

**Figure 21.17.** **A:** Short-axis view of the descending aorta demonstrating an acute aortic dissection. Note that the true lumen is much smaller in size than the false lumen. **B:** Color flow within the true lumen

section include complete separation of intimal layers secondary to thrombus, complete thrombosis of the false lumen, and central displacement of intimal calcification or bright echogenic densities within the aorta.

### Location of Entry Sites

An entry site of an intimal tear is defined as a distinct disruption in the continuity of the flap that is often identified by 2-D or color Doppler. Color Doppler is superior to two-dimensional Doppler in identifying small intimal tears (54). Figure 21.18 demonstrates a turbulent jet of bright mosaic color transversing from the true to the false lumen.

Greater than 70% of cases will demonstrate the intimal tear occurring in the ascending aorta 1 to 3 cm above the right or left sinus of Valsalva. The remaining 20%–30% will demonstrate the intimal flap at the site of the ligamentum arteriosum in the descending thoracic aorta (52,56). It is important to give an estimate of the location of the intimal tear from both the patient's incisors, that is, the depth of probe insertion and from a major anatomical landmark, such as the sinus of Valsalva or the left subclavian artery. Adachi has proven that Type B dissection entry sites can be identified in 90% of cases, compared to only 83% for Type A dissections. The combined frequency of entry site identification was 88% in his study (57). Identification and localization of the primary tear is extremely important to the ultimate success of the surgical repair because resection of the primary entry site will decrease the occurrence of late reoperations and complications.

### Identification of True versus False Lumen

There are multiple 2-D echo findings that can be utilized to differentiate the true from the false lumen. The true lumen usually expands during systole and is compressed during diastole (54). The true lumen has a thin, less echogenic inner layer, while the false lumen has a bright echogenic layer adjacent to the aortic lumen. Spontaneous echo contrast and/or thrombus are frequently present in the false lumen secondary to stagnant flow. The false lumen will typically be larger in size, especially with chronic dissections (Figs. 21.19A and 21.19B) (58,59).

Color flow Doppler can provide additional clues on the identification of the true versus false lumen. The true lumen will have flow immediately at the onset of systole whereas the false lumen will typically have delayed systolic flow, which is complicated and variable. How-

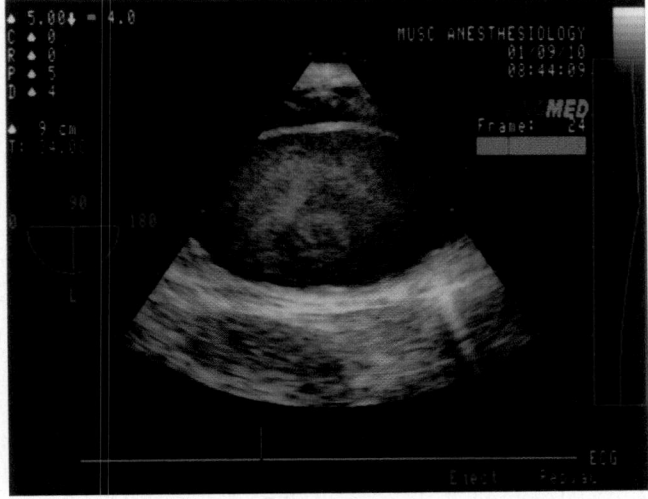

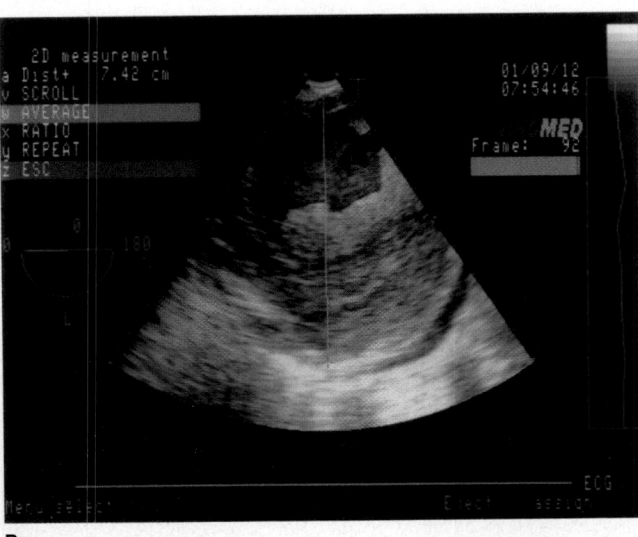

**FIGURE 21.19. A:** Spontaneous echo contrast within the false lumen in a patient with acute aortic dissection. **B:** Profound thrombus formation in a patient with a chronic aortic dissection within the false lumen.

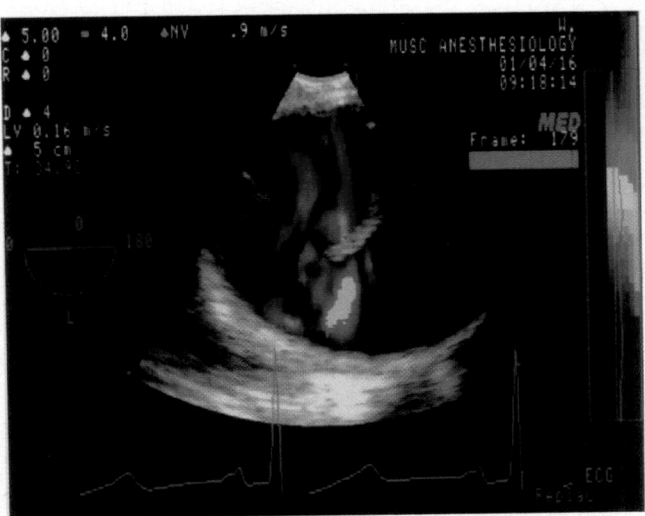

***Figure 21.18.*** A color flow image demonstrating flow from the true lumen to the false lumen through the entry site.

ever, with large proximal entry tears, flow in the nearby segments of the false lumen may be equal in direction and timing to the true lumen (56).

### Aortic Insufficiency

Up to 70% of proximal dissections and 10% of descending thoracic aortic dissections will have aortic insufficiency complicating the acute aortic dissection (60). Therefore, TEE evaluation of aortic valve structure and function is integral in the assessment of aortic dissection. TEE is more sensitive than aortography in the detection of mild aortic insufficiency.

Aortic insufficiency is diagnosed with color flow Doppler as previously described. The ratio of the regurgitation jet width to the left ventricular outflow tract width may be used to grade aortic insufficiency into mild, moderate, moderate to severe, and severe.

Transesophageal echocardiography is also useful in demonstrating and defining the causes of aortic insufficiency. The mechanisms of aortic insufficiency include disturbance of cusp closure by hematoma at the annulus (Fig. 21.20), destruction of the annular support of the cusp with subsequent cusp prolapse, dilatation of the aortic root leading to widening of the aortic annulus and disturbance of aortic valve cusp coaptation (Figs. 21.21A and 21.21B), and prolapse of the dissection flap into the aortic valve orifice and left ventricular outflow tract with interference of aortic cusp motion. Figure 21.22 summarizes the mechanisms for acquiring aortic insuffiency in acute aortic dissections. Aortic insufficiency has a negative effect on outcome in aortic dissection and may dictate the surgical approach. In 86% of Type A dissections, native aortic valve repair and resuspension may be possible (61).

### Coronary Artery Involvement

Coronary artery involvement in acute aortic dissection has been estimated to occur in 10%-20% of cases (52,69).

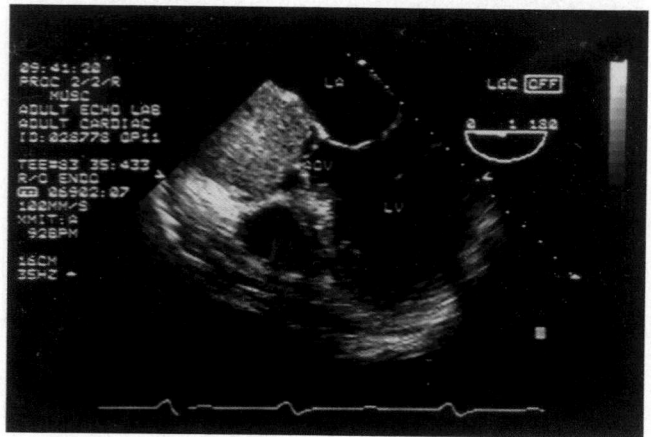

**FIGURE 21.20.** A proximal aortic hematoma that would cause significant aortic insufficiency.

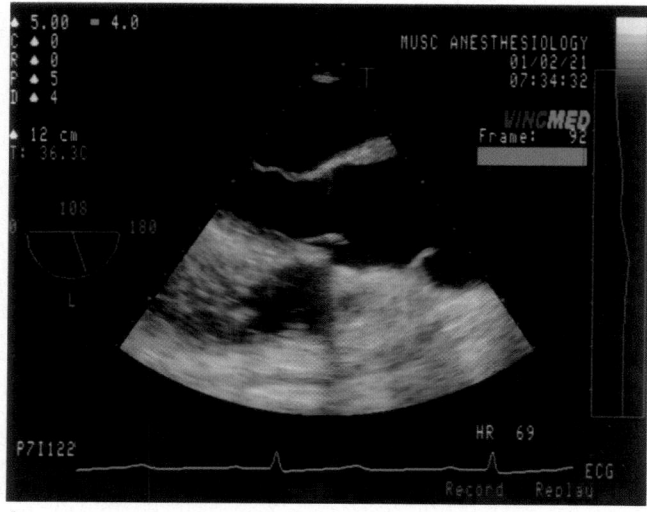

**A**

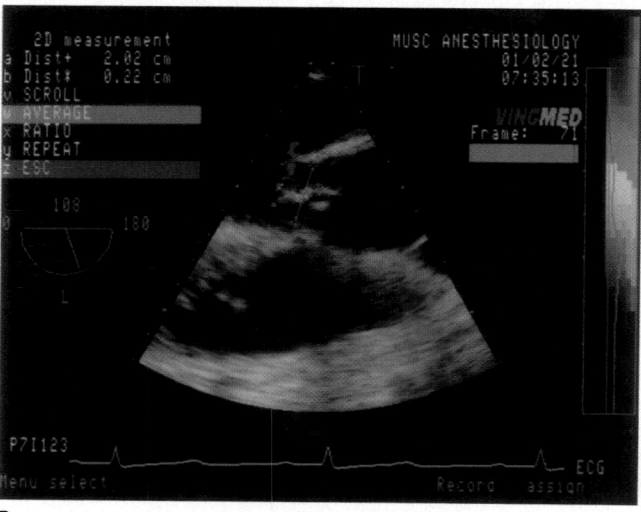

**B**

**FIGURE 21.21. A:** A Debakey Type I proximal aortic dissection with dilatation of the proximal ascending aorta resulting in poor coadaptation of the aortic valve leaflets and **(B)** a central jet of aortic regurgitation.

TEE has been shown to be a reliable tool in the evaluation of proximal coronary anatomy. In a series of 34 aortic dissection patients, Ballard detected coronary artery involvement with TEE in six out of seven surgically documented dissected coronaries. Adequate views of the ostea and proximal vessels were obtained for 88% of left main coronary arteries and 50% of right coronary arteries (62). The relationship of the dissection flap to the proximal left and right coronary arteries, the extent of dissection into the coronary artery, and coronary blood flow obstruction produced by the flap should be evaluated via TEE. Presence of segmental regional wall motion abnormalities may be an additional clue to the presence of coronary artery involvement.

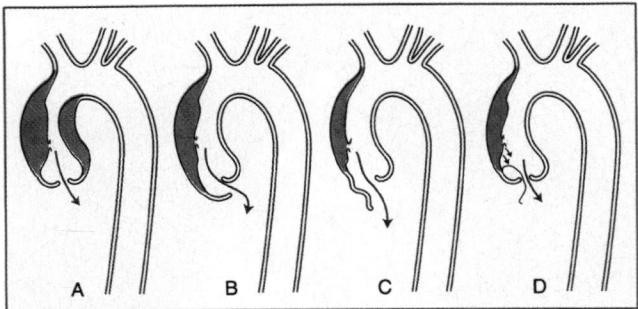

**FIGURE 21.22.** Mechanism of aortic regurgitation in proximal aortic dissection. **A:** An extensive or circumferential tear dilates the aortic root and annulus, causing failure of coaptation of aortic valve leaflets. **B:** With asymmetric dissection, pressure from the false lumen depresses one aortic leaflet below the coaptation line of the other leaflets. **C:** The annular support is disrupted, resulting in a flail aortic leaflet. **D:** Prolapse of a mobile intimal flap through the aortic valve during diastole, which permits leaflet coaptation. From Braunwald E, ed. *Heart Disease: a textbook of cardiovascular medicine,* 5th ed., Vol 2. Philadelphia: WB Saunders Co 1997;1557, with permission.

### Left Ventricular Function

The heart may experience significant ischemia in the face of aortic dissection and subsequent coronary dissection. Acute LV global dysfunction may be due to ischemia with dissection of both coronary arteries or aortic insufficiency related left ventricular decompensation. As previously discussed, the presence of segmental wall motion abnormalities may indicate coronary artery involvement. The patient's overall LV ejection fraction may be the primary factor used in determining whether or not the patient can tolerate a surgical repair procedure without the assistance of cardiopulmonary bypass.

### Pericardial and Pleural Effusion

In the face of aortic dissection, the aortic wall may rupture through the adventitia at the site of the dissection. Proximal extension of the dissection with the rupture at the aortic root may result in acute cardiac tamponade. In the descending thoracic aorta, blood will enter the left pleural space creating a hemothorax. Uncontained rupture within the mediastinum or pleural spaces will result in sudden death (63).

### Transesophageal Echocardiography Image Artifacts

All ultrasound imaging techniques can lead to artifacts. The multitude of fluid and tissue interfaces that occur during echocardiographic examinations of the heart and aorta produce an ideal setting for the development of imaging artifacts. Any artifacts involving the ascending

**TABLE 21.9. Linear Artifacts versus Intimal Flaps**

a. Indistinct borders of the artifact
b. The lack of rapid oscillatory movement associated with intimal flaps
c. The extension of the artifact through the aortic wall as a straight line
d. The linear artifact may be extrapolated to the starting point of the transducer
e. Color Doppler imaging will frequently demonstrate homogenous color on both sides of the linear artifact without any transverse or communicating jets.

aorta, which can be misinterpreted as a Type I or Type II aortic dissection, may result in unnecessary surgery. Appelbe demonstrated that linear artifacts were detected in the ascending aorta in 40% of patients leading to false-positive diagnoses and decreased specificity of TEE (64). These artifacts are secondary to reverberation artifacts of the aortic wall and the presence of atherosclerosis, a sclerotic aortic root, or calcific aortic disease. They produce echo images that resemble an intimal flap. Side-lobe artifacts from the aortic valve can also simulate an intimal flap. In addition, extreme care must be taken if a Swan-Ganz catheter is present, as it may frequently present as an artifact within the ascending aorta. While the question arises regarding the diagnosis of an intimal flap versus an artifact, our motto is *"When in doubt, pull the Swan out."* Table 21.9 clarifies the difference between linear artifacts of the ascending aorta and intimal flaps.

## PENETRATING CARDIAC INJURIES

Patients who have sustained a penetrating injury, such as a gun or knife wound, require careful evaluation. The entry site may not be close to the heart but cardiac involvement may occur secondary to a change in the projectile's path once it enters the body. These cases can be difficult to diagnose and a high index of suspicion for cardiac involvement is imperative. The right ventricle and atrium are most frequently involved. TTE is extremely useful at evaluating these anterior structures. If a pericardial effusion is visualized, a detailed evaluation must be performed. Figures 21.23A and 21.23B show a knife injury to the RVOT and its postsurgical repair.

## TRAUMA WITH CARDIAC COMPLICATIONS

### Acute Pulmonary Embolism and Paradoxical Embolism

Acute massive pulmonary embolism is a life-threatening condition and requires emergent diagnosis and treatment. In the trauma situation, massive pulmonary embolism is

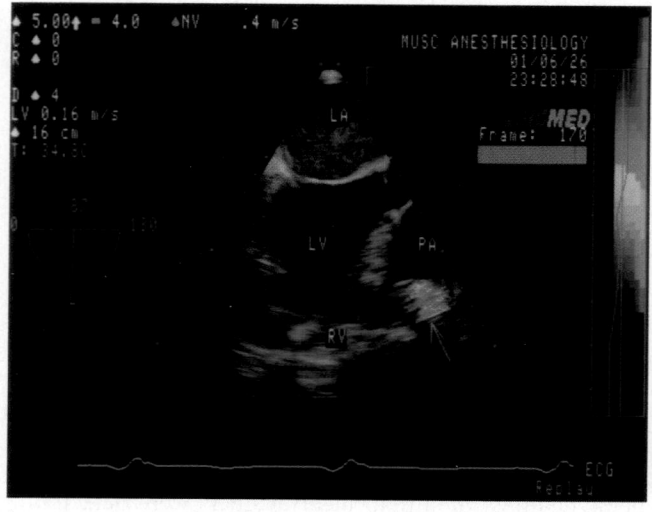
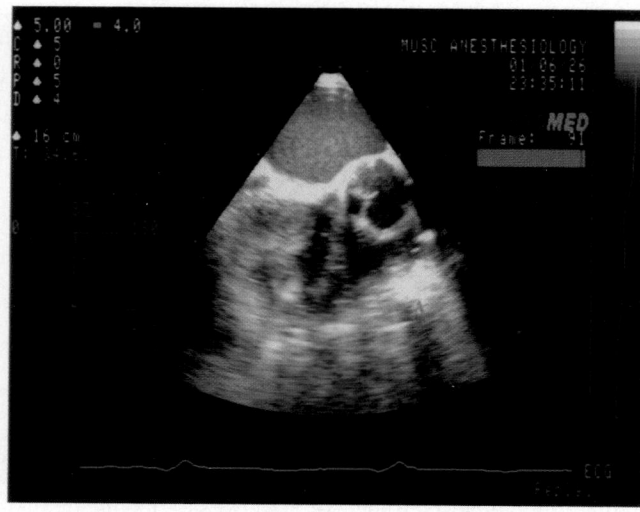

**FIGURE 21.23.** **A:** A color flow disturbance in the distal right ventricle and the proximal pulmonary artery indicative of a knife wound to the chest. **B:** The same patient following pledget repair of the injury.

frequent, especially in association with femur and pelvic fractures. The diagnosis of pulmonary embolism in these critically ill patients would be facilitated if an inexpensive and rapid standard bedside diagnostic test were available. Unfortunately, such a test does not exist.

Selective pulmonary angiography remains the gold standard; however, it requires transport of the patient from the ICU or the ER to the angiography suite, which is time-consuming. It requires contrast dye, which frequently cannot be tolerated by patients with blunt trauma secondary to renal insufficiency.

Recently, spiral CT has become popular for the acute diagnosis of pulmonary embolism. Spiral CT can image from the aortic knob to the diaphragm within 20–30 seconds and has the potential to image the pulmonary vasculature extending from the right and main pulmonary arteries to the segmental arteries. An intraluminal filling defect or vascular occlusion characterizes a positive test. Its major drawback is that the expertise required to interpret a spiral CT is not readily available at all institutions. In addition the cost, need for patient transport, use of iodinated contrast material, and radiation exposure may be problematic (65).

Transesophageal echocardiography is emerging as one means to diagnose suspected hemodynamically significant pulmonary embolism. It allows direct visualization of emboli in the right ventricular outflow tract and right main pulmonary artery up to the point of the interlobar trunks and lobar arteries. The left main pulmonary artery may be difficult to image secondary to its location anterior to the left main bronchus. Table 21.10 summarizes the sensitivity and specificity of the available noninvasive confirmatory tests for pulmonary embolism (65,66).

There remains no optimal noninvasive diagnostic test for pulmonary embolism.

### Echocardiography Evaluation

Transthoracic echocardiography should be used as an initial rapid diagnostic test in patients suspected of having pulmonary embolism. Four distinct findings may be found during this initial TTE evaluation.

1. Normal examination that would make the possibility of acute pulmonary embolism extremely unlikely
2. Right heart thrombus that confirms the diagnosis of right pulmonary embolism
3. Some diagnosis other than pulmonary embolism
4. Findings of right ventricular dysfunction, which would support a diagnosis of pulmonary embolism, and if it were absent, would make hemodynamically significant pulmonary embolism extremely unlikely (67)

When number 4 above occurs, Pruszczyk has proposed that patients have three of the following five criteria of right ventricular pressure overload in order to proceed to transesophageal echocardiography. The criteria include

1. A peak velocity of tricuspid valve insufficiency corresponding to a right ventricular to a right atrial pressure gradient of more than 30 mm Hg
2. An enlargement of the right ventricle of more than 27 mm in diameter measured in the peristernal long axis
3. A shortened, less than 80 msec, pulmonary ejection acceleration time measured at the right ventricular outflow tract
4. Flattening of the intraventricular septum

▶ TABLE 21.10. Pooled Diagnostic Data for Confirmatory Test for Pulmonary Embolism

| Imaging Test | No. Patients | Sensitivity | Specificity |
|---|---|---|---|
| I. Ventilation/Perfusion Scan (30) (All Class I Data) | 931 | | |
|   High Probability | | 41 | 97 |
|   High, Intermediate, or Low Probability | | 82 | 52 |
|   High or Intermediate Probability | | 98 | 10 |
| II. Spiral CT | | | |
|   TOTAL | 935 | 86 | 93 |
|   Class I | 324 | 77 | 89 |
|   Class II | 586 | 91 | 95 |
|   Class III | 25 | 95 | 67 |
| III. MRI | | | |
|   Class I | 150 | 77 | 87 |
| IV. Echocardiography | | | |
|   TOTAL | 480 | | |
|   TTE–Class II | 366 | 68 | 89 |
|   TEE–Class II | 114 | 70 | 81 |

Modified from Kline (65) of 28 studies utilizing spinal CT, MRI, TTE, and TEE for the confirmation of pulmonary embolism and the Prospective Investigation of Pulmonary Embolism Diagnosis Trial (66).
*Class I* included prospective, blinded, cohort studies using angiography or autopsy as the reference standard.
*Class II* included prospective, blinded cohort studies utilizing combinations of clinical suspicion, V/Q scans, selective use of ultrasonography of the lower extremities, and pulmonary angiography together with clinical follow-up.
*Class III* included blinded studies using only the V/Q scan as the reference standard without corroborative studies or follow-up.
*Kline JA, Johns KL, Colucciello SA, Israel EG. New diagnostic tests for pulmonary embolism. Ann Emerg Med 2000;35:175 (printed with permission).

5. Distention of the inferior vena cava of > 20 mm in diameter.

If three of these five criteria are met, then transesophageal echocardiography should be performed at the bedside (67).

### Direct Echo Manifestations of Thrombus

The following echo manifestations of thrombus have been proposed in order to minimize false-positive diagnoses of pulmonary embolism.

1. An unequivocal thrombus that has distinct borders and has a different echo density than blood in the adjacent vascular walls.
2. The thrombus may protrude into the arterial lumen and will thus alter the blood flow by Doppler imaging.
3. The thrombus must be imaged in more than one plane.
4. The thrombus may have distinct movement separate from the vascular wall and blood flow (67,68).

When used as a prompt bedside diagnostic test in the presence of right ventricular overload, TEE can rapidly detect clots in 80% of cases. It may be the method of choice for hemodynamically compromised patients who would require urgent thrombolytic treatment or surgery. Equally important is that an alternative diagnosis will occur in approximately one-third of patients without pulmonary embolism when transesophageal echocardiography is utilized. The most common alternative diagnoses include left ventricular dysfunction and valvular insufficiency (65,67). The TEE manifestations of pulmonary embolism are summarized in Table 21.11. Figure 21.24 demonstrates a pulmonary embolism well visualized within the right atrium with paradoxical embolization across a patent foramen ovale into the left atrium.

▶ TABLE 21.11. Pulmonary Embolism Echo Findings

Direct
• Evidence of clot
Indirect–"Right Heart Strain"
• RV dilation
• Abnormal septal motion
• Tricuspid regurgitation
• Pulmonary hypertension
• Inferior vena cava dilatation
• Pulmonary artery dilatation

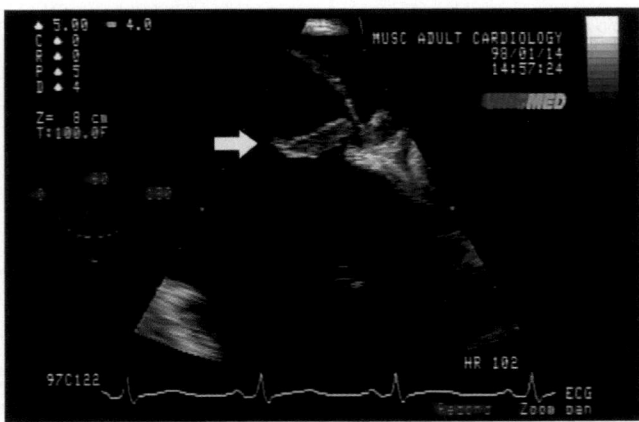

**FIGURE 21.24.** A pulmonary embolism well visualized within the right atrium with paradoxical embolization across a patent foramen ovale into the left atrium.

Both transthoracic echocardiography and transesophageal echocardiography have been used to evaluate the therapeutic response of patients undergoing intravenous tissue plasminogen activator for clot lysis following significant pulmonary embolism. One expects to see a decline in the pulmonary artery systolic pressure, a decrease in right ventricular diameter, and an increase in left ventricular diameter following the onset of thrombolytic treatment. Right ventricular wall movement will typically improve over time with resolution of hypokinetic wall motion abnormalities.

### Paradoxical Pulmonary Embolism (PFO)

The incidence of a patent foramen ovale has been reported to be as high as 35% in the normal population. If a massive pulmonary embolism occurs in the presence of a patent foramen ovale, the resultant sudden increase in right atrial pressure can cause the PFO to open and result in a right-to-left atrial shunt. The incidence of paradoxical embolism in patients with known PFOs and pulmonary embolism is up to 16% (69). In addition, the presence of a PFO in the setting of a major pulmonary embolism is a predictor of adverse outcomes. Death rates in these patients will approach 33% compared to 14% in patients without a PFO (70). TEE is far superior to transthoracic echocardiography in evaluation of patients with PFOs and paradoxical embolism (Fig. 21.24).

### KEY POINTS

- Echocardiography is a Class 1 indication in the setting of hemodynamic instability and suspected aortic dissection.

- Transesophageal echocardiography provides superior resolution and overcomes the technical difficulties encountered with transthoracic echocardiography in the evaluation of the critically ill or injured patient.
- Transesophageal echocardiography leads to changes in management in approximately 50% of critically ill and injured patients, regardless of whether a pulmonary artery catheter is present.
- Unexplained hypoxemia in a critically ill patient should prompt an echocardiographic assessment for patent foramen ovale.
- Positive contrast echocardiography for PFO requires opacification of the right atrium and visualization of contrast in the left atrium within a few cardiac cycles.
- Transesophageal echocardiography is more sensitive and equally specific to transthoracic echocardiography in diagnosis of infective endocarditis.
- Endocarditic valve lesions are usually on the upstream side of a valve leaflet.
- Mitral valve vegetations greater than 10 mm in size are associated with an almost 50% risk of embolization.
- Fifty-six percent of patients following blunt chest trauma will have a pathologic diagnosis established following a transesophageal echocardiography evaluation.
- The most sensitive 2-D manifestation of cardiac tamponade is right ventricular collapse during diastole.
- Acute valve injury may occur following blunt chest trauma, with injury to the aortic valve being most common.
- Acute aortic dissection has a mortality of 1% per hour for the first 48 hours.
- An intimal flap must be observed in two image planes to reliably make the diagnosis of aortic dissection.
- Transesophageal echocardiography is emerging as one means to diagnose suspected hemodynamically significant pulmonary embolism.

### REFERENCES

1. Cheitlin MD, Armstrong WF, Aurigemma GP, et al. ACC/AHA/ASE 2003 guideline update for the clinical application of echocardiography—summary article: a report of the American College of Cardiology/American Heart Association Task Force on Practice Guidelines (ACC/AHA/ASE Committee to update the 1997 guidelines on the clinical application of Echocardiography). Circulation 2003;108:1146–62.

2. Khandhiera BK, Seward JB, Tajik AJ. Critical appraisal of transesophageal echocardiography. Crit Care Clin 1996;12:235–51.
3. Parker MM, Cunnion RE, Parrillo JE. Echocardiography and nuclear cardiac imaging in the critical care unit. JAMA 1985;254:2935–39.
4. Heidenreich PA, Stainback RF, Redberg RF, et al. TEE predicts mortality in critically ill patients with unexplained hypotension. J Am Coll Cardiol 1995;26:152–58.
5. Hwang JJ, Shyu KG, Chen JJ, et al. Usefulness of transesophageal echocardiography in the treatment of critically ill patients. Chest 1993;104:861–66.
6. Pearson AC. Noninvasive evaluation of the hemodynamically unstable patient: the advantages of seeing clearly (editorial). Mayo Clin Proc 1995;70:1012–14.
7. Slama MA, Novara A, Van De Putte P, et al. Diagnostic and therapeutic implications of transespohageal echocardiography in medical ICU patients with unexplained shock, hypoxemia, or suspected endocarditis. Intensive Care Med 1996;22:916–22.
8. Cook CH, Praba AC, Beery PR, Martin LC. Transthoracic echocardiography is not cost-effective in critically ill surgical patients. J Trauma 2002;52:280–84.
9. Mohsin A. Transesophageal echocardiography in critical care units: Henry Ford Hospital experience and review of the literature. Prog Cardiovasc Dis 1996;38:315–28.
10. Oh JK, Seward JB, Khandheria BK, et al. Transesophageal echocardiography in critically ill patients. Am J Cardiol 1990;66:1492–95.
11. Sohn DW, Shin GL, Oh JK, et al. Role of transesophageal echocardiography in hemodynamically unstable patients. Mayo Clin Proc 1995;70:925–31.
12. Khoury AF, Afridi I, Quinones MA. Transesophageal echocardiography in critically ill patients: feasibility, safety, and impact on management. Am Heart J 1994;127:1363–71.
13. Pearson AC, Castello R, Labovitz AJ. Safety and utility of transesophageal echocardiography in the critically ill patient. Am Heart J 1990;119:1083.
14. Seward JB, Douglas PS, Erbel R, et al. Hand-carried ultrasound (HSU) device: recommendations regarding new technology. A report from the echocardiography task force on new technology of the nomenclature and standards committee of the American society of echocardiography. J Am Soc Echocardiogr 2002;15:369–73.
15. Reichert CLA, Visser CA, Koolen JJ, et al. Transesophageal echocardiography in hypotensive patients after cardiac operations. J Thorac Cardiovasc Surg 1992;104:321–6.
16. Chan K-L. Transesophageal echocardiography for assessing cause of hypotension after cardiac surgery. Am J Cardiol 1988;62:1142–3.
17. Costachescu T, Denault A, Guimond JG, et al. The hemodynamically unstable patient in the intensive care unit: hemodynamic vs TEE monitoring. Crit Care Med 2002;30:1214–223.
18. Denault A, Ferrar P, Couture P, et al. Transesophageal echocardiography monitoring in the intensive care department: the management of hemodynamic instability secondary to thoracic tamponade after single lung transplantation. J Am Soc Echocardiogr 2003;16:688–92.
19. Swenson JD, Harkin C, Pace NL, et al. Transesophageal echocardiography: an objective tool defining maximum ventricular response to intravenous fluid therapy. Anesth Analg 1996;83:1149–53.
20. Poelaert JI, Trouerbach J, De Buyzere M, et al. Evaluation of transesophageal echocardiography as a diagnostic and therapeutic aid in a critical care setting. Chest 1995;107:774–9.
21. Bouchard MJ, Denault A, Couture P, et al. Poor correlation between hemodynamic and echocardiographic indexes of left ventricular performance in the operating room and intensive care unit. Crit Care Med 2004;32:644–48.
22. Nacht A, Kronzon I. "Intracardiac Shunts" in Critical Care Clinics, Porembka DT (guest ed.). Philadelphia: WB Saunders, Vol 12, no. 2 (April 1996), 295–319.
23. Kronzon I, Tunick PA, Freedberg RS, et al. Transesophageal echocardiography is superior to transthoracic echocardiography in the diagnosis of sinus venosus atrial septal defect. J Am Coll Cardiol 1991;17:537.
24. Hagen PT, Schulz DG, Edwards WD. Incidence and size of patent foramen ovale during the first ten decades of life: An autopsy study of 965 normal hearts. Mayo Clin Proc 1984;59:17.
25. Sukernik MR, Mets B, Bennett-Guerrero E. Patent foramen ovale and its significance in the perioperative period. Anesth Analg 2001;93:1137–46.
26. Louie Ek, Konstadt SN, Rao TK, et al. Transesophageal echocardiographic diagnosis of right to left shunting across the patent foramen ovale in adults without prior stroke. J Am Coll Cardiol 1993;21:1231.
27. Konstadt SN, Louie EK, Balack S, et al. Intraoperative detection of patent foramen ovale by transesophageal echocardiography. Anesthesiology 1991;74:212.
28. Stewart M. Contrast echocardiography. Heart 2003;89(3):342–48.
29. Heidenreich PA, Masoudi FA, Maini B, et al. Echocardiography in patients with suspected endocarditis: a cost-effectiveness analysis. Am J Med 1999;107:198-208.
30. Von Reyn CF, Levy BS, Arbeit RD, et al. Infective endocarditis: an analysis based on strict case definitions. Ann Int Med 1981;94:505-18.
31. Durak DT, Lukes AS, Bright DK. New criteria for diagnosis of infective endocarditis: utilization of specific echocardiographic findings. Am J Med 1994;96:200–9.
32. Roe MT, Abramson MA, Li J, et al. Clinical information determines the impact of transesophageal echocardiography on the diagnosis of infective endocarditis by the Duke criteria. Am Heart J 2000;139:945–51.
33. Shanewise JS, Martin RP. Assessment of endocarditis and associated complications with transesophageal echocardiography. Crit Care Clin 1996;12:411–27.
34. Reynolds HR, Jagen MA, Tunick PA, Kronzon I. Sensitivity of transthoracic versus transesophageal echocardiography for the detection of native valve vegetations in the modern era. J Am Soc Echocardiogr 2003;16:67–70.
35. Mugge A, Daniel WG, Frank G, et al. Echocardiography in infective endocarditis: reassessment of prognostic implications of vegetation size determined by the transthoracic and transesophageal approach. J Am Coll Cardiol 1989;14:631–8.
36. Rohmann S, Erbel R, Gorge G, et al. Clinical relevance of vegetation localization by transesophageal echocardiography in infective endocarditis by monitoring vegetation size. Eur Heart J 1992;12:446–52.
37. O'Connor C. Chest trauma: the role of transesophageal echocardiography. J Clin Anes 1996;8:605–13.
38. Garcia-Fernandez MA, Lopez-Perez JM, Perez-Castellano N, et al. Role of transesophageal echocardiography in the assessment of patients with blunt chest trauma: Correlation of echocardiographic findings with the electrocardiogram and creatine kinase monoclonal antibody measurements. Am Heart J 1998;135:476–81.
39. Johnson SB, Kearney PA, Smith MD. Echocardiography in the evaluation of thoracic trauma. Surg Clin North Am 1995;75:193–205.
40. Chirillo F, Totis O, Cavarzerani A, et al. Usefulness of transthoracic and transesophageal echocardiography in recognition and management of cardiovascular injuries after blunt chest trauma. Heart 1996;75:301–6.
41. Beck CS. Two cardiac compression trials. JAMA 1935;104:714–6.
42. Tsang TSM, Oh JK, Seward JM. Diagnosis and management of cardiac tamponade in the era of echocardiography. Clin Cardiol 1999;22:446–52.
43. Merce J, Sagrista-Sauleda J, Permanyer-Miralda G, Evangelista A, Soler-Soler J. Imaging/diagnostic testing. Correlation between clinical and Doppler echocardiographic findings in patients with moderate and large pericardial effusion: Impli-

cations for the diagnosis of cardiac tamponade. Am Heart J 1999;138:759–64.

44. Pandian NG, Skorton DJ, Doty DB. Immediate diagnosis of acute myocardial contusion by two-dimensional echocardiography: Studies in a canine model of blunt chest trauma. J Am Coll Cardiol 1983;2:488–96.

45. Weiss RL, Brier JA, O'Connor W, Ross S, Brathwaite CM. The usefulness of transesophageal echocardiography in diagnosing cardiac contusions. Chest 1996;109:73–7.

46. Hiatt JR, Yeatman Jr LA, Child JS. The value of echocardiography in blunt chest trauma. J Trauma 1988;28:914–22.

47. Krasna MJ, Flancbaum L. Blunt cardiac trauma: clinical manifestations and management. Sem Thorac Cardiovasc Surg 1992;4:195–202.

48. Symbas PN. Cardiac heart disease. Curr Prob Cardiol 1991; 537–82.

49. Devineni R, McKenzie FN. Avulsion of a normal aortic valve cusp due to blunt chest injury. J Trauma 1984;24(10);910–12.

50. Debakey ME, Henly WS, Cooley DA, Morris GC, Crawford ES, Beall AC. Surgical management of dissecting aneurysms of the aorta. J Thorac Cardiovasc Surg 1965;49:130–41.

51. Daily PO, Trueblood HW, Stinson EB, Wuerflein RD, Shumway NE. Management of acute aortic dissections. Ann Thorac Surg 1970;10:237–47.

52. Hirst AE, Jr., Johns VJ, Jr., Kime SW, Jr. Dissecting aneurysm of the aorta: a review of 585 cases. Medicine (Baltimore) 1985;37:217–79.

53. Erbel R, Engberding R, Daniel W, Roelandt J, Visser C, Rennollett H. Echocardiography in diagnosis of aortic dissection. Lancet 1989;451–57.

54. Iliceto S, Nanda NC, Rizzon P, et al. Color Doppler evaluation of aortic dissection. Circulation 1987;75:748–55.

55. Matthew T, Nanda NC. Two-dimensional and Doppler echocardiographic evaluation of aortic aneurysm and dissection. Am J Cardiol 1984;54:379–85.

56. Erbel K, Mohr-Kahaly S, Rennullet H, et al. Diagnosis of aortic dissection: the value of transesophageal echocardiography. Thorac Cardiovasc Surg 1987;35(Special Issue 1):126–33.

57. Adachi H, Kyo S, Takamoto S, Yokoto Y, Omoto K. Early diagnosis and surgical intervention of acute aortic dissection by transesophageal color flow mapping. Circulation 1990;82 (Suppl IV):19–23.

58. Erbel R, Mohr-Kahaly S, Oelert H, et al. Diagnostic strategies in suspected aortic dissection: comparison of computed tomography, aortography, and transesophageal echocardiography. Am J Cardiac Imaging 1990;4:157–72.

59. Mohr-Kahaly S, Erbel R, Rennollet H, et al. Ambulatory follow-up of aortic dissection by transesophageal two-dimensional and color-coded Doppler echocardiography. Circulation 1989;80:24–33.

60. Slater EE, DeSanctis RW. The clinical recognition of dissecting aortic aneurysm. Am J Med 1976;60:625–33.

61. Mazzucotelli JP, Deleuze PH, Baufreton C, et al. Preservation of the aortic valve in acute aortic dissection: long-term echocardiographic assessment and clinical outcome. Ann Thorac Surg. 1993;55:1513–17.

62. Ballard RS, Nanda NC, Gatewood R, et al. Usefulness of transesophageal echocardiography in assessment of aortic dissection. Circulation 1991;84:1903–14.

63. Erbel R, Oelert H, Meyer J, et al. Effect of medical and surgical therapy on aortic dissection evaluated by transesophageal echocardiography. Circulation 1993;87:1604–15.

64. Appelbe AF, Walker PG, Yeoh JK, Bonitatibus A, Yoganthan AP, Martin RP. Clinical significance and origin of artifacts in transesophageal endocardiography of the thoracic aorta. J Am Coll Cardiol 1993;21:754–60.

65. Kline JA, Johns KL, Colucciello SA, Israel EG. New diagnostic tests for pulmonary embolism. Ann Emerg Med 2000;35:168–80.

66. The PIOPED Investigators. Value of the ventilation/perfusion scan in acute pulmonary embolism: results of the prospective investigation of pulmonary embolism diagnosis (PIOPED). JAMA 1990;260:2753–59.

67. Pruszczyk A, Torbicki A, Kuch-Wocial A, Szulc M, Pacho R. Diagnostic value of transesophageal echocardiography in suspected haemodynamically significant pulmonary embolism. Heart 2001;85:628–34.

68. Riedel M. Emergency diagnosis of pulmonary embolism (editorial). Heart 2001;85:628–34.

69. Chaikof EL, Campbell DE, Smith RB. Paradoxical embolism in acute arterial occlusion: rare or unsuspected? J Vasc Surg 1994;20:377–84.

70. Konstantinides S, Geibel A, Kasper W, Olschewski M, Blumel L, Just H. Patent foramen ovale is an important predictor of adverse outcome in patients with major pulmonary embolism. Circulation 1998;97:1946–51.

## QUESTIONS

1. All of the following transthoracic echocardiographic findings are indicative of right ventricular overload and would support the decision to proceed to a transesophageal echocardiography evaluation of a patient suspected of having an acute pulmonary embolism *except*:
   A. A peak velocity of tricuspid valve insufficiency corresponding to a right ventricular to a right atrial pressure gradient of more than 20 mm Hg
   B. An enlargement of the right ventricle of more than 27 mm diameter measured in the peristernal long axis
   C. A shortened, less than 80 msec, pulmonary ejection acceleration time measured at the right ventricular outflow tract
   D. Flattening of the intraventricular septum
   E. Distention of the inferior vena cava of > 20 mm in diameter

2. The following statements are true regarding myocardial contusions *except*:
   A. Most patients with RV contusions are asymptomatic at presentation.
   B. The RV is involved in more than 30% of patients.
   C. The echo diagnostic criterion is the presence of impaired regional wall systolic function following blunt trauma in the absence of a transmural myocardial infarction on EKG.
   D. Significant reductions in cardiac output of 30%–40% may occur but rarely persist for more than a few days.

3. The following are 2-D manifestations of pericardial tamponade:
   A. RA collapse in diastole
   B. RV collapse in diastole
   C. LA collapse in late diastole and early systole
   D. Dilated IVC without inspiratory collapse
   E. All the above

# Assessment of Perioperative Hemodynamics

## *Lee Wallace, Michael Licina, and Ahmad Adi*

While M-mode and two-dimensional (2-D) echocardiography can provide indirect evidence of hemodynamic abnormalities, 2-D echocardiography combined with Doppler echocardiography can be used to perform a quantitative hemodynamic assessment. Quantitative hemodynamic data that can be obtained with 2-D Doppler echocardiography are listed in Table 22.1.

The accuracy of many of these Doppler-derived measurements has been validated in the cardiac catheterization laboratory using transthoracic echocardiography (1–4). The principles on which these measurements are based hold as true for transesophageal echocardiography (TEE) as they do for transthoracic echocardiography. The accuracy of a hemodynamic assessment performed using either transthoracic echocardiography or TEE is dependent on the ability of a knowledgeable and skilled echocardiographer to acquire accurate data. The accuracy of the hemodynamic data acquired using either approach depends on the following: parallel alignment of the ultrasound beam with the blood flow of interest, minimal interference from adjacent blood flows, and for many calculations, an accurate determination of area or diameter.

Prior to the introduction of multiplane TEE probes, transthoracic echocardiography was considered a superior approach because it offered far more echocardiographic windows for interrogation of blood flow. The introduction of multiplane TEE probes has significantly increased the number of windows and angles from which blood flows may be interrogated. Furthermore, the introduction of high frequency transducers into multiplane TEE probes has aided in the accurate measurement of areas and diameters such that TEE may be superior to transthoracic echocardiography in many instances. Nevertheless, in order to avoid misdiagnosis, Doppler-derived measurements must be considered in the context of the quality of the acquired data as well as the overall hemodynamic status of the patient. This is especially true when using the transesophageal approach in the operating room setting. This chapter will focus on quantitative he-modynamic assessment using 2-D Doppler echocardiography. M-mode and 2-D echocardiographic signs of hemodynamic abnormalities, determination of diastolic function with Doppler, and estimation of cardiac-filling pressures based on diastolic parameters will be discussed in more detail in other chapters.

## DOPPLER MEASUREMENTS OF STROKE VOLUME AND CARDIAC OUTPUT

### Calculation of Stroke Volume

The flow rate of a fluid through a fixed orifice is directly proportional to the product of the cross-sectional area (CSA) of the orifice and the flow velocity of the fluid

▶ TABLE 22.1. Hemodynamic Data Obtainable with 2-D Doppler Echocardiography

Volumetric measurements
    Stroke volume
    Cardiac output
    Pulmonary-to-systemic flow ratio (Qp/Qs)
    Regurgitant volume and fraction
Pressure gradients
    Maximum gradient
    Mean gradient
Valve area
    Stenotic valve area
    Regurgitant orifice area
Intracardiac and pulmonary artery pressures
    Right ventricular systolic pressure
    Pulmonary artery systolic pressure
    Pulmonary artery mean pressure
    Pulmonary artery diastolic pressure
    Left atrial pressure
    Left ventricular end-diastolic pressure
Ventricular dp/dt

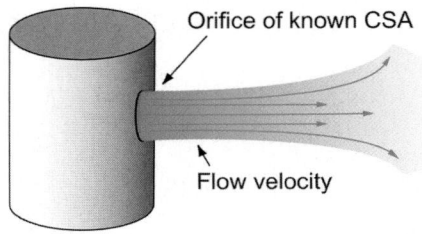

Flow rate (cm$^3$/s) = CSA (cm$^2$) x flow velocity (cm/s)

**FIGURE 22.1.** The hydraulic orifice formula. The volumetric flow rate through an orifice is equal to the product of the cross-sectional area of the orifice and the flow velocity of the fluid through the orifice. If flow velocity is constant, so is flow rate; however, if flow velocity varies, so will flow rate. *CSA*, cross-sectional area.

within the orifice as given by the *hydraulic orifice formula* (Fig. 22.1):

$$\text{Flow rate (cm}^3/\text{s)} = \text{CSA (cm}^2) \times \text{Flow velocity (cm/s)}$$

Because the cardiovascular system is pulsatile, blood flow velocity varies. Nevertheless, the instantaneous flow rate of blood going through an orifice or blood vessel of constant cross-sectional area is directly proportional to the product of the cross-sectional area (CSA) of the orifice or blood vessel and the instantaneous blood flow velocity.

The acceleration and deceleration of blood flow velocity during the ejection period (or filling period) provides a distinct Doppler profile for a given orifice. The summation of velocities over the entire flow period is correctly called the *velocity-time integral* (VTI), although it is also commonly referred to as the time-velocity integral (TVI). The VTI is equal to the area bounded by the Doppler flow velocity profile and the zero velocity baseline (Fig. 22.2). It is measured by tracing the Doppler velocity signal using the calculation package built in the ultrasound machine. The VTI can be conceptually thought of as the distance that blood travels with each beat of the heart and is thus also called the stroke distance.

Stroke volume (SV) can be calculated as the product of the cross-sectional area and VTI (Fig. 22.3):

$$\text{SV (cm}^3) = \text{CSA (cm}^2) \times \text{VTI (cm)}$$

Stroke volume can be calculated at many different locations within the heart or great vessels by using the appropriate Doppler velocity signal to determine the VTI at the same location that 2-D imaging is used to determine cross-sectional area. Accordingly, the VTI is usually measured with pulse wave Doppler. However, continuous wave Doppler may be utilized to determine the aortic

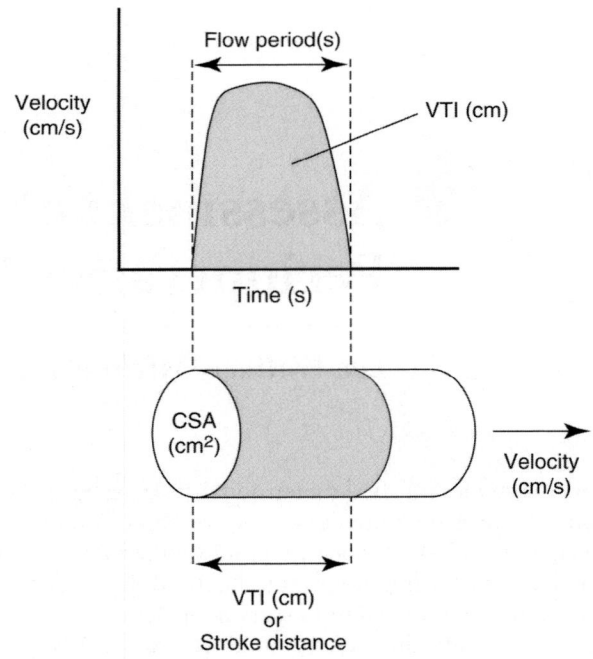

**FIGURE 22.2.** The Doppler velocity-time integral and stroke distance. As flow in the heart and great vessels is pulsatile, blood flow velocity varies during the period of ejection (or filling) as shown by the Doppler velocity curve. The area under the Doppler velocity curve (the velocity-time integral) is equivalent to the distance blood flow travels with one beat of the heart (stroke distance). *VTI*, velocity-time integral; *CSA*, cross-sectional area.

valve VTI in the absence of subvalvular or supravalvular aortic obstruction. In this case, the velocity signal obtained by continuous wave Doppler across the aortic valve should be the same as that obtained by pulse wave Doppler within the aortic valve.

Most often the cross-sectional area of the "orifice" to be measured is assumed to be circular and thus can be calculated using the formula for the area of a circle (of radius r) after measuring the orifice diameter (D) in cm:

$$\text{CSA (cm}^2) = \Pi \times r^2 = \Pi \times (D/2)^2 = 0.785 \times D^2$$

The Doppler method for determining stroke volume at a particular site is based on the following four assumptions, which are listed in Table 22.2. First, blood flow is assumed to be laminar and the spatial flow velocity profile is assumed to be flat, as is generally the case in the LVOT (Fig. 22.4). The narrow band of velocities and smooth spectral signal obtained with pulsed wave Doppler is evidence of laminar flow in the great vessels and across normal cardiac valves. A flat flow velocity profile can be demonstrated by showing uniform velocities while moving the pulsed wave Doppler sample volume from side to side within the flow of interest from two orthogonal views.

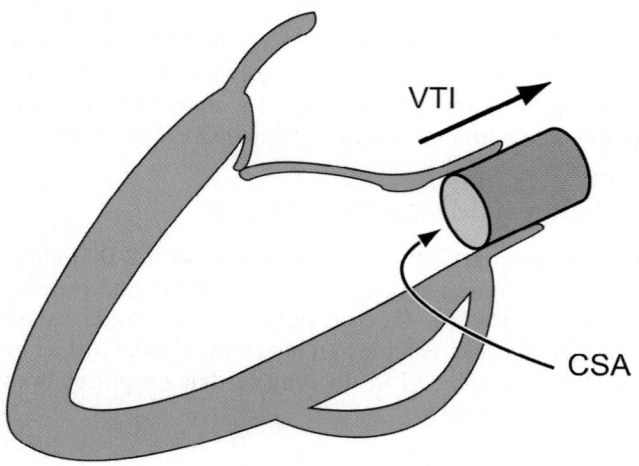

$$SV\ (cm^3) = CSA\ (cm^2) \times VTI\ (cm)$$

**FIGURE 22.3.** Doppler stroke volume calculation. The velocity-time integral of the Doppler velocity curve can be conceptualized as the length of a cylinder of blood (stroke distance) ejected through a cross-sectional area on one beat of the heart. Stroke volume is calculated as the product of cross-sectional area and the velocity-time integral. *SV*, stroke volume; *CSA*, cross-sectional area; *VTI*, velocity-time integral.

Second, cross-sectional area (i.e., diameter) and VTI measurements are assumed to be made *at the same time and at the same anatomic location.* Diameter is measured most accurately when the ultrasound beam is perpendicular to the blood-tissue interface, while VTI is measured most accurately when the ultrasound beam is parallel to blood flow. Thus, diameter measurements and Doppler velocity profiles are usually not recorded from the same imaging plane. Nevertheless, every effort should be made to perform these measurements *at the same anatomic location* and *in close sequence* in order to minimize error in the calculated stroke volume.

▶ **TABLE 22.2. Assumptions for Accurate Doppler Stroke Volume Calculations**

1. Blood flow is laminar with a spatially flat flow velocity profile.
2. Measurements of the velocity-time integral and cross-sectional area (i.e., diameter) are made at the same time and at the same anatomic location.
3. The velocity-time integral measurement represents the average velocity-time integral (several measurements should be averaged for a patient in normal sinus rhythm, whereas 8 to 10 should be averaged for a patient in atrial fibrillation).
4. Cross-sectional area (i.e., diameter) measurement is accurate.
5. The velocity-time integral is measured with the Doppler beam parallel to blood flow (i.e., $\Theta = 0$ in the Doppler equation) in order to avoid underestimation.

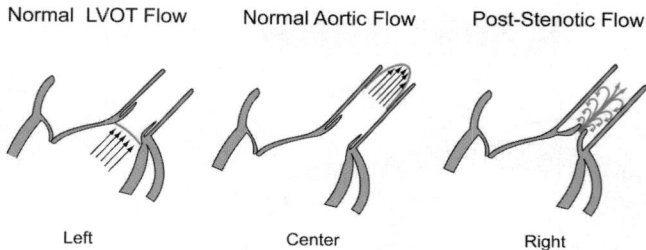

**FIGURE 22.4.** Common flow patterns. **Left:** Acceleration of blood within the left ventricular outflow tract leads to laminar flow with a flat velocity profile. **Center:** Friction along the wall of the ascending aorta leads to laminar flow with a parabolic flow profile. **Right:** Aortic stenosis results in a narrow, high velocity laminar jet originating from the stenotic orifice surrounded by turbulent flow.

Third, the VTI used in calculating stroke volume is assumed to represent the average VTI. Therefore, several measurements should be averaged for a patient in normal sinus rhythm, whereas between 8 and 10 measurements should be averaged for a patient in atrial fibrillation, in order to most accurately estimate the average VTI.

Fourth, determination of cross-sectional area is assumed to be accurate. Changes in cross-sectional area during the flow period, or deviations from an assumed geometry (usually circular) are inherent problems in Doppler stroke volume calculations. Accurate determination of 2-D measurements for calculation of cross-sectional area is essential. In the case of an assumed circular orifice, a small error in diameter measurement will result in a large error in the calculated cross-sectional area due to the quadratic relationship between the radius and area of a circle (i.e., $CSA = \prod \times r^2$). The use of high frequency multiplane TEE probes for measuring diameters (or areas) undoubtedly increases the reliability of these measurements when compared to the use of lower frequency monoplane or biplane TEE probes.

Fifth, the VTI is assumed to be recorded with the ultrasound beam parallel to the flow (i.e., the intercept angle $\Theta = 0$). In this case the velocities measured by Doppler are accurate based on a cosine $\Theta = 1$ in the Doppler equation (Fig. 22.5). However, as $\Theta$ increases from 20° to 60°, the error in the calculated Doppler velocity increases from 6% to 50% (Fig. 22.6). Small adjustments in the TEE probe transducer position and the pulsed wave Doppler sample volume (or continuous wave Doppler beam) are necessary to obtain the highest velocity signal. Multiple imaging planes should be utilized when possible to ensure that the highest velocity signal is obtained. Use of the audio Doppler signal in addition to the visual Doppler display may aid the echocardiographer in optimal alignment of the ultrasound beam with the flow of interest. The highest velocity signal obtained (the loudest audio signal) will correlate with the most parallel align-

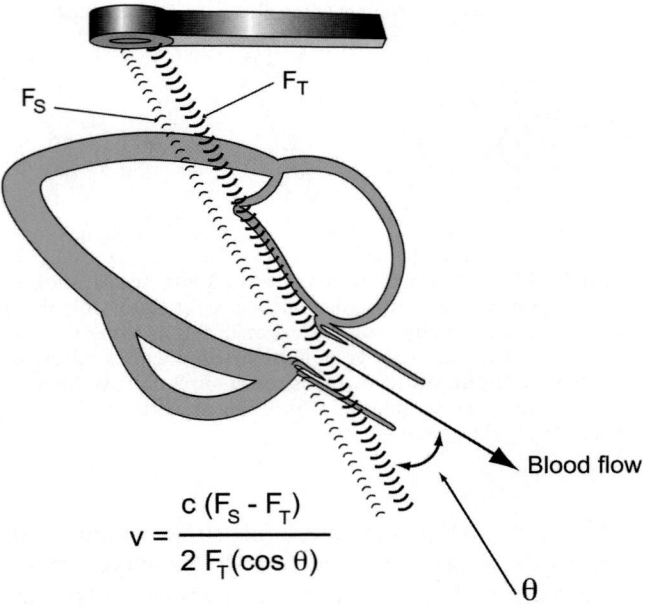

$$v = \frac{c(F_S - F_T)}{2F_T(\cos\theta)}$$

**FIGURE 22.5.** The Doppler equation. Blood flow velocity can be calculated based on the Doppler shift, which is the change in frequency between transmitted and backscattered ultrasound. *v*, blood flow velocity; *c*, the speed of sound in blood; $F_T$, the frequency of transmitted ultrasound; $F_S$, the frequency of backscattered ultrasound (the ultrasound reflected from moving red blood cells); $\theta$, the angle between the blood flow and interrogating ultrasound beam.

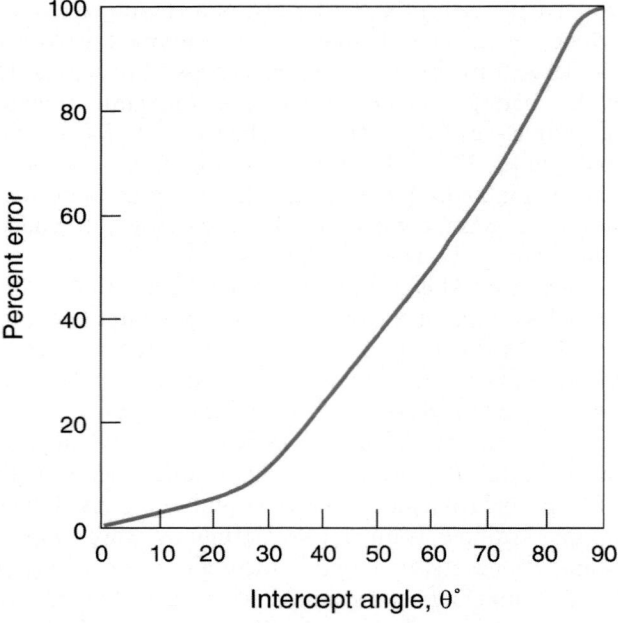

**FIGURE 22.6.** Velocity measurement error due to a nonparallel intercept angle. This graph shows the percentage error in the velocity calculation using the Doppler equation if the intercept angle between blood flow and the ultrasound beam is erroneously assumed to be zero. $\theta$, the true angle between blood flow and the interrogating ultrasound beam.

ment of the Doppler beam with blood flow. While underestimation of velocities is always a potential source of error in Doppler stroke volume determination with TEE imaging, it is undoubtedly less of a concern with multiplane than with monoplane or biplane TEE imaging.

## Calculation of Cardiac Output

Cardiac output (CO) can be estimated with 2-D Doppler after determining a Doppler stroke volume and measuring heart rate (5). Cardiac output is calculated as the product of stroke volume and heart rate (HR). Cardiac index (CI) is calculated by dividing cardiac output by body surface area (BSA):

$$CO \text{ (l/min)} = SV \text{ (cm}^3\text{)} \times (1 \text{ liter} / 1000 \text{ cm}^3) \times HR \text{ (bpm)}$$
$$CI \text{ (l/min/m}^2\text{)} = CO \text{ (l/min)} / BSA \text{ (m}^2\text{)}$$

Cardiac output measurements performed with TEE, usually measured at the LVOT or aortic valve in the absence of aortic regurgitation, have been shown to correlate well with measurements made by thermodilution (6–11). An accurate estimation of cardiac output depends on accurate determinations of the VTI and cross-sectional area. It is advisable to interrogate from multiple windows when possible. Accuracy is improved by assessing multiple Doppler flow profiles, typically 3–5 for a regular rhythm and 10 for an irregular rhythm. Furthermore, accuracy is improved if multiple diameter measurements are averaged prior to calculation of cross-sectional area as any error in this measurement is squared as previously discussed.

Stroke volume calculations for estimation of cardiac output are preferably made with multiplane TEE at the LVOT or aortic valve for three reasons. First, the acceleration of blood through the LVOT or aortic valve during systole favors laminar flow with a flat flow velocity profile, in contrast to the parabolic flow velocity profile present in the ascending aorta or pulmonary artery. Doppler determination of the VTI within a small sample of the cross-sectional area will be more representative of that throughout the cross-sectional area when the flow velocity profile is flat. Second, multiplane TEE provides excellent views of the LVOT and aortic valve for accurate determinations of LVOT diameter and aortic valve cross-sectional area. Third, the LVOT is more circular and changes shape very little during the cardiac cycle when compared to the main pulmonary artery or mitral valve. Measurements made at the main pulmonary artery or mitral valve are less reliable than those made at the LVOT and aortic valve (12). Although the cross-sectional area of the aortic valve orifice changes dramatically throughout systole, the cross-sectional area of the aortic valve during midsystole can be used to provide a good estimate of transaortic stroke volume by Doppler.

## Data for LVOT Stroke Volume Calculation (Fig. 22.7)

The pulsed wave Doppler sample volume is placed in the LVOT just proximal to the aortic valve (approximately 1 cm), using either the transgastric long-axis view or the deep transgastric long-axis view for determination of the $VTI_{LVOT}$. The diameter (cm) of the LVOT is best obtained from the midesophageal long-axis view of the aortic valve (approximately 1 cm proximal to the valve) for determination of cross-sectional area using the formula for the area of a circle:

$$CSA_{LVOT} \ (cm^2) = 0.785 \times D_{LVOT}{}^2$$

## Data for Transaortic Valve Stroke Volume Calculation (Fig. 22.8)

The *continuous wave* Doppler beam is placed through the aortic valve from either the transgastric long-axis view or the deep transgastric long-axis view for determination of

the $VTI_{AV}$. The cross-sectional area of the aortic valve can be determined by one of two methods. Planemetry can be used to measure the area ($cm^2$) of the aortic valve orifice *during midsystole* from a cine of the midesophageal short-axis view of the aortic valve (9).

Alternatively, a cine of a normal aortic valve from the same midesophageal short-axis view is used to measure the side (S) in cm of the equilateral opening of the valve *during midsystole*. Several measurements may be made and then averaged in order to improve accuracy. The formula for the area of an equilateral triangle is then used to calculate the cross-sectional area of the aortic valve:

$$CSA_{AV} \ (cm^2) = 0.433 \times (S)^2$$

## Data for Main PA Stroke Volume Calculation (Fig. 22.9)

The pulsed wave Doppler sample volume is placed in the main pulmonary artery using the upper esophageal short-axis view of the aortic arch (with the transducer rotated

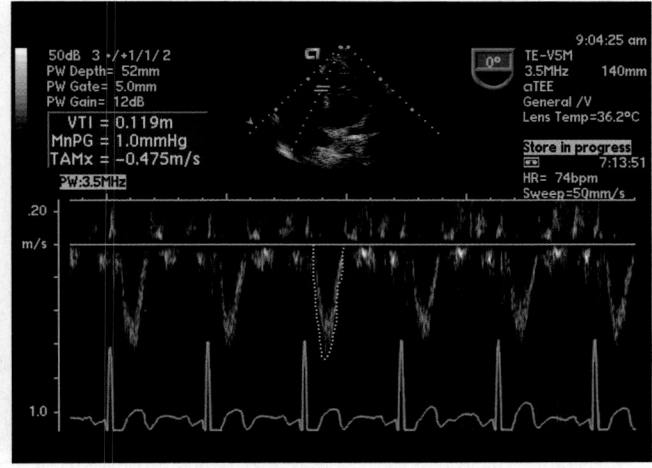

**B**

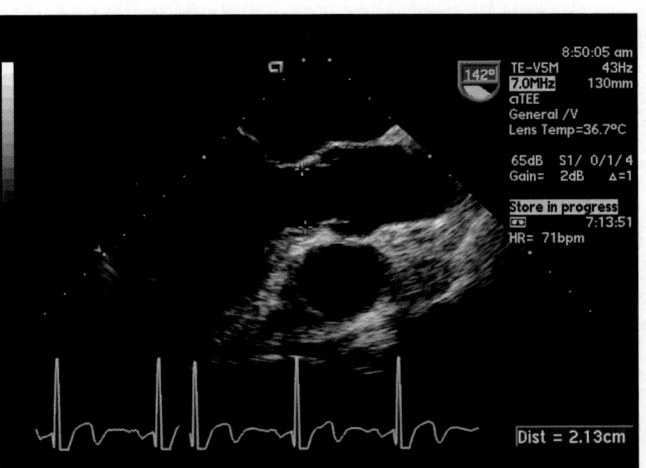

**A**

**C**

*FIGURE 22.7.* Data for LVOT stroke volume calculation. **A:** The $VTI_{LVOT}$ can be measured using pulsed wave Doppler with the sample volume in the LVOT just proximal to the aortic valve from a transgastric long-axis view. **B:** Alternatively, the $VTI_{LVOT}$ can be measured using pulsed wave Doppler with the sample volume in the LVOT just proximal to the aortic valve from a deep transgastric long-axis view. **C:** The diameter of the LVOT is usually measured from the midesophageal long-axis view of the aortic valve. *VTI,* velocity-time integral; *LVOT,* left ventricular outflow tract.

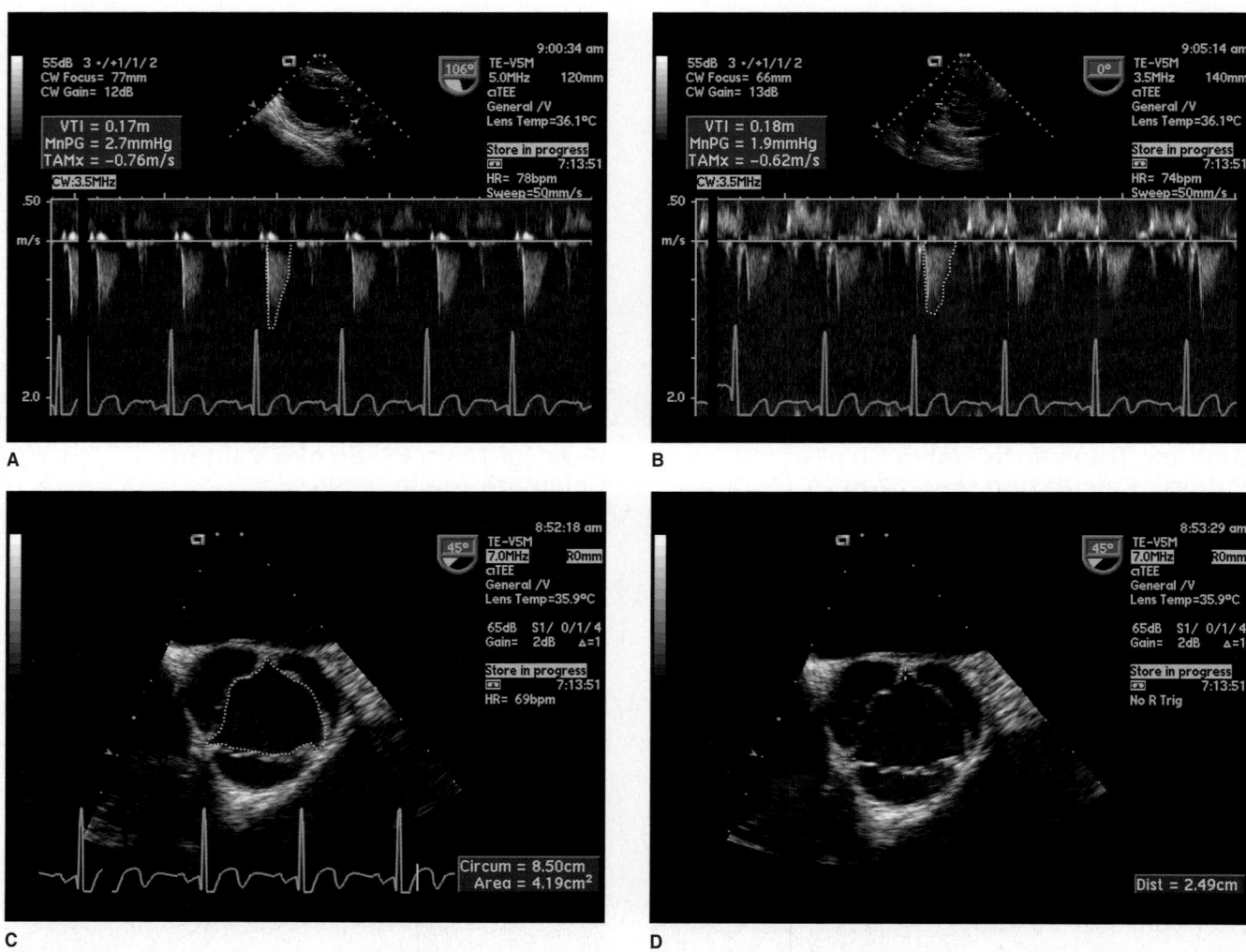

**FIGURE 22.8.** Data for transaortic valve stroke volume calculation. **A:** The $VTI_{AV}$ can be measured with the continuous wave Doppler beam placed through the aortic valve from a transgastric long-axis view. **B:** Alternatively, the $VTI_{AV}$ can be measured with the continuous wave Doppler beam placed through the aortic valve from a deep transgastric long-axis view. **C:** Planimetry can be used to measure the cross-sectional area of the aortic valve orifice during midsystole from a cine of the midesophageal short-axis view of the aortic valve. **D:** Alternatively, the length of a side of the aortic valve can be measured in midsystole for calculating the aortic valve area. *VTI*, velocity-time integral; *AV*, aortic valve; *S*, length of side of aortic valve.

from 80° to 90°) or the midesophageal short-axis view of the aorta for determination of the $VTI_{PA}$. The diameter (cm) of the main pulmonary artery is obtained from either view *at the same location* for determination of the cross-sectional area using the formula for the area of a circle:

$$CSA_{PA} (cm^2) = 0.785 \times D_{PA}{}^2$$

In either case, fluctuation in the diameter of the main pulmonary artery during the cardiac cycle makes stroke volume measurement at this location less reliable than at the LVOT or aortic valve (12).

## Data for RVOT Stroke Volume Calculation (Fig. 22.10)

The RVOT may be visualized using a transgastric RV inflow-outflow view with the transducer rotated from 110° to 150° and the probe turned to the right. The pulsed wave Doppler sample volume is placed in the RVOT just proximal to the pulmonic valve for determination of the $VTI_{RVOT}$. The diameter (cm) of the RVOT is best obtained from the same view *at the same location* for determination of cross-sectional area, using the formula for the area of a circle:

$$CSA_{RVOT} (cm^2) = 0.785 \times D_{RVOT}{}^2$$

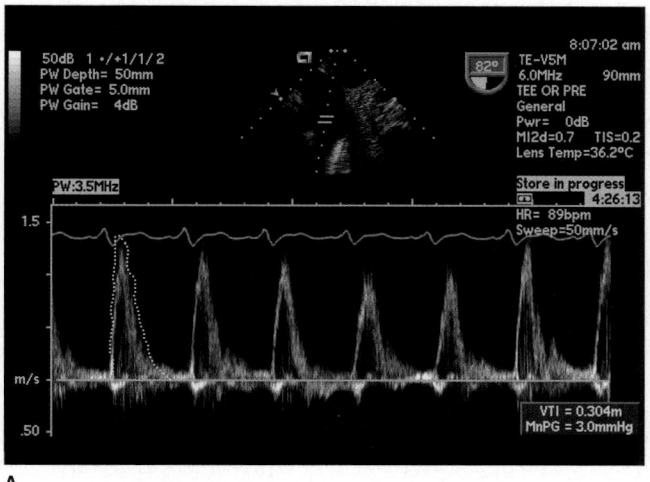

A

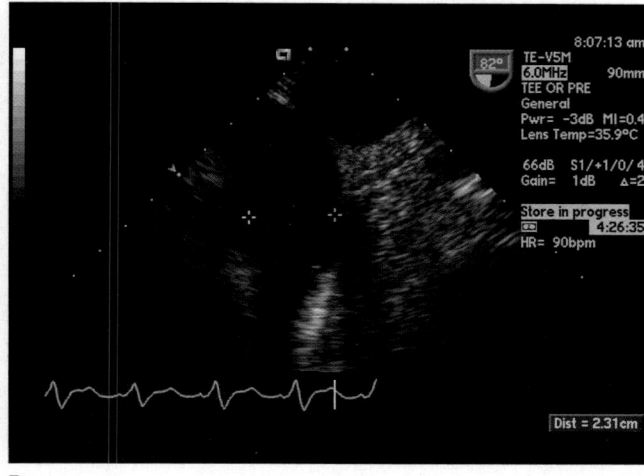

B

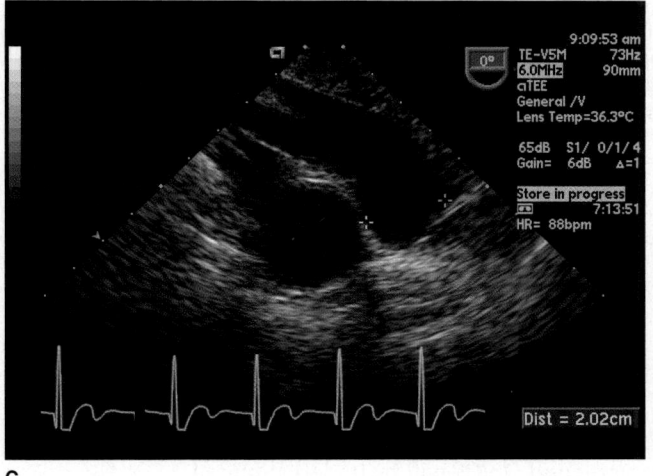

C

**FIGURE 22.9.** Data for main PA stroke volume calculation. **A:** The $VTI_{PA}$ can be measured using pulsed wave Doppler with the sample volume in the main pulmonary artery using the upper-esophageal short-axis view of the aortic arch. **B:** The diameter of the main pulmonary artery can be measured from the same view at the same location. **C:** Alternatively, the diameter of the main pulmonary artery (as well as the $VTI_{PA}$) can be measured using the midesophageal short-axis view of the ascending aorta (the $VTI_{PA}$ may also be obtained from this view). *VTI*, velocity-time integral; *PA*, pulmonary artery.

Alternatively, the diameter (cm) of the RVOT can be measured from the upperesophageal short-axis view of the aortic arch in some patients.

## Data for Transmitral Stroke Volume Calculation (Fig. 22.11)

The pulsed wave Doppler sample volume is placed at the level of the mitral valve annulus, using the midesophageal four-chamber view (alternatively, the midesophageal two-chamber view or midesophageal long-axis view may be used) for determination of the $VTI_{MV}$. While the mitral valve orifice is not truly elliptical during diastole, it is more elliptical than circular. The American Society of Echocardiography concluded in its document on quantitation of Doppler echocardiography that assumption of a circular orifice has generally worked well for all valves other than the tricuspid (13). Nevertheless, it may be preferable to estimate the cross-sectional area of the mitral valve, using the formula for an ellipse. The long and short diameters (cm) of the mitral valve annulus can be approximated using measurements from the midesophageal four-chamber and two-chamber views. The formula for an ellipse can then be used to calculate the cross-sectional area of the mitral valve:

$$CSA_{MV} (cm^2) = 0.785 \times D_1 \times D_2$$

The irregular semielliptical shape of the mitral valve orifice and the fluctuation in its size during diastole make stroke volume measurement at this location less reliable than at the LVOT or aortic valve (12).

## DOPPLER MEASUREMENT OF PULMONARY-TO-SYSTEMIC FLOW RATIO (Qp/Qs)

The ratio of pulmonic-to-systemic blood flow, Qp/Qs usually indicates the magnitude of a shunt (i.e., atrial septal defect, ventricular septal defect, or patent pulmonary ductus arteriosus) and may be useful information in determining

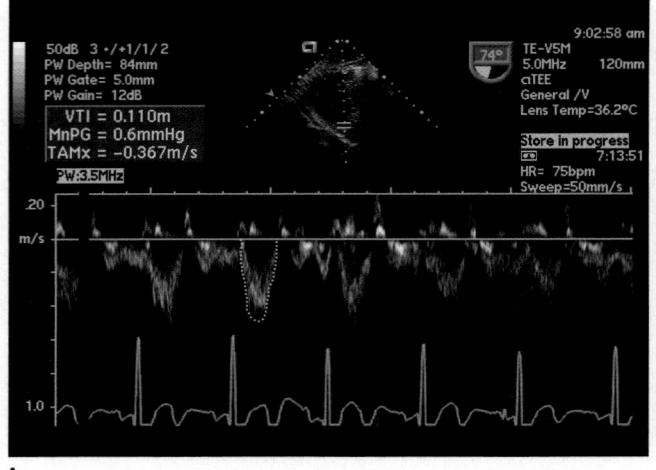

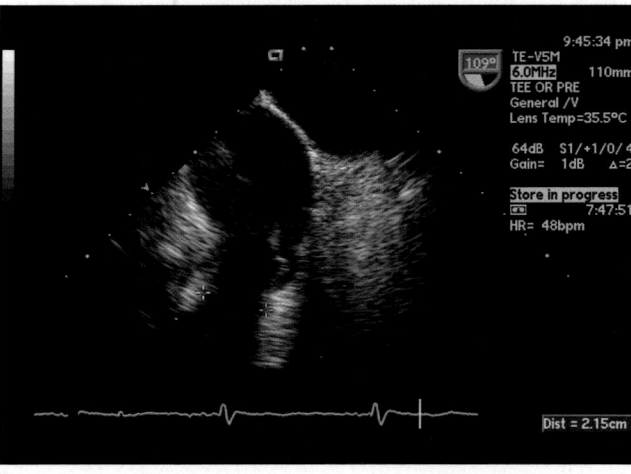

**FIGURE 22.10.** Data for RVOT stroke volume calculation. **A:** The VTI$_{RVOT}$ can be measured using pulsed wave Doppler with the sample volume placed just proximal to the pulmonic valve from a transgastric RV inflow-outflow view (transducer usually rotated from 110° to 150° and the probe turned to the right). **B:** The diameter of the RVOT may be obtained from this same view or the upper esophageal short-axis view of the aortic arch. *VTI,* velocity-time integral; *RVOT,* right ventricular outflow tract.

the need for surgery or the timing of surgery. Qp/Qs can be calculated once the systemic stroke volume (measured at the LVOT or aortic valve) and pulmonic stroke volume (measured at the PA or RVOT) have been determined (14):

$$Qp/Qs = (SV_{PA} \times HR) / (SV_{LVOT} \times HR)$$
$$Qp/Qs = SV_{PA} / SV_{LVOT}$$

Potential errors in the estimation of Qp/Qs are the same as for other Doppler determinations of stroke volume. It should be noted that there is also the possibility of compounding calculated Doppler stroke volume errors in the calculation of Qp/Qs with this formula (i.e., if SV$_{PA}$ is overestimated and SV$_{LVOT}$ is underestimated, then Qp/Qs may be significantly overestimated). This potential propagation of errors will lead to a range in the confidence intervals for Qp/Qs, which is unacceptable to many clinicians using TEE. Furthermore, in the presence of significant aortic regurgitation this calculation is not accurate and Qp/Qs will be underestimated.

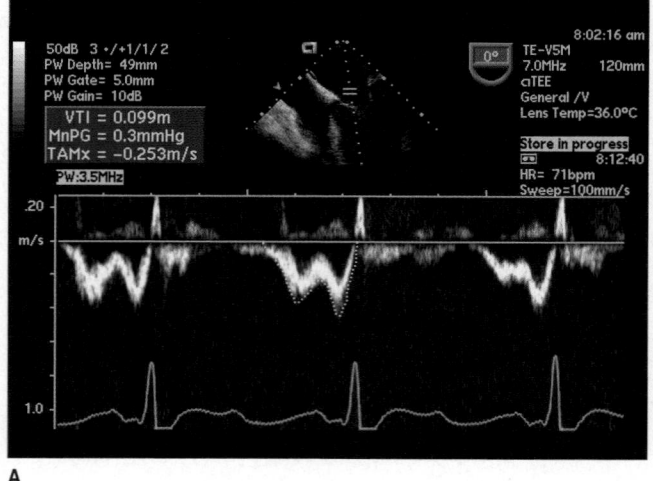

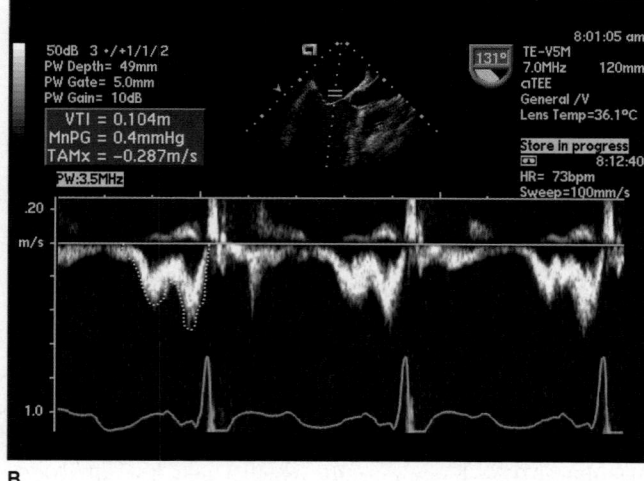

**FIGURE 22.11.** Data for transmitral stroke volume calculation. The VTI$_{MV}$ can be measured using pulsed wave Doppler with the sample volume placed within the mitral valve annulus using any midesophageal view of the mitral valve. **A:** The VTI$_{MV}$ measured from the midesophageal four-chamber view. **B:** The VTI$_{MV}$ measured from the midesophageal long-axis view in the same patient.   *(continued)*

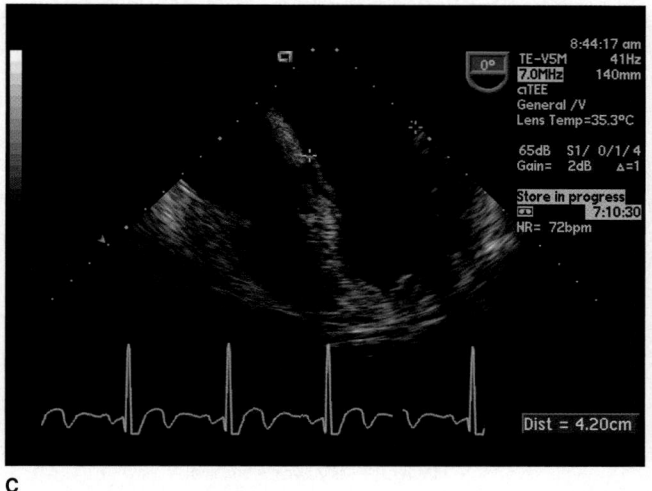

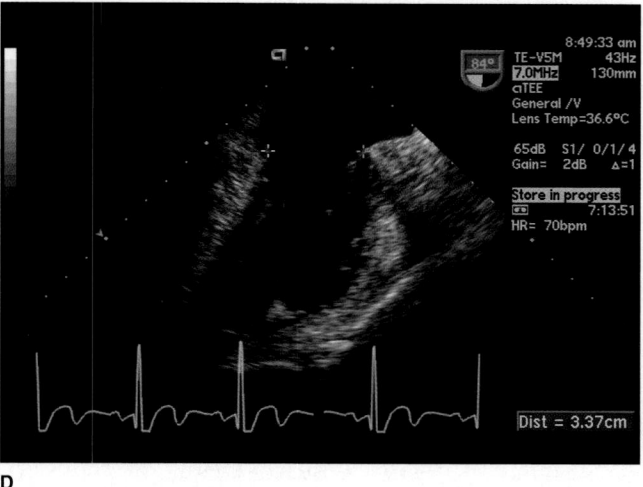

**C**  **D**

**FIGURE 22.11.** *(Continued)* **C:** The long diameter ($D_1$) of the mitral valve annulus can be approximated using measurements from the midesophageal four-chamber view. **D:** The short diameter ($D_2$) of the mitral valve annulus can be approximated using measurements from the midesophageal two-chamber view. *VTI,* velocity-time integral; *MV,* mitral valve.

# DOPPLER MEASUREMENT OF REGURGITANT VOLUME AND FRACTION

## Volumetric Method (Fig. 22.12)

Regurgitant volume (RV) is the volume of blood that flows backwards through a regurgitant valve during one cardiac cycle. Conservation of mass says that the stroke volume delivered to the systemic circulation ($SV_{SYSTEMIC}$) must equal the total forward stroke volume across a regurgitant valve ($SV_{TOTAL}$) minus the regurgitant volume:

$$SV_{SYSTEMIC} = SV_{TOTAL} - RV$$

Thus, regurgitant volume can be calculated once $SV_{TOTAL}$ and $SV_{SYSTEMIC}$ have been determined:

$$RV = SV_{TOTAL} - SV_{SYSTEMIC}$$

The regurgitant fraction (RF) for any valve is calculated as the ratio of regurgitant volume to total forward flow across the regurgitant valve expressed as a percentage.

$$RF\ (\%) = (RV\ /\ SV_{TOTAL}) \times 100\%$$

## Assessment of Mitral Regurgitation (Fig. 22.13)

In mitral regurgitation, the $SV_{TOTAL}$ is the mitral inflow stroke volume and the $SV_{SYSTEMIC}$ is the LVOT stroke volume. Thus, the mitral valve regurgitant volume can be estimated by subtracting the LVOT stroke volume from the

mitral valve inflow stroke volume and then the mitral regurgitant fraction can be calculated (15):

$$RV_{MV} = SV_{MVI} - SV_{LVOT}$$
$$RF_{MV}\ (\%) = (RV_{MV}\ /\ SV_{MVI}) \times 100\%$$

This method of assessing mitral regurgitation is performed infrequently during TEE examinations due to the time required to acquire the data and the possibility of compounding calculated Doppler stroke volume errors during the calculation of mitral regurgitant volume or

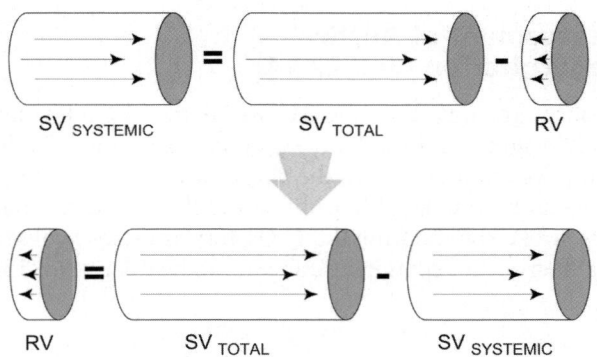

**FIGURE 22.12.** The volumetric method for calculation of regurgitant volume. Conservation of mass dictates that regurgitant volume must be equal to the difference between the total forward stroke volume across the regurgitant valve and the systemically delivered stroke volume. *RV,* regurgitant volume; *$SV_{TOTAL}$,* total forward stroke volume across the regurgitant valve; *$SV_{SYSTEMIC}$,* systemically delivered stroke volume.

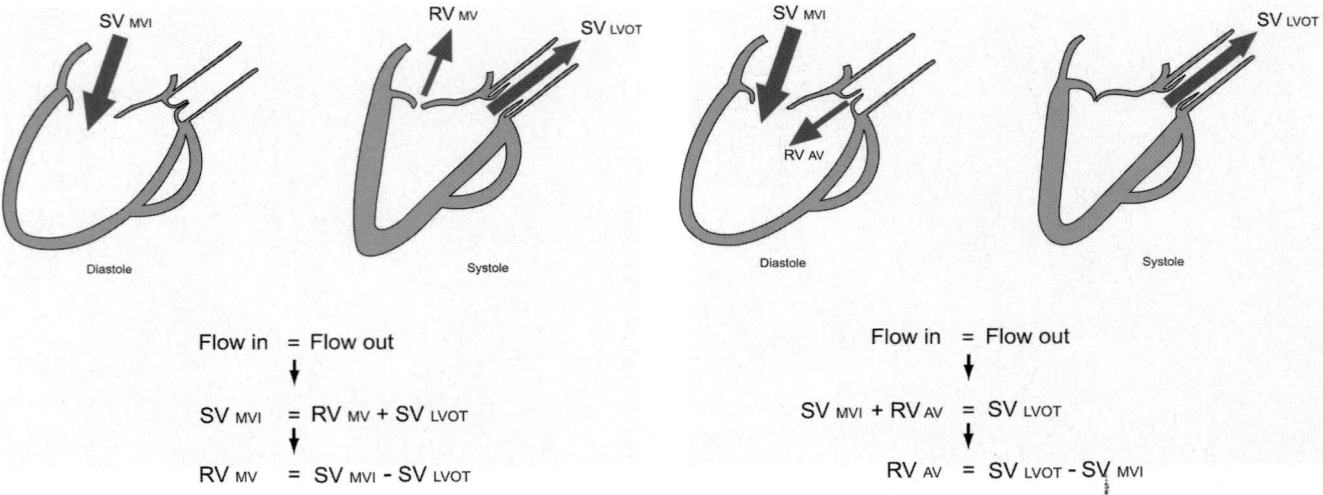

**Flow in = Flow out**

$SV_{MVI} = RV_{MV} + SV_{LVOT}$

$RV_{MV} = SV_{MVI} - SV_{LVOT}$

**Flow in = Flow out**

$SV_{MVI} + RV_{AV} = SV_{LVOT}$

$RV_{AV} = SV_{LVOT} - SV_{MVI}$

**FIGURE 22.13.** Assessment of mitral regurgitant volume using the volumetric method. Diastolic flow into the left ventricle must equal systolic flow out. Therefore, the mitral regurgitant volume must equal the difference between the mitral valve inflow stroke volume and the LVOT stroke volume. This method will underestimate mitral regurgitant volume in the presence of significant aortic regurgitation. $RV_{MV}$, mitral regurgitant volume; $SV_{MVI}$, mitral valve inflow stroke volume; $SV_{LVOT}$, left ventricular outflow tract stroke volume.

**FIGURE 22.14.** Assessment of aortic regurgitant volume using the volumetric method. Diastolic flow into the left ventricle must equal systolic flow out. Therefore, the aortic regurgitant volume must be equal to the difference between the LVOT stroke volume and the mitral valve inflow stroke volume. This method will underestimate aortic regurgitant volume in the presence of significant mitral regurgitation. $RV_{AV}$, aortic regurgitant volume; $SV_{LVOT}$, left ventricular outflow tract stroke volume; $SV_{MVI}$, mitral valve inflow stroke volume.

fraction. This potential propagation of errors will lead to a range in the confidence intervals for the mitral valve regurgitant volume, which is unacceptable to many clinicians. A particular problem exists with reliably measuring the mitral valve inflow stroke volume due to the irregular shape of the mitral valve orifice (semielliptical) and the fluctuation in its size during diastole (12). Furthermore, in the presence of significant aortic regurgitation this calculation is not accurate and mitral regurgitant volume will be underestimated.

## Assessment of Aortic Regurgitation (Fig. 22.14)

In aortic regurgitation, the $SV_{TOTAL}$ is the LVOT forward stroke volume and the $SV_{SYSTEMIC}$ is the mitral valve inflow stroke volume. Thus, the aortic valve regurgitant volume can be estimated by subtracting the mitral valve inflow stroke volume from the LVOT forward stroke volume and then aortic regurgitant fraction can be calculated (15):

$$RV_{AV} = SV_{LVOT} - SV_{MVI}$$
$$RF_{AV} (\%) = (RV_{AV} / SV_{LVOT}) \times 100\%$$

This method of assessing aortic regurgitation is also performed infrequently during TEE examinations due to the time required to acquire the data and the possibility of compounding calculated Doppler stroke volume errors during the calculation of aortic regurgitant volume or fraction. This potential propagation of errors will lead to

a range in the confidence intervals for the aortic valve regurgitant volume that is unacceptable to many clinicians. A particular problem exists with reliably measuring the mitral valve inflow stroke volume due to the irregular semielliptical shape of the mitral valve orifice and the fluctuation in its size during diastole (12). Furthermore, in the presence of significant mitral regurgitation this calculation is not accurate and aortic regurgitant volume will be underestimated.

## Proximal Convergence Method

As blood flows towards a regurgitant orifice (i.e., mitral regurgitation), or in some cases a stenotic orifice (i.e., mitral stenosis), blood flow velocity increases with the formation of multiple concentric "isovelocity" shells (Fig. 22.15) (16,17). These "isovelocity" shells can be "seen" with color flow imaging, as seen in Fig. 22.16, and have been termed proximal isovelocity surface areas (PISAs). The size of a PISA proximal to a regurgitant orifice can be altered by adjusting the Nyquist limit of the color flow map. As the negative aliasing velocity is reduced (in the case of mitral regurgitation), the transition from red to blue will occur farther from the regurgitant orifice resulting in a hemispheric shell with a larger radius (r). The instantaneous velocity of blood at the PISA is the same as the aliasing velocity on the color flow map. The instantaneous flow rate through a PISA that is a *hemispheric shell* is equal to the product of the area of the PISA and the instantaneous velocity of blood at the PISA:

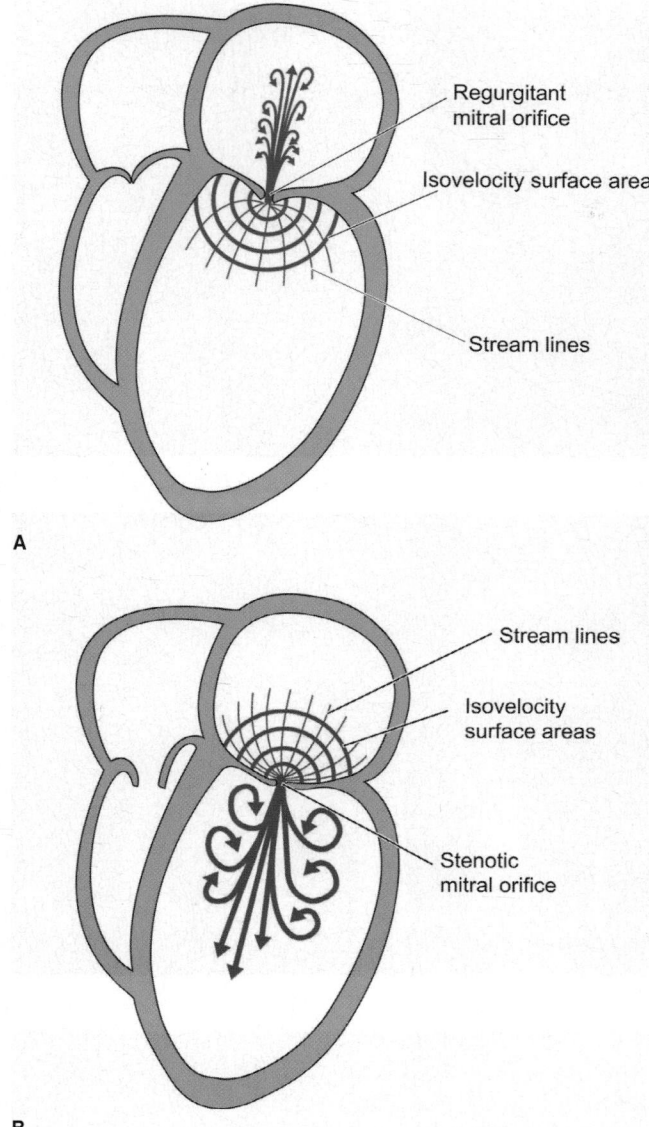

**A**

**B**

**FIGURE 22.15.** Proximal flow convergence. The slow acceleration of blood from within a large chamber towards a small orifice results in the formation of multiple concentric "isovelocity" shells with decreasing radius. **A:** In mitral regurgitation, these isovelocity shells occur in the left ventricle. **B:** In mitral stenosis, these isovelocity shells occur in the left atrium.

$$PISA \text{ flow rate} = PISA \text{ area} \times \text{Blood velocity at } PISA$$
$$PISA \text{ flow rate} = 2\Pi \times r^2 \times \text{Aliasing velocity}$$
$$PISA \text{ flow rate} = 6.28 \times r^2 \times \text{Aliasing velocity}$$

Conservation of mass says that the flow rate at the surface of each of these isovelocity shells should be equal to the flow rate through the regurgitant orifice. In other words, the PISA flow rate must be equal to the product of the effective regurgitant orifice area (EROA) and the instantaneous regurgitant velocity (Fig. 22.17):

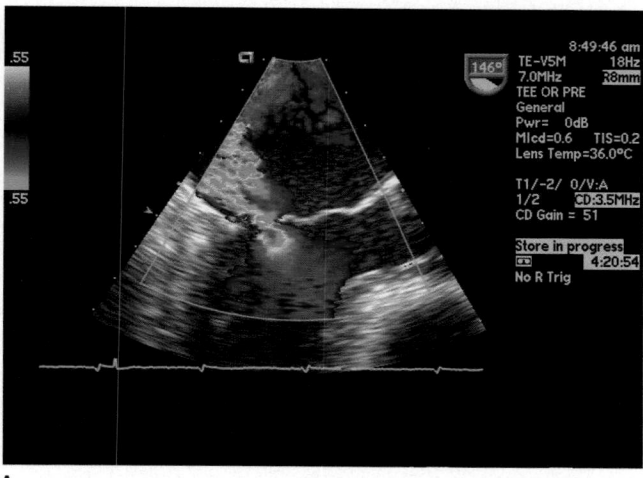

**A**

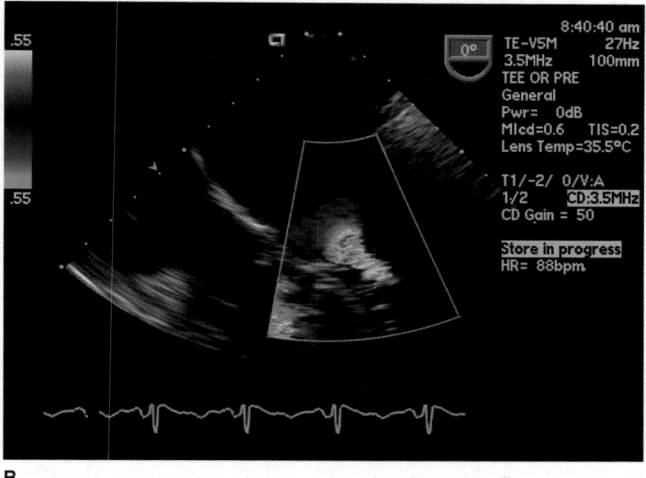

**B**

**FIGURE 22.16.** Proximal isovelocity surface area (PISA) by color flow imaging. **A:** These proximal isovelocity surface areas (or PISAs) can be demonstrated with Doppler color flow imaging within the left ventricle in the setting of mitral regurgitation. **B:** Similarly, PISAs can be demonstrated with Doppler color flow imaging within the left atrium in the setting of mitral stenosis.

$$PISA \text{ flow rate} = \text{Regurgitant flow rate}$$
$$PISA \text{ flow rate} = EROA \times \text{Regurgitant velocity}$$

The effective regurgitant orifice area can therefore be calculated at midsystole as the PISA flow rate *at* midsystole divided by the regurgitant velocity *at* midsystole (which is the peak velocity of the regurgitant jet):

$$EROA = PISA \text{ flow rate} / \text{Regurgitant velocity}$$
$$EROA = (6.28 \times r^2 \times \text{Aliasing velocity}) / V_{RJ}$$

where r is in cm and the aliasing velocity and peak regurgitant jet velocity (peak $V_{RJ}$) are in cm/s.

Just as forward stroke volume is equal to the product of cross-sectional area and the forward flow velocity-time

## Proximal Flow Convergence Method

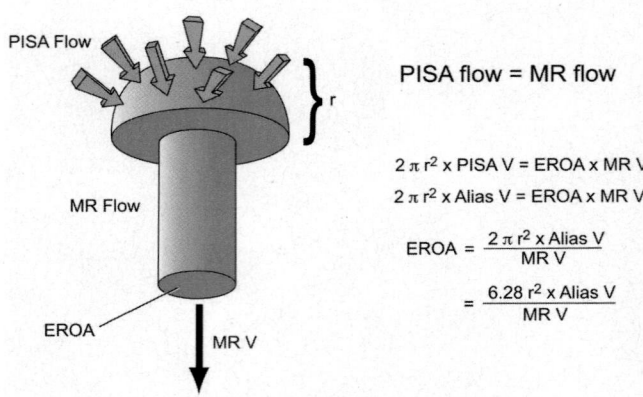

PISA flow = MR flow

$$2 \pi r^2 \times \text{PISA V} = \text{EROA} \times \text{MR V}$$

$$2 \pi r^2 \times \text{Alias V} = \text{EROA} \times \text{MR V}$$

$$\text{EROA} = \frac{2 \pi r^2 \times \text{Alias V}}{\text{MR V}}$$

$$= \frac{6.28 \, r^2 \times \text{Alias V}}{\text{MR V}}$$

**FIGURE 22.17.** The proximal flow convergence method for calculating ERO in mitral regurgitation. Conservation of mass dictates that PISA flow rate must equal regurgitant flow rate across the mitral regurgitant orifice. Thus, the effective regurgitant orifice area (EROA) in mitral regurgitation can be calculated using the PISA method. *PISA,* proximal isovelocity surface area; *r,* PISA radius; *v,* velocity.

integral, regurgitant volume is equal to the product of the effective regurgitant orifice area and the velocity-time integral of the regurgitant jet ($\text{VTI}_{RJ}$):

$$\text{RV} = \text{EROA} \times \text{VTI}_{RJ}$$

The formula for regurgitant volume using the flow convergence method is thus given by substituting the formula for effective regurgitant orifice area using the PISA method into the above formula for regurgitant volume:

$$\text{RV} = (6.28 \times r^2 \times \text{Aliasing velocity} \times \text{VTI}_{RJ}) / \text{V}_{RJ}$$

where r and $\text{VTI}_{RJ}$ are in cm and the aliasing velocity and peak regurgitant jet velocity (peak $\text{V}_{RJ}$) are in cm/s.

Thus, in the case of mitral regurgitation, the calculation of regurgitant volume using the flow convergence method is dependent on determining four pieces of data (Fig. 22.18). First, following color-flow imaging of the PISA resulting from mitral regurgitation, the PISA radius must be measured and the aliasing velocity noted (after shifting the baseline towards the TEE transducer). Second, a continuous wave Doppler examination of the mitral regurgitant jet must be performed to measure the peak velocity and velocity-time integral of the mitral regurgitant jet.

The proximal convergence method has been validated for assessing mitral regurgitation in many experimental and clinical studies (18). Advantages of the proximal flow convergence method over the volumetric method include the ability to make all necessary measurements from a single imaging window and the fact that flow rate is mea-

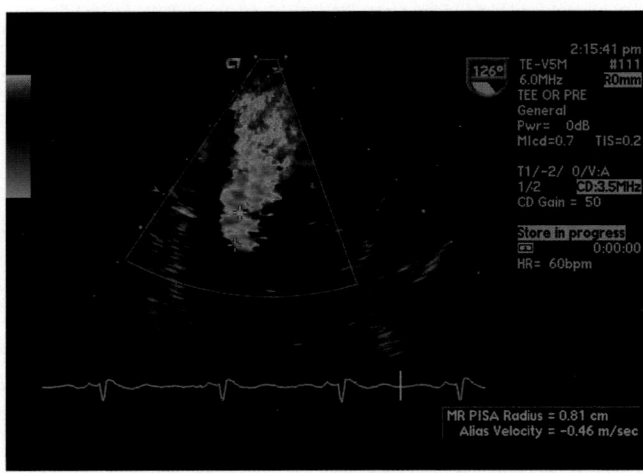

**A**

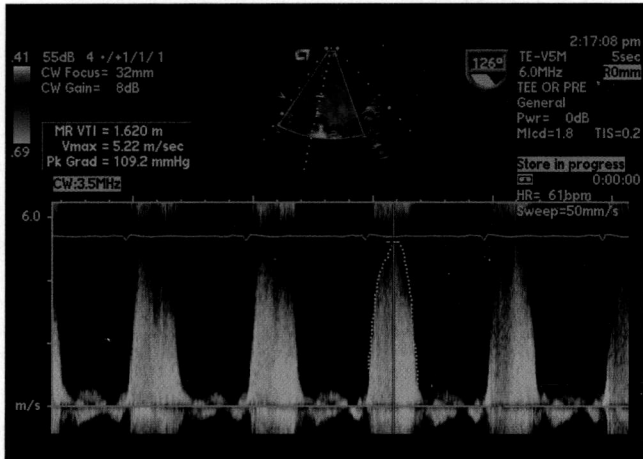

**B**

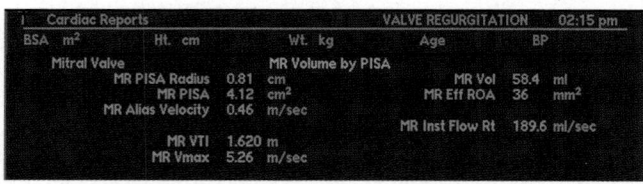

**C**

**FIGURE 22.18.** Data necessary for calculation of mitral regurgitant volume using the PISA method. **A:** The mitral regurgitant jet is visualized using color flow imaging. After appropriate baseline shifting, the PISA radius must be measured from a cine of the mitral regurgitant jet frozen during midsystole and the aliasing velocity noted. **B:** The VTI and peak velocity of the mitral regurgitant jet are measured from a continuous wave Doppler velocity tracing. **C:** Report of mitral regurgitant volume and regurgitant orifice area using PISA method. *PISA,* proximal isovelocity surface area; *VTI,* velocity-time integral.

sured directly (not requiring the subtraction of one large quantity from another). Nevertheless, there are four potentially significant limitations to the proximal flow convergence method.

First, as the regurgitant orifice is not infinitely small, the hemispheric shape of PISAs is not maintained all the way to the orifice and using the standard formula, flow underestimation may occur (19). A correction factor has been determined, but, fortunately, it is not typically necessary for mitral or aortic regurgitation. Second, flow may be constrained by structures proximal to the regurgitant orifice such that the PISAs are not full hemispheres leading to flow overestimation if the standard formula is used. Most of this overestimation can be eliminated by simply excluding from the calculations an amount of flow proportional to the reduction of the PISA from a full hemisphere (see the section on the Continuity Equation and Fig. 22.23) (20). Third, while it is generally easy to identify where the color Doppler changes from blue to red, it is often difficult to locate the exact center of the regurgitant orifice (the center of the PISA radius) (21). As the radius is squared in the proximal flow convergence formula, a 10% error in radius measurement may lead to a 20% error in calculated flow rate and regurgitant orifice area. Fourth, the degree of regurgitation is not constant throughout systole in many patients and determining regurgitant severity based on the maximal regurgitant orifice area may overestimate the actual hemodynamic impact of the regurgitant lesion (22). In spite of these limitations, the flow convergence method is quantitative, relatively simple to perform, and applicable in a large number of patients with valvular regurgitation.

### Simplified Proximal Convergence Method

Although the proximal flow convergence method is considerably more practical than previous volumetric methods, it is still considered to be too complex for routine intraoperative use by many. A simplified proximal convergence method has been developed for estimating mitral regurgitant orifice area with only one measurement (23). This simplified method is based on the assumption that the pressure difference between the left ventricle and left atrium is 100 mm Hg during systole, which would result in a 5 m/s mitral regurgitant jet. With this assumption, if the aliasing velocity is set to *approximately* 40 cm/s and the radius of the first PISA (r) is measured, then the mitral effective regurgitant orifice area can be estimated as follows:

$$EROA = r^2 / 2$$

Results using the simplified method are almost the same as those determined using the standard proximal flow convergence method. Obviously, the error created by using the simplified method will increase as the pressure difference between the left ventricle and left atrium differs from 100 mm Hg. Nevertheless, this error should not exceed 20% to 25% as long as the pressure difference

between the left ventricle and left atrium ranges between 64 mm Hg and 144 mm Hg.

## DOPPLER MEASUREMENT OF PRESSURE GRADIENTS

Doppler echocardiography can measure blood flow velocities using the principle of the Doppler shift to assess conditions, such as valvular stenosis, left ventricular outflow tract obstruction, septal defects, and coarctation of the aorta (24,25). Each of these conditions effectively produces a "stenosis" through which blood flow velocity is increased. This increase in blood flow velocity is related to the degree of "stenosis."

The Bernoulli equation describes the relationship between the increase in the velocity of a fluid (i.e., blood) across a narrowed orifice (i.e., a stenotic valve) and the pressure gradient across that narrowed orifice (Fig. 22.19):

$$\Delta P = P_1 - P_2 = \frac{1}{2}\rho(v_2^2 - v_1^2) + \rho(dv/dt)ds + R(v)$$

where the first term describes convective acceleration ($\rho$ = the density of the fluid, $v_1$ = the peak velocity of fluid proximal to the narrowed orifice, and $v_2$ = the peak velocity of fluid through the narrowed orifice), the second term describes flow acceleration, and the third term describes viscous friction.

Since pressure gradients are most often determined at peak flow, the effects of flow acceleration can be ignored.

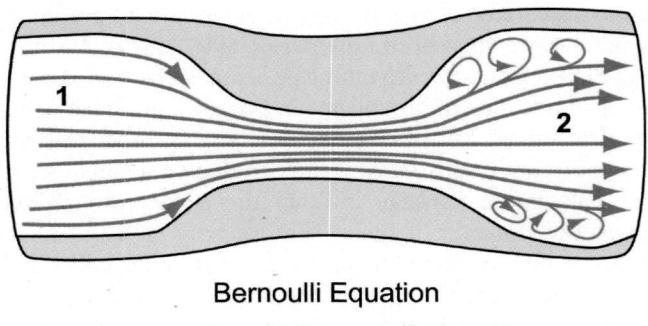

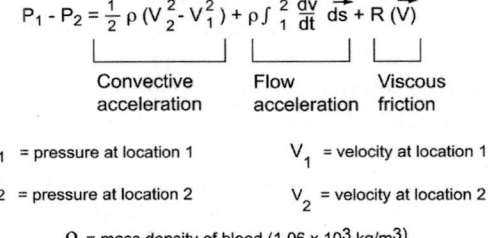

**Bernoulli Equation**

$$P_1 - P_2 = \frac{1}{2}\rho (V_2^2 - V_1^2) + \rho \int_1^2 \frac{d\vec{v}}{dt}\,\vec{ds} + R(\vec{V})$$

Convective acceleration    Flow acceleration    Viscous friction

$P_1$ = pressure at location 1      $V_1$ = velocity at location 1

$P_2$ = pressure at location 2      $V_2$ = velocity at location 2

$\rho$ = mass density of blood ($1.06 \times 10^3$ kg/m$^3$)

*FIGURE 22.19.* The Bernoulli equation. The Bernoulli equation describes the relationship between the increase in the velocity of a fluid across a narrowed orifice and the pressure gradient across that narrowed orifice.

Furthermore, the effects of viscous friction are only significant in orifices with an area less than 0.25 cm² (26). Thus, in clinical echocardiography, the Bernoulli equation can be simplified by ignoring the effects of flow acceleration and viscous friction:

$$\Delta P = \frac{1}{2} \rho(v_2{}^2 - v_1{}^2)$$

Furthermore, since the distal blood flow velocity ($v_2$) is substantially greater than the proximal blood flow velocity ($v_1$) for most clinically significant lesions, $v_2{}^2 - v_1{}^2$ can be approximated by $v_2{}^2$ alone. Thus, assuming the density of blood to be $1.06 \times 10^3$ kg/m³, the Bernoulli equation can be simplified even further:

$$\Delta P = 4v_2{}^2$$

where $\Delta P$ is the pressure gradient across the obstruction in mm Hg and $v_2$ is the peak blood flow velocity across the obstruction in m/s. The simplified Bernoulli equation is the basis for virtually all pressure gradient calculations in clinical echocardiography. However, there are occasions when this equation is invalid. For example, in the setting of aortic stenosis and significant LVOT obstruction (dynamic or fixed), the simplified Bernoulli equation would overestimate the aortic valve pressure gradient because $v_2{}^2$ would overestimate $v_2{}^2 - v_1{}^2$.

As Doppler echocardiography measures instantaneous blood flow velocities, the pressure gradients derived from Doppler velocities using the simplified Bernoulli equation are instantaneous pressure gradients. The maximum instantaneous pressure gradient will therefore always be given by the maximum Doppler velocity. The mean gradient is calculated as the average Doppler-derived pressure gradient over the entire flow period (Fig. 22.20). Assuming the Doppler sample volume or beam is positioned correctly, both maximum and mean pressure gradients can be determined from low velocity jets with either pulsed wave or continuous wave Doppler velocity signals using the calculation package built in the echocardiography machine. However, if blood flow velocity is $\geq$ 1.4 m/s, aliasing may occur with pulsed wave Doppler and thus continuous wave Doppler is preferable. In general, it is common practice to use continuous wave Doppler when determining maximum and mean valvular pressure gradients, keeping in mind that the wrong flow signal could erroneously be interrogated as a result of range ambiguity (i.e., in the case of coexisting LVOT obstruction and aortic stenosis).

The Doppler beam must be positioned so that it can interrogate the highest velocity jet or the pressure gradient may be significantly underestimated. Velocity underestimation is of most concern when measuring high velocity jets due to valve stenosis or regurgitation or other intracardiac abnormalities. Accuracy is improved by assessing

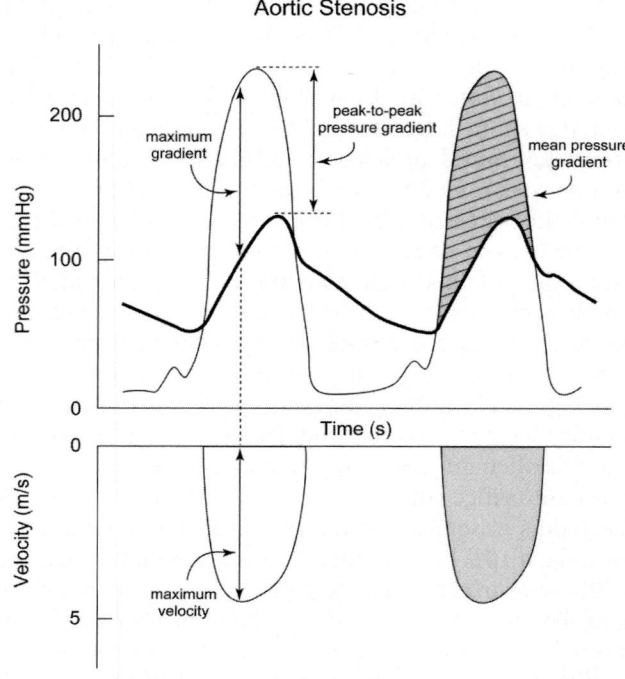

**FIGURE 22.20.** Maximum and mean pressure gradients. As seen in this diagram of left ventricular and left atrial pressure tracings and the Doppler velocity spectrum in aortic stenosis, the maximum instantaneous pressure gradient corresponds to the maximum Doppler velocity. The maximum aortic valve instantaneous pressure gradient determined by Doppler is greater than the peak-to-peak gradient sometimes reported following cardiac catheterization. The mean pressure gradient determined by Doppler, the average of pressure gradients determined by Doppler over the entire flow period (see *shaded area*), correlates well with the mean gradient determined by cardiac catheterization (see *hatched area*).

multiple Doppler flow profiles, typically 3 to 5 for a regular rhythm and 10 for an irregular rhythm. Furthermore, small adjustments in the TEE probe transducer position and the Doppler beam are necessary to obtain the highest velocity signal. It is advisable to interrogate from multiple windows when possible. While underestimation of velocities is always a potential source of error in Doppler determination of pressure gradients with TEE, it is undoubtedly of greater concern with either monoplane or biplane TEE than with multiplane TEE. However, regardless of the type of TEE imaging probe used, the inability to adequately align the interrogating Doppler beam parallel with the blood flow of interest can lead to significant underestimation of pressure gradients (a common concern in the setting of aortic stenosis or LVOT obstruction).

Some cardiac catheterization laboratories report the peak-to-peak gradient in aortic stenosis. As this is the pressure difference between the peak left ventricular pressure and the peak aortic pressure, which occur at different times, this is a nonphysiologic measurement (Fig. 22.20). However, the Doppler-derived maximum instantaneous gradient can provide clinicians with an accurate estimate of the true physiologic maximum pressure gradient in aortic stenosis. Mean gradients determined by Doppler have correlated well with those simultaneously measured by cardiac catheterization.

Many studies have shown an excellent correlation with Doppler-derived pressure gradients using transthoracic echocardiography and catheter-derived pressure gradients across mitral valve stenosis, various prosthetic valves, LVOT obstruction, and RVOT obstruction (2–4,27,28). However, the transmitral pressure gradient may be overestimated by cardiac catheterization if pulmonary capillary wedge pressure is used instead of direct left atrial pressure measurement (29). Doppler echocardiography is thus considered the optimal method for determining the transmitral pressure gradient. As TEE generally provides excellent windows for mitral valve interrogation using the midesophageal views, it should also provide accurate estimates of transmitral pressure gradients.

## DOPPLER DETERMINATION OF VALVE AREA

### Continuity Equation (Fig. 22.21)

The continuity equation is another expression of the principle of conservation of mass. Simply stated, it says flow in must equal flow out. Most commonly it is used in echocardiography to determine the area of a stenotic valve (i.e., aortic valve area in aortic stenosis). However, it can also be used to determine effective regurgitant orifice area (i.e., effective regurgitant orifice area in mitral regurgitation). More specifically, the continuity equation states that flow or stroke volume ($SV_2$) across a stenotic (or regurgitant) orifice is equal to the flow or stroke volume ($SV_1$) across a proximal (or upstream) flow of known area and velocity. Thus, using the Doppler formula for stroke volume, the unknown area of a stenotic valve ($CSA_2$) can be calculated as shown:

$$SV_1 = SV_2$$
$$CSA_1 \times VTI_1 = CSA_2 \times VTI_2$$
$$CSA_2 = CSA_1 \times (VTI_1 / VTI_2)$$

### Continuity Equation in Aortic Stenosis (Fig. 22.22)

In aortic stenosis, stroke volume across the aortic valve must equal the stroke volume across the LVOT. Thus, aortic valve area (AVA) may be calculated using the continuity equation as follows, with either transthoracic echocardiography or multiplane TEE (30,31):

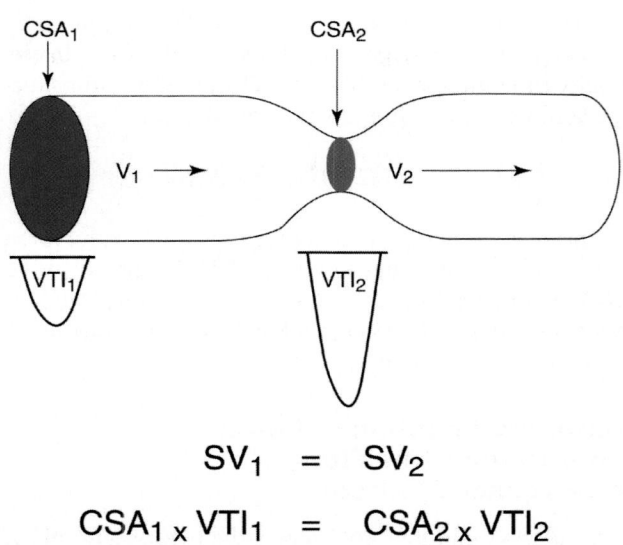

$$SV_1 = SV_2$$
$$CSA_1 \times VTI_1 = CSA_2 \times VTI_2$$

**FIGURE 22.21.** The continuity equation. Stroke volume proximal to a stenosis ($SV_1$) must equal stroke volume across a stenosis ($SV_2$). *A*, area; *VTI*, velocity-time integral.

$$AVA = CSA_{LVOT} \times (VTI_{LVOT} / VTI_{AV})$$
$$AVA \, (cm^2) = 0.785 \times D_{LVOT}^2 \times (VTI_{LVOT} / VTI_{AV})$$

where the $D_{LVOT}$ is measured in cm, the $VTI_{LVOT}$ is measured in cm using pulsed wave Doppler, and the $VTI_{AV}$ is measured in cm using continuous wave Doppler. Because the shapes of the $VTI_{LVOT}$ and $VTI_{AV}$ Doppler profiles are

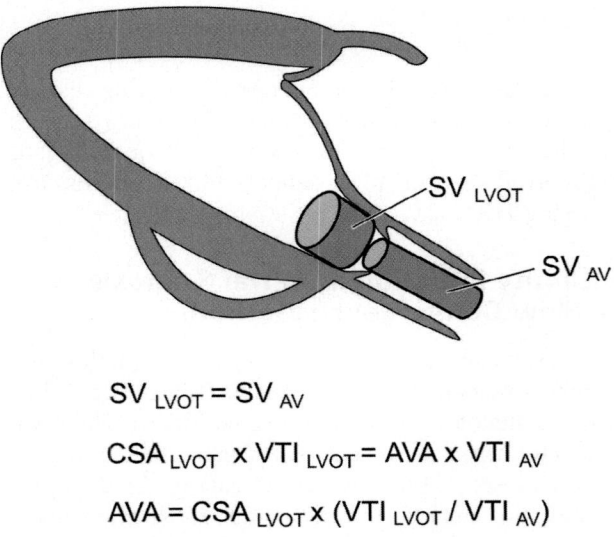

$$SV_{LVOT} = SV_{AV}$$
$$CSA_{LVOT} \times VTI_{LVOT} = AVA \times VTI_{AV}$$
$$AVA = CSA_{LVOT} \times (VTI_{LVOT} / VTI_{AV})$$

**FIGURE 22.22.** The continuity equation in aortic stenosis. Stroke volume across the LVOT must equal stroke volume across the aortic valve. *SV*, stroke volume; *CSA*, cross-sectional area; *VTI*, velocity-time integral; *v*, peak velocity; *LVOT*, left ventricular outflow tract; *AV*, aortic valve; *AVA*, aortic valve area.

similar in aortic stenosis, the ratio of the maximum velocities ($V_{LVOT}/V_{AV}$) may be substituted for the ratio of the velocity-time integrals ($VTI_{LVOT}/VTI_{AV}$) without introducing significant error into the AVA calculation:

$$AVA\ (cm^2) = 0.785 \times D_{LVOT}^2 \times (V_{LVOT} / V_{AV})$$

The primary concern in determining aortic valve area with the continuity equation using TEE is related to the possible underestimation of time-velocity integrals (or peak velocities) in the LVOT and/or aortic valve due to inadequate beam alignment.

## Continuity Equation in Mitral Regurgitation (the Flow Convergence Method)

In mitral regurgitation, flow across the regurgitant mitral orifice ($CSA_2$) must equal flow at a proximal isovelocity surface area ($CSA_1$). However, here the continuity equation is used in the form that states that two instantaneous flows, rather than two stroke volumes, must be equal:

$$Flow_1 = Flow_2$$
$$CSA_1 \times V_1 = CSA_2 \times V_2$$
$$CSA_2 = CSA_1 \times (V_1 / V_2)$$

Thus, the effective regurgitant orifice area for mitral regurgitation may be calculated using the continuity equation (as seen earlier in the section on the flow convergence method for calculation of regurgitant volume) (16):

$$EROA = PISA\ area \times (Aliasing\ velocity\ /\ Regurgitant\ velocity)$$
$$EROA\ (cm^2) = 6.28 \times r^2 \times (Aliasing\ velocity\ /\ V_{RJ})$$

where r is the PISA radius in cm and the aliasing velocity and the peak mitral regurgitant jet velocity ($V_{RJ}$) are in cm/s. This same technique has been used to quantify left-to-right atrial shunting after balloon mitral commissurotomy using TEE (32).

## Continuity Equation in Mitral Stenosis (the Flow Convergence Method)

In mitral stenosis, just as in mitral regurgitation, flow at a proximal isovelocity surface area ($CSA_1$) must equal flow across the stenotic mitral valve orifice ($CSA_2$). Thus, the mitral valve area may be calculated using the continuity equation as seen above, with one caveat. As the PISA proximal to a stenotic mitral valve is most often not a complete hemisphere, an angle correction factor is usually necessary (Fig. 22.23). The mitral valve area (MVA) is thus given by the following equation where r is the PISA radius, $V_{MS}$ is the peak velocity of the mitral stenosis jet, and $\alpha$ is the angle between the mitral leaflets (17):

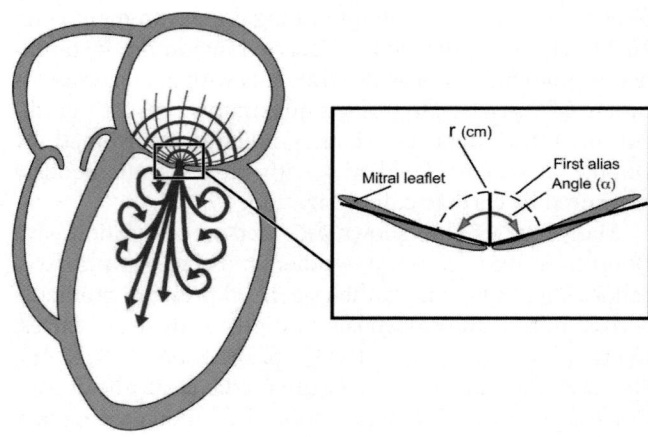

$$PISA = \frac{\alpha}{180} \times hemispheric\ area$$

**FIGURE 22.23.** Proximal isovelocity surface area (PISA) correction in mitral stenosis. The proximal flow convergence method may be used to calculate mitral valve area in mitral stenosis. However, because the PISA is not a complete hemisphere, an angle correction is necessary. r, PISA radius; $\alpha$, angle between mitral valve leaflets.

$$MVA = PISA\ area \times (Aliasing\ velocity\ /\ V_{MS}) \times (\alpha°/180°)$$
$$MVA\ (cm^2) = 6.28 \times r^2 \times (Aliasing\ velocity\ /\ V_{MS}) \times (\alpha°/180°)$$

where r is in cm and the aliasing velocity and peak mitral stenosis jet velocity ($V_{MS}$) are in cm/s.

## Pressure Half-time

The rate of decline in the pressure gradient across a diseased valve is related to the severity of the valvular abnormality (33). With valvular stenosis a slower rate of decline indicates more severe stenosis (Fig. 22.24), whereas with

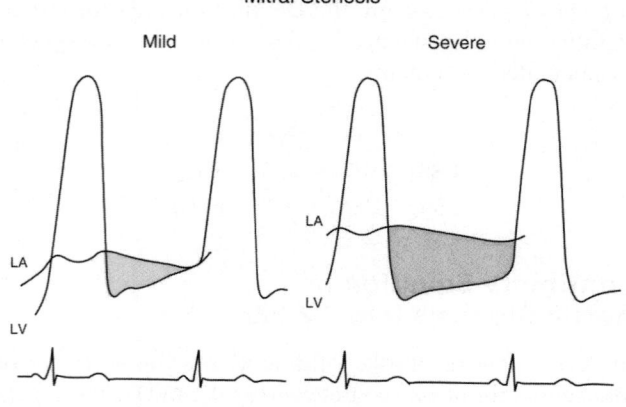

**FIGURE 22.24.** Rate of pressure decline across a stenotic valve. In mitral stenosis, a slower rate of pressure decline indicates more severe stenosis.

Aortic Regurgitation

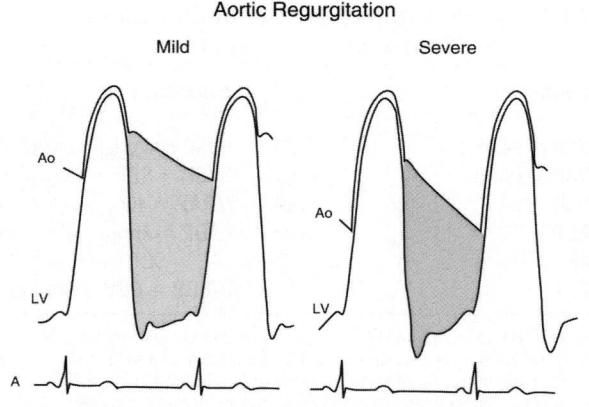

FIGURE 22.25. Rate of pressure decline across a regurgitant valve. In aortic regurgitation, a faster rate of pressure decline indicates more severe regurgitation.

valvular regurgitation a faster rate of decline indicates more severe regurgitation (Fig. 22.25). This rate of decline in the pressure gradient across a valve can be described by the pressure half-time.

The pressure half-time (PHT) is defined as the time required for the peak pressure gradient to decline by 50% (Fig. 22.26) (34). Due to the fixed relationship between velocity and pressure gradient, the pressure half-time will also be equal to the time required for the peak Doppler velocity to decline to that velocity divided by the $\sqrt{2}$ (35,36). Furthermore, the pressure half-time is also proportional to the deceleration time (DT), which is defined as the time required for the deceleration slope to reach the zero velocity baseline (Fig. 22.27):

$$\text{PHT (msec)} = 0.29 \times \text{DT (msec)}$$

The pressure half-time can be used to estimate the mitral valve area of stenotic native mitral valves using an empirically determined constant of 220:

$$\text{MVA (cm}^2) = 220 / \text{PHT (msec)}$$

Pressure half-time cannot be used for estimating the area of a normal mitral valve, as it is more dependent on LV compliance than the area of the valve. Furthermore, in patients with mitral stenosis, the pressure half-time will overestimate or underestimate valve area in a wide variety of circumstances (37). The pressure half-time will be decreased by an increase in cardiac output, an increase in LVEDP, more than mild aortic regurgitation, tachycardia, or restrictive LV filling, and therefore will overestimate mitral valve area. The pressure half-time may be increased by severe aortic regurgitation directed at the anterior mitral leaflet (causing a functional mitral stenosis) or impaired LV relaxation and therefore may underestimate

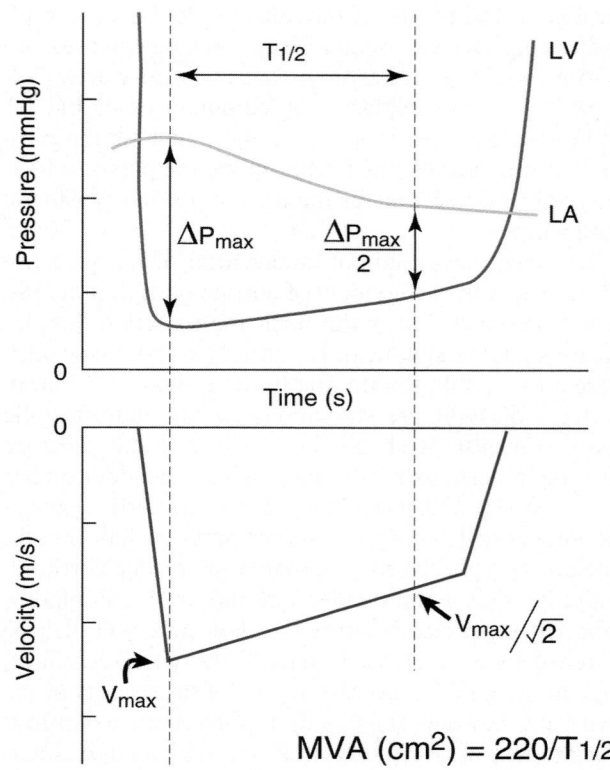

$$\text{MVA (cm}^2) = 220/T_{1/2}$$

FIGURE 22.26. The pressure half-time in mitral stenosis. The pressure half-time is the time interval required for the pressure gradient to drop by half. On the Doppler velocity curve it is the time interval required for the maximum velocity to drop to the maximum velocity/$\sqrt{2}$. *LA,* left atrium; *LV,* left ventricle; $T_{\frac{1}{2}}$, pressure half-time; *P,* pressure; *v,* peak velocity; *MVA,* mitral valve area.

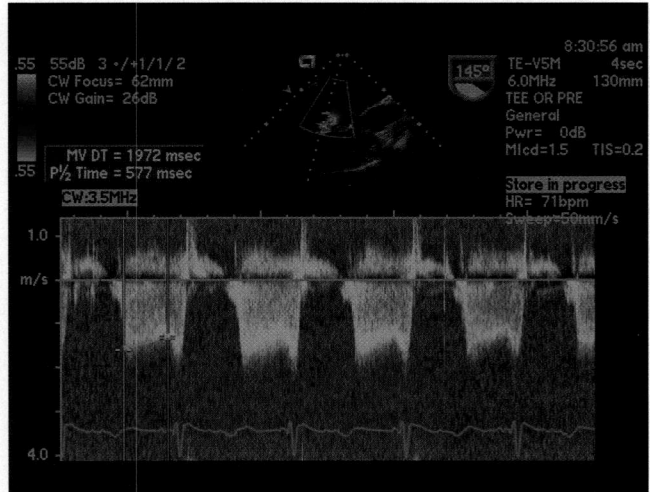

FIGURE 22.27. The deceleration time in mitral stenosis. The deceleration time is the time interval required for the deceleration slope of the Doppler velocity curve to reach the zero baseline. The deceleration time (as well as pressure half-time) can be measured using continuous wave Doppler from any midesophageal view of the mitral valve.

mitral area. The profile of the mitral inflow E wave is altered during atrioventricular block, making the pressure half-time an unreliable estimate of mitral valve area. Following mitral valvuloplasty the compliances of the LA and LV may be altered for several days, making the pressure half-time unreliable. Furthermore, the pressure half-time method overestimates the area of normal prosthetic mitral valves.

The other most common application of the pressure half-time is in the assessment of aortic regurgitation (38). The pressure half-time of the aortic regurgitation Doppler velocity signal is significantly shorter (< 250 msec) with severe aortic regurgitation due to the rapid equilibration of arterial diastolic pressure and left ventricular diastolic pressure (39,40). It should be noted that the pressure half-time in aortic regurgitation is also dependent on left ventricular size and compliance. The same aortic regurgitant volume will result in a shorter pressure half-time in acute aortic regurgitation compared to chronic aortic regurgitation due to the smaller size and lower compliance of the left ventricle. The pressure half-time will also be shortened by an increased systemic vascular resistance, which may lead to an overestimation of the severity of the aortic valve disease (41). Finally, in the presence of mitral regurgitation, pressure half-time is unreliable in estimating the severity of aortic regurgitation.

## DOPPLER DETERMINATION OF INTRACARDIAC PRESSURES

Estimation of an intracardiac or pulmonary pressure is possible by combining a pressure gradient calculated from a Doppler velocity using the simplified Bernoulli equation with a known or estimated pressure from a proximal or distal chamber (Table 22.3). Accuracy depends on proper alignment of the Doppler beam with the regurgitant jet, as well as a reliable determination or estimation of the pressure in the proximal or distal chambers.

### Estimation of RVSP (Fig. 22.28)

The peak velocity of the tricuspid regurgitant jet can be used to calculate the pressure difference between the right atrium and right ventricle using the simplified Bernoulli equation (42). The peak tricuspid regurgitant jet velocity can be obtained with continuous wave Doppler, using TEE from either the midesophageal RV inflow-outflow view, a modified midesophageal bicaval view, or the midesophageal four-chamber view. The right ventricular systolic pressure (RVSP) can be estimated by adding a known or estimated right atrial pressure (RAP) to the calculated RA-RV pressure gradient (43,44).

$$\text{RVSP} = \text{RA} = \text{RV systolic gradient} + \text{RA systolic pressure}$$
$$\text{RVSP (mm Hg)} = 4(v_{TR})^2 + \text{RAP (mm Hg)}$$

▶ **TABLE 22.3. Estimation of Pulmonary and Intracardiac Pressures**

| _Pressure_ | | _Equation_ |
|---|---|---|
| RVSP or PASP | (1) | $\text{RVSP} = 4(v_{TR})^2 + \text{RAP}$ |
| RVSP or PASP | (2) | $\text{RVSP} = \text{SBP} - 4(v_{VSD})^2$ |
| MPAP | (3) | $\text{MPAP} = 4(v_{early\,PR})^2 + \text{RAP}$ |
| PADP | (4) | $\text{PADP} = 4(v_{late\,PR})^2 + \text{RAP}$ |
| LAP | (5) | $\text{LAP} = \text{SBP} - 4(v_{MR})^2$ |
| LVEDP | (6) | $\text{LVEDP} = \text{DBP} - 4(v_{end\,AR})^2$ |

Equations (1) and (2) are invalid in the presence of pulmonic stenosis or RVOT obstruction for estimation of PASP. Equations (2) and (5) are invalid in the presence of aortic stenosis or LVOT obstruction. _RVSP,_ right ventricular systolic pressure; _PASP,_ pulmonary artery systolic pressure; _MPAP,_ mean pulmonary artery pressure; _PADP,_ pulmonary artery diastolic pressure; _LAP,_ left atrial pressure; _RAP,_ right atrial pressure; _LVEDP,_ left ventricular end-diastolic pressure; _v,_ peak velocity; _TR,_ tricuspid regurgitation; _PR,_ pulmonic regurgitation; _MR,_ mitral regurgitation; _AR,_ aortic regurgitation; _SBP,_ systolic blood pressure; _DBP,_ diastolic blood pressure; _RVOT,_ right ventricular outflow tract; _LVOT,_ left ventricular outflow tract.

where the peak tricuspid regurgitant jet velocity ($v_{TR}$) is given in m/s. If a direct measurement of right atrial pressure (or central venous pressure) is not available, it may be estimated in spontaneously breathing patients as seen in Table 22.4.

Alternatively, RVSP may be calculated in a patient with a VSD and a left-to-right shunt by subtracting the LV-RV pressure difference from the systolic blood pressure,

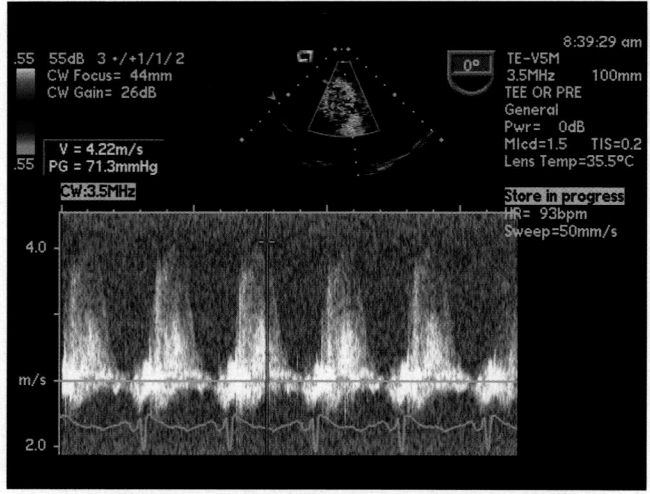

**FIGURE 22.28.** Measurement of tricuspid regurgitant jet velocity for estimation of RVSP or PASP. The peak tricuspid regurgitant jet velocity can be obtained with continuous wave Doppler using TEE from either the midesophageal RV inflow-outflow view, a modified midesophageal bicaval view, or the midesophageal four-chamber view as seen in this example of a patient with pulmonary hypertension. _RVSP,_ right ventricular systolic pressure; _PASP,_ pulmonary artery systolic pressure.

▶ **TABLE 22.4. Estimation of Right Atrial Pressure**

| Inferior Vena Cava | Change with Negative Inspiration (i.e., sniff) | Estimated Right Atrial Pressure |
|---|---|---|
| Small (< 1.5 cm) | Collapse | 0–5 mm Hg |
| Normal (1.5–2.5 cm) | Decrease by > 50% | 5–10 mm Hg |
| Normal (1.5–2.5 cm) | Decrease by < 50% | 10–15 mm Hg |
| Dilated (> 2.5 cm) | Decrease by < 50% | 15–20 mm Hg |
| Dilated (with dilated hepatic veins) | No change | > 20 mm Hg |

which is a good estimate of LV systolic pressure in most patients:

$$RVSP = \text{LV systolic pressure} - \text{VSD systolic gradient}$$
$$RVSP \text{ (mm Hg)} = \text{systolic blood pressure (mm Hg)} - 4(v_{VSD})^2$$

where the peak velocity across the VSD ($v_{VSD}$) is given in m/s. In the presence of aortic stenosis or LVOT obstruction, systolic blood pressure will not approximate LV systolic pressure and this formula is invalid.

## Estimation of PASP

In the absence of pulmonic stenosis or RVOT obstruction, RV systolic pressure and pulmonary artery systolic pressure (PASP) are essentially identical, giving the formula commonly used to estimate pulmonary artery systolic pressure (42):

$$PASP \text{ (mm Hg)} = RVSP \text{ (mm Hg)} = 4(v_{TR})^2 + RAP \text{ (mm Hg)}$$

where the peak tricuspid regurgitant jet velocity ($v_{TR}$) is given in m/s.

## Estimation of PADP

The late peak velocity of the pulmonic regurgitant jet can be used to calculate the pressure difference between the pulmonary artery and right ventricle at end-diastole using the simplified Bernoulli equation. The late peak pulmonic regurgitant jet velocity is obtained with continuous wave Doppler using multiplane TEE from a transgastric RV inflow-outflow view with the transducer rotated from 110° to 150° and the probe turned to the right. (Alternatively, it can be obtained from a short-axis view of the aortic arch or ascending aorta if the pulmonic regurgitant jet is visualized adequately to be interrogated with continuous wave Doppler.) The pulmonary artery diastolic pressure (PADP) can be estimated by adding a known or estimated

right atrial pressure, which is equal to RV pressure during diastole, to the calculated PA-RV pressure gradient during late diastole (45):

$$PADP = \text{PA-RV late diastolic gradient} + \text{RV diastolic pressure}$$
$$PADP \text{ (mm Hg)} = 4(v_{late\ PR})^2 + RAP \text{ (mm Hg)}$$

where the late peak velocity of the pulmonic regurgitant ($v_{late\ PR}$) is given in m/s.

## Estimation of MPAP

The early peak velocity of the pulmonic regurgitant jet can be used to calculate the pressure difference between the pulmonary artery and right ventricle in early diastole using the simplified Bernoulli equation. The early peak pulmonic regurgitant jet velocity is obtained with continuous wave Doppler using multiplane TEE from a transgastric RV inflow-outflow view with the transducer rotated from 110° to 150° and the probe turned to the right. (Alternatively, it can be obtained from a short-axis view of the aortic arch or ascending aorta if the pulmonic regurgitant jet is well visualized in the RVOT.) The mean pulmonary artery pressure (MPAP) can be estimated by adding a known or estimated right atrial pressure, which is equal to RV pressure during diastole, to the calculated PA-RV pressure gradient during early diastole (42):

$$MPAP = \text{PA-RV early diastolic gradient} + \text{RV diastolic pressure}$$
$$MPAP \text{ (mm Hg)} = 4(v_{early\ PR})^2 + RAP \text{ (mm Hg)}$$

where the early peak velocity of the pulmonic regurgitant jet ($v_{early\ PR}$) is given in m/s.

## Estimation of LAP (Fig. 22.29)

The peak velocity of the mitral regurgitant jet can be used to calculate the pressure difference between the left atrium and left ventricle using the simplified Bernoulli equation. The peak mitral regurgitant jet velocity is obtained with continuous wave Doppler by TEE from any midesophageal view of the mitral valve. The left atrial pressure (LAP) can be estimated by subtracting the LA-LV pressure gradient from the LV systolic pressure (46,47):

$$LAP = \text{LV systolic pressure} - \text{LA-LV systolic gradient}$$
$$LAP \text{ (mm Hg)} = \text{systolic blood pressure (mm Hg)} - 4(v_{MR})^2$$

where the peak velocity of the mitral regurgitant ($v_{MR}$) is given in m/s. In the presence of aortic stenosis or LVOT obstruction, systolic blood pressure will not approximate LV systolic pressure and this formula is invalid.

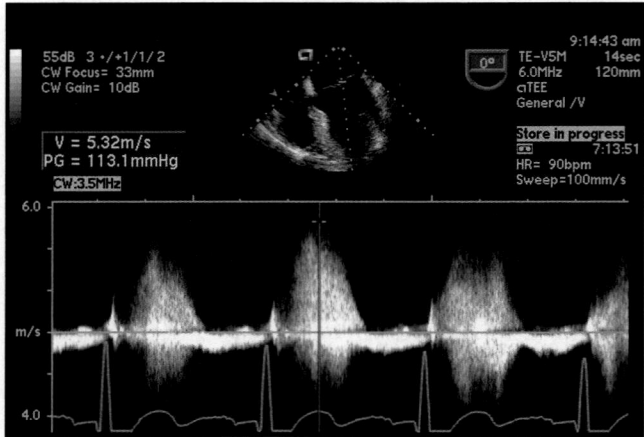

**FIGURE 22.29.** Measurement of mitral regurgitant jet velocity for estimation of LAP. The peak mitral regurgitant jet velocity is obtained with continuous wave Doppler by TEE from any midesophageal view of the mitral valve. *LAP,* left atrial pressure.

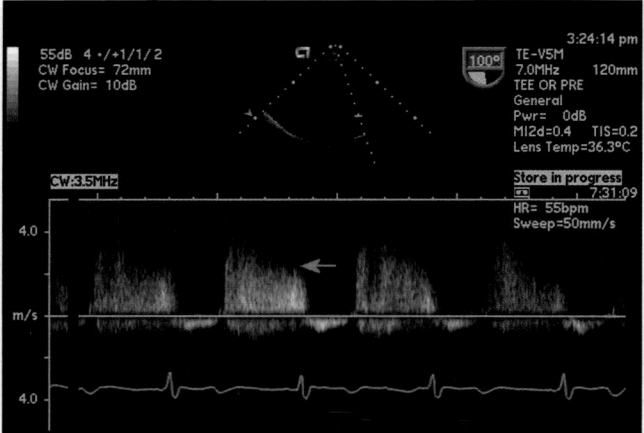

**FIGURE 22.30.** Measurement of the late peak velocity of the aortic regurgitant jet for estimation of LVEDP. The peak end-diastolic velocity of the aortic regurgitation jet (located at the *arrow* in this figure) is determined with the continuous wave Doppler beam placed through the aortic valve from a transgastric long-axis or deep transgastric long-axis view using TEE. *LVEDP,* left ventricular end-diastolic pressure.

## Estimation of LVEDP (Fig. 22.30)

The peak end-diastolic velocity of the aortic regurgitation jet can be used to calculate the difference between the diastolic aortic pressure and the left ventricular end-diastolic pressure using the simplified Bernoulli equation. The peak end-diastolic velocity of the aortic regurgitation jet is determined with the continuous wave Doppler beam placed through the aortic valve from a transgastric long-axis or deep transgastric long-axis view using TEE. The left ventricular end-diastolic pressure (LVEDP) is estimated by subtracting the end-diastolic aortic-LV pressure gradient from the aortic diastolic pressure (47):

$$LVEDP = \text{aortic diastolic pressure} - \text{end-diastolic aortic-LV}$$
$$\text{pressure gradient}$$
$$LVEDP \text{ (mm Hg)} = \text{diastolic blood pressure (mm Hg)} - 4(v_{end\,AR})^2$$

where the peak end-diastolic velocity of the aortic regurgitation jet ($v_{end}$ AR) is given in m/s.

## DOPPLER MEASUREMENT OF dp/dt

The rate of pressure increase within the left ventricle during isovolumic contraction, LV dp/dt, has been used as a measure of left ventricular systolic function. As left atrial pressure does not change significantly during isovolumic contraction, changes in the velocity of the mitral regurgitation jet reflect changes in left ventricular pressure. Thus, a continuous-wave Doppler interrogation of the mitral regurgitant jet can be used to determine LV dp/dt. Usually, LV dp/dt is calculated from the time interval be-

tween 1 m/s and 3 m/s on the mitral regurgitation Doppler velocity profile using the simplified Bernoulli equation to calculate the LA-LV pressure gradients (Fig. 22.31). The following formula is used to calculate LV dp/dt:

$$LV \ dp/dt = [4(3 \ m/s)^2 - 4(1 \ m/s)^2] / dt$$
$$LV \ dp/dt = [36 \ mm \ Hg - 4 \ mm \ Hg] / dt$$
$$LV \ dp/dt = 32 \ mm \ Hg / dt$$

where dt is the time interval in sec for the mitral regurgitant jet velocity to increase from 1 m/s to 3 m/s. Thus, a longer time interval indicates a reduced LV dp/dt and reduced systolic function. LV dp/dt is normally ≥ 1,200 mm Hg/sec with values < 1000 mm Hg/sec corresponding to reduced left ventricular systolic function. Doppler-derived LV dp/dt appears to correlate well with catheter-derived LV dp/dt (48,49). Postoperative LV systolic function has been correlated with preoperative LV dp/dt in patients undergoing mitral valve surgery (50).

RV dp/dt can also be calculated from a continuous wave Doppler interrogation of the tricuspid regurgitant jet; however, the following formula is used:

$$RV \ dp/dt = [4(2 \ m/s)^2 - 4(1 \ m/s)^2] / dt$$
$$RV \ dp/dt = [16 \ mm \ Hg - 4 \ mm \ Hg] / dt$$
$$RV \ dp/dt = 12 \ mm \ Hg / dt$$

where dt is the time interval in sec for the mitral regurgitant jet to increase from 1 m/s to 2 m/s.

▶ TABLE 22.5. **Classic M-Mode and 2-D Echocardiographic Signs of Hemodynamic Abnormalities**

| M-mode or 2-D finding | Hemodynamic abnormality |
|---|---|
| Systolic anterior motion of mitral valve | Dynamic LVOT obstruction |
| Midsystolic aortic valve closure | Dynamic LVOT obstruction |
| Systolic fluttering of aortic valve | Fixed LVOT obstruction (i.e., subaortic membrane) |
| Diastolic fluttering of mitral valve | Aortic regurgitation |
| Midsystolic pulmonary valve closure | Pulmonary hypertension |
| Dilated RV with D-shaped LV | Elevated RV systolic pressure |
| Abnormal ventricular septal motion | Constrictive pericarditis |
| Diastolic RA and RV wall collapse | Cardiac tamponade |
| Spontaneous echo contrast in LA | Low cardiac output |
| Dilated IVC without inspiratory collapse | Increased RA pressure |
| Constant atrial septal bowing into LA | RA pressure ≫ LA pressure |
| Constant atrial septal bowing into RA | LA pressure ≫ RA pressure |

*LVOT,* left ventricular outflow tract; *RV,* right ventricle; *LV,* left ventricle; *RA,* right atrium; *LA,* left atrium; *IVC,* inferior vena cava.

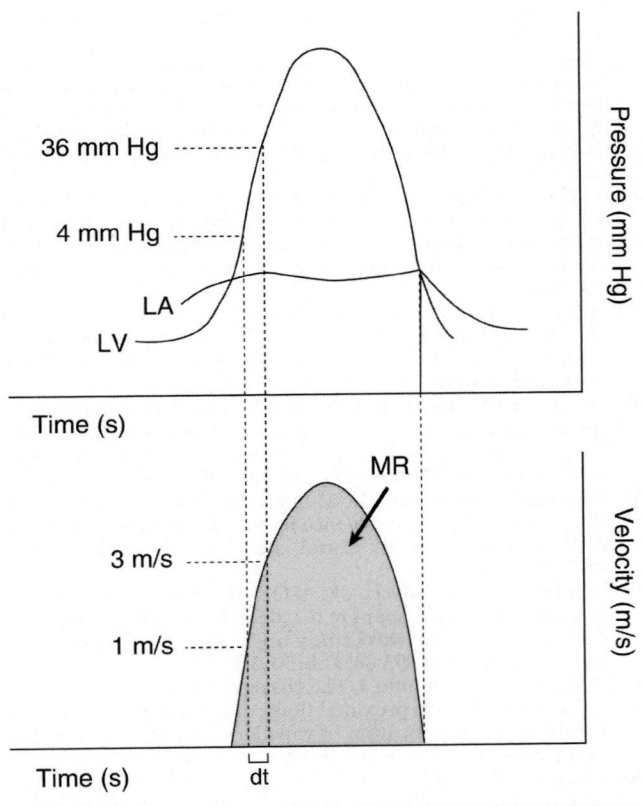

**FIGURE 22.31.** Left ventricular dp/dt. Left ventricular and left atrial pressure tracings are shown along with the corresponding Doppler velocity tracing for mitral regurgitation (as from a midesophageal view). Dp/dt is calculated from the time interval it takes the mitral regurgitant jet to increase from 1 m/s to 3 m/s. *dp/dt,* rate of pressure increase (in the left ventricle) during isovolumic contraction.

## ECHOCARDIOGRAPHIC SIGNS OF HEMODYNAMIC ABNORMALITIES

There are numerous M-mode and 2-D echocardiographic signs of hemodynamic abnormalities (51). Some of these "classic" echocardiographic signs are listed in Table 22.5. Furthermore, pulsed wave Doppler velocity patterns from the mitral valve inflow and pulmonary veins can be used to estimate left atrial and left ventricular pressures (52–58). These techniques will be discussed further in other chapters.

### KEY POINTS

- The Doppler velocity-time integral can be used to calculate stroke volume at a specific location:

$$SV = CSA \times VTI$$

- Doppler-derived stroke volumes can be used to determine cardiac output, the pulmonary-to-systemic shunt ratio (Qp/Qs), and regurgitant volume. However, propagation of errors may lead to a significant error in either the pulmonary-to-systemic shunt ratio (Qp/Qs) or a regurgitant volume calculated using Doppler stroke volumes using TEE.
- The proximal flow convergence method can be used to determine regurgitant severity based on the maximal regurgitant orifice area:

$$EROA = (6.28 \times r^2 \times \text{Aliasing velocity}) / V_{RJ}$$

This method may overestimate the actual hemodynamic impact of the regurgitant lesion as the degree of regurgitation is not constant throughout systole in many patients. In spite of this and other limitations, the flow convergence method is useful in evaluating regurgitation as it is quantitative, relatively simple to perform, and applicable in a large number of patients with valvular regurgitation.

- The continuity equation is another expression of the principle of conservation of mass (flow through the LVOT must equal flow through the aortic valve):

$$AVA = CSA_{LVOT} \times (VTI_{LVOT} / VTI_{AV})$$

The primary concern in determining aortic valve area with the continuity equation using TEE is related to the possible underestimation of time-velocity integrals (or peak velocities) in the LVOT and/or aortic valve due to inadequate beam alignment.

- With valvular stenosis a longer pressure half-time indicates more severe stenosis, whereas with valvular regurgitation a shorter pressure half-time indicates more severe regurgitation. The pressure half-time can be used to estimate the mitral valve area of a stenotic native mitral valve using the following empirically derived formula:

$$MVA \ (cm^2) = 220 / PHT \ (msec)$$

- Estimation of an intracardiac or pulmonary pressure is possible by combining a pressure gradient calculated from a Doppler velocity using the simplified Bernoulli equation with a known or estimated pressure from a proximal or distal chamber. Example:

$$RVSP \ (mm \ Hg) = 4(v_{TR})^2 + RAP \ (mm \ Hg)$$

## REFERENCES

1. Callahan MJ, Tajik AJ, Su-Fan Q, et al. Validation of instantaneous pressure gradients measured by continuous wave Doppler in experimentally induced aortic stenosis. Am J Cardiol 1985;56:989–93.
2. Currie PJ, Seward JB, Chan KL. Continuous wave Doppler determination of right ventricular pressure: a simultaneous Doppler-catheterization study in 127 patients. J Am Coll Cardiol 1985;6:750–56.
3. Currie PJ, Hagler DJ, Seward JB, et al. Instantaneous pressure gradient: a simultaneous Doppler and dual catheter correlative study. J Am Coll Cardiol 1986;7:800–6.
4. Burstow DJ, Nishimura RA, Bailey KR, et al. Continuous wave Doppler echocardiographic measurement of prosthetic valve gradients: a simultaneous Doppler-catheter correlative study. Circulation 1989;80:504–14.
5. Zoghbi WA, Quinones MA. Determination of cardiac output by Doppler echocardiography: a critical appraisal. Herz 1986;11:258–68.
6. Savino JS, Troianos CA, Aukburg S, et al. Measurements of pulmonary blood flow with transesophageal two-dimensional and Doppler echocardiography. Anesthesiology 1991; 75:445–51.
7. Muhiuden IA, Kuecherer HF, Lee E, et al. Intraoperative estimation of cardiac output by transesophageal pulsed Doppler echocardiography. Anesthesiology 1991;74:9–14.
8. Gorcsan III J, Diana P, Ball BS, et al. Intraoperative determination of cardiac output by transesophageal continuous wave Doppler. Am Heart J 1992;123:171–76.
9. Darmon PL, Hillel Z, Mogtader, et al. Cardiac output by transesophageal echocardiography using continuous-wave Doppler across the aortic valve. Anesthesiology 1994;80: 796–805.
10. Maslow AD, Haering J, Comunale M, et al. Measurement of cardiac output by pulsed wave Doppler of the right ventricular outflow tract. Anesth Analg 1996;83:466–71.
11. Perrino AC, Harris SN, Luther MA. Intraoperative determination of cardiac output using multiplane transesophageal echocardiography: a comparison to thermodilution. Anesthesiology 1998;89:350–57.
12. Stewart WJ, Jiang L, Mich R, et al. Variable effects of changes in flow rate through the aortic, pulmonary, and mitral valves on valve area and flow velocity; impact on quantitative Doppler flow calculations. J Am Coll Cardiol 1985; 6:653–62.
13. Quinones MA, Otto CM, Stoddard M, et al. Recommendations for the quantification of Doppler echocardiography: a report from the Doppler Quantification Task Force of the Nomenclature and Standards Committee of the American Society of Echocardiography. J Am Soc Echocardiogr 2002;15:167–84.
14. Valdes-Cruz LM, Horowitz S, Mesel E, et al. A pulsed Doppler echocardiographic method for calculating pulmonary and systemic blood flow in trial level shunts: validation studies in animals and initial human experience. Circulation 1984; 69:80–86.
15. Rokey R, Sterling LL, Zohgbi WA, et al. Determination of regurgitation fraction in isolated mitral or aortic regurgitation by pulsed Doppler two-dimensional echocardiography. J Am Coll Cardiol 1986;7:1273–78.
16. Bargiggia GS, Tronconi L, Sahn DJ, et al. A new method for quantitation of mitral regurgitation based on color flow Doppler imaging of flow convergence proximal to regurgitant orifice. Circulation 1991;84:1481–89.
17. Rodriguez L, Thomas, JD, Monterroso V, et al. Validation of the proximal flow convergence method: calculation of orifice area in patients with mitral stenosis. Circulation 1993; 88:1157–65.
18. Vandervoort PM, Rivera JM, Mele D, et al. Application of color Doppler flow mapping to calculate effective regurgitant orifice area. An in vitro study and initial clinical observations. Circulation 1993;88(3):1150–56.
19. Rodriguez L, Anconina J, Flaschskampf FA, et al. Impact of finite orifice size on proximal flow convergence. Implications for Doppler quantification of valvular regurgitation. Circulation Research 1992;70(5):923–30.
20. Pu M, Vandervoort P, Griffin BP, Leung DY, et al. Quantification of mitral regurgitation by the proximal convergence method using transesophageal echocardiography. Clinical validation of a geometric correction for proximal flow constraint. Circulation 1995;92(8):2169–77.
21. Vandervoort PM, Thoreau DH, Rivera JM, et al. Automated flow rate calculations based on digital analysis of flow convergence proximal to regurgitant orifices. J Am Coll Card 1993;22(2):535–41.
22. Schwammenthal E, Chen C, Benning F, Block M, et al. Dynamics of mitral regurgitant flow and orifice area. Physiologic application of the proximal flow convergence method:

clinical data and experimental testing. Circulation 1994; 90(1):307–22.

23. Pu M, Prior DL, Fan X, et al. Calculation of mitral regurgitant orifice area with the use of the simplified proximal convergence method: initial clinical application. J Am Soc Echocardiogr 2001;14(3):180–85.

24. Hatle L, Angleson B. Doppler ultrasound in cardiology: physical principles and clinical applications. 2nd ed. Philadelphia: Lea & Febiger, 1985.

25. Nishimura RA, Miller FA Jr, Callahan MJ, et al. Doppler echocardiography: theory, instrumentation, technique, and application. Mayo Clin Proc 1985;60:321–43.

26. Perrino AC, Reeves ST. A practical approach to transesophageal echocardiography. 1st ed, Philadelphia: Lippincott Williams & Wilkins, 2003.

27. Hatle L, Brubakk A, Tromsdal A, et al. Noninvasive assessment of pressure drop in mitral stenosis by Doppler ultrasound. Br Heart J 1978;40:131–40.

28. Teirstein PS, Yock PG, Popp RL. The accuracy of Doppler ultrasound measurements of pressure gradients across irregular, dual, and tunnel-like obstructions to blood flow. Circulation 1985;72:577–84.

29. Nishimura RA, Rihal CS, Tajik AJ, et al. Accurate measurement of the transmitral gradient in patients with mitral stenosis: a simultaneous catheterization and Doppler echocardiographic study. J Am Coll Cardiol 1994;24:152–58.

30. Skjaerpe T, Hegrenaese L, Hatle L. Noninvasive estimation of valve area in patients with aortic stenosis by Doppler ultrasound and two-dimensional echocardiography. Circulation 1985;72:810–18.

31. Blumberg FC, Pfeifer M, Holmer SR, et al. Quantification of aortic stenosis in mechanically ventilated patients using multiplane transesophageal Doppler echocardiography. Chest 1998;114:94–97.

32. Rittoo D, Sutherland GR, Shaw TR. Quantification of left-to-right atrial shunting defect size after balloon mitral commissurotomy using biplane transesophageal echocardiography, color flow Doppler mapping, and the principle of proximal flow convergence. Circulation 1993;87:1591–1603.

33. Nakatani S, Masuyama T, Kodama K, et al. Value and limitations of Doppler echocardiography in the quantification of stenotic mitral valve area: comparison of the pressure half-time and the continuity equation methods. Circulation 1988; 77:78–85.

34. Libanoff AJ, Rodbard S. Atrioventricular pressure half-time: measurement of mitral valve orifice area. Circulation 1968; 38:144–50.

35. Hatle L, Angelson B, Tromsdal A. Noninvasive assessment of atrioventricular pressure half-time by Doppler ultrasound. Circulation 1979;60:1096–1104.

36. Thomas JD, Weyman AE. Doppler mitral pressure half-time: a clinical tool in search of theoretical justification. J Am Coll Cardiol 1987;10:923–29.

37. Sidebotham D, Merry A, Legget M. Practical perioperative transesophageal echocardiography. 1st ed. London: Butterworth-Heinemann, 2003.

38. Teague SM, Heinsimer JA, Anderson JL, et al. Quantification of aortic regurgitation utilizing continuous wave Doppler ultrasound. J Am Coll Cardiol 1986;8(3)592–99.

39. Samstad SO, Hegrenaes L, Skjaerpe T, et al. Half-time of the diastolic aortoventricular pressure difference by continuous wave Doppler ultrasound: a measure of the severity of aortic regurgitation? Br Heart J 1989;61:336–43.

40. Grayburn PA, Handshoe R, Smith MD, et al. Quantitative assessment of the hemodynamic consequences of aortic regurgitation by means of continuous wave Doppler recordings. J Am Coll Cardiol 1987;10:135–41.

41. Griffin BP, Flaschskampf FA, Reinold SC, et al. Relationship of aortic regurgitant velocity slope and pressure half-time to severity of aortic regurgitation under changing hemodynamic conditions. Eur Heart J 1994;15(5):681–85.

42. Come PC. Echocardiographic recognition of pulmonary arterial disease and determination of its cause. Am J Med 1988; 84:384–93.

43. Yock PG, Popp RL. Noninvasive estimation of right ventricular systolic pressure by Doppler ultrasound in patients with tricuspid regurgitation. Circulation 1984;70:657–62.

44. Chan KL, Currie PJ, Seward JB, et al. Comparison of three Doppler ultrasound methods in the prediction of pulmonary artery pressure. J Am Coll Cardiol 1987;9:549–54.

45. Lee RT, Lord CP, Plappert T, et al. Prospective Doppler echocardiographic evaluation of pulmonary artery diastolic pressure in the medical intensive care unit. Am J Cardiol 1989;64:1366–77.

46. Gorcsan III J, Snow FR, Paulsen W, et al. Noninvasive estimation of left atrial pressure in patients with congestive heart failure and mitral regurgitation by Doppler echocardiography. AM Heart J 1991;121:858–63.

47. Nishimura RA, Tajik AJ. Determination of left-sided pressure gradients by utilizing Doppler aortic and mitral regurgitation signals: validation by simultaneous dual catheter and Doppler studies. J Am Coll Cardiol 1988;11:317–21.

48. Bargiggia GS, Bertucci C, Recusani F, et al. A new method for estimating left ventricular dp/dt by continuous wave Doppler echocardiography: validation studies at cardiac catheterization. Circulation 1989;80:1287–92.

49. Chung NS, Nishimura RA, Holmes DR Jr, et al. Measurement of left ventricular dp/dt by simultaneous Doppler echocardiography and cardiac catheterization. J Am Soc Echocardiogr 1992;5:147–52.

50. Leung DY, Griffin BP, Stewart WJ, et al. Left ventricular function after valve repair for chronic mitral regurgitation: predictive value of preoperative assessment of contractile reserve by exercise echocardiography. J Am Coll Cardiol 1996;28:1198–1205.

51. Oh JK, Seward JB, Tajik AJ. The echo manual, 2nd ed. Philadelphia: Lippincott-Raven, 1999.

52. Moller JE, Poulsen SH, Songderfaard E, et al. Preload dependence of color M-mode Doppler flow propagation velocity in controls and in patients with left ventricular dysfunction. J Am Soc Echocardiogr 2000;13:902–9.

53. Gonzalez-Viaches F, Ares M, Ayeula J, et al. Combined use of pulsed and color M-mode Doppler echocardiography for the estimation of pulmonary capillary wedge pressure: an empirical approach based on an analytical relation. J Am Coll Cardiol 1999;34:515–23.

54. Garcia MJ, Ares MA, Asher C, et al. An index of early left ventricular filling that combined with pulsed Doppler peak E velocity may estimate capillary wedge pressure. J Am Coll Cardiol 1997;29:448–54.

55. Oh JK, Appleton CP, Hatle LK, et al. The noninvasive assessment of left ventricular diastolic function with two-dimensional and Doppler echocardiography. J Am Soc Echocardiogr 1997;10:246–70.

56. Nagueh SF, Kopelen HA, Quinones MA. Assessment of left ventricular filling pressures by Doppler in the presence of atrial fibrillation. Circulation 1996;94:1238–2145.

57. Nishimura RA, Housmans PR, Hatle LK, et al. Assessment of diastolic function of the heart: background and current applications of Doppler echocardiography. Part 2. Clinical studies. Mayo Clin Proc 1989;64:181–294.

58. Temporelli PL, Scapellato F, Corra U, et al. Estimation of pulmonary wedge pressure by transmitral Doppler in patients with chronic heart failure and atrial fibrillation. Am J Cardiol 1999;83:724–7.

## QUESTIONS

1. Which of the following statements concerning determination of stroke volume using Doppler is *incorrect*?

   A. VTI and area should be determined at the same location.

   B. The spatial flow velocity profile should be flat.

C. VTI should be determined with the ultrasound beam parallel to blood flow.

D. VTI and area should both be determined during systole.

2. Which of the following statements regarding determination of mitral regurgitation severity using the proximal flow convergence method is *incorrect*?

A. Because the regurgitant orifice is not infinitely small, the hemispheric shape of PISAs is not maintained all the way to the orifice and thus, flow underestimation may occur.

B. Flow may be constrained by structures proximal to the regurgitant orifice such that PISAs are not full hemispheres leading to flow overestimation.

C. It is often difficult to locate the exact center of the regurgitant orifice resulting in an error in the measured PISA radius.

D. Results using the simplified method significantly overestimate mitral regurgitation severity compared with the standard method.

3. Which of the following statements related to the determination of aortic stenosis severity is *incorrect*?

A. In the setting of aortic stenosis and significant LVOT obstruction (dynamic or fixed), the simplified Bernoulli equation will overestimate the aortic valve pressure gradient.

B. Mean gradients determined by Doppler have correlated well with those simultaneously measured by cardiac catheterization.

C. The primary concern in determining aortic valve area with the continuity equation using TEE is related to the possible underestimation of the area of the LVOT.

D. Since the shapes of the $VTI_{LVOT}$ and $VTI_{AV}$ Doppler profiles are similar, the ratio of the maximum velocities ($V_{LVOT}/V_{AV}$) may be substituted for the ratio of the velocity-time integrals ($VTI_{LVOT}/VTI_{AV}$) in the continuity equation without introducing significant errors into the aortic valve area calculation.

4. Which of the following statements concerning determination of mitral valve area using the pressure half-time method is *incorrect*?

A. Pressure half-time cannot be used for estimating the area of a normal mitral valve as it is more dependent on LV compliance than the area of the valve.

B. The pressure half-time will be decreased by more than mild aortic regurgitation and therefore will overestimate mitral valve area.

C. Following mitral valvuloplasty the compliances of the LA and LV may be altered for several days, making the pressure half-time method unreliable.

D. The pressure half-time method underestimates the area of normal prosthetic mitral valves.

5. Which of the following statements regarding estimation of an intracardiac or pulmonary pressure is *incorrect*?

A. Estimation of the PASP using an estimated (or measured) RAP and the peak velocity of the tricuspid regurgitant jet is not valid in the setting of RVOT obstruction.

B. Estimation of RVSP from the systemic systolic blood pressure and the peak velocity across the VSD is not valid in the setting of significant aortic regurgitation.

C. Estimations of LAP from the systemic systolic blood pressure and the peak velocity of the mitral regurgitant jet are not valid in the setting of significant LVOT obstruction.

D. LVEDP can be estimated from the peak end-diastolic velocity of the aortic regurgitation jet and the systemic diastolic pressure.

# Surgical Decision Making in Coronary Artery Disease

# Assessment of Myocardial Viability

*Frank W. Dupont and Solomon Aronson*

## DEFINITIONS

*Viable* means capable of living. One definition of myocardial viability is histological because viability is defined by the presence of living myocytes (1). During myocardial infarction viability is lost. A nonviable myocardium is one with infarcted (necrosed) tissue. Viable myocardium may be normal or dysfunctional in the reversible state of acute ischemia, stunning, or hibernation.

### Myocardial Ischemia

As early as 1935, it was known that total ischemia stops myocardial contraction (2). Four abnormal contraction patterns develop in sequence: *dyssynchrony*—dissociation of adjacent segments in the course of contraction; hypokinesis; akinesis; and dyskinesis (3). The proportional decrease in regional myocardial blood flow and contractility is typical of acute myocardial ischemia (perfusion–contraction match). Reperfusion within less than 10 minutes after coronary occlusion restores cardiac performance completely.

### Myocardial Stunning

In the classic model of myocardial stunning, reperfusion after coronary occlusion lasting less than 15–20 minutes is associated with postischemic contractile dysfunction (4). Myocardial stunning is the fully reversible mechanical dysfunction that persists up to 24 hours after reperfusion despite restoration of normal or near-normal coronary blood flow (perfusion–contraction mismatch) (5–7). The severity of stunning is always greater in the subendocardial layers of the left ventricular wall than in the subepicardial layers (8). The diagnosis of stunning requires demonstration of two conditions: reversibility of the contractile abnormality and evidence of normal or near-normal coronary blood flow in the dysfunctional myocardium. Myocardial stunning is caused in part by injurious events during ischemia and reperfusion, so this contractile dysfunction can be considered a form of ischemia-reperfusion injury.

### Hibernating Myocardium

Resting wall-motion abnormalities in patients with coronary artery disease (CAD) improve after administration of an inotropic agent (9). In 1978, Diamond et al. (10) introduced the concept of hibernating myocardium: Sometimes dramatic improvement in segmental left ventricular function after coronary artery bypass surgery suggested that the "ischemic non-infarcted myocardium can exist in a state of function hibernation." In 1985, Rahimtoola (11) used the phrase *hibernating myocardium* to describe impaired ventricular function at rest because of reduced coronary blood flow that was restored when blood flow was improved or oxygen demand was reduced (12).

Myocardial hibernation can be defined as reversible left ventricular dysfunction due to chronic CAD (13). It is a complex, progressive, and dynamic phenomenon that is initiated by repeat episodes of ischemia. Patients with hibernating myocardium have normal or slightly reduced myocardial blood flow and limited coronary flow reserve. Hibernation involves repetitive postischemic dysfunction, perpetuated by renewed episodes of ischemia and changes in cell phenotype induced by ischemia-reperfusion, which eventually culminates in dramatic morphological alterations. Tissue necrosis is not substantial, although pathognomonic morphological changes have been found. A hibernating myocardium reveals residual contractile reserve with adrenergic stimulation. Regional and global ventricular function can improve in a hibernating myocardium after revascularization.

## THE CLINICAL IMPORTANCE OF ASSESSING MYOCARDIAL VIABILITY

The assessment of myocardial viability in the perioperative setting has two applications:

- To differentiate hibernating myocardium (reversible) from one with necrotic tissue (irreversible) for risk stratification and guidance of therapeutic decisions
- To differentiate acute myocardial ischemia from stunning

CAD is the most common cause of heart failure in the Western world, accounting for up to 60% of cases (14). Because of new therapeutic strategies that reduce the mortality associated with acute coronary syndromes, more patients suffer from the long-term sequelae of this condition. For many years, the functional sequelae of chronic CAD were considered irreversible and amenable only to palliative therapy; however, chronic left ventricular dysfunction is not necessarily caused by a myocardial infarction. It can be an effect of myocardial hibernation. The extent and severity of hibernating myocardium in patients with CAD varies considerably. The dysfunction may be limited to regional wall-motion abnormalities (RWMA) ranging from hypokinesia to akinesia or dyskinesia, with a relatively normal ejection fraction, or may involve global impairment of left ventricular function. In patients with CAD and no electrocardiographic evidence of previous myocardial infarction, prevalence of hibernating myocardium has been reported at 33% (15). Up to 50% of patients with a previous infarction may have areas of hibernating tissue mixed with areas of scar tissue, even in the presence of Q waves on the electrocardiogram (16). Noninvasive imaging to determine the presence and extent of viable myocardium distal to coronary stenoses is of considerable clinical importance because selection of patients for coronary revascularization depends on it (Fig. 23.1).

Coronary artery bypass graft (CABG) surgery contributes to improved regional and global left ventricular function in patients with left ventricular dysfunction with or without infarction (17–22). In patients with CAD without previous myocardial infarction, revascularization is important both to reperfuse hibernating myocardium and to remove the source of repeated hypoperfusion. Of the asynergic myocardial segments that are revascularized, function will improve in 85% (23). In patients with CAD and previous myocardial infarction, functional recovery varies from 24% to 82% of segments (21). Recovery of function depends on a number of factors, including the severity of global left ventricular dysfunction preoperatively, the technique for myocardial protection during surgery, the presence or absence of perioperative myocardial infarction, and the adequacy of revascularization.

Revascularization is also associated with improved survival rates compared with medical therapy for patients

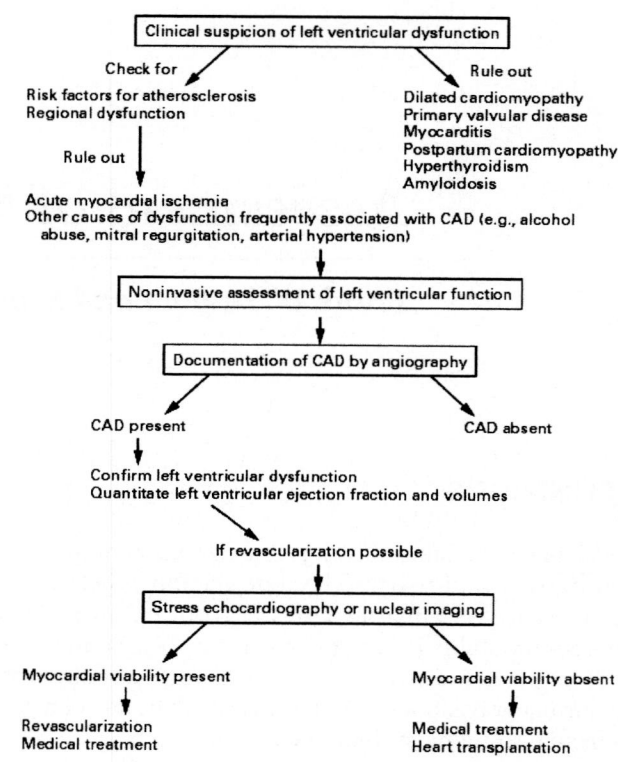

**FIGURE 23.1.** Algorithm for the identification of patients with hibernating myocardium. In addition to the evaluation of the viability of myocardial segments, the final choice of treatment is guided by many factors, such as coexisting conditions, age, and coronary anatomy. In most cases, medical treatment complements revascularization. *CAD,* coronary artery disease. With permission from Wijns W, Vatner SF, Camici PG. Hibernating myocardium. N Engl J Med 1998;339:173–81 (94).

with a left ventricular dysfunction caused by CAD (20,22,24,25). For patients with a left ventricular ejection fraction (LVEF) < 35%, five-year survival rate for the surgical group was 68% compared with 54% for the group treated medically (20). In a surgical subgroup of patients with LVEF < 26%, five-year survival rate was 63% compared with 43% for the group treated medically (24–28). The results of surgical revascularization in patients with chronic left ventricular dysfunction is strongly affected by the presence of viable myocardium (15,29–33). After revascularization of a hibernating myocardium, improvement in the ejection fraction correlated with the number of dysfunctional but viable segments (34–36). Mortality was associated with a low-viability index; survival, both short- and long-term, was significantly better in patients with a high-viability index (6,16,22,37). Therefore, the presence of viable myocardium identifies patients most likely to benefit from coronary revascularization by postoperative improvement in LV systolic function, exercise capacity, quality of life, or survival. Identifying patients without viable myocardium is equally important in view of the high morbidity and mortality rates associated with surgery in such patients (38–40).

Reperfusion of viable myocardium may have beneficial effects other than improving LV function. With an admixture of scarred and viable myocardium (nontransmural infarct), reperfusion may not improve regional function. The presence of viable myocardium in the outer layers of the ventricular wall, however, maintains the left ventricular shape and size by preventing infarct expansion with subsequent heart failure (Figure 23.2) (41–45). A patent infarct-related artery reduces late mortality in patients after acute myocardial infarction independent of left ventricular systolic function (46–49). In addition, revascularization of nonsubendocardial tissue may reduce the likelihood of irritable electrical foci and arrhythmias, thereby reducing late mortality. Table 23.1 summarizes the implications of assessing myocardial viability in patients with chronic ischemic LV dysfunction.

Myocardial stunning, that is, reversible postoperative ventricular contractile dysfunction unrelated to a continuing source of ischemia, may follow CABG surgery (6). Distinguishing ventricular dysfunction caused by acute ischemia or infarction from stunned myocardium remains critical for determining perioperative management strategies (return to cardiopulmonary bypass, utilization of a mechanical assist device, administration of vasoactive drugs) and long-term prognosis (37,50,51). Improvement in regional function after an ischemic event or

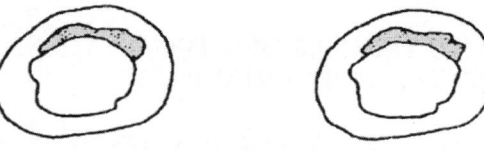
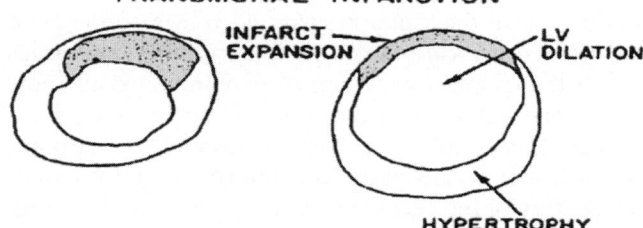

**FIGURE 23.2.** Relation between the transmurality of infarction and infarct expansion. **A:** There are fewer transmural infarcts because they are surrounded by normal myocardium, which will not expand, and the left ventricle will not dilate. **B:** In contrast, large infarcts, which have less normal tissue to buttress them, will expand and result in left ventricular (LV) dilation. With permission from Lindner JR, Kaul S. Assessment of myocardial viability with two-dimensional echo and magnetic resonance imaging. J Nucl Cardiol 1996;3:167–82 (41).

▶ **TABLE 23.1.** Clinical and Economic Implications of Assessing Myocardial Viability in Patients with Chronic Ischemic Left Ventricular Dysfunction

| | Presence of Viable Myocardium | Absence of Viable Myocardium |
|---|---|---|
| **Clinical Implications** | | |
| Advantage | Lower perioperative risk associated with PTCA or CABG | |
| | Improved LVSF after PTCA or CABG | Avoidance of PTCA or CABG in high-risk patients |
| | Lower long-term cardiac morbidity and mortality after PTCA or CABG | |
| Disadvantage | Higher long-term cardiac morbidity and mortality without PTCA or CABG | Higher perioperative risk associated with PTCA or CABG |
| **Economic Implications** | | |
| Cost Savings | Lower cost with PTCA or CABG | |
| | Lower costs for medical treatment after PTCA or CABG | Selective use of PTCA or CABG |
| | Avoidance of heart transplantation | |
| Cost Expenditures | Medical treatment of future cardiac complications | Treatment of perioperative complications or need for heart transplant |

*CABG,* coronary artery bypass graft; *PTCA,* percutaneous coronary angioplasty

acute myocardial infarction may require days to weeks after the initial compromising episode, despite adequate restoration of coronary blood flow (52).

## DIAGNOSTIC TECHNIQUES TO ASSESS MYOCARDIAL VIABILITY

A "bull's-eye" model can describe the three-dimensional anatomy of an infarcted myocardium. Anatomically, the infarct zone at the center is surrounded by a border zone and normal myocardium in the outer zone. The border zone is thought to contain a mixture of infarcted and normal tissue, scattered in the form of "peninsulas" of infarcted myocardium in a "sea" of normal myocardium (53). The area of the infarct is confined within the vascular territory of the occluded coronary artery. The severity of ischemia is always maximal in the endocardial and minimal in the epicardial layers. Pathophysiologically, the severity of the injury is uniform, progressing from the center of the infarct laterally toward normally perfused tissue, except for an area at the lateral edge where overlapping portions of normally perfused and ischemic myocardium are mixed together.

Because assessing myocardial viability by histological methods is not practical, a number of diagnostic techniques are used. Diagnostic techniques are used to detect myocardial contractility, metabolic activity, or the persistence of microvascular integrity (Table 23.2). To differentiate hibernating from infarcted tissues and stunned from ischemic myocardium, the ideal imaging method should delineate infarcted from noninfarcted (viable) tissue and perfused from underperfused dysfunctional myocardium, respectively.

Serum markers, such as creatine kinase and troponin T or I, have limited value in the assessment of myocardial viability after an acute myocardial infarction. They are elevated only in the early period after an infarction and cannot localize the infarct territory. Assessment of myocardial viability with ECG is most helpful during an episode of chest discomfort to observe ST-segment elevation; otherwise, ST-T abnormalities are not specific for a viable but ischemic myocardium. Resolution of ST-segment elevation can be helpful in determining successful reperfusion (54), but the absence of ST-segment resolution does not exclude reperfusion. ST-segment elevation resolves slowly in acute myocardial infarction even in the absence of reperfusion. The presence of Q waves on the ECG correlates poorly with the transmurality of infarction after successful reperfusion. The presence of Q waves does not rule out viable myocardium (55).

Resting echocardiography assists in the assessment of both regional and global myocardial viability. Most left ventricular wall thickening occurs as a result of endocardial thickening; the middle layer of the myocardium contributes only modestly to thickening, and the contribution of the epicardium is negligible (56). In patients with CAD, a hypokinetic region at rest is a clue to viability. But whether hypocontractility is caused by acute ischemia, stunning, hibernation, or altered loading conditions cannot be determined. On the other hand, akinetic or dyskinetic segments are not necessarily nonviable. The overall contraction of a region after a myocardial infarction depends on how much subepicardial myocardium survives. When infarction involves < 20% of wall thickness, hypokinesia can be observed. When 20% of wall thickness is infarcted, akinesia or dyskinesia is seen (57). Thus, if the endocardium is necrosed, wall thickening is akinetic or even dyskinetic, but the middle and outer thirds of the ventricular wall may still be perfused and viable (42,56).

Thallium scintigraphy is used to measure cell membrane integrity. The Na/K–ATPase system transports thallium like potassium across the myocyte sarcolemmal membrane. Cellular extraction of thallium across the cell membrane is unaffected in hypoxic, stunned, or hibernat-

▶ TABLE 23.2. **Diagnostic Techniques for the Assessment of Myocardial Viability**

| Contractile Integrity | Metabolic Integrity | Microvascular Integrity |
|---|---|---|
| Echocardiography: Regional wall motion | Electrocardiogram: ST-segments, Q-waves | Myocardial contrast echocardiography: Myocardial perfusion |
| Dobutamine echocardiography: Recruitable contractility | Thallium scintigraphy: Myocardial perfusion and integrity of cell membranes | |
| | Positron emission tomography: Myocardial metabolism and perfusion | |

ing myocardium, but thallium does not penetrate scarred tissue (58). Single-photon emission computerized tomography (SPECT) imaging at stress, redistribution (early and late), and reinjection at rest can assess myocardial viability. Assessment with technetium-99m sestamibi (Tc-99m MIBI) is still under active investigation. Positive and negative predictive accuracy for reversal of wall-motion abnormalities after revascularization varies, as do results after direct comparison with thallium scintigraphy.

Positron emission tomography (PET) imaging is regarded as the gold standard and final arbiter in decisions regarding viability (59). PET scanning tracks markers of perfusion ($NH_3$) and metabolism of (18F-fluorodeoxyglucose) to compare blood flow and metabolism activity. Under normal conditions flow and metabolic activity match, and distribution of each tracer is homogeneous. Regional blood flow may be decreased while glucose utilization is normal or increased. This pattern of blood flow–metabolism mismatch signals myocardial viability in the presence of ventricular dysfunction. Decreases in blood flow and glucose utilization are a marker of myocardial scarring and irreversible damage. Measurement of myocardial blood flow by PET has several limitations, however. In the presence of spatial tissue heterogeneity with ischemic injury, the flow value may represent a transmural average between low values in necrotic areas to normal values in well-perfused zones. During flow restriction, subendocardial layers tend to have less flow than subepicardial layers. Therefore, a small reduction in average flow across the wall may correspond to a more severe reduction in subendocardial blood flow. Whether or not subendocardial blood flow is reduced in patients with hibernating myocardium awaits verification by direct measurement.

Dobutamine echocardiography and myocardial contrast echocardiography can be used in the operating room to differentiate hibernating myocardium from necrotic tissue and acute myocardial ischemia from stunning, respectively.

## Dobutamine Echocardiography

Resting two-dimensional echocardiography cannot differentiate hibernating from irreversibly damaged myocardium because it does not account for coronary blood flow reserve. Provocative testing is necessary to find viable segments. Dobutamine echocardiography is a safe, noninvasive, and accurate diagnostic technique to identify viable myocardium in chronically dysfunctional regions (51,60–64). In the standard protocol for dobutamine stress echocardiography, increments of dobutamine from 5 to 40 μg/kg/min are added at three-minute intervals with intravenous atropine if 85% of the maximum predicted heart rate is not achieved. In a low-dose dobut-

amine protocol, which assesses left ventricular systolic function at baseline and at doses from between 5 and 10 μg/kg/min, the different contractile response in hibernating and infarcted myocardium distinguishes reversible from irreversible tissue injury.

Dobutamine is a synthetic catecholamine with strong $\beta_1$-receptor and mild $\alpha_1$- and $\beta_2$-receptor agonist activity (65). Dobutamine also may have a minor direct vasodilatative effect on coronary vessels. It has a plasma half-life of approximately 2 minutes and is metabolized rapidly by the liver.

In normal myocardium, the response of regional left ventricular function to dobutamine is dose-dependent. A low-dose of up to 10 μg/kg/min produces marked inotropic effects independent of endogenous norepinephrine stores (mediated by both $\alpha_1$- and $\beta_1$-receptor stimulation). At doses up to 40 μg/kg/min, heart rate is progressively increased (mediated by $\beta_1$-receptor stimulation). Then demand for oxygen increases, coronary arteries dilate, and coronary blood flow increases three-fold (66). Despite an increase in cardiac output, systemic blood pressure increases only minimally because systemic vascular resistance decreases. Peripheral vasoconstrictive effects (mediated by $\alpha_1$-receptor stimulation) are overwhelmed by vasodilative effects (mediated by $\beta_2$-receptor stimulation). In a normally perfused myocardium, resting wall motion is normal; hyperdynamic function develops because oxygen demand is matched by blood flow.

In patients with chronic CAD, five factors influence the response of the myocardium to dobutamine:

1. Extent of viable tissue
2. Degree of coronary artery stenosis
3. Size of risk area
4. Spatial extent and magnitude of collateral blood flow
5. Effect of beta-blockade (67)

Figure 23.3 depicts the first two factors for interpretation of dobutamine echocardiography. Regions with chronically abnormal baseline function may respond to dobutamine with progressive worsening, a biphasic response, or no change. Worsening of baseline regional wall-motion abnormalities with escalating doses of dobutamine indicates myocardial ischemia; the increase in oxygen demand cannot be met by an adequate increase in blood flow. In a biphasic response, after low-dose dobutamine augments contractile function (contractile reserve), systolic dysfunction worsens with higher doses (ischemic response) (68). Dobutamine stimulation augments function at a dose of 5–10 μg/kg/min before ischemia is engendered by increased work and metabolic demands at the higher dose of > 10 μg/kg/min. Regional segments that remain akinetic or dyskinetic despite dobutamine infusion likely reflect scarring (Fig. 23.4).

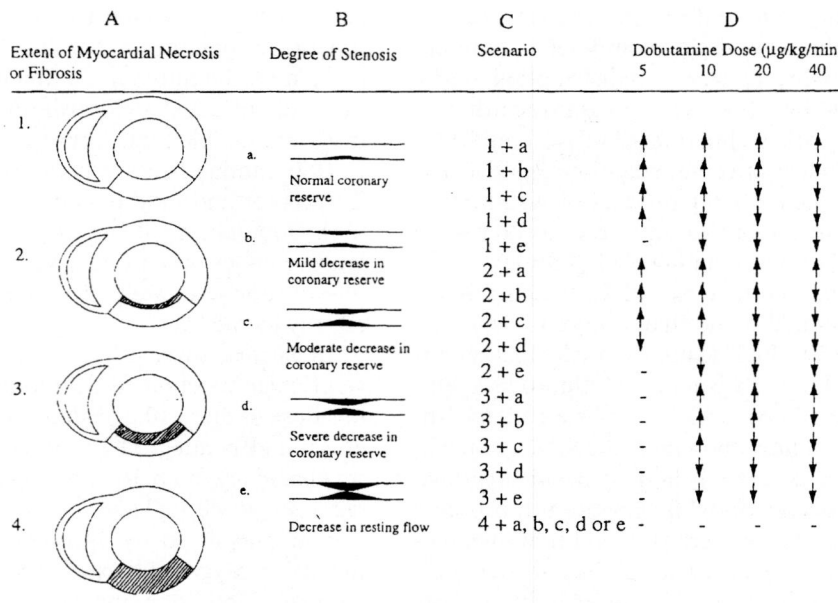

**FIGURE 23.3.** Expected response to different doses of dobutamine after reflow has been achieved in patients with acute myocardial infarction and abnormal function within the infarct zone. **Panel A** depicts the extent of necrosis: 1 = none; 2 = minimal; 3 = moderate; 4 = extensive. **Panel B** illustrates the severity of stenosis whereby the degree of stenosis is defined in terms of its ability to reduce coronary flow reserve: a = normal flow reserve; b = mildly reduced flow reserve; c = moderately reduced flow reserve; d = severely reduced flow reserve; e = reduced rest flow. **Panel C** denotes the possible combination of the extent of necrosis (**panel A**) and degree of stenosis (**panel B**). **Panel D** shows the expected response to dobutamine according to the scenario shown in **panel C.** Arrows in the same direction indicate a greater response than that at the previous stage. The responses in chronic coronary artery disease could be different from those depicted here, depending on the extent of myocardial downregulation and collateral perfusion — = no change. With permission from Kaul S. Response of dysfunctional myocardium to dobutamine, "The eyes see what the mind knows!" J Am Coll Cardiol 1996;27:1608–11.

## Prediction of Regional Improvement after Revascularization

Table 23.3 summarizes the diagnostic accuracy of dobutamine echocardiography for the prediction of reversible regional dysfunction in patients with chronic ischemic left ventricular dysfunction. The overall sensitivity of a contractile response to low-dose dobutamine for predicting recovery of regional function after revascularization is 84%; specificity is 81%. A biphasic response had the highest predictive value (72%) for recovery of function followed by worsening of function (35%). In segments with a biphasic response, the low dose at which improvement in RWMA was most prevalent (84%) was 7.5 μg/kg/min; improvement increased to 94% when the 5 and 7.5 μg/kg/min doses were displayed. The reworsening phase of the biphasic response was usually seen with doses ≥ 20 μg/kg/min, but was also observed with doses of 7.5 μg/kg/min (69).

Sensitivity of dobutamine echocardiography may be affected by the following factors:

- Premature termination of dobutamine infusion will not elicit a contractile response in myocardium that is largely necrotic; hence greater inotropic stimulation may be required.
- Severe reduction of myocardial blood flow and coronary flow reserve will preclude the contractile response.
- Resting tachycardia will sometimes render the myocardium ischemic, and dobutamine stimulation will only augment ischemia.

Specificity of dobutamine echocardiography may be affected by the following factors:

- A false-positive response to dobutamine can be observed when nonviable myocardium is dragged along with normal segments (tethering effect).
- Regional akinesis may reflect the presence of subendocardial infarction. The injured subendocardium does not respond to dobutamine, but because the mid- and epicardial myocardium do respond, overall regional

*(text continues on page 358)*

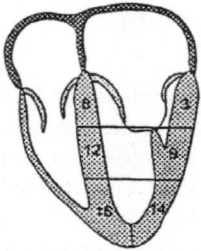
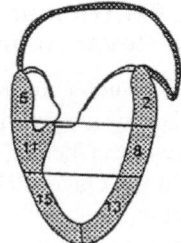

a. four chamber view     b. two chamber view

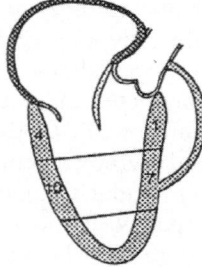
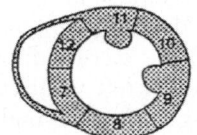

d. mid short axis view

c. long axis view

e. basal short axis view

| Basal Segments | Mid Segments | Apical Segments |
|---|---|---|
| 1= Basal Anteroseptal | 7= Mid Anteroseptal | 13= Apical Anterior |
| 2= Basal Anterior | 8= Mid Anterior | 14= Apical Lateral |
| 3= Basal Lateral | 9= Mid Lateral | 15= Apical Inferior |
| 4= Basal Posterior | 10= Mid Posterior | 16= Apical Septal |
| 5= Basal Inferior | 11= Mid Inferior | |
| 6= Basal Septal | 12= Mid Septal | |

**FIGURE 23.4.** A 16-segment model of the left ventricle for analysis of regional wall motion abnormalities. With permission from Shanewise JS, Cheung AT, Aronson S, et al. ASE/SCA guidelines for performing a comprehensive intraoperative multiplane transesophageal echocardiography examination: recommendations of the American Society of Echocardiography Council for Intraoperative Echocardiography and the Society of Cardiovascular Anesthesiologists Task Force for Certification in Perioperative Transesophageal Echocardiography. Anesth Analg 1999;89:870–84 (95).

▶ **TABLE 23.3. Sensitivity, Specificity, and Diagnostic Accuracy of Dobutamine Echocardiography in the Prediction of Reversible Dysfunction**

| Study | No. patients | Mean EF (SD) | No. segments | Sensitivity | | Specificity | | Accuracy | |
|---|---|---|---|---|---|---|---|---|---|
| Marzullo et al. (94) | 14 | 39 (7) | 75 | 40/49 | 82% | 24/26 | 92% | 64/75 | 85% |
| Alfieri et al. (95) | 14 | 35 (8) | 125 | 85/93 | 91% | 25/32 | 78% | 110/125 | 88% |
| Cigarroa (51) | 25 | NA | — | 9/11 | 82% | 12/14 | 86% | 21/25 | 84% |
| La Canna et al. (61) | 33 | 33 (8) | 314 | 178/205 | 87% | 89/169 | 82% | 267/314 | 85% |
| Charney et al. (62) | 26 | 46 (9) | 58 | 22/31 | 71% | 25/27 | 93% | 47/58 | 81% |
| Perrone-Filardi et al. (64) | 18 | 39 (14) | 81 | 42/48 | 88% | 27/31 | 87% | 69/81 | 85% |
| Senior et al. (74) | 22 | 26 (8) | 168 | 103/118 | 87% | 41/50 | 82% | 144/168 | 86% |
| Afridi et al. (77) | 20 | NA | 114 | 28/38 | 74% | 55/76 | 73% | 83/114 | 73% |
| Arnese et al. (63) | 38 | 31 | 170 | 24/33 | 74% | 150/137 | 95% | 154/170 | 91% |
| Haque et al. (96) | 26 | 43 (14) | 43 | 31/33 | 94% | 8/10 | 80% | 39/43 | 91% |
| Vanoverschelde et al. (75) | 73 | 36 (12) | 444 | 123/167 | 76% | 238/277 | 86% | 361/444 | 81% |
| Qureshi et al. (97) | 34 | 39 (14) | 148 | 31/42 | 74% | 94/106 | 89% | 125/148 | 84% |
| Perrone-Filardi et al. (98) | 40 | 43 (12) | 109 | 58/73 | 79% | 30/36 | 83% | 88/109 | 81% |
| Bax et al. (35) | 17 | 36 (11) | 92 | 23/27 | 85% | 41/65 | 63% | 64/92 | 70% |
| Baer et al. (99) | 42 | 40 (13) | 42 | 25/26 | 96% | 11/16 | 69% | 36/42 | 86% |
| de Filippi et al. (100) | 23 | 38 (10) | 152 | 94/97 | 97% | 41/55 | 75% | 135/152 | 89% |
| Gerber et al. (101) | 39 | 33 (10) | 39 | 17/24 | 71% | 13/15 | 89% | 30/39 | 77% |
| Total/mean | 504 | | | 933/1,115 | 84% | 924/1,142 | 81% | 1,857/2,257 | 82% |

EF, left ventricular ejection fraction; NA, not available. With permission from Vanoverschelde J-L, Pasquet A, Gerber B, Melin JA. Pathophysiology of myocardial hibernation: implications for the use of dobutamine echocardiography to identify myocardial viability. Heart 1999;82(Suppl III) III1-7 (13).

function may improve. After revascularization, however, the myocardium may remain akinetic because the subendocardium is necrotic and mid- and subepicardial thickening remains unchanged. This akinesis explains the lower positive predictive value of dobutamine-induced contractile response from hypokinetic segments. Because most myocardial thickening is a consequence of subendocardial thickening, an extensive subendocardial scar may prevent improvement in regional wall motion after revascularization. Because hypokinetic segments are viable, further evaluation of viability by dobutamine is unnecessary.

- Specificity may be reduced in ischemic myocardial regions in which the subtending artery is not flow-limiting. Resting dyssynergy improves during dobutamine infusion, but function rarely improves after revascularization.

Low-dose dobutamine echocardiography is slightly more specific than thallium scintigraphy and PET for predicting recovery of regional function; however, it is slightly less sensitive (35). Hibernating myocardium often loses contractile myofilaments, which prevents a positive response to inotropic stimulation even though myocytes are still viable (70–73). Therefore, a higher level of functional myocyte integrity is necessary to show contractile reserve with dobutamine echocardiography than with thallium uptake.

## Improvement of Global Systolic Function

Several studies confirm the predictive value of dobutamine echocardiography for improvement of global left ventricular systolic function (74–76). In patients with chronic ischemic left ventricular dysfunction, left ventricular ejection fraction (LVEF) increased from 27% ± 8% to 38% ± 9% after revascularization in the group with contractile reserve (shown with dobutamine infusion 10 μg/kg/min), but not in those without contractile reserve (77).

Results were similar with low doses of dobutamine. LVEF improved after CABG or angioplasty in patients with contractile reserve (38 ± 5% to 42 ± 5%, p < 0.01), but not in patients without contractile reserve (38 ± 7% to 39 ± 8%, p = NS). In the group with contractile reserve, linear correlation between the number of segments with contractile reserve and the improvement in LVEF (r = 0.91, p < 0.0001) was significant, indicating that the extent of jeopardized but viable tissue determines the magnitude of improvement after revascularization (76).

In a study examining the diagnostic value of low doses of dobutamine, changes in global wall-motion score during dobutamine correlated with global ejection fraction (r = 0.81, p < 0.001) or end-systolic volume (r = 0.75, p < 0.001) after revascularization (75).

## Left Ventricular Remodeling after Revascularization

With subendocardial infarction, regional function may not recover after revascularization despite myocardial viability. Nevertheless, revascularization may restore perfusion in the epicardial half and prevent left ventricular remodeling.

Among 70 patients with severe left ventricular dysfunction caused by ischemic cardiomyopathy, in those with viability in ≥ 5 of 12 segments (predicted by low-dose dobutamine), left ventricular volumes and myocardial mass were reduced significantly after revascularization, and left ventricular shape was altered (78). These changes went beyond those predicted for both regional and global left ventricular function. In those with myocardial viability under medical therapy, ejection fraction did not deteriorate, but left ventricular volume and mass increased significantly, accompanied by abnormal alteration in the shape of the left ventricle. The mortality rate in the group that received medical therapy was greater than that of the revascularized group. Regression of left ventricular remodeling with relief of ischemia, prevention of reinfarction, and reduction in the rates of heart failure contributes to improved survival rates.

## Survival Rates

Several studies have demonstrated the value of dobutamine echocardiography for predicting survival (79–81). In 274 consecutive patients with CAD and LVEF ≤ 40%, 118 had CABG surgery and 15 patients had coronary angioplasty. The mean period for follow-up was 20 ± 12 months. Of the 133 patients who had revascularization, 29 had dysfunctional but viable myocardium in ≥ 6 segments, 60 patients had dysfunctional but viable myocardium in 2 to 5 segments, and 44 patients had dysfunctional myocardium irreversibly damaged. Patients with the greatest functional improvement after revascularization had a lower rate of cardiac events during follow-up and better cardiac event-free survival (81).

In another study of 318 patients with CAD and a LV ejection fraction ≤ 35%, follow-up was for 18 ± 10 months. Of the two groups with myocardial viability, group I (n = 85) underwent revascularization and group II (n = 119) did not. Of the two groups without myocardial viability, group III (n = 30) underwent revascularization, and group IV (n = 84) did not. Mortality rates were 6% in group I, 20% in group II, 17% in group III, and 20% in group IV (p = 0.01, group I versus the other groups) (80).

When 87 patients with LVEF of 25 ± 9% and symptomatic heart failure were followed up 40 ± 17 months later, mortality was reduced by 93% in patients with > 5 viable segments (12-segment model) who underwent revascularization. Mortality rates for those with > 5 viable segments who were treated medically were higher than for those who had revascularization (p = 0.01) (79). Patients with fewer viable segments did poorly with revascularization or medical treatment.

## Intraoperative Use of Low-Dose Dobutamine Echocardiography

Low-dose dobutamine predicts improvement in regional wall motion after CABG (82). When 560 segments in 40 patients were analyzed for regional wall motion according to a 16-segment model (Fig. 23.5) at baseline (after induction and intubation), with administration of low-dose dobutamine before cardiopulmonary bypass, after separation from cardiopulmonary bypass (early), and after administration of protamine (late), response to dobutamine was recorded as improved or not improved from baseline and analyzed with logistic regression. The influence of ejection fraction, myocardial infarction, diabetes mellitus, and beta-blockers was also determined. Changes in myocardial function after low-dose dobutamine were highly predictive for early (p < 0.0001) and late (p < 0.0001) changes in myocardial function from baseline regional scores. The overall odds ratio for early and late improvement increased by 20.7 and 34.6, respectively, when improvement was observed after low-dose dobutamine was administered. The overall positive predictive value of improved regional wall motion after CABG did not vary with left ventricular ejection fraction, a history of myocardial infarction, or beta-blocker use, and it varied little with diabetic status (range, 0.86–0.96) if regional wall motion improved with low-dose dobutamine before CABG. The overall negative predictive value was 0.70; however, the range varied with diabetic status (range 0.54–0.81).

A response to low-dose dobutamine intraoperatively predicted changes in regional function at one year (83).

The overall odds of improvement in myocardial function were 2.66 times greater (95% CI = 1.30, 5.45; p = 0.0074) with a positive response than without. The positive predictive value for improvement in myocardial function was 0.81, and the negative predictive value was 0.32, too low to make predictions about regional myocardial function in nonresponding segments. Of segments with unexpected deterioration of RWM after cardiopulmonary bypass, 87% recovered on the one-year follow-up echocardiogram. This result means that most of unexpected regional dysfunction after CABG surgery can be attributed to stunning.

## Myocardial Contrast Echocardiography

Myocardial contrast echocardiography is a diagnostic technique that utilizes an ultrasound contrast agent and adapted ultrasound systems to provide a safe, noninvasive means of assessing perfusion directly (84). The flow of contrast microbubbles can be visualized through vessels < 100 μm in diameter to verify microvascular integrity, which is a marker for viability.

The relationship between function and flow has been evaluated in patients with CAD by contrast echocardiography. In patients with acute myocardial infarction and occlusion of the infarct-related artery, collateral flow that was identified with contrast echocardiography correlated with improvement in regional wall motion one month after successful coronary angioplasty (85). In another study of patients with acute infarction, confirmation of reflow by contrast echocardiography after reperfusion therapy meant greater improvement in global and regional left ventricular function on follow-up than in patients with no reflow (86). With respect to chronic ischemia, perfusion observed with contrast echocardiography correlated with improvement in regional wall motion and global left ventricular function after revascularization. These patients

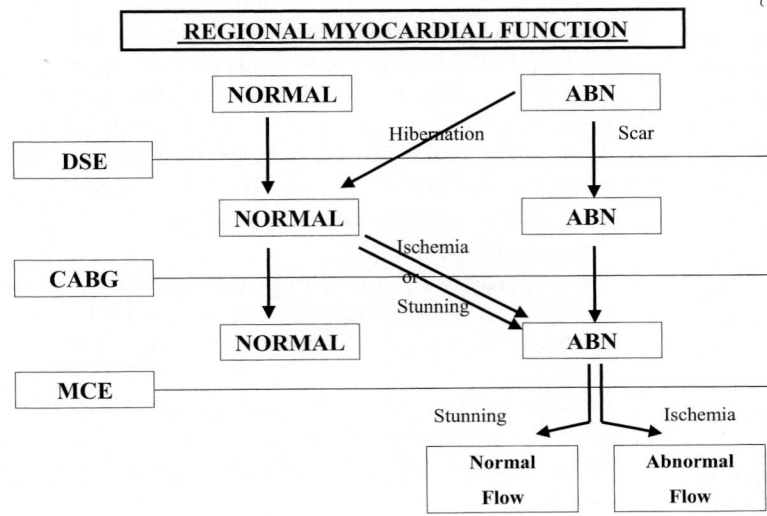

**FIGURE 23.5.** Intraoperative assessment of myocardial function during coronary artery bypass graft surgery. *DSE*, dobutamine stress echocardiography; *MCE*, myocardial contrast echocardiography; *ABN*, abnormal.

had a previous myocardial infarction and reduced left ventricular ejection fraction (87). Assessment of myocardial perfusion in the operating room with contrast ultrasonography has been reported (88–90). The availability of commercially produced ultrasound contrast agents has greatly enhanced the ease of intraoperative application of this technique (91–93). In one study, transesophageal echocardiography and sonicated Renografin-76 microbubbles were used to determine the distribution of myocardial blood flow during CABG surgery (91). The contrast agent was injected into the aortic root after cardiopulmonary bypass and aortic clamping and again after anastomosis of the bypass graft. Contrast echocardiography predicted myocardial perfusion patterns, based on preoperative evaluation of the distribution in epicardial vessels derived from coronary angiography. Regional myocardial perfusion deficits detected after CAPG were associated with RWMA detected after separation from cardiopulmonary bypass.

In another application, transesophageal echocardiography with injection of the contrast agent Albunex was used to evaluate regional myocardial perfusion during minimally invasive CABG surgery (91). The contrast agent was injected after anastomosis of the internal mammary artery to the left anterior descending artery. Evidence of graft patency and adequacy of revascularization were confirmed.

Intraoperative myocardial contrast echocardiography has also been used to determine whether regional flow patterns during revascularization can predict contractile function after CABG surgery (92). Opacification of flow was graded from echocardiographic images after injection of Albunex into the aortic root during cardiopulmonary bypass. Three groups of patients were defined according to the relationship between flow and function in the myocardium: normal flow with normal function immediately after separation from bypass and at one month after surgery; normal flow with abnormal function immediately after bypass and normal function at one month (i.e., stunning); and abnormal flow with abnormal function immediately after bypass and at one month, (i.e., old infarction). Myocardial contrast opacification predicted regional function at one week (p ≤ 0.05) and at one month (p ≤ 0.01) after CABG surgery.

During CABG surgery, delineation of myocardial perfusion patterns may have an impact on pharmacological and surgical treatment options. Before cardiopulmonary bypass, contrast echocardiography may aid in the differential diagnosis of baseline RWMA to distinguish hibernating myocardium (presence of perfusion) from infarcted myocardium (absence of perfusion). After separation from cardiopulmonary bypass, assessment of perfusion may show that the cause of a new RWMA is graft incompetence (decreased perfusion and contractility) or stunning (decreased perfusion but normal contractility). The application of contrast echocardiography in the operating room continues to evolve along with the technology itself.

## CONCLUSIONS

Dobutamine stress and contrast echocardiography can be used in the operating room suite. Combined they are a diagnostic aid in the perioperative assessment of myocardial viability, perfusion-contraction mismatching, and contractile reserve (Fig. 23.4). Understanding how to identify reversible contractile dysfunction (stunning, hibernation, and ischemia) is critical during ischemic heart surgery for optimal revascularization.

### KEY POINTS

- Viable myocardium may be dysfunctional in the state of acute ischemia, stunning, or hibernation.
- The proportional decrease in regional myocardial blood flow and contractility is typical of acute myocardial ischemia (perfusion–contraction match).
- Myocardial stunning is the fully reversible dysfunction that persists up to 24 hours after reperfusion despite restoration of normal or near-normal coronary blood flow (perfusion-contraction mismatch).
- Myocardial hibernation can be defined as reversible left ventricular dysfunction due to chronic CAD with normal or slightly reduced myocardial blood flow and limited coronary flow reserve.
- Differentiating hibernating from infarcted myocardium is important because revascularization of hibernating myocardium decreases perioperative and long-term morbidity and mortality, and improves left ventricular systolic function.
- Differentiation of acutely ischemic from stunned myocardium is critical after separation from cardiopulmonary bypass to select appropriate management strategies because therapeutic interventions will affect long-term outcome.
- Ambulatory dobutamine echocardiography predicts global and regional improvement, left ventricular remodeling, and survival after revascularization.
- Intraoperative low-dose dobutamine echocardiography predicts recovery of regional myocardial function immediately after CABG surgery.
- Myocardial contrast echocardiography may aid to distinguish acutely ischemic from stunned myocardium in the operating room.

# REFERENCES

1. Kaul S. There may be more to myocardial viability than meets the eye. Circulation 1995;92:2790–3.
2. Tennant R, Wiggers CJ. The effects of coronary occlusion on myocardial contraction. Am J Physiol 1935;112:351–61.
3. Herman MV, Heinle RA, Klein MD, Gorlin R. Localized disorders in myocardial contraction. Asynergy and its role in congestive heart failure. N Engl J Med 1967;277:222–32.
4. Bolli R. Mechanism of myocardial "stunning." Circulation 1990;82:723–38.
5. Braunwald E, Kloner RA. The stunned myocardium: prolonged, postischemic ventricular dysfunction. Circulation 1982;66:1146–9.
6. Bolli R. Myocardial "stunning" in man. Circulation 1992;86:1671–91.
7. Bolli R, Marban E. Molecular and cellular mechanisms of myocardial stunning (review). Physiol Rev 1999;79:609–34.
8. Bolli R, Patel BS, Hartley CJ, et al. Nonuniform transmural recovery of contractile function in stunned myocardium. Am J Physiol 1989;257:H375–85.
9. Horn HR, Teichholz LE, Cohn PF, Herman MV, Gorlin R. Augmentation of left ventricular contraction pattern in coronary artery disease by an inotropic catecholamine: the epinephrine ventriculogram. Circulation 1974;49:1063–71.
10. Diamond GA, Forrester JS, deLuz PL, Wyatt HL, Swan HJC. Post-extrasystolic potentiation of ischemic myocardium by atrial stimulation. Am Heart J 1978;95:204–9.
11. Rahimtoola SH. A perspective on the three large multicenter randomized clinical trials of coronary bypass for chronic stable angina. Circulation 1985;72 (Suppl V): V123–35.
12. Rahimtoola SH. From coronary artery disease to heart failure: role of the hibernating myocardium. Am J Cardiol 1995;75:16E–22E.
13. Vanoverschelde J-L, Pasquet A, Gerber B, Melin JA. Pathophysiology of myocardial hibernation: implications for the use of dobutamine echocardiography to identify myocardial viability. Heart 1999;82 (Suppl III) III1–7.
14. Terrlink J, Goldhaber S, Pfeffer M. An overview of contemporary etiologies of congestive heart failure. Am Heart J 1991;121:1852–3.
15. Lee KS, Marwick TH, Cook SA. Prognosis of patients with left ventricular dysfunction, with and without viable myocardium after myocardial infarction. Relative efficacy of medical therapy and revascularization. Circulation 1994;90:2687–94.
16. Pagley PR, Beller GA, Watson DD, Gimple LW, Ragosta M. Improved outcome after coronary bypass surgery in patients with ischemic cardiomyopathy and residual myocardial viability. Circulation 1997;96:793–800.
17. Brundage BH, Massie BM, Botvinick EH. Improved regional ventricular function after successful surgical revascularization. J Am Coll Cardiol 1984;3:902–8.
18. Rees G, Bistow JD, Kremkau EL, et al. Influence of aorto-coronary bypass surgery on left ventricular performance. N Engl J Med 1971;284:1116–20.
19. Chatterjee K, Swan HJC, Parmley WW, et al. Influence of direct myocardial revascularization on left ventricular asynergy and function in patients with coronary heart disease: with and without previous myocardial infarction. Circulation 1973;47:276–86.
20. Alderman EL, Fisher LD, Litwin P, et al. Results of coronary artery surgery in patients with poor left ventricular function (CASS). Circulation 1983;68:785–95.
21. Bax JJ, Wijns W, Cornel JH, et al. Accuracy of currently available techniques for prediction of functional recovery after revascularization in patients with left ventricular dysfunction due to chronic coronary artery disease: comparison of pooled data. J Am Coll Cardiol 1997;30:1451–60.
22. Nesto RW, Cohn LH, Collins JJ Jr, et al. Inotropic contractile reserve: a useful predictor of increased 5 year survival and improved postoperative left ventricular function in patients with coronary artery disease and reduced ejection fraction. Am J Cardiol 1982;50:39–44.
23. Lewis SJ, Sawada SG, Ryal T, et al. Segmental wall motion abnormalities in the absence of clinically documented myocardial infarction: clinical significance and evidence of hibernating myocardium. Am Heart J 1991;121:1088–94.
24. Bounous EP, Mark Db, Pollock BG, et al. Surgical survival benefit for coronary disease in patients with left ventricular dysfunction. Circulation 1988;78 (Suppl I):151–7.
25. Pagano D, Camici PG, Bonser RS. Revascularization for chronic heart failure: a valid option? Eur J Heart Fail 1999;1:69–73.
26. Hochberg MS, Parsonnet V, Gielchinksy I, Hussain SM. Coronary artery bypass grafting in patients with ejection fractions below forty percent. Early and late results in 466 patients. J Thorac Cardiovasc Surg 1983;86:519–27.
27. Pigott JD, Kouchoukos NT, Oberman A, Cutter GR. Late results of surgical and medical therapy for patients with coronary artery disease and depressed left ventricular function. J Am Coll Cardiol 1985;5:1036–45.
28. Passamani E, Davis KB, Gillespie MJ, Killip T. A randomized trial of coronary artery bypass surgery. Survival of patients with a low ejection fraction. N Engl J Med 1985;312:1665–71.
29. Eitzman D, Al-Aouar ZR, Kanter HL, et al. Clinical outcome of patients with advanced coronary artery disease after viability studies with positron emission tomography. J Am Coll Cardiol 1992;20:559–65.
30. DiCarli MF, Davidson M, Little R, et al. Value of metabolic imaging with positron emission tomography for evaluating prognosis in patients with coronary artery disease and left ventricular dysfunction. Am J Cardiol 1994;73:527–33.
31. Yoshida K. Gould KL. Quantitative relation of myocardial infarct size and myocardial viability by positron emission tomography to left ventricular ejection fraction and 3–year mortality with and without revascularization. J Am Coll Cardiol 1993;22:984–7.
32. Gioia G, Powers J, Heo J, Iskandrian AS. Prognostic value of rest-redistribution tomographic thallium-201 imaging in ischemic cardiomyopathy. Am J Cardiol 1995;75:759–62.
33. Williams MJ, Odabashian J, Lauer MS, Thomas JD, Marwick TH. Prognostic value of dobutamine echocardiography in patients with left ventricular dysfunction. J Am Coll Cardiol 1996;27:132–9.
34. Tillisch J, Brunken R, Marshall R, et al. Reversibility of cardiac wall motion abnormalities predicted by positron tomography. N Engl J Med 1986;314:884–8.
35. Bax JJ, Cornel JH, Visser FC, et al. Prediction of recovery of myocardial dysfunction after revascularization. Comparison of fluorine-18 fluorodeoxyglucose/thallium-201 SPECT, thallium-201 stress-reinjection SPECT and dobutamine echocardiography. J Am Coll Cardiol 1996;28:558–64.
36. Vanoverschelde JL, Gerber BL, D'Hondt AM, et al. Preoperative selection of patients with severely impaired left ventricular function for coronary revascularization: role of low-dose dobutamine echocardiography and exercise-redistriubtion-reinjection thallium SPECT. Circulation 1995;92 (Suppl II):37–44.
37. van den Berg EK, Popma JJ, Dehmer GJ, et al. Reversible segmental left ventricular dysfunction after coronary angioplasty. Circulation 1990;81:1210–16.
38. Louie HW, Laks H, Milgalter E, et al. Ischemic cardiomyopathy: criteria for coronary revascularization and cardiac transplantation. Circulation 1991;84 (Suppl III):290–5.
39. Luciani GB, Faggian G, Razzolini R, et al. Severe ischemic left ventricular failure: coronary operation or heart transplantation? Ann Thorac Surg 1993;55:719–23.
40. Milano CA, White WD, Smith LR, et al. Coronary artery bypass in patients with severely depressed ventricular function. Ann Thorac Surg 1993;56:487–93.
41. Lindner JR, Kaul S. Assessment of myocardial viability with two-dimensional echo and magnetic resonance imaging. J Nucl Cardiol 1996;3:167–82.
42. Touchstone DA, Beller GA, Nygaard TW, Tedesco C, Kaul S. Effects of successful intravenous reperfusion therapy on regional myocardial function and geometry in man: a tomographic assessment using two-dimensional echocardiography. J Am Coll Cardiol 1989;13:1506–13.

43. Eaton LW, Weiss JL, Bulkley BH, Garrison JB, Weisfeldt ML. Regional cardiac dilatation after acute myocardial infarction. N Engl J Med 1979;300:57–62.

44. Pirolo JS Hutchins GM, Moore GW. Infarct expansion: pathologic analysis of 204 patients with a single myocardial infarct. J Am Coll Cardiol 1986;7:349–54.

45. Marino P, Zanolla L, Zardini P. Effect of streptokinase on left ventricular modeling and function after myocardial infarction: the GISSI (Gruppo Italiano per lo Studio della Streptochinasi nell'Infarto Miocardico) Trial. J Am Coll Cardiol 1989;14:1149–58.

46. Cigarroa RG, Lange RA, Hillis LD. Prognosis after acute myocardial infarction in patients with and without residual anterograde coronary blood flow. Am J Cardiol 1989;64:155–60.

47. Schroder R, Neuhaus KL, Linderer T, et al. Impact of late coronary artery reperfusion on left ventricular function one month after acute myocardial infarction (results from the ISAM study). Am J Cardiol 1989;64:878–84.

48. Galvani M, Ottani F, Ferrini D, Sorbellow F, Rusticali F. Patency of the infarct-related artery and left ventricular function as the major determinants of survival after Q-wave acute myocardial infarction. Am J Cardiol 1993;71:1–7.

49. Braunwald E. Myocardial reperfusion, limitation of infarct size, reduction of left ventricular dysfunction, and improved survival; should the paradigm be expanded? Circulation 1989;70:441–4.

50. Marwick TH, Mehta R, Arheart K, Lauer MS. Use of exercise echocardiography for prognosis evaluation of patients with known or suspected coronary artery disease. J Am Coll Cardiol 1997;30:83–90.

51. Cigarroa CG, deFilippi CR, Brickner ME, et al. Dobutamine stress echocardiography identifies hibernating myocardium and predicts recovery of left ventricular function after coronary revascularization. Circulation 1993;88:430–6.

52. Bush LR, Buja LM, Samowitz W, et al. Recovery of left ventricular segmental function after long-term reperfusion following temporary coronary occlusion in conscious dogs: comparison of 2- and 4-hour occlusions. Circ Res 1983;53:248–63.

53. Factor SM, Sonnenblick EH, Kirk ES. The histologic border zone of acute myocardial infarction—islands or peninsulas? Am J Pathol 1978;92:111–24.

54. Weintraub WS, Hattori S, Aggarwal JB, et al. The relationship between myocardial blood flow and contraction by myocardial layer in the canine left ventricle during ischemia. Cir Res 1981;48:430–8.

55. Brunken R, Tillisch J, Schwaiger M, et al. Regional perfusion, glucose metabolism, and wall motion in patients with chronic electrocardiographic Q wave infarctions: evidence for persistence of viable tissue in some infarct regions by positron emission tomography. Circulation 1986;73:951–63.

56. Myers JH, Stirling MC, Choy M, Buda AJ, Gallagher KP. Direct measurement of inner and outer wall thickening dynamics with epicardial echocardiography. Circulation 1986;74:164–72.

57. Lieberman AN, Weiss JL, Jugdutt BI, et al. Two-dimensional echocardiography and infarct size: relationship of regional wall motion and thinning to the extent of myocardial infarction in the dog. Circulation 1981;63:739–46.

58. Al-Khouri F, Narula J. Radionuclide imaging for the assessment of myocardial viability in chronic LV dysfunction. Echocardiography 2000;17:605–12.

59. Schelbert HR. PET contributions to understanding normal and abnormal cardiac perfusion and metabolism. Ann Biomed Eng 2000;28:922–9.

60. Lualdi JC, Douglas PS. Echocardiography for the assessment of myocardial viability. J Am Soc Echocardiogr 1997;10:772–80.

61. La Canna G, Alfieri O, Giubbini R, et al. Echocardiography during infusion of dobutamine for identification of reversible dysfunction in patients with coronary artery disease. J Am Coll Cardiol 1994;23:617–26.

62. Charney R, Schwinger ME, Chun J, et al. Dobutamine echocardiography and resting-redistribution thallium-201 scintigraphy predicts recovery of hibernating myocardium after coronary revascularization. Am Heart J 1994;128:864–9.

63. Arnese M, Cornel JH, Salustri A, et al. Prediction of improvement of regional left ventricular function after surgical revascularization. A comparison of low-dose dobutamine echocardiography with $^{201}$T1 single photon emission computed tomography. Circulation 1995;91:2748–52.

64. Perrone-Filardi P, Pace L, Prastaro M, et al. Dobutamine echocardiography predicts improvement of hypoperfused dysfunctional myocardium after revascularization in patients with coronary artery disease. Circulation 1995;91:2556–65.

65. Willerson JT, Hutton I, Watson JT, et al. Influence of dobutamine on regional myocardial blood flow and ventricular performance during acute and chronic myocardial ischemia in dogs. Circulation 1976;53:828–33.

66. Krivokapich J, Huang SC, Schelbert HR. Assessment of the effects of dobutamine on myocardial blood flow and oxidative metabolism in normal human subjects using nitrogen-13 ammonia and carbon-11 acetate. Am J Cardiol 1993;71:1351–6.

67. Kaul S. Response of dysfunctional myocardium to dobutamine, "The eyes see what the mind knows!" J Am Coll Cardiol 1996;27:1608–11.

68. Senior R, Lahiri A. Enhanced detection of myocardial ischemia by stress dobutamine echocardiography utilizing the "biphasic" response of wall thickening during low and high dose dobutamine infusion. J Am Coll Cardiol 1995;26:26–32.

69. Afridi I, Kleiman NS, Raizner AE, Zoghbi WA. Dobutamine echocardiography in myocardial hibernation. Optimal dose and accuracy in predicting recovery of ventricular function after coronary angioplasty. Circulation 1995;91:663–70.

70. Flameng W, Suy R, Schwarz F, et al. Ultrastructural correlates of the ventricular contraction abnormalities in patients with chronic ischemic heart disease: determinants of reversible segmental asynergy postrevascularization surgery. Am Heart J 1981;102:846–57.

71. Borgers M, Thone F, Wouters L, et al. Structural correlates of regional myocardial dysfunction in patients with critical coronary artery stenosis: chronic hibernation? Cardiovasc Pathol 1993;2:237–45.

72. Maes A, Flameng W, Nuyts J, et al. Histological alterations in chronically hypoperfused myocardium: correlation with PET findings. Circulation 1994;90:735–45.

73. Pagano D, Bonser RS, Townend JN, Parums D, Camici PG. Histopathological correlates of dobutamine echocardiography in hibernating myocardium. Circulation 1996;94 (Suppl I):543.

74. Senior R, Glenville B, Basu S, et al. Dobutamine echocardiography and thallium-201 imaging predict functional improvement after revascularization in severe ischemic left ventricular dysfunction. Br Heart J 1995;74:358–64.

75. Vanoverschelde J-L, d'Hondt A-M, Marwick T, et al. Head-to-head comparison of exercise-redistribution-reinjection thallium SPECT and low-dose dobutamine echocardiography for prediction of the reversibility of chronic left ventricular ischemic dysfunction. J Am Coll Cardiol 1996;28:432–42.

76. Meluzin J, Cigarroa CG, Brickner ME, et al. Dobutamine echocardiography in predicting improvement in global left ventricular systolic function after coronary bypass or angioplasty in patients with healed myocardial infarcts. Am J Cardiol 1995;76:877–80.

77. Afridi I, Kleiman NS, Raizner AE, Zoghbi WA. Dobutamine echocardiography in myocardial hibernation. Optimal dose and accuracy in predicting recovery of ventricular function after coronary angioplasty. Circulation 1995;91:663–70.

78. Senior R, Lahiri A. Role of dobutamine echocardiography in detection of myocardial viability for predicting outcome after revascularization in ischemic cardiomyopathy. J Am Soc Echocardiogr 2001;14:240–8.

79. Senior R, Kaul S, Lahiri A. Myocardial viability on echocardiography predicts long-term survival after revascularization

in patients with ischemic congestive heart failure. J Am Coll Cardiol 1999;33:1848–54.

80. Afridi I, Grayburn PA, Panza JA, et al. Myocardial viability during dobutamine echocardiography predicts survival in patients with coronary artery disease and severe left ventricular dysfunction. J Am Coll Cardiol 1998;32:921–6.

81. Meluzin J, Cerny J, Frelich M, et al. Prognostic value of the amount of dysfunctional but viable myocardium in revascularized patients with coronary artery disease and left ventricular dysfunction. J Am Coll Cardiol 1998;32:912–20.

82. Aronson S, Dupont F, Savage R, et al. Changes in regional myocardial function after coronary artery bypass graft surgery are predicted by intraoperative low-dose dobutamine echocardiography. Anesthesiology 2000;93:685–92.

83. Dupont FW, Lang R, Dean K, et al. Myocardial function changes one year following CABG are predicted with intraoperative dobutamine stress echocardiography. Anesthesiology 2000;92:A-241.

84. Kaul S. Myocardial contrast echocardiography: 15 years of research and development. Circulation 1997;96:3745–60.

85. Sabia PJ, Power ER, Ragosta M, et al. An association between collateral blood flow and myocardial viability in patients with recent myocardial infarction. N Engl J Med 1992;327:1825–31.

86. Ito H, Tomooka T, Sakai N, et al. Lack of myocardial perfusion immediately after successful thrombolysis. A predictor of poor recovery of left ventricular function in anterior myocardial infarction. Circulation 1992;85:1699–705.

87. Iliceto S, Galiuto L, Marchese A, et al. Analysis of microvascular integrity, contractile reserve, and myocardial viability after acute myocardial infarction by dobutamine echocardiography and myocardial contrast echocardiography. Am J Cardiol 1996;77:441–5.

88. Kabas JS, Kisslo J, Flick CL, et al. Intraoperative perfusion contrast echocardiography. Initial experience during coronary artery bypass grafting. J Thorac Cardiovasc Surg 1990;99:536–42.

89. Spotnitz WD, Kaul S. Intraoperative assessment of myocardial perfusion using contrast echocardiography. Echocardiography 1990;7:209–28.

90. Aronson S, Lee BK, Wiencek JG, et al. Assesment of myocardial perfusion during CABG surgery with two-dimensional transesophageal contrast echocardiography. Anesthesiology 1991;75:433–40.

91. Aronson S, Savage R, Fernandez A, et al. Assessing myocardial perfusion with Albunex during coronary artery bypass surgery: technical considerations and safety of aortic root injections. J Cardiothorac Vasc Anesth 1996;10:713.

92. Jacobsohn E, Aronson S, Young CJ, Ferdinand FD, Albertucci M. Case 2—1997. On-line contrast echocardiographic assessment of myocardial perfusion: its role in minimally invasive coronary artery bypass procedures. J Cardiothorac Vasc Anesth 1997;1:517–21.

93. Aronson S, Savage R, Toledano A, et al. Identifying the cause of left ventricular systolic dysfunction after coronary artery bypass surgery; the role of myocardial contrast echocardiography. J Cardiothorac Vasc Anesth 1998;12:512–8.

94. Marzullo P, Parodi O, Reisenhofer B, et al. Value of rest thallium-201 technetium-99m sestamibi scans and dobutamine echocardiography in detecting myocardial viability. Am J Cardiol 1993;71:166–72.

95. Alfieri O, La Canna G, Giubbini R, et al. Recovery of myocardial function: the ultimate target of coronary revascularization. Eur J Cardiothorac Surg 1993;7:325–30.

96. Haque T, Furukawa T, Takahashi M, et al. Identification of hibernating myocardium by dobutamine stress echocardiography: comparison with thallium-201 reinjection imaging. Am Heart J 1995;130:553–63.

97. Qureshi U, Nagueh SF, Afridi I, et al. Dobutamine echocardiography and quantitative rest-redistribution [201]T1 tomography in myocardial hibernation. Relation of contractile reserve to [201]T1 uptake and comparative prediction of recovery of function. Circulation 1997;95:626–35.

98. Perrone-Filardi P, Pace L, Prastaro M, et al. Assessment of myocardial viability in patients with chronic coronary disease. Rest-4-hour-24-hour [201]T1 tomography versus dobutamine echocardiography. Circulation 1996;97:2712–19.

99. Baer FM, Voth E, Deutsch HJ, et al. Assessment of viable myocardium by dobutamine transesophageal echocardiography and comparison with fluorine-18 fluorodeoxyglucose PET. J Am Coll Cardiol 1994;24:343–53.

100. de Fillipi CR, Willett DWL, Irani WN, et al. Comparison of myocardial contrast echocardiography and low-dose dobutamine stress echocardiography in predicting recovery of left ventricular function after coronary revascularization in chronic ischemia heart disease. Circulation 1995;92:2863–8.

101. Gerber BL Vanoverschelde J-L, Bol A, et al. Myocardial blood flow, glucose uptake and recruitment of inotropic reserve in chronic left ventricular ischemic dysfunction. Implications for the pathophysiology of chronic myocardial hibernation. Circulation 1996;94:651–9.

102. Wijns W, Vatner SF, Camici PG. Hibernating myocardium. N Engl J Med 1998;339:173–81.

103. Shanewise JS, Cheung AT, Aronson S, et al. ASE/SCA guidelines for performing a comprehensive intraoperative multiplane transesophageal echocardiography examination: recommendations of the American Society of Echocardiography Council for Intraoperative Echocardiography and the Society of Cardiovascular Anesthesiologists Task Force for Certification in Perioperative Transesophageal Echocardiography. Anesth Analg 1999;89:870–84.

## QUESTIONS

1. Viable myocardium can exist in all of the following states, *except*:
   A. Acute ischemic contractile dysfunction
   B. Regional akinesis without recruitable reserve during low-dose dobutamine
   C. Myocardial stunning
   D. Myocardial hibernation

2. What is *not* characteristic of myocardial stunning?
   A. A perfusion-contraction mismatch
   B. The reversibility of regional contractile dysfunction
   C. Decreased coronary blood flow
   D. Injurious events during ischemia and reperfusion

3. What is *not* characteristic of myocardial hibernation?
   A. A normal or slightly reduced myocardial blood flow
   B. A limited coronary flow reserve
   C. Residual contractile reserve with low-dose dobutamine stimulation
   D. Improvement of regional, but not global, left ventricular function after coronary revascularization

4. Which statement is *false*?

   Preoperative differentiation of hibernating from infarcted myocardium is important because revascularization of hibernating myocardium
   A. increases perioperative morbidity and mortality associated with coronary revascularization procedures.
   B. improves left ventricular regional and global systolic function.
   C. maintains the left ventricular shape and size by preventing infarct expansion with subsequent heart failure.
   D. decreases long-term morbidity and mortality.

**5.** Which statement is *false*?

   Differentiation of acutely ischemic myocardium from stunned myocardium is critical after separation from cardiopulmonary bypass because

   A. it may initiate the return to cardiopulmonary bypass for reexploration of the coronary bypass graft.

   B. it may necessitate the administration of vasoactive drugs to improve contractile function.

   C. it will determine the dosage of vasoactive drugs .

   D. the selection of appropriate management strategies will affect long-term outcome.

**6.** Which statement about dobutamine echocardiography is *true*?

A. Preoperative low-dose dobutamine echocardiography predicts regional but not global improvement after coronary revascularization.

B. Preoperative low-dose dobutamine echocardiography cannot predict left ventricular remodeling after coronary revascularization.

C. Preoperative low-dose dobutamine echocardiography cannot predict survival after coronary revascularization.

D. Intraoperative low-dose dobutamine echocardiography predicts recovery of regional myocardial function immediately after CABG surgery

# Assessment in Higher Risk Myocardial Revascularization and Complications of Ischemic Heart Disease

*Robert M. Savage, Gonzalo Gonzalez-Stawinski, Jacek Cywinski, David Vener, and Bruce W. Lytle*

## HISTORICAL PERSPECTIVES

The first association between coronary artery disease and myocardial dysfunction was suggested in 1779 by Caleb Hillier Parry who described his autopsy findings of hardened "ossified" blockages in the coronary arteries and death associated with "syncope anginos" (1). It was three years later that William Heberden provided his classic description of the syndrome of pectoralis dolor as "a disagreeable sensation in the breast" associated with exertion (2). In 1856, Rudolf Virchow described the evolution of fibrous thickening in the arterial wall into arterial atheroma because of a reactive inflammatory process resulting in fibrotic proliferation cells (3). Since these early characterizations of coronary artery disease, remarkable advances have been made in our understanding of this disease process and its management. In 1910, Alexis Carrell performed the first aortocoronary bypass surgery in a dog, using a preserved carotid artery between the ascending aorta and left anterior descending coronary artery (4). However, it was not until early 1958 that Longmire was credited with performing the first internal mammary to coronary artery anastomosis following a right coronary endarterectomy, which had "disintegrated" (5). As seen in Tables 24.1 and 24.2, the management of coronary artery disease has been driven by numerous factors and spans more than two centuries from initial scientific observations to the advanced direct surgical and percutaneous approaches to myocardial revascularization. While there may be a number of surgical teams credited with performing the first coronary artery bypass surgery, it was René Favaloro's report, in 1968, of 171 patients undergoing direct surgical myocardial revascularization that ushered in the modern era of coronary bypass surgery (Fig. 24.1) (6). Since that time, there have been number of milestones in the evolution of myocardial revascularization.

1. The introduction of myocardial protection strategies
2. Demonstration of long-term advantages of IMA conduits
3. Advances in cardiovascular anesthetic management
4. Introduction of percutaneous approaches to revascularization
5. Introduction of intraoperative echocardiography into patient management
6. Improved management of the complications of ischemic heart disease
7. Identification of the variables improving repeat coronary bypass surgery
8. Development of ventricular support devices
9. Development of ventricular reconstruction surgery

## INDICATIONS FOR MYOCARDIAL REVASCULARIZATION

The American College of Cardiology recently revised their Guidelines for Coronary Artery Bypass Graft Surgery (CABG) (Table 24.3) (7). A number of factors created an evolution in the current indications for myocardial revascularization by traditional surgical CABG or percutaneous coronary intervention (PCI). The factors are related to patient selection, differences in institutional CABG and PCI capabilities, temporal differences in recurrence for CABG and PCI, accelerated pace of innovations affecting the scientific study relevancy, and the inherent difficulties in comparing CABG and PCI due to the inability to account for all of the definable and less definable outcome risks in randomized studies (7,8). While the pace may slow, physicians involved in the care of patients with coronary artery disease will need to stay current with the scientific literature and ongoing innovations in revascularization.

## DEFINITION OF HIGHER RISKS IN PATIENTS UNDERGOING CORONARY ARTERY BYPASS GRAFT SURGERY

To assist patients in making an informed decision and enable the surgical team to develop optimal perioperative strategies, it is important to identify factors that may affect a patient's perioperative outcome. To identify risks of morbidity and mortality, patient- and disease-related features from patient's history, physical examination, or diagnostic evaluation are subjected to statistical analysis to determine the degree of correlation with adverse clinical events. Such risks are related to the severity and extent of ischemic heart disease or other comorbid chronic disease processes. While many factors are associated with higher morbidity and mortality, it is typically only those commonly occurring that permit a statistical correlation with outcomes. From these studies, outcome prediction

▶ **TABLE 24.1.  History of Coronary Artery Disease and Its Management**

| Year | Investigator | Milestone |
|------|--------------|-----------|
| **1770–1935** | | **Observations Considerations for Treatment** |
| 1779 | Caleb Hillier Parry | Discovered relation between angina and coronary ossification |
| 1856 | Rudolf Virchow | Described inflammatory process of atheroma development |
| 1856 | William Heberden | Characterized classic angina |
| 1880 | Langer | Described coronary collateral communications |
| 1899 | Francois-Franck | Described sympathetic innervation |
| 1902 | Kocher | Absence of angina in thyroidectomy patient |
| **1910** | **Alexis Carrell** | **Experimental aortocoronary bypass with preserved carotid artery** |
| 1916 | Jonnesco | Performed first cardiac sympathetectomy |
| 1926 | Boas | Subtotal thyroidectomy for treatment of angina |
| 1929 | Richardson and White | Series of patients undergoing ganglionic sympathetectomy |
| 1930 | Sussman | Performed cardiac irradiation for sympathetic denervation |
| 1930s | Carrell and Lindberg | Developed primitive heart lung machine |
| **1935–1953** | | **Indirect myocardial revascularization** |
| **1930** | **Claude S. Beck** | **Performed epicardial abrasion to increase collateral flow** |
| 1934 | Robertson | Ligated coronary sinus to redirect coronary flow |
| 1937 | O'Shaughnessy | Used omental flap to epicardium for revascularization |
| 1937 | John Gibbon, Jr. | Bypassed a dog's heart during pulmonary artery occlusion |
| 1938 | Griffith and Bates | Direct implantation of blood vessels into myocardium |
| **1946** | **Arthur Vineberg** | **Reported internal mammary implants directly into myocardium** |
| 1946 | Beck | Arterialized coronary sinus |
| 1951 | Gordon Murray | Direct arterial repair and venous interposition homografts |
| 1953 | William Mustard | Carotid to coronary bypass |
| **1953** | **John Gibbon** | **First effective heart-lung bypass machinery** |
| **1954–1966** | | **Early direct coronary artery bypass** |
| 1954 | Murray | First successful bypass on beating heart of a dog |
| 1955 | Melrose | Elective potassium-induced arrest |
| **1957** | **F. Mason Sones** | **First cineangiogram of coronary artery** |
| **1958** | **William Longmire** | **Grafted IMA to coronary vessel** |
| 1958 | Senning | Coronary endartectomy with plaque excision and graft |
| 1960 (reported 1964) | Robert Goetz | IMA to right coronary anastomosis |
| **1962 (reported 1974)** | **David Sabiston** | **First saphenous vein CABG** |
| 1964 | Vasilii Kolesov | Performed internal mammary to LAD graft without CPB |
| **1964 (reported 1973)** | **Garrett and DeBakey** | **First successful saphenous vein bypass graft** |
| 1966 | Bailey | Gastroepiploic artery implantation into myocardium |
| **1967–present** | | **Modern era of revascularization** |
| **1967** | **René Favaloro** | **First series of free SVG and end-to-side anastomosis** |
| 1968 | Dudley Johnson | Other saphenous vein grafting series |
| 1970 | René Favaloro | Double IMA grafts alone or in combination with SVG |
| 1968 | René Favaloro | Aortocoronary bypass for unstable angina and AMI |
| 1968 | René Favaloro | Combined CABG and valve replacement or aneurysmectomy |
| 1973 | Alan Carpentier | Free radial artery grafts |
| **1974** | **Gerald Buckberg** | **Myocardial protection strategies using cardioplegia** |
| **1976–1986** | **Floyd Loop** | **Reported survival benefit IMA-LAD graft** |

Mueller RL, Rosengart TK, Isom W. The history of surgery for ischemic heart disease. Ann Thorac Surg 1997;63:869–78.

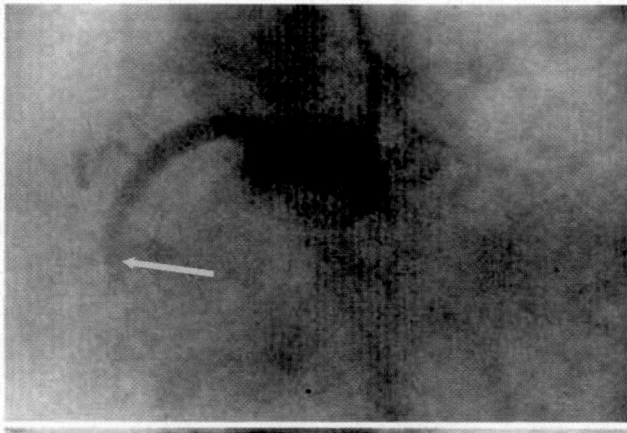
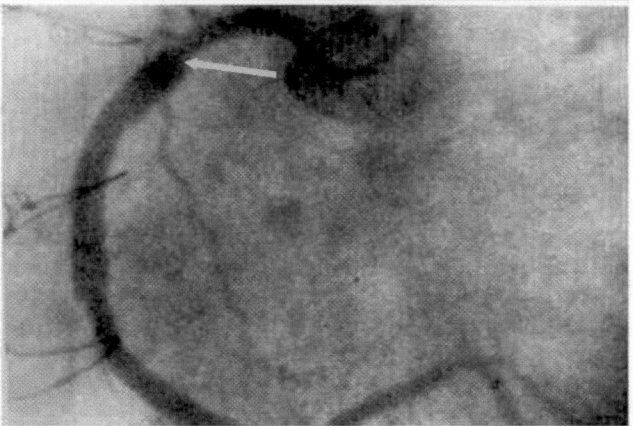

**FIGURE 24.1.** René Favaloro and Mason Sones of the Cleveland Clinic united as a team in demonstrating the feasibility of safely performing saphenous vein interposition and aortocoronary bypass grafts. In May of 1967, this angiogram demonstrated the intersegmental graft with end-to-end anastomoses. In December of 1968, Favaloro, Sones, and Effler summarized the advances in the first large series of 171 patients. Favaloro, RG. Landmarks in the development of coronary bypass surgery. Circulation. 1998;98(5):466–78.

may be based on cumulative risks (7). While many of these risks are easily defined (Table 24.3), others are more difficult to define objectively. Yet, many of these issues have a significant impact on the patient's outcome. Included in these more difficult to define risks are:

1. Availability of suitable bypass conduits
2. Diffuseness of distal coronary atherosclerosis (reducing distal coronary blood flow)
3. Presense of noncardiac atherosclerosis
4. Uncommon combinations of patient comorbidities (9,10)

## Risk Factors and Mortality

There have been a number of studies evaluating the clinical variables associated with perioperative death (11–13). They are difficult to compare due to differences in the definitions of clinical or disease variables, clinical end-

▶ **TABLE 24.2. Challenges with Guideline Indications for Myocardial Revascularization Using CABG and PCI**

1. Rapid pace of technology
2. Time between scientific investigation and technology
3. Time difference in disease recurrence for CABG and PCI
4. Comparability of CABG-PCI study groups (selection bias, non-randomized patient, and disease risk factors)
5. Randomized trials for degree of risk
6. Initial therapy studies include crossover success
7. Differences in definitions of re-stenosis in CABG and PCI
8. Secondary prevention in studies differs
9. High volume center studies not as relevant to low volume practices
10. Unique capabilities of individual centers in CABG and PCI
11. Difficulties of informed consent

points, institutional differences in clinical practices, and clinical outcomes. Jones et al. combined the data from seven large studies to evaluate recurring factors that contribute to in-hospital mortality following CABG (14a). This resulted in a clinical study population of more than 172,000 patients, enabling the identification of two levels of variables. Those variables having the strongest correlation with outcome included:

1. Patient's age
2. Gender
3. Previous cardiac surgery
4. Operation urgency
5. Ventricular ejection fraction
6. Characterization of coronary anatomy (left main > 50% stenosis, number of vessels with > 70% stenosis)

Age, urgency of procedure, and reoperation were the variables most strongly correlated with mortality. There were other variables identified that influenced mortality but they were not as strongly correlated (Table 24.4).

Trials that were initiated in the first decade of coronary bypass surgery demonstrated that patients with left main or triple vessel disease and abnormal LV function had an improved long-term survival when coupled with an aggressive strategy of complete revascularization (14b,14c). Since then, there have been remarkable improvements in the management of this unique group of higher risk patients with the advent of myocardial protection strategies, integrated perioperative care, secondary prevention, use of arterial grafts, and the increased collective experience of the surgical community. This has led to a growing consensus, as outlined by the recent ACC Guidelines for Coronary Artery Bypass Surgery, that left main equivalent or triple vessel disease combined with abnormal LV function are indications for surgical revascularization (Table 24.2) (7). Despite recent improvements in the medical management of this group of patients, the yearly mortality remains at 12%, indicating

▶ TABLE 24.3 **Indications for Coronary Artery Bypass Surgery**

**Asymptomatic or Mild Angina**
**Class I**
1. Left main disease (A)
2. Left main equivalent (A)
3. 3-vessel disease, EF < 0.50 and/or large ischemic areas (C)
4. Prox LAD Dz + 1–2 vessel Dz + EF < 0.50 +/or large at-risk ischemic area (A)
**Class IIa**
Prox LAD Dz + 1–2-vessel disease (A)
**Class IIb**
1- or 2-vessel Dz + large at-risk viable area (B)
**Stable Angina**
**Class I**
1. Left main Dz (A)
2. Left main equivalent (A)
3. 3-vessel Dz (benefit greater with LVEF < 0.50.) (A)
4. 2-vessel Dz with prox LAD stenosis + either EF < 0.50 or ischemia (A)
5. 1- or 2-vessel Dz (no prox LAD stenosis) + large at-risk area (B)
6. Disabling angina on max med Rx and acceptable risk (B)
**Class IIa**
1. Prox LAD Dz + 1-vessel disease (A)
2. 1- or 2-vessel Dz (no prox LAD Dz ) mod viable ischemic area at-risk (B)
**Class III (not recommended)**
1. 1–2 vessel Dz (no prox LAD Dz) symptoms not ischemia, < max med Rx, small ischemia viable area (B)
2. Borderline coronary Dz (50%–60% or left main < 40%) + no ischemia (B)
3. Insignificant coronary Dz (< 50%) (B)
**Unstable Angina (Non-STEMI)**
**Class I**
1. Left main stenosis (A)
2. Left main equivalent: (> 70% prox LAD + prox LCx)(A)
3. Active ischemia not responsive to med Rx + PCI not possible (B)
**Class IIa**
1. Prox LAD Dz with 1- or 2-vessel Dz (A)
**Class IIb**
1- or 2-vessel disease not involving the proximal LAD when PCI not possible/optimal
**Emergent / Urgent CABG STEMI**
**Class I**
1. Failed PCI + persistent pain or unstable hemodynamics + suitable Sx anatomy (B)
2. Persistent recurrent ischemia on max med Rx and suitable Sx anatomy + significant area at risk + not PCI candidates (B)
3. During surgery for VSD or ischemic MR (B)
4. Cardiogenic shock < 36 hrs of MI (age < 75) + ST elevation, LBBB, posterior MI + suitable Sx anatomy (A)
5. Life-threatening ventricular arrhythmias and left main Dz (> 40%) or equivalent (B)
**Class IIa**
1. < 6–12 MI + suitable anatomy not candidates or failed fibrinolysis/PCI (B)
2. CABG mortality elevated (< 3 to 7 days MI); benefit CABG by risk-benefit (B)
**Class III (not recommended)**
1. Persistent angina + small area myocardium at-risk and stable hemodynamics (C)
2. Successful epicardial reperfusion + poor microvascular reperfusion (C)
**Poor LV Function**
**Class I**
1. Left main Dz (B)
2. Left main equivalent (B)
3. Prox LAD Dz + 2- or 3-vessel Dz (B)
**Class IIa**
Significant viable noncontracting revascularizable myocardium (B)
**Class III (not recommended)**
No evidence of ischemia or significant revascularizable viable myocardium (B)

**Classification of Recommendations**
**Class I:** Conditions for which there is evidence and/or general agreement that a procedure is beneficial and effective.
**Class II:** Conditions for which there is conflicting evidence and/or a divergence of opinion about the usefulness of a procedure or treatment.
**IIa:** Conflicting evidence but weight of evidence/opinion is in favor of benefit/ efficacy.
**IIb:** Conflicting evidence and  benefit/efficacy is less well established by evidence/opinion.
**Class III:** Conditions for which there is evidence and/or general agreement that the procedure/ treatment is not useful or effective.
**Level of Evidence**
**A:** Data from multiple randomized trials or metaanalysis
**B:** Data from single randomized trial or nonrandomized studies
**C:** Concensus opinion of experts only or standard of care

▶ **TABLE 24.3** (continued)

**Life Threatening Ventricular Arrhythmias**
**Class I**
1. Left main stenosis (B)
2. Left main equivalent (B)
**Class IIa**
1. 1–2 vessel Dz causing the arrhythmias (B)
2. Prox LAD Dz + 1–2 vessel Dz (B)
**Class III (not recommended)**
1. VT with scar + no ischemia (B)
2. CABG after failed PCI
**Class I**
1. Ischemia or threatened occlusion with significant at-risk area (B)
2. Hemodynamic compromise (B)
**Class IIa**
1. Foreign body crucial anatomic position (C)
2. Unstable hemodynamics + impaired coagulation + no previous sternotomy (C)
**Class IIb**
Unstable hemodynamics + impaired coagulation + previous sternotomy (C)
**Class III**
1. Absence of ischemia (C)
2. Inability to revascularize target anatomy or no-reflow state (C)
**Previous CABG**
**Class I**
1. Disabling angina with max med Rx or atypical angina with ischemia (B)
2. No patent grafts + left main Dz or equivalent (B)
**Class IIa**
1. Bypassable distal vessel(s) with large area threatened myocardium (B)
2. Atherosclerotic LAD vein graft (Dz > 50%) or large at risk areas (B)
**Valve Surgery at Time of CABG**
**Class I**
Severe AS 1 criteria for AVR (B)
**Class IIa**
1. Mod MR correction probably indicated (B)
2. Mod AS acceptable combined risks (B)
**Class IIb**
1. Mild AS if acceptable combined risk (C)
2. Arterial conduits
**Class I**
In all CABG, the LAD Dz should considered for left IMA graft (B)
**Transmyocardial revascularization (laser)**
**Class IIa**
Angina refractory to Rx 1 not candidates for PCI-CABG (A)

Adapted from Eagle KA, Guyton RA, Davidoff R, et al. ACC/AHA guidelines for coronary artery bypass graft surgery: a report of the American College of Cardiology/American Heart Association task force on practice guidelines (committee to revise the 1991 guidelines for coronary artery bypass graft surgery). J Am Coll Cardiol 1993;34:1262–1346.

that surgical management of this high-risk group is warranted (14d). This strategy is further supported by an understanding that:

1. Ischemia is the inciting event of death when these patients are treated medically.
2. Revascularization results in decreased incidence of ischemic-related sudden death.
3. The low mortality rate of patients with poor LV function undergoing CABG is 0.8% to 3.2% in experienced centers (9).

Allman et al. performed a metaanalysis of 24 studies, representing a total of 3,088 patients, with an average ejection fraction of 32%. They demonstrated that surgical revascularization in patients with viable myocardium reduced the mortality by 80% (without) 3.2% compared to 16% with CABG (14e). Patients without areas of viable myocardium did not demonstrate a survival benefit, regardless of the severity of ventricular dysfunction. With 6% to 9% of patients over age 65 exhibiting ischemic cardiomyopathy, this higher risk population will continue to challeng the medical community to develop

▶ **TABLE 24.4. Coronary Artery Bypass Surgery Relative Mortality Risks**

| Risk Factor | Relative Risk | Risk Score |
|---|---|---|
| **Core Variables** | | |
| Age | add 1.01–1.05 per yr > 50 | |
| 60–69 | | 1.5 |
| 70–79 | | 2.5 |
| > 80 | | 6 |
| **Previous CABG** | 1.39–3.6 | 5 |
| **Urgency** | | |
| Elective | 1 | 0 |
| Urgent (required to stay in hospital) | 1.2–3.5 | 2 |
| Emergent (refractory compromise) | 2–7.4 | 5 |
| Salvage (ongoing CPR) | 6.7–29 | 5 |
| **Sex** | 1.2–1.63 for female | |
| Female | | |
| **LV Ejection Fraction** | | |
| 40%–60% | 1 | |
| < 40% | | 2 |
| 30%–39% | 1.6 | |
| 20%–29% | 2.2 | |
| < 20% | 4.1 | |
| Left main stenosis | | |
| 50%–89% | | 1.5 |
| > 90% | | 2 |
| **Number of Major Coronaries > 70%** | | |
| 3-vessel disease | 1.5 | 1.5 |
| 2-vessel disease | 1.3 | 1.3 |
| 1-vessel disease | 1 | 1 |
| **Influencing Variables** | | |
| History of angina | | |
| CHF | | |
| Recent MI (< 1 week) | 1.5 | 1.5 |
| PCI index | | |
| Ventricular arrhythmia | | |
| Mitral regurgitation | | |
| **Comorbidities** | | |
| Diabetes | 1 | 1 |
| Cerebrovascular disease | | |
| Peripheral vascular Dz | 1.5 | 1.5 |
| Renal dysfunction | | |
| Hemodialysis | 4 | 4 |
| Creatinine > 2.0 | 2 | 2 |
| **Other Variables** | | |
| COPD | | 2 |
| WBC > 12K | | 2.5 |
| **Total Point Score** | | **Mortality Risk** |
| 0–5 | | 0.2–0.7% |
| 6–10 | | 1–3 % |
| 11–15 | | 4–11.5% |
| 16–17 | | 14.1–18.7% |
| 18 | | > 23% |

innovative strategies to meet this growing concern (22–24).

## Risk Factors and Morbidity

Clinical studies have been performed evaluating those variables influencing the perioperative morbidity (Table 24.5) (15–18). Many have evaluated specific morbidities, including central nervous system dysfunction, cardiac morbidity (recurrence of angina, LV dysfunction, perioperative MI, and dysrhythmias), and renal dysfunction. Neurologic dysfunction following CABG surgery is considered in two broad categories. Type 1 deficits involve major focal neurologic deficits, stupor, and coma. Type 2 deficits are characterized as alterations in cognitive function. In a multicenter study involving 2,108 patients, Roach et al. identified CNS dysfunction in 6% of patients, which was evenly distributed between type 1 and type 2 deficits (19). Predictors of both types of neurologic dysfunction included age > 70 and a history of hypertension. Risk factors associated with type 1 deficits included diabetes, use of an IABP, prior neurologic event, perioperative hypotension, use of an LV vent, and a history of unstable angina. Atheromatous disease involving the proximal ascending aorta, as detected by intraoperative echo (TEE and epivascular imaging) has also been closely associated with type 1 neurologic events. Risk factors associated with type 2 deficits include a history of previous CABG, CHF, peripheral vascular disease (PVDz), alcohol consumption, or dysrhythmias (19).

Renal dysfunction is a significant contributor to perioperative morbidity. Mangano et al., in 1998, evaluated more than 2,200 CABG patients for factors associated

▶ **TABLE 24.5 Coronary Artery Bypass Surgery Morbidity Risk Factors**

| Risk Factor |
|---|
| Patient |
| Age |
| Sex |
| **Cardiac-Related Factors** |
| Previous CABG |
| Left main stenosis |
| Triple vessel disease |
| Recent mi (< 1 week) |
| Ejection fraction |
| Urgency |
| **Comorbidities** |
| Obesity |
| Diabetes |
| Cerebrovascular disease |
| Peripheral vascular DZ |
| Renal dysfunction |
| COPD |
| WBC > 12 k |

with the development of perioperative renal dysfunction (creatinine > 2 mg/dl or increase of 0.7 mg/dl) (20). Renal dysfunction occurred in 7.7% of this patient population postoperatively with a mortality of 19% compared to 1% of those patients with no renal dysfunction. Risk factors associated with post-CABG renal dysfunction included age, type 1 diabetes, preexisting renal dysfunction, CHF, and previous CABG surgery.

In looking at factors associated with a higher risk of death and postoperative morbidity, Higgins et al. developed and validated a severity scoring system using measurable factors that defined a patient population at increased risk (Table 24.6) (Figs. 24.2A–24.2C) (21). This Cleveland Clinic Preoperative Cardiac Surgical Severity Score assigned points (from 1 to 6), for the factors most closely associated with mortality and morbidity (21). As the severity score index became greater than 4, the incidence of morbidity and mortality markedly increased. The highest number of points was assigned to emergent surgery (6) while serum creatinine > 1.9 mg/dl was given 4 points. Severe LV dysfunction, prior cardiac surgery, and mitral valve insufficiency were assigned 3 points each. In correlating the total severity score with morbidity and mortality outcomes, patients with a total score ≥ 4, have a higher risk for postoperative morbidity and mortality when undergoing myocardial revascularization (21).

## IMPORTANCE OF ISCHEMIC HEART DISEASE IN FUTURE HEALTH-CARE DELIVERY

Despite recent advances in the management of ischemic heart disease, the National Center for Health Statistics and World Health Organization report that it

▶ **TABLE 24.6.  Coronary Artery Bypass Surgery Cleveland Clinic Severity Score (21)**

| | |
|---|---|
| Age 65 to 74 years | 1 |
| Age 75 years or older | 2 |
| Weight ≤ 65 kg | 1 |
| Emergency | 6 |
| Severe LV dysfunction | 3 |
| Operative AV stenosis | 1 |
| Operative MV insufficiency | 3 |
| Prior cardiovascular surgery | 2 |
| Prior cardiac operation | 3 |
| Diabetes on medication | 1 |
| COPD on medication | 2 |
| Cerebrovascular | 1 |
| Serum creatinine 1.6–1.8 mg | 1 |
| Serum creatinine >1.9 mg | 4 |
| Anemia (Hct ≤ 34%) | 2 |
| **Maximum score:** | **31** |

## Cleveland Clinic Preoperative Cardiac Surgical Severity Score

| | | | |
|---|---|---|---|
| Emergency | 6 | Prior vascular surgery | 2 |
| Serum creatinine > 1.9 mg | 4 | COPD on medication | 2 |
| Serum creatinine 1.6–1.8 | 1 | Anemia (Hct ≤ 34%) | 2 |
| Severe LV dysfunction | 3 | Operative AV stenosis | 1 |
| Prior cardiac operation | 3 | Weight ≤ 65 kg | 1 |
| Operation MV insufficiency | 3 | Diabetes on medication | 1 |
| Age 75 years or older | 2 | Cerebrovascular | 1 |
| Age 65 to 74 years | 1 | | |

| | |
|---|---|
| Maximum score: | 31 |
| Clinically relevant range: | 0 to 13+ |

**A**

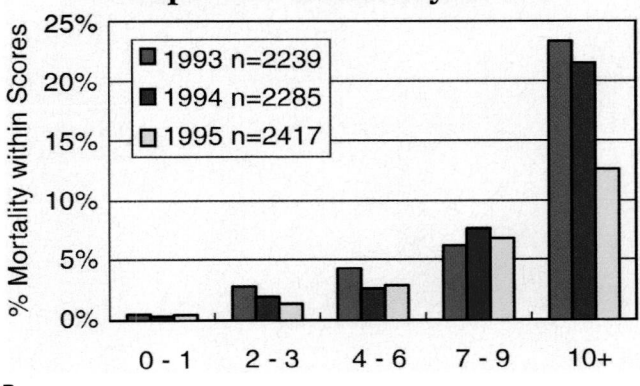

**B**

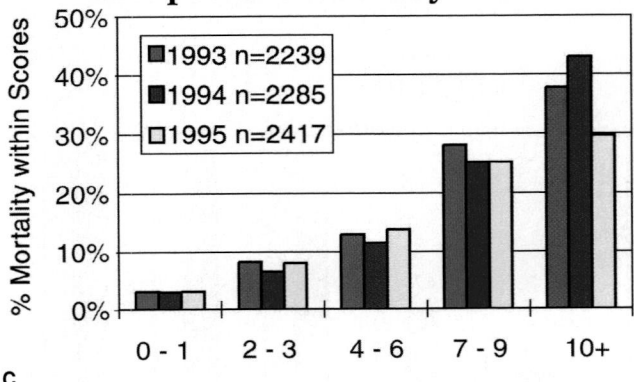

**C**

*FIGURE 24.2.* **A.** The Cleveland Clinic Severity Score was developed and validated in 1992 to predict those patients who were at risk for significant morbidity and mortality based on preoperative risk factors. **B and C.** Those patients with a severity score of 4 represent a patient population at higher risk of developing significant perioperative morbidity and increased mortality.

remains the leading cause of death throughout the world and will remain so through the year 2020 (22,23). The factors behind these trends are related to the increased incidence of coronary artery disease and associated risk factors in aging patients (for example, diabetes, hypertension, and obesity). The number of individuals over the age of 65 is expected to increase from 35 million to 71 million by the year 2030 in the United States alone (Fig. 24.3) (24). Of individuals over the age of 65, greater than 65% have cardiovascular disease (Fig. 24.4) (22,25). This age group has an increasing incidence of atherosclerotic vascular disease. More alarming is the increasing incidence of these factors in younger generations, suggesting that the cardiovascular epidemic will continue for years

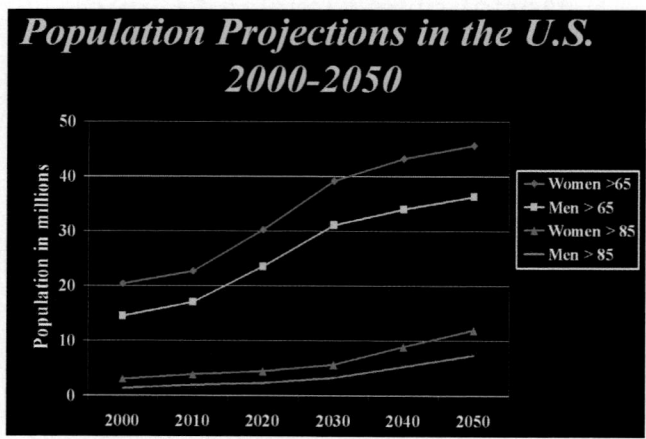

**FIGURE 24.3.** The aging of the United States population. It is estimated by the Center for Health Statistics that there will be more than 52 million individuals over the age of 65 living in the United States.

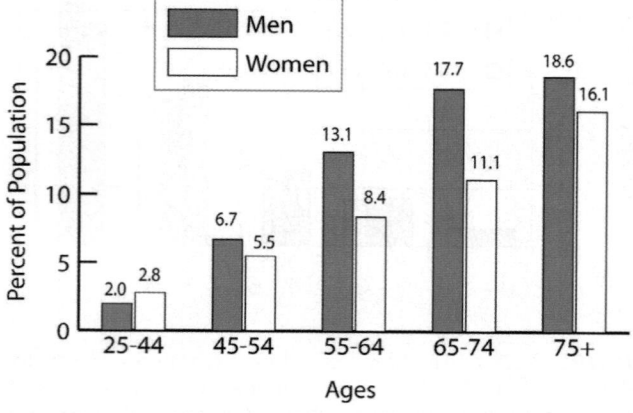

**FIGURE 24.4.** Age and incidence of coronary artery disease in men and women. The Center for Disease Control and Prevention reports that there is an age-related increase in the incidence of coronary artery disease.

to come. Consequently, we find ourselves in the midst of a growing cardiovascular pandemic in the United States and throughout the world, with ischemic heart disease constituting the major cause of significant cardiovascular morbidity and mortality (26). In addition, 80% of the elderly over 60 years old have at least one chronic disease and 50% have two chronic diseases (23). In addition to these demographic trends, the number of percutaneous revascularizations will continue to increase. Patients with coronary artery disease are living longer. This has resulted in a surgical revascularization population that is older, has more diffuse coronary disease, more frequent complications associated with chronic ischemic disease, and a more frequent history of previous surgical interventions (PCI and CABG).

The morbidity and mortality associated with myocardial revascularization has steadily declined over the last 35 years (28). If we are to maintain this trend, it will be necessary to develop strategies for addressing those critical issues that guide the intraoperative decision-making process. The purpose of this chapter is to provide an overview of the role of intraoperative echocardiography in the management of patients undergoing surgical revascularization of the myocardium. The principles of the intraoperative echo exam will be identified. The critical issues that must be addressed to insure the successful management of higher risk patients who are undergoing surgical myocardial revascularization will be examined, followed by outcome studies characterizing the effectiveness of such perioperative strategies. We will then focus on the complications of ischemic heart disease and their echocardiographic diagnosis and intraoperative management as guided by TEE. This discussion will conclude with an examination of future clinical applications of intraoperative TEE.

## PRINCIPLES OF PERFORMING INTRAOPERATIVE ECHO EXAM IN CABG SURGERY

The intraoperative echo examination for higher risk patients undergoing myocardial revascularization is guided by principles related to the unique demands of the environment and the potential for sudden changes in the patient's cardiovascular function (Table 24.7). Because of this potential for change in cardiovascular function throughout the procedure, complete diagnostic TEE exams are performed at each of the progressive phases of the surgical procedure:

1. Pre-CPB
2. Pre-Sep from CPB
3. Post-Sep CPB
4. Post-chest closure

▶ **TABLE 24.7. Principles of Intraoperative Echo Exam Higher Risk Coronary Artery Bypass Surgery**

1. Addresses critical issues
2. Systematic examination
   - Organized by priority
   - Initial overview exam
   - Focused diagnostic exam
   - Comprehensive exam documented
3. Efficient
4. Severity assessment by weighted integration
5. Study results recorded and discussed with surgeon
6. Comprehensive digital study archived
7. Results compared to preoperative data
   - Variances addressed
   - Communicated with surgical team
   - Potential Rx alterations discussed with cardiologist
8. Qualified personnel trained and credentialed
9. IOE exam under CQI process
10. Equipment maintained and updated

In addition, should the patient encounter hemodynamic instability at any point during the course of the procedure, an overview is performed followed by a more "focused diagnostic exam" directed by the clinical course and overview exam. The examination following chest closure insures that grafts are not kinked, interrupting flow and impeding an accurate determination of the effect of chest closure on preload.

The intraoperative TEE exam is performed at each of the stages in a sequence that first resolves those critical issues guiding the patient's management, yet, recognizes the ongoing management of the patient and the need to document a complete examination for future comparison. To prevent significant mid-exam revelations from occurring, an abbreviated 60-second overview exam may be performed followed by the remainder of the exam. In addition to the diagnostic issues that are already on the agenda, the abbreviated overview exam provides an up-to-date assessment of additional issues that might be addressed.

Because of the inherent difficulties in distinguishing degrees of degenerative calcification and fibrosis of the aorta and heart, subdued lighting in the OR reduces monitor glare, enabling a more accurate assessment of aortic arteriosclerosis, myocardial fibrosis, and calcification of cardiovascular structures. Periods without electrocautery interference during critical portions of the intraoperative exam also contribute to the acquisition of quality two-dimensional (2-D) images and Doppler-derived hemodynamic data. Such an atmosphere permits the precise recognition of intricate structural abnormalities (vegetation, thrombi, right-to-left shunts), which may have potentially devastating consequences if missed. It also enables the acquisition of the quality of diagnostic infor-

mation, which may confidently guide the pivotal surgical and hemodynamic decisions.

The conclusions of the TEE exam are communicated directly to the surgical team in addition to being documented in the patient's permanent medical record. Digital loops and images, which support the diagnostic conclusions and constitute the complete systematic examination, are achieved for future retrieval for comparison and reviewed under an organized CQI process.

## Critical Issues in CABG Surgery Addressed by Intraoperative Echo (Tables 24.8A and 24.8B)

The purpose of the intraoperative echo is not to replace the patient's preoperation assessment, but to confirm and refine it. Due to the clinical dynamic associated with ischemic heart disease, it is always possible that new ventricular or valve dysfunction may occur as a consequence of intervening ischemia or infarction. In addition to providing an ongoing method of monitoring the patients' cardiovascular function, intraoperative echocardiography is used to address a number of critical issues that may influence the outcome of coronary bypass surgery. These

▶ **TABLE 24.8A. Critical Issues in Higher Risk Coronary Artery Bypass Surgery**

1. Intraoperative monitoring
2. Diagnosis of unrecognized abnormalities changing management
   - Unplanned surgical procedures
   - Anesthetic-hemodynamic management
3. Cannulation and perfusion strategy
4. Predict post-CPB complications
5. Surgical results and potential complications
   - Global and regional function
     - Functioning bypass grafts
     - Inotropic support
     - Mechanical support (IABP or LVAD / RVAD ECMO)
   - Valve function
     - Ischemic MR
     - TR
     - AR (LV distension prior to separation)
   - Complications of cannulation
     - Aortic dissection
     - Plaque disruption
   - Complications of myocardial protection
     - Regional dysfunction (septal)
     - RV dysfunction
     - Coronary sinus trauma
6. Documentation of comprehensive study (future reference)
   - Global and regional (LV and RV) function
   - Valve function
   - LA, RA, and shunt potential
   - Aorta (ascending, arch, and descending)

▶ TABLE 24.8B.  Critical Surgical Decisions in Higher Risk Coronary Artery Bypass Surgery

**Impact of Echo on Surgical Decision Making**

| Echo Finding | Surgical Decisions |
|---|---|
| Proximal aortic mobile atheroma | Off pump vs. on CPB |
| | Alternative arterial cannulation (axillary, femoral) |
| | Identify cross-clamp site (epiaortic echo) |
| | Identify ascending aortic cannulation site |
| | Identify site for antegrade cardioplegia insertion |
| Calcified atheromatous aorta | Off-pump CABG |
| | All arterial grafts (IMA, gastroepiploic) |
| | Axillary cannulation |
| | Circulatory arrest |
| Significant aortic regurgitation | LV venting |
| | Direct coronary administration of cardioplegia |
| Demonstrable regional viability | Coronary bypass graft of anatomy suitable |
| Pre-CPB | Additional unplanned bypass grafts |
| New regional wall motion abnormalities | Pre-CPB IABP, additional grafts, check angio |
| New valve dysfunction | Unplanned MVREP or MVR |
| | Unplanned AVR, TVREP, or TVR |
| Post-CPB new regional wall motion abnormalities | Delayed wean from CPB, revision of grafts |
| | IABP |
| Postbypass global LV dysfunction | Return to CPB |
| | Additional grafts |
| | Graft revision |
| | IABP |
| | LVAD |
| Post-CPB localized aortic dissection | Localized repair |
| Post-CPB extensive type I or II aortic dissection | Replace ascending aorta |
| Reduced celiac axis flow (metabolic acidosis) | Explore abdomen for gut ischemia |
| Mechanical complications of ischemic heart disease | |
| — VSD, aneurysm, pseudoaneurysm | Repair of structural defect |
| — LV or LA thrombus | Thrombus removal |
| — ischemic MR (ruptured papillary muscle) | MVR or MVRep |

critical issues include the diagnosis of previously unrecognized cardiovascular abnormalities requiring additional unplanned surgical intervention or altering the patient's anesthetic-hemodynamic management, development of the cannulation-perfusion strategy to prevent neurologic dysfunction, an assessment of the results of the surgical procedure and potential complications, and a final documentation of a comprehensive baseline study for future comparison. Each phase of the procedure has issues that are important to address depending on the extent of the patient's preoperative assessment. If there is a concern regarding the viability of a specific region of myocardium, a pre-CPB dobutamine stress test may be performed as discussed in Chapter 23, Assessment of Myocardial Viability (29,30).

## Intraoperative Monitoring

There are a number of determinants of cardiac function that may be monitored intraoperatively by TEE (Table 24.9A), including preload, diastolic function, contractility, regional myocardial function, valve function, and afterload. Compared with the hemodynamics and calculations derived from measurements obtained with the pulmonary artery thermodilution catheter, TEE provides a more direct physiologic assessment of each determinant of cardiac function (Table 24.9B). Hemodynamic instability is more often encountered in higher risk patients. It may be caused by hypovolemia, ventricular dysfunction, or low systemic vascular resistance. In these circumstances, the intraoperative echo provides a rapid method of assessing global (LV and RV) ventricular function, preload, presence of segmental dysfunction indicating myocardial ischemia, and an indication of lower systemic vascular resistance (low MAP with hypercontractile LV).

Two-dimensional echocardiography provides both qualitative and quantitative evaluation of systolic ventricular function. The midesophageal four-chamber (ME 4-chamber) and two-chamber (ME 2-chamber) views,

▶ TABLE 24.9A. **Intraoperative Assessment of Cardiac Function**

| Determinant | TEE | PA Catheter |
|---|---|---|
| Preload | Direct volume assessment | PAOP |
| | PW Doppler pulmonary veins | RVEDP |
| | Interatrial septum shift | CVP |
| Diastolic Function | Inflow patterns | Indirect PAOP |
| | Tissue Doppler | |
| Global Contractility | LV/RV 2-D image | Cardiac output |
| | Cardiac output by volumetric flow | Stroke volume |
| Regional Function | Systolic thickening | NA |
| | Contraction pattern | |
| Valve Function | 2-D imaging of structure | cv wave |
| | CF Doppler assessment | |
| Afterload | Calculation regional wall stress | SVR calculation |
| | Tissue Doppler imaging | |

the midesophageal long-axis (ME LAX) view and transgastric short-axis (TG SAX) views (basal, midpapillary, and apical), and the transgastric long-axis view (TG LAX) allow assessment of global and regional ventricular function. Two-dimensional quantitative measures of LV systolic function include ventricular dimensions, volume, stroke volume (SV), cardiac output (CO), ejection fraction (EF), and regional wall motion abnormalities. Left ventricular ejection fraction (LVEF) can be calculated

from LV end-systolic volume (LVESV) and end-diastolic volume (LVEDV) as the ratio (LVEDV-LVESV)/LVEDV. Cardiac output can be calculated using the area-length formula across a cardiac valve (most commonly the aortic valve): $CO = 0.785 \times LVOT\ D^2 \times LVOT_{VTI} \times HR$ (*LVOT* = left ventricular outflow tract; *D* = LVOT diameter; $LVOT_{VTI}$ = velocity time integral, measured with Doppler spectrum across the aortic valve; and *HR* = heart rate). IOE determination of CO using TEE is helpful even when a pulmonary artery catheter is used, because the thermodilution technique is inaccurate in patients with significant tricuspid valve regurgitation (31).

### Preload

Preload has been indirectly assessed utilizing either the pulmonary artery catheter (PAOP, PAEDP) or left atrial catheter (LAP). Because preload recruitment is dependent upon end-diastolic volume, compliance of the ventricle is an integral component of normal systolic function. In circumstances of a noncompliant ventricular chamber, the LV end-diastolic pressure may not accurately reflect the volume of the LV. Clements et al. reported on 14 patients undergoing surgery for abdominal aortic aneurysms in which TEE, pulmonary artery catheterization, and portable radionuclide measurements of end-diastolic volume were simultaneously determined (32). There was a very close correlation between the TEE (end-diastolic diameter and area) and the accepted gold standard of radionuclide measurement of end-diastolic volume. Interestingly, there was no correlation between PA catheter and the ultrasound or nuclear methods of preload assessment. Standard criteria for diagnosing hypovolemia include an end-diastolic diameter less than

▶ TABLE 24.9B. **Intraoperative TEE Assessment of Hemodynamic Instability**

| | MAP | LV EDD | RV EDD | RV Fx | LV Fx | RWMA |
|---|---|---|---|---|---|---|
| Hypovolemia | Low | Decreased | Decreased | Variable | Systolic collapse | No |
| Low SVR | Low | Normal | Variable | Variable | Systolic collapse | No |
| Low SVR and Ischemia | Low | Variable | Variable | Decreased with RCA ischemia | Variable depending on extent | Yes |
| LV Ischemia | Low | Dilated | Increased with global LV dysfunction | RCA ischemia decreased | Variable | Yes |
| Increased RV Afterload | Increased PAM | Dilated | Increased | Variable | Systolic collapse | No |
| RV Ischemia | Variable | Decreased | Increased | Decreased | Systolic collapse | No; except distal RCA |
| Tamponade | Variable | Compressed LV with left-sided tamponade | Collapsed with right-sided tamponade | Variable | Systolic collapse | No |

25 mm, systolic obliteration of the LV cavity, and a LV end-diastolic area of less than 55 cm² (33).

### Diastolic Function

Diastole is the period between aortic valve closure and mitral valve closure and is divided into four phases:

1. Isovolumic relaxation
2. Early rapid diastolic filling
3. Diastasis
4. Late diastolic filling caused by atrial contraction (Fig. 24.5)

Ventricular relaxation may be assessed by the isovolumic relaxation time (IVRT), the rate of pressure decline (–Dp/dt), and a time constant of relaxation (τ). Compliance is estimated by the early diastolic LV filling (*E* wave), deceleration time (DT), late diastolic LV filling ($A_M$ wave), E:A ratio, the $A_P$ wave (reversed) of LA contraction, the *s* wave of the systolic LA filling phase, and the *d* wave of the LA diastolic filling phase.

Diastolic dysfunction is often the earliest marker of ischemia and, in the more advanced stages is predictive of a poorer long-term prognosis. The earliest stage of abnormal diastolic filling is impaired or abnormal relaxation with inverse E/A ratio < 1.0. With progression of the disease, pseudonormalization of diastolic filling flow occurs as a result of impaired myocardial relaxation balanced by elevation of mean LA pressures. The diagnosis is confirmed by abnormal pulmonary venous flow or response to Valsalva maneuver. The restrictive filling pattern is the most advanced form of diastolic dysfunction. Bernard et

al. evaluated the diastolic function in 52 consecutive CABG patients. Thirty percent of their study population had diastolic dysfunction, including patterns of abnormal relaxation (50%), pseudonormal (40%), and restrictive physiology (10%) (34). Patients with diastolic dysfunction more frequently required initial inotropic support with restrictive physiology (100%), pseudonormal (88%), and abnormal relaxation (75%). The need for inotropic support at 12 hours postoperative was similarly increased for these patterns at 100%, 75%, and 50% (34).

### Contractility

Assessment of contractility may be performed using visual estimations of global LV function or more volumetric methods based on Simpson's formula. While gross detection of subtle changes in overall ventricular performance may be difficult, detection of more substantial alterations in function lie within the capabilities of trained echocardiographers. The LV may be assessed utilizing the midesophageal four- or two-chamber views or the TG mid SAX or LAX views. The percentage of two-dimensional area change between end-diastole (measure at the ECG R-wave) and end systole is estimated. Global LV function may be classified as normal (estimated ejection fraction > 50%), mild global LV dysfunction (estimated ejection fraction 30% to 50%), moderate global LV dysfunction (estimated ejection fraction > 15% to 30%), and severe global LV dysfunction (estimated ejection fraction < 15%). Ejection fraction measurements represent the stroke volume as a percentage of the end-diastolic volume (EF = EDV − ESV/EDV). If there are no regional wall motional abnormalities simple LV diameters, measured at the mid PM level, may be used to estimate ejection fraction (EF = EDD² − ESD²/EDD²). The volumes may also be calculated utilizing the modified Simpson method whereby the length of the LV cavity and the diameter of individual discs are used to calculate and summate the volume in each of a series of discs comprising the LV cavity. With modern ultrasound platforms, these measurements may be either determined on-line (using the automated backscatter technique described above) or off-line. The LV end-diastolic volume (LVEDV) and LV end-systolic volume (LVESV) are determined automatically and the ejection fraction is calculated as in the formula expressed above.

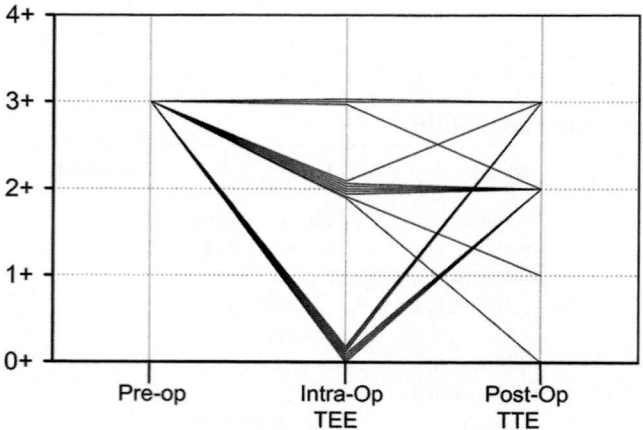

**FIGURE 24.5.** In a group of 18 patients with moderate (3+) ischemic MR undergoing CABG, Cohen et al. reported that 7 were down graded to no significant (0) MR by intraoperative TEE following induction of anesthesia. Post-operative transthoracic echo demonstrated that 4 of these patients had mild to moderate (2+) MR and 3 had returned to moderate (3+) MR (39).

### Myocardial Ischemia

One of the earliest manifestations of myocardial ischemia occurring with coronary occlusion is reduction in systolic thickening of the myocardium supplied by the occluded artery. This is followed by increase in diastolic dysfunction and, about 45 seconds after, by the ST segment changes on surface ECG (35). Minutes later, if there is a large enough perfusion defect, global ventricular dysfunction develops and manifests as elevated filling pressures. The segmental wall motion is assessed by evaluating two variables: the wall thickening and the local change of radius (movement of the myocardium toward the center of the heart). Consequently, the assessment of new regional wall motion abnormalities by intraoperative transesophageal echocardiography is a very sensitive marker to detect myocardial ischemia. However, there are other causes of wall motion abnormalities including ventricular pacing, interventricular conduction disturbances, alterations in afterload, ventricular systolic translocation, and tethering associated with adjacent wall motion abnormalities. Under normal conditions, there is marked wall thickening, usually greater than 30% increase in wall thickness during systole, whereas the decrease in radius is usually greater than 30% during systole. Mild hypokinesia corresponds with moderate wall thickening and a 10%–30% decrease in the local radius, while in severe hypokinesia there is only minimal wall thickening and a 0%–10% decrease in the local radius. Akinesia is characterized by the absence of wall thickening and no change in the radius and dyskinesia corresponds with thinning and a protruding of myocardial wall away from the heart center. Using radioactive microspheres and ultrasonic dimension crystals, Savage et al. quantified transmural myocardial perfusion and compared it with the various degree of wall motion abnormalities (35). It was determined that hypokinesia was associated with 25%–50% decrease in the transmural blood flow, while akinesia was related to a decrease of blood flow in three-quarters of the wall thickness. With dyskinesia, there was 100% reduction in blood flow to a dyskinetic region of myocardium.

van Daele et al. (36) monitored 98 patients undergoing cardiac surgery with transesophageal echocardiography, electrocardiogram, and the pulmonary artery catheter. Myocardial ischemia was diagnosed in 14 of 98 patients based on the presence of wall motion abnormalities. Interestingly, in only 10 of these 14 patients were there electrocardiographic changes indicating ischemia. The pulmonary artery catheter wedge pressure increased in the 14 patients by 3.5 mm Hg. This was an insignificant change in the wedge pressure compared with the baseline and only provided an overall sensitivity of 33% and a predictive value of 16%. Smith et al. (37) compared assessment of myocardial ischemia with the ECG vs. transesophageal echo. The authors evaluated 50 patients undergoing myocardial revascularization surgery who were monitored with TEE and multilead ECG. They found that 24 of the patients had echocardiographic evidence of ischemia compared to only 6 by ECG. All the patients who had ECG evidence of ischemia had regional wall motion abnormalities visible on TEE images, whereas there were numerous patients who had regional wall motion abnormalities and did not have ECG changes indicating myocardial ischemia. In all cases, segmental wall motion abnormalities occurred before ECG changes. Three of the patients had myocardial infarction.

### *Afterload*

While afterload may be estimated by calculation of systemic vascular resistance, it is more accurately characterized by determination of systolic wall stress. Systolic wall stress may be calculated using a combination of ultrasound and blood pressure measurements. Wall stress is represented by the Laplace formula, which expresses the direct proportionality between stress and systolic blood pressure and the LV end-diastolic diameter and the inverse relation to the LV wall thickness (WTh). This relation is expressed in the simplified equation:

$$\text{Wall stress} = (P)\,(\text{LVEDD}^2\,/\,(\text{WTh}))$$

Where P = systolic pressure, WTh = wall thickness, and LVEDD = LV end-diastolic diameter

## Unplanned Surgical Intervention or Alteration of Hemodynamic Management

Because of the thoroughness of the preoperative assessment for patients undergoing surgical myocardial revascularization, it is unusual today to find significantly undiagnosed or underdiagnosed cardiovascular disease. However, in circumstances where there has been an intervening clinical event, such as a recent silent myocardial infarction or the patient being rushed for surgery, it is possible for such intraoperative revelations to lead to alterations in the surgical or anesthetic-hemodynamic management. In a retrospective analysis of 3,245 cardiac surgery patients, Click et al. reported that intraoperative echo was utilized in 292 (9%) undergoing CABG surgery (38). In this patient subset, intraoperative echocardiography was most commonly used to evaluate suspected valve abnormalities. The largest percentage (33%) of new pre-CPB findings occurred in the CABG subset of patients. Some patients were found to have less MR intraoperatively than their preoperative evaluation with the result that their mitral valve was not inspected. Mitral annular dilation caused by LV dilation and mitral apparatus dysfunction is the most common mechanism of mitral regurgitation in patients with ischemic heart disease. Remodeling leads to changes in the shape and size of the ventricle and may alter the structural integrity of the mitral valve apparatus. While ischemic MR may be either transient or chronic, it is clear that the hemodynamic perturbations of the anesthetic agents and effects of positive pressure ventilation may alter the severity of mitral or tricuspid regurgitation.

In a similar group of patients undergoing CABG with ischemic MR, Cohn et al. reported that 90% were downgraded from moderate to less than mild to moderate MR by IOE exam (Fig. 24.6) (39). Seven of the patients went from moderate MR to no MR intraoperatively and consequently did not receive a MVRep or MVR. Postoperatively 3 out of 7 patients returned to their original 3+ MR and 4 returned to moderate MR on their postoperative TTE (39).

Grewal et al. (40) demonstrated that 51% of patients with MR improve by at least one MR severity grade when assessed under general anesthesia. The most significant changes occurred in patients with ischemic MR with normal MV leaflets (40). Bach et al. compared the severity of preoperative MR with the IOE (41), discovering that patients with structural valve leaflet abnormalities (flail) did not have a significant change in their severity assessment, whereas those with functional ischemic MR decreased significantly (41).

In a prospective study of 82 consecutive higher risk CABG patients performed at the Cleveland Clinic, there were a total of 7 patients who underwent unplanned valve

surgery. Two received an aortic valve replacement for underdiagnosed aortic stenosis, 1 patient had a pulmonic valve replacement for undiagnosed stenosis, and 3 patients underwent mitral valve repair procedures for MR of greater severity (> moderate) than the preoperative evaluation (Table 24.10A) (34). Consistent with the findings of Cohn, Grewal, and Bach, there were no cancellations of a planned mitral valve procedure because of a finding of less MR than was present preoperatively. Sheikh et al. found a 2% incidence of CABG patients demonstrating greater MR leading to MV surgery (42). Interestingly they found 11% of their CABG patients had less MR than their preoperative evaluation and the MV procedure was cancelled. From a clinical perspective, if the variance in the OR is more than two grades less, the potential exists that the patient may have indolent ischemia at the time of the original exam. In these circumstances, if canceling the MV procedure is a consideration, altering the loading conditions with neosynephrine or challenging with a bolus of intravenous fluid may duplicate the MV dysfunction seen preoperatively. Other undi-

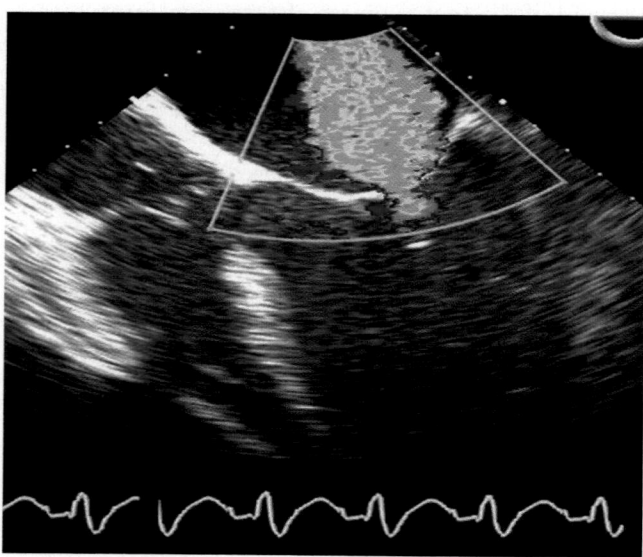

**FIGURE 24.6.** Patients with an ischemic cardiomyopathy, may develop eccentric remodeling. The development of a more spherically shaped ventricle results in a subvalvular apparatus that symmetrically restricts the AMVL and PMVL equally, resulting in a central regurgitant jet.

▶ **TABLE 24.10A. Cleveland Clinic Higher Risk CABG Study Surgical Management Alterations**

|  | Pre-CPB | Pre-SEP CPB | Post-SEP CPBP | Post-CC | #PTS |
|---|---|---|---|---|---|
| **MV Repair** | 3 | 0 | 0 | 0 | 3 |
| **AO VR** | 2 | 0 | 0 | 0 | 2 |
| **PVR** | 1 | 0 | 0 | 0 | 1 |
| **LV Vent** | 7 | 0 | 0 | 0 | 7 |

▶ **TABLE 24.10B. Cleveland Clinic Higher Risk CABG Study Surgical Management Alterations**

|  | Pre-CPB | Pre-SEP CPB | Post-SEP CPBP | Post-CC | #PTS |
|---|---|---|---|---|---|
| **Off-Pump CABG** | 3 | NA | NA | NA | 3 |
| **Axillary Cannulation** | 6 | NA | NA | NA | 6 |
| **Circulatory Arrest** | 1 | NA | NA | NA | 1 |
| **GLOBAL DYSFX** | 6 | 25 | 37 | 37 | 37 |
| **RWMA** | 8 | 18 | 8 | 1 | 35 |
| **RV DYSFX** | 2 | 12 | 15 | 15 | 15 |
| **Diastolic DYSFX** | 13 | 5 | 12 | 15 | 15 |
| **UN-DX Valve DZ** | 13 | 3 | 2 | 3 | 16 |
| **Under-DX Valve** | 15 | 0 | 0 | 0 | 16 |

agnosed findings that may lead to alterations in the patient's surgical management include complications of ischemic heart disease (see Assessment of Complications of Ischemic Heart Disease). These include LV or LA thrombi, atrial fibrillation, pseudoaneurysms, ruptured papillary muscle, ischemic VSD, and LV aneurysms.

Previous studies have demonstrated the ability of pre-CPB diagnostic intraoperative echocardiography to alter the anesthetic management of patients undergoing CABG surgery. Couture et al. utilized IOE in 624 patients undergoing CABG and found that it altered the anesthetic-hemodynamic management in 53% of this population (43). Berquist et al. evaluated the impact of IOE on the management of 75 patients undergoing CABG procedures (44). In 17% of patients, IOE was critical in the decision-making process and supportive in 43% with the management of ischemia and guidance of fluid administration being predominant (44). In our study of 82 consecutive CABG patients, global LV dysfunction was diagnosed in 37 (45%) patients and characterized as mild (18.5%), moderate (35%), or severe (59%). RV dysfunction was diagnosed in 15 (18%) patients with predominant moderate (47%) and severe (53%) dysfunction (34). There were 35 patients with new or increased regional wall motion abnormalities (42.6%) detected by intraoperative echocardiography. Electrocardiographic evidence of myocardial ischemia was noted in only 7 patients, and in all patients, the electrocardiographic changes followed the regional wall motion changes. Postoperative persistence of the regional wall motion abnormality remained in 3 of these patients, and 1 of these 3 patients sustained a myocardial infarction documented by creatine kinase level and electrocardiogram. Intraoperative TEE demonstrated significant valve disease that had not been previously reported and led to alteration in the hemodynamic management in 32 patients (34).

## Cannulation and Perfusion Strategy to Prevent Neurologic Dysfunction

Neurologic dysfunction occurs in up to 30% to 80% of patients following coronary bypass surgery (45,46,48). It has been classified as either Type 1 (focal neurologic deficit) or Type 2 (cognitive dysfunction or encephalopathy). While both types may be associated with aortic atherosclerosis, type 1 has the strongest correlation. Newman et al. also defined a higher risk population for developing perioperative CNS dysfunction (47,48). They reviewed 2,417 patients undergoing CABG surgery, looking for predictors and risk factors of perioperative neurologic events, such as a stroke, TIA, or coma (Table 24.11A). It was found that the predictors of the neurologic events included:

1. Age over 65 years
2. Diabetes

3. Previous neurologic event
4. Previous cardiac surgery
5. Pulmonary disease
6. Unstable angina at the time of presentation

The more elderly and debilitated patients benefit most from cardiac surgery yet they sustain greater overall risk for morbidity and mortality after cardiac surgery.

In a multicentered study of more than 2,100 patients undergoing CABG, Roach et al. reported an incidence of 3.1% type 1 (focal cerebrovascular accident, transient ischemic attack (TIA), or persistent coma) and 3% type 2 neurologic dysfunction (neurocognitive dysfunction or encephalopathy) (48). In addition to those factors associate with both types (increased age and hypertension), there were factors uniquely associated with type 1 (previous neurologic deficit, IABP, perioperative hypotension, IABP, and ventricular venting) and type 2 neurologic dysfunction (alcohol consumption, dysrhythmias, CHF, peripheral vascular disease, and previous CABG).

The strongest predictor of type 1 neurologic dysfunction post-CABG remains the presence of significant atheroma in the proximal aorta. Currently the indications for epiaortic echo include the presence of atheroma (grade 3 or higher in the descending aorta), any palpable aortic atheroma or calcified aorta, age > 65–70 years, a history of previous neurologic event, history of coronary artery bypass grafting, presence of peripheral vascular disease, and presenting with one or more risk factors for atherosclerosis (34). If those factors reported by Newman and Roach in Table 24.11A (history of diabetes, COPD, unstable angina, prior CNS event, need for LV vent, prior

▶ **TABLE 24.11A. Predictors of Neurologic Dysfunction**

| Variable | Type 1 Deficit, Stupor Coma | Type 2 Cognitive |
|---|---|---|
| Increased age >65–70 | X | X |
| Proximal aortic atheroma | X (strongest) | |
| Hypertension | X | X |
| History of diabetes | X | |
| COPD | X | |
| Unstable angina | X | |
| Prior CNS event | X | |
| Periop hypotension | X | X |
| IABP | X | |
| LV venting | X | |
| Alcohol history | | X |
| Dysrhythmia | | X |
| Prior CABG | | X |
| Peripheral vascular disease | | X |
| Macroemboli | X | |
| Macroemboli and microperfusion | | X |

CABG, and peripheral vascular disease) are combined with current practices, it may assist in identifying patients at higher risk. The use of intraoperative echo (TEE and epiaortic imaging) in the higher risk population provides a strategy to reduce perioperative neurologic dysfunction (Table 24.11B).

Transesophageal echocardiography can image the descending aorta, arch, and proximal ascending aorta. The site of aortic cannulation is not visualized by TEE, necessitating epiaortic scanning. Importantly palpation of the aorta is not as accurate in assessing severity of atherosclerotic changes in the aorta. Wareing et al. demonstrated that palpation alone was only able to identify 38% of protruding plaques in the aorta (49). The study population included 500 patients older than 50, undergoing cardiac surgery. The same findings were confirmed by Konstadt et al. (50). The authors demonstrated that palpation of the aorta by the surgeon missed 83% of aortic atheroma detected by TEE or epiaortic scanning. Davila-Roman et al. showed that when compared with epiaortic scanning and TEE, palpation of the aorta significantly underestimates the presence and severity of arteriosclerosis (51).

Blauth et al. analyzed the autopsies in 221 patients undergoing myocardial revascularization or valve operations (52). Complete autopsies were performed in 129 patients (58.4%) and limited to the chest and abdomen in the remainder. Embolic disease was identified in 69 patients (31.2%). Atheroemboli or abnormalities consistent with atheroemboli were identified in 48 patients (21.7%). Atheroembolic disease was found in the brain in 16.3% of patients, there was a high correlation of atheroemboli with severe atherosclerosis of the ascending aorta. Atheroembolic events occurred in 46 of 123 patients (37.4%) with severe disease of the ascending aorta but in only 2 of 98 patients (2%) without significant ascending aortic disease (p < 0.0001) (52). There was a direct correlation between age, severe atherosclerosis of the ascending aorta, and atheroemboli. Incremental risk factors for atheroembolic disease are peripheral vascular disease and severe atherosclerosis of the ascending aorta.

## Assessment of the Surgical Results

The purpose of the preseparation CPB examination is to assess the degree of recovery of cardiac function and exclude the potential for complications. Issues that are clarified by the TEE examination prior to separation from cardiopulmonary bypass include:

1. Assessment of the regional myocardial function in the perfusion beds of the bypassed coronary vessels
2. Detection of significant complications related to cannulation and myocardial protection strategy
3. Assessment of the valve function of valves
4. Guidance of the de-airing process

▶ **TABLE 24.11B.  Cannulation and Perfusion Strategy**

| *Intraoperative Echo Finding* | *Surgical Options* |
|---|---|
| Proximal ascending atheroma | Off-pump CABG |
| | Axillary or femoral cannulation |
| | Identify cross-clamp site or circulatory arrest |
| | Identify site for antegrade cardioplegia |
| | Identify site for proximal grafts or all IMA grafts |
| | Single cross clamp |
| | Higher perfusion pressures |
| Ascending and descending atheroma | Axillary cannulation only |
| | Potential morbidity with IABP |
| | Higher perfusion pressures |
| Calcified arteriosclerotic ascending aorta | Off-pump CABG |
| | Axillary cannulation and circulatory arrest |
| | Replace ascending aorta |
| | All arterial grafts |
| | TMR |
| | PCI accepting incomplete revascularization |
| ≥ mild aortic regurgitation | Monitor for LV distension |
| | LV venting |
| | Consider intercoronary antegrade cardioplegia |
| | Retrograde cardioplegia more important |
| | Cooling of heart for added protection |
| Post-pump localized dissection | Localized repair |
| | Replace ascending aorta with circulatory arrest |

TEE helps identify the optimal time to separate from cardiopulmonary bypass once the heart is completely de-aired and ejecting effectively.

As soon as the cross clamp is removed, intraoperative echo may be utilized to evaluate potential distensibility of the LV caused by aortic regurgitation. Until the LVOT is pressurized and the heart is actively ejecting, there may not be complete coaptation of the aortic valve leaflets. If the heart is slow to initiate an intrinsic rhythm and eject on its own, placement of an LV vent may be indicated with significant aortic regurgitation. Intraoperative TEE provides a reliable method for assessing micro-air that may be distributed to the cerebral circulation or coronary. When simultaneous recordings of intracranial Doppler and TEE visualizing the descending aorta are performed, detection of micro-air emboli in the cerebral circulation is simultaneous with micro-air visualization in the descending thoracic aorta (53). Strategies to prevent further embolization to the coronary arteries or cerebral circulation include: increasing the aortic vent flow, emptying the heart, and increasing pump flow, in addition to lowering the head with Trendelenburg positioning so that micro-air will accumulate at the ventricular apex more readily permitting needle aspiration. If waves of air cycle with the ventilator, ventilation may be transiently disrupted until the micro-air clears. Air may also collect at the dome of the LA adjacent to the aortic sinotubular junction or in the left atrial appendage. Micro-air may be visualized in the proximal right or left main coronary arteries. If this happens, the perfusion pressure can be increased to hasten passage of the micro-air through the circulation.

### Aortic Dissection

Aortic dissection is a recognized complication of aortic cannulation and is readily identified by the post-CPB TEE or epicardial imaging. While most cannulation-related dissections are self-limiting, if not detected intraoperatively, they can present catastrophic challenges. Significant ulcerated plaques or ascending aortic disease may lead to the use of alternative cannulation sites.

### Post-CPB LV Dysfunction

LV dysfunction following myocardial revascularization is usually associated with pre-CPB LV dysfunction and higher stages of diastolic dysfunction. Poor LV function post-CPB may be predicted by the pre-CPB IOE exam's assessment of diastolic and systolic parameters of LV function in addition to the completeness of myocardial revascularization and length of time spent on the heart-lung machine. Small changes in regional wall function may be indicative of alterations in coronary blood flow to the perfusion bed of the grafted vessels. Micro-air bub-bles do cause regional wall motion abnormalities, usually in the more superiorly originating right coronary artery.

### Valve Dysfunction

Transiently, ischemic mitral regurgitation may occur in the periods preceding and following separation from cardiopulmonary bypass. After a period of equilibration, if the severity of MR persists, standard methods of severity assessment are utilized to direct the surgical decision-making process. If improvement of the underlying ventricular function, regional wall motion, or structural integrity of the MV apparatus is unlikely to improve, returning to CPB and repair or replacement of the MV may be indicated.

Prior to separation from cardiopulmonary bypass, more significant levels of aortic regurgitation may be noted until the heart is completely filled and ejecting. If the heart remains in asystole or is bradycardic with an inability to capture with pacing, the ventricle may distend. Ventricular distension may further contribute to post-CPB LV dysfunction.

### Other Applications

Intraoperative echocardiography may be used to determine the need for or direct the placement of mechanical support device placement such as intraaortic balloon pump (IABP) or left ventricular assist device (LVAD) (54). When a balloon is placed intraoperatively, the placement wire must be visualized in the aorta to prevent the development of an iatrogenic aortic dissection. Also, correct position of the balloon in the aorta (tip of the balloon below the left subclavian artery) can be verified with TEE.

## Outcome Studies

### Neurologic Dysfunction

Duda et al. compared 195 consecutive CABG patients evaluated by intraoperative surface aortic ultrasonography with 164 control patients in whom the ascending aorta was assessed by inspection and palpation only (55). Findings from the epiaortic echo led to a modification of the cannulation and perfusion strategy in 19 (10%) patients with hypothermic fibrillatory arrest with no cross-clamping of the aorta and left ventricular venting in 14 patients, modification in the aortic cannulation site or single cross-clamping in three patients, and modification in placement of proximal anastomoses or all arterial grafts in two patients. No strokes occurred in this group and 3 patients died, yielding an operative mortality rate of 2.6%. In those patients whose cannulation and perfusion strategy was guided by palpation of the aorta only, there were 5 strokes (3.0%), and 6 patients died

(3.6%) with stroke contributing to the cause of death in 1 patient (55). They concluded that intraoperative echocardiography (TEE and epivascular imaging) reduced the stroke rate in CABG compared to inspection and palpation of the aorta alone.

Kouchoukos et al. evaluated intraoperative epiaortic detection and treatment of the severely atherosclerotic ascending aorta, which included epiaortic imaging and resection, and graft replacement of the involved segment using hypothermic ischemic arrest (56). Forty-seven CABG patients had resection and graft replacement of the ascending aorta. It was associated with lower mortality and stroke rates than those that were observed in patients with moderate or severe atherosclerosis in whom only minor modifications in technique were made to avoid embolization of atheroma.

Wareing et al. evaluated 1,200 of 1,334 consecutive patients (> 65 years old) with epiaortic scanning of the aorta. Coronary artery disease was present is 88% of the patients and moderate and severe atherosclerosis of the ascending aorta was found in 19.3% of the patients (57). Strategies for the prevention of perioperative neurologic dysfunction included alteration of the site of arterial cannulation, proximal graft anastomosis, antegrade cardioplegia administration, and replacement of the ascending aorta. There were 33 patients out of 1,200 who had carotid disease. They underwent combined carotid and cardiac surgery. 1,200 patients had 4% 30-day mortality; the stroke rate was 1.6% (57). Type 1 neurologic dysfunction was correlated with the degree of atherosclerosis in the ascending aorta. Interestingly, those patients who underwent replacement of the ascending aorta had no strokes. The stroke rates were higher for 111 patients with moderate or severe ascending aortic disease who had only minor interventions (6.3%) and for 16 patients with severe carotid artery disease who did not have carotid endarterectomy.

Davila-Roman et al. performed epiaortic scanning on 1,200 patients undergoing heart surgery and demonstrated ascending aorta atherosclerosis in 19.3% of patients (58). Predictors of ascending aorta atherosclerosis were smoking, diffuse coronary disease, and increased age (> 50 years old). Patients with neurologic dysfunction were more likely to have significant atherosclerosis in the ascending aorta. In a separate report of epiaortic scanning in 472 patients undergoing on-pump coronary artery bypass grafting surgery following CPB new lesions in the aorta were found in 3.4% of patients (58). Of the 10 patients with mobile or intramural disruptions postbypass, 60% were at the site of aortic cross-clamp application and 40% at the point of cannulation of the ascending aorta. Interestingly, atheroma < 3 mm were associated with a 0.8% incidence of new lesions postbypass, whereas in patients with atheromas 3 mm–4 mm (11.8%) and > 4 mm (33%) neurologic deficits correlated with the presence of

atherosclerosis and new aortic lesions postbypass (58). Evidence from these studies suggest that TEE and epiaortic echocardiography predict stroke rate and help to stratify patient risk for adverse neurologic events in the perioperative period.

Using TEE, Hartman et al. examined the descending aorta of 189 patients undergoing elective CABG surgery (59a). As seen in Table 24.11C, they graded the severity of atheromatous disease as Grade 1 normal (mild intimal thickening), grade 2 (severe thickening < 3 mm), grade 3 (atheroma 3 mm–5 mm), grade 4 (protruding atheroma greater than 5 mm), and grade 5 (mobile atheroma). Nine of the 189 patients had stroke within one week of surgery. Patients with grade 1 or 2 atheromatous disease on TEE of their descending aorta had no strokes, whereas grade 3 had 5.5%, grade 4 had 10.5%, and grade 5 had 45.5% incidence of stroke. The one-week stroke rate was 5.5% (2/36), 10.5% (2/19), and 45.5% (5/11) for grades 3, 4, and 5 (59). For six-month outcome, advancing aortic atheroma grade was a predictor of stroke (59). Atheromatous disease of the descending aorta was a strong predictor of stroke and death after CABG (59).

In the higher risk CABG population study performed at the Cleveland Clinic, epiaortic scanning was performed if the descending aorta demonstrated ≥ grade 3 in the descending aorta on TEE or the patient was in the high-risk group (34). If there were mobile plaques in the descending aorta and protruding plagues in the ascending aorta, axillary cannulation was performed. If the aorta was calcified with protruding plaques, axillary cannulation was utilized with circulatory arrest or the patient underwent off-pump coronary bypass. The changes in cannulation and profusion strategy in the 82 consecutive patients based on echocardiographic exam included 3 patients who received coronary bypass surgery off pump because of the presence of significant protruding atheroma in the ascending aorta. There were 6 patients who had axillary cannulation because of concomitant protruding plaques in the descending aorta and ascending aorta (34). One of these patients underwent circulatory arrest because of the coexistence of a calcified aorta that would preclude cross-clamp. When this study population was compared with a similar high-risk group of patients, without having

▶ **TABLE 24.11C. Grading of Aortic Atheroma and Risk of Stroke (59a–59d)**

| Grade | Stroke | Definition |
|---|---|---|
| 1 | 0% | Normal or mild aortic thickening |
| 2 | 0% | Severe aortic thickening |
| 3 | 5.6% | Protruding atheroma less than 5 mm in width |
| 4 | 10.5% | Protruding atheroma over 5 mm in width |
| 5 | 45.5% | Mobile atheroma |

intraoperative TEE, it was found that the incidence of stroke was three times greater than those patients in whom the cannulation site was based solely on palpation of the ascending aorta (3.8% vs. 1.2%). Epiaortic echocardiography helps to develop the cannulation and perfusion strategy, helps to make an educated decision regarding the need for circulatory arrest or femoral or axillary cannulation, and also guides the need for higher perfusion pressures during cardiopulmonary bypass. It also helps to determine the best location for the placement of the aortic cross clamp, the need for off-pump CABG, and to localize the best site for the proximal coronary graft and cardioplegia cannula.

Leung et al. continuously monitored 50 patients undergoing elective coronary artery bypass graft (CABG) surgery with continuous TEE, ECG, and hemodynamic measurements during the pre-CPB, post-CPB, and 4 hours postoperatively (60). TEE and ECG evidence of ischemia were characterized during each of the periods and were associated with adverse clinical outcomes (postoperative myocardial infarction, ventricular failure, and cardiac death). Myocardial ischemia detected by TEE was predictive of poor outcome with 6 of 18 patients demonstrating ischemia by TEE having adverse cardiac outcomes compared with none of the 32 without such evidence (60). Seventy-six percent of the TEE ischemic episodes occurred without acute change in heart rate, BP, or PA pressure. It was concluded that the incidence of ECG and TEE ischemia was highest in the postbypass period and postbypass RWMA were related to postoperative myocardial infarction, ventricular failure, and cardiac death.

Mishra et al. (61) have reported on the value of TEE in 5,016 patients (3,660 CABG patients). Pre-CPB TEE demonstrated findings that helped or modified the surgical plan in 993 of 3,660 CABG patients (27.13%). They reported 3,217 TEE-guided anesthetic-hemodynamic interventions in 944 CABG patients (25.79%) (61). Postbypass TEE identified the need for graft revision in 29 patients (0.8%) and the need for intraaortic balloon pump (IABP) in 29 patients (0.8%). Overall, 38.78% of patients benefited from pre-CPB and 39.16% from post-CPB use of TEE with an alteration of management in 26.7% of CABG patients as compared to 12.5% of those undergoing valve surgery (61).

Couture et al. evaluated the use of IOE in 851 patients, 624 (73.3%) of the patients were undergoing CABG (43). TEE was used to modify therapy in 10% of isolated CABG patients (higher in repeat and MIDCAB) and included 4 patients who returned to CPB for revision of their bypass grafts, additional valve procedure, ventricular aneurysm resection, LVAD, and detection of micro-air. The clinical impact was higher (39%) in patients undergoing combined CABG and valve procedures compared to isolated CABG (10%). There were unplanned surgical interventions in 30% of the study population and confirmation of

the preoperative diagnosis in 34%. The anesthetic-hemodynamic management was altered in 53% of patients including treatment of hypovolemia, myocardial ischemia, and global dysfunction. Interestingly, evaluation of the aorta for atheroma and potential alteration of cannulation and perfusion strategy was not a part of this study (53).

Berquist et al. performed intraoperative TEE in 75 patients undergoing CABG (44). There were 584 interventions, TEE was most important in 17%, contributed to guidance of fluid administration in 30%, and guided antiischemic therapy in 21%. TEE was found to direct critical surgical intervention in 3% of patients (44). Overall, 17% of all interventions were predominantly guided by intraoperative echocardiography. The use of TEE and epiaortic imaging for guidance of the cannulation and perfusion strategy was not part of this study. Deutch et al. evaluated 50 consecutive nonrisk stratified patients undergoing CABG surgery and found that it was dispensable in 33 patients (66%), informative (22%), valuable (8%), and essential (4%) (62). This included 2 patients who had graft occlusion detected post-CPB by new regional wall motion abnormalities. Benson and Cahalan provided a projected cost savings of $300 per patient if routinely used in patients undergoing myocardial revascularization (63).

In the higher risk Cleveland Clinic study involving 82 consecutive patients, there were 16 (19.5%) patients with undiagnosed valve disease and 16 patients with underdiagnosed valve disease (34). This led to the adjustment of the anesthetic-hemodynamic management in 34% of the study population. Major alterations in the surgical management of patients occurred in 33% of patients, including performing CABG off-CPB (3 patients), axillary cannulation (6 patients), circulatory arrest (1 patient), rush to bypass (2 patients), return to CPB (4 patients), and reopening the chest (2 patients). Additional valve procedures were precipitated by intraoperative TEE findings in 6 patients, including mitral valve repair, aortic valve replacement, and pulmonic valve replacement. A transmitral pulmonary vein LV vent was placed in 7 patients due to the finding of significant aortic regurgitation. When the higher risk study group, whose management was guided by intraoperative TEE and epivascular imaging, was compared with a similar group who did not receive routine intraoperative echo the outcomes noted in Table 24.12 were obtained. The incidence of hospital deaths, CNS morbidity, and cardiac morbidity were three times greater in those patients who did not receive intraoperative echocardiography.

There are a variety of studies that provide a similar analysis of the frequency with which intraoperative echo altered the intraoperative management of patients undergoing CABG surgery. Click et al. reported that only 8% of their patients undergoing CABG received intraoperative echocardiography (38). Thirty-three percent of these patients had new findings pre-CPB and 8% post-CPB. The

▶ TABLE 24.12. Cleveland Clinic Higher Risk CABG Study Intraoperative Echo vs. No Intraoperative Echo Comparison

| Patient and Outcome Variables | No Intraoperative TEE | Diagnostic Intraoperative TEE at Each Stage |
|---|---|---|
| Age | 64.8 | 68.4 |
| Number of Patients | 397 | 82 |
| Average CCF Severity Score | 5.9 | 6.1 |
| In-hospital Mortality | 18 (3.8%) | 1 (1.2%)* |
| Perioperative MI | 14 (3.5%) | 1 (1.2%)* |
| Focal Neurologic Deficit | 18 (3.8%) | 1 (1.2%)* |

* Study was not a randomized comparison, but relied on retrospective data comparison of similar high risk patients undergoing CABG surgery during period of study.

majority of these patients were those in whom valve function was to be assessed intraoperatively. No mention was made in this study regarding the risk stratification of their CABG patient population or the cannulation and perfusion strategy guidance by intraoperative echo. Sheikh et al. (42) demonstrated that 2% of patients undergoing CABG had more significant MR than expected.

With the exception of the Mishra study, these studies would seem to indicate that intraoperative echocardiography may not have a similar impact on the clinical management as the Cleveland Clinic study. Or do they? The remarkable studies referred to above were performed in leading cardiac centers and are extremely valuable contributions to our understanding of the potential impact of intraoperative echo. However, the information that they provide does not apply directly to the prospective Cleveland Clinic study, which was performed by a surgical team utilizing intraoperative echo as a "gold standard" (34). It is consistently used as a reliable guide in many of the surgical and anesthetic-hemodynamic decisions related to cannulation and myocardial protection, myocardial viability, valve dysfunction, need for off-pump CABG, and mechanical support (LVAD or IABP). The study reported by Click et al. was a retrospective review that included mostly those CABG patients who required an intraoperative assessment of valve dysfunction (38). In addition, the risk stratification of patients undergoing CABG receiving intraoperative echo was not part of their retrospective analysis. The study reported by Berquist et al. similarly did not include risk stratification or detection of aortic atheroma for modification of the cannulation and perfusion strategy (44).

For intraoperative echocardiography to have an influential impact on patient management and outcome, a number of requirements must be met. These include:

1. The need for reliably performed and interpreted intraoperative examination
2. Accurate communication of the information to the surgical and anesthetic-hemodynamic management
3. A correct understanding of the information in conjunction with the patient preoperative evaluation
4. The correct choice of therapeutic intervention
5. Accurate execution of the surgical intervention

Because of institutional and individual variations in the use of information derived from the intraoperative TEE, it is difficult to accurately compare such decision-making and outcome impact data. Ultimately, as our patient population ages and develops greater comorbidity, the perioperative team managing patients undergoing myocardial revascularization will require management strategies that more accurately guide the decision-making process and improve the outcome of our patients.

## COMPLICATIONS OF ISCHEMIC HEART DISEASE

There are a number of complications of ischemic heart disease that are seen throughout the perioperative period. Complications that are commonly seen include atrial fibrillation, ischemic mitral regurgitation, rupture of the ventricular septum, LV aneurysm, ventricular pseudoaneurysm, RV infarction, and LV thrombus (Table 24.13).

### Atrial Fibrillation

Postoperative atrial fibrillation in CABG surgery occurs in up to 40% of patients and is associated with a significant morbidity (64). Shore-Lesserson et al. evaluated patients undergoing coronary artery bypass with TEE to determine if there are identifiable risk factors for atrial fibrillation (65a). Univariate predictors of atrial fibrillation include advanced age, precardiopulmonary bypass left atrial appendage area, postcardiopulmonary bypass, and left upper pulmonary vein systole/diastole velocity ratio (65a). Because the entire LA is poorly visualized by TEE, the LAA area serves as a marker for LA enlargement. Patients who are in atrial fibrillation at the

▶ TABLE 24.13.  **Complications of Ischemic Heart Disease Intraoperative Echocardiographic Assessment**

| Complication | Pre-CPB IOE | Post-CPB IOE |
|---|---|---|
| **Atrial fibrillation** | LA or LAA thrombi | Residual LAA thrombi or ligation-flow |
| **LAA thrombus** | Spontaneous contrast | Spontaneous contrast |
| | LAA PW Doppler velocities | LAA PW Doppler velocities |
| | Increased thrombus < 20–30 cm/sec | Increased thrombus < 20–30 cm/sec |
| | Increased thrombus > 5.0 cm | Increased thrombus > 5.0 cm$^2$ |
| | Determine cause LAE | PV Doppler velocities |
| | MV inflow PW Doppler | LV/RV global-regional Fx |
| | Pulmonary vein PW Doppler | Cannulation-perfusion complications |
| | LVH | Document comprehensive exam |
| **Ischemic MR** | Severity of MR | Success of MVRep or MVR |
| | Mechanism of MR (I, IIIb, and or II) | Post-MVRep SAM |
| | Annulus diameter (ME 4, LAX, Comm) | Residual 2nd mechanism MR |
| | Height PMVL:AMVL | RV/LV global-regional Fx |
| | Coaptation-septal distance | Bypass graft Fx |
| | Ventricularization of coaptation | Pulmonary HTN reversal |
| | | Document comprehensive exam |
| **LV aneurysm** | Location and size aneurysm | LV/RV global and regional Fx |
| | Presence of mural thrombus | Bypass graft function |
| | Interference with MV apparatus | Need for IABP or LVAD |
| | Interpapillary distance | Pulmonary HTN |
| | Global and regional LV and RV Fx | Mitral regurgitation—2nd to resection |
| | Tricuspid regurgitation | - Ischemic |
| | LA size, LAA thrombi/contrast | Interpapillary distance |
| | Diastolic function assessment | Complications cannulation-perfusion |
| | Cannulation perfusion strategy | Residual thrombus |
| | Suitability of aorta for IABP | Document comprehensive exam |
| | Necessity for LVAD support | |
| | Shunt, AR, RVfx, TR | |
| **Pseudoaneurysm** | Location and number of communications | Residual communication |
| | Pseudoaneurysm flow volume | LV/RV global and regional Fx |
| | Viability of adjacent myocardium | Mitral or tricuspid regurgitation—2nd to resection |
| | Global-regional LV/RV Fx | |
| | Ischemic MR | - Ischemic MR |
| | Cannulation and perfusion strategy | Interpapillary distance |
| | Aortic or tricuspid regurgitation | Complications cannulation-perfusion |
| | Necessity for LVAD support | LV/RV global and regional Fx |
| | - Shunt, AR, apical thrombi | Pulmonary HTN |
| | - Aortic atheroma | Document comprehensive exam |
| **VSD** | Number, size, and location(s) | Residual VSD flow |
| | Calculate shunt flow | Residual communication |
| | LV/RV global-regional Fx | LV/RV global and regional Fx |
| | Adjacent myocardial viability | Mitral or tricuspid regurgitation—2nd to resection |
| | | - Ischemic MR |
| | | Interpapillary distance |
| | | Complications cannulation-perfusion |
| | | Pulmonary HTN |
| | | Document comprehensive exam |
| **RV infarction** | RV global and regional Fx | RV global and regional Fx |
| | Tricuspid regurgitation | Tricuspid regurgitation |
| | Pulmonary HTN | Complications cannulation-perfusion |
| | Hepatic congestion-plethora | Pulmonary HTN |
| | Shunt potential | LV filling, global and regional Fx |
| | LV global and regional Fx | Need IABP or RVAD (ECMO) support |
| | - Inferior and septal segmental Fx | Document comprehensive exam |

time of surgery undergo interventions to interrupt the macro- or micro-reentry circuit. In patients with paroxysmal atrial fibrillation and without left atrial enlargement, pulmonary vein isolation is usually performed using radiofrequency ablation. In patients with enlarged left atria, a macro-reentry circuit may emerge. Such patients often require a more comprehensive approach, including the classic Maze operation in addition to pulmonary vein isolation. Atrial fibrillation secondary to ischemic heart disease, may be associated with left atrial enlargement and stagnant blood flow in the left atrial appendage. For patients undergoing CABG, as seen in Table 24.13, the goal is to determine the propensity for developing atrial fibrillation postoperatively. Because TEE cannot visualize the entire LA consistently, it is difficult to obtain a consistent diameter measurement. Despite these limitations, a LA diameter in the anterior-posterior plane (ME 2 Chamber) with a LA diameter > 40 cm or indexed area measurement of > 2.0 cm/m², reduced LAA outflow velocities, presence of spontaneous contrast or thrombi may suggest the need for ligation of the LAA. For patients in atrial fibrillation scheduled for pulmonary vein isolation or Maze, additional measurements also include the LA/RA diameter and circumference as well as PV Doppler velocities are documented for comparison to post-CPB findings. The pulmonary vein PW Doppler velocities are documented for future comparison with suspected pulmonary vein stenosis though more commonly associated with percutaneous ablation procedures. Reduced left atrial appendage contractility in patients with AF has been associated with thrombus formation. Left atrial appendage function, represented by PW Doppler measurement of LAA outflow velocity, is an important predictor for thrombus formation in patients with nonrheumatic atrial fibrillation. The extent of blood stasis and propensity for thrombus can be assessed during TEE by measurement of the peak PW Doppler velocity of outflow from the LAA. Spontaneous echocardiographic contrast, a swirling pattern of increased blood echogenicity, may be detected by TEE in the left atrium in patients with AF and is associated with blood stasis and a prothrombotic state. SEC is associated with an increased risk of systemic thromboembolic events. LA thrombi are associated with a larger LAA, and decreased LAA outflow velocities (< 20 cm/sec–30 cm/sec), and a higher prevalence of severe spontaneous LA contrast (65b). Interestingly, patients with atrial fibrillation less than 2 weeks have peak ejection velocities of 40 cm/sec compared to 10 cm/sec for those in atrial fibrillation > 2 weeks. Both spontaneous contrast and left atrial thrombi are associated with reduced outflow velocities of 18 cm/sec vs. 33 cm/sec and 10 cm/sec, respectively vs. 22 cm/sec (65b). LAA thrombi were also associated with larger LAA area (5.4 cm² vs. 3.9 cm²). In patients with spontaneous contrast, reduced peak outflow velocities, and increased LAA area, ligation of the LAA may be considered.

## Ischemic Mitral Regurgitation

For a more comprehensive discussion, please refer to Chapters 25, 27, and 28. By definition, ischemic mitral regurgitation is due to myocardial ischemia or infarction with structurally normal valvular leaflets and chordae (66). It occurs in 10%–50% of the cases of myocardial infarction (66). However, ischemic MR may also be associated with transient ischemia. The intraoperative echo exam in patients with ischemic MR focuses on determining the mechanism of MV dysfunction in addition to its severity (Table 24.13). There are a number of different mechanisms of ischemic MR (67). Included among these mechanisms are papillary muscle rupture (type II mechanism), apical tethering associated with ischemic cardiomyopathy (symmetrical bileaflet type IIIb), posterior wall infarcts (asymmetrical PMVL type IIIb), and transient ischemia leading to global dysfunction (central MR, symmetrical type IIIb) or posterior or anterolateral wall motion abnormality with asymmetrical restriction of the mitral apparatus (asymmetrical IIIb) (68). There are number of different mechanisms responsible for ischemic mitral regurgitation, including ventricular remodeling leading to a dilated spherical-shaped heart (eccentric remodeling) and/or global dysfunction of the left ventricle with distending of the mitral apparatus and the tethering effect, in these patients tenting of the mitral valve by the secondary chordae is seen. The risk factors for ischemic mitral regurgitation include an inferior and posterior myocardial infarction causing posterior leaflet restriction and left ventricle dysfunction. The severity of mitral regurgitation depends on left ventricle function; if regurgitation is secondary to a spherical LV remodeling there is tethering of both mitral leaflets and this tends to produce a central jet of regurgitation (Fig. 24.6). Posterior, inferior, or posterolateral myocardial infarction can produce mitral regurgitation whose mechanism is related to an isolated restriction of the posterior leaflet and an override of the anterior leaflet with a posteriorly directed jet. It is important to keep in mind the influence of left ventricle afterload and the color Doppler gain setting when judging and grading mitral regurgitation. The patients, who have trivial mitral regurgitation, are routinely given a pressor agent to see if this maneuver increases the mitral insufficiency. Intraoperative echo should be utilized to confirm the presence of mitral regurgitation; however, it should not be used to determine whether a mitral valve repair needs to be performed when the patient has documented significant mitral regurgitation. If, however, there is no mitral regurgitation in the preoperative evaluation and one finds greater than 2–3⁺ mitral regurgitation, these patients will routinely undergo mitral valve annuloplasty or depending on what the structural abnormality is, other types of repair.

Papillary muscle rupture, an extreme subset of ischemic MR, occurs in 1% of patients with acute myocar-

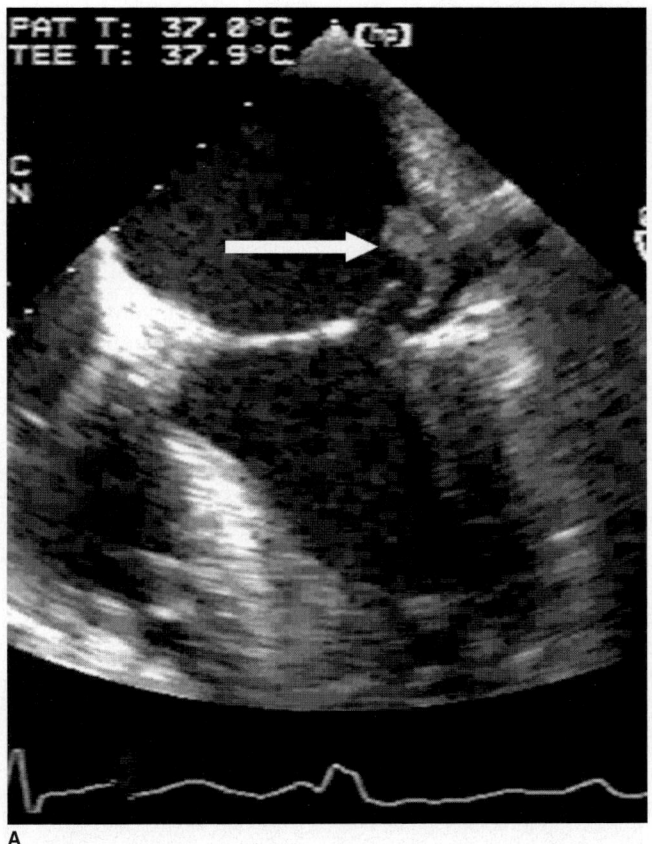

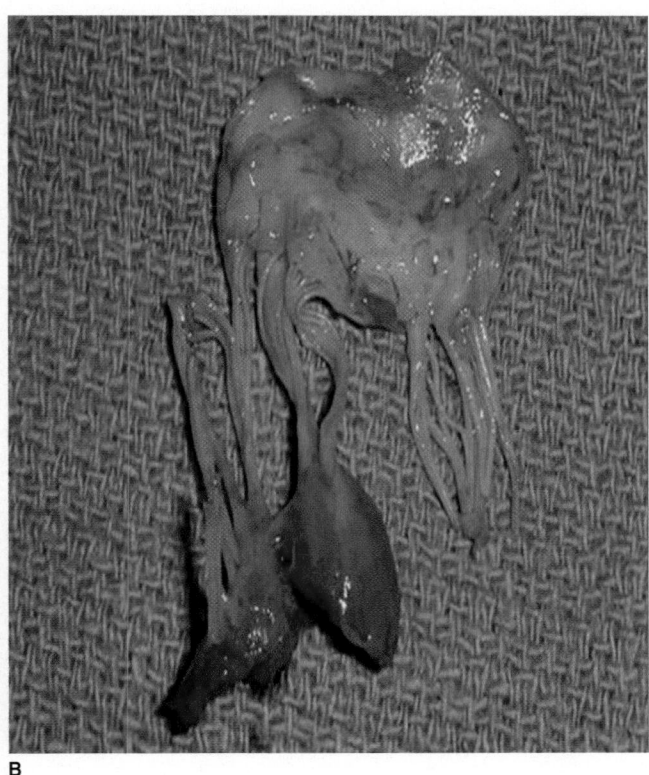

**FIGURE 24.7.** Rupture of an ischemic papillary muscle is a rare complication of ischemic heart disease. When it occurs, it most frequently involves the posteromedial papillary muscle due to its solitary blood supply from the posterolateral branch of the circumflex coronary artery.

dial infarction (Fig. 24.7) (69). It is seen 6 to 12 times more frequently in patients with infarcts involving the mid and apical inferior and posterior segments due to the single coronary artery perfusing the posteromedial papillary muscle (69). In contrast, the anterolateral papillary muscle is supplied by a dual blood supply from the circumflex (anterolateral obtuse marginal branch) and LAD (diagonal branch). If there is complete rupture, it usually involves both, because the posteromedial papillary muscle provides chordae to both the medial halves of the anterior and posterior mitral valve leaflets. Patients with ruptured papillary muscles develop the acute onset of pulmonary edema due to severe regurgitation into a noncompliant left atrium. Prior to the era of aggressive surgical management of these patients, the mortality approached 50% (66,67b,69).

An acute infarct of the tip of the papillary muscle may also lead to an elongation or "ribboning" of the tip of the papillary muscle, which results in elongation of the overall tensile apparatus. This may result in a small focal prolapse of either the anterior or posterior MV leaflet. It is distinguished from that associated with myxomatous de-

generation by its association with coronary disease, a small regional wall motion abnormality, or focal fibrosis of the tip of the papillary muscle head (69).

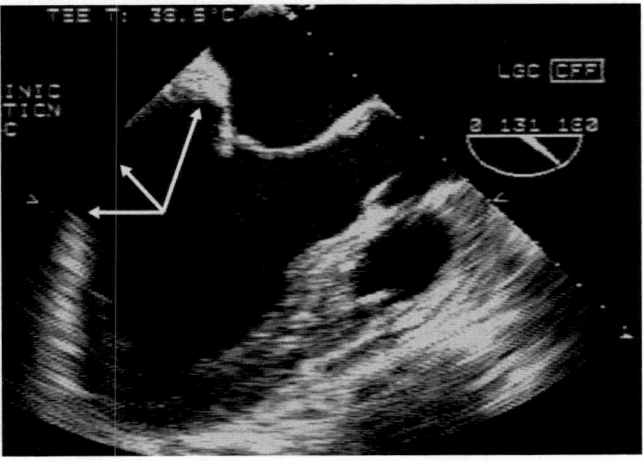

**FIGURE 24.8.** Posterobasal Aneurysm. Aneurysms of the LV are associated with transmural infarcts in regions of the heart that are not well collateralized.

## LV Aneurysm

Aneurysms of the left ventricle are associated with transmural myocardial infarction and commonly occur in regions of the heart not usually provided with collateralized blood flow. Loop et al. reported a series of patients with true aneurysms and found only 3% to be posterior (71). In contrast, in a report characterizing 65 consecutive au-topsies of true aneurysms, 15 (23%) involved only the posterior wall (66,71–73). Because such infarcts usually involve the posteromedial papillary muscle, the difference may be due to a more fulminate course leading to cardiogenic shock. In autopsy series, Roeske et al. demonstrated an increased likelihood of permission for autopsy in circumstances of more rapid progression of cardiogenic shock (72). Massive inferoposterior myocardial infarctions are more frequently fatal than extensive anterior infarctions, and patients don't live long enough for aneurysm formation.

Despite their more frequent occurrence in the anteroapical and anteroseptal regions of the heart, they may be seen in the posterobasal and inferoapical segments (Fig. 24.8). An anteroapical aneurysm is an example of mechanical complications following an anterior myocar-

dial infarction in which there is actual thinning of the myocardium and scar formation in the apical region of the left ventricle. It tends to occur in the transmural myocardial infarction and may be associated with the presence of apical thrombus. The apical aneurysm is commonly associated with LAD disease and anterior myocardial infarction (73). The intraoperative TEE exam may be used to guide the resection of the aneurysm. Depending on the size and location of the aneurysm, the ventricle may undergo significant reconstruction. It is important to maintain the various anatomic relations of the components of the mitral apparatus. To guide this process the relation of the aneurysm to the papillary muscles, size of the mitral annulus, interpapillary muscle distance, and regional function adjacent to the aneurysm are important considerations when determining the success of resection of the aneurysm. The echocardiographic characteristics of ventricular aneurysms include thin walled of the myocardium and a very wide neck to the aneurysm as opposed to a pseudoaneurysm, in which the narrowest portion or the aneurysm is at its neck. Usually there is dyskinetic motion of the aneurysmal wall and there may be a thrombus over that dyskinetic region inside the left ventricle. If

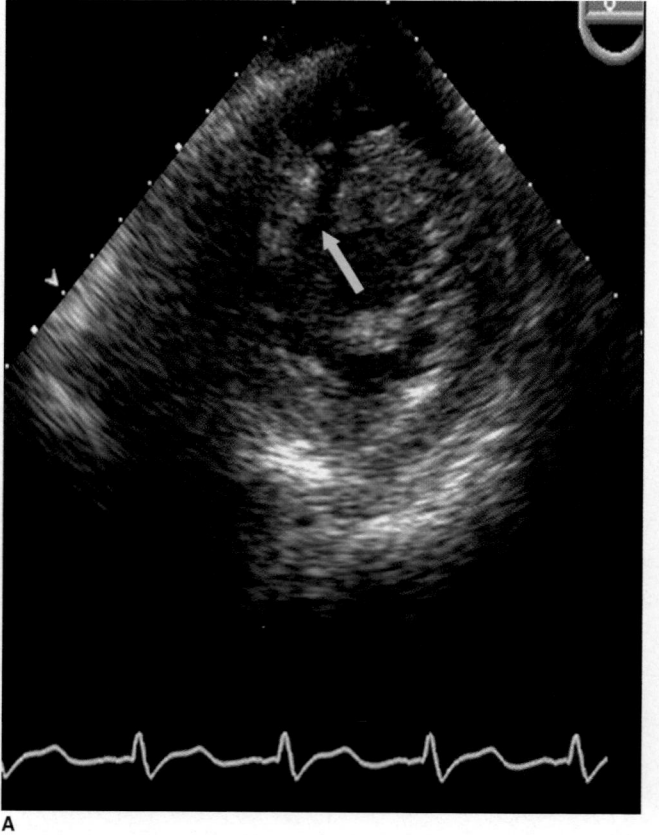 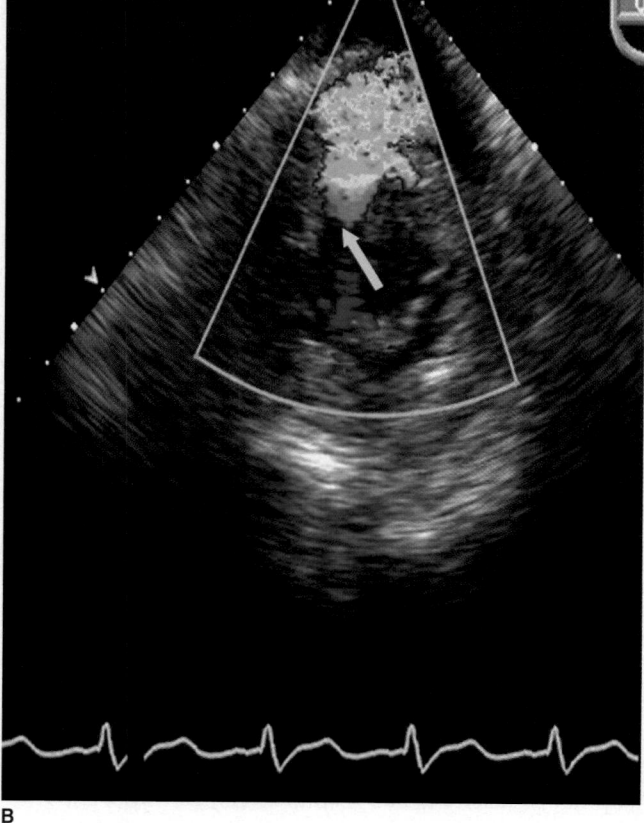

A                                          B

*FIGURE 24.9.* Pseudoaneurysm. Postmyocardial infarction LV pseudoaneurysms occur when the ventricular rupture is contained by overlying adherent pericardium.

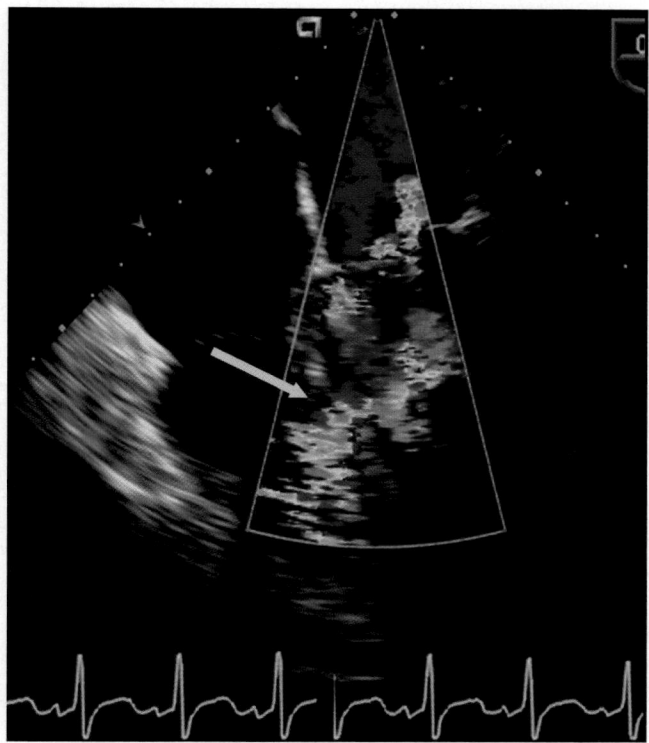

**FIGURE 24.10.** Ischemic ventricular septal defects (VSD) occur in 1%–3% of infarctions (usually within 7 days) and account for 5% of all postinfarction deaths.

there is a thrombus present and the apex is hard and there is no segmented wall motion abnormality, consideration should be given to an eosinophilic syndrome. Also, patients who develop posterobasal aneurysm are prone to develop a thrombus in the aneurysm. Maneuvers that may increase sensitivity of the echocardiography in detecting LV thrombi include the use of echo contrast or B-mode imaging, the use of the highest transducer frequency, focused imaging of the region of interest, and color Doppler imaging.

## Pseudoaneurysms

Clinically, pseudoaneurysms usually occur in patients who have ongoing or recurrent angina and hypotension, following a myocardial infarction. Signs of cardiac tamponade may or may not be present. It may be associated with or without cardiac tamponade. Postmyocardial infarction LV pseudoaneurysms occur when the LV rupture is contained by an overlying adherent pericardium (73). Ischemic pseudoaneurysms more frequently occur in the inferior and inferoposterior segments of the LV due to the solitary coronary blood supply frequently seen in this region of the heart. Figure 24.9 illustrates a rupture of the inferior myocardium with associated pericardial effusion

and thrombus. As seen in Table 24.13, the intraoperative echo examination in patients with pseudoaneurysms provides the surgical team with insight into the viability of the myocardium adjacent to the ventricular rupture. Such would permit a decision to either repair or patch the defect.

## Ventricular Septal Defect

Ischemic rupture of the ventricular septum occurs in 1% to 3% of acute myocardial infarctions being evenly distributed between anterior and inferior septal ruptures (66a,66b,73). Figure 24.10 shows an example of a ventricular septum defect after posterior infarction. The risk factors for developing postinfarction VSD include old age, female gender, previous myocardial infarction, history of hypertension, and presentation 3 to 6 days post-MI (74). There may be single or multiple defects in the ventricular septum, and usually is associated with RV dilatation and pulmonary artery hypertension. The short term survival of ischemic ventricular septal defects is reported within a very wide range between 42% to 75% (74,75). The intraoperative echo examination in patients with an ischemic VSD, is valuable in confirming the number, location, and size of the interventricular communications (Table 24.13). In addition to issues addressed in patients undergoing CABG surgery, determining the viability of myocardium adjacent to the VSD provides the surgical team with an understanding of the extent of the repair and propensity for additional necrotic myocardium, which may undermine the repair.

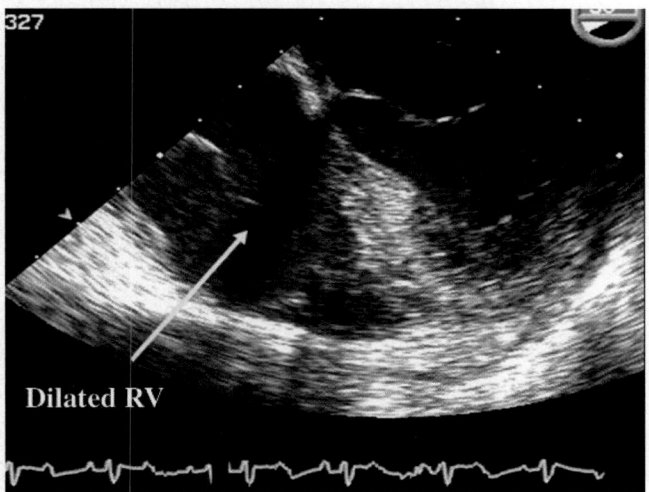

**FIGURE 24.11.** Right ventricular infarcts occur in 30% of inferior wall myocardial infarcts. Depending on the degree of LV dysfunction, pulmonary hypertension, and RV ischemia or infarction, the clinical manifestations may vary.

## RV Infarction

Right ventricle infarction (Fig. 24.11) occurs in 30% of patients with inferior wall infarction and 25% of patients with posterior wall infarction, and is associated with lesions in the right coronary artery (76). RV infarction may be associated with pulmonary hypertension and, depending on the degree of involvement of the left ventricle, may result in a dilated left ventricle cavity, which may cause mitral regurgitation. Echocardiographic signs of right ventricle infarct include RV dilatation, decreased function (may be segmental), decreased TV annular motion, bowing of interatrial septum (R to L), and increased RA (76). Because RV infarcts are commonly associated with infarcts of the inferior LV, an understanding of the global and regional function provides the perioperative team with a better understanding of potential issues that will become manifest in the perioperative period. If the patient has LV dysfunction leading to pulmonary hypertension, the increased RV afterload will accelerate development of RV dysfunction, tricuspid regurgitation, and hepatic congestion.

## FUTURE APPLICATIONS (TABLE 24.14)

While we have made great advances in the intraoperative management of our patients, with the increasingly older population with associated comorbidities, our health-care system will be challenged as never before. To meet this challenge in a way that permits us to continue to provide the level of care that is demanded by the public, we will need to provide wiser and more efficient health care to either avoid the costly perioperative complications or recognize those patients who would not benefit from costly medical interventions. Michael Porter of the Harvard Business School understands that innovation is the one affordable solution of the future. Advances that are already in practice in the echocardiography laboratory may provide solutions to many of the most pressing concerns, including the intraoperative assessment of myocardial viability, monitoring of myocardial protection, prevention of neurologic dysfunction, more accurate assessment of renal perfusion, and the prediction of the long-term patency of bypass grafts.

## Myocardial Viability

Accurate prediction of myocardial viability following revascularization is important in the higher risk patient for three reasons:

1. It is a predictor of long-term outcome.
2. Additional "wasted" time on cardiopulmonary bypass is required for unnecessary coronary grafts to nonviable tissue.

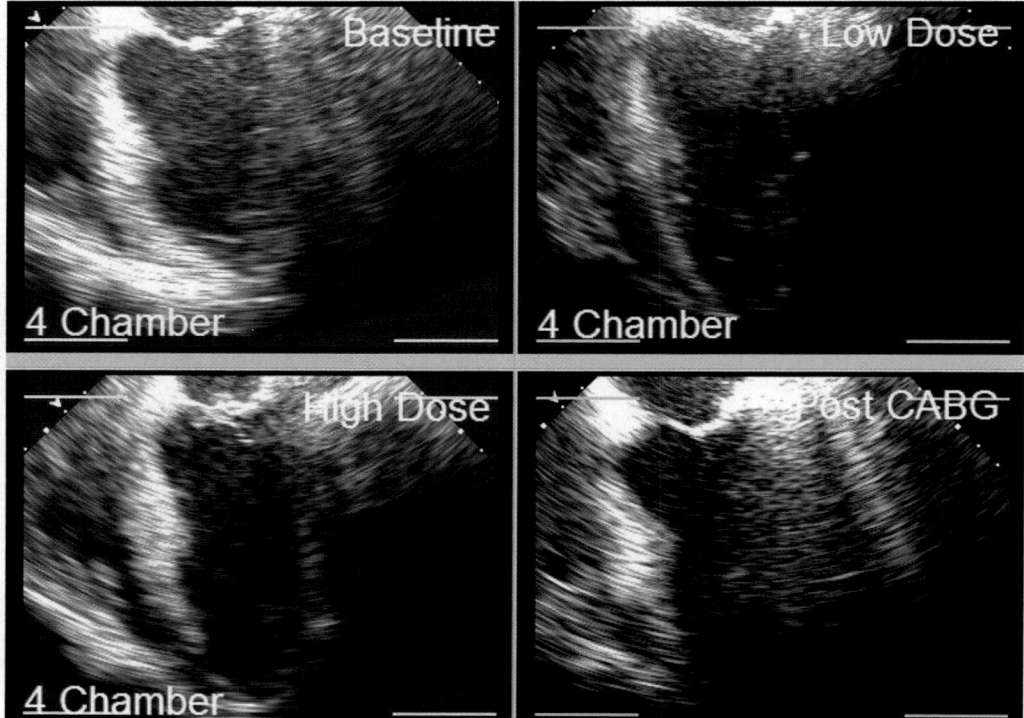

**FIGURE 24.12.** Intraoperative dobutamine stress echocardiography may provide an efficient strategy for determining myocardial viability in higher risk patients undergoing surgical revascularization.

▶ TABLE 24.14.  **Future Applications of Intraoperative Echo**

| *Concern* | *Current* | *Future* |
|---|---|---|
| Type 1 neurologic dysfunction | Palpation of aorta and inconsistent epiaortic scanning | Consistent epivascular scanning and intervention |
| Type 2 neurologic dysfunction | Palpation of aorta | Epivascular scanning |
| | TEE guided micro-air clearance | Transcranial Doppler |
| Myocardial viability | Preoperative MRI, nuclear or dobutamine stress, spect scan | Intraoperative dobutamine stress test and contrast perfusion |
| Renal perfusion | Urine output | Renal ultrasound-guided intervention |
| Myocardial protection | Retrograde pressures | Contrast demonstration of myocardial plegia flow |
| | Appearance of retrograde blood | |
| | Antegrade resistance | |
| Prediction of long-term graft patency | RWMA or ischemia | Graft doppler flow velocities and resistances |
| | | Contrast perfusion intensity and washout |

**3.** An accurate assessment of postbypass ventricular function is helpful.

Afridi et al. reported on 318 patients undergoing revascularization with severe LV dysfunction, and demonstrated that the presence of contractile reserve by dobutamine stress testing was a reliable predictor of survivability following surgical revascularization (77). During the past decade, stress echocardiography has emerged as a safe and sensitive method for the detection of coronary artery disease and it has been used to provide data for risk stratification during the perioperative period (77,78). The response of regional left ventricular function to dobutamine is useful to characterize myocardium. In the therapeutic dose range, (5 μg/kg/min–20 μg/kg/min) cardiac output is augmented by an increase in ventricular contractility, heart rate, and stroke volume, and a β2-mediated decrease in systemic vascular resistance. Contractility increases at higher doses (20 μg/kg/min–40 μg/kg/ min). Normal resting wall motion and the development of hyperdynamic function with increasing doses of dobutamine are hallmarks of normally perfused myocardium. The development of new wall motion abnormalities or the worsening of baseline systolic dysfunction with escalating doses of dobutamine increases myocardial ischemia. Contractile reserve, on the other hand, is consistent with viability and characterized by baseline wall motion abnormalities that improve with low-dose dobutamine (79,80). When such a low-dose augmentation of function is followed by progressive systolic dysfunction with higher doses (biphasic response), the accuracy of predicting postoperative cardiac morbidity or changes in regional function after revascularization is enhanced (77). Regional segments that remain akinetic (or dyskinetic) despite dobutamine infusion are nonviable. Dobutamine stress echocardiography has a high sensitivity (85%) and specificity (88%) when compared to angiography in patients with recent myocardial infarction (77).

Aronson et al. performed intraoperative low-dose dobutamine stress echocardiography in 40 patients scheduled for elective CABG surgery for regional wall motion evaluation at four stages: baseline (after induction and intubation), with administration of low-dose dobutamine before cardiopulmonary bypass, after separation from cardiopulmonary bypass (early), and after administration of protamine (late) (81). They analyzed 560 segments for 40 patients corresponding to these stages. Changes in myocardial function following low-dose dobutamine were highly predictive for early ($p < 0.0001$) and late ($p < 0.0001$) changes in myocardial function from baseline regional scores (85). It was also found that the positive predictive value of improved regional wall motion after CABG did not vary with left ventricular ejection fraction, a history of myocardial infarction, or beta blocker use. This study demonstrated the potential value of intraoperative dobutamine stress echocardiography to fine tune the placement of grafts in patients in whom a decision has been made to proceed with CABG surgery without preoperative viability testing (Fig. 24.12). When combined with myocardial contrast perfusion imaging, this will permit the identification of hypoperfused regions prior to the patient's leaving the operating room (Fig. 24.13).

## Cardioplegia Administration

To demonstrate the ability of intraoperative contrast echocardiography to accurately predict antegrade cardioplegia distribution in patients undergoing CABG procedures, Aronson et al. recorded intraoperative TEE im-

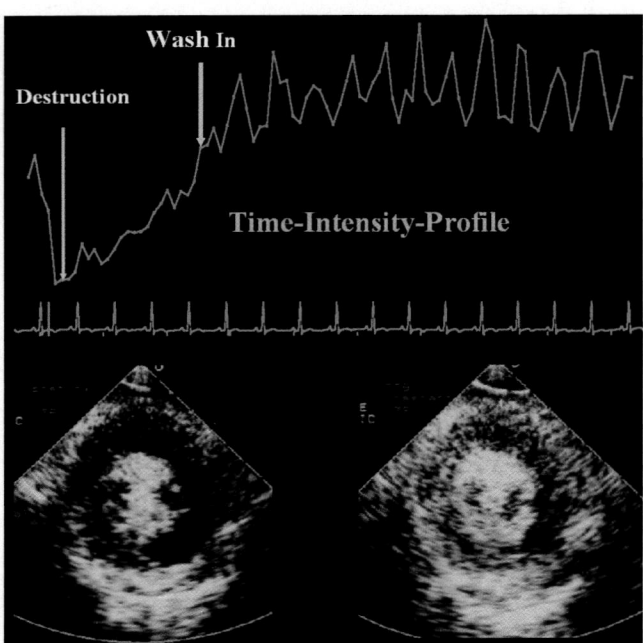

**FIGURE 24.13.** Intraoperative myocardial contrast echocardiography (MCE) may provide an opportunity to verify immediate and long-term graft patency by assessing various MCE parameters. These include baseline perfusion, wash-in flow rate, flow, and degree of collateralization.

ages of the RV free wall, apex, and intraventricular septum (82). This was done before and following the injection of 4 cc of contrast into antegrade and retrograde cardioplegic catheters during cardioplegia delivery. When the observed cardioplegia distribution (by myocardial contrast echocardiography) was compared to the predicted cardioplegia distribution, it was shown that antegrade cardioplegia delivery was distributed to the RV in 31% of patients, despite 100% occlusion of the right coronary artery (86). Interestingly retrograde cardioplegia delivery to the right ventricle occurred only 20% of the time (82). This study demonstrated the potential for myocardial contrast echocardiography to guide the intraoperative administration of cardioplegia in the higher risk patient in whom myocardial protection may determine the success or failure of the patient's surgical intervention.

## End Organ Perfusion

### Renal Perfusion

Despite the many advances in nephrology and renal ultrasound, the intraoperative assessment of renal perfusion continues to rely on the historic indicator of urine output. Given the increased complexity of patients with chronic hypertension and diffuse noncoronary atherosclerosis, we will need to consider methods to continuously assess renal blood flow to initiate therapeutic measures in low flow

states (Fig. 24.14). Garwood et al. performed renal ultrasound utilizing intraoperative TEE (83). They obtained Doppler-derived indices of renal blood flow (pulsatility index and resistive index) by obtaining 2-D images of renal parenchyma and Doppler measurement of intrarenal arterial blood flow during IMA dissection before and after a 20-minute infusion of 2 mcg/kg/min dopamine. Following infusion of dopamine, they demonstrated an increased

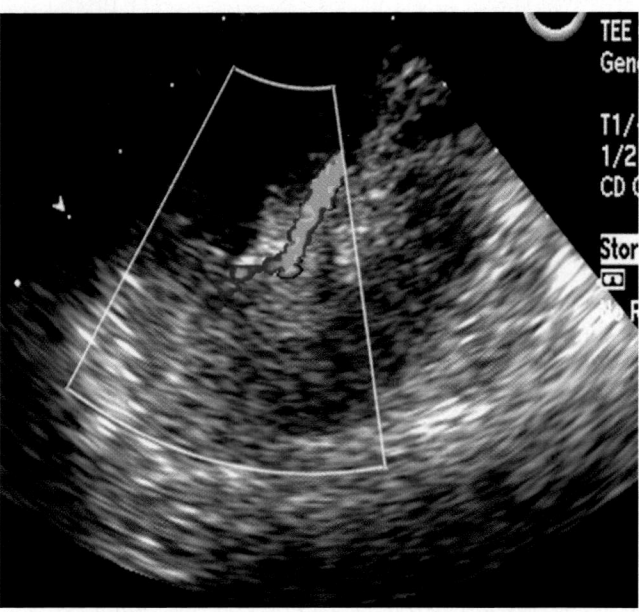

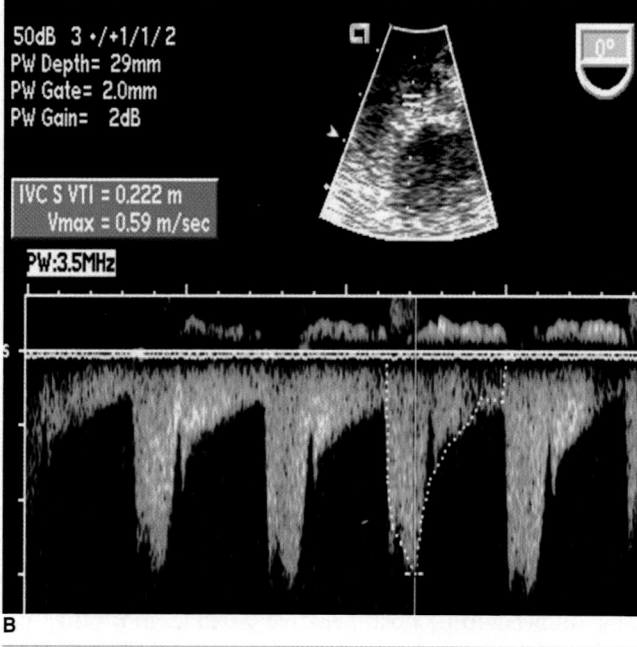

**FIGURE 24.14.** Intraoperative monitoring of renal perfusion, utilizing PW Doppler, may provide a means of assessing optimal renal perfusion pressure and response to pharmacologic interventions to improve perioperative renal function.

velocity of systolic, diastolic, and mean renal blood flow velocity indicating an increase in renal blood flow from baseline (83). The pulsatility and resistive index decreased indicating a reduction in renal vascular resistance. This study clearly demonstrated the potential to utilize intraoperative TEE to acquire two-dimensional images of the kidney and monitor renal arterial Doppler velocities during cardiac surgery. By providing a guide during such interventions, MAP and pump, flow may be optimized while on CPB. In addition, renal perfusion may be assessed following the initiation of dopamine or other vasoactive medications.

### Transcranial Doppler and CNS Function

Intraoperative transcranial Doppler monitoring has been used to detect microembolic phenomena during various stages of coronary artery bypass grafting. To determine the relation between transcranial Doppler and early neuropsychologic deficits, Sylivris et al. correlated MRI findings with microembolic numbers during the bypass period in 41 consecutive patients undergoing coronary bypass grafting (84). Transcranial Doppler monitoring confirmed that most microemboli occurred during cardiopulmonary bypass and demonstrated a correlation between early neuropsychological deficit post-CABG with total microembolic load during bypass (85). This study indicates the potential that transcranial Doppler may some day be used to routinely monitor the intraoperative detection of microemboli during surgical manipulation of the aorta and events related to cannulation and perfusion strategy.

### KEY POINTS

- Despite the many remarkable advances in the management of patients with coronary artery disease, ischemic heart disease remains the leading cause of death in the United States and the world. It is projected to remain so at least through 2020.
- The concept of myocardial revascularization has gone through a number of evolutionary phases from initial observations detailing the coronary anatomy and microvasculature to early experimental coronary artery bypass, early attempts at indirect and direct myocardial revascularization, the modern era of surgical coronary artery bypass relying on arterial conduits, and percutaneous coronary interventions.
- Patient decisions regarding the mode of revascularization are driven by multiple factors, including the scientific body of evidence comparing surgical and percutaneous revascu-

larization, the public's perception equating the most recent technology with better care, the patient's innate desire to avoid traditional surgery, and variation of institutional capabilities in surgical and percutaneous revascularization.
- Because of the rapid evolution of myocardial revascularization technology and the numbers of ongoing trials comparing the different approaches, the physicians responsible for patients' perioperative care need to stay abreast of the scientific information and latest innovations that serve as the basis for our patients' decisions.
- There are inherent difficulties in established indication guidelines for surgical and percutaneous revascularization. For example:
  - Randomized trials comparing these approaches are lengthy due to the different time intervals for recurrent disease requiring repeat revascularization for CABG (8–10 years) compared to PCI (1–5 years).
  - Trials are overpowered with lower risk patients with a low incidence of hard outcomes (death, MI, or stroke).
  - The ongoing evolution of new developments in both approaches to revascularization translate into the results of randomized trials always lagging behind the current generation of technology.
  - Difficulties in having comparable patient groups in randomized trials comparing revascularization approaches due to the many definable and indefinable risk factors that impact patient outcome.
- Factors contributing to higher patient risk in myocardial revascularization include those factors related to a characterization of their manifestations of ischemic heart disease and the patients overall health. While some risk factors are easily defined and more readily subjected to statistical correlation with outcome (ejection fraction, number of coronary arteries involved, history of diabetes, etc.), others are more difficult to define but often are extremely important in determining the patient's eventual outcome (suitable conduits, diffuseness of distal disease, and collateral coronary flow).
- Definable cardiovascular risk factors include age, ventricular function, number and location of coronary disease, peripheral vascular disease, disease emergent operation, diabetes (insulin and non-insulin dependent) degree of

aortic atherosclerosis, and the presence of structural complications of ischemic heart disease (mitral regurgitation, aneurysms, VSD, and pseudoaneurysm). Among the cardiac risk factors that are more difficult to define are degree of collateral, distal coronary flow, diffuseness of coronary disease, availability and quality of conduits, extent of noncoronary atherosclerosis, institutional experience, and operator dependent risks.

- In addition to providing an ongoing method of monitoring the patient's cardiovascular function, intraoperative echocardiography is used to address a number of critical issues that may influence the outcome of the coronary bypass surgery. These critical issues include the development of the cannulation-perfusion strategy to prevent neurologic dysfunction, the diagnosis of previously unrecognized cardiovascular abnormalities requiring surgical intervention or alteration of the patient's anesthetic-hemodynamic management, an assessment of the surgical procedure, and a final documentation of a comprehensive baseline study for future comparison.

- Future daily applications of intraoperative echo in the higher risk coronary bypass patient may include intraoperative viability assessment, assessment of the effectiveness of cardioplegia administration, monitoring of renal perfusion and CNS embolic load, and an immediate prediction of long-term graft survival by coronary flow characterization.

# REFERENCES

1. Parry CH. An inquiry into the symptoms and causes of the syncope anginosa commonly called angina pectoris, illustrated by dissections. Bath: R. Cruttwell; London: Cadell and Davis, 1799.
2. Heberden W. Commentaries on the history and cure of diseases. News-gate: London: T. Payne. 1802. Pectoris dolor in chapter 70, 362–8.
3. Schoen FJ, Padera RF Jr. Cardiac surgical pathology in Cohn LH, Edmunds LH Jr, eds. Cardiac surgery in the adult. New York: McGraw-Hill, 2003: 119–85.
4. Carrell A. On the experimental surgery of the thoracic aorta and the heart. Ann Surg 1910;52:83.
5. Shumacker HB Jr. The evolution of cardiac surgery. Bloomington: Indiana University Press, 1992.
6a. Favaloro RG. Saphenous vein autograft replacement of severe segmental coronary artery occlusion: operative technique. Ann Thorac Surg 1968; 5:334.
6b. Effler DB, Favaloro RG, Groves LK. Coronary artery surgery utilizing saphenous vein graft techniques. Clinical experience with 224 operations. J Thorac Cardiovasc Surg 1970;59(1):147–54.

6c. Favaloro RG, Effler DB, Groves LK, Sheldon WC, Riahi M. Direct myocardial revascularization with saphenous vein autograft. Clinical experience in 100 cases. Diseases of the Chest 1969;56(4):279–83.
7. Eagle KA, Guyton RA, Davidoff R, et al. ACC/AHA guidelines for coronary artery bypass graft surgery: a report of the American College of Cardiology/American Heart Association task force on practice guidelines (committee to revise the 1991 guidelines for coronary artery bypass graft surgery). J Am Coll Cardiol 1999;34:1262–1346.
8. Sundt TM III, Gersh BJ, Smith HC. Indications for coronary revascularization. In: Cohn LH, Edmunds LH Jr, eds. Cardiac surgery in the adult. New York: McGraw-Hill; 2003:541–59.
9. Lytle BW. The role of coronary revascularization in the treatment of ischemic cardiomyopathy. Ann Thorac Surg 2003;75:S2–S5.
10. Lytle BW. Coronary artery reoperations. In: Cohn LH, Edmunds LH Jr, eds. Cardiac surgery in the adult. New York: McGraw-Hill, 2003:659–79.
11. Herlitz J, Brandrup G, Haglid M, et al. Death, mode of death, morbidity, and rehospitalization after coronary artery bypass grafting in relation to occurrence of and time since a previous myocardial infarction. Thorac Cardiovasc Surg 1997 Jun;45(3):109–13.
12. Tu JV, Sykora K, Naylor CD for the Steering Committee of the Cardiac Care Network of Ontario. Assessing the outcomes of coronary artery bypass graft surgery: how many risk factors are enough? J Am Coll Cardiol 1997;30: 1317–23.
13. Hannan EL, Kilburn H, O'Donnell JF, Lukacik G, Shields EP. Adult open heart surgery in New York State: an analysis of risk factors and hospital mortality rates. JAMA 1990;264:2768–74.
14a. Jones RH, Hannan EL, Hammermeister KE, et al. for the Working Group Panel on the Cooperative CABG Database Project. Identification of preoperative variables needed for risk adjustment of short-term mortality after coronary artery bypass graft surgery. J Am Coll Cardiol 1996;28: 1478–87.
14b. The VA Cooperative Study Group. Eighteen-year follow-up in the Veterans Affairs Cooperative Study of coronary artery bypass surgery for stable angina. Circulation 1992; 86:121–130.
14c. Alderman E.L., Bourassa M.G., Cohen L.S., et al. Ten year follow-up of survival and myocardial infarction in the randomized Coronary Artery Surgery Study. Circulation 1990;82:1629–46.
14d. Uretsky BF, Thygesen K, Armstrong PW, et al. Acute coronary findings at autopsy in heart failure patients with sudden death. Results from the assessment of treatment with lisinopril and survival (ATLAS) trial. Circulation 2000;102:611–16.
14e. Allman KC, Shaw LJ, Hachamovitch R, Udelson JE. Myocardial viability testing and impact of revascularization on prognosis in patients with coronary artery disease and left ventricular dysfunction: a meta-analysis. J Am Coll Cardiol 2002;39:1151–8.
15. Frye RL, Kronmal R, Schaff HV, Myers WO, Gersh BJ, for the participants in the Coronary Artery Surgery Study. Stroke in coronary artery bypass graft surgery: an analysis of the CASS experience. Int J Cardiol 1992;36:213–21.
16. Mangano CM, Diamondstone LS, Ramsay JG, et al. The Multicenter Study of Perioperative Ischemia Research Group. Renal dysfunction after myocardial revascularization: risk factors, adverse outcomes, and hospital resource utilization. Ann Intern Med 1998;128:194–203.
17. Gardner TJ, Horneffer PJ, Manolio TA, et al. Stroke following coronary artery bypass grafting: a ten-year study. Ann Thorac Surg 1985;40:574–81.
18. Mangano DT. Cardiovascular morbidity and CABG surgery—a perspective: epidemiology, costs, and potential therapeutic solutions. J Card Surg 1995;10:366–8.

19. Roach GW, Kanchuger M, Mangano CM, et al, for the Multicenter Study of Perioperative Ischemia Research Group and the Ischemia Research and Education Foundation Investigators. Adverse cerebral outcomes after coronary bypass surgery. N Engl J Med 1996;335:1857–63.

20. Mangano CM, Diamondstone LS, Ramsay JG, et al. for the Multicenter Study of Perioperative Ischemia Research Group. Renal dysfunction after myocardial revascularization: risk factors, adverse outcomes, and hospital resource utilization. Ann Intern Med 1998;128:194–203.

21. Higgins T, Estafanous FG, Loop FD, et al. Stratification of morbidity and mortality by preoperative risk factors in coronary artery bypass patients. JAMA 1992;267:2344–8.

22. National Center for Health Statistics, Owings MF, Lawrence L. Detailed diagnosis and procedures: National Hospital Discharge Survey, 1997. Vital and health statistics. Series 13. No. 145. Washington, DC: Government Printing Office, December 1999.

23. Pearson TA, Smith SC, Poole-Wilson P. Cardiovascular specialty societies and the emerging global burden of cardiovascular disease: a call to action. Circulation 1998;97:602–04.

24. From the Centers for Disease Control and Prevention. Public health and aging: trends in aging—United States and worldwide. JAMA 2003;289(11):1371–3.

25. US Census Bureau. US Population Estimates by Age, Sex, Race, and Hispanic Origin: 1990 to 1999. Washington, DC: US Census Bureau, April 11, 2000

26. Bonow RO, Smaha LA, Smith SC, et al. , World Heart Day 2002: the international burden of cardiovascular disease: responding to the emerging global epidemic. Circulation 2002 Sep 24;106(13):1602–5.

27. Committee on Quality of Health Care in America, Institute of Medicine. Crossing the Quality Chasm: A New Health System for the 21st Century. Washington, DC: National Academy Press; 2001.

28. Ferguson BT, Hammill BG, Peterson ED, et al. A decade of change—risk profiles and outcomes for isolated coronary artery bypass grafting procedures, 1990–1999: a report from the STS National Database Committee and the Duke Clinical Research Institute. Ann. Thorac. Surg 2002 Feb; 73:480–9.

29. Marwick TH. Use of standard imaging techniques for prediction of post revascularization functional recovery in patients with heart failure. J Cardiac Failure 1999;5:334–46.

30. Bonow RO. Myocardial viability and prognosis in patients with ischemic left ventricular dysfunction. J Am Coll Cardiol 2002;39:1159–62.

31. Rafferty T, Durkin M, Hines RL, et al. The relationship between "normal" transesophageal color-flow Doppler-defined tricuspid regurgitation and thermodilution right ventricular ejection fraction measurements. J Cardiothorac Vasc Anesth 1993 Apr;7(2):167–74.

32. Clements FM, Harpole DH, Quill T, et al. Estimation of left ventricular volume and ejection fraction by two-dimensional transesophageal echocardiography: comparison of short axis imaging and simultaneous radionuclide angiography. Br J Anaesth 1990;64:331.

33. Sohn DW, Shin GJ. Oh JK. Tajik AJ, et al. Role of transesophageal echocardiography in hemodynamically unstable patients. Mayo Clinic Proc1995 Oct;70(10):925–31.

34. Savage RM, Lytle BW, Aronson S, et al. Intraoperative echocardiography is indicated in high-risk coronary artery bypass grafting. Ann Thorac Surg 1997;64:368–73.

35. Savage RM, Guth B, White F, Hagan AD, Bloor CM: Correlation of regional myocardial blood flow and function with myocardial infarct size during acute ischemia in the conscious pig. Circulation 1981; 64:284–90.

36. van Daele ME, Sutherland GR, Mitchell MM, et al. Do changes in pulmonary capillary wedge pressure adequately reflect myocardial ischemia during anesthesia? A correla-

tive preoperative hemodynamic, electrocardiographic, and transesophageal echocardiographic study. Circulation 1990 Mar; 81(3):865–71.

37. Smith JS, Cahalan MK, Benefiel DJ, et al. Intraoperative detection of myocardial ischemia in high-risk patients: electrocardiography versus two-dimensional transesophageal echocardiography. Circulation 1985 Nov; 72(5): 1015–21.

38. Click RL, Abel MD, Schaff HV Intraoperative transesophageal echocardiography: 5-year prospective review of impact on surgical management. Mayo Clin Proc 2000(Mar);75(3):241–7.

39. Cohn LH, Rizzo RJ, Adams DH, et al. The effect of pathophysiology on the surgical treatment of ischemic mitral regurgitation: operative and late risks of repair versus replacement. Eur J Cardiothorac Surg 1995;9:568–74.

40. Grewal KS, Malkowski MJ, Kramer CM, et al. Multiplane transesophageal echocardiographic identification of the involved scallop in patients with flail mitral valve leaflet: intraoperative correlation. J Am Soc Echocardiogr 1998; 11:966–71.

41. Bach DS, Deeb GM, Bolling SF. Accuracy of intraoperative transesophageal echocardiography for estimating the severity of functional mitral regurgitation. Am J Cardiol 1995 Sep 1;76(7):508–12.

42. Sheikh KH, de Bruijn NP, Rankin JS, et al. The utility of transesophageal echocardiography and Doppler color flow imaging in patients undergoing cardiac valve surgery. J Am Coll Cardiol 1990;15:363–72.

43. Couture P, Denault AY, McKenty S, et al. Impact of routine use of intraoperative transesophageal echocardiography during cardiac surgery. Can J Anesth 2000; 47: 20–6.

44. Bergquist BD, Bellows WH, Leung JM. Transesophageal echocardiography in myocardial revascularization: II. Influence on intraoperative decision making. Anesth Analg 1996;82:1139–45.

45. Gardner TJ, Horneffer PJ, Manolio D, et al. Stroke following coronary artery bypass grafting: a ten year study. Ann Thorac Surg 1985;40:574–81.

46. Murkin JM, Martzke JS, Buchan AM. A randomized study of the influence of perfusion technique and pH management strategy in 316 patients undergoing coronary artery bypass surgery. II. Neurologic and cognitive outcomes. J Thorac Cardiovasc Surg 1995 Aug;110(2):349–62.

47. Newman MF, Wolman R, Kanchuger M, et al. .Multicenter preoperative stroke risk index for patients undergoing coronary artery bypass graft surgery. Multicenter Study of Perioperative Ischemia (McSPI) Research Group.Circulation 1996 Nov 1;94(9 Suppl):II74–80.

48. Roach GW, Kanchuger M, Mangano CM, et al, for the Multicenter Study of Perioperative Ischemia Research Group and the Ischemia Research and Education Foundation Investigators. Adverse cerebral outcomes after coronary bypass surgery. N Engl J Med 1996;335:1857–63.

49. Wareing TH, Davila-Roman VG, Daily BB, et al. Strategy for the reduction of stroke incidence in cardiac surgical patients. Ann Thorac Surg 1993 Jun;55(6):1400–7; discussion 1407–8.

50. Konstadt SN, Reich DL, Quintana C et al, The ascending aorta: how much does transesophageal echocardiography see? Anesth Analg 1994;78:240–4.

51. Davila-Roman VG, Barzilai B, Wareing TH, et al. Atherosclerosis of the ascending aorta. Prevalence and role as an independent predictor of cerebrovascular events in cardiac patients. Stroke 1994;25(10):2010–6.

52. Blauth CI, Cosgrove DM, Webb BW, et al. Atheroembolism from the ascending aorta. An emerging problem in cardiac surgery, J Thorac Cardiovasc Surg 1992 Jun:103(6): 1104–11; discussion 1111–2.

53. Abu-Omar Y, Balacumaraswami L, Pigott DW, et al. . Solid and gaseous cerebral microembolization during off-pump, on-pump, and open cardiac surgery procedures. J Thorac Cardiovasc Surg 2004 Jun;127(6):1759–65.

54. Scalia GM, McCarthy PM, Savage RM, et al. Clinical utility of echocardiography in the management of implantable ventricular assist devices. J Am Soc Echocardiogr. 2000 Aug;13(8):754–63.

55. Duda AM, Letwin LB, Sutter FP, Goldman SM. Does routine use of aortic ultrasonography decrease the stroke rate in coronary artery bypass surgery? J Vasc Surg 1995;21:98–107.

56. Kouchoukos NT, Wareing TH, Daily BB, et al. .Management of the severely atherosclerotic aorta during cardiac operations. J Cardiac Surg 1994;9(5):490–4.

57. Wareing TH, Davila-Roman VG, Daily BB, et al., Strategy for the reduction of stroke incidence in cardiac surgical patients. Ann Thorac Surg 1993 Jun;55(6):1400–7; discussion 1407–8.

58. Davila-Roman VG, Barzilai TH, Wareing TH et al: Atherosclerosis of the ascending aorta: prevalence and role as an independent predictor of cerebrovascular events in cardiac patients. Stroke 1994;25:2010–6.

59a. Hartman GS, Yao FS, Bruefach M 3rd, Barbut D, et al. Severity of aortic atheromatous disease diagnosed by transesophageal echocardiography predicts stroke and other outcomes associated with coronary artery surgery: a prospective study. Anesth Analg. 1996 Oct;83(4):701–8.

59b. Katz ES, Tunick PA, Rusinek H, et al. Protruding aortic atheroma predicts stroke in elderly patients undergoing cardiopulmonary bypass; experience with intraoperative transesophageal echocardiography. J Am Coll Cardiol 1992;20:70-77.

59c. Ribakove GH, Katz ES, Galloway AC, et al: Surgical implications of transesophageal echocardiography to grade the atheromatous aortic arch. Ann Thorac Surg 53:758-63, 1992.

59d. Tunick PA, Perez JL, Kronzon I: Protruding atheromas in the thoracic aorta and systemic embolization. Ann Int Med 115:423-427, 1991.

60. Leung JM, O'Kelly B, Browner WS, et al. Prognostic importance of post bypass regional wall motion abnormalities in patients undergoing coronary artery bypass surgery. Anesthesiology 1989;71:16.

61. Mishra M, Chauhan R, Sharma KK, et al. Real-time intraoperative transesophageal echocardiography--how useful? Experience of 5,016 cases. J Cardiothorac Vasc Anesth 1998 Dec;12(6):625–32.

62. Deutsch J II, Curtius JM, Leischik R, et al. Diagnostic value of transesophageal echocardiography in cardiac surgery. Thorac Cardiovasc Surg 1991;39:199–204.

63. Benson MJ, Cahalan MK. Cost-benefit analysis of transesophageal echocardiography in cardiac surgery. Echocardiography 1995;12:171–83.

64. Cox JL. A perspective of postoperative atrial fibrillation in cardiac operations. Ann Thorac Surg 1993;56:405–9.

65a. Shore-Lesserson L, Moskowitz D, Hametz C, et al. .Use of intraoperative transesophageal echocardiography to predict atrial fibrillation after coronary artery bypass grafting. Anesthesiology 2001 Sep;95(3):652–8.

65b. Rubin DN, Katz SE, Riley MF, et al. Evaluation of left atrial appendage anatomy and function in recent-onset atrial fibrillation by transesophageal echocardiography. Am J Cardiol 71996 Oct 1;8(7):774–8.

66a. Agnihotri AK, Madsen JC, Daggett WM Jr. Surgical Treatment of complications of acute myocardial infarction: postinfarction ventricular septal defect and free wall rupture. In: Cohn LH, Edmunds LH Jr , eds. Cardiac surgery in the adult. New York: McGraw-Hill, 2003:681–714.

66b. Reeder GS Identification and treatment of complications of myocardial infarction, Mayo Clin Proc 1995;70:880–4.

67a. Gillinov AM, Wierup PN, Blackstone EH, et al: Is repair preferable to replacement for ischemic mitral regurgitation? J Thorac Cardiovasc Surg 2001;122:1125.

67b. Barbour DJ, Roberts WC: Rupture of a left ventricular papillary muscle during acute myocardial infarction; analysis of 22 necropsy patients. J Am Coll Cardiol 1986; 8(3):558.

68. Carpentier A. Cardiac valve surgery: the French correction. J Thorac Cardiovasc Surg 1983; 86:323.

69. Gorman RC, Gorman JH III, Edmunds LH Jr. Ischemic Mitral Regurgitation. In: Cohn LH, Edmunds LH Jr, eds. Cardiac Surgery in the Adult. New York: McGraw-Hill, 2003: 751–69.

70. Smith RC, Goldberg H, Bailey CP. Pseudoaneurysm of the left ventricle: diagnosis by direct cardioangiography. Surgery 1957; 42:496–510.

71. Loop FD, Effler DB, Webster JS, et al. Posterior ventricular aneurysms: etiologic factors and results of surgical treatment. N Engl J Med 1973; 288:237–3.

72. Roeske WR, Savage RM, O'Rourke R, Bloor CM: Clinicopathologic correlation in patients after myocardial infarction. Circulation 1981;63:36–45.

73. Brown, SL, Gropler RJ, Harris KM, et al. Distinguishing left ventricular aneurysm from pseudoaneurysm: a review of the literature. Chest 1997;111:1403–9.

74. Kitamura S, Mendez A, Kay JH. Ventricular septal defect following myocardial infarction: experience with surgical repair through a left ventriculotomy and review of the literature. J Thorac Cardiovasc Surg 1971; 61:186.

75. Lundberg S, Sodestrom J. Perforation of the interventricular septum in myocardial infarction: a study based on autopsy material. Acta Med Scand 1962; 172:413.

76. Zehender MK, Kauder ES, Schonthaler M, et al. Right ventricular infarction as an independent predictor of prognosis after acute inferior myocardial infarction. N Engl J Med 1993; 328:981–8.

77. Afridi I, Grayburn PA, Panza JA, et al. Myocardial viability during dobutamine echocardiography predicts survival in patients with coronary artery disease and severe left ventricular systolic dysfunction. J Am Coll Cardiol 1998;32: 921–6.

78. Allman KC, Shaw LJ, Hachamovitch R, Udelson JE. Myocardial viability testing and impact of revascularization on prognosis in patients with coronary artery disease and left ventricular dysfunction: a meta-analysis. J Am Coll Cardiol 2002;39:1151–8.

79. Seeberger MD, Skarvan K, Buser P, et al. Dobutamine stress echocardiography to detect inducible demand ischemia in anesthetized patients with coronary artery disease. Anesthesiology.1998;88(5):1233–9.

80. Leung JM, Bellows WH, Pastor D. Does intraoperative evaluation of left ventricular contractile reserve predict myocardial viability? A clinical study using dobutamine stress echocardiography in patients undergoing coronary artery bypass graft surgery. Anesth Analg 2004;99:647–54.

81. Aronson S. Dupont F. Savage R, et al. Changes in regional myocardial function after coronary artery bypass graft surgery are predicted by intraoperative low-dose dobutamine echocardiography. Anesthesiology 2000;93(3):685–92.

82. Aronson S, Jacobsohn E, Savage R, et al. The influence of collateral flow on the antegrade and retrograde distribution of cardioplegia in patients with an occluded right coronary artery. Anesthesiology 1998;89(5):1099–107.

83. Garwood S, Davis E, Harris SN. Intraoperative transesophageal ultrasonography can measure renal blood flow. J Cardiothorac Vasc Anesth 2001;15(1):65–71.

84. Sylivris S, Levi C, Matalanis G, et al. Pattern and significance of cerebral microemboli during coronary artery bypass grafting. Ann Thorac Surg 1998;66(5):1674–8.

85. Edmonds HL Jr, Rodriguez RA, Audenaert SM, et al. The role of neuromonitoringin cardiovascular surgery. J Cardiothorac Vasc Anesth 1996;10:15–23.

86. Mueller RL, Rosengart TK, Isom W. The history of surgery for ischemic heart disease. Ann Thorac Surg 1997;63: 869–78.

## QUESTIONS

**1.** Which of the following factors are the strongest predictors of death following coronary bypass surgery?

A. Increased age, emergency surgery, reoperation
B. Increased age, hypertension, LV ejection fraction
C. Emergency surgery, ejection fraction, LAD disease
D. Female gender, ejection fraction, left main stenosis
E. Renal dysfunction, left main disease, ejection fraction

2. Which of the following uses of intraoperative echo findings is most likely to impact patient mortality following CABG in the higher risk patient?
   A. Moderate MR with central jet direction
   B. Grade V atheroma in ascending aorta
   C. Moderate tricuspid regurgitation
   D. Pre-CPB anteroseptal dyskinesia
   E. Mitral inflow e wave deceleration time of 150 msec

3. Based on current projections by the National Center for Health Statistics and the U.S. Census Bureau, the number of individuals over the age of 65 with clinically significant coronary artery disease in the year 2020 will be what?
   A. 5,000,000
   B. 1,500,000
   C. 750,000
   D. 250,000
   E. 500,000

4. Myocardial protection strategies for patients with mild to moderate aortic regurgitation include which of the following
   A. LV venting
   B. Direct intercornary cardioplegia
   C. Retrograde cardioplegia
   D. Antegrade cardioplegia
   E. Aortic valve replacement

5. Patients with an ischemic cardiomyopathy and mitral regurgitation may have which of the following mechanisms of mitral valve dysfunction?
   A. Type I
   B. Type II
   C. Type IIIa
   D. Asymmetrical Type IIIb
   E. Symmetrical Type IIIb

## Chapter 25

# Assessment of the Mitral Valve in Ischemic Heart Disease[1]

*Alexander N. Chapochnikov, Solomon Aronson, and David Jayakar*

Mitral regurgitation (MR) that accompanies acute myocardial ischemia or infarction is associated with an unfavorable prognosis for both medical and surgical treatment. It has been reported that up to 41% of coronary artery bypass-grafting (CABG) candidates may also have chronic ischemic mitral insufficiency (1). When the severity of ischemic mitral regurgitation (IMR) necessitates CABG and mitral valve repair or replacement, the combined procedure may lead to significantly increased in-hospital mortality compared with that for CABG alone. This risk is further enhanced in patients over 80 years of age (2). It has previously been demonstrated that CABG alone can lead to reduction of IMR severity (3). On the other hand, significant residual MR after revascularization is associated with increased immediate postoperative and long-term morbidity and mortality (4,5).

The intraoperative severity assessment of residual MR is further complicated by hemodynamic changes related to the effect of general anesthesia and is often underestimated (6). Intraoperative transesophageal echocardiography (TEE) in experienced hands enables precise assessment of the mechanism and may improve intraoperative decision making and patient outcome. This chapter discusses the anatomic and physiologic principles of IMR and reviews the use of TEE in the diagnosis of this condition (7,8).

## SCIENTIFIC PRINCIPLES

### Prevalence and Outcome

Ischemic MR is present in 7% to 31% of patients undergoing coronary angiography (4,9). In a series of 140 patients with mitral insufficiency, 26% had IMR (10), with other reported causes of MR in that series being 41% myxomatous degeneration, 17% rheumatic valvular disease, 12% endocarditis, and 2% congenital pathology

(Fig. 25.1). The same group reported that among 755 patients who had undergone a primary operation for MR (11), the total operative mortality rate was 4%, whereas the mortality rate in the group of patients with combined repair and CABG was 6.6%. Analysis of 150 consecutive patients with IMR undergoing either repair (63%) or replacement has been reported to result in different long-term outcome based on the underlying pathophysiology, rather than the type of procedure (12). It was found that the functional subset of IMR (annular dilatation or restrictive leaflet motion) had the worse long-term (5-year) survival rate (43%) compared with the structural IMR (ruptured chordae or papillary muscle) repair (76%) or structural/replacement groups (89%). The predictor of worse long-term survival (repair of functional IMR) indicates that pathophysiologic mechanisms may be the major determinants of survival rather than the type of surgi-

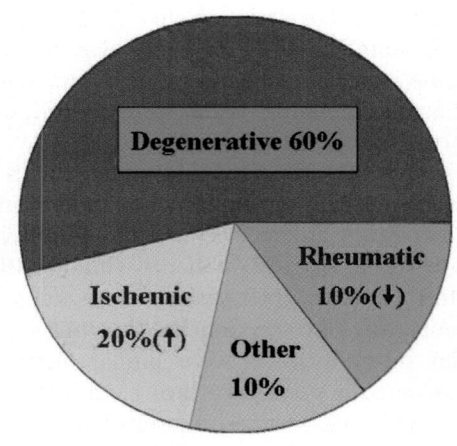

**FIGURE 25.1.** Prevalence of mitral valve disease. Ischemic etiology is increasing while rheumatic etiology is decreasing in the U.S. population.

---

[1]This chapter is reprinted in its entirety from Konstadt SN, Shernan S, Oka, Y. Clinical Transesophageal Echocardiography: A Problem-Oriented Approach, 2nd ed. Philadelphia: Lippincott Williams & Wilkins, 2003:299–318.

cal intervention (12). Retrospective analysis of 1,292 patients at the Cleveland Clinic over a 5-year period revealed an overall incidence of IMR of 6.5%, of which 40% had valve prolapse and 60% had restrictive leaflet motion due to regional or global left ventricular (LV) dilatation (13). Forty-two percent of the patients had rheumatic valvular disease; 44% had degenerative valvular disease; and 6% had endocarditis or congenital valve malformation. A mean follow-up (3 ± 1.6 years) interval after repair revealed a superior survival in the patients with valve leaflet prolapse (96%) versus 48% for those with restricted valvular motion (13,14).

In a reported series by Seipelt and colleagues, 262 patients underwent mitral valve operations (replacement, 198; repair, 64) in combination with coronary revascularization. MR was determined to be secondary to coronary artery disease (CAD) in 31% of patients (19.5% in-hospital mortality), whereas 53% of cases had a rheumatic etiology and 16% were attributed to degenerative changes, with a combined in-hospital mortality rate of 6.7% (15). Mitral valve repair was performed in 37% of the patients with IMR versus 19% with rheumatic or degenerative disease. The survival rates (valve-related, event-free survival) in the first, fifth, and tenth years were 94%, 66%, and 53% in the IMR group, compared with 95%, 76%, and 41% in the rheumatic or degenerative groups.

The reported in-hospital mortality rate for isolated CABG is 3%, whereas isolated mitral valve procedures carry a reported in-hospital mortality rate of 3% to 7% (16,17).

Combined mitral valve surgery and CABG is associated with a reported in-hospital mortality rate of 7% to 20% (2,16–18), with advanced age of the patients (≥ 80 years) being described as an independent risk factor leading to increased in-hospital mortality (19.6% vs. 12.2% in younger patients) as well as congestive heart failure (CHF), acute onset of ischemia requiring intensive care, LV end-diastolic pressure greater than 15 Torr, and New York Heart Association class IV (2,8).

Investigators have reported that patients with grade 2 or less ischemic MR (group I) who underwent CABG alone had reduced angina pectoris and improved functional status equal to CABG patients without MR (group II) (19). In that series, IMR patients were older and had lower preoperative LV ejection fraction (42% vs. 58%). The 30-day mortality rates were similar (4.5% in both groups), as were the survival rates at 1 year (91% vs. 93%) and 3 years (84% vs. 88%). The severity grade of MR increased in 2% of the patients and was unchanged in 36% (19).

At the Society of Cardiovascular Anesthesiologists (SCA) Annual Meeting in April 2002, it was reported that isolated off-pump coronary artery bypass (OPCAB) may offer improvement and resolution of mild IMR (20). A total of 144 patients undergoing OPCAB were evaluated ret-rospectively. Sixteen of 144 required conversion to cardiopulmonary bypass (CPB), and 5 patients among them had moderate IMR. Of the remaining 128 patients who tolerated the OPCAB procedure, 109 were examined by preoperative, intraoperative, and postoperative echocardiography. Fourteen patients were excluded from the study because nonischemic mitral valve pathology was found. Forty-eight of 109 patients (44%) had varied degrees of IMR, 11 patients (10%) had moderate IMR, 37 patients (34%) had mild or trace IMR, and none had severe IMR. Three of five patients with moderate IMR who required conversion to CPB died postoperatively due to low output syndrome and respiratory failure. Postoperative transthoracic echocardiography (TTE) or TEE revealed no improvement in IMR degree in four of these five patients. The patients with moderate IMR who tolerated OPCAB had postoperative TTE at 1 to 35 weeks, which showed improvement in MR severity in 9 of 11. All had functional improvement. No deaths were reported in the moderate IMR OPCAB group. The researchers concluded that OPCAB patients with moderate IMR who required conversion to on-pump CABG represented a high-risk group, whereas patients with moderate or less IMR who tolerated OPCAB appeared to benefit from revascularization alone. This may be important in the subgroup of patients with IMR and perioperative risk, which strongly preclude aortic occlusion and initiation of CPB (20).

## Anatomy

The mitral valve (MV) is a complex structure consisting of two leaflets (posterior and anterior), the chordal structures (primary, secondary, and tertiary), the papillary muscles [anterolateral (AL) and posteromedial (PM)], and the ventricular wall extending between the base of the PM papillary muscle insertion and the annulus of the MV. While the LV remains in systole, the leaflets come together, forming the coaptation point, which—along with AL and PM commissures—create a "line of coaptation."

The posterior leaflet consists of three scallops: medial, middle, and lateral. The corresponding portions of the anterior leaflet are medial, middle, and lateral thirds. The chordae, which consist of connective tissue (mainly collagen bundles), extend from the head of each papillary muscle to the nearest half of each leaflet.

The primary chordae attach to the tip of the leaflet, the secondary chordae attach to the mid-portion of the leaflet, and the tertiary chordae attach to the base of the leaflet or mitral annulus. These tertiary chordae (also referred to as "stay" chordae) form a posterior chordal structure that has a stabilizing function. Interruption of the tertiary chordae due to ischemic/necrotic rupture in the corresponding myocardial zone (including papillary muscle) will have a significant impact on the maintenance of normal LV geometry and ventricular function. The number of papillary muscle heads varies from one to five.

The blood supply to the PM papillary muscle was provided by one vessel (either right coronary artery or obtuse marginal artery) in 63% of the patients and two vessels in 37% (21). The AL papillary muscle had a double-vessel blood supply (obtuse marginal and diagonal) in 71% and single-vessel supply in 29%. In a study that included 20 patients monitored by TEE during coronary surgery, selective coronary graft injections of sonicated albumin microbubbles were performed to assess graft patency and papillary muscle perfusion. It was demonstrated that in the subgroup of 10 patients with an old inferior myocardial infarction (MI), MR was present only among those 6 with a single rather than a double blood supply.

Presently used nomenclature systems include both Carpentier classification, where the posterior MV leaflet is divided into P1, P2, and P3 (lateral, middle, and medial) scallops, and the Duran classification (22). The latter uses a P1, PM, P2 for the same scallops, respectively, where the middle scallop is subdivided into the PM1 and PM2 with regard to the chordae that come from the corresponding AL papillary muscle (PM I) or the PM papillary muscle (PM2). The anterior leaflet (comprising 60%–70% of the mitral valve area and 30% of the annular circumference) is also divided differently. The Carpentier classification provides Al, A2, and A3 nomenclature (lateral, middle, medial) segments, respectively, versus a division into Al and A2 portions (by Duran classification) with the corresponding papillary muscles attached via chordae. The specific approach to the anterior leaflet division may reflect different mitral regurgitant pathophysiology and a different approach from the surgical standpoint. The American Society of Echocardiography and the SCA incorporate the anatomic classification represented by the Carpentier scheme. Mitral valve regurgitation may be caused by malfunctioning of any component of the mitral valve apparatus. Chronic regurgitation leads to dilatation of the left atrium (LA) and the annulus, which loses its physiologic elliptoid shape during systole. The resulting circular annulus portends poor leaflet coaptation and MR. Increased LA dimension suggests an advanced degree of MR, although smaller dimensions do not exclude insufficiency.

## Mechanism

Mitral regurgitation as a primary complication of ischemic heart disease was initially described by Burch and De Pasquale in 1963, when they recognized papillary muscle dysfunction as a primary consequence of ischemia (23).

There are many ways to classify IMR, for example, acute versus chronic, or by underlying pathology, such as CAD with annular dilatation, CAD with ischemic or infarcted papillary muscles, or CAD with restrictive chordae or leaflet pathology with or without annular dilatation (24). The classification of mitral valve insufficiency proposed by Alain Carpentier included a description as follows: Type I: pure dilatation of the annulus, leaflet motion normal, leaflet perforation may be present; Type II: leaflet prolapse due to chordal rupture or elongation or papillary muscle rupture or elongation; and Type III: restricted leaflet motion due to posterior papillary muscle dysfunction in conjunction with LV dysfunction (25).

Acute transient MR during ischemic episode occurs primarily due to leaflet restriction as a result of ventricular dyskinesia, rather than of annular dilatation (26). Segmental asynergy of the LV wall was found in up to 96% of

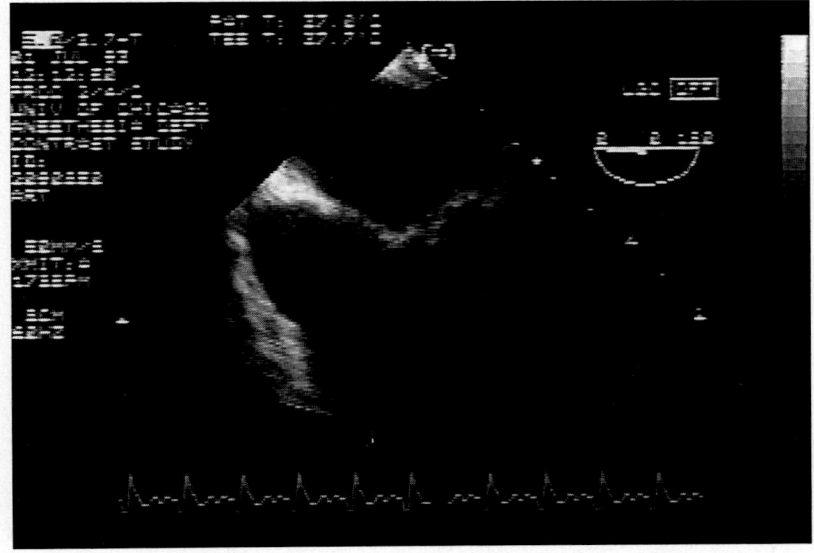

**FIGURE 25.2.** Prolapsed posterior leaflet of the mitral valve. Magnified view of left atrium and coapted mitral valve leaflets forming a chevron shape.

the patients with acute severe MR. The inferior wall was impaired in 86% (Fig. 25.2) (27).

It is important to distinguish IMR that is described in the context of other organic causes of MR from the IMR described among patients with CAD and no primary organic mitral valve disease. The latter type may be as high as 57%, with prevalence up to 90% represented by incomplete mitral leaflet closure in patients with acute MI and acute IMR (14).

The current understanding about the mechanism of IMR after acute MI involves consideration of unbalanced ventricular forces, changes in papillary muscle geometry, asymmetric widening of the annulus, expansion of the border zone myocardium, and early systolic leaflet loitering.

The normal saddle shape of the valve promotes caudal opening, with less force required to open the valve than to close it (Fig. 25.3) (28). The diastolic LA pressure to LV pressure gradient determines the rate of mitral valve leaflet opening. The rate of change of the early systolic LV to LA pressure gradient affects (in part) the degree of mitral leaflet closure. If this gradient is low (as seen with LV dysfunction), then MR will occur. This principle was examined by Dent et al. (28) when global LV function was changed by altering the left main coronary artery flow while maintaining constant LA pressure. Left ventricular end-systolic dimension and peak positive LV rate of pressure development (dP/dt) correlated well with the degrees of mitral leaflet opening and closure. They concluded that LV systolic function determines the extent (both opening and closure) of mitral leaflet excursion (28).

Papillary muscle dynamics also play a significant role in proper mitral leaflet closure in normal hearts. In a diseased heart, even a preexisting single blood supply to the PM papillary muscle can uncommonly lead to its necrosis. On the other hand, the consequent LV systolic dysfunction of ischemia may significantly contribute to the geometry changes of the mitral valve apparatus. The tethering distance (Fig. 25.4) between an ischemic PM papillary muscle tip and the anterior annulus has been measured experimentally. Initial inferior ischemia alone produced papillary muscle tip retraction with restricted closure and mild to moderate MR (regurgitant fraction, 25%), whereas the addition of papillary muscle ischemia consistently decreased MR and tethering distance. It was concluded that papillary muscle contractile dysfunction paradoxically decreased MR because the inferobasal ischemia reduced leaflet tethering and improved coaptation (29).

The otherwise normal constant distance between the tip of the papillary muscle and the annulus may become variable in ischemic heart disease, whereas the papillary muscle tip to the leaflet edge distance (determined by the length of the primary chorda) remains constant despite the presence of ischemic changes. If the primary chorda is intact, tethering of the leaflet edges occur, which leads to restrictive leaflet closure and MR (Fig. 25.5). The annulus area normally decreases by 25% during systole and preserves its physiologic elliptoid shape. Most changes in annulus shape are posterior.

Komeda and associates used an acute ischemic dog model along with radiopaque markers and simultaneous

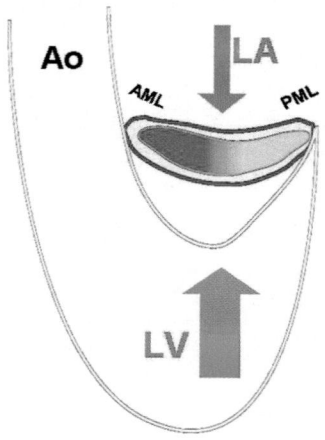

**FIGURE 25.3.** The saddle-shaped mitral valve requires greater force to move the leaflets cephalad than caudad. Ischemic mitral regurgitation also may occur when the pressure gradient between the left ventricle and the left atria during early systole is low due to increased left atrial end-diastolic pressure, or diminished left ventricular early-systolic pressure. *AML,* anterior mitral leaflet; *PML,* posterior mitral leaflet; *LA,* left atrium; *LV,* left ventricle; *Ao,* aorta.

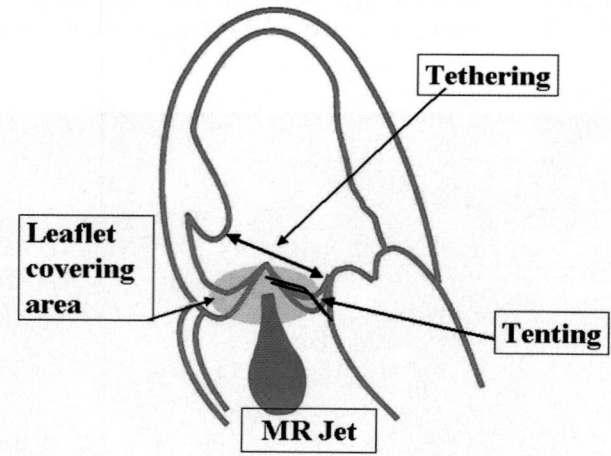

**FIGURE 25.4.** Echocardiography-derived indices to assess ischemic mitral regurgitation include tethering (the distance between the posteromedial papillary muscle and the anterior annulus), tenting height (the distance of the mitral valve leaflet from the tip to the hinge point of restrictive motion), leaflet covering area, and mitral valve regurgitant jet area. *MR,* mitral regurgitation.

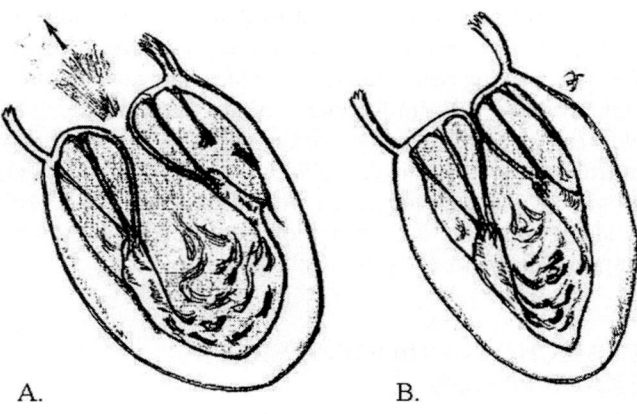

A.                                    B.

**FIGURE 25.5.** Mechanisms of ischemic mitral regurgitation are attributable to apical tethering of the left ventricle resulting in restricted mitral valve leaflet motion and poor leaflet coaptation. The annulus is apically displaced due to chordae tendineae retaining their length constant between the tips of the leaflets and the papillary muscles **(A)**. The normal mitral valve apparatus is demonstrated **(B)**.

biplane videofluoroscopy to evaluate annular dimensions during regional (posterolateral wall) LV ischemia (30). They demonstrated that end-systolic mitral annulus area increased (4.9 vs. 5.9 cm²) and IMR occurred in an asymmetric manner, with the most anterior annular segment lengths not changed. Markedly increased radial dislocation of PM papillary muscle at end-systole, dilatation (in the septal-lateral direction) of the mitral annulus, and AL apical motion (tethering) of the posterior mitral leaflet all led to MR. Based on these data, it might seem that an initial procedure of choice would be a ring annuloplasty provided that TEE assessment revealed no leaflet prolapse. The ring annuloplasty, although causing augmentation of leaflet coaptation, may in some circumstances not completely eliminate MR due to the fact that it does not normalize the radial displacement of the posterior mitral leaflet and the PM papillary tips in the radial direction. Thus, the tethering effect may not be eliminated, and an additional procedure, such as chordal extension (or replacement with expanded synthetic chordae), posterior papillary muscle elongation, or even excision of the posterior LV wall between the PM bases may be necessary.

The Surgical Anterior Ventricular Endocardial Restoration (SAVER) trial has demonstrated that surgical anterior ventricular endocardial restoration can be used for remodeling the dysfunctional and dilated anterior portion of the LV after anterior MI (31). In this important series of 439 patients, concomitant CABG was performed in 89% and mitral repair in 22%. Mitral valve replacement was necessary in 4% of the patients.

Gorman and associates in an acute infarction sheep model demonstrated that circumflex coronary artery occlusion (which subtended 32% of the posterior LV) produced acute 2 to 3+ MR. Sonomicrometry transducers implanted around the mitral annulus and the tips and bases of papillary muscles revealed that the mitral annulus was dilated asymmetrically orthogonal to the line of leaflet coaptation. Although annular area increase was rather small (9.2%), when combined with tethering of the leaflet scallops, it was sufficient to produce moderate to severe MR (32).

Radiopaque markers sutured around the mitral annulus, to the central free mitral leaflet edges, and to both papillary muscle tips and bases again helped reveal changes in mitral annular dimensions and leaflet closing dynamics in pre- and postinduction of acute ischemia (33). During control (preischemic phase), leaflet coaptation occurred 23 msec after end-diastole, whereas during ischemia (with LV dysfunction) coaptation was delayed to 115 msec after end-diastole with MR occurring. Mitral annulus area was also 14% larger during ischemic conditions compared with control measurements. In that experimental model, the posterior papillary muscle tip was displaced laterally and posteriorly, but no apical displacement was noted. "Loitering" of the leaflets associated with posterior mitral annulus enlargement and circularization led to incomplete mitral leaflet coaptation during early systole, not at end-systole (33). This early systolic mitral annular dilatation and shape change, as well as altered posterior papillary muscle motion, should be considered as one of the mechanisms by which incomplete mitral leaflet coaptation occurs during acute IMR.

Carpentier and associates showed that mitral valve incompetence could not be produced by infiltrating the papillary muscle with formaldehyde. In order to get MR, it was also necessary to infiltrate the myocardial wall that supports the papillary muscle. These experimental findings were revealed when Carpentier commented on a similar conclusion made by Llaneras et al. (34).

The role of an LV shape in the development of functional MR in heart failure was demonstrated by Sabbah and associates (35). Global LV shape changes were induced in dogs by multiple sequential intracoronary microembolizations. Sixty-one percent of animals developed 1+ to 3+ MR during heart failure. End-systolic sphericity index increased 72%. Animals without MR were found with only a 30% increase of the same index. These data support the concept of spherical LV shape as a determinant of functional MR (35–37). The same group of researchers (35) commented on the mechanism of functional MR with the emphasis on the LV chamber enlargement and LV reshaping along with papillary muscle dysfunction, regional LV wall motion abnormalities, and dilatation of the mitral valve annulus (38).

The concept of simultaneous ischemic impairment of the anterior papillary muscle and mitral annulus dilatation contributing to clinically significant MR remains controversial. In a sheep model, it was shown that simultaneous mitral annular dilatation and anterior papillary muscle dislocation produced no MR (39). Implanted radiopaque markers with biplane videofluoroscopy revealed significantly increased, (11%–13%) mitral valve area 1 week after chemical obliteration of the anterior annular and leaflet muscles. Exclusive intercommissural axis increase and AL displacement of the anterior papillary muscle tip were noted at end-systole with displacement toward the mitral annulus. The posterior papillary muscle geometry remained unchanged. The presence of biaxial annular enlargement resulted in MR, which suggested that septolateral axis elongation (as observed with proximal circumflex coronary artery occlusion) may play a role in the development of clinically significant IMR. It was reported that ischemia delays leaflet coaptation and shifts it to the late end-diastole (40). Ischemia was also associated with a significant increase in end-diastolic annular area (8.0 vs. 6.7 cm$^2$) and septal-lateral annular diameter (2.9 vs. 2.5 cm, $p = 0.02$).

The importance of mitral annulus dynamics was described during rapid atrial pacing as a close link was shown to exist between mitral annulus area reduction and LA volume reduction during diastole. Rapid pacing at 140 per minute helped to reliably couple a minimum mitral annulus area and LA volume (41). Annuloplasty has been shown in animal models to decrease the distance from the papillary muscle tip to the annulus in control and ischemic conditions (42).

The chronic phase seen in postinfarcted myocardium is characterized by its dilatation and an increased distance from the tip of papillary muscles to the tip of the leaflets. Progression of MR parallels changes in LV geometry where increased leaflet tethering, leaflet tenting, and leaflet restriction take place. Restoring this tethering geometry toward normal, using ventricular remodeling procedures, has been demonstrated (43). During 8 weeks of observation following ligation of the circumflex coronary artery, LV dilatation was noted, as was a shift of the papillary muscles posteriorly and mediolaterally. The leaflet tethering distance increased with the progression of MR. By multiple regression analysis it was shown that the only independent predictor of MR was tethering distance.

The paradoxic decrease in IMR with papillary muscle dysfunction was reported in an animal model (29). Three-dimensional (3D) echocardiography was used to measure the tethering distance between the ischemic PM papillary muscle tip and anterior annulus. Initial inferior ischemia alone produced papillary muscle tip retraction with restricted closure and mild to moderate MR (regurgitant fraction, 25%). However, adding papillary muscle ischemia consistently decreased MR and tethering distance. It was concluded that papillary muscle contractile dysfunction could paradoxically decrease MR from inferobasal ischemia by reducing leaflet tethering and improving coaptation.

The multiple mechanisms of IMR suggest that our understanding of this subject continues to evolve. Clinical decision making regarding the type of repair may be difficult. Annular ring implantation alone (rigid vs. flexible with the intention to preserve the elliptoid shape during mitral annular dynamics) or with the addition of leaflet or subvalvular procedures, as well as possible LV wall remodeling all should be based on comprehensive understanding of the underlying mechanisms.

## THE ECHOCARDIOGRAPHIC EXAMINATION

Two-dimensional (2D) TEE enables the mitral valve to be seen in several tomographic planes [midesophageal (ME) four-chamber, commissural, two-chamber, long-axis, and transgastric short-axis (TG SAX) views] (Fig. 25.6).

Pulsed-wave (PW) Doppler and color flow Doppler imaging of the LA will delineate the regurgitant jet. Fine manipulation of the TEE probe allows inspection of the mitral valve in the aforementioned planes. Transgastric short-axis reveals the mitral valve and mitral annulus with the P3 scallop as the uppermost on the screen (the closest to the TEE probe). The ME images (two- and four-chamber views) allow focusing on the specific scallops of the posterior leaflet and the specific regions of the anterior leaflet. These views also survey the motion of the leaflets relative to the annulus. In these views, the leaflet coaptation point below the annulus gives the classic appearance of the chevron (Fig. 25.7).

A systematic study of these views often reveals the mechanism of injury. Elongated chordae may lead to prolapse of one or both leaflets. Marked prolapse of the affected leaflet may have a "flail" appearance in the direction of the LA. Flail leaflets are commonly caused by ruptured chordae and less commonly by infarcted and ruptured papillary muscle. Ruptured primary or secondary chordae may be seen as a fluttering thin structure in the LA during systole. In contrast, shorter tertiary chordae or just elongated chordae do not prolapse into the LA during systole, but rather appear as an excessively mobile structure near the tip of the leaflets during diastole. The presence of a flail leaflet helps to distinguish isolated severe mitral leaflet prolapse with intact chordae from the ruptured subvalvular structures.

Infarcted papillary muscle in combination with infarction of the nearest LV myocardium also may lead to the regurgitation. This happens secondary to a lack of the tethering function normally performed by this myocardial structure. On the other hand, when this dilated myocardial segment is moving dyskinetically, it prevents proper coaptation of the leaflets during systole. Echocardiographic findings, such as papillary muscle atrophy with increased echogenicity on the SAX view, thinning

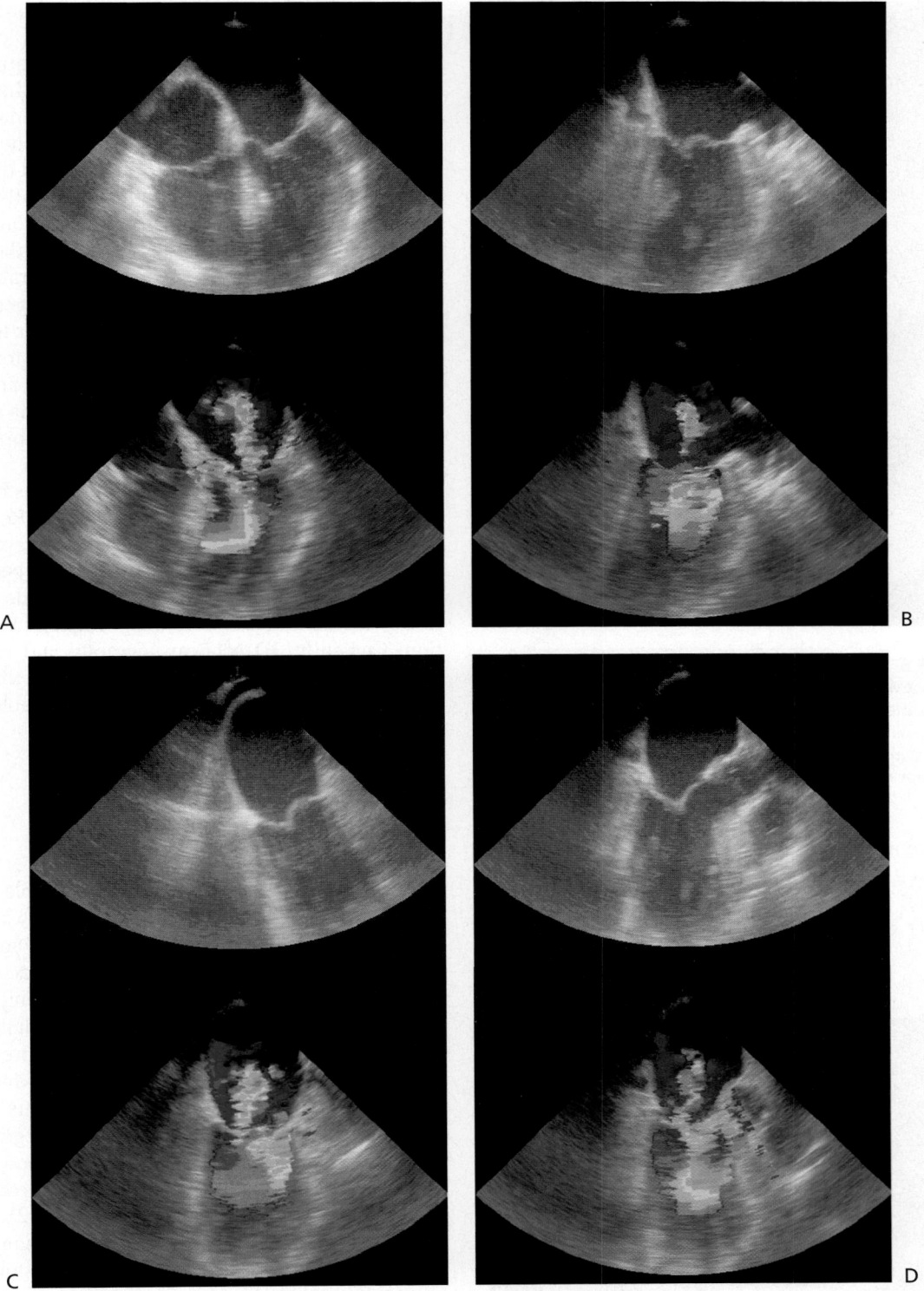

**FIGURE 25.6.** Tomographic planes of the mitral valve apparatus with corresponding color flow Doppler (*CFD*) images are demonstrated. There are midesophageal (*ME*) four-chamber view **(A)**, ME commissural view **(B)**, ME two-chamber view **(C)**, ME long-axis view **(D)**, and transgastric short-axis view (*TG SAX*) **(E).**   *(Continued)*

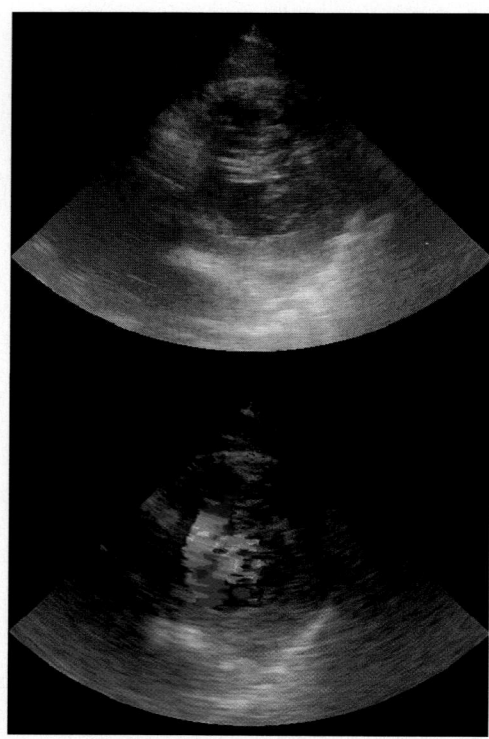

**E**

**FIGURE 25.6.** *(continued)* The central regurgitant jet is visualized in all views. The TG SAX CFD image may suggest the anatomic location of the jet regarding the posterior leaflet scallops. Of note, complete analysis of the severity of the regurgitant jet requires evaluation of the proximal isovelocity surface area and pulmonary vein flow pattern.

of the adjacent myocardium, or akinetic or dyskinetic motion during systole, indicate a previously infarcted state. Of note, postinfarction changes (connective tissue development) of papillary muscle with its subsequent

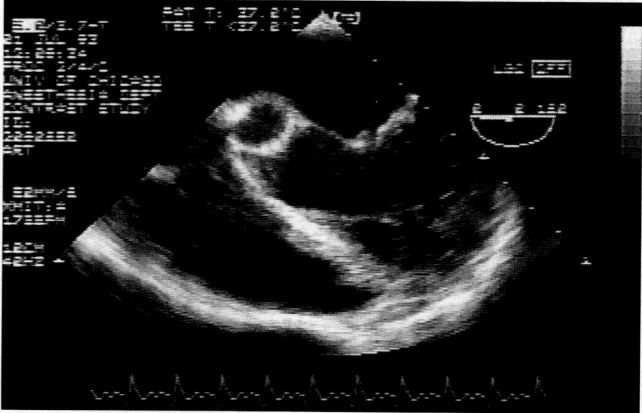

**FIGURE 25.7.** Classic chevron shape of coapted mitral valve leaflets in a long-axis view. The posterior leaflet prolapses into the left atrium.

shrinkage may lead to the retraction of chordal structure and regurgitation.

Severity of MR assessed with intraoperative TEE and postoperative TTE has been compared. Intraoperative TEE assessment tends to downgrade evaluation of MR severity (5). It has been observed that systolic blood pressure, mean arterial pressure, and LV end-diastolic and end-systolic dimensions become significantly lower during the intraoperative TEE examination compared with the preoperative TEE examination (5,6). Although preoperative assessment of severity may be preferable when deciding whether to perform mitral valve surgery (6), intraoperative TEE evaluation is critical in order to determine the mechanism of MR and guide a strategy for repair.

Phenylephrine may help increase the patient's blood pressures to preoperative values and provide an adequate hemodynamic environment for the intraoperative MR grading.

Three-dimensional echocardiography has been used to evaluate mechanism of disease (44). Real-time 3D echocardiography of LV function after infarct exclusion surgery for ischemic cardiomyopathy has been reported as an excellent quantitative assessment mode for changes in LV volume and function after complex LV reconstruction. Currently, 3D echocardiography and real-time 3D echocardiography are labor-intensive and time-consuming manipulations and are not yet available for widespread intraoperative application.

## CLINICAL INFORMATION

### Case 1

A 75-year-old man with hypertension, unstable angina, and diabetes mellitus had a history of inferior wall MI and a preoperative electrocardiogram (ECG) showing a Q wave in leads II, III, and aVF. Preoperative cardiac catheterization revealed 80% stenosis of the left ascending artery, total stenosis of the first marginal artery, and total stenosis of the proximal right coronary artery. Before cardiopulmonary bypass, TEE revealed severely hypokinetic inferior septal, inferior, and inferoposterior segments in the SAX view and apical, middle, and inferobasal segments in the long-axis view. Color Doppler imaging showed mild to moderate MR originating from the site of the PM commissure shown in the two-chamber view (Fig. 25.8). The mitral annulus was slightly dilated (3.5-cm diameter in the three-chamber view). Pulmonary venous systolic flow was normal. The patient underwent CABG to the left anterior descending artery, the first marginal artery, and the posterior descending artery. The patient was weaned from bypass without inotropic therapy. After CABG, TEE showed improvement of all inferior segments and only trivial MR (Fig. 25.9). The postoperative course was uneventful.

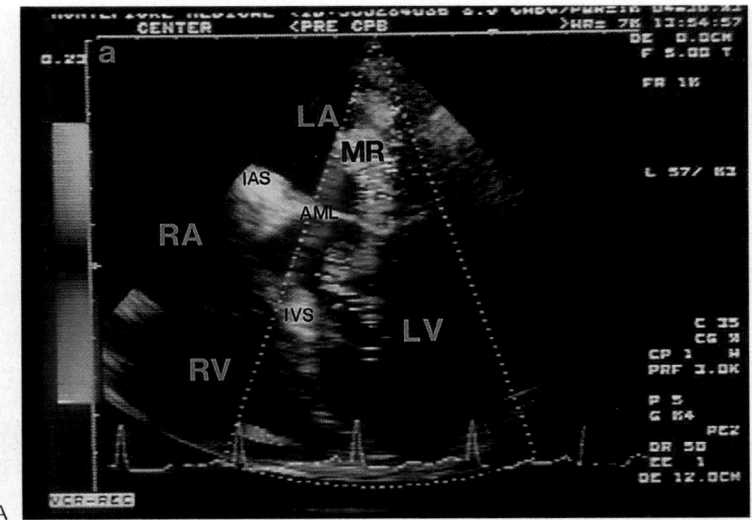

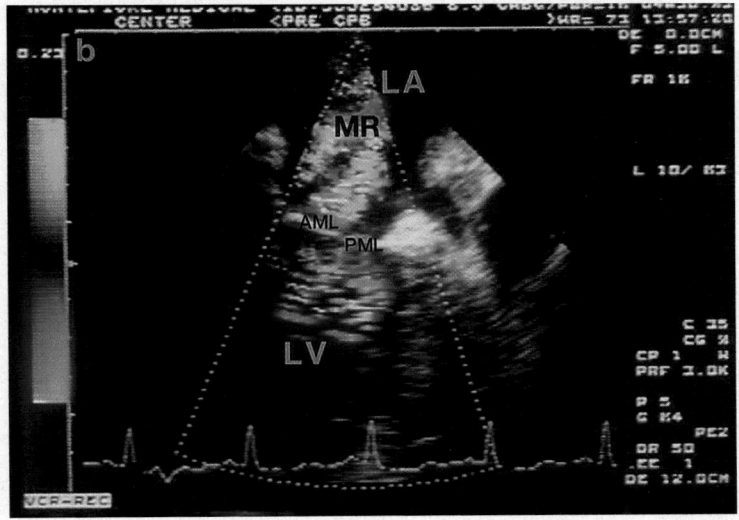

*FIGURE 25.8.* Color Doppler imaging shows mild to moderate mitral regurgitation in the three-chamber view **(A)** originating from the site of the posteromedial commissure in the two-chamber view **(B).** *MR,* mitral regurgitation; *LA,* left atrium; *RA,* right atrium; *LV,* left ventricle; *RV,* right ventricle; *IAS,* interatrial septum; *IVS,* interventricular septum; *AML,* anterior mitral leaflet; *PML,* posterior mitral leaflet.

## Case 2

A 73-year-old woman had a history of inferior wall MI and a preoperative ECG showing a Q wave in leads II, III, and aVF; preoperative cardiac catheterization revealed 80% stenosis of the left main trunk, 90% stenosis of the left circumflex artery, and 90% stenosis of the proximal right coronary artery. Ejection fraction was 50%. Before CPB, TEE revealed an akinetic inferior septal segment; hypokinetic inferior, inferoposterior, and posterolateral segments in the SAX view (Fig. 25.10); and akinetic apical, middle, and inferobasal segments in the long-axis view (Fig. 25.11). Color Doppler imaging showed severe MR originating from the site of the PM commissure (Fig. 25.12), and decreased pulmonary venous systolic flow (systolic < diastolic) was noted in PW Doppler mode (Fig. 25.13). The mitral annulus was mildly dilated (3.7 cm diameter in the three-chamber view). An intraaortic balloon

pump was placed before the CPB, but akinetic wall motion and severe MR did not improve. The patient underwent CABG using veins to the left anterior descending artery and the first marginal artery. After the patient was initially weaned from bypass, MR was still severe (Fig. 25.14) and wall motion of all inferior segments was still akinetic. The patient underwent another bypass and annuloplasty was added. She was weaned from bypass with inotropic therapy (epinephrine, amrinone) and intraaortic balloon pump. After CABG, color Doppler imaging showed remarkably reduced MR (Fig. 25.15) associated with normalization (systolic > diastolic) of the pulmonary venous systolic flow (Fig. 25.16). Transesophageal echocardiography also revealed a little improvement of inferior septal and posterolateral segments in the SAX view and the inferobasal segment in the long-axis view, but other inferior segments were still akinetic. The diam-

*(text continues on page 414)*

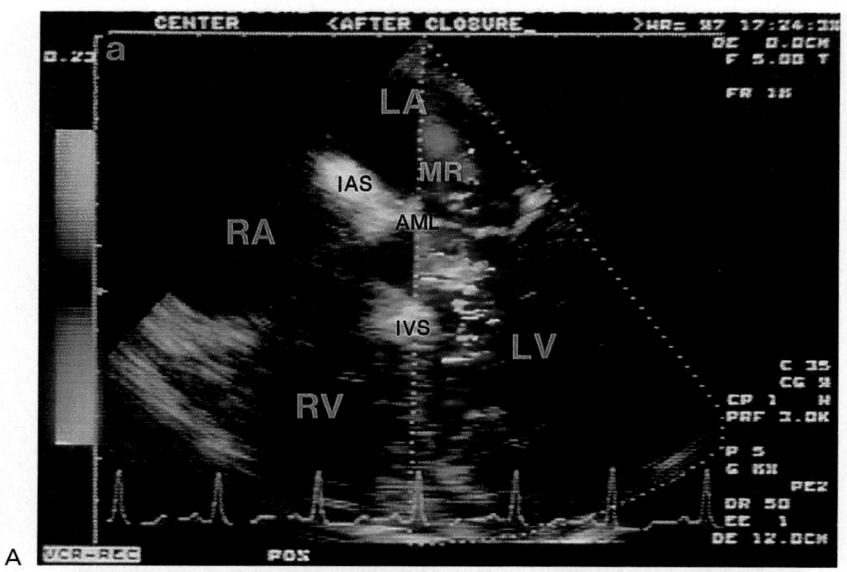

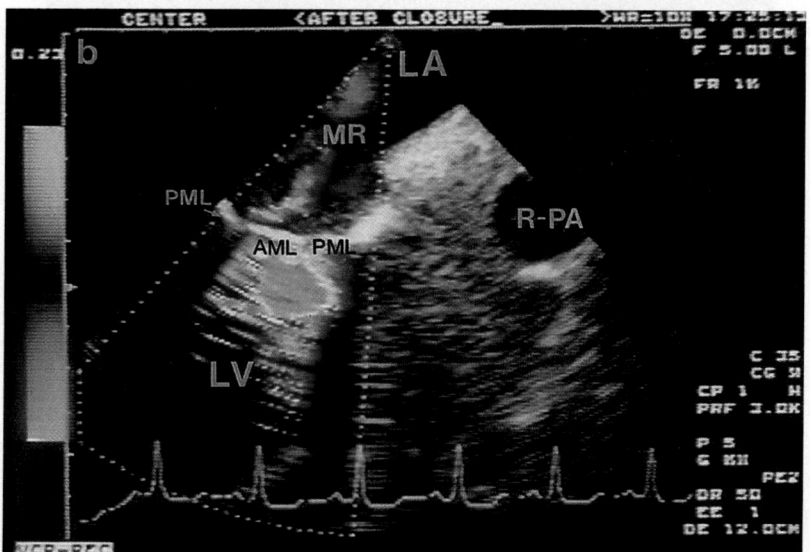

**FIGURE 25.9.** Color Doppler imaging shows trivial mitral regurgitation in the three-chamber view **(A)** originating from the site of the posteromedial commissure in the two-chamber view **(B)**. *MR*, mitral regurgitation; *LA*, left atrium; *RA*, right atrium; *RV*, right ventricle; *LV*, left ventricle; *IAS*, interatrial septum; *IVS*, interventricular septum; *AML*, anterior mitral leaflet; *PML*, posterior mitral leaflet; *R-PA*, right pulmonary artery.

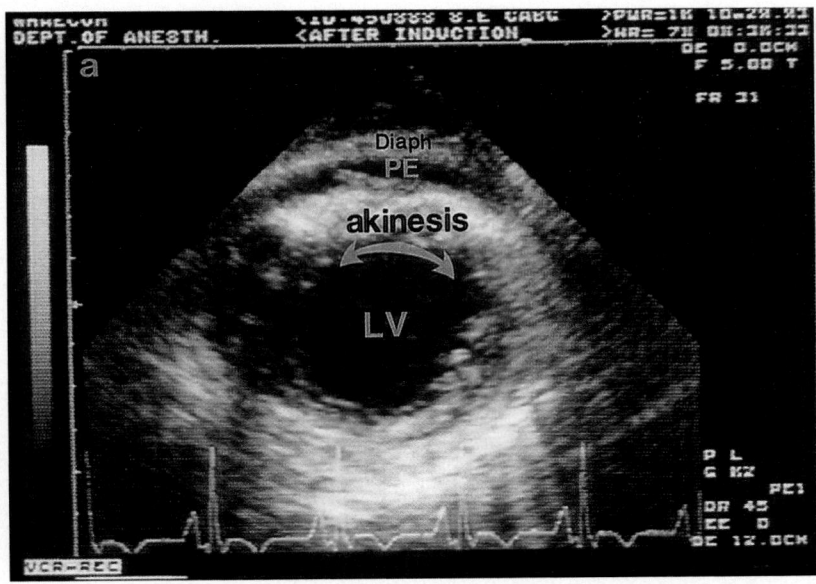

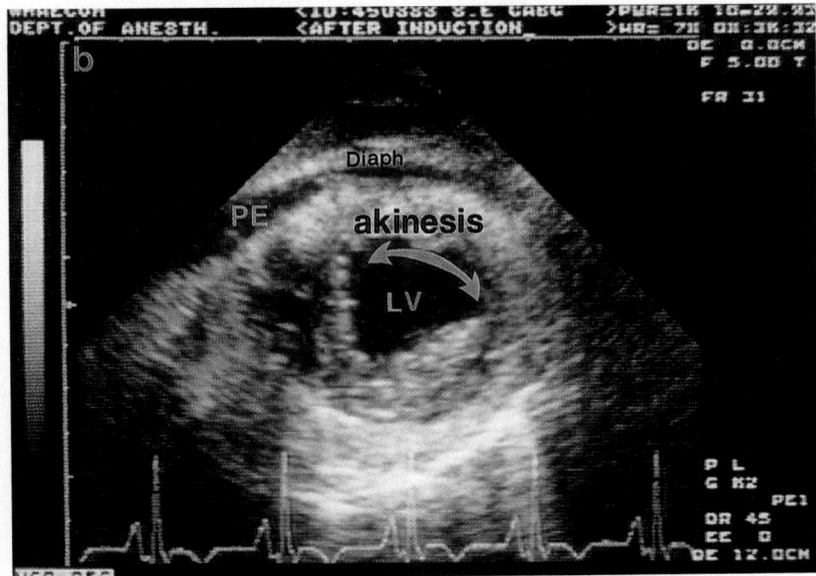

**FIGURE 25.10.** Short-axis view of the left ventricle (*LV*) in the transverse scan at end-diastole **(A)** and end-systole **(B).** *Arrow* shows akinetic inferior septum (IS), inferior (I), inferoposterior (IP), and posterolateral segments of the LV. *Diaph,* diaphragm; *PE,* pericardial effusion.

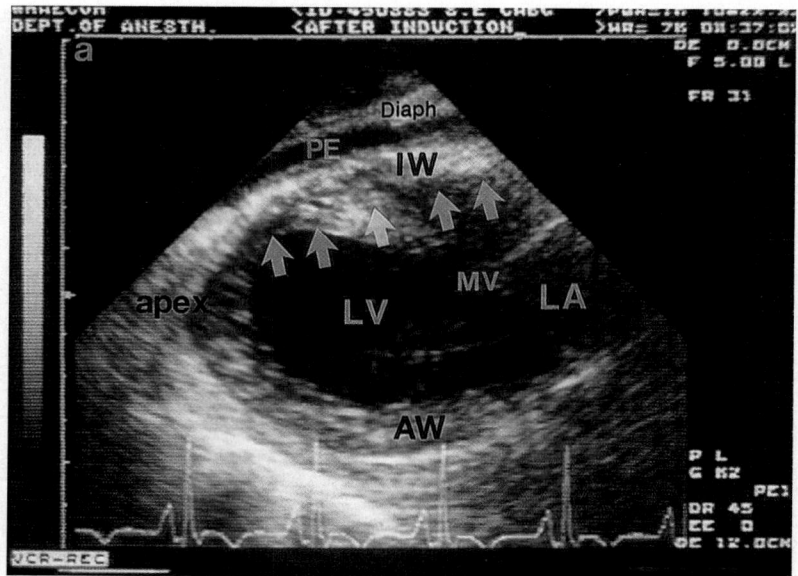

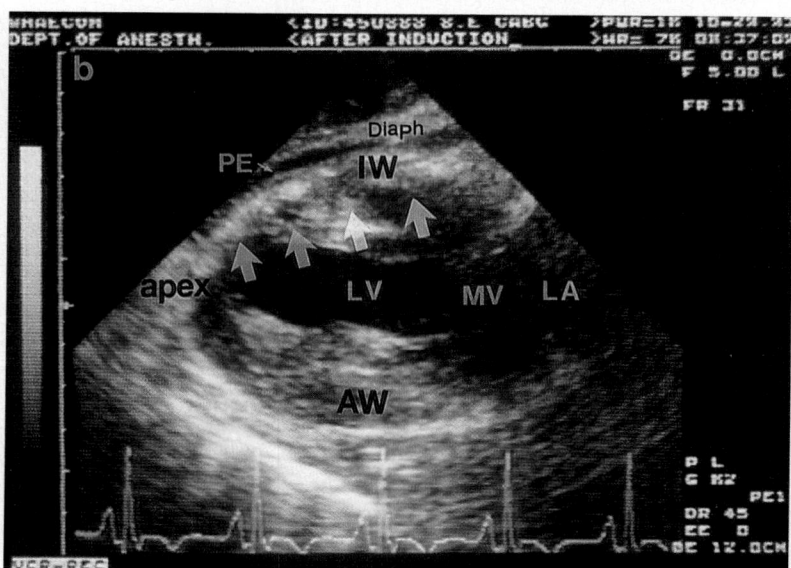

**FIGURE 25.11.** Long-axis view of the left ventricle (*LV*) in the longitudinal scan at end-diastole (**A**) and end-systole (**B**). Arrows show akinetic apical, middle, and basal-inferior segments of the LV. *LA,* left atrium; *LV,* left ventricle; *MV,* mitral valve; *AW,* anterior wall; *IW,* inferior wall; PE, pericardial effusion; *Diaph,* diaphragm.

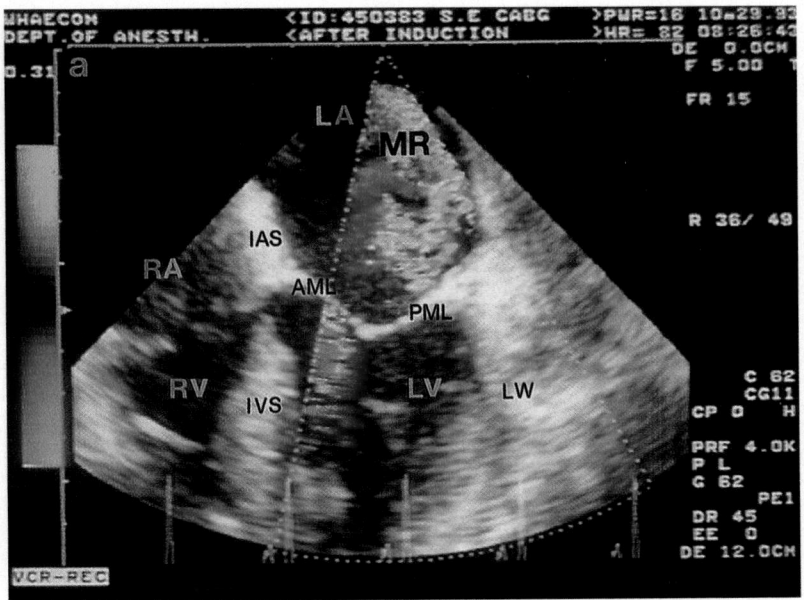

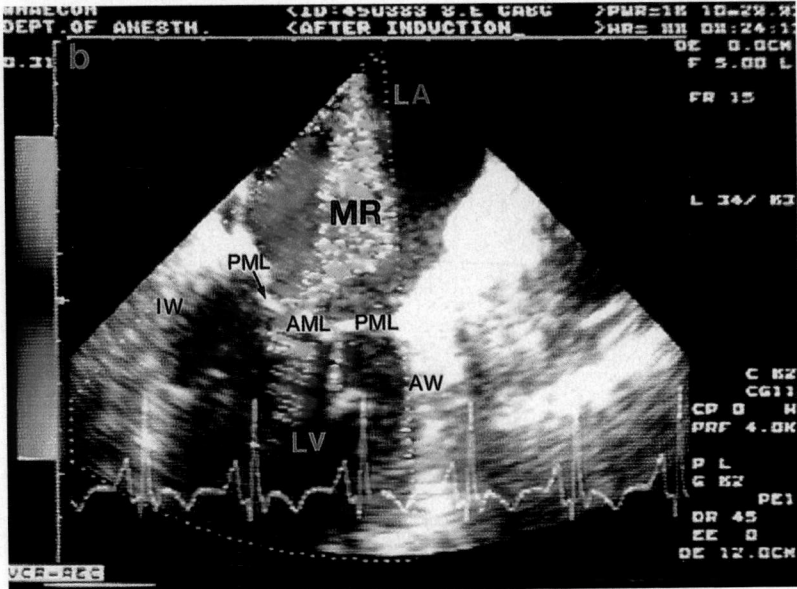

**FIGURE 25.12.** Color Doppler imaging shows severe mitral regurgitation originating from the posteromedial commissure in the three-chamber view **(A)** and the two-chamber view **(B).** *MR,* mitral regurgitation; *LA,* left atrium; *RA,* right atrium; *RV,* right ventricle; *LV,* left ventricle; *IAS,* interatrial septum; *IVS,* interventricular septum; *AML,* anterior mitral leaflet; *PML,* posterior mitral leaflet; *LW,* lateral wall; *AW,* anterior wall; *IM,* inferior wall.

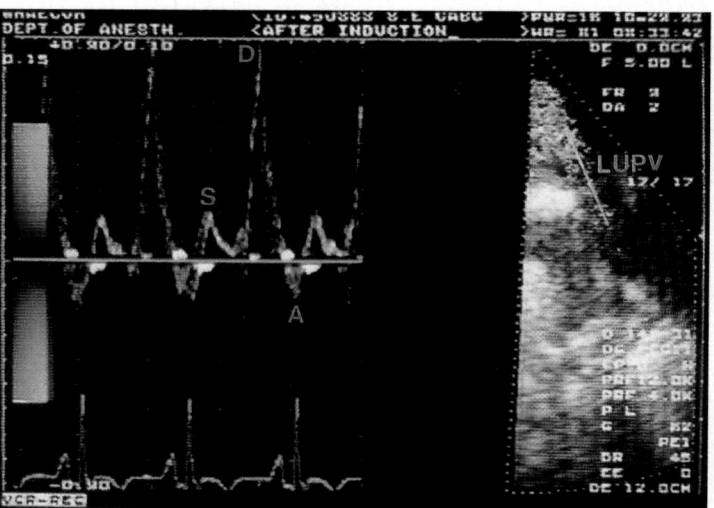

**FIGURE 25.13.** Decreased left pulmonary venous systolic flow compared with diastolic flow in the pulsed-wave mode. Negative velocity **(A)** is seen just after the D wave. *S,* peak pulmonary venous systolic filling; *D,* peak pulmonary venous diastolic filling; *LUPV,* left upper pulmonary vein.

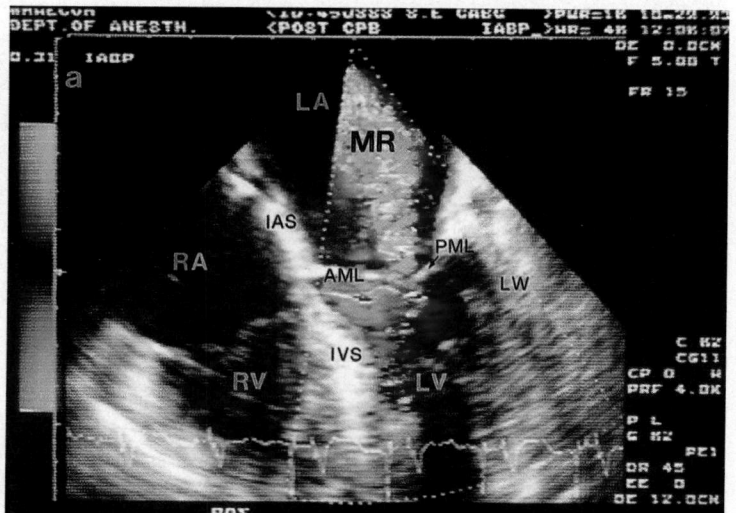

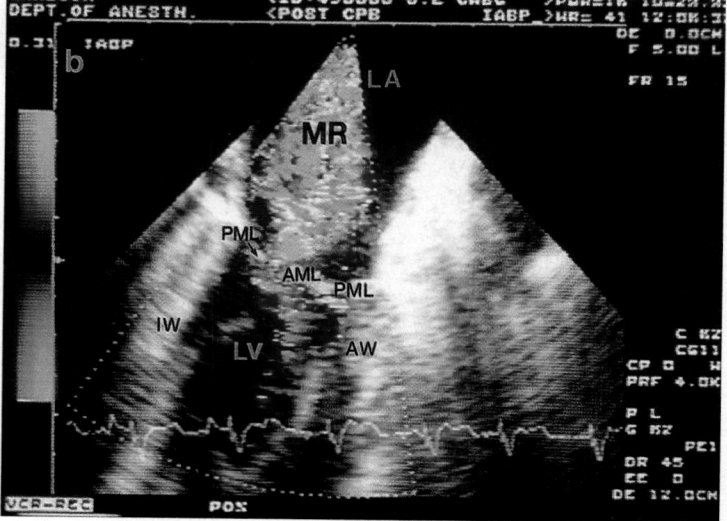

**FIGURE 25.14.** After revascularization, color Doppler imaging continues to show severe mitral regurgitation originating from the site of posteromedial commissure in the four-chamber view **(A)** and the two-chamber view **(B)** after initial weaning from the bypass. *MR,* mitral regurgitation; *LA,* left atrium; *RA,* right atrium; *RV,* right ventricle; *LV,* left ventricle; *IAS,* interatrial septum; *IVS,* interventricular septum; *AML,* anterior mitral leaflet; *PML,* posterior mitral leaflet; *LW,* lateral wall; *AW,* anterior wall; *IW,* inferior wall.

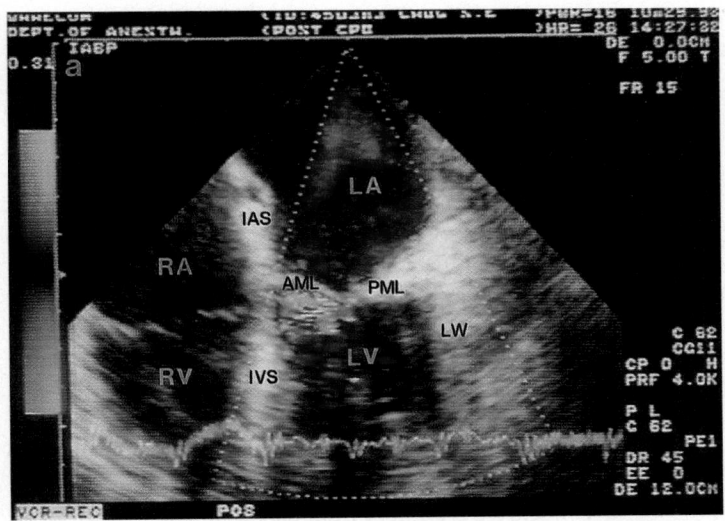

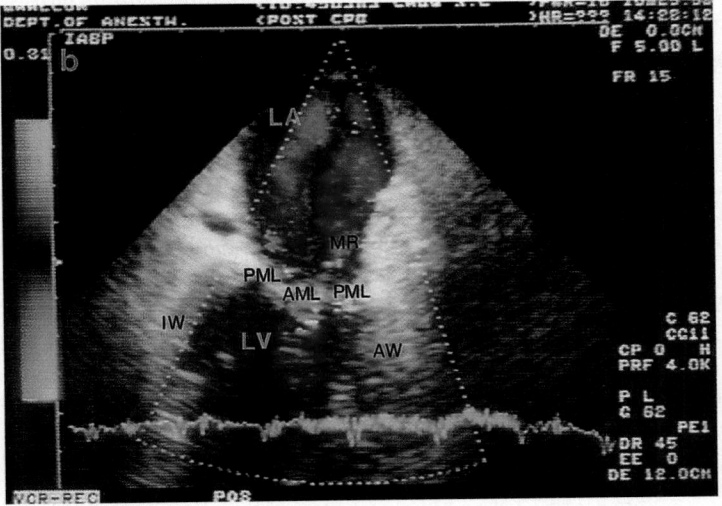

**FIGURE 25.15.** Color Doppler imaging shows trivial mitral regurgitation in the four-chamber view **(A)** and the two-chamber view **(B)** after annuloplasty. *MR*, mitral regurgitation; *LA*, left atrium; *RA*, right atrium; *RV*, right ventricle; *LV*, left ventricle; *AML*, anterior mitral leaflet; *PML*, posterior mitral leaflet; *IAS*, interatrial septum; *IVS*, interventricular septum; *LW*, lateral wall; *AW*, anterior wall; *IW*, inferior wall.

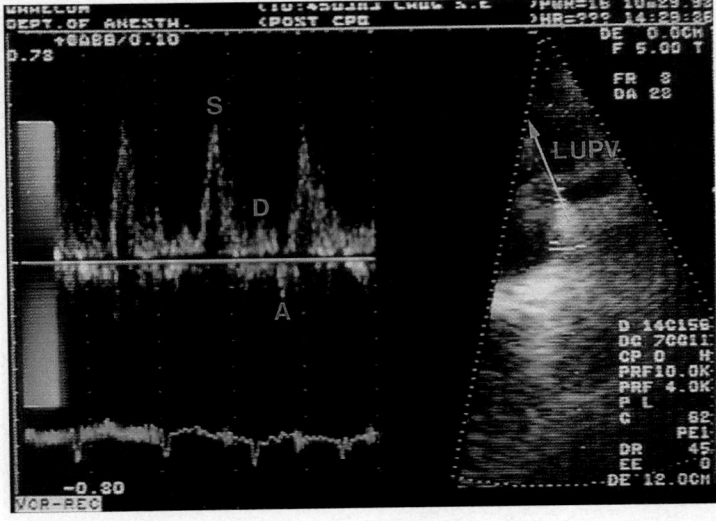

**FIGURE 25.16.** Normalization of left pulmonary venous systolic flow (PVSF) in pulsed-wave mode after annuloplasty. *LUPV*, left upper pulmonary vein; *S*, peak pulmonary venous systolic filling; *D*, peak pulmonary diastolic filling; *A*, negative velocity seen just before the S wave.

eter of the mitral annulus was shown as 3.1 cm in the three-chamber view. The postoperative course was uneventful, without complications.

## CLINICAL DECISION MAKING

Because of the increased risks associated with mitral valve surgery in ischemic heart disease, TEE has been used to assess the underlying mechanisms of injury of the mitral valve apparatus and to guide the formulation of a surgical plan (45–47). Before intraoperative TEE became routinely available, surgeons relied on the filling of the arrested LV with fluid to test the competency of the repaired mitral valve. The parallel line of leaflet closure to the posterior part of the ring also indicated a good apposition of the leaflets (25).

These techniques were less sensitive than using TEE during beating heart conditions, because testing an arrested heart may not accurately reflect physiologic changes.

Assessment of residual mitral incompetence (after unclamping the aorta) by digital palpation of the LA for a systolic thrill or by identification of a V wave of the LA pressure tracing are also unreliable due to variations in preload, LA size, and chamber compliance. Two-dimensional TEE with color-flow imaging allows evaluation of the function of the valve. The presence and severity of MR and the location of the regurgitant jet can be clearly ascertained.

The severity of regurgitation can be measured by the size of the jet relative to the atrium. Data obtained from this technique correlate well with angiographic data (4), but overestimation of the mitral regurgitant central jet is possible. The color Doppler flow method is not a quantitative approach. Entrained nonregurgitant blood flow within the LA may increase the overall color jet area, which may be important in the estimation of ischemic/functional MR. In addition, an eccentric regurgitant jet may be attenuated by viscous forces within the wall of the LA, as well as increased heart rate. Other methods to assess the severity of MR include pulmonary venous flow velocity, vena contracta, regurgitant fraction, and proximal isovelocity surface area (PISA) analysis.

Anesthetic technique, hemodilution, temperature, and the use of vasoactive drugs influence the hemodynamic variables that determine the severity of MR during surgery. These factors can affect preload, afterload, heart rate, and rhythm, which significantly influence the degree of MR at a given time. Discordance between angiographic and echocardiographic evidence of mitral insufficiency may involve patients with unstable hemodynamics during angiography and those with high LV end-diastolic pressures whose disease has been palliated with thrombolytic therapy (4).

In a study comparing echocardiographic assessment with surgical inspection of the mitral valve, the direction of the regurgitant jet elucidated the mechanism of MR (14). In general, the jet is directed away from an excessively mobile leaflet and toward a leaflet with restricted mobility. For example, a posteriorly displaced jet can be seen in the presence of a flail or prolapsed (excessive mobility) anterior leaflet or a fibrotic or calcified (restricted mobility) posterior leaflet (Fig. 25.17). Mitral regurgitation with normal leaflet motion as manifested by a central Doppler jet is usually seen with annular dilatation associated with ischemic disease. Less commonly, a central jet is seen with bileaflet prolapse secondary to papillary

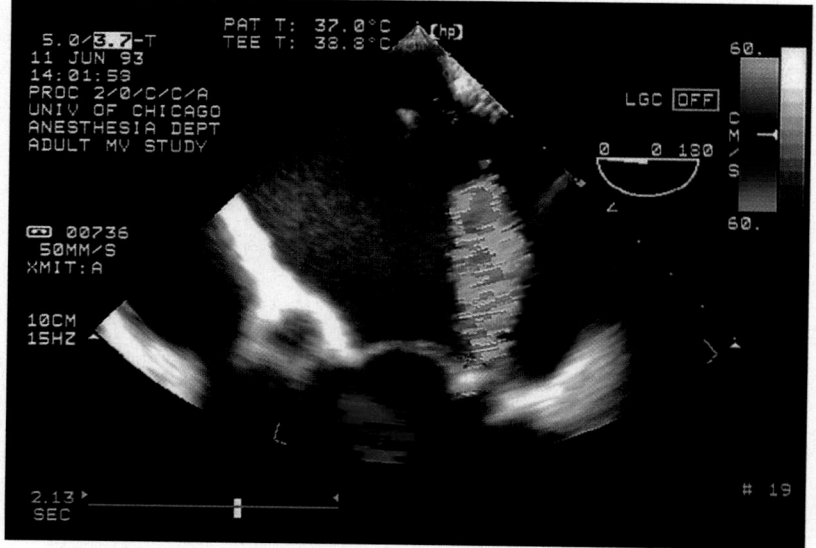

**FIGURE 25.17.** A posteriorly displaced regurgitant jet in a patient with a prolapsed anterior valve leaflet. Note the aliasing of the color hues, demonstrating high-velocity flow.

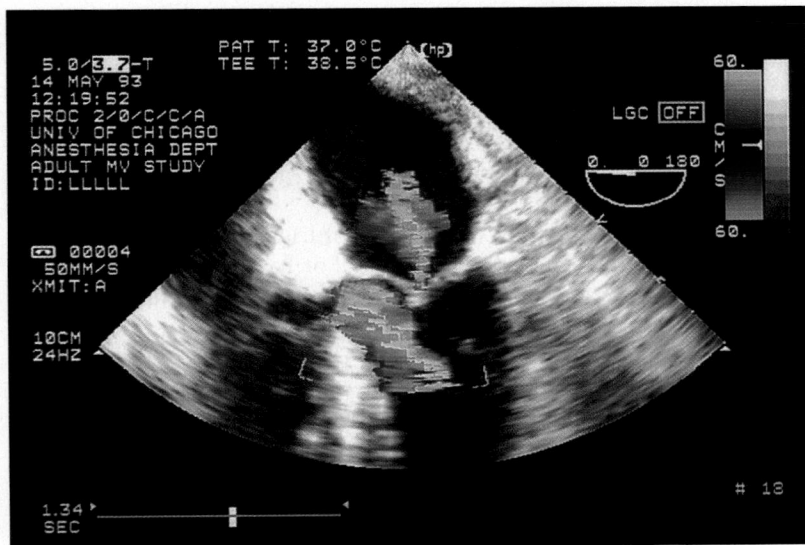

**FIGURE 25.18.** Central regurgitant jet in a patient with diffuse coronary disease. This type of jet is seen in patients with bileaflet restricted mobility or with either restricted or excessive mobility of both mitral valve leaflets.

muscle rupture or with restricted leaflet motion as in rheumatic heart disease (Fig. 25.18).

Interrogation of the mitral valve apparatus in multiple planes before using color Doppler is useful to visualize and diagnose the mechanism of injury causing insufficiency. Tomographic images of all components of the mitral valve apparatus should be obtained and recorded, recognizing that 2D and Doppler determination of leaflet dysfunction and jet direction correctly diagnoses the mechanism of disease in up to 85% of patients (14). A useful way to differentiate severe from moderate or mild mitral insufficiency is to examine flow patterns in the pulmonary vein during systole. At the ME level, the echocardiographic probe is positioned posterior to the LA. Rotation of the omniplane allows interrogation of the left upper pulmonary vein. Color Doppler helps locate the maximum flow for the subsequent use of the P-W mode. The PW cursor positioned 1 cm into the vein will permit a high-quality signal. Left upper pulmonary vein flow is the easiest to image with TEE. Mitral regurgitation is graded on a scale of 1 to 4, depending on the direction and ratio of the systolic and diastolic components of pulmonary venous velocity tracings. The presence of systolic flow reversal in the pulmonary vein has been shown to be 93% sensitive and 100% specific for detecting mitral insufficiency graded at 4 or more. A problem of many noninvasive techniques is their inability to directly measure regurgitant flow rate at the lesion.

The power-velocity integral at the vena contracta was described as a method for direct quantification of regurgitant volume flow. Flow rate is a product of velocity and area, where the Doppler signal can produce backscattered acoustic power that can be used as an estimation of flow rate:

$$Velocity \times Power = Flow\ Rate$$

Backscattered power returning to the ultrasound transducer is a nonlinear function of hematocrit, and the backscattered power in the Doppler spectrum of flow velocities is linearly proportional to the cross-sectional area of flow within the beam. The power-velocity integral at the vena contracta provides an accurate direct measurement of regurgitant flow.

Regurgitant volume can be indirectly measured as a difference between SV through the MV (SVmv) and a nonregurgitant reference valve, such as the aortic valve (AV) (SVav). Further calculation of the regurgitant fraction (RFmv = SVmv – SVav/SVmv) can grade MR severity, where 30% to 50% is considered moderate. Limitations of this method include assumption that the left ventricular outflow tract (LVOT) and AV orifice and mitral annulus are circular, aortic regurgitation is absent, and no ventricular septal defect is present. Furthermore, the calculation error is squared if the LVOT or MV annulus area is not measured accurately.

Proximal isovelocity surface area analysis was introduced as a quantitative Color Doppler flow measurement approach. Laminar flow stream narrows and accelerates proximal to a regurgitant valve orifice. This creates a hemispheric flow convergence region (FCR), where at each point the flow has the same velocity. Volume flow rate (mL/s) can be calculated as PISA ($cm^2$) multiplied by the isovelocity of the PISA (cm/s). The first PISA, with an isovelocity corresponding to the "aliasing" velocity (at one half the Nyquist sampling limit) is identified as blue and red color interface proximal to the orifice. The instantaneous flow rate (Q) at the FCR can be calculated as: $Q = 2\pi r^2 Vr$. The grading of MR by using FCR radius correlates with angiographic MR.

Measurements of effective mitral regurgitant orifice area (ROA) and regurgitant volume are derived from the PISA method. ROA is equal to Q/V, where Q is the maximum instantaneous regurgitant flow rate in mL/min and V is measured by CVM in cm/s. The ROA grade of MR is as follows: 1+ (mild) degree, ROA (cm$^2$) < 0.1; 2+ (moderate), 0.1 to 0.25 cm$^2$ (with regurgitant volume of 25–40 mL); 3+ (moderate-severe), 0.25 to 0.5 cm$^2$ (40–55 mL); 4+ (severe), > 0.5 cm$^2$ (or > 55 mL).

Recent experimental findings suggest that a simplified formula can reliably estimate regurgitant volume and that blood viscosity does not affect the grade of regurgitation by the PISA method.

When evaluating mitral annuloplasty procedures, there are two primary complications: functional stenosis and dynamic obstruction of the LVOT ring annuloplasty, which uses a downsized ring may result in functional stenosis. In patients requiring ring annuloplasty, the valve area can be assessed with planimetric measurements. PW or continuous-wave Doppler measurement of flow velocity can be used to obtain the pressure half-time ($t\frac{1}{2}$) or (PHT) of diastolic flow, which can be used to calculate the effective valve area as follows:

$$\text{Mitral valve area (cm}^2) = 220 / t\tfrac{1}{2}$$

The normal range of PHT is 50 to 70 msec. Tachycardia, prolonged PR interval, and aortic insufficiency may alter its measurement. Of note, the mitral valve area is approximately 1 cm$^2$ when the PHT is 220 msec, so mitral valve area is equal to $220 / t\frac{1}{2}$.

Echocardiographic evidence of systolic anterior motion (SAM) of the mitral leaflets in the presence of normal septal thickness is associated with the high-velocity flow disturbance seen in dynamic obstruction of the LVOT. With a rigid Carpentier-Edwards ring for annuloplasty, the risk of the LVOT obstruction is 4.5% to 17%. Freeman and colleagues reported that severe SAM of the anterior leaflet could cause moderate to severe MR in 9.1% of patients during separation from CPB after mitral valve repair.

Experimental research of ring annuloplasty in an animal model indicated that its implantation can reliably prevent delayed leaflet coaptation, which occurs after acute LV ischemia. Preischemic implantation of both the Duran and the Physio rings facilitated timely coaptation after induction of ischemia (40).

Preischemic implantation of either ring also preserved papillary-annular distances, which invariably tended to increase after the induction of ischemia in the control group (42). In a chronic ischemia animal model, reduction of MR was achieved by restoring tethering geometry toward normal by plication of the infarct region. Myocardial bulging was reduced without muscle excision or CPB. Immediately and up to 2 months after plication, mi-tral insufficiency was reduced (trace to mild) as tethering distance decreased (43).

In this experiment, implantation of a ring before induction of ischemia not only prevented delayed coaptation and preserved tethering distance as above, but also prevented disturbances in the geometry of both mitral valve leaflets (48).

Neither flexible nor semirigid mitral annuloplasty rings appear to affect global or basal regional LV systolic function (48). It has been shown that rigid fixation of the mitral annulus does not result in regional systolic dysfunction at the base of the LV (49).

A recent report of how mitral annular area and intercommissural and anteroseptal dimensions change throughout the cardiac cycle in a sheep model has demonstrated that a flexible Tailor partial ring preserves physiologic mitral annular folding dynamics (50).

A double-orifice technique in mitral valve repair (51) may represent a simple solution for complex problems associated with bileaflet prolapse, prolapse of either leaflet, lack of leaflet coaptation for restricted motion, or erosion of the free edge. In a series of 260 patients, a 5-year freedom from reoperation was achieved in 90% with this procedure. However, an ischemic cause of MR was only attributed to 2.3% of the patients, whereas degeneration was found in 81% of the patients. The group of patients without annuloplasty (20%, when annulus was not dilated or it was severely calcified) showed an inferior rate of freedom from reoperation (70%). None of the six patients with IMR required reoperation during the follow-up period. Although overall survival at 5 years was 94.4%, in this series outcome data for IMR were not as positive.

Dilated cardiomyopathy with functional mitral insufficiency required repair of MR in 59% in a reported series of 49 patients, with 75% of the patients having an ischemic etiology (52). The importance of mitral valve coaptation depth (MVCD), which is defined as the distance between the annulus and the coaptation point of the leaflets and is equivalent to the Mayo term *coaptation height*, was emphasized. As compared with healthy individuals with an average distance of 4.1 mm, the cardiomyopathic patients with an MVCD of less than 10 mm had postoperative functional MR of 1.2 degree. If preoperative MVCD was greater than 11 mm, it led to an average postrepaired MR degree of 2.5. In this series, late survival was similar in both repair and replacement groups, with functional class also similar in those who survived (73%) at a mean follow-up period of 24 months.

It has been suggested that surgeons be more aggressive and not ignore substantial degrees of IMR at the time of CABG (45). Whether to perform a simple ring annuloplasty or a more reliable chordal-preserving mitral valve replacement (MVR) remains a challenging question. In one recent report, patients who underwent mitral repair (although not as sick as those who required MVR) had survival rates similar to those of the MVR group (52).

Valve repair with a down-sized annuloplasty ring, in order to enhance coaptation, works satisfactorily in most cases of functional IMR, but the surgeon must pay attention to the interpretation of the associated mechanism and direction of the regurgitation. Simple ring annuloplasty may be sufficient if a Carpentier type I pathology is present, but it is not a remedy in cases of type III restricted systolic leaflet motion. Reduction of septal-lateral but not the intercommissural dimension should be performed. Both partial or complete and flexible or rigid rings perform well (46,47). Do all patients undergoing CABG who have more than mild MR need a concomitant mitral annuloplasty? This question remains to be answered, but preliminary data suggest that patients with moderate or less IMR who tolerated off-pump CABG appear to benefit from revascularization alone (20).

In summary, ischemic mitral insufficiency carries a worse prognosis than MR from other causes (4,9,13). The use of TEE enables the assessment of valvular function in real time so that surgical plans and techniques can be adopted.

## KEY POINTS

- Up to 41% of CABG candidates also may have chronic ischemic mitral insufficiency.
- Coronary artery bypass grafting alone can lead to reduction of IMR severity.
- Significant residual MR after revascularization is associated with increased immediate postoperative and long-term morbidity and mortality.
- Combined mitral valve surgery and CABG is associated with a reported in-hospital mortality rate of 7% to 20%.
- The intraoperative severity assessment of residual MR is further complicated by hemodynamic changes related to the effect of general anesthesia and is often underestimated.
- Intraoperative TEE evaluation is critical in order to determine the mechanism of MR and guide a strategy for repair.
- Acute transient MR during an ischemic episode occurs primarily due to leaflet restriction as a result of ventricular dyskinesia, rather than of annular dilatation (type IIIb).
- Valve repair with a down-sized annuloplasty ring, in order to enhance coaptation, works satisfactorily in most cases of functional IMR.
- Patients with moderate or less severe IMR who tolerated off-pump CABG appear to benefit from revascularization alone.

## REFERENCES

1. Izhar U, Daly R, Dearani J, et al. Mitral valve replacement or repair after previous coronary artery bypass grafting. Circulation 1999;100(suppl II):84–9.
2. Alexander K, Anstrom K, Muhlbaier L, et al. Outcomes of cardiac surgery in patients age ≥ 80 years: results from the national cardiovascular network. J Am Coll Cardiol 2000;35: 731–38.
3. Duarte I, Shen Y, MacDonald M, et al. Treatment of moderate regurgitation and coronary disease by coronary bypass alone: late results. Ann Thorac Surg 1999;68:426–30.
4. Sheikh KH, Bengtson JR, Rankin JS, et al. Intraoperative transesophageal Doppler color flow imaging used to guide patient selection and operative treatment of ischemic mitral regurgitation. Circulation 1991;84:594–604.
5. Aklog L, Filsoufi F, Flores K, et al. Does coronary artery bypass grafting alone correct moderate ischemic mitral regurgitation? Circulation 2001;104(suppl 1):68–75.
6. Grewal K, Malkowski M, Piracha A, et al. Effect of general anesthesia on the severity of mitral regurgitation by transesophageal echocardiography. Am J Cardiol 2000;85: 199–203.
7. Shanewise J, Cheung A, Aronson S, et al. ASE/SCA guidelines for performing a comprehensive intraoperative multiplane transesophageal echocardiographic examination: recommendations of the American Society of Echocardiography Council for intraoperative echocardiography and the Society of Cardiovascular Anesthesiologists Task Force for certification in perioperative transesophageal echocardiography. J Am Soc Echocardiogr 1999;12:884–900.
8. Miller J, Lambert A, Shapiro W, et al. The adequacy of basic intraoperative transesophageal echocardiography performed by experienced anesthesiologists. Anesth Analg 2001;92: 1103–10.
9. Hickey M, Smith L, Muhlbaier L, et al. Current prognosis of ischemic mitral regurgitation. Implications for future management. Circulation 1988;78(suppl I):51–9.
10. Cohn L, Kowalker W, Bhatia S, et al. Comparative morbidity of mitral valve repair versus replacement for mitral regurgitation with and without coronary artery disease. Ann Thorac Surg 1988;45:284–90.
11. Cohn L, Kowalker W, Bhatia S, et al. Comparative morbidity of mitral valve repair versus replacement for mitral regurgitation with and without coronary artery disease. 1988. Updated in 1995. Ann Thorac Surg 1995;60:1452–53.
12. Cohn L, Rizzo R, Adams D, et al. The effect of pathophysiology on the surgical treatment of ischemic mitral regurgitation: operative and late risks of repair versus replacement. Eur J Cardiothorac Surg 1995;9:568–74.
13. Hendren W, Nemec J, Lytle B, et al. Mitral valve repair for ischemic mitral insufficiency. Ann Thorac Surg 1991;52: 1246–51.
14. Stewart W, Currie P, Salcedo E, et al. Evaluation of mitral leaflet motion by echocardiography and jet direction by Doppler color flow mapping to determine the mechanism of mitral regurgitation. J Am Coll Cardiol 1992;20:1353–61.
15. Seipelt R, Schoendube F, Vazquez-Jimenez J, et al. Combined mitral valve and coronary surgery: ischemic versus non-ischemic mitral valve disease. Eur J Cardiothorac Surg 2001; 20(2):270–75.
16. Ferguson T, Dziuban F, Edwards F, et al. STS National Database: current changes and challenges for the new millennium. Ann Thorac Surg 2000;69:680–91.
17. Andrade I, Cartier R, Panisi P, et al. Factors influencing early and late survival in patients with combined mitral valve replacement and myocardial revascularization and in those with isolated replacement. Ann Thorac Surg 1987;44:607–13.
18. Lytle B, Cosgrove D, Gill C, et al. Mitral valve replacement combined with myocardial revascularization: early and late results for 300 patients, 1970 to 1983. Circulation 1987;44: 1179–90.
19. Ryden T, Bech-Hanssen O, Brandrup-Wognsen G, et al. The importance of grade 2 ischemic mitral regurgitation in coro-

nary artery bypass grafting. Eur J Cardiothorac Surg 2001; 20:276–81.

20. Chapochnikov A, Jayakar D, Jeevanandam V, et al. Off pump coronary artery bypass alone can remedy ischemic mitral regurgitation of moderate degree. 24th Annual Meeting of the Society of Cardiovascular Anesthesiologists, April 2002.

21. Voci P, Bilotta F, Caretta Q, et al. Papillary muscle perfusion pattern. A hypothesis for ischemic papillary muscle dysfunction. Circulation 1995;91(6):1714–18.

22. Bollen B, Luo H, Oury J, et al. A systematic approach to intraoperative transesophageal echocardiographic evaluation of the mitral valve apparatus with anatomic correlation. J Cardiothorac Vasc Anesth 2000;14(3):330–38.

23. Burch G, De Pasquale N, Phillips J. Clinical manifestations of papillary muscle dysfunction. Arch Intern Med 1963;59: 508–20.

24. Grigioni F, Enriquez-Sarano M, Zehr K, et al. Ischemic mitral regurgitation. Long-term outcome and prognostic implications with quantitative Doppler assessment. Circulation 2001;103:1759–64.

25. Carpentier A. Cardiac valve surgery—the "French correction." J Thorac Cardiovasc Surg 1983;86:323–37.

26. Fehrenbacher G, Schmidt D, Bommer W. Evaluation of transient mitral regurgitation in coronary artery disease. Am J Cardiol 1991;68:868–73.

27. Sharma S, Secker J, Israel D, et al. Clinical, angiographic and anatomic findings in acute severe ischemic mitral regurgitation. Am J Cardiol 1992;70:277–80.

28. Dent J, Spotnitz W, Nolan S, et al. Mechanism of mitral leaflet excursion. Am J Physiol 1995;269:H2100-H2108.

29. Messas E, Guerrero J, Handschumacher M, et al. Paradoxic decrease in ischemic mitral regurgitation with papillary muscle dysfunction. Insights from three-dimensional and contrast echocardiography with strain rate measurement. Circulation 2001:104;1952–60.

30. Glasson J, Komeda M, Daughters G, et al. Three-dimensional dynamics of the canine mitral annulus during ischemic mitral regurgitation. Ann Thorac Surg 1996;62:1059–68.

31. Athanasuleas C, Stanley A, Buckberg G, et al. Surgical anterior ventricular endocardial restoration (SAVER) in the dilated remodeled ventricle after anterior myocardial infarction. J Am Coll Cardiol 2001;37:1199–209.

32. Gorman J 3rd, Gorman R, Jackson B, et al. Distortions of the mitral valve in acute ischemic mitral regurgitation. Ann Thorac Surg 1997;64:1026–31.

33. Glasson J, Komeda M, Daughters G, et al. Early systolic mitral leaflet "loitering" during acute ischemic mitral regurgitation. J Thorac Cardiovasc Surg 1998;116:193–205.

34. Llaneras M, Nance M, Streicher J, et al. Pathogenesis of ischemic mitral insufficiency. J Thorac Cardiovasc Surg 1993; 105:439–43.

35. Sabbah H, Kono T, Rosman H, et al. Left ventricular shape: a factor in the etiology of functional mitral regurgitation in heart failure. Am Heart J 1992;123:961–66.

36. Lamas G, Mitchell G, Flaker G. Clinical significance of mitral regurgitation after acute myocardial infarction. Circulation 1997;96:827–33.

37. Di Donato M, Sabatier M, Dor V. Effects of the Dor procedure on left ventricular dimension and shape and geometric correlates of mitral regurgitation one year after surgery. J Thorac Cardiovasc Surg 2001;121:91–6.

38. Kono T, Sabbah H, Rosman H, et al. Mechanism of functional mitral regurgitation during acute myocardial ischemia. J Am Coll Cardiol 1992;19:1101–5.

39. Green G, Dagum P, Glasson J, et al. Mitral annular dilatation and papillary muscle dislocation without mitral regurgitation in sheep. Circulation 1999;100(suppl II):95–102.

40. Timek T, Glasson JR, Dagum P, et al. Ring annuloplasty prevents delayed leaflet coaptation and mitral regurgitation dur-

ing acute left ventricular ischemia. J Thorac Cardiovasc Surg 2000;119:774–83.

41. Timek T, Lai D, Dagum P, et al. Mitral annular dynamics during rapid atrial pacing. Surgery 2000;128:361–7.

42. Dagum P, Timek T, Green R, et al. Coordinate-free analysis of mitral valve dynamics in normal and ischemic hearts. Circulation 2000;102(suppl III1):62–9.

43. Liel-Cohen N, Guerrero J, Otsuji Y, et al. Design of a new surgical approach for ventricular remodeling to relieve ischemic mitral regurgitation. Circulation 2000;101:2756–63.

44. Otsuji Y, Handschumacher M, Schwammenthal E, et al. Insights from three-dimensional echocardiography into the mechanism of functional mitral regurgitation: direct in vivo demonstration of altered leaflet tethering geometry. Circulation 1997;96:1826–34.

45. Miller DC. Ischemic mitral regurgitation redux—to repair or to replace? J Thorac Cardiovasc Surg 2001;122:1059–62.

46. Gillinov A, Wierup P, Blackstone E, et al. Is repair preferable to replacement for ischemic mitral regurgitation? J Thorac Cardiovasc Surg 2001;122:1125–41.

47. Grossi E, Goldberg J, LaPietra A, et al. Ischemic mitral valve reconstruction and replacement: comparison of long-term survival and complications. J Thorac Cardiovasc Surg 2001;122:1107–24.

48. Lai D, Timek T, Dagum P. The effects of ring annuloplasty on mitral leaflet geometry during acute left ventricular ischemia. J Thorac Cardiovasc Surg 2000;120:966–75.

49. Green G, Dagum P, Glasson J. Semirigid or flexible mitral annuloplasty rings do not affect global or basal regional left ventricular systolic function. Circulation 1998;98(suppl 11): 128–36.

50. Dagum P, Timek T, Green G, et al. Three-dimensional geometric comparison of partial and complete flexible mitral annuloplasty rings. J Thorac Cardiovasc Surg 2001;122:665–73.

51. Alfieri O, Maisano F, De Bonis M. The double-orifice technique in mitral valve repair: a simple solution for a complex problem. J Thorac Cardiovasc Surg 2001;122:674–81.

52. Calafiore A, Gallina S, Di Mauro M. Mitral valve procedure in dilated cardiomyopathy: repair or replacement? Ann Thorac Surg 2001;71:1146–53.

## QUESTIONS

**1.** Among the following underlying causes of IMR, which carries the most promising 5-year prognosis after mitral valve surgery?
   A. Mitral valve dilation
   B. Restrictive anterior leaflet motion
   C. Ruptured papillary muscle

**2.** The least likely cause of IMR is
   A. infarction of the posterior medial papillary muscle due to single coronary blood supply.
   B. ventricular regional wall motion abnormality without anterior mitral annular dilation.
   C. early versus late systolic mitral leaflet loitering.

**3.** Which of the following best explains why mitral valve ring annuloplasty reduces the severity of IMR?
   A. It modifies the anterior displacement of the posterior mitral leaflet and posterior medial papillary muscle.
   B. It reduces radial displacement of the anterior and posterior papillary muscles.
   C. It reduces annular diameter.
   D. All of the above

# Assessment in Off Pump Myocardial Revascularization

## Jack S. Shanewise

Over the past several years, there has been a great increase in interest in performing coronary artery bypass graft (CABG) surgery without cardiopulmonary bypass (CPB). Initially in the United States efforts were primarily directed at "minimally invasive" direct coronary artery bypass (MIDCAB), a procedure in which an in situ left internal mammary artery (LIMA) graft is anastomosed to the left anterior descending (LAD) artery through a small left anterior thoracotomy. This procedure was developed to compete with angioplasty for LAD lesions, its proponents emphasizing the decreased cost and time of recovery compared to conventional CABG, usually performing it on younger, healthier patients. However, as time passed, the more widely adopted approach has been to perform CABG surgery on one or more vessels through a full median sternotomy but without CPB, a procedure called off-pump CABG (OPCAB). Its purpose is to provide adequate coronary revascularization while avoiding the morbidity associated with CPB, such as coagulopathy, pulmonary dysfunction, renal insufficiency, and CNS injury. This chapter will discuss how echocardiography can facilitate the management of patients undergoing these procedures.

A few surgeons have performed CABG without CPB for many years (1–3). But its widespread application of OPCAB occurred with the development of techniques that enable the performance of distal coronary anastomoses on a beating heart. Early on, drugs such as beta antagonists were used to decrease the heart rate and contractility to help provide a quiet surgical field. But more recently, retracting and stabilizing devices have been developed that usually provide an immobile surgical field without the need for pharmacological intervention (Fig. 26.1).

There are several theoretical advantages of performing CABG surgery without CPB compared to conventional CABG. Proponents of OPCAB claim that it costs less than CABG with CPB. While one might think the cost for disposable equipment might be less, in fact, most of the disposable epicardial stabilization devices actually cost more than the disposables needed to put a patient on

cardiopulmonary bypass. Costs for personnel are the same because OPCAB is done with a bypass pump and perfusionist standing by. OPCAB would cost less if patients recover more quickly, are extubated sooner, spend less time in the ICU, and are discharged sooner from the hospital than conventional CABG patients. Reports in the literature suggest that this is the case (4,5). The main theoretical advantage of OPCAB, however, is its lack of the untoward effects of CPB, especially in patients with existing impairment of pulmonary, renal, or central nervous system function. OPCAB may be especially beneficial for patients with atherosclerosis of the ascending aorta. Atheroembolism from cannulation and clamping of the ascending aorta for CPB is an important cause of perioperative stroke in these patients (6). With the use of in situ internal mammary artery grafts, OPCAB allows revascularization of the coronaries without touching the aorta. Using a partially occluding aortic clamp ("j" clamp) to

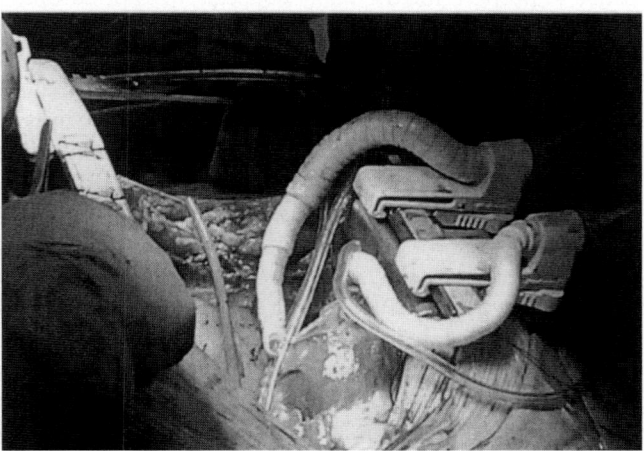

**FIGURE 26.1.** Typical positioning and stabilizing of the heart for performance of a distal anastomosis on a marginal branch of the circumflex coronary artery. The LV apex is displaced up and to the right and the stabilizer applied to the lateral wall.

construct proximal anastomoses for grafts would largely negate this advantage of OPCAB. There are at least two theoretical disadvantages of OPCAB compared to CABG with CPB. First, the positioning and stabilization of the heart and the occlusion of the coronary arteries required to construct grafts with this technique may cause hemodynamic instability, especially in patients with poor ventricular function. Second, the quality of distal coronary artery anastomoses performed on a beating heart may not be as good as those made with the quiet, clear field provided by CPB, possibly causing a lower rate of graft patency. Reports suggest comparable patency rates for the two techniques in the short term, but it will be some time before long-term patency rates can be compared.

## HEMODYNAMIC CONSEQUENCES OF OPCAB

Two features of OPCAB can lead to hemodynamic instability: transient occlusion of coronary arteries during distal anastomosis construction and displacement of the heart to provide access to the distal coronary arteries (7). During OPCAB, the ability of the patient to tolerate occlusion of the artery being grafted is critically dependent on both the severity of the lesion in the artery and the presence of collateral flow into it or from it. For example, grafting of an LAD with a high-grade distal lesion is likely to be well tolerated for two reasons: only a small area of myocardium is supplied by the vessel distal to the obstruction, and collaterals into this region are likely to have developed. On the other hand, occlusion of an LAD with a less severe obstruction may cause hemodynamic instability, especially if this artery supplies collateral flow to another vessel with a high-grade obstruction. Thus, in order to prepare for the likely consequences of coronary occlusion, it is critical to know precisely the severity and location of the coronary lesions, as well as the surgical plan: which vessels will be occluded in what order, including plans for the use of shunts or other means to support the circulation during graft construction. When multiple grafts are to be performed with OPCAB, the order in which they are performed is important. Highly obstructed vessels supplied by collateral flow are usually grafted first to provide flow into more critical vessels before they are grafted. Performing the proximal anastomosis before the distal allows flow to be directed through the graft to the vessel as soon as the distal anastomosis is completed, and can minimize the time a critical portion of myocardium is ischemic during graft construction. To avoid any unnecessary confusion during the operation, the plan should be discussed directly with the surgeon.

In both clinical practice and in the laboratory, augmenting the preload by volume loading and/or use of the head-down position can help maintain cardiac output

and perfusion pressure when the heart is displaced (8). TEE is a good means of assessing adequacy of the volume status before displacement for graft construction is attempted (9). Making an incision in the pleura to the right of the heart allows the heart to be elevated without as much compression of the right heart and the vena cava, improving hemodynamic stability. As the heart is positioned, TEE can often provide an indication as to how much compression of the right or left ventricle has occurred. If either chamber is not filling, repositioning of the heart will be necessary. Close observation of the heart with TEE during periods of coronary occlusion may facilitate detection of worsening cardiac function as evidenced by weakening contraction, ventricular dilatation, or increasing mitral or tricuspid regurgitation. Seeing such changes should prompt aggressive interventions to support the circulation or insertion of an intracoronary shunt. On occasion, stopping in the midst of anastomosis to let the heart down to rest may restore stability to the circulation. Hemodynamic changes are more pronounced with displacement of the heart to access posterior coronary arteries than anterior vessels (10,11).

## INTRAOPERATIVE ECHOCARDIOGRAPHY FOR OPCAB

Intraoperative monitoring with transesophageal echocardiography (TEE) during OPCAB is interesting and useful. Information obtained before, during, and after graft construction can be important, and a systematic approach should be used (Table 26.1). A careful and thorough examination is completed and recorded at the beginning of the procedure to establish a baseline for later comparison. Particular attention is placed on documenting LV function and regional wall motion, but it is important to assess right heart function and the valves, as well. Mitral regurgitation (MR) and tricuspid regurgitation (TR) can be dynamic, so their presence and severity are documented at the start of the procedure. Detection of severely impaired cardiac function at this point of the procedure may prompt intervention with drugs or mechanical devices to support the cardiovascular system or even lead to the decision to go on CPB. The aorta is assessed for the presence of atherosclerosis before it is clamped. Epiaortic echocardiography is the best way to detect atherosclerosis in the ascending aorta (12,13) and only takes a few minutes to perform.

Next, TEE can be used to assess the effects of displacement of the heart to gain access to the coronary arteries. With multiplane imaging, the three midesophageal views (four-chamber, two-chamber, and long-axis) allow assessment of all 16 segments of the LV and provide the ability to detect MR with color-flow Doppler, as well as assess right heart function (Fig. 26.2) (14). If the TEE imaging

▶ **TABLE 26.1.** **Approach to Intraoperative Echocardiography during OPCAB**

Baseline TEE examination (record images for comparison)
    Global LV function
    Regional LV function
    Global RV function
    Valvular function
        Mitral, aortic, tricuspid, pulmonic
    Intravascular volume status
Epiaortic examination of ascending aorta
    Consider modification of manipulation of aorta if atherosclerosis
      present
During graft construction
    Effects of heart displacement
      Compression of right heart
      Mitral or aortic regurgitation
    Effects of stabilizer placement
      Compression of LV
      Change in wall motion due to stabilizer
    Effects of vessel occlusion
      New RWMA usually but not always seen
      TEE signs of "impending doom"
        Deteriorating global LV or RV function
        Increasing MR or TR
After graft completion
    Return of regional LV function
After protamine and chest closure
    New RWMA suggesting graft occlusion
    Global LV and RV function
    If aorta clamped, check for dissection

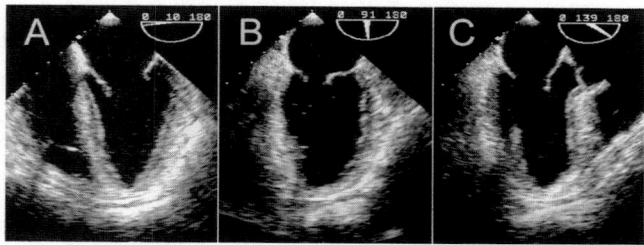

**FIGURE 26.2.** The three midesophageal views of the heart obtained by directing the imaging plane simultaneously through the MV annulus and the LV apex, and then rotating the multiplane angle while holding the probe still. **A:** Four-chamber view showing the inferoseptal and anterolateral segments of the LV, the RV, the MV, and the TV. **B:** Two-chamber view showing the anterior and inferior segments of the LV and the MV. **C:** Long-axis view showing the anteroseptal and inferolateral segments of the LV, the MV, and the AV.

plane is properly oriented to pass simultaneously through the middle of the MV annulus and the LV apex and held in that position by a clamp, the entire LV may be examined very quickly by just rotating the multiplane angle from zero to 180 degrees. Color-flow Doppler may be activated and the angle decreased back to zero to quickly assess changes in MR, and the RV and TR then examined in the four-chamber view, accomplishing a thorough assessment of the heart in just a few seconds. It is usually not possible to obtain transgastric views of the LV when the heart is displaced for graft construction to the right and circumflex coronary arteries because of loss of contact of the heart with the diaphragm, obscuring the transgastric echocardiographic window. Also, elevation of the heart by placing a lap pad underneath it will obscure the transgastric window. Changes, such as compression of the RV with underfilling of the LV or aggravation of valvular regurgitation, are sought. Placement of the vessel stabilizer may also cause changes in the TEE appearance of the heart, such as compression and underfilling of the LV. Tethering of the myocardium in the region of the stabilizer makes interpretation of wall motion changes more difficult in this area (Fig. 26.3) (15). Once positioning of

the heart is completed for grafting, the LV is examined again to establish a baseline for comparison to detect changes during vessel occlusion.

TEE examination during vessel occlusion should focus on changes in global and regional LV function, which can be quite variable. RV function can be affected by vessel occlusion as well, especially of the right coronary artery. Change in ventricular function may result in an acute increase in MR or TR, as well. While new, small regional wall motion abnormalities (RWMA) are often seen, the primary change to watch for during vessel occlusion is steadily decreasing ventricular function, either of the LV or the RV. This is often accompanied by increasing MR or TR, and may be a TEE sign of "impending doom" detected earlier than major hemodynamic changes, allowing timelier intervention before cardiovascular collapse or cardiac arrest occurs. After restoration of flow to the occluded vessel, rapid improvement in any new RWMA

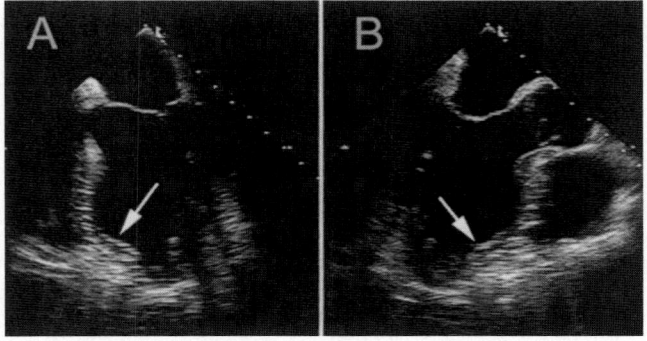

**FIGURE 26.3.** Deformity of the anteroapical LV caused by application of a stabilizing device during OPCAB (arrows). **A:** Midesophageal four-chamber view. **B:** Midesophageal long-axis view.

should be seen. It is important to complete another TEE assessment after protamine is given and the chest is closed, as these may cause acute occlusion of a graft warranting immediate intervention, such as reopening of the chest to check for kinked grafts. Ideally, the global and regional LV function should be back to baseline or better at this point; if not, there is cause for concern.

## ECHO FINDINGS DURING OPCAB

Our early experience with TEE, used during 152 cases of MIDCAB and OPCAB, allow some conclusions to be reached (16). Most patients developed a new, transient RWMA in the territory of the occluded vessel that quickly returned to baseline after restoration of flow. However, almost 30% showed no change in wall motion with TEE during vessel occlusion, typically because the vessel being grafted was already completely or nearly occluded. Ten patients had a new RWMA develop during vessel occlusion that persisted after reperfusion and through the end of surgery. Six of these patients had a significant cardiac complication, with four requiring further surgical intervention. But five of the 142 patients in this group without a persistent RWMA in the operating room subsequently were shown to have graft occlusion postoperatively, so the return of RWMA to baseline does not guarantee a perfect result. Typically, transient RWMAs seen during vessel occlusion disappear within 30 seconds, although more gradual recovery may be seen. Moises et al. reported a similar experience in 27 patients undergoing OPCAB (17). In 36% of their vessel occlusions, no new RWMAs were seen with TEE. Eighty-three percent of the RWMAs that were detected during vessel occlusion showed improvement by the end of the operation. The RWMAs that persisted to the end of surgery (17%) were still present on transthoracic echocardiography a week later, and those patients had more enzyme release, ECG changes, and clinical problems. A persistent, new RWMA after OPCAB should be cause for concern and may be an indication of a technically flawed or occluded graft.

There are limitations to all monitoring techniques. Often when the heart is displaced, the voltage of the ECG is often too low to provide useful information regarding myocardial ischemia because of loss of contact of the heart with the chest wall. In this situation, TEE may be used to detect a new RWMA suggesting ischemia. At least a limited view of the LV can be developed in most patients from the midesophageal window even when the heart is displaced by directing the imaging plane through the left atrium towards the LV. There are some patients, however, in whom no usable TEE views of the heart can be developed once the heart is displaced. While interesting, detecting signs of ischemia with ECG or TEE during vessel occlusion is not surprising. The main point is to observe

resolution of these changes by the end of the case. Failure of these changes to clear quickly once flow is restored should be cause for concern, and a graft occlusion should be considered.

Intraaortic balloon counterpulsation has been used to support the cardiovascular system during graft construction in high risk OPCAB patients with left main coronary artery disease, unstable angina, and/or poor ventricular function (18). TEE can be used to facilitate insertion of the balloon pump by ensuring that the guidewire is in the thoracic aorta before attempting to advance the balloon catheter and in positioning the tip of the catheter just distal to the left subclavian artery (19). Quest Medical, Inc., has developed a device designed to maintain normal or high levels of blood flow through vein grafts, independent of the patient's blood pressure, after the distal anastomosis, but before the proximal anastomosis has been completed. This allows the surgeon to perform the distal grafts first, which is the traditional approach for on-pump surgery, and permits not only supraphysiologic flow but also provides the potential for additives (such as vasodilators or inotropic drugs). Use of the pump requires full heparinization, and a nine-gauge arterial cannula inserted into the ascending aorta or the femoral artery to provide a source of arterial blood. There is an anecdotal report that the device facilitated off-pump surgery in which TEE demonstrated improved myocardial function in the region perfused with the pump (20). Another approach to mechanically supporting the heart during vessel occlusion is to place intracoronary shunts that provide some distal perfusion during graft construction (21). TEE would be expected to demonstrate improved thickening of the myocardium perfused through the shunt. TEE has also been used to evaluate the effect of OPCAB on patients with a patent foramen ovale (22). No significant problems were encountered in 11 such patients.

## THE FUTURE OF OPCAB

Conventional CABG using CPB was first performed over 35 years ago (23) and is one of the most extensively studied operations in history. It has very clearly defined results and risks. Numerous uncontrolled studies in the scientific literature suggest that OPCAB can be performed with at least similar results, many indicating that OPCAB has decreased morbidity and costs compared to conventional CABG (24). A few small, but well-controlled trials, comparing the two procedures have recently been published (25–27). To date, there has been no clear advantage proven in mortality and freedom from subsequent cardiac events for OPCAB. But long-term, large, and well-controlled studies will be needed to conclusively settle the issue. In the meantime, it is likely that OPCAB will continue to be performed on a large number of patients. Echocardiography can be an important tool for managing these patients during surgery.

## KEY POINTS

- Although performed by relatively few surgeons since the beginning of CABG surgery, OPCAB has been much more commonly performed in the past 10 years.
- The theoretical advantage of OPCAB over conventional CABG using CPB is the avoidance of the adverse effects of CPB.
- The disadvantages of OPCAB are hemodynamic instability during graft construction and concern about the long-term patency of bypass grafts constructed on a beating heart.
- Intraoperative TEE for OPCAB should start with a comprehensive baseline exam.
- While the heart is displaced, midesophageal TEE views are usually more obtainable than transgastric views.
- Epiaortic examination of the ascending aorta for atherosclerosis allows modification of surgical techniques to avoid atheroembolism during OPCAB surgery.
- Most patients undergoing OPCAB develop transient, high grade wall motion abnormalities during graft construction.
- Persistence of a new wall motion abnormality after flow is restored may indicate a problem with the graft.
- Increasing MR or TR, deteriorating LV or RV function are TEE signs of impending hemodynamic collapse during graft construction.

## REFERENCES

1. Kolessov VI. Mammary artery-coronary artery anastomosis as method of treatment for angina pectoris. J Thorac Cardiovasc Surg 1967;54(4):535–44.
2. Ankeny JL. Editorial: To use or not to use the pump oxygenator in coronary bypass operations. Ann Thorac Surg 1975;19(1):108–9.
3. Buffolo E, Andrade JC, Branco JN, Aguiar LF, Ribeiro EE, Jatene AD. Myocardial revascularization without extracorporeal circulation. Seven-year experience in 593 cases. Eur J Cardiothoracic Surg. 1990;4(9):504–7; discussion 507–8.
4. Puskas JD, Thourani VH, Marshall JJ, et al. Clinical outcomes, angiographic patency, and resource utilization in 200 consecutive off-pump coronary bypass patients. Ann Thorac Surg 2001;71(5):1477–83; discussion 1483–4.
5. Lee JH, Abdelhady K, Capdeville M. Clinical outcomes and resource usage in 100 consecutive patients after off-pump coronary bypass procedures. Surgery 2000;128(4):548–55.
6. Blauth CI, Cosgrove DM, Webb BW, et al. Atheroembolism from the ascending aorta. An emerging problem in cardiac surgery. J Thorac Cardiovasc Surg 1992;103(6):1104-11; discussion 1111–2.
7. Couture P, Denault A, Limoges P, Sheridan P, Babin D, Cartier R. Mechanisms of hemodynamic changes during off-pump coronary artery bypass surgery. Canadian J Anaesthesia. 2002;49(8):835–49.
8. Grundeman PF, Borst C, van Herwaarden JA, Verlaan CW, Jansen EW. Vertical displacement of the beating heart by the octopus tissue stabilizer: influence on coronary flow. Ann Thorac Surg 1998;65(5):1348–52.
9. Cheung AT, Savino JS, Weiss SJ, Aukburg SJ, Berlin JA. Echocardiographic and hemodynamic indexes of left ventricular preload in patients with normal and abnormal ventricular function. Anesthesiology 1994;81(2):376–87.
10. Biswas S, Clements F, Diodato L, Hughes GC, Landolfo K. Changes in systolic and diastolic function during multivessel off-pump coronary bypass grafting. Eur J Cardiothorac Surg 2001;20(5):913–7.
11. Mishra M, Malhotra R, Mishra A, Meharwal ZS, Trehan N. Hemodynamic changes during displacement of the beating heart using epicardial stabilization for off-pump coronary artery bypass graft surgery. J Cardiothorac Vasc Anesth 2002;16(6):685–90.
12. Shimokawa T, Minato N, Yamada N, Takeda Y, Hisamatsu Y, Itoh M. Assessment of ascending aorta using epiaortic ultrasonography during off-pump coronary artery bypass grafting. Ann Thorac Surg 2002;74(6):2097–100.
13. Wilson MJ, Boyd SY, Lisagor PG, Rubal BJ, Cohen DJ. Ascending aortic atheroma assessed intraoperatively by epiaortic and transesophageal echocardiography. Ann Thorac Surg 2000;70(1):25–30.
14. Shanewise JS, Cheung AT, Aronson S, et al. ASE/SCA guidelines for performing a comprehensive intraoperative multiplane transesophageal echocardiography examination: recommendations of the American Society of Echocardiography Council for Intraoperative Echocardiography and the Society of Cardiovascular Anesthesiologists Task Force for Certification in Perioperative Transesophageal Echocardiography. Anesth Analg 1999;89(4):870–84.
15. Shiga T, Terajima K, Matsumura J, Sakamoto A, Ogawa R. Local cardiac wall stabilization influences the reproducibility of regional wall motion during off-pump coronary artery bypass surgery. J Clin Monit Comput 2000;16(1):25–31.
16. Shanewise JS, Zaffer R, Martin RP. Intraoperative echocardiography and minimally invasive cardiac surgery. Echocardiography 2002;19(7):579–82.
17. Moises VA, Mesquita CB, Campos O, et al. Importance of intraoperative transesophageal echocardiography during coronary artery surgery without cardiopulmonary bypass. J Am Soc Echocardiogr 1998;11(12):1139–44.
18. Kim KB, Lim C, Ahn H, Yang JK. Intraaortic balloon pump therapy facilitates posterior vessel off-pump coronary artery bypass grafting in high-risk patients. Ann Thorac Surg 2001;71(6):1964–8.
19. Shanewise JS, Sadel SM. Intraoperative transesophageal echocardiography to assist the insertion and positioning of the intraaortic balloon pump. Anesth Analg 1994;79(3):577–80.
20. Guyton RA, Thourani VH, Puskas JD, et al. Perfusion-assisted direct coronary artery bypass: selective graft perfusion in off-pump cases. Ann Thorac Surg 2000;69(1):171–5.
21. Lucchetti V, Capasso F, Caputo M, et al. Intracoronary shunt prevents left ventricular function impairment during beating heart coronary revascularization. Eur J Cardiothorac Surg 1999;15(3):255–59.
22. Sukernik MR, Mets B, Kachulis B, Oz MC, Bennett-Guerrero E. The impact of newly diagnosed patent foramen ovale in patients undergoing off-pump coronary artery bypass grafting: case series of eleven patients. Anesth Analg 2002; 95(5):1142–6.
23. Favaloro RG. Landmarks in the development of coronary artery bypass surgery. Circulation 1998;98(5):466–78.
24. Hart JC, Spooner T, Edgerton J, Milsteen SA. Off-pump multivessel coronary artery bypass utilizing the Octopus tissue stabilization system: initial experience in 374 patients from

three separate centers. Heart Surgery Forum 1999;2(1): 15–28.

25. Ascione R, Lloyd CT, Gomes WJ, Caputo M, Bryan AJ, Angelini GD. Beating versus arrested heart revascularization: evaluation of myocardial function in a prospective randomized study. Eur J Cardiothoracic Surg 1999;15(5):685–90.

26. van Dijk D, Nierich AP, Jansen EW, et al. Octopus Study Group. Early outcome after off-pump versus on-pump coronary bypass surgery: results from a randomized study. Circulation 2001;104(15):1761–6.

27. Angelini GD, Taylor FC, Reeves BC, Ascione R. Early and midterm outcome after off-pump and on-pump surgery in Beating Heart Against Cardioplegic Arrest Studies (BHACAS 1 and 2): a pooled analysis of two randomised controlled trials. Lancet 2002;359(9313):1194–9.

## QUESTIONS

1. The major advantage of OPCAB over CABG with CPB is
   A. More stable hemodynamics during graft construction
   B. Avoidance of the adverse consequences of CPB
   C. Higher quality distal coronary anastomoses
   D. Avoidance of heparin administration
   E. Fewer grafts need to be constructed

2. Which of the following patients would most likely benefit from OPCAB rather than CABG with CPB?
   A. A 65-year-old man who previously had CABG 12 years ago
   B. A 55-year-old insulin dependent diabetic woman needing five bypass grafts
   C. A 64-year-old man with moderate mitral regurgitation needing four grafts
   D. A 78-year-old man with atherosclerosis of the ascending aorta
   E. A 43-year-old man needing a single graft to an intramyocardial LAD

3. For monitoring during OPCAB, the advantage of the transgastric mid short-axis TEE view over midesophageal views is that it
   A. Simultaneously shows myocardium supplied by all three major coronary arteries
   B. Allows assessment of mitral regurgitation
   C. Shows all 16 segments of the left ventricle
   D. Provides a clear view of the left ventricle when the heart is displaced
   E. Allows assessment of right ventricular function

4. When monitoring with TEE during OPCAB, a problem is most likely present when
   A. A wall motion abnormality present on the baseline exam is not improved on the chest closed exam
   B. There is no change seen in the wall motion during vessel occlusion
   C. A new, high grade wall motion abnormality is seen during vessel occlusion
   D. The mitral and tricuspid regurgitation increase from mild to moderate while the heart is displaced
   E. A new wall motion abnormality persists after the chest is closed

# Surgical Decision Making in Valvular Heart Disease

Chapter 27

# Surgical Considerations in Mitral and Tricuspid Valve Surgery

*Erik A.K. Beyer, Gonzalo Gonzalez-Stawinski, and A. Marc Gillinov*

## PRIMARY MITRAL VALVE DISEASE

The most common cause of mitral regurgitation in North America is degenerative mitral valve disease (1–4). In recent surgical series, myxomatous degeneration of the mitral valve accounted for more than 50% of the cases (5). Rheumatic heart disease, though rare in industrialized nations, is still a frequent cause of mitral regurgitation and stenosis, requiring surgical correction in developing countries (4). Mitral regurgitation caused by coronary artery disease, termed ischemic mitral regurgitation, is increasingly common. Of patients evaluated for surgery for coronary artery disease, approximately one-third will have some degree of mitral regurgitation (6). Infective endocarditis remains a problem and is the etiology of pure mitral regurgitation in 2% to 8% of patients presenting for surgical correction of mitral regurgitation (7). Severe endocarditic mitral regurgitation is related to ruptured chordae and/or leaflet perforation (8). Other diseases that can affect the mitral valve include idiopathic calcification of the mitral annulus; systemic diseases, such as Marfan's and Ehlers-Danlos syndromes; and hypertrophic cardiomyopathy.

Preoperative evaluation of mitral valve pathology is performed with transthoracic echo. Doppler echocardiography is the primary tool for assessing mitral valve disease. It identifies the morphologic lesions, the degree of mitral regurgitation/stenosis, and quantifies ventricular function. During mitral valve surgery, transesophageal echocardiography (TEE) is essential. It allows identification of the lesion and mechanisms of mitral valve dysfunction (Tables 27.1 and 27.2). It also determines whether the valve is regurgitant, stenotic, or a combination of both. TEE is valuable in determining the likelihood of repair versus replacement. Intraoperative TEE delineates dynamic abnormalities related to valve opening and closing. It also characterizes leaflet abnormalities and regurgitant jet size and duration. Characteristics of the regurgitant jet help clarify the nature of the mitral valve dysfunction. Usually, leaflet flail directs the regurgi-

tant jet in the opposite direction of the flail segment, whereas restricted leaflets generally cause jets on the ipsilateral side of the pathologic segment. TEE therefore guides the surgeon's approach to reestablish effective coaptation in regurgitant valves and to improve opening in stenotic ones (9). Echocardiography is also necessary to assess the other valves and quantify ventricular function. Finally, TEE assesses the results of surgical intervention. Late durability of MV repair in degenerative disease is enhanced by TEE (10). Technical errors at surgery are identified accurately in the operating room, thereby allowing immediate correction.

## PROSTHETIC MITRAL DISEASE

Since the first prosthetic heart valve was placed in 1960, millions of valves have been implanted. Although most patients do well following mitral valve replacement, they are subject to a variety of complications (11,12). These complications include prosthetic valve endocarditis (PVE), periprosthetic leak, structural valve degeneration (SVD), valve thrombosis, and thromboembolism. PVE most frequently occurs in the first several months postoperatively, with an early incidence of up to 2% (13). The incidence then decreases to 0.17% to 1% per patient year (14). Periprosthetic leaks occur when the seal between the sewing ring and the host tissue is inadequate. The incidence of periprosthetic leaks ranges between 0.3% and 2.2% per year (15,16). Structural failure related to valve design or material selection is rare with currently available mechanical valves. However, bioprosthetic valves have limited durability due to SVD (17).

## TRICUSPID VALVE

Tricuspid regurgitation is most commonly caused by volume overload attributable to chronic left-sided valvular lesions (Table 27.3). Right ventricular and atrial volume

▶ TABLE 27.1. Mitral Regurgitation: Etiology and Pathologic Changes

| Etiology | Pathologic Changes |
|---|---|
| Degenerative or myxomatous | 1. Asymmetric dilatation of the posterior two-thirds of the mitral annulus, resulting in posterior leaflet prolapse<br>2. Chordae elongation or rupture |
| Rheumatic heart disease | 1. Annular dilatation at the posteromedial commissure<br>2. Leaflet shortening<br>3. Cleft obliteration and scallop fusion |
| Ischemic mitral regurgitation | 1. Alterations in ventricular and papillary muscle geometry, with tethering of mitral leaflets resulting in failure of leaflet coaptation<br>2. Unruptured/infarcted papillary muscle, causing papillary muscle elongation<br>3. Ruptured papillary muscle resultant leaflet flail |
| Infective endocarditis | 1. Infective valvular vegetations commonly on the atrial aspect of the leaflet at the line of valve closure<br>2. Tissue necrosis, thus leaflet ulceration/perforation<br>3. Annular abscesses<br>4. Annular fistulae |
| Idiopathic calcification of the annulus | 1. Calcification involving the hinge point of the leaflets, commonly involving the posterior leaflet. |
| Connective tissue disorders (e.g., Marfan's syndrome and Ehlers-Danlos syndrome) | 1. Excessive elongation of the papillary muscles<br>2. Billowing and redundant leaflets |

▶ TABLE 27.2. Mitral Stenosis: Etiology and Pathologic Changes

| Etiology | Pathologic Changes |
|---|---|
| Rheumatic heart disease (most common) | 1. Leaflet thickening and fibrosis<br>2. Commissural fusion<br>3. Chordal fusion and shortening |
| Massive mitral annular calcification | 1. Restrictive leaflet motion from invasive calcification disease |
| Congenital mitral stenosis | 1. Congenital slit-like orifice in line of a mitral valve |
| Infective endocarditis | 1. Large vegetations obstructing the mitral orifice |
| Inborn errors in metabolism (e.g., Fabry's disease, Hurler-Scheie syndrome) | 1. Polysaccharide deposits within the valve structure, leading to leaflet thickening and eventual fibrosis |
| Cor triatriatum (rare) | 1. Abnormal subdivision of the left atrium, partially obstructing the outflow of the pulmonary veins to the mitral orifice |

▶ TABLE 27.3. Tricuspid Valve Disease: Etiology and Pathologic Changes

| Etiology | Pathologic Changes |
|---|---|
| Functional regurgitation | 1. Asymmetric annular dilatation universally involving the anterior and posterior leaflets |
| Rheumatic | 1. Leaflet thickening and fibrosis<br>2. Commissural fusion (commonly the anteroseptal commissural)<br>3. Chordal fusion and shortening |
| Endocarditis | 1. Vegetations usually on the atrial side of the valves |
| Carcinoid | 1. Endocardial fibrous thickening on the ventricular surface of the valve |

overload causes annular dilatation and tricuspid regurgitation. Ten to fifty percent of patients with severe mitral valve dysfunction have significant tricuspid regurgitation (18). Functional tricuspid regurgitation is frequently accompanied by pulmonary hypertension and right ventricular dilatation and dysfunction (19). Organic involvement of the tricuspid valve by rheumatic disease can also result in tricuspid regurgitation. Another major etiology of tricuspid regurgitation is endocarditis. Endocarditis of the tricuspid valve is prevalent in IV drug abusers and in patients with chronic indwelling venous catheters. Other less common causes of tricuspid regurgitation include fibrosis secondary to carcinoid disease and degenerative disease.

## STRUCTURE AND ANATOMY

### Mitral Valve

The components of the mitral valve include the annulus, leaflets, chordae, and papillary muscles. A review of the anatomic and functional aspects as they pertain to mitral valve surgery will be presented. The mitral annulus is composed of muscular and fibrous tissue that anchors the base of the mitral valve leaflets (20,21). The annular ring extends between the endocardium of the left atrium and the endocardium of the left ventricle and incorporates within its boundaries the valve tissue itself. In an average adult, the orifice area of the mitral valve at the level of the annulus is approximately 6.5 cm$^2$ for women and 8 cm$^2$ for men (22). Diastolic and systolic annulus sizes differ by 23% to 40% (23). The annulus itself is extremely dynamic and changes in size, shape, and position throughout the cardiac cycle. During diastole, the annulus moves outward with the posterior wall of the left ventricle, allowing the shape of the annulus to become more circular (22).

### Leaflets

The mitral valve has two leaflets, the anterior and posterior. The anterior leaflet is triangular and the posterior leaflet is rectangular. The length of the basal attachments of the posterior leaflet is 0.5 cm longer than the basal attachment of the anterior leaflet (22). The posterior leaflet edge has multiple indentations or clefts, which are connected by fanlike cords. The commissures separate the anterior and posterior leaflets. Commissural cusps (leaflets) are also present and can vary in size with the posterior commissural cusp being more prominent. During diastole, the combined surface area of the two leaflets is 1.5 to 2 times the surface area of the functional mitral orifice. During systole, the anterior leaflet alone could cover the mitral orifice.

### The Chords

The chordae are tendinous, stringlike structures connecting the valvular tissue to the papillary muscles or the myocardium. The chords do not stretch more than 10% under physiologic conditions. They vary in length from approximately 3 to 0.2 cm from the valvular to the ventricular insertion (20). Chords arise as single projections from the ventricle and then divide in succession until attaching to the valve as small chords. The chords insert into the papillary muscle in a semicircular fashion. Chords arising from the lowest portion of the papillary muscle are known as strut chords because they support the central portion of the leaflets. Chords are further divided anatomically into marginal, intermediate, and basal chords based on their attachment to the ventricular surface of the leaflets in a perpendicular plane to the edge of the valve leaflet. Marginal or first-order chordae attach to the edge of the valve leaflet and thereby prevent eversion of the free marginal component of the valve. The intermediate or second-order ("strut") chordae attach to the midsection/rough zone of the ventricular leaflet and prevent billowing or doming of the cusp. Finally the basal, or third-order chordae, which represent the largest chords morphologically, insert at the annulus and help maintain ventricular geometry (22).

### Papillary Muscles

There are two distinct papillary muscles arising from the free wall of the left ventricle. The anterolateral papillary muscle is single and usually larger than the posteromedial muscle. It is located posterior and to the left on the left ventricle. The posteromedial papillary muscle is U-shaped and located near the septal border of the posterior wall. It can have two or more subheads. The posteromedial papillary muscle usually derives its blood supply from the right coronary artery, whereas the anterolateral papillary muscle has dual blood supply from the left anterior descending and circumflex coronary arteries (24). Therefore, the posterior papillary muscle is more susceptible to ischemic insults, which can directly affect valvular competence.

### Tricuspid Valve

The tricuspid valve is composed of an annulus, leaflets, chordae, and papillary muscles. The tricuspid valve does not have a well-formed collagenous annulus. The normal annulus circumference is 10 cm in women and 11.2 cm in men (25). The atrioventricular groove folds into the tricuspid valve leaflets. There are three leaflets of the tricuspid valve that are named based on their anatomic locations: anterior, posterior, and septal. The leaflets are separated at the commissures and are tethered by chordae tendineae. The anterior leaflet is usually the longest, measuring on average 2.2 cm in length. The posterior leaflet typically has two or three scallops separated by cleft or indentations at its free edge (26). Chordae arise from three papillary muscles and consist of five different types, the fan-shaped, rough zone, basal, free-edge, and deep (26). On average, there are 25 chordae to the tricuspid valve.

## PATHOLOGY

### Mitral Valve

#### Degenerative Myxomatous Disease of the Mitral Valve

Dilatation of the mitral annulus is a major factor in mitral insufficiency caused by degenerative disease. It is the sole cause of mitral insufficiency in 15% of degenerative cases (27). The dilatation is asymmetric, causing the anterior to posterior diameter to become greater than the transverse diameter. Dilatation only affects the posterior two-thirds of the annulus, which corresponds to the area of the posterior leaflet.

The most commonly encountered lesion in degenerative mitral valve disease is posterior chordal rupture (5). Prolapse of the posterior leaflet because of elongated or ruptured chords is the cause of mitral regurgitation in the majority of cases (4). Of degenerative mitral valves operated on in one surgical series, 41% had ruptured posterior chords, 30% had elongated chords, and 10% had ruptured anterior chords (27). Other features of myxomatous mitral valves found on echocardiogram include billowing and redundant leaflets. The leaflet tissue is thinned and increased in size. In 16% of patients, annular and leaflet calcification is seen in myxomatous disease of the mitral valve. Prolapse of the mitral valve leaflets is generally present in myxomatous mitral valve disease. Intraoperative TEE determines the site of leaflet involvement and therefore dictates techniques of repair.

Left ventricular outflow tract obstruction (LVOTO) caused by abnormal systolic anterior motion (SAM) of the anterior leaflet of the mitral valve occurs in 4%–10% of patients having mitral valve repair for myxomatous disease (28). Intraoperative transesophageal echocardiography is essential in diagnosing this complication following repair. TEE can also help determine valvular pathology that would lend to the potential for SAM and thereby guide surgical decision making. Excess valvular tissue is associated with a higher risk of LVOTO. A posterior leaflet with a significant redundant central portion pushes the anterior leaflet against the septum after correction of the mitral regurgitation (3). Therefore, a sliding leaflet repair is applied to floppy valves with large posterior leaflets in order to restore a more normal ratio of the anterior to posterior leaflet surface area. The incidence of SAM has been reduced in several recent surgical series to as low as 0%–2% (28).

### Rheumatic Disease of the Mitral Valve

Rheumatic mitral valve disease remains a surgical challenge because of the progressive nature of its pathology and the young patient population affected. It is not repaired as frequently as myxomatous disease due to the very nature of the disease. Rheumatic mitral valve disease can result in stenosis, regurgitation, or a combination of the two.

The cardinal anatomic changes of mitral valve stenosis are leaflet thickening and fibrosis, commissural fusion, and chordal fusion and shortening (29). Chordae tendineae can become shortened to the point that they appear to insert directly into the papillary muscle. As the disease progresses a stenosed, slitlike orifice, termed "fishmouth," is produced. Surgical candidates for valve repair or replacement have valve areas less than 1.4 cm². 

Isolated mitral valve regurgitation secondary to rheumatic valvular disease is the result of leaflet shortening caused by scarring. Often the posterior leaflet is affected when the clefts are obliterated and the scallops become fused. In longstanding regurgitation, the leaflet free margin becomes thickened and folded in the direction of regurgitant flow. However, rheumatic mitral regurgitation is more often associated with valve stenosis caused by commissural fusion. Leaflet and annular calcification are also seen in longstanding rheumatic heart disease. This is readily seen on TEE as echodense areas. Also, annular dilatation in rheumatic disease is asymmetric and is often greatest toward the posteromedial commissure (30).

Intraoperative TEE helps establish repairability or the need for valve replacement in rheumatic heart disease. Some centers report a 65% repair rate for rheumatic mitral disease (31). For mitral stenosis, commissurotomy and valve debridement are often used. Generally it is unnecessary to place an annuloplasty ring following a commissurotomy. However, when a central leak is observed and when the annulus is dilated, as shown by a circular rather than an oval shape, an annuloplasty ring should be considered. The ability to repair a stenotic rheumatic mitral valve rests on the thickness of the valve leaflets and the presence of chordae tendineae. Patients with anterior leaflet and chordal pliability should be considered for repair (32). A regurgitant rheumatic mitral valve should likewise be considered for repair if there is annular dilatation and the leaflets are thickened but mobile and the chords are thickened and elongated. Severe commissural fusion and subvalvular fibrosis are a contraindication to repair (32).

## Ischemic Disease of the Mitral Valve

Ischemic mitral valve disease represents approximately 11%–27% of patients undergoing surgery for mitral valve disease. Compared to other etiologies of mitral valve disease, surgery for ischemic mitral valve disease is associated with higher mortality rates, ranging between 10% and 48% (33). This is clearly related to the underlying cause of mitral regurgitation—coronary artery disease.

Ischemic mitral valve disease lacks a widely accepted classification scheme. This makes comparing studies difficult. For our purposes, ischemic mitral valve disease will be divided into the three categories based on the mechanisms causing regurgitation. These categories include functional, infarcted but unruptured papillary muscle, and ruptured papillary muscle (34).

The most common cause of regurgitation in ischemic disease is functional. In a recent review by Gillinov, 76% of patients undergoing surgery for ischemic mitral regurgitation had functional impairment. In these patients, the leaflets and subvalvular apparatus appear morphologically normal at echo and upon direct inspection. The cause of regurgitation is failure of leaflet coaptation during ventricular systole. This produces a regurgitant jet on echo that is usually central but can be eccentric or complex (34).

The mechanism of functional ischemic mitral regurgitation is complex. Changes in annular, ventricular, and papillary muscle geometry and function appear to all contribute. The primary pathology likely involves alterations in ventricular and papillary muscle geometry that produce a tethering effect on the mitral leaflets. There is considerable debate whether annular dilatation is an important component of functional ischemic mitral regurgitation.

Patients in the functional group are amenable to treatment by annuloplasty alone. An undersized annuloplasty produces excellent results in this subgroup of patients. The rationale for this is that by reducing annular size, the leaflet contact area is increased and thereby compensates for papillary muscle and left ventricular wall dyskinesis (33). Furthermore, this may result in ventricular remodeling over time (35).

The next most common subgroup of ischemic mitral regurgitation is the infarcted or elongated papillary muscle. Papillary muscle infarction represents approximately 24% of IMR. On echo, the valve leaflet prolapses secondary to the elongated papillary muscle. Repair techniques can be performed for this process and include shortening of the papillary muscles. However, the tendency by most surgeons is to replace rather than repair the valve (33).

The least prevalent subgroup of ischemic mitral regurgitation is papillary muscle rupture. This is usually an acute and catastrophic event that presents differently from papillary muscle infarction without rupture. This usually occurs 2 to 7 days after MI and without urgent surgery, 50%-75% of these patients may die (36). Echo

findings of a ruptured papillary muscle include a flail leaflet, which is easily visualized (37). Surgical repair by papillary muscle reimplantation or by resecting the prolapsing portion of the posterior leaflet is feasible. As is seen with infarcted papillary muscles, surgeons more often opt to replace the valve in these situations.

Pre- and postoperative echo are essential when evaluating ischemic mitral regurgitation. The cause of regurgitation in ischemic disease must be determined preoperatively in order to assess for repairability. Echocardiography can also identify crucial components of mitral valve dysfunction that further guide therapy. A recent study showed the beneficial effects of mitral repair in ischemic mitral regurgitation were reduced if a complex regurgitant jet pattern was present on preop echo. It was also noted that late survival was reduced in the repair versus the replacement group when lateral wall motion abnormalities were identified on echo.

## Endocarditis

Valve dysfunction as a result of bacterial endocarditis is an uncommon form of mitral valve disease. In one large surgical series, only 3.4% of mitral valve procedures were related to bacterial endocarditis (38). TEE plays a major role in the diagnosis and management of mitral valve endocarditis. Echocardiographic features of bacterial endocarditis that suggest a need for surgical intervention include vegetation, perforation, annular abscess with sinus and fistula formation, and less commonly ruptured chords and papillary muscles (39). Most cases of acute endocarditis can be repaired and early valve repair is recommended (40). Postoperative TEE is essential in order to determine the adequacy of repair.

Vegetations appear as echodense masses with irregular margins attached to the leaflet. They are most commonly found attached to the atrial side aspect of the mitral valve leaflets and are related to the lines of valve closure. Vegetations can vary in size, where TEE resolution easily reaches 2 mm–3 mm in diameter. Vegetation removal or partial leaflet resection is performed when isolated lesions are identified.

Tissue necrosis as a result of the infectious process can cause destruction of the mitral valve leaflet. Ulcerations at the edge of the mitral leaflets and perforations of the body of the leaflets are manifestations of this process. Valvular regurgitation results and is demonstrated by TEE. Pericardial patches are used to repair perforations if the surrounding mitral valve tissue is well preserved and the subvalvular apparatus is intact. Local progression of the infection into the annular tissue can produce an annular abscess. Though annular abscesses are uncommon, they may spread into the atrium, ventricle, and pericardial space. Mitral annular abscesses represent a great challenge to the surgeon. Thorough debridement of the abscess cavity is essential and repair undertaken with a pericardial patch (41). Fistulae also arise from abscess cavities and these are visible on TEE. The fistulae should be delineated carefully because this dictates the surgical approach to closing them (42).

## Prosthetic Dysfunction

TEE allows superb visualization of prosthetic valves in the mitral position. Origins of prosthetic valve dysfunction and paraprosthetic pathology can be detailed with TEE. Structural valve dysfunction, paravalvular leaks, endocarditis, and thrombus are complications of prosthetic valves that often require surgical attention.

Prosthetic valves are predisposed to structural dysfunction and outright failure. Mechanical stresses that come with repeated opening and closing can take their toll. Failure of a bioprosthesis is usually related to leaflet fracture with subsequent regurgitation. On TEE this presents as an eccentric regurgitant jet (43). Mechanical prosthetic valves are more durable than bioprostheses, but are nonetheless subject to structural dysfunction. A severe regurgitant jet noted on TEE is indicative of occluder dysfunction.

Paravalvular regurgitation is the result of an incomplete seal of the sewing ring and annulus. This typically occurs as a result of a failed suture line or an infectious process. Immediately following surgery a small amount of paravalvular leak is common and tends to resolve over time once the suture line heals. However, identification of a large paravalvular leak on the postoperative TEE requires surgical intervention. A new paravalvular leak occurring months after surgery should alert the surgeon to an infectious process.

Prosthetic valve endocarditis (PVE) is a serious complication associated with prosthetic mitral valves. Vegetations identified on echocardiogram are pathognomonic of PVE and typically occur on the atrial side of the mitral prosthesis. TEE demonstrates vegetations in 80% of PVE cases (44). Bulky vegetations may interfere with opening and closure of mechanical prosthesis, causing either stenosis or regurgitation. Paravalvular abscesses are more common in patients with PVE than with native valve endocarditis and are seen as areas of low echodensity adjacent to the sewing ring of the prosthesis. Furthermore, progression of the infection may cause partial or complete dehiscence of the valve and results in paraprosthetic regurgitation. Surgical therapy is directed at radical debridement of infected tissue with reconstruction of cardiac structures with biologic materials (45).

Mechanical prostheses are prone to thrombus formation. TEE allows excellent visualization of thrombus on prosthetic mitral valves. Thrombi can occur on the sewing cuff, as well as on the occluder mechanism. On TEE, transvalvular gradients are increased when thrombus occludes the valve orifice. Regurgitation can also de-

velop if the thrombus prevents complete closure of the valve leaflets.

## Tricuspid Valve

### Rheumatic Disease of Tricuspid Valve

Rheumatic fever is the most common cause of organic tricuspid regurgitation worldwide. Endocarditis of the tricuspid valve is becoming increasingly prevalent in industrialized nations, secondary to drug abuse and chronically hospitalized patients with long-term central venous catheters. In the United States the most common etiology of tricuspid regurgitation is related to annular dilatation, often referred to as functional TR.

### Functional Tricuspid Regurgitation

Functional TR is related to increases in pulmonary artery pressure caused by left ventricular failure or pulmonary vascular or interstitial disease. Diseases of the left-sided heart valves are frequently the cause of functional TR. Ten to fifty percent of patients with severe mitral valve dysfunction have significant TR (46). Therefore, the tricuspid valve should be evaluated thoroughly during echocardiographic evaluation of the mitral valve.

In functional TR, the valve leaflets are normal but the annulus is dilated. Annular dilatation is asymmetric and develops at the portion of the annulus that corresponds to the anterior and posterior leaflets.

Early and late clinical outcomes are adversely affected when functional tricuspid insufficiency is left untreated. Therefore, it is important to address these lesions and aggressively treat them (47). Moderate-to-severe tricuspid regurgitation is easily visualized on TEE and should be surgically corrected. Common surgical repair techniques used to address TR are the suture annuloplasty, such as the Kay or DeVega method, and placement of either a rigid or soft annuloplasty ring. The annuloplasty ring remodels the annulus, decreases tension on the suture lines, increases leaflet coaptation, and prevents recurrent annular dilatation (48).

Following tricuspid valve repair, TEE is essential so that the repair may be evaluated. Following tricuspid annuloplasty, residual TR of 2+ or more is associated with late tricuspid reoperation (49).

### Rheumatic Disease of the Tricuspid Valve

Rheumatic postinflammatory scarring can result in combined tricuspid stenosis and regurgitation. Rheumatic tricuspid valve disease is rarely an isolated lesion and as with rheumatic mitral disease, it is more common in the developing world. Echocardiographic evaluation of tricuspid rheumatic disease reveals leaflet thickening, commissural fusion, and chordal thickening. Anteroseptal commissural fusion is commonly pronounced. Coaptation of the tricuspid valve leaflets is often incomplete, resulting in tricuspid regurgitation (50). In distinction to mitral valve disease, secondary annular calcification is rare in tricuspid valve disease. Symptomatic patients with rheumatic tricuspid valve disease are usually managed by replacing the valve.

### Endocarditis of the Tricuspid Valve

Tricuspid endocarditis has been increasing in frequency over the last two decades, primarily because of increased IV drug abuse and more liberal use of long-term indwelling venous catheters. Primary infection accounts for only 1% of all bacterial infective endocarditis (51). Vegetations, which usually appear on the atrial side of the tricuspid valve, are the hallmark of infective tricuspid valve endocarditis. On TEE, they appear as sessile or pedunculated echodensities attached to the valve surface or margins (50). Unlike mitral endocarditis, annular abscess is a rare complication of tricuspid endocarditis. Again, TEE is critical in determining the cause of tricuspid insufficiency and in guiding surgical correction. Surgical options for tricuspid endocarditis range from excising the valve to replacement. A recent study suggests that if the infectious process is limited to one leaflet, surgical excision with suture annuloplasty provides excellent results (52).

### Carcinoid Disease of the Tricuspid Valve

Carcinoid heart disease occurs in patients with carcinoid tumors of the gastrointestinal tract that have metastasized to the liver and with carcinoid tumors in other sites that drain directly into the systemic venous circulation. The valvular lesions associated with carcinoid syndrome are usually limited to the right side of the heart. The predominant valve abnormality is tricuspid regurgitation. Patients with carcinoid heart disease present with right heart failure. Tricuspid valve lesions consist of endocardial fibrous thickening occurring on the ventricular aspect of the TV. TEE reveals leaflet thickening and chordal fusion (50). Surgical management of carcinoid tricuspid valve disease relies mainly on replacing the diseased valve once symptoms become evident or echocardiographic evidence of right heart failure is revealed (53).

## SURGICAL MANAGEMENT OF MITRAL VALVE DISEASE

In the current era, the main objective of surgeons operating on patients with mitral valve disease is to correct the pathology at hand to provide relief of signs and symptoms of the disease. The choice of intervention is dictated by the pathology. While in the past most patients were treated with valve replacement, presently every effort is made to preserve the mitral valve apparatus. This results

in the preservation of ventricular geometry, which is critical for ventriucular function, while at the same time rendering patients anticoagulation-free. Every attempt should be made to conserve the mitral valve; techniques for its repair are described in the following section.

## SURGICAL PROCEDURES FOR MITRAL VALVE REGURGITATION

### Operative Approach

For isolated mitral valve disease our approach of choice is through a mini skin incision and a hemisternotomy (Figs. 27.1A and 27.1B). Some technical points are key to maximizing such an approach. The incision is initiated on the skin over the sternum about a centimeter below the sternal angle of Louis. It is then extended towards the xiphoid for a distance of 7 cm. Once the subcutaneous tissues and pectoralis fascia overlying the sternum are divided, the surgeon proceeds to develop a subcutaneous flap over the sternum towards the sternal notch. With the aid of a small finger retractor, this plane is developed, dissecting over the notch and dividing all strap muscles' attachments to it (Fig. 27.2). The anterior mediastinum is entered bluntly and the anterior plate of the sternum is scored with electrocautery. A gentle curve is carried towards the left fourth intercostal space. Using a small sternotomy saw, the hemisternotomy is completed from the sternal notch curving towards the left fourth intercostal. The anterior mediastinum is packed with a laparotomy pad and hemostasis is achieved with electrocautery and topical hemostatics. The pericardium is opened, exposing the upper portion of the heart. It becomes evident with this approach that the key elements for a mitral valve repair are within the operative field (Fig. 27.2). A second technical point is the creation of the pericardial cradle. Six 2-0 silk stitches are placed at equal intervals on either side of the free edge of the pericardium. After removing the ministernal retractor, the pericardium is stretched over the sternum with the aid of the silk stitches and these are then clamped with hemostats to the drapes. The miniretractor is replaced and the sternum reopened. This allows the heart to be pulled further into the operative field.

Finally, cardiopulmonary bypass (CPB) cannulation is performed in the standard fashion. We use small, flexible pediatric cannulas for cannulation (Fig. 27.3). After aortic cannulation the superior vena cava is cannulated with a small right-angled cannula, and then, with the patient on CPB, a small right-angled cannula is introduced into the inferior vena cava (Fig. 27.4). With the patient completely cannulated and on CPB, the left atrium is approached using a transseptal technique (Fig. 27.5). Excellent exposure to the mitral valve is facilitated with a mitral valve retractor. The choice of surgical procedure is guided by the

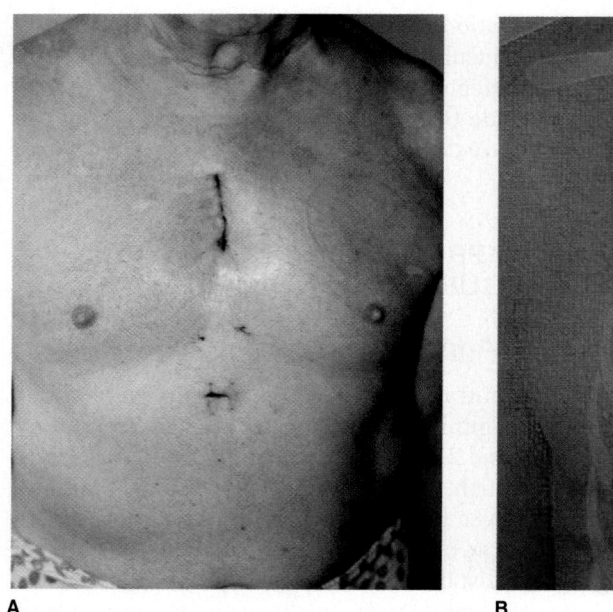 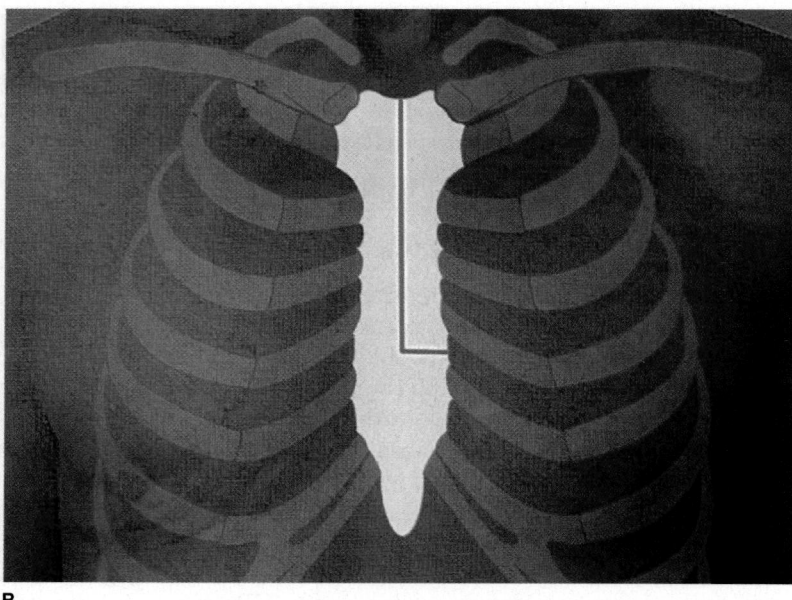

**A**                                         **B**

**FIGURE 27.1. A:** Healed skin incision of a patient who has undergone a hemisternotomy through a miniexposure. **B:** Typical hemisternotomy to access the mitral valve.

precardiopulmonary bypass echocardiogram, as well as the direct inspection of the anatomy of the mitral valve (Table 27.4).

## RING ANNULOPLASTY

Ischemic mitral regurgitation from annular dilatation and leaflet restriction from papillary-chordal tethering are best treated by an annuloplasty ring. Once access and exposure to the mitral valve are gained the valve is care-

fully inspected for any concomitant pathology. Ring selection is done by measuring the anterior mitral valve leaflet with a Cosgrove-Edwards annuloplasty ring sizer (Fig. 27.6). With appropriate ring selection, six to eight annuloplasty ring sutures are placed on the posterior annulus from trigone to trigone (Fig. 27.7). These are evenly spaced just outside the muscular annulus. The sutures are passed through the ring using the same spacing ratio as on the annulus (Fig. 27.8). Sutures are securely tied and the repair is tested by filling the left ventricle with saline (Fig. 27.9). Once the adequacy of the repair is ascertained, the septal atriotomy is closed with a running prolene suture. The right atriotomy is repaired in a similar fashion. Warm cardioplegia is administered at this point, and the patient weaned from CPB. Intraoperative echo is used to confirm the repair.

## QUADRANGULAR RESECTION AND ANNULOPLASTY RING FOR POSTERIOR LEAFLET PROLAPSE OR FLAIL

The most common use of a quadrangular resection is a prolapsed middle scallop of the posterior leaflet, resulting from chordal rupture or elongation. A quadrangular resection is accomplished by initially identifying the margins of resection, and surrounding the normal chordae with silk ties. The flail scallop and its associated chordae are sharply resected with an 11-blade (Fig. 27.10). If primary repair of the remaining scallops is judged to result

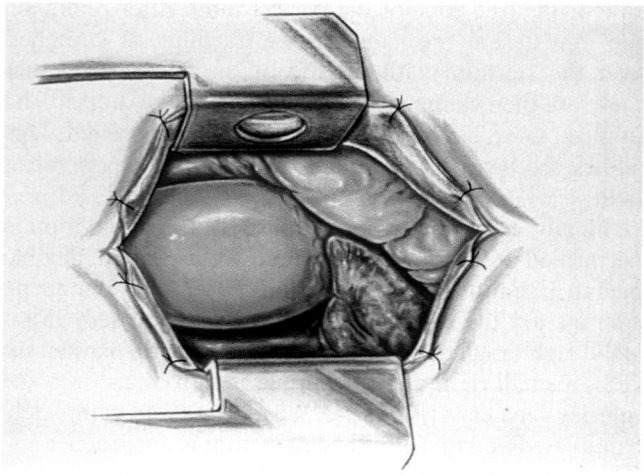

**FIGURE 27.2.** Exposure provided by hemisternotomy.

*(text continues on page 437)*

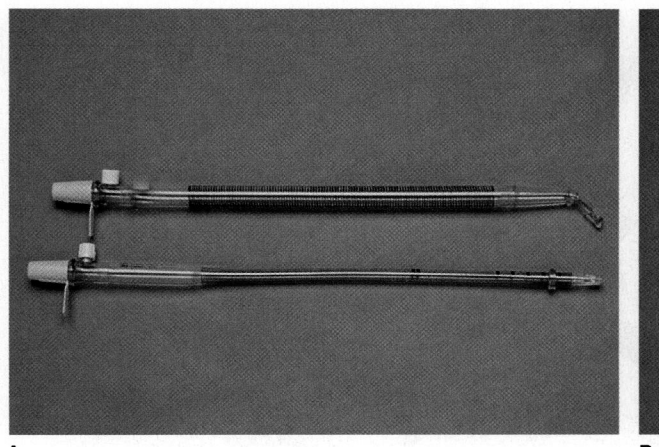
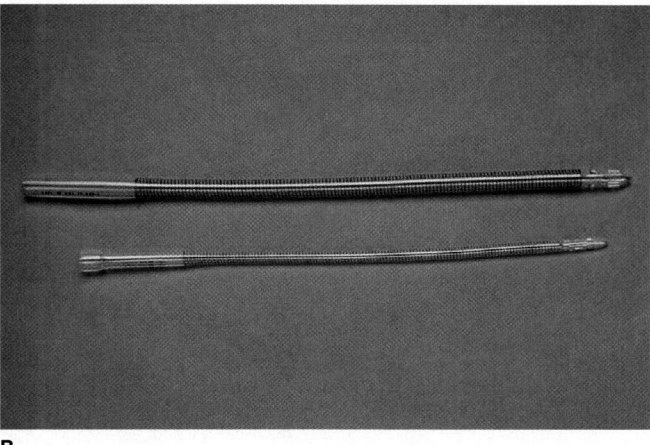

**A**                                                 **B**

**FIGURE 27.3. A:** Comparison of size of standard adult aortic cannula and pediatric aortic cannula. **B:** Comparison of size of standard adult venous cannula and pediatric venous cannula.

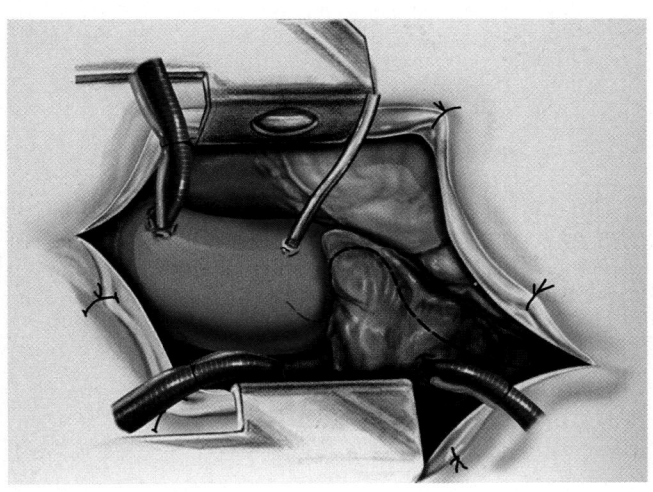

**FIGURE 27.4.** Typical cannulation for cardiopulmonary bypass through a ministernotomy. The *dotted line* on the right atrium (RA) represents the location of a future incision.

▶ TABLE 27.4.  **Surgically Relevant Echocardiographic Information in Mitral Valve Disease**

| Echocardiographic Parameter | Relevant Surgical Information |
|---|---|
| Annular diameter | 1. Annular dilatation may be solely correctable with an annuloplasty ring |
| Direction of the regurgitant jet | 1. Central jets correlate with functional regurgitation and thus ischemic annular dilatation<br>2. Anterior jets correlate with posterior leaflet prolapse<br>3. Posterior jets correlate with anterior leaflet prolapse |
| Anatomy of the leaflets | 1. Flail leaflets can be evaluated, aiding in planning the type of repair (i.e., quadrangular resection for posterior leaflet flail vs. choral transfer for anterior leaflet prolapse)<br>2. Restricted leaflet motion and calcium deposition suggest the need for potential valve replacement in stenosis<br>3. Leaflet vegetation or perforations secondary to endocarditis, which might require resection |
| Calcification of the annulus | 1. Aids in planning intraoperative annular debridement |
| Shunts | 1. Unsuspected septal defects, or fistulas, complicating abscess, requiring repair |
| Left atrial thrombus | 1. Concomitant thrombectomy |
| Ventricular dimensions and function | 1. Prognostic indicator |

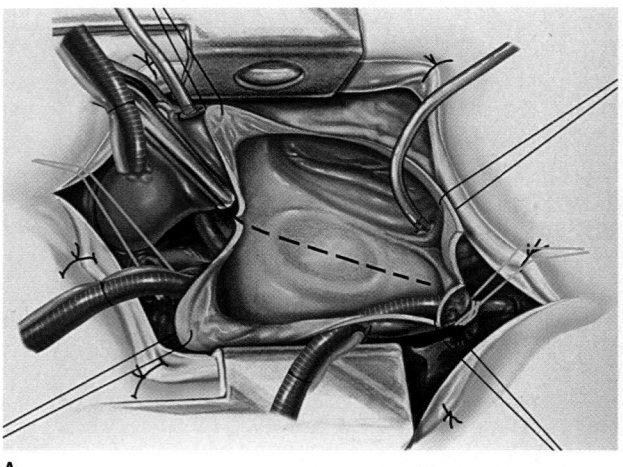

A

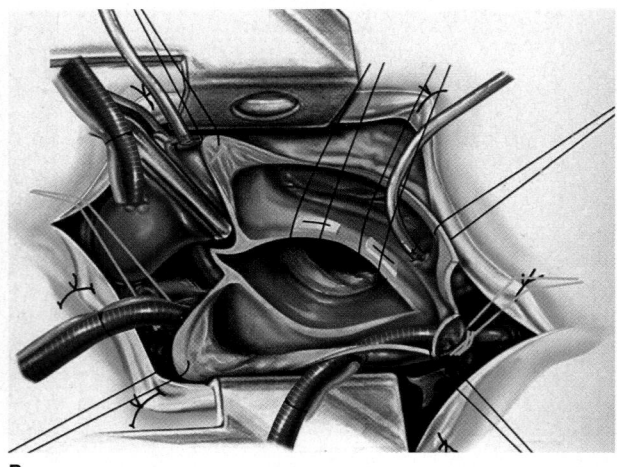

B

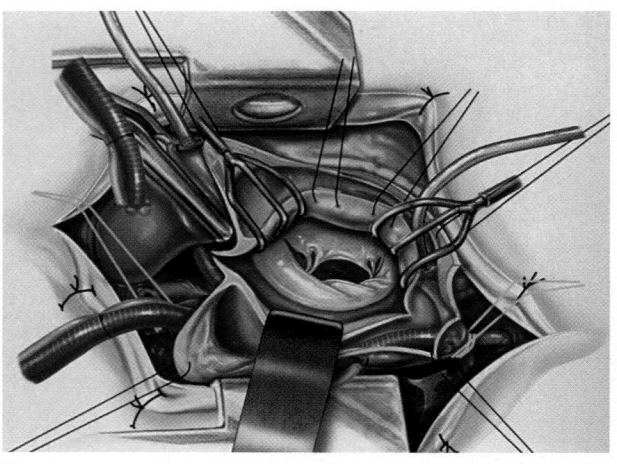

C

**FIGURE 27.5. A:** Right atriotomy. The dotted line represents the orientation of the incision for a transeptal approach to the mitral valve (MV). **B:** Pledgetted sutures aid in retracting the septum for a MV exposure. **C:** Exposure provided by the transeptal approach.

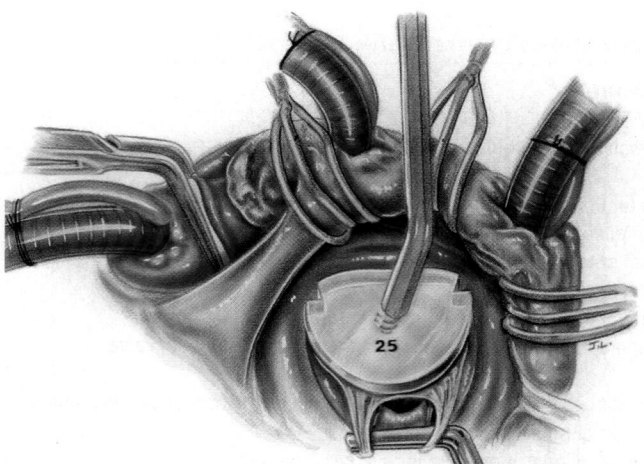

**FIGURE 27.6.** Measuring the anterior MV leaflet area to choose an annuloplasty ring.

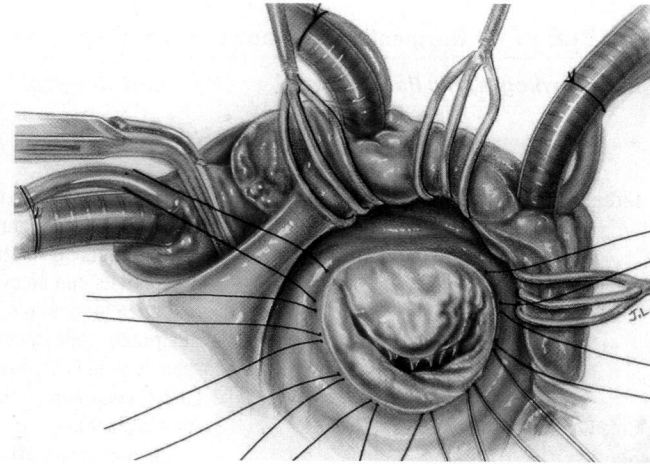

**FIGURE 27.7.** Annuloplasty ring sutures are placed on the posterior MV annulus for subsequent repair.

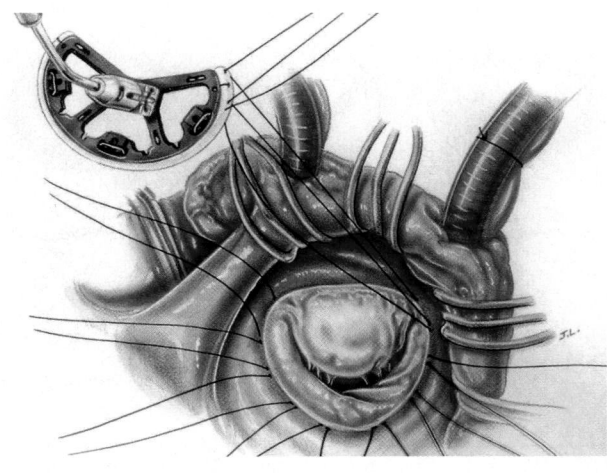

**FIGURE 27.8.** Threading individual stitches through a selected annuloplasty ring.

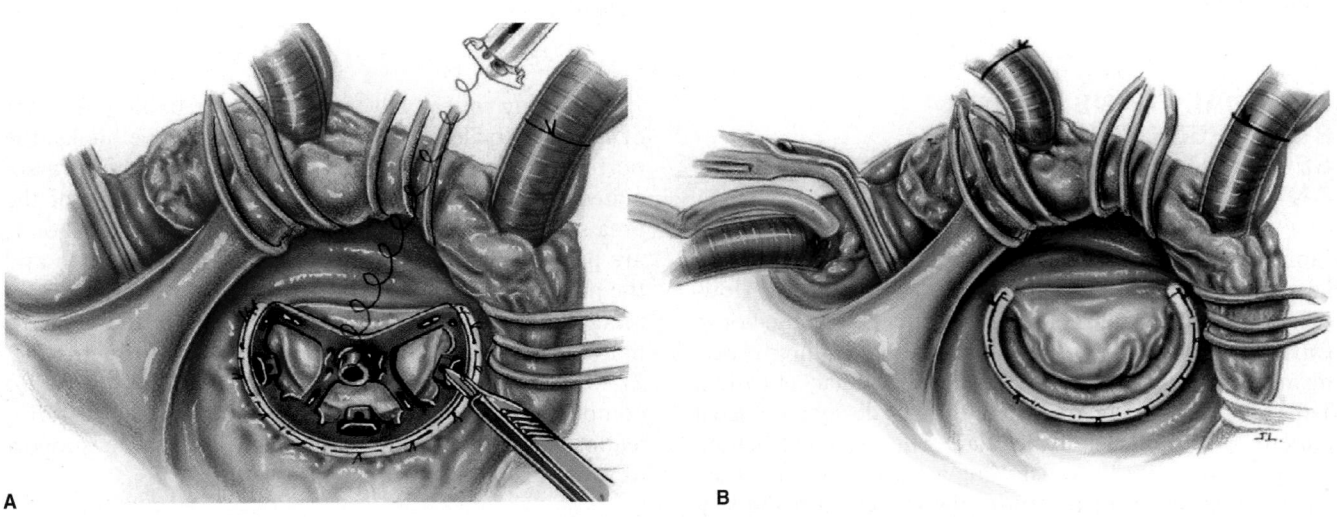

A                                                            B

**FIGURE 27.9. A:** Sutures are tied securely and the annuloplasty is uncoupled from the ring holder. **B:** Representation of final repair of an ischemic MV regurgitation with an annuloplasty ring.

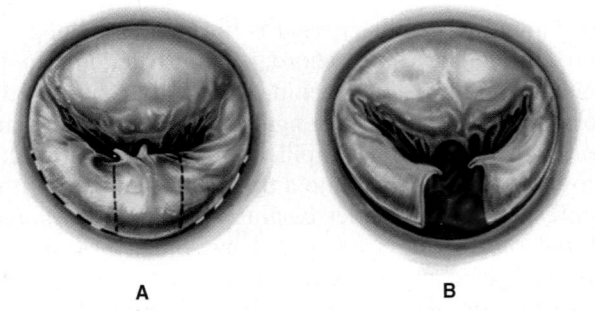

A                          B

**FIGURE 27.10. A:** Depiction of a P2 flail with the limits of resection represented by *vertical dotted lines.* Notice on the posterior annulus another set of *dotted lines* representing the site of a second incision to create advancement flaps for a sliding MV repair, following the quadrangular resection. **B:** Complete quadrangular resection of prolapsing scallop. Notice the incision on the posterior annulus created for a sliding repair.

in excessive tension, then posterior advancement flaps are created by an incision along the posterior annulus towards each commissure for the final repair.

Because we believe that longevity of the repair depends on the support of the surrounding annulus, every patient receives an annuloplasty ring. Following the resection and advancement flaps annuloplasty sutures are placed (Fig. 27.11). The realignment of the posterior leaflet is then performed using a running 5-0 suture. A similar suture is used to re-approximate the free margins of the remaining scallops. Finally the annuloplasty sutures are placed through an annuloplasty ring, which was previously chosen by measuring the area of the anterior mitral leaflet. These sutures are tied securely and the repair tested (Fig. 27.12).

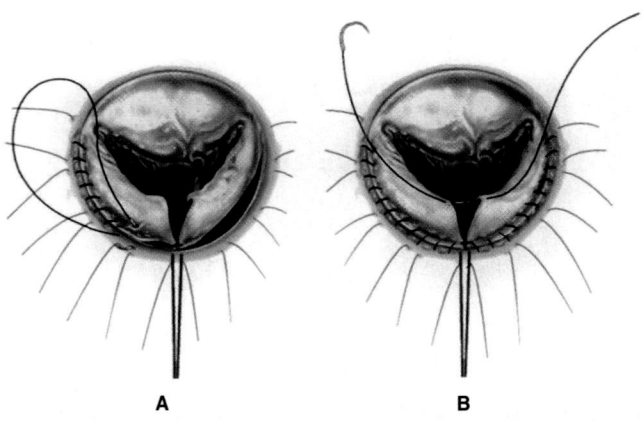

**FIGURE 27.11. A:** Following the placement of annuloplasty rings, the sliding repair is completed with a running suture. **B:** The free edges of P1 and P3 scallops are approximated with a running suture.

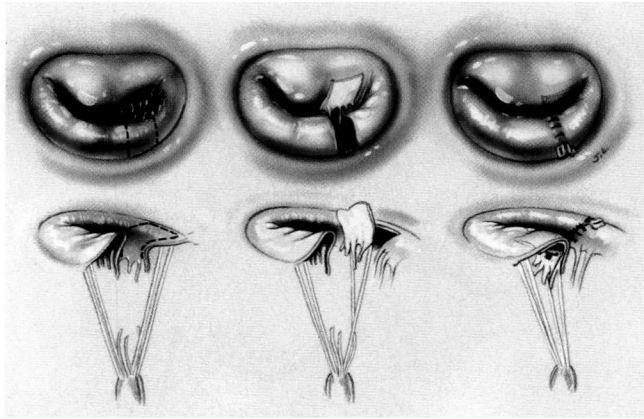

**FIGURE 27.13.** Steps for an anterior MV segment prolapse repair using the chordal-transferring technique. Notice the ruptured chordae and how the segment of posterior leaflet serves as a chordae donor.

## CHORDAL TRANSFER FOR RUPTURED OR ELONGATED SEGMENT OF THE ANTERIOR LEAFLET

Similar to posterior leaflet prolapse, anterior leaflet prolapse is caused by chordal elongation or rupture. However, because the anterior leaflet is attached to the aortic valve annulus, repair of the anterior leaflet cannot be performed by segmental resection and annular plication. Thus chordal transfer, or "flip over," was designed to treat patients with anterior leaflet flail. The principle behind this procedure lies in transposing a scallop, and its associated chordae, from the posterior leaflet onto the segment of diseased anterior leaflet.

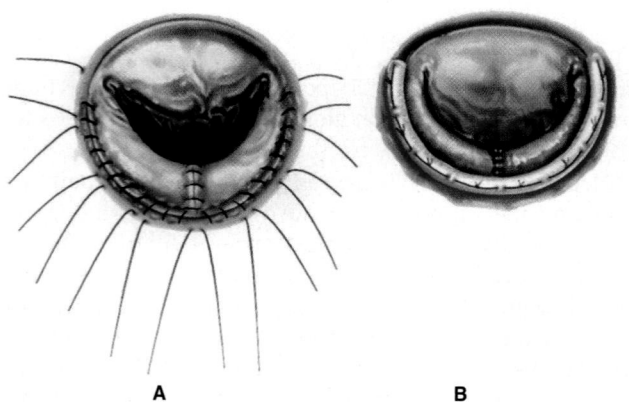
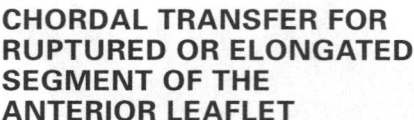

**FIGURE 27.12. A:** Completed quadrangular resection with a sliding repair. **B:** Completed MV repair with an annuloplasty ring.

Following mitral valve exposure, the flailing segment of the anterior leaflet is isolated. Using nerve hooks, the portion of posterior leaflet to be transferred with its associated chordae is identified. The margin chordae of the area selected are encircled with silks. Two 5-0 Ethibonds are placed through the free edge of the selected area and the prolapsing segment. The area of posterior leaflet is resected, and each suture is tied, resulting in the approximation of the chordae to the prolapsing segment (Fig. 27.13). Additional sutures are placed onto the transfer to complete the repair. The remaining defect in the posterior leaflet is repaired with an annuloplasty ring for support as previously described.

## CHORDAL RECONSTRUCTION AND PAPILLARY MUSCLE REIMPLANTATION

When an entire papillary head is fibrosed and elongated from chronic ischemia, chordal reconstruction can be achieved by chordal shortening. For this technique the prolapsing segment and elongated papillary muscle are identified. The tip of the papillary muscle is either folded onto itself or embedded into a trench created within it to restore the normal leaflet height (Fig. 27.14). Although chordal shortening is advocated by some, these procedures lack good long-term outcomes.

Mitral insufficiency may result from chronic or acute ventricular ischemia. With papillary muscle infarction and subsequent papillary muscle rupture, acute mitral valve leaflet prolapse with resultant severe mitral regurgitation may occur. This injury commonly involves the posterior medial muscle rather than the anterior lateral mus-

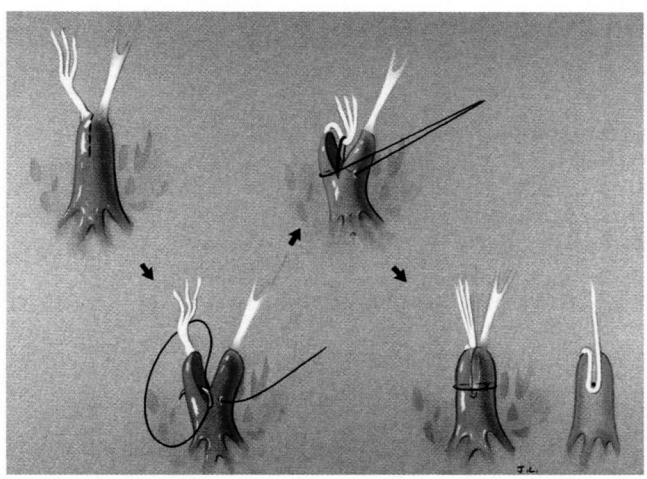

**FIGURE 27.14.** Graphic depiction of a chordal shortening procedure to treat mitral valve regurgitation in a case of chordae elongation.

cle. A ruptured papillary muscle may be repaired by suturing it to the immediately adjacent papillary muscle or left ventricular wall. For both procedures care must be taken to ensure proper chordal lengths in the dependent reattached leaflet segments.

## SURGICAL PROCEDURES FOR MITRAL VALVE STENOSIS

### Mitral Valve Replacement

For mitral valve replacement there are two types of valves: bioprosthetic and prosthetic valves. While superb durability has been reported with mechanical valves, patients receiving them require lifelong anticoagulation to prevent thromboembolic events. Thus an attractive alternative is a bioprosthetic valve. While these valves protect the patient from the untoward effects of anticoagulation, they are flawed by their lack of durability. However, in patients over the age of 70, structural deterioration is rare. Furthermore, results from clinical trials suggest that bovine pericardial mitral valves have a better long-term durability when compared with their porcine counterparts.

Despite good attempts to establish guidelines to help surgeons in choosing the right valve for the right patient, valve selection must be individualized for each patient. It depends on weighing the disadvantages of anticoagulation-related complications associated to mechanical valve against the disadvantages of decreased longevity of the bioprosthetic valves. Thus mechanical valves are placed in young patients, lacking contraindications to anticoagulation or patients who already take anticoagulants. Alter-

natively, older patients (> 70), or patients in whom anticoagulation is contraindicated, a bioprosthetic valve should be the valve of choice.

To replace the mitral valve we use the same approach as previously described, unless other pathology (i.e., coronary artery disease or endocarditis) precludes this technique. The diseased mitral valve should be debrided of all calcium deposits and fibrous material. It is essential to preserve the mitral leaflets and chordae tendineae to preserve ventricular function when replacing the mitral valve. Debridement restores leaflet flexibility and allows insertion of an artificial valve. While inserting a prosthetic valve, it is essential to ensure that the remaining mitral valve leaflets or chordae do not obstruct, or become caught in, the valve mechanism, preventing proper valve functioning.

Selection of the appropriate size valve is facilitated using commercially available sizers. To insert the valve, sutures are initially placed through the valve annulus and then the sewing ring. Our preference is to use pledges with our valve sutures placed on the atrial side of the annulus to avoid interfering with valve function. Once the valve is seated in the annulus the sutures are tied. As with repairs, the replaced valve is tested both directly and with echocardiography.

## SURGICAL MANAGEMENT OF TRICUSPID VALVE DISEASE

### Surgical Therapy for Functional Tricuspid Valve Disease

The surgical approach for functional tricuspid valve disease can be performed as above. Functional tricuspid regurgitation is seldom the only indication for operation. Again, as with mitral valve disease, the surgical plan for management of tricuspid valve dysfunction is guided by the findings of the intraoperative echocardiographic examination, as well as direct inspection of the tricuspid valve (Table 27.5). Thus, commonly, functional tricuspid insufficiency is repaired with an additional surgical procedure. Key to this procedure is the fact that it can be performed as the last part of a case without the use of an aortic cross-clamp. Regardless, the tricuspid valve is approached through a lateral right atriotomy. A mitral valve retractor can be used to aid exposure. Once tricuspid insufficiency is confirmed, a valve sizer is used to determine ring size (Fig. 27.15). The commissures of the sizer should equal the extreme attachments of the septal leaflet. For patients with tricuspid regurgitation, the chosen ring should be one to two sizes smaller than the measured distance. The first suture is placed along the anterior leaflet just above the anterior/septal commissure.

▶ TABLE 27.5. **Surgically Relevant Echocardiographic Information in Tricuspid Valve Disease**

| *Echocardiographic Parameter* | *Relevant Surgical Information* |
| --- | --- |
| Annular diameter | 1. Functional tricuspid regurgitation: valves are normal but dilated annulus. Findings would allow its repair rather than replacement. |
| Anatomy of the leaflets | 1. Leaflet thickening, commissural fusion, and chordal thickening suggest rheumatic or carcinoid valve disease and the need for replacement.<br>2. Valve vegetations (pedunculated or sessile echodensities) suggest endocarditis and the need for replacement. |
| Right ventricular function | 1. Right ventricular failure in a patient with carcinoid and valve disease suggests the need for valve replacement. |

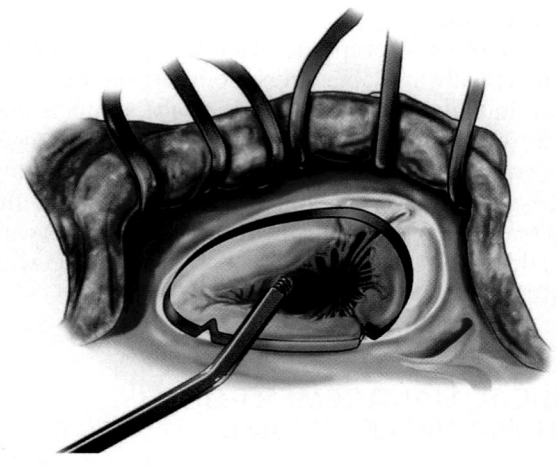

*FIGURE 27.15.* Measuring the septal area in a case depicting function tricuspid valve (TV) insufficiency.

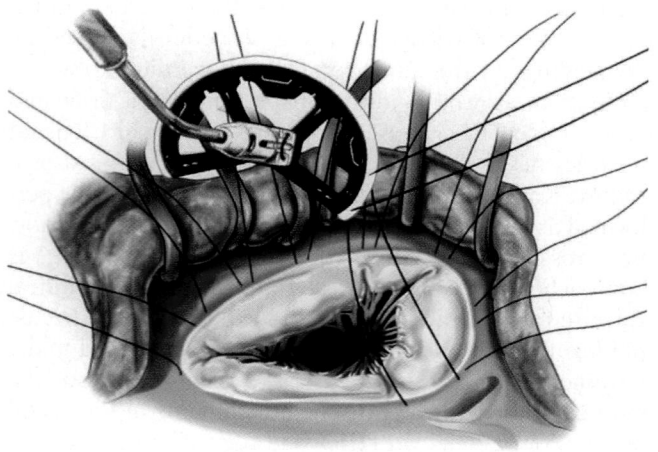

*FIGURE 27.16.* With the annuloplasty ring sutures in place, each individual suture is threaded through an annuloplasty ring.

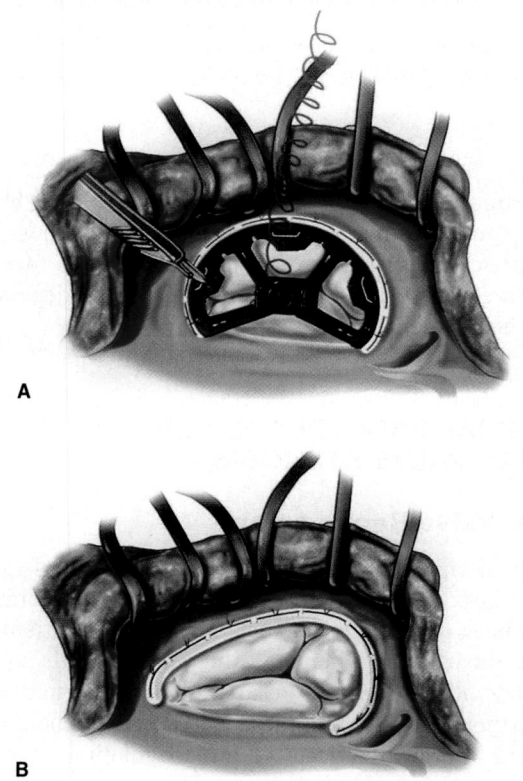

*FIGURE 27.17.* **A:** After each suture is tied, the ring is uncoupled from its holder. **B:** Completed TV repair with an annuloplasty ring.

Suture placement continues clockwise until the medial aspect of the coronary sinus, approximately half-way across the septal leaflet. After completing the annular sutures the stitches are placed through the annuloplasty ring (Fig. 27.16). Sutures are tied, the repair tested, and the atriotomy closed with a permanent running suture (Fig. 27.17). Intraoperative echocardiography is used to confirm the adequacy of repair.

## TRICUSPID VALVE REPLACEMENT

Surgical replacement of the tricuspid valve is reserved for rheumatic tricuspid valve disease with its accompanying stenosis, tricuspid valve endocarditis, and carcinoid-linked tricuspid valve disease. Common to these etiologies is the consequential valve destruction not amenable to repair.

For all the previous entities the leaflets are excised, and the orifice of the valve is measured with valve sizers to choose the correct valve. With the appropriate valve, selected valve sutures are placed around the tricuspid annulus and then through the valve. Similar to all other techniques, the atriotomy is closed with a running suture and TEE confirms the adequacy of the repair.

## KEY POINTS

- Prolapse of the posterior leaflet secondary to elongated or ruptured chords is the most common cause of mitral regurgitation in degenerative disease of the mitral valve.
- Systolic anterior motion occurs following repair of a degenerative mitral valve and is caused by a tall posterior leaflet, displacing the anterior leaflet toward the septum during systole.
- Patients with rheumatic mitral valve disease who should be considered for repair are those with anterior leaflet and chordal pliability.
- The most common cause of mitral regurgitation in ischemic disease is failure of leaflet coaptation during ventricular systole.
- In patients with bacterial endocarditis, vegetations, leaflet perforation, annular abscess, and ruptured chords or papillary muscles found on TEE suggest the need for surgical intervention.
- Periprosthetic valve regurgitation is the result of an incomplete seal of the sewing ring and annulus caused by either a failed suture line (early) or an infectious process.
- Clinical outcomes are adversely affected when moderate-to-severe functional tricuspid regurgitation is not corrected surgically.
- Tricuspid valve endocarditis is increasing in frequency secondary to the increased use of long-term venous catheters and the rise in IV drug abuse.

## REFERENCES

1. Cosgrove DM. Mitral valve repair in patients with elongated chordae tendineae. J Card Surg 1989;4:247–53.
2. Reul RM, Cohn LH. Mitral valve reconstruction for mitral insufficiency. Prog Cardiovasc Dis 1997;39:567–99.
3. David TE, Armstrong S, Sun Z, Daniel L. Late results of mitral valve repair for mitral regurgitation due to degenerative disease. Ann Thorac Surg 1993;56:7–14.
4. Olson LJ, Subramanian R, Ackerman DM, Orszulak TA, Edwards W. Surgical pathology of the mitral valve: a study of 712 cases spanning 21 years. Mayo Clin Proc 1987;62:22–34.
5. Gillinov AM, Cosgrove DM. Mitral valve repair. Oper Tech Thor Cardiovasc Surg 1998;3:95–108.
6. Fenster MS, Feldman MD. Mitral regurgitation: an overview. Curr Prob Cardiol. 1995;20:193–228.
7. Waller BF, Morrow AG, Maron BJ, et al. Etiology of clinically isolated, severe, chronic, pure mitral regurgitation: analysis of 97 patients over 30 years of age having mitral valve replacement. Am Heart J 1982;104:276–88.
8. Buchbinder NA, Roberts WC. Left-sided valvular active infective endocarditis. A study of forty-five necropsy patients. Am J Med 1972;53:20–35.
9. Stewart WJ, Salcedo EE. Echocardiography in patients undergoing mitral valve surgery. Semin Thorac Cardiovasc Surg 1989;1:194–202.
10. Gillinov AM, Cosgrove DM, Blackstone EH, et al. Durability of mitral valve repair for degenerative disease. J Thorac Cardiovasc Surg 1998;116:734–43.
11. Roberts WC. Complications of cardiac valve replacement: characteristic abnormalities of prostheses pertaining to any or specific site. Am Heart J 1982; 103:113–22.
12. Zabalgoitia M. Echocardiographic assessment of prosthetic heart valves. Curr Probl Cardiol 2000;25(3):157–218.
13. Calderwood SB, Swinski LA, Waternaux CM, Karchmer AW, Buckley MJ. Risk factors for the development of PVE. Circulation 1985;72:31–7.
14. Rutledge R, Kim BJ, Applebaum RE. Actuarial analysis of the risk of prosthetic valve endocarditis in 1598 patients with mechanical and bioprosthetic valves. Arch Surg 1985;120:469–72.
15. Czer LS, Chaux A, Matloff JM, et al. Ten-year experience with the St. Jude Medical valve for primary valve replacement. J Thorac Cardiovasc Surg 1990;100:44–54.
16. Copeland JG 3rd, Sethi GK. Four-year experience with the CarboMedics valve: the North American experience. North American team of clinical investigators for the CarboMedics prosthetic heart valve. Ann Thorac Surg 1994;58:630–7.
17. Fann JI, Burdon TA. Are the indications for tissue valves different in 2001 and how do we communicate these changes to our cardiology colleagues? Curr Opin Cardiol 2001;16(2):126–35.
18. Breyer RH, McClenathan JH, Michaelis LL, McIntosh CL, Morrow AG. Tricuspid regurgitation: a comparison of nonoperative management, tricuspid annuloplasty, and tricuspid valve replacement. J Thorac Cardiovasc Surg 1976;72:867–74.
19. Carpentier A, Deloche A, Hanania G, Forman J, et al. Surgical management of acquired tricuspid valve disease. J Thorac Cardiovasc Surg 1974;67:53–6.
20. Davila JC, Palmer TE. The mitral valve: anatomy and pathology for the surgeon. Arch Surg 1962;84:38–62.
21. Silverman ME, Hurst JW. The mitral complex: interaction of the anatomy, physiology, and pathology of the mitral annulus, mitral valve leaflets, chordae tendineae, and papillary muscles. Am Heart J 1968;76:399–418.
22. van Rijk-Zwikker GL, Delemarre BJ, Huysmans HA. Mitral valve anatomy and morphology: relevance to mitral valve replacement and valve reconstruction. J Card Surg 1994;9(2 Suppl):255–61.
23. Ormiston JA, Shah PM, Tei C, Wong M. Size and motion of the mitral valve annulus in man. II. Abnormalities in mitral valve prolapse. Circulation 1982;65:713–9.
24. Voci P, Bilotta F, Caretta Q, Mercanti C, Marino B. Papillary muscle perfusion pattern: hypothesis for ischemic papillary muscle dysfunction. Circulation 1995;91:1714–8.

25. Kitzman DW, Scholz DG, Hagen PT, Ilstrup DM, Edwards WD. Age-related changes in normal human hearts during the first 10 decades of life. Part II (Maturity): a quantitative anatomic study of 765 specimens from subjects 20 to 99 years old. Mayo Clin Proc 1988;63(2):137–46.

26. Silver MD, Lam JH, Ranganathan N, Wigle ED. Morphology of the human tricuspid valve. Circulation 1971;43:333–48.

27. Loop FD, Cosgrove DM, Stewart WJ. Mitral valve repair for mitral insufficiency. Eur Heart J 1991;12 Suppl B:30–3.

28. Gillinov AM, Cosgrove DM 3rd. Modified sliding leaflet technique for repair of the mitral valve. Ann Thorac Surg 1999;68:2356–7.

29. Spencer FC. A plea for early, open mitral commissurotomy. Am Heart J 1978;95:668–70.

30. Galloway AC, Colvin SB, Baumann FG, Harty S, Spencer FC. Current concepts of mitral valve reconstruction for mitral insufficiency. Circulation 1988;78:1087–98.

31. Duran CM, Gometza B, De Vol EB. Valve repair in rheumatic mitral disease. Circulation 1991;84[supp 5]:III125132.

32. Yau TM, El-Ghoneimi YA, Armstrong S, Ivanov J, David TE. Mitral valve repair and replacement for rheumatic disease. J Thorac Cardiovasc Surg 2000;119:53–60.

33. Oury JH, Cleveland JC, Duran CG, Angell WW. Ischemic mitral valve disease: classification and systemic approach to management. J Card Surg 1994;9(supp2)262–73.

34. Gillinov AM, Wierup PN, Blackstone EH, et al. Is repair preferable to replacement for ischemic mitral regurgitation? J Thorac Cardiovasc Surg 2001;122:1125–41.

35. Bolling SF, Pagani FD, Deeb GM, Bach DS. Intermediate-term outcome of mitral reconstruction in cardiomyopathy. J Thorac Cardiovasc Surg 1998;115:381–88.

36. Kishon Y, Oh JK, Schaff HV, Mullany CJ, Tajik AJ, Gersh BJ. Mitral valve operation in postinfarction rupture of a papillary muscle: immediate results and long-term follow-up of 22 patients. Mayo Clin Proc 1992;67:1023–30.

37. Moursi MH, Bhatnagar SK, Vilacosta I, San Roman JA, Espinal MA, Nanda NC. Transesophageal echocardiographic assessment of papillary muscle rupture. Circulation 1996;94:1003–9.

38. Hendren WG, Morris AS, Rosenkranz E, et al. Mitral valve repair for bacterial endocarditis. J Thorac Cardiovasc Surg 1992;103:124–29.

39. Bayer AS, Bolger A, Taubert K, et al. Diagnosis and management of infective endocarditis and its complications. Circulation 1998;98:2936–48.

40. Dreyfus G, Serref A, Jebara V, et al. Valve repair in acute endocarditis. Ann Thorac Surg 1990; 49:706–13.

41. David TE, Bos J, Christakis GT, Brofman PR, Wong D, Feindel C. Heart valve operations in patients with active infective endocarditis. Ann Thorac Surg 1990;49:701–5.

42. Ryan EW, Bolger A. TEE in the evaluation of infective endocarditis. Card Clinic 2000;18:773–87.

43. Zabalgoitia M, Herrera CJ, Chaundhry FA, et al. Improvement in the diagnosis of bioprosthetic valve dysfunction by TEE. J Heart Valve Dis 1993;2:595.

44. Shulz R, Werener GS, Fuchs JB, et al. Clinical outcome and echocardiographic findings of native and prosthetic valve endocarditis in the 1990s. Euro Heart J 1996;17:281–8.

45. Lytle BW, Priest BP, Taylor PC, et al. Surgical treatment of prosthetic valve endocarditis. J Thorac Cardiovasc Surg 1996;111:198–207.

46. Gillinov AM, Cosgrove DM. Tricuspid valve repair for functional TR. Op Tech Thor CV Surg 1998;3:2;134–39.

47. Frater R. Tricuspid insufficiency. J Thorac Cardiovasc Surg 2001;122:427–9.

48. Gatti G, Maffei G, Lusa AM, Pugliese P. Tricuspid valve repair with the Cosgrove-Edwards annuloplasty system: early clinic and echocardiographic results. Ann Thor Surg 2001; 72:764–7.

49. Kuwaki K, Morishita K, Tsukamoto M, Abe T. Tricuspid valve surgery for functional tricuspid valve regurgitation associated with left-sided valvular disease. Euro J Cardiothorac Surg 2001;20:577–82.

50. Blaustein AS, Ramanathan A. Tricuspid valve disease. Clinical evaluation, physiopathology, and management. Cardiol Clin 1998;16:551–72.

51. Chan P, Ogilby JD, Segal B. Tricuspid valve endocarditis. Am Heart J 1989;117:1140–6.

52. Carozza A, Renzulli A, DeFeo M, et al. Tricuspid repair for infective endocarditis: clinical and echocardiographic results. Tex Heart Inst J 2001;28:96–101.

53. Connolly HM, Schaff HV, Mullany CJ, Rubin J, Abel MD, Pellikka PA. Surgical management of left-sided carcinoid heart disease. Circulation 2001;104(12 Supp):I36–40.

## QUESTIONS

1. What is the direction of the regurgitant jet on Doppler TEE for prolapse of the posterior mitral valve leaflet?
   A. Posterior
   B. Lateral
   C. Anterior
   D. Central
   E. Distal

2. The most common cause of tricuspid regurgitation in the United States is
   A. a carcinoid tumor.
   B. rheumatic disease.
   C. Ehlers-Danlos syndrome.
   D. functional secondary to mitral dysfunction.
   E. endocarditis.

3. Third-order chordae of the mitral valve
   A. prevent billowing of the leaflets.
   B. attach to the free margin of the leaflet.
   C. arise from the lowest portion of the papillary muscle.
   D. are the smallest chords morphologically.
   E. insert into the annulus and maintain ventricular geometry.

4. The most commonly encountered lesion in degenerative mitral valve disease is
   A. restricted motion of the anterior leaflet.
   B. prolapse of the posterior leaflet.
   C. prolapse of the anterior leaflet.
   D. restricted motion of the posterior leaflet.
   E. annular calcification.

5. Systolic anterior motion (SAM) occurs in what percentage of patients following mitral valve repair for myxomatous disease?
   A. 5%
   B. 15%
   C. 20%
   D. 30%
   E. 45%

# Assessment in Mitral Valve Surgery

*Robert M. Savage, Taka Shiota, William J. Stewart,*
*Lee Wallace, and A. Marc Gillinov*

## HISTORICAL PERSPECTIVES

Over the last three decades, there have been great advances in mitral valve (MV) surgery closely affiliated with innovations in the intraoperative applications of echocardiography. In 1972, Johnson et al. reported the first use of echocardiography in MV surgery by demonstrating a successful open mitral commissurotomy using epicardial m-mode (1). Frazin, Talano, and Stephanides subsequently demonstrated the ability to accurately measure valve size and flow velocities using a transducer passed into the esophagus on a thin cable (2). In the late 1970s, Hisanga et al. placed a two-dimensional (2-D) ultrasound transducer prototype on a flexible gastroscope (3). Kremer, Hanrath, Roizen et al. first reported the intraoperative use of transesophageal echocardiography for monitoring patients undergoing abdominal aortic aneurysm resections in 1982 (4,5). Goldman and colleagues demonstrated the potential intraoperative impact of echocardiography by detecting mitral regurgitation (MR), utilizing contrast-enhanced epicardial imaging in valve surgery (6). Takamoto et al. demonstrated the use of real-time color flow mapping during valve surgery (7).

## IMPORTANCE OF INTRAOPERATIVE ECHOCARDIOGRAPHY (IOE) IN MV SURGERY

Early use of intraoperative guidance during MV repair surgery using Doppler color flow mapping was reported by Stewart and colleagues in 1986 (8). Since then, its use in guiding the intraoperative management of patients undergoing MV surgery has continued to expand. Intraoperative echocardiography (IOE) has demonstrated a unique ability to yield new diagnostic information impacting the surgical and hemodynamic management of patients in MV surgery (9–13). Based on such scientific evidence and expert opinion, the American College of Cardiology and the American Heart Association classified mitral valve repair and MV replacement (MVR) as Class I and IIA indications for intraoperative echocardiography (19). The ability of IOE to impact the outcome of surgical procedures involving the MV has established it as a universal diagnostic and monitoring standard of care for the intraoperative management of patients undergoing MV surgery (14–18).

## IMPORTANCE OF MV SURGERY IN THE FUTURE OF CARDIAC SURGERY

Consequently, there is a growing demand for clinicians with an experienced understanding of the echocardiographic assessment of the MV and its use in the intraoperative decision-making process (20). Because of the increasing numbers of patients projected to undergo surgical interventions for MV dysfunction over the next 20 years, this demand will continue (21–25). These projections are based on our aging population (Fig. 28.1), the high incidence of significant MV disease in the elderly, and

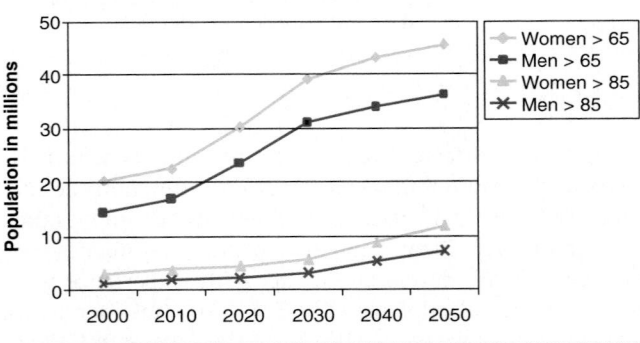

**FIGURE 28.1.** Population projections forecast the aging of America. By the year 2030, the United States Census Bureau estimates that 20% of individuals living in the United States will be over the age of 65.

| Variable | Men (n = 554) No. (%) | Women (n = 1,243) No. (%) |
|---|---|---|
| Rheumatic mitral stenosis | 2 (0.4) | 20 (2) |
| Mitral annular calcium | 194 (35) | 665 (53) |
| ≥ 1 + mitral regurgitation | 176 (32) | 415 (33) |
| Aortic stenosis | 79 (14) | 222 (18) |
| ≥ 1 + aortic regurgitation | 174 (31) | 352 (28) |
| Hypertrophic cardiomyopathy | 5 (3) | 47 (4) |
| Idiopathic dilated cardiomyopathy | 6 (1) | 10 (1) |
| Left atrial enlargement | 159 (29) | 460 (37) |
| LV hypertrophy | 226 (41) | 539 (43) |
| Abnormal LV ejection fraction | 159 (29) | 263 (21) |

**FIGURE 28.2A.** Aronow et al. demonstrated that more than 30% of individuals over the age of 60 have greater than mild mitral insufficiency. Understanding that some patients have significant structural abnormalities of the valve and supporting apparatus, the incidence of clinical disease involving the mitral valve will likely increase. Aronow WS, Ahn C, Kronzon I of Echocardiographic Abnormalities in African-American, Hispanic, and White Men and Women Aged > 60 Years. Am J Cardiol 2001: 87(9):1131–33.

| | Age (yr) | | | | |
|---|---|---|---|---|---|
| | 26–39 | 40–49 | 50–59 | 60–69 | 70–83 |
| Mitral regurgitation | (n = 93) | (n = 452) | (n = 515) | (n = 395) | (n = 90) |
| None (%) | 14.0 | 8.6 | 9.0 | 7.2 | 5.6 |
| Trace (%) | 76.3 | 75.0 | 74.0 | 66.5 | 70.8 |
| Mild (%) | 9.7 | 15.5 | 16.0 | 24.0 | 23.6 |
| ≥ Moderate (%) | 0.0 | 0.9 | 1.0 | 2.3 | 0.0 |

**FIGURE 28.2B.** The Framingham study population has demonstrated an increased incidence of mitral regurgitation associated with aging. More than 25% of individuals over the age of 60 demonstrated greater than mild mitral insufficiency.

the large percentage of patients having surgery within 10 years of their initial diagnosis of MV dysfunction (26–29) (Figs. 28.2 and 28.3). Because of the many advantages that MV repair offers the patient, an expanding number of cardiac centers are developing a successful experience with MV repair in all etiologies (30–32). With this increasing probability of successful MV repair, the American College of Cardiology (ACC) and American Heart Association (AHA) Task Force on Practice Guidelines for the Management of Patients with Valvular Heart Disease have recommended earlier surgical referral for patients with MV

dysfunction who are candidates with a high probability of successful MV repairs (MVRep) (33). Currently, the Society of Thoracic Surgeons STS database reports that only 33% of isolated MV procedures from reporting cardiac surgery programs are MV repairs (34). This is in contrast to the 90% incidence of MV repair reported by some cardiac centers experienced with MV repair (Fig. 28.4) (30–32). If the number of advanced MVRep procedures is to grow, it will require an increased availability of echocardiographic expertise throughout for the duration of such surgical procedures (20,33).

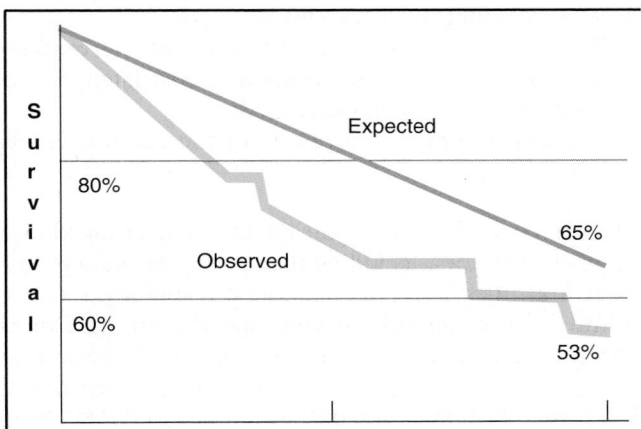

**FIGURE 28.3A.** There are wide ranges of long-term survival and freedom from operation in patients with MR. Enriquez-Sariano et al. compared the cardiac morbidity and long-term survival at 5 and 10 years in patients diagnosed with flail MV leaflet to normal survival for age. There was over a 6.0% excess mortality per year, with a 5- and 10-year survival of 65% and 53%, respectively. Patients with ejection fractions < 50% had a 10-year survival of 32%. Over 90% of patients had either received surgical intervention or expired at the end of 10 years. Timing of mitral valve surgery. Br Heart J; 28:79-85, Jan.

| EVENT | | OVERALL POPULATION | | |
|---|---|---|---|---|
| | NO. OF EVENTS | 5-YEAR RATE | 10-YEAR RATE | LINEARIZED YEARLY RATE |
| | | | | percent |
| Death from any cause | 45 | 28 ± 4 | 43 ± 7 | 6.3 |
| Death from cardiac cause | 31 | 21 ± 4 | 33 ± 7 | 4.3 |
| Congestive heart failure | 55 | 30 ± 4 | 63 ± 8 | 8.2 |
| Chronic atrial fibrillation† | 13 | 8 ± 3 | 30 ± 12 | 2.2 |
| Thromboembolism | 13 | 12 ± 3 | 12 ± 3 | 1.9 |
| Hemorrhage | 3 | 1 ± 1 | 3 ± 2 | 0.4 |
| Endocarditis | 10 | 5 ± 2 | 8 ± 3 | 1.5 |
| Mitral-valve surgery | 143 | 57 ± 3 | 82 ± 47 | 20.0 |
| Mitral-valve surgery or death | 188 | 69 ± 3 | 90 ± 3 | 26.3 |
| Outcome in subgroups of patients | | | | |

**FIGURE 28.3B.** Ling et al. and Enriquez-Sariano et al. have demonstrated that a high percentage of patients with structural mitral regurgitation either expire or have surgery within 10 years of their initial diagnosis. Timing of mitral valve surgery. Br Heart J; 28:79-85, Jan.

## INTRAOPERATIVE ECHOCARDIOGRAPHY (IOE) AND CRITICAL ISSUES IN MV SURGERY

For patients who are scheduled for elective MV surgery, the purpose of the IOE exam is not to replace the preoperative diagnostic evaluation of the patient. The purpose of the pre-cardiopulmonary bypass (pre-CPB) IOE exam is to confirm the severity of MV dysfunction and to refine the understanding of the mechanism of dysfunction, in addition to

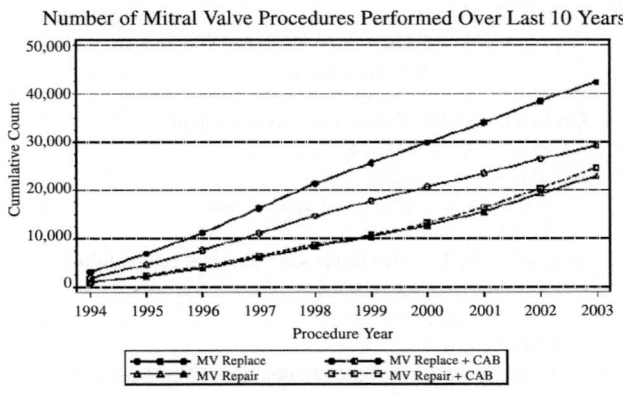

**FIGURE 28.4A.** The 2003 Executive Summary of the Society of Thoracic Surgeons documents the continued growth of mitral valve surgery. More than 30% of all mitral valve surgeries since 1994 involved a reconstructive approach to MV dysfunction (34). The percentage of MVRep versus replacements continues to increase.

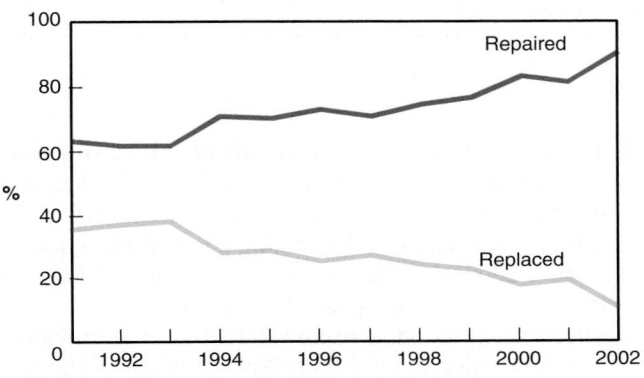

**FIGURE 28.4B.** The percentage of mitral valve repair procedures performed in patients undergoing isolated mitral valve surgery at the Cleveland Clinic has consistently increased since 1995.

addressing those critical issues that guide the intraoperative management of the patient and ensure the results of the surgical intervention (Table 28.1). However, there are some unusual scenarios where decisions to perform, or not perform, MV surgery are made following the results of the IOE exam.

1. The first of these involves patients with preoperative mild to moderate MR or MS who are undergoing another cardiac surgical procedure and confirmation of the decision to avoid MV surgery is desired. In these circumstances, customary monitors are placed, prior to induction, to better understand the patient's baseline hemodynamics. During the intraoperative assessment, hemodynamics similar to those recorded at a preoperative echocardiographic exam or just prior to induction are reproduced.

▶ **TABLE 28.1.    Intraoperative Echocardiography Exam and Critical Issues in MV Surgery**

1. **Confirm and Refine Preoperative Assessment**
   • Confirm MV dysfunction and severity
   • Determine repairability of valve
      • Refine pathoanatomy and mechanism
      • Explain variances
2. **Determine the Need for Unplanned Surgical Intervention**
   • Secondary pathophysiology
   • Associated abnormality
   • Unrelated process
3. **Determine Cardiac Dysfunction Impacting Management**
   • Secondary pathophysiology
   • Dysfunction associated with primary etiology
   • Coexisting dysfunction
4. **Cannulation and Perfusion Strategy**
5. **Address Surgical Procedure-Specific Issues**
6. **Predict Complications**
7. **Assess Surgical Results**
   • Initial and ongoing patient management
   • Results of surgery
   • Complications

2. The second such scenario is significant MV dysfunction that was either undiagnosed or is more severe than was determined by the preoperative evaluation. When the MR is of surgical severity, adding a mitral procedure is often a good idea, as long as it does not prohibitively increase the surgical risk-to-benefit ratio.
3. The final situation is finding MR that is significantly less than expected or absent. When findings of the pre-CPB IOE suggest a change in the operative plan, considerable thought must be given to the reasons for this discrepancy. However, intraoperative conditions may underestimate the amount of MR present under "street conditions" that have led to the well-established plan to perform MV surgery. We often challenge such patients with afterload stress (volume loading and phenylephrine) to see if the underrepresentation of MR might be a transient or misleading issue. When the operative mission is changed substantially, it is helpful to contact the consultative clinicians who have been involved in the long-term management of the patient. These are also situations where it is advisable to use the most quantitative assessments of severity, such as those recommended by the ASE Nomenclature and Standards Committee Task Force on Native Valve Regurgitation (35).

Because MV repair is the preferred treatment for MV dysfunction of all etiologies, every patient is considered a potential candidate for repair. The most significant surgical issues that the initial intraoperative exam assists in resolving are:

1. The probability of successful MV repair
2. The necessity to perform other surgical interventions related to the patient's secondary, associated, or co-existing cardiovascular dysfunction.
3. The assessment of the results of the surgical procedure

The surgeon's ability to repair the MV is determined by a number of factors, including the underlying etiology, the structural integrity of the anatomic components of the mitral valve apparatus (MVAp), and the mechanism of dysfunction caused by the underlying pathologic process (36,37). The surgeon's strategy for repair or replacement is a result of examination of the anatomy of the MVAp in correlation with the functional assessment of the MVAp provided by the IOE exam. The direct inspection of the MVAp includes an evaluation of the left atrium (size and secondary regurgitant lesions), annulus (secondary jet lesions, degree dilatation, scarring, and deformity), valve leaflets (thickness, motion, and coaptation), chordae (redundancy, thickness, and presence of fusion or rupture), papillary muscle (elongation, infarct, or rupture), and the free wall of the left ventricle (LV). From this information, the surgeon establishes the most effective line of attack, incorporating a variety of MVRep techniques or replacing the valve.

For the surgeon who is less experienced in mitral valve repair surgery, the IOE exam contributes to an accelerated learning curve enabling him or her to immediately compare the findings of their direct inspection with those of the echocardiography examination. For the more accomplished surgeon who can develop a strategy from what he has learned from experience with the IOE exam, the echocardiographer provides greater assistance with the post-CPB assessment of the repair and, if necessary, determining the mechanism(s) of an initially unsuccessful MVRep or other potential post-CPB complications. However, even with the experienced surgeon, the IOE exam serves as a final preintervention diagnostic screen for previously undiagnosed but significant valve or other cardiac dysfunction.

The decision to perform additional surgical interventions is made during the pre-CPB evaluation for significant secondary pathophysiology and associated or coexisting cardiovascular disease. Chaliki et al. discovered that in 1,265 patients undergoing MV surgery, 146 (12%) had new precardiopulmonary bypass (pre-CPB) findings that altered their intraoperative management (38). Sheikh et al. evaluated 154 consecutive patients who had IOE assessment in conjunction with a valve operation. The IOE yielded unsuspected findings prior to cardiopulmonary bypass that either modified or changed the planned operation in 19% of patients (39). Other important issues that the IOE exam addresses include the cannulation-perfusion and myocardial protection strategy, specific surgical procedure-related issues (i.e., need for sliding annuloplasty), determination of the probability of certain post-CPB complications, and assessment of the results of surgical intervention. The information provided from the systematic IOE exam provides the intraoperative team with an up-to-date road map, which will guide the surgical decision-making process and direct the hemodynamic management of the patient throughout the operation (40).

## ORGANIZATION OF CHAPTER

Intraoperative echocardiography has become an integral part of the comprehensive management of the patient undergoing MV surgery. As we will see, it has a direct influence on the intraoperative decision-making process for the surgical and hemodynamic management of the patient. It has a lasting impact on long-term outcome. The majority of patients having MV surgery are customarily scheduled following a thorough and extensive evaluation. Consequently, the intraoperative focus shifts from one of exhaustive assessment of severity of MV dysfunction to those essential issues that will impact the course of the surgical intervention and, ultimately, patient outcome. These issues include an understanding of the mechanism(s) of MV dysfunction, the potential repairability of the valve, and the patient's intraoperative management. Consequently, we will emphasize the technique of the intraoperative exam used for developing a three-dimensional understanding of the etiology and mechanics causing dysfunction of the MVAp. This chapter will provide an understanding of how echocardiography is incorporated into the daily management of patients undergoing MV surgery. It will focus on those aspects of the intraoperative examination that permit an accurate and efficient assessment of the critical issues that must be addressed for patients undergoing MV surgery. To reinforce the fundamental considerations in the chapter, a summary of "Key Concepts" is provided at the beginning and a brief review at the conclusion. An overview of the surgical anatomy of the mitral valve apparatus (MVAp) and the imaging planes that are used in its intraoperative assessment are provided. We will then concentrate on the efficient approach to the systematic echocardiographic exam for patients undergoing MV surgery; this includes the evaluation of MV pathology, secondary pathophysiology, as well as associated or coexisting cardiovascular disease. Finally, we concentrate on specific additional details that are required from the intraoperative examination to ensure the successful outcome of patients undergoing the wide range of MV surgical interventions.

## KEY CONCEPTS

- The MVAp is a complex structure consisting of the fibrous cardiac skeleton, saddle-shaped mitral annulus, mitral valve leaflets, chordae, papillary muscles, and ventricular wall complex. Pathologic processes that lead to structural damage to the anatomic integrity of the components of the MVAp may result in mitral valve dysfunction.

- The purpose of the intraoperative echocardiographic IOE exam is to confirm and refine the patient's preoperative assessment as issues that are critical to their intraoperative management are resolved.

- Mitral valve repair is the treatment of choice for MV dysfunction resulting from all etiologies because of its superior long-term survival, preservation of ventricular function, and greater freedom from thromboembolism, endocarditis, and anticoagulant related complications.

- For patients scheduled for elective MV surgery, the most significant surgical issues that the IOE exam assists in resolving include the repairability of the MV apparatus (MVAp), the necessity to perform other surgical interventions, and the postcardiopulmonary bypass assessment of the surgical procedure and complications.

- The feasibility of MVRep is guided by the real-time assessment of the mitral valve apparatus and the mechanism of dysfunction by the IOE exam, in conjunction with the surgeon's direct inspection of the MVAp.

- The IOE exam is performed according to the unique demands of the cardiac surgical environment, with the pre-CPB and post-CPB exams organized by priority to ensure that critical issues are addressed should the patient require the initiation of CPB.

- The pre-CPB IOE exam determines the severity and anatomic mechanism of MV dysfunction, in addition to assessing secondary or associated pathophysiology, cannulation-perfusion strategy, the potential for post-CPB complications, and providing an ongoing assessment of cardiac function.

- The post-CPB IOE exam provides a quality assurance safety net with immediate assessment of the surgical procedure and diagnosis of complications related to the surgery or disease process.

- The IOE exam relies upon integrated methods of severity assessment that may be efficiently performed in a multitasking environment. The methods included here are those recommended by the American Society of Echocardiography's Task Force on Native Valvular Regurgitation. They have been validated by accepted standards to ensure their ability to reliably guide the intraoperative decision-making process.

- The severity of mitral valve dysfunction is evaluated intraoperatively by the integration of multiple two-dimensional and Doppler parameters. The reliance on any one method of assessing severity is weighted by dependability of the specific data acquired and the quantitative reliability of a particular technique. Such an integrated approach minimizes the individual measurement error inherent to each.

■ Color flow Doppler is a method to screen for severe MV dysfunction. Its use as a stand-alone method of severity assessment to guide the intraoperative decision-making process is not recommended (35).

## MITRAL VALVE APPARATUS (MVAp)

### Normal Anatomy of the Mitral Valve Apparatus

The mitral valve apparatus is the anatomical term describing the structures associated with MV function. It consists of the fibrous skeleton of the heart, the mitral annulus, mitral leaflets, mitral chordae, and the papillary muscle-ventricular wall complex (Fig. 28.5) (41–45). This complex structure is comprised of the tensor apparatus (fibrous annulus, left ventricular myocardium from the fibrous MV annulus to the base of papillary muscle insertion, the papillary muscles, and the chordae) and the valvular apparatus (valve leaflets). Maintenance of the continuity of the tensor and valvular apparatus is essential for normal ventricular and MV function (41,42).

### Fibrous Skeleton

The fibrous skeleton of the heart is formed by the three U-shaped cords of the aortic annulus and their extensions, forming the right trigone, left trigone, and a smaller fibrous structure from the right aortic coronary cusp to the root of the pulmonary artery (42,44,46). This skeleton plays a primary function in structural support of the heart. The U-shaped cords of the aortic annulus merge to form the right and left fibrous trigone (46). A fibrous skeleton extends between the aortic and mitral annulus and is referred to as the intervalvular fibrosa (44–46).

### Mitral Annulus (Fig. 28.7 A,B, C, and D)

Fibrous tissue extends from the left and right atrioventricular orifices, forming the annulus of the mitral and tricuspid valves (41,43,47,48). The mitral annulus serves as a transition between the left atrium, mitral leaflets, and left ventricle. The base of the anterior mitral valve leaflet (AMVL) is closely associated with the left trigone, inter-trigonal space, and right trigone area (Fig. 28.6) (44). The fibrous mitral annulus is an ellipsoidal, three-dimensional, saddle-shaped structure that thins posteriorly where it is more prone to dilatation in pathologic conditions (Figs. 28.7A–28.7C) (48). The resulting increased tension on the posterior valve leaflet at its thinnest region contributes to the 60% incidence of chordal tears. The annulus is saddle-shaped during systole but changes to a circular shape in diastole (Fig. 28.7B) (36). The anterior mitral annulus is more rigid. It undergoes less change in shape during the cardiac cycle and is less prone to dilation (47,48). The U-shaped minor axis of the ellipsoid annulus is best visualized and measured in the midesophageal long-axis (LAX) imaging plane, whereas the U-shaped major axis is best visualized and measured in the ME commissural imaging plane

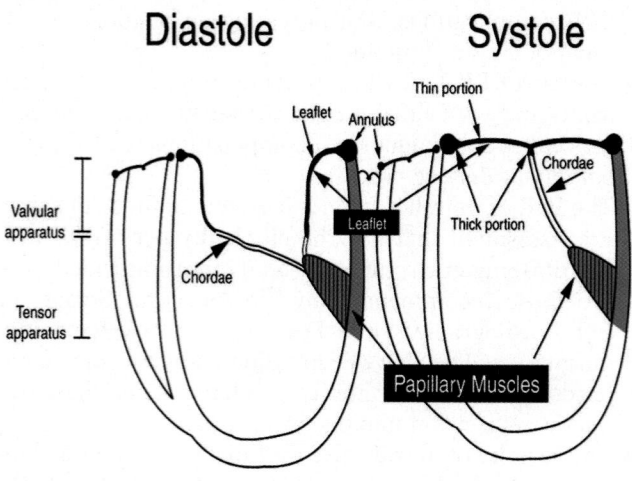

**FIGURE 28.5.** The mitral valve is composed of five distinct anatomic structures including the mitral annulus, valve leaflets, chordae, papillary muscles and ventricular wall. Dysfunction of any one of these structures will eventually interfere with the effective coaptation of the valve leaflets with associated valve regurgitation and its associated sequelae.

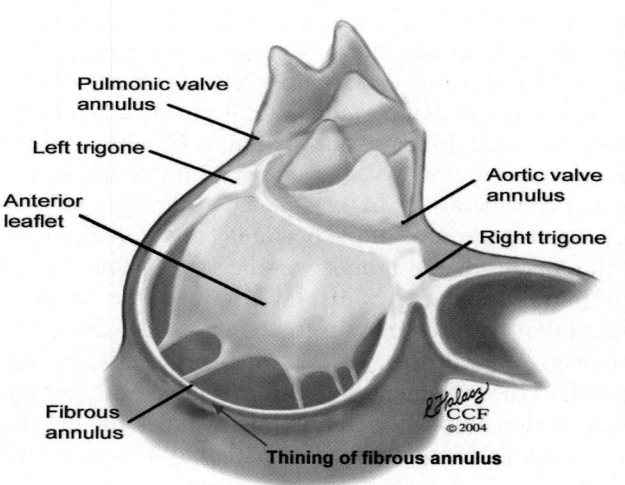

**FIGURE 28.6.** The fibrous skeleton of the heart is formed by the three U-shaped cords of the aortic annulus and by extensions forming the right trigone, left trigone and a smaller fibrous structure from the right aortic coronary cusp to the root of the pulmonary artery. The skeleton provides a rigid structural foundation for the valves and chambers of the heart. The anterior leaflet attaches to the fibrous skeleton at the rigid intervalvular fibrosa, giving it less flexibility and a tendency to dilate anteriorly. The fibrous tissue of the annulus thins posteriorly (*red arrow*).

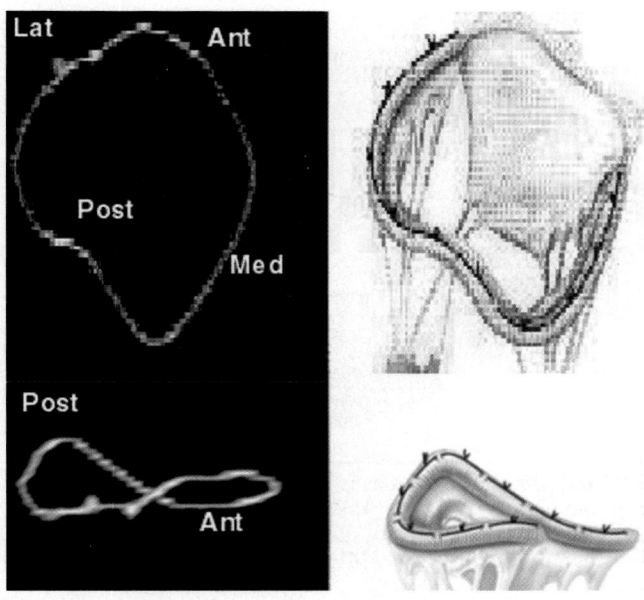

**FIGURE 28.7A.** Three-dimensional shape of MV annulus and with a three-dimensional annuloplasty ring.

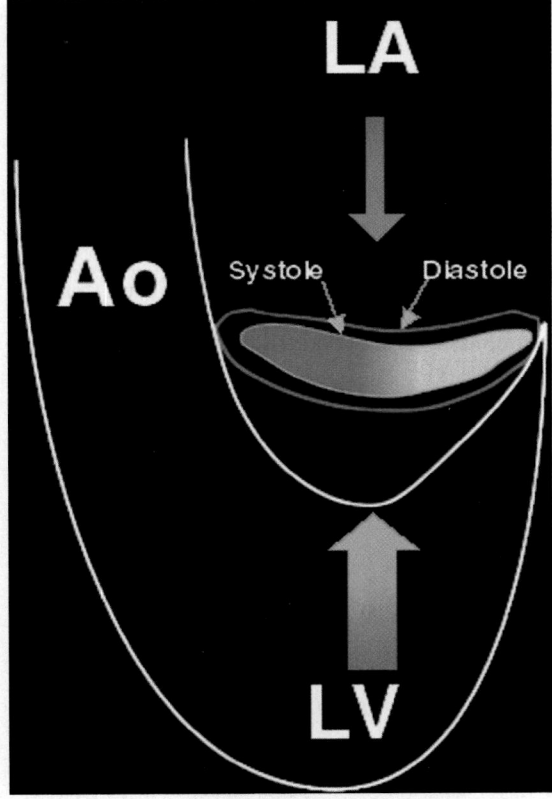

**FIGURE 28.7B.** During systole, the circular annulus circumferentially narrows, becoming a 3-dimensional saddle-shaped annulus. This effectively decreases the size of the MV orifice. Fibrosis or calcification of the annulus interferes with its mobility and effectively increases the area requiring leaflet apposition to prevent regurgitant flow.

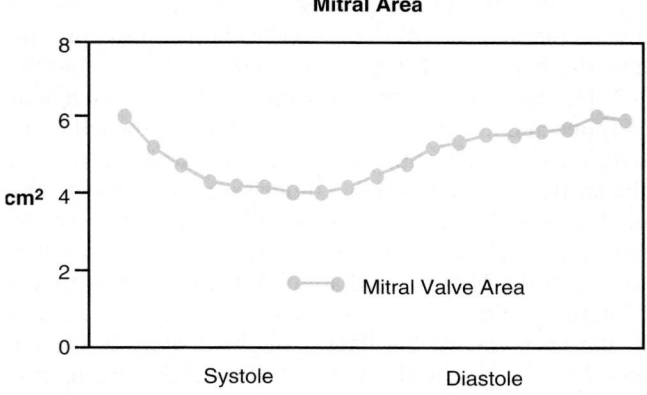

**FIGURE 28.7C.** The fibrous mitral annulus is an ellipsoidal saddle-shaped structure, which thins posteriorly where it is more prone to dilatation in pathologic conditions. During systole the annulus decreases in size and becomes saddle-shaped. In diastole it changes to a circular shape. The anterior mitral annulus is more rigid and has minimal change in shape during the cardiac cycle.

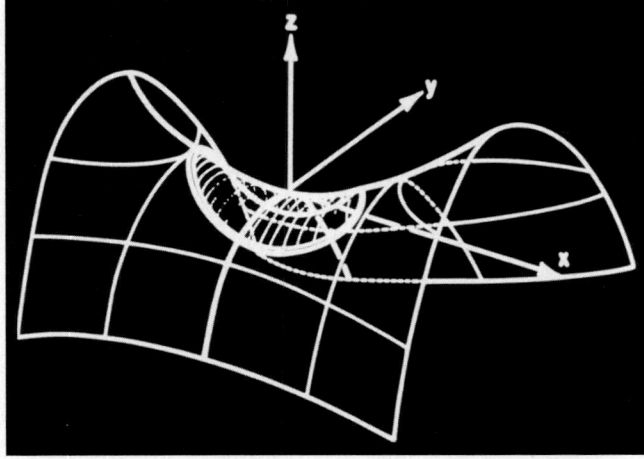

**FIGURE 28.7D.** The 3-dimensional shape of the annulus demonstrating the most superior (farthest from apex) points in the anterior-posterior orientation (ME LAX TEE plane). The most inferior (nearest the apex) points of the annulus are in the inferoseptal and anterolateral plane (ME Com TEE plane). Using the ME Com imaging plane will result in lower specificity in the diagnosis of MV prolapse or excessive leaflet motion.

(Fig. 28.7C). Accordingly, prolapse of valve leaflets (extension above the plane of the mitral annulus) is more accurately assessed in the long-axis imaging plane due to its more basal position compared to the commissural imaging plane (41,46,48).

### Mitral Valve Leaflets

Morphologically, the MV has two leaflets referred to as the anterior and posterior leaflets (AMVL and PMVL).

The mitral leaflets are attached to the fibrous annulus and to the free wall of the ventricle via papillary muscles and the primary edge and secondary midvalve chordae (43–45). The anterior mitral leaflet (AMVL) is triangular in shape and attached to the fibrous body at the left coronary cusp and anterior half of the noncoronary cusp of the aortic valve. The AMVL comprises about 55% to 60% of the total MV area and about 30% of the annular circumference (42,43). The posterior leaflet comprises 40% to 45% of the MV area and attaches to the mitral annulus posteriorly (Fig. 28.8) (41,42). As the heart normally lies in the chest cavity, the PMVL height (length) is usually less than the height of the AMVL (Fig. 28.9). During systole, the leaflets come together along a "line of coaptation," which extends anteriorly to the anterolateral commissure and posteriorly to the posteromedial commissure (Fig. 28.10). During diastole, the middle of the leaflet initially moves toward the ventricle followed by opening of the valve at the leaflet edges (44,48) (Fig. 28.11). The middle of the leaflet opens before the commissures. Once the leaflet extends fully it may flutter and drift upwards until the atrial contraction. The surface of each leaflet is divided into a rough zone (coapting surface where primary and secondary chords attach), clear zone (midportion of leaflet, secondary chordae attachments), and basal zone (leaflet attachment to the annulus, insertion of posterior tertiary chordae) (49). The basal two-thirds of each leaflet are smoother than the distal third. The combined surface area of the mitral leaflets is twice that of the mitral orifice. This permits large areas of coaptation with a normal 3 mm to 5 mm of residual leaflet apposition distal to the point of coaptation (43–45). This line of coaptation

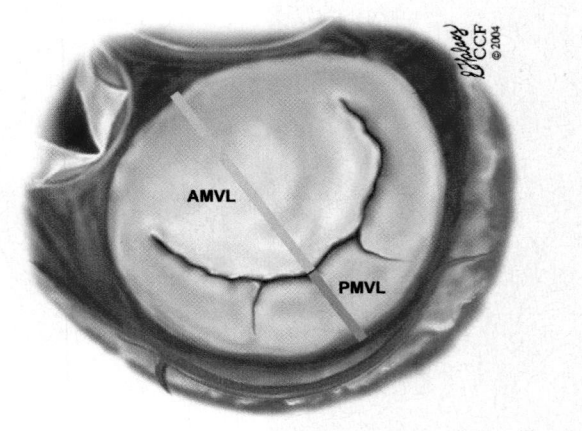

**FIGURE 28.9.** The MV has two leaflets referred to as the anterior and posterior leaflets (AMVL and PMVL). As the heart normally lies in the chest cavity, the PMVL height (length) is usually less than the height of the AMVL.

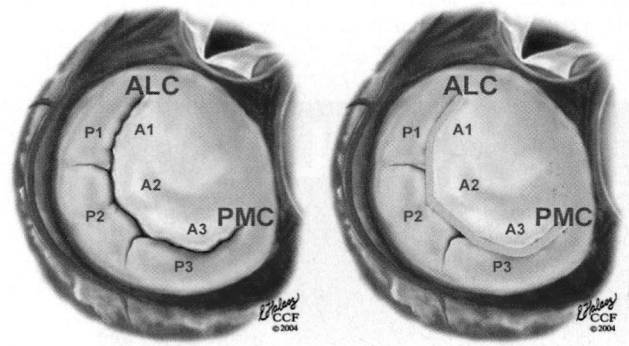

**FIGURE 28.10.** During systole, the leaflets come together along a "line of coaptation," which extends anteriorly to the anterolateral commissure (ALC ) and posteriorly to the posteromedial commissure (PMC).

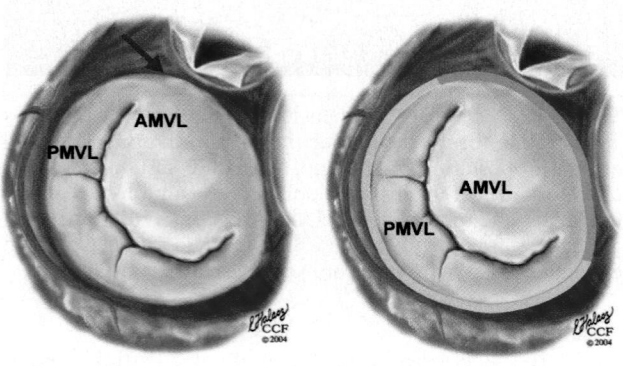

**FIGURE 28.8.** The MV has two leaflets referred to as the anterior and posterior leaflets (AMVL and PMVL). The mitral leaflets are circumferentially attached to the fibrous annulus. The anterior mitral leaflet (AMVL) is attached to the same fibrous body as the left coronary cusp (→). The anterior mitral valve leaflet (AMVL) comprises about 55% to 60% of the total MV area and about 30% to 40% of the annular circumference (—). The posterior leaflet comprises 40% to 45% of the MV area, and 60% to 70% of the circumference attaches to the mitral annulus posteriorly.

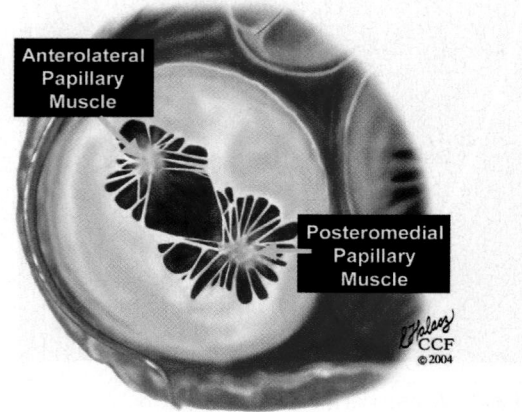

**FIGURE 28.11.** During diastole, the middle of the leaflet moves toward the ventricle with opening of the valve at the leaflet edges. The middle of the leaflet opens before the commissures. Once the leaflet extends fully, it may loiter until atrial contraction.

between the two leaflets is semicircular and influences the segments of the valve leaflets, which are visualized in the standard imaging planes (Fig. 28.12). There is a range of mitral commissural orientations due to variation in the degree of annular size and rotation of the heart caused by individual variations and enlargement of chambers. Consequently, the commissure may be oriented more clockwise in some individuals, explaining the variability of segmental mitral anatomy visualized at the same transducer rotation in different patients (Fig. 28.13). The posterior MV leaflet consists of three scallops that are separated by prominently distinct indentations called clefts (Fig. 28.14). These scallops are referred to as lateral, middle, and medial. The lateral scallop is closest to the left atrial appendage (43,45). The anterior leaflet, for purely descriptive purposes, is segmented into the corresponding lateral, middle, and medial thirds.

### Chordae Tendineae

Chordae are fibrous attachments extending from the leaflet to the papillary muscles and posterior ventricular wall. During systole, the papillary muscles contract and keep the chordae taut, preventing prolapse of the leaflets into the left atrium. The spaces between the chordae also serve as secondary orifices between the left atrium and left ventricle (41,43). With rheumatic fusion of the chordae, subvalvular narrowing of the ventricular inflow may be more pronounced than that caused by leaflet fusion

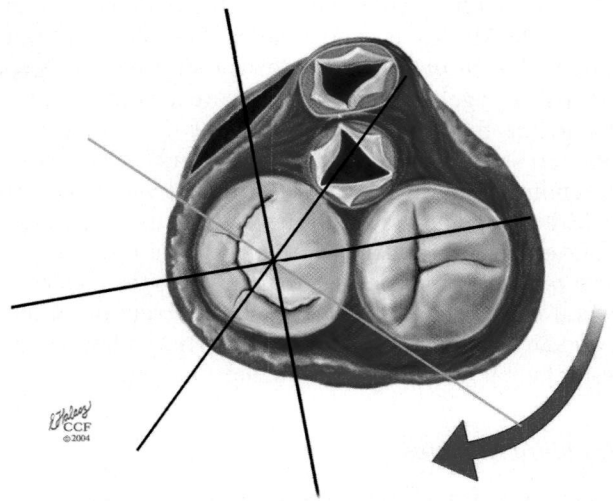

**FIGURE 28.13.** There is a range of mitral commissural shapes and orientations due to variation in annular size and rotation of the heart. This may be caused by individual variations and/or by enlargement of chambers that rotate the orientation of the commissure. Because of the fibrous skeleton, the rotation between the mitral valve and aortic valve is consistent.

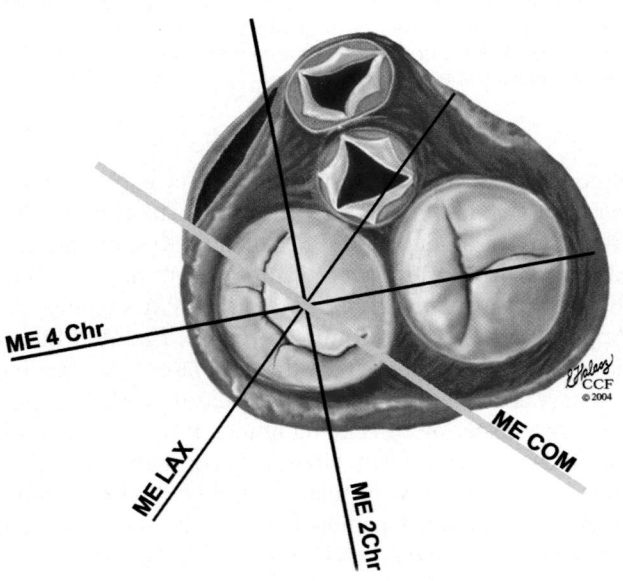

**FIGURE 28.12.** The line of coaptation between the two leaflets is semicircular, and the orientation of the commissure determines the segments of the valve leaflets that are visualized in the standard imaging planes.

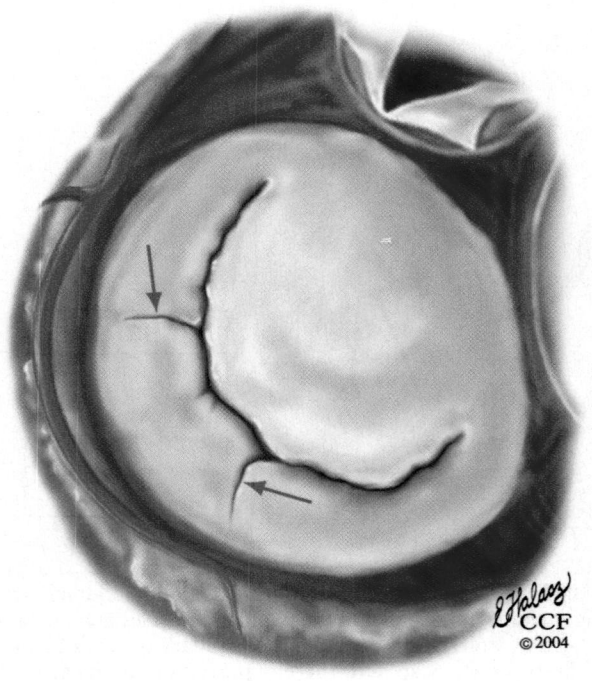

**FIGURE 28.14.** The posterior MV leaflet consists of three scallops that are separated by prominently distinct indentations called clefts (→). These scallops are referred to as the (antero) lateral, middle, and (postero) medial. The (antero) lateral scallop is closest to the left atrial appendage. The anterior leaflet, for purely descriptive purposes, is segmented into the corresponding lateral, middle, and medial thirds.

(45). Up to 120 chordae attach to the undersurface and edge of the MV leaflets and annulus (Fig. 28.15). They are classified as *primary chordae* (extending from the PM to the leaflet edge), *secondary chordae* (extending from the PM to the mid-undersurface belly of the leaflet at the junction of the rough and clear zone), and *tertiary chordae* (extending from the posterior ventricular wall to the base of leaflet or annulus) (49). There are usually two dominant anterior secondary chordae that are referred to as strut or stabilizing, chordae, that attach to the medial and lateral halves of the AMVL (49,50). Interruption of these secondary stabilizing or posterior tertiary chordae may result in deterioration of ventricular function.

### Papillary Muscles

Originating from the anterolateral and posteromedial walls of the left ventricle, (between the middle and apical segments), are the two papillary muscles named due to their segmental ventricular origin, *anterolateral papillary* (ALPM) and *posteromedial papillary muscles* (PMPM) (41–43,49). These papillary muscles run parallel to the adjacent ventricular wall. The larger ALPM usually has one or two heads, whereas the smaller PLPM may have two or

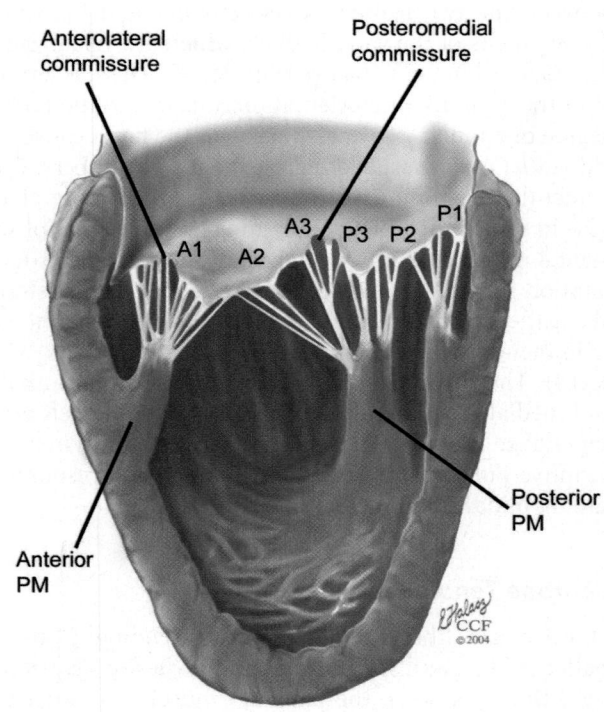

**FIGURE 28.16.** Originating from the anterolateral and posteromedial walls of the left ventricle (between the middle and apical segments) are the two papillary muscles called by their segmental ventricular origin: *anterolateral papillary muscle* (ALPM) and *posteromedial papillary muscle* (PMPM). These papillary muscles run parallel to the adjacent ventricular wall. The larger ALPM usually has one or two heads whereas the smaller PLPM may have two or three. Chordal tendons from the head of each papillary muscle attach to both of the MV leaflets. The chordae that arise from the anterolateral PM extend to the lateral halves of the posterior and anterior MV leaflets. Consequently the ALPM and PMPM subtend and support their respective commissure (49).

three. Chordal tendons from the head of each papillary muscle attach to both of the MV leaflets. The chordae that arise from the anterolateral PM extend to the anterolateral halves of the posterior and anterior MV leaflets (Fig. 28.17). Consequently the ALPM and PMPM subtend and support their respective commissure (49). The ALPM muscle is perfused by blood from the left anterior descending coronary artery and circumflex, whereas the PMPM is supplied by a posterior descending branch from a right dominant RCA or left dominant circumflex coronary artery (51). Consequently, isolated papillary muscle infarct or rupture of the posteromedial papillary muscle is more common than a rupture of the anterolateral papillary muscle.

### Left Ventricle

The anterolateral and posteromedial papillary muscles are inserted into the anterolateral and posteroinferior

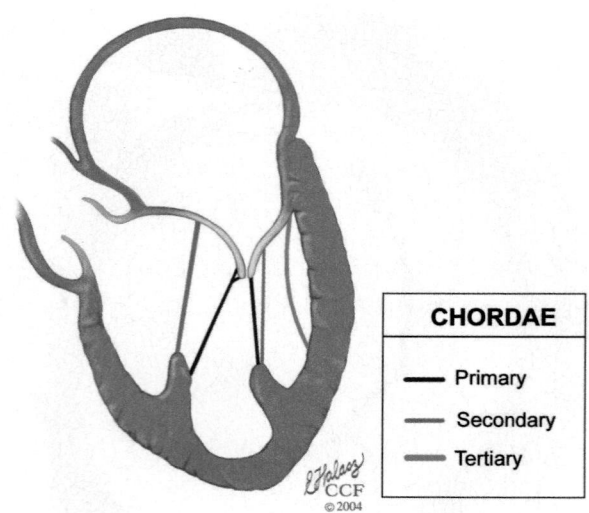

**FIGURE 28.15.** Chordae are fibrous tendon-like attachments extending from the leaflet to the papillary muscles and posterior ventricular wall. During systole, the papillary muscles contract and keep the chordae taut, thereby preventing prolapse of the leaflets into the left atrium. Tandler and Quain classified chordae as first, second, and third order. The first order attach to the leaflet edges adjacent to the commissure. Secondary rough zone chordae insert 8 mm from the free margin. There are two dominant secondary chordae (strut or stay chordae) going to the medial and lateral halves of the AMVL. Third order basal chordae only extend to the base of the PMVL. And maintain annular ventricular relation during the cardiac cycle.

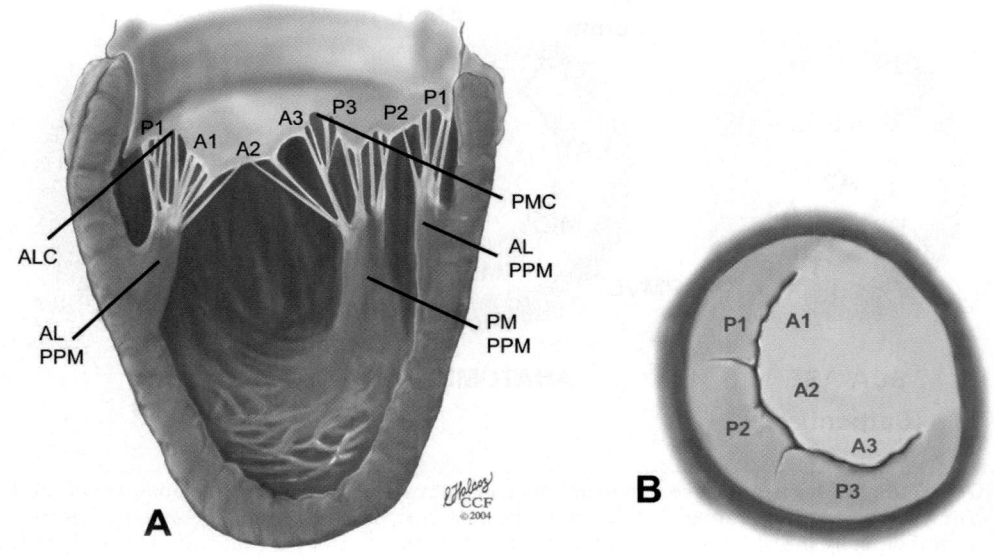

**FIGURE 28.17. A:** The posterior mitral valve leaflet (PMVL) and its supporting chordae are illustrated in blue. The anterior mitral valve leaflet (AMVL) and its supporting chordae are shown in beige. The anterolateral papillary muscle (ALPM) provides chordae to the lateral half of the PMVL and the lateral half of the AMVL. The posteromedial papillary muscle (PMPM) provides chordae to the medial half of the PMVL and the medial half of the AMVL. **B:** The PMVL and its 3 scallops are illustrated in blue coloration. The AMVL and its 3 segments are illustrated in beige.

segments of the left ventricle in the region near the interface between the middle and apical thirds of the ventricular chamber (41,44,51). The mechanical tensor function of the MVAp is maintained through the continuity that the ventricular walls provide in connecting the papillary muscles with the MV annulus (41). If there is scarring in the anterolateral or posteromedial free walls of the left ventricle, this may result in traction on the MV annulus and deformity throughout the cardiac cycle. This may lead to restriction of the PMVL during systole, with a resulting override of the AMVL and a posteriorly directed regurgitant jet.

### Nomenclature of the Mitral Valve Apparatus (MVAp)

There are three segmental nomenclatures commonly employed to describe the anatomy of the MVAp: the ASE-SCA (Carpentier), the anatomic, and the Duran (Fig. 28.18). The American Society of Echocardiography (ASE) Nomenclature and Standards Committee and the Society of Cardiovascular Anesthesiologists (SCA) adopted the Carpentier system for standardizing the segmental leaflet nomenclature (52). The Duran nomenclature system is an extremely valuable contribution to our understanding of

the MVAp because it is established on the chordal distribution between the papillary muscles and the valve leaflet segments (43).

The ASE-SCA nomenclature (Carpentier) defines the three scallops of the posterior leaflet as P1 (lateral), P2 (middle), and P3 (medial) (Figs. 28.18 and 28.19). The P1 (lateral) scallop is adjacent to the anterolateral commissure and is closest to the left atrial appendage. The P3 scallop is adjacent to the posteromedial commissure (52). This nomenclature defines the three corresponding areas of the anterior leaflet and A1 (opposite P1), A2 (opposite P2), and A3 (opposite P3).

With the anatomic nomenclature (Fig. 28.18), the posterior leaflet consists of three scallops: lateral (antero), middle, and medial (postero) as described above (52). The (antero) lateral scallop is closest to the left atrial appendage. The anterior leaflet, for purely descriptive purposes, is divided into the corresponding lateral, middle, and medial thirds. The anterolateral papillary muscle provides chordae to the lateral halves of the AMVL and PMVL (53). Consequently, the middle scallop of the posterior leaflet and middle segment of the anterior leaflet receive chordae from both papillary muscles (Figs. 28.17–28.19).

The Duran nomenclature system is based on the chordal distribution and refers to the three scallops of the

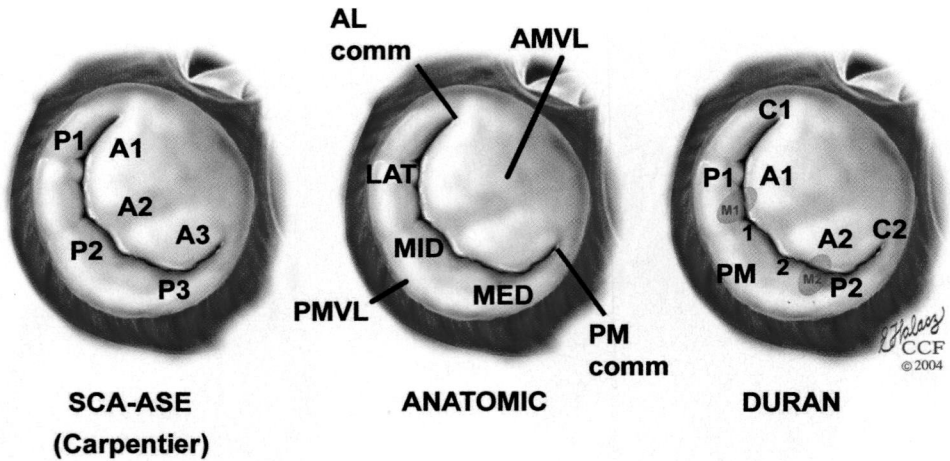

**FIGURE 28.18.** There are three segmental nomenclatures used to describe the anatomy of the MV apparatus: the ASE-SCA (Carpentier adoption), the anatomic, and the Duran. The American Society of Echocardiography (ASE) Nomenclature and Standards Committee of the ASE and the Society of Cardiovascular Anesthesiologists (SCA) adopted the Carpentier system for standardizing the segmental leaflet nomenclature. The Duran nomenclature is an extremely valuable contribution to our understanding of the MV apparatus because it is established on the chordal distribution between the papillary muscles and the valve leaflet segments.

*SCA-ASE standardized nomenclature:* P = PMVL segments (P1 = lateral scallop, P2 = middle scallop, P3 = medial scallop). A = AMVL segments (A1 = lateral segment, A2 = middle segment, A3 = medial segment). Chordae, commissures use anatomic descriptors (PMPM = posteromedial papillary muscle, ALPM = anterolateral papillary muscle)

*Duran nomenclature:* P = PMVL [(P1 = lateral scallop, PM = middle scallop, PM1 = lateral portion of middle scallop receiving chordae from ALPM (M1), PM2 = medial portion of middle scallop receiving chordae from PMPM (M2)]. The ALC is referred to as C1 and the PMC is C2.

## ASE/SCA Terminology
### (per Carpentier)

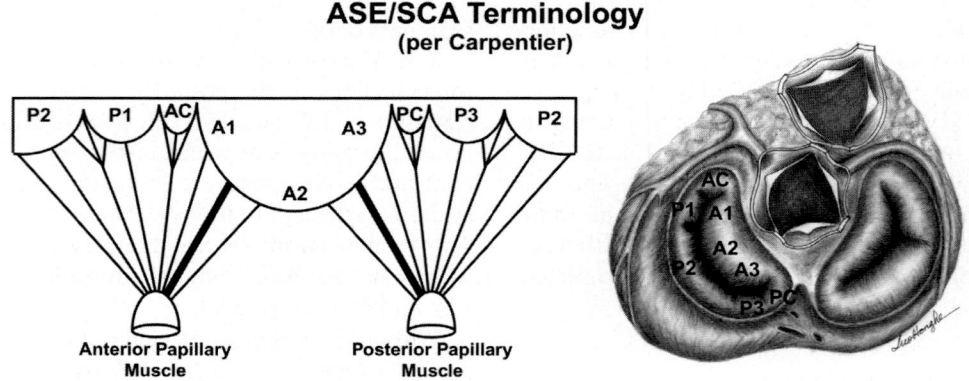

**FIGURE 28.19.** The *SCA-ASE nomenclature* (Carpentier) defines the three scallops of the posterior leaflet as P1 (lateral), P2 (middle), and P3 (medial). The P1 (lateral) scallop is adjacent to the anterolateral commissure and is closest to the left atrial appendage. The P3 scallop is adjacent to the posteromedial commissure. This nomenclature defines the three corresponding areas of the anterior leaflet and A1 (opposite P1), A2 (opposite P2), and A3 (opposite P3). Originating from the anterolateral and posteromedial walls of the left ventricle (between the middle and apical segments) are the two **papillary muscles** called by their segmental ventricular origin, *anterolateral papillary muscle* (ALPM) and *posteromedial papillary muscle* (PMPM). These papillary muscles run parallel to the adjacent ventricular wall. The larger ALPM usually has one or two heads, whereas the smaller PLPM may have two or three. Chordal tendons from the head of each papillary muscle attach to both of the MV leaflets. The chordae that arise from the anterolateral PM extend to the lateral halves of the posterior and anterior MV leaflets. The ALPM and PMPM subtend and support their respective commissure (49).

# Duran Terminology

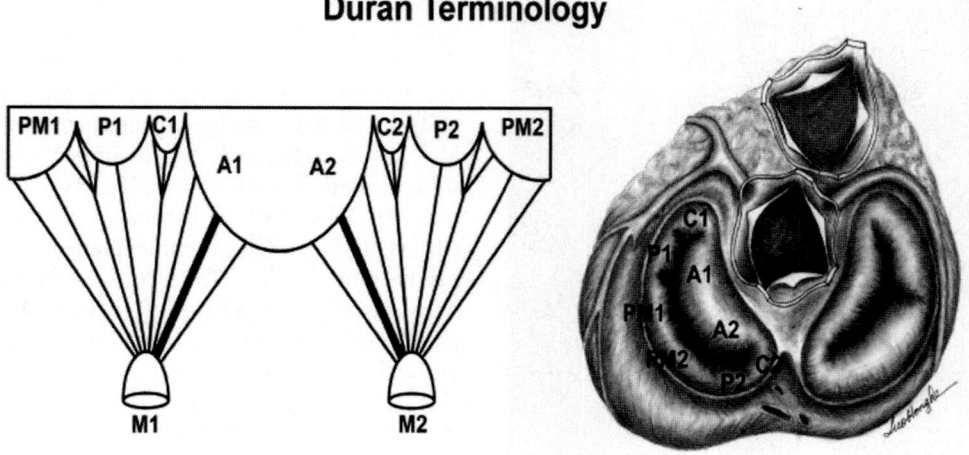

**FIGURE 28.20.** The *Duran nomenclature* system is based on the chordal distribution and refers to the three scallops of the posterior leaflet as P1 (lateral and closest to the left atrial appendage), PM (middle), and P2 (medial and adjacent to the posteromedial commissure) (53). The middle scallop (PM) is further subdivided into the PM1 and PM2, corresponding to the portion of the middle scallop that receives chordae from the anterolateral (M1) and posteromedial (M2) papillary muscles. The anterior leaflet is divided into two areas, A1 and A2, corresponding to the areas subtended by the corresponding chordal attachments from the anterolateral (M1) and posteromedial (M2) papillary muscles. In addition, the two commissural areas of the valve are defined as C1 (anterolateral, between A1 and P1) and C2 (posteromedial, between A2 and P2).

posterior leaflet as P1 (lateral and closest to the left atrial appendage), PM (middle), and P2 (medial and adjacent to the posteromedial commissure) (Figs. 28.17–28.20) (53). The middle scallop (PM) is further subdivided into the PM1 and PM2, corresponding to the portion of the middle scallop that receives chordae from the anterolateral (M1) and posteromedial (M2) papillary muscles. The anterior leaflet is divided into two areas, A1 and A2, corresponding to the areas subtended by the corresponding chordal attachments from the anterolateral (M1) and posteromedial (M2) papillary muscles (53). In addition, the two commissural areas of the valve are defined as C1 (anterolateral, between A1 and P1) and C2 (posteromedial, between A2 and P2).

## CORRELATION WITH IMAGING PLANES

The goal of the two-dimensional echocardiographic exam of the MVAp is to develop a three-dimensional understanding of the anatomy of the dysfunctional MV. While this may be routinely accomplished with three-dimensional transesophageal echocardiography in the future (Fig. 28.21), such an understanding is routinely available through a cognitive reconstruction of three-dimensional anatomy utilizing multiplane two-dimensional TEE imaging. The posterior and superior location of the midesophagus in relation to the adjacent blood-filled left

atrium and MV annulus enable detailed 360° imaging of the MV leaflets and apparatus utilizing a two-dimensional multiplane transducer (Fig. 28.22). If the rotational axis of the transducer is positioned in the center of the

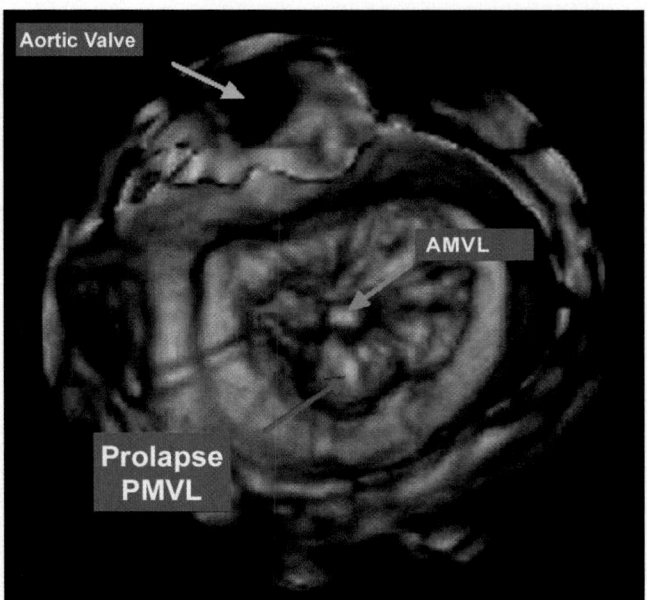

**FIGURE 28.21.** Three-dimensional visualization of a severe prolapse of the PMVL (red →) performed by TEE in the cardiac operating room. Calcified A2 of the AMVL (green →) and aortic valve are noted.

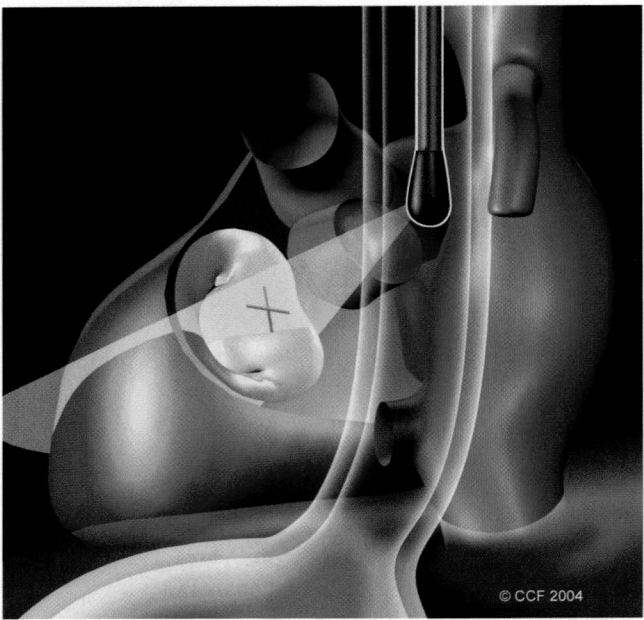

**FIGURE 28.22.** The posterior and superior location of the mid-esophagus in relation to the adjacent blood-filled left atrium and MV annulus enable ideal detailed 360° imaging of the MV leaflets and apparatus utilizing a two-dimensional multiplane transducer.

AMVL, it enables up to 360° imaging of the MV leaflets and an understanding of the three-dimensional structure of the MVAp (Fig. 28.23).

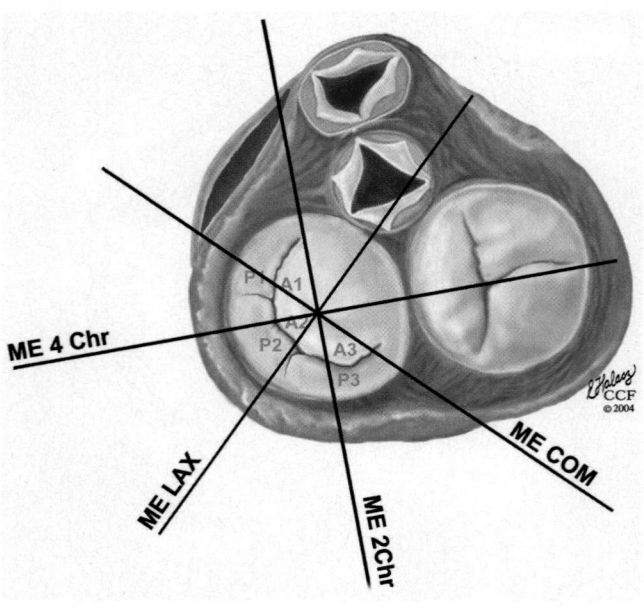

**FIGURE 28.23.** If the rotational axis of the transducer is positioned in the center of the anterior mitral valve leaflet (AMVL), it enables 360° imaging of the MV leaflets and an understanding of the three-dimensional structure of the MV apparatus.

The MV may be examined utilizing up to 10 or more variations of 6 of the recommended ASE-SCA imaging planes frequently used in evaluating the MVAp (Table 28.2). These include the midesophageal four-chamber (ME 4 Chr MV), midesophageal commissural (ME Com MV), midesophageal two-chamber (ME 2 Chr MV), midesophageal LAX (ME LAX MV), transgastric short-axis (TG SAX MV), and transgastric two-chamber (TG 2 Chr MV) planes. These image planes are obtained by manipulations of the TEE probe including advancing or withdrawing, turning right (clockwise) and left (counter-clockwise), rotating the transducer angulations forward or backward, and flexing the probe to the right or left (Fig. 28.24). For an expanded description of the probe manipulations for each of the standard imaging planes and their variations, please see the section on "Comprehensive Examination in MV Surgery" or Chapter 6, "Comprehensive and Abbreviated Intraoperative TEE Examination."

The following section lists the standard imaging planes and their variations in the sequence in which they are commonly utilized in the evaluation of the MVAp. The probe manipulation required to obtain an image plane, which is a variation of the "ASE-SCA recommended cross-sectional view," is included with the description of the visualized MV anatomy (52). The anatomic description for these imaging planes is always dependent on the three-dimensional orientation of the line of coaptation and the extent of probe manipulation.

## Midesophageal Four-Chamber MV and Variations

**Midesophageal Five-Chamber MV (ME 5 Chr MV)**
**Lower-Esophageal Four-Chamber MV (LE Four Chr MV) (Table 28.2, Figs. 28.25–28.27 and 28.55)**

### Midesophageal Four-Chamber MV (ME 4 Chr MV)

**Transducer Depth:** 30 cm
**Transducer Rotation:** 0°–15°
Depending on the orientation of the MV commissure and transducer rotation angle, the 2-D plane may cut through the A2 and P2 and/or P1 segments of the MV. On the monitor in this imaging plane, the anterior leaflet is displayed on the left and the posterior leaflet on the right. Proceeding from left to right are A2, midcommissure, and P2 and/or P1.

### Midesophageal Five-Chamber MV (ME 5 Chr MV)

**Variation of ME 4 Chr MV**
**Transducer Depth:** 30 cm

**Probe Manipulation: Withdraw from ME 4 Chr MV**
This imaging plane cuts through the left ventricular outflow tract. Depending on the orientation of the MV commissure and transducer rotation angle, the 2-D plane may cut through the A1 segment, anterolateral commissure, and P1 segments of the MV. On the monitor in this imaging plane, the anterior leaflet is displayed on the left and the posterior leaflet on the right. Proceeding from left to right are A1, anterolateral commissure, and P1.

*Lower-Esophageal Four-Chamber MV*
*(LE Four Chr MV)*

**Variation of ME 4 Chr**
**Transducer Depth:** 32 cm
**Probe Manipulation:** Advance
Depending on the orientation of the MV commissure and transducer rotation angle, the 2-D plane may cut through the A3 segment, posteromedial commissure, and the P3

scallop of the MV. On the monitor in this imaging plane, the anterior leaflet is displayed on the left and the posterior leaflet on the right. Proceeding from left to right are A3, posteromedial commissure, and P3.

## Midesophageal Commissural MV and Variations

*Midesophageal Commissural Right MV*
*(Table 28.2 and Fig. 28.29)*

*Midesophageal Commissural Left MV (Table 28.2 and Fig. 28.30) (Table 28.2, Figs. 28.28–28.30 and 28.47)*

*Midesophageal Commissural MV (ME Com MV) (Table 28.2 and Fig. 28.28)*

**Transducer Depth:** 30 cm
**Transducer Rotation:** 45°–70°

*(text continues on page 463)*

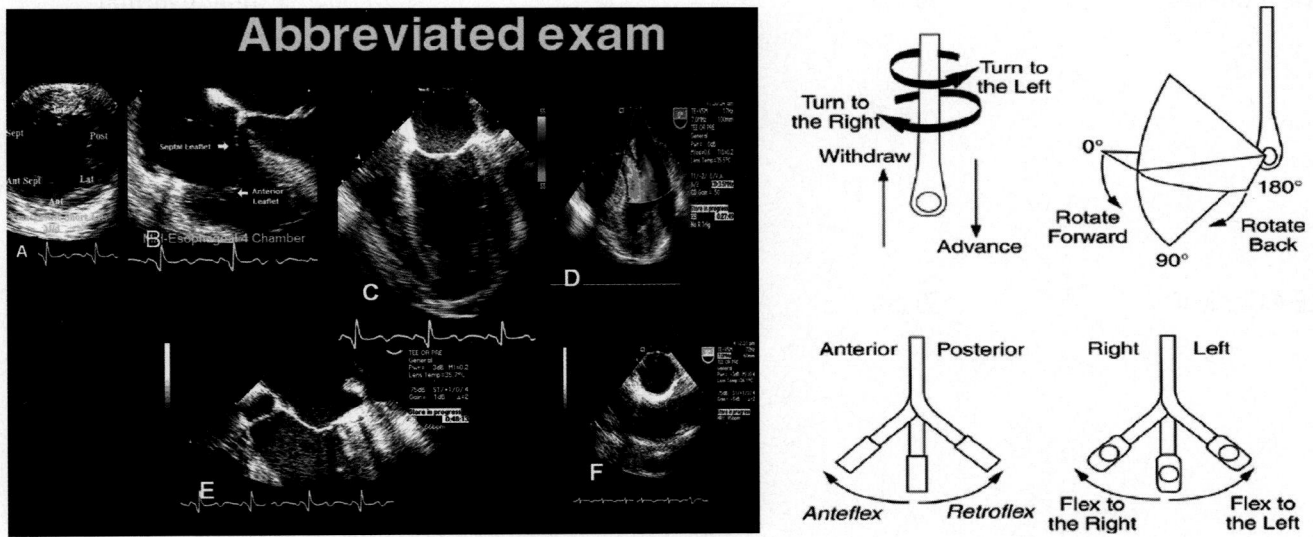

**FIGURE 28.24.** Standard image planes and their variations are obtained by manipulations of the TEE probe, including advancing or withdrawing, turning right (clockwise) and left (counterclockwise), rotating the transducer angulations forward or back, and flexing the probe to the right or left.

▶ TABLE 28.2.  Correlation of Image Plane and Cardiac Anatomy

| Imaging Plane Nomenclature | Probe Depth | Transducer Angle | Probe Maneuver |
|---|---|---|---|
| ME 5 Chr MV | 28 cm | 0–15° | Withdraw |
| ME 4 Chr MV | 30 cm | 0–15° | Probe Insertion |
| LE 4 Chr MV | 30 cm | 0–15° | Advance |
| ME Com MV | 30 cm | 45–70° | Rotate Transducer Angle Forward |
| ME Com Right MV | 30 cm | 45–70° | Turn Right (Clockwise) |

▶ TABLE 28.2.   **Correlation of Image Plane and Cardiac Anatomy** (Continued)

| 3 D Imaging Plane View | 2 D Anatomic Imaging Plane | Corrresponding Segmental Anatomy |
|---|---|---|
| | | |
| | | |
| | | |
| | | |
| | | |

*(continued)*

▶ TABLE 28.2.  **Correlation of Image Plane and Cardiac Anatomy** (Continued)

| Imaging Plane Nomenclature | Probe Depth | Transducer Angle | Probe Maneuver |
|---|---|---|---|
| ME Com Left MV | 30 cm | 45–70° | Turn Left (Counter–Clockwise) |
| ME 2 Chr MV | 30 cm | 80–110° | Rotate Transducer Angle Forward |
| ME LAX MV | 30 cm | 110–150° | Rotate Transducer Angle Forward |
| TG SAX$_B$ | 35 cm | 0–5° | Advance probe Rotate Transducer Angle Forward |
| TG 2 Chr | 35 cm | 70–90° | Rotate Transducer Angle Forward |

**TABLE 28.2.   Correlation of Image Plane and Cardiac Anatomy** (Continued)

| 3 D Imaging Plane View | 2 D Anatomic Imaging Plane | Corresponding Segmental Anatomy |
|---|---|---|
| | | |
| | | |
| | | |
| | | |
| | | |

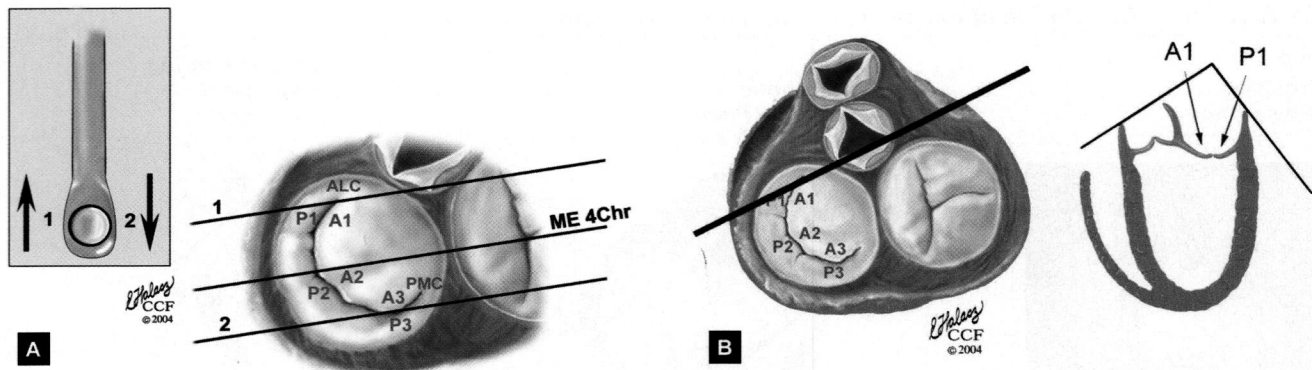

**FIGURE 28.25 A and B.** Midesophageal Five Chamber MV (ME 5 Chr MV). Variation of ME 4 Chr MV; Transducer Depth: 30 cm; Probe Manipulation: Withdraw from ME 4 Chr MV. **A:** The TEE probe is slowly withdrawn 1-2 cm from the ME 4 Chr imaging plane to obtain the ME 5 Chr view. The LE 4 Chr imaging plane is obtained by advancing the probe 1-2 cm from the ME 4 Chr plane. **B:** This imaging plane cuts through the left ventricular outflow tract. Depending on the orientation of the MV commissure and transducer rotation angle, the 2-D plane may pass through the A1 segment, anterolateral commissure, and P1 segments of the MV.

**FIGURE 28.26.** Four Chamber MV (LE Four Chr MV). Variation of ME 4 Chr transducer; Depth: 32 cm; Probe Manipulation: Advance depending on the orientation of the MV commissure and transducer rotation angle. The 2-D plane may pass through the A2 segment, middle commissure, and the P2 scallop of the MV. The height of the P2 and A2 may be measured in this plane for comparison with the ME LAX MV measurements.

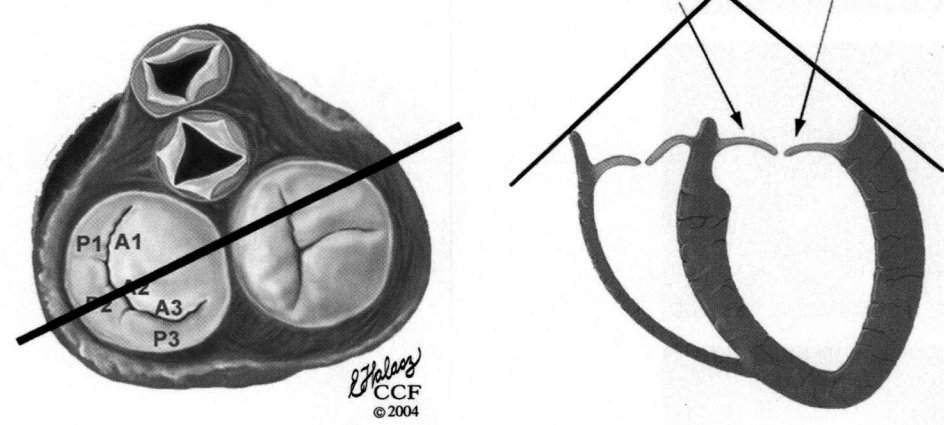

**FIGURE 28.27.** Lower-esophageal Four Chamber MV (LE Four Chr MV). Variation of ME 4 Chr transducer; Depth: 32 cm; Probe Manipulation: Advance depending on the orientation of the MV commissure and transducer rotation angle. The 2-D plane may pass through the A3 segment, posteromedial commissure, and the P3 scallop of the MV.

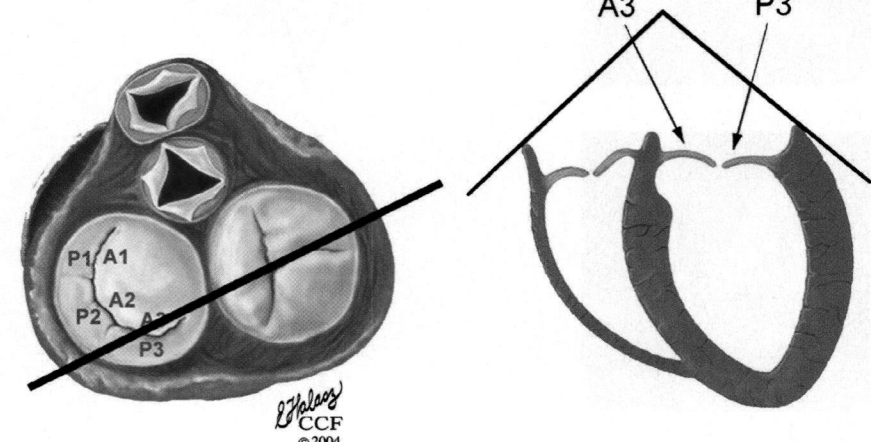

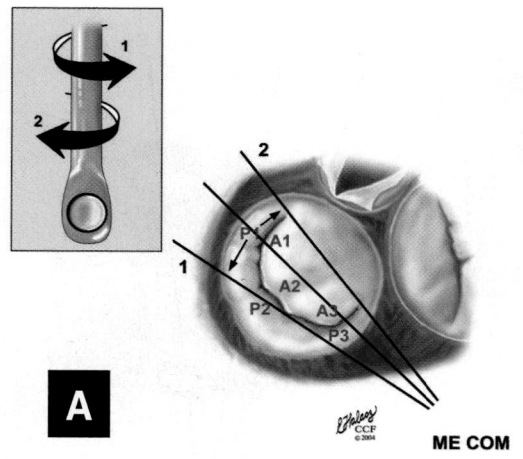

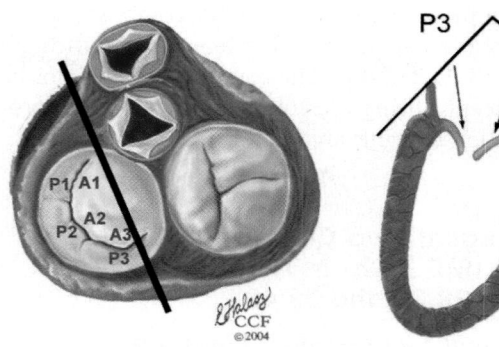

**FIGURE 28.29.** Midesophageal Commissural Right MV (Probe Turned Right) (ME Com_R MV). Variation of ME Com; Transducer Depth: 30 cm; Probe Manipulation: Turn left or counterclockwise; Transducer Rotation: 45-70°. Depending on the orientation of the MV commissure and transducer rotation angle, the 2-D plane may pass through the P3, A3, A2, and A1 segments.

**Transducer Rotation:** 45°–70°
**Probe Manipulation:** Turn right or clockwise
Depending on the orientation of the MV commissure and transducer rotation angle, the 2-D plane may cut through the P3 scallop, the posteromedial commissure, the A3 segment, the A2 segment, and the A1 segment. On the monitor (proceeding from left to right) are P3, the posteromedial commissure, A3, A2, and A1.

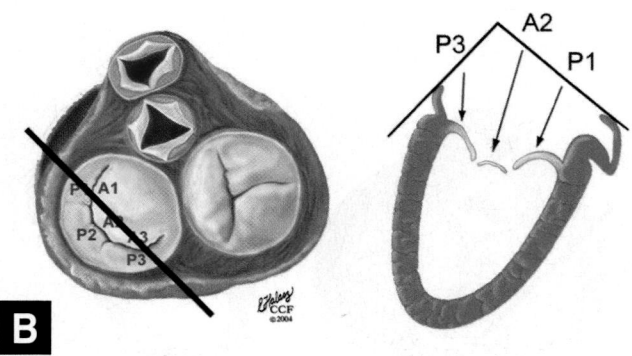

**FIGURE 28.28.** Midesophageal Commissural MV (ME Com MV). Transducer Depth: 30 cm; Transducer Rotation: 45-70° **A:** The ME Com MV is obtained by rotating the transducer forward to 45-70°. Turning the probe to the right (clockwise) and to the left (counterclockwise) enable visualization of the variations of this imaging plane. **B:** Depending on the orientation of the MV commissure and transducer rotation angle, the 2-D plane may cut through the P3 scallop, the posteromedial commissure, tip of A2, anterolateral commissure, and the P1 segments of the MV.

### Midesophageal Commissural Left MV (ME Com_L MV) (Table 28.2 and Fig. 28.30)

**Variation of ME Com**
**Transducer Depth:** 30 cm
**Transducer Rotation:** 45°–70°

Depending on the orientation of the MV commissure and transducer rotation angle, the 2-D plane may cut through the P3 scallop, the posteromedial commissure, tip of A2, anterolateral commissure, and the P1 segments of the MV. On the monitor (from left to right) are P3, posteromedial commissure, A2, anterolateral commissure, and P1. The annular plane drawn between the MV annulus on the left of the screen and the MV annulus on the right usually represents the most inferior (closest to the apex) aspects of the saddle-shaped annulus. A plane drawn between these points consequently may overcall MV prolapse.

### Midesophageal Commissural Right MV (ME Com_R MV) (Table 28.2 and Fig. 28.29)

**Variation of ME Com MV**
**Transducer Depth:** 30 cm

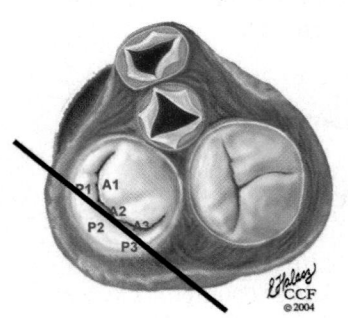
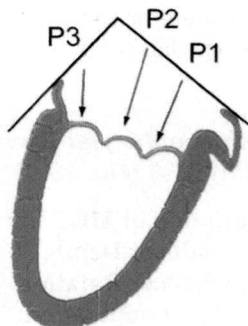

**FIGURE 28.30.** Midesophageal Commissural Left MV (Probe Turned Left) (ME Com_L MV): Variation of ME Com; Transducer Depth: 30 cm; Probe Manipulation: Turn left or counterclockwise; Transducer Rotation: 45-70°. Depending on the orientation of the MV commissure and transducer rotation angle, the 2-D plane may pass through the P3, P2, and P1 scallops.

**Probe Manipulation:** Turn left or counterclockwise
Depending on the orientation of the MV commissure and
transducer rotation angle, the 2-D plane may cut through
the P3, P2, and P1 scallops. The commissure may not be
visualized except during diastole. On the monitor (proceeding from left to right) are P3, P2, and P1.

## Midesophageal Two-Chamber MV and Variations (ME 2 Chr MV) (Table 28.2, Figs. 28.31–28.33 and 28.48)

### Midesophageal Two-Chamber Right MV

### Midesophageal Two-Chamber Left MV

### Midesophageal Two-Chamber MV (ME 2 Chr MV)

**Transducer Depth:** 30 cm
**Transducer Rotation:** 80°–110°
**Probe Manipulation:** Midline
Depending on the orientation of the MV commissure and
transducer rotation angle, the 2-D plane may cut through
the P3 scallop, the posteromedial commissure, and the
A3, A2, and A1 segments. On the monitor (proceeding
from left to right) are P3, posteromedial commissure, A3,
A2, and A1.

### Midesophageal Two-Chamber Right MV (ME 2 Chr_R MV) (Fig. 28.32)

**Variation of ME 2 Chr MV**
**Transducer Depth:** 30 cm
**Transducer Rotation:** (80°–110°)
**Probe Manipulation:** Turn right (clockwise)
Depending on the orientation of the MV commissure and
transducer rotation angle, the 2-D plane may cut through
the P3 scallop, the apex of the posteromedial commissure, the A3 segment, and the base of the A2 segment. On
the monitor (proceeding from left to right) are P3, posteromedial commissure, A3, and A2.

### Midesophageal Two-Chamber Left MV (ME 2 Chr_L MV) (Fig. 28.33)

**Variation of ME 2 Chr MV**
**Transducer Depth:** 30 cm
**Transducer Rotation:** 80°–110°
**Probe Manipulation:** Turn left or counterclockwise
Depending on the orientation of the MV commissure
and transducer rotation angle, the 2-D plane may cut
through the P3, P2, and P1 scallops. The commissure
may not be visualized except during diastole. On the
monitor (proceeding from left to right) are P3, P2,
and P1.

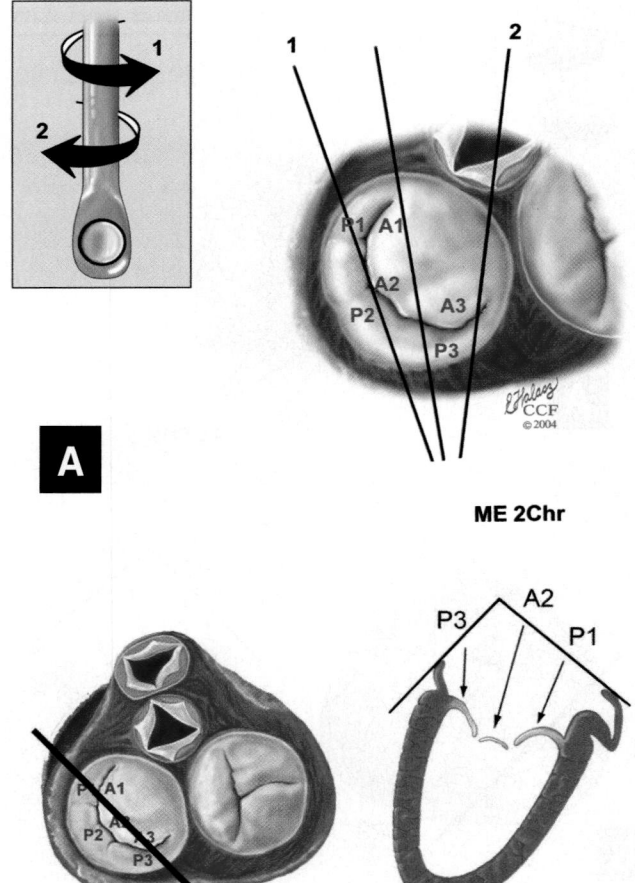

**ME 2Chr**

**FIGURE 28.31.** Midesophageal Two Chamber MV (ME 2 Chr
MV). Transducer Depth: 30 cm; Probe Manipulation: Midline;
Transducer Rotation: 80-110°. **A:** The ME 2 Chr imaging plane is
obtained by rotating the transducer forward to 80-110°. Variations of this plan are obtained by turning the probe to the right
and left. **B:** Depending on the orientation of the MV commissure
and transducer rotation angle, the 2-D plane may cut through
the P3 scallop, the posteromedial commissure, the A3 segment,
the A2 segment, and the A1 segment.

## Midesophageal Long-Axis MV and Variations (Table 28.2, Figs. 28.34–28.36 and 28.49)

### Midesophageal Long-Axis Right MV

### Midesophageal Long-Axis Left MV

### Midesophageal Long-Axis MV (ME LAX MV) (Table 28.2, Fig. 28.34)

**Transducer Depth:** 30 cm
**Transducer Rotation:** 110°–150°
Depending on the orientation of the MV commissure and
transducer rotation angle, the 2-D plane passes through
the minor axis of the MV annulus and aortic valve. The 2-D

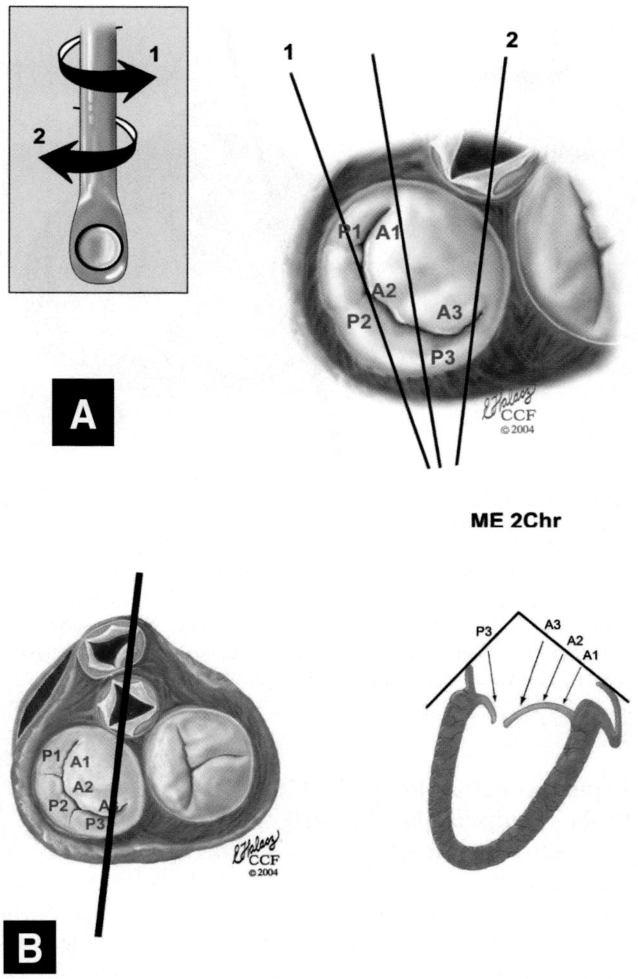

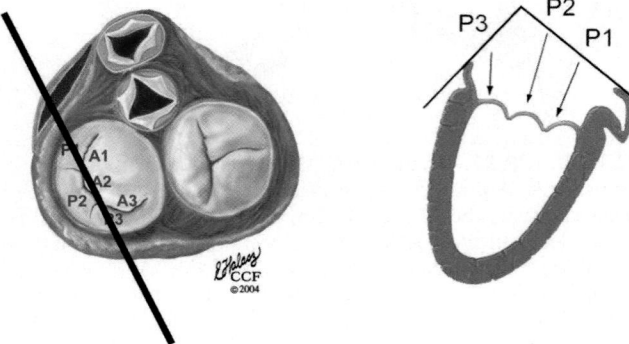

**ME 2Chr**

**ME LAX**

**FIGURE 28.32.** Midesophageal Two Chamber Right MV (Turned Right) (ME 2 Chr$_R$ MV). Variation of ME 2 Chr MV; Transducer Depth: 30 cm; Transducer Rotation: 80-110°; Probe Manipulation: Turn right (clockwise). Depending on the orientation of the MV commissure and transducer rotation angle, the 2-D plane may cut through the P3 scallop, the apex of the posteromedial commissure, the A3 segment, and base of the A2 segment.

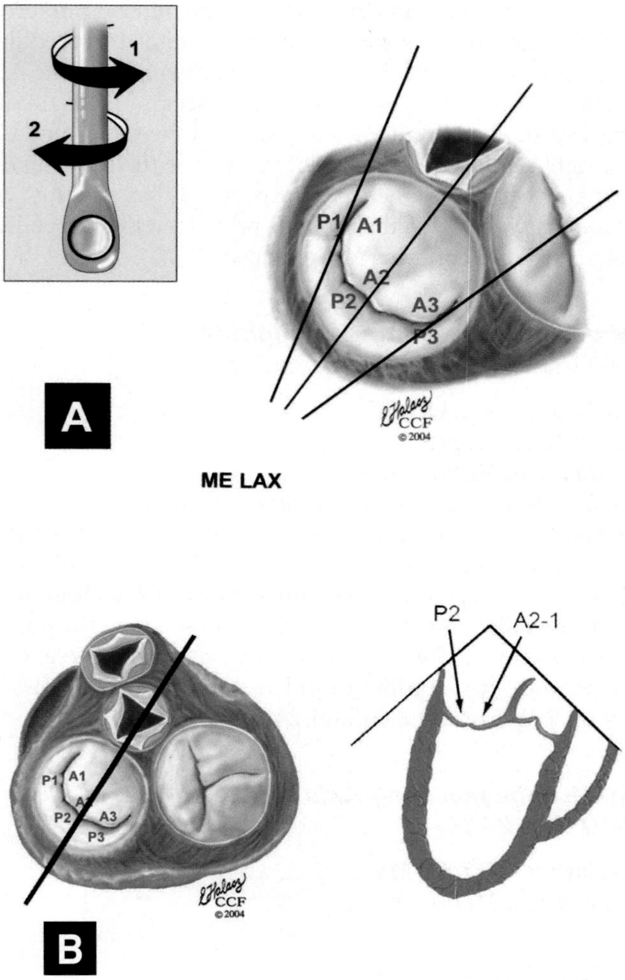

**FIGURE 28.34.** Midesophageal Long Axis MV (ME LAX MV). Transducer Depth: 30 cm; Transducer Rotation: 110-150°. **A:** The ME LAX MV imaging plane is obtained by rotating the transducer forward to 110-150°. Variations of this plan are obtained by turning the probe to the right and left. **B:** Depending on the orientation of the MV commissure and transducer rotation angle, the 2-D plane passes through the minor axis of the MV annulus and aortic valve. The 2-D plane may cut through the P2 scallop, the midcommissure, and through the A2 segment. Height of the PMVL, AMVL, and C-sept are measured in this plane and compared to the ME 4 Chr MV measurements. This plane demonstrates the most superior aspects of the MV annulus.

**FIGURE 28.33.** Midesophageal Two Chamber Left MV (Turned Left) (ME 2 Chr$_L$ MV). Variation of ME 2 Chr MV; Transducer Depth: 30 cm. Probe Manipulation: Turn left or counterclockwise; Transducer Rotation: 80-110°. Depending on the orientation of the MV commissure and transducer rotation angle, the 2-D plane may cut through the P3, P2, and P1 scallops. The commissure may not be visualized except during diastole.

plane may cut through the P2 scallop, the midcommissure, and through the A2 segment. On the monitor (proceeding from left to right) are P2, the midcommissure, and the A2 segment of the MV. The aortic valve is seen of the right of the screen. The MV annulus to the left of the screen and to the right—adjacent to the aortic valve—are the most superior (farthest from the apex) aspects of the annulus. A plane drawn between these points provides a more specific reference for diagnosing MV prolapse.

### Midesophageal Long-Axis Right MV (ME LAX_R MV) (Fig. 28.35)

**Variation ME LAX MV**
**Transducer Depth:** 30 cm
**Transducer Rotation:** 110°–150°
**Probe Manipulation:** Turn right or clockwise
Depending on the orientation of the MV commissure, transducer rotation angle, and extent of probe manipulation, the 2-D plane may cut through the P2 scallop, the posteromedial commissure, and the P3 scallop. The commissure may not be visualized except during diastole. On the monitor (proceeding from left to right) are P2, possibly the posteromedial commissure, and P1.

### Midesophageal Long-Axis Left MV (ME LAX_L MV) (Fig. 28.36)

**Variation ME LAX MV**
**Transducer Depth:** 30 cm

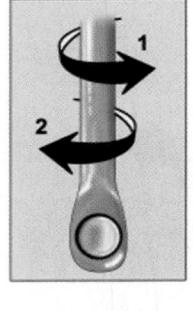
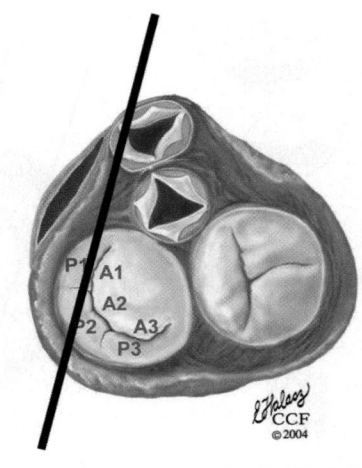

**FIGURE 28.36.** Midesophageal Long-Axis Left MV (ME LAX_L MV). Variation ME LAX MV; Transducer Depth: 30 cm Probe Manipulation: Turn left or counterclockwise; Transducer Rotation; 110-150°. Depending on the orientation of the MV commissure, transducer rotation angle, and extent of probe manipulation, the 2-D plane may cut through the P2 scallop, the anterolateral commissure, and P1 scallops. The commissure may not be visualized except during diastole.

**Transducer Rotation:** 110°–150°
**Probe Manipulation:** Turn left or counterclockwise
Depending on the orientation of the MV commissure, transducer rotation angle, and extent of probe manipulation, the 2-D plane may cut through the P2 scallop, the anterolateral commissure, and the P1 scallop. The commissure may not be visualized except during diastole. On the monitor (proceeding from left to right) are P2, possibly the anterolateral commissure, and P1.

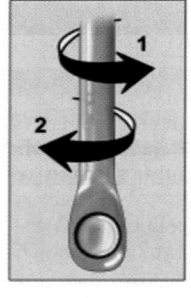
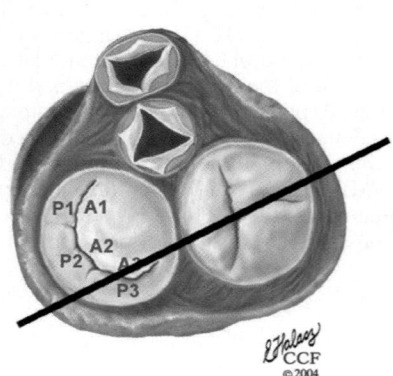

**FIGURE 28.35.** Midesophageal Long-Axis Right MV (Probe Turned Right) MV ME LAX_R MV. Variation ME LAX MV; Transducer Depth: 30 cm; Probe Manipulation: Turn right clockwise; Transducer Rotation: 110-150°. Depending on the orientation of the MV commissure, transducer rotation angle, and extent of probe manipulation, the 2-D plane may cut through the P2 scallop, the posteromedial commissure, and P3 scallops. The commissure may not be visualized except during diastole.

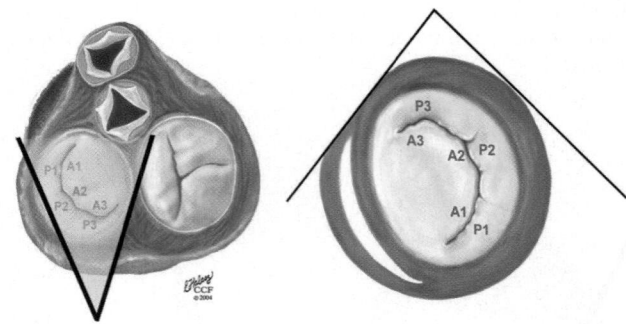

**FIGURE 28.37.** Transgastric Basal Short Axis (TG SAX_B). Transducer Depth: 35 cm; Transducer Rotation: 0-5°. In this imaging plane, the AMVL (A1-2-3, bottom to top) is visualized on the left and the PMVL (P1-2-3, bottom to top) is visualized on the right. The clear space to the left of the AMVL edge and toward the bottom of the screen is the left ventricular outflow tract (LVOT), which is shaded in gray. Systolic turbulence in this area suggests SAM with LVOTO.

### Transgastric Basal Short Axis (TG SAX_B) (Table 28.2 and Fig. 28.37)

**Transducer Depth:** 35 cm
**Transducer Rotation:** 0°–5°
In this imaging plane, the AMVL (A1-2-3, bottom to top) is visualized on the left and the PMVL (P1-2-3, bottom to top) is visualized on the right. The clear space to the left of the AMVL edge and toward the bottom of the screen is the left ventricular outflow tract (LVOT).

### Transgastric Two Chamber (TG 2 Chr) (Table 28.2 and Fig. 28.38)

**Transducer Depth:** 35 cm
**Transducer Rotation:** 70°–90°
This image is similar to the ME 2 Chr imaging plane except that the ventricle is horizontally oriented. Depending on the orientation of the MV commissure and transducer rotation angle, the 2-D plane may cut through the P3 scallop, the posteromedial commissure, and the A3, A2, and A1 segments. On the monitor (proceeding from top to bottom) are P3, posteromedial commissure, A3, A2, and A1.

## Intraoperative Examination Approach

### Principles of Intraoperative Examination (Table 28.3)

The principles of the intraoperative echocardiographic (IOE) examination for patients undergoing MV surgery are guided by the unique demands of the cardiac surgery environment. By the very nature of this atmosphere, the IOE exam is performed in a sequence that first resolves

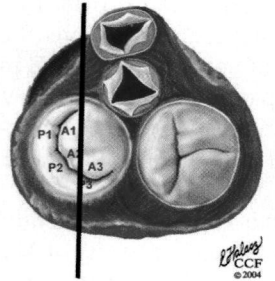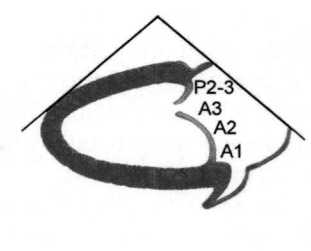

**FIGURE 28.38.** Transgastric Two Chamber (TG 2 Chr). Transducer Depth: 35 cm; Transducer Rotation 70-90°. This image is similar to the ME 2 Chr imaging plane except that the ventricle is horizontally oriented. Depending on the orientation of the MV commissure and transducer rotation angle, the 2-D plane may cut through the P3 scallop, the posteromedial commissure, the A3 segment, the A2 segment, and the A1 segment.

the issues guiding patient management. Yet it also acknowledges the more comprehensive aspects of active patient management and the need to provide digitally archived documentation of the patient's complete examination for future comparison. While these may appear to be conflicting objectives, eventually every echocardiographer incorporates both into the daily routine of an efficiently organized IOE exam with which they feel comfortable. To accomplish these goals (Table 28.4), the systematic IOE exam may be structured into a priority ordered exam and a more general comprehensive exam (54). To prevent significant midexam revelations from occurring and reordering priorities, the priority ordered exam is initiated by a brief abbreviated overview exam followed by the more complete focused diagnostic exam.

▶ **TABLE 28.3. Principles of Intraoperative Echo Exam in Mitral Valve Surgery**

1. **Addresses Critical Issues of MV Surgery (Table 28.1)**
2. **Systematic Examination**
   - Organized by priority
   - Initial overview exam (patient management and exam organization)
   - Focused diagnostic exam (priority issues)
   - Comprehensive exam documented
3. **Efficient (critical issues and comprehensive exam in prebypass period)**
4. **Severity by Weighted Integration 2-D Imaging and Doppler**
5. **Study Results Discussed with Surgeon and Documented in Record**
6. **Comprehensive Digital Study Achieved**
7. **Compares Results with Pre-OR Data and Addresses Variances**
   - Variance explained to extent possible
   - Communicated with surgical team
   - Communicated with patient's primary physician
8. **IOE Exam under CQI Process**
9. **Training and Hospital Credentialing of Qualified Personnel**
10. **Equipment Maintained and Updated**

▶ **TABLE 28.4. Systematic Intraoperative Echo Exam in MV Surgery**

| *Systematic IOE Exam Components* |
|---|
| • Priority Ordered Examination |
| • Abbreviated overview examination |
| • Rapid assessment of cardiac function (patient management) |
| • Diagnostic screen for organizing focused study |
| • Focused diagnostic examinaion |
| • General comprehensive examination |
| • Remaining ASE-SCA |

| *Stages of IOE Exam in MV Surgery* |
|---|
| • Precardiopulmonary bypass (pre-CPB) |
| • Postcardiopulmonary bypass (post-CPB) |
| • Preseparation CPB (pre-sep CPB) |
| • Postseparation CPB (post- CPB) |

In addition to the diagnostic issues that are already on the agenda, the abbreviated overview exam provides an up-to-date assessment of additional issues that must be addressed. It also recognizes the important role of IOE in the ongoing management of the patient and, if necessary, permits the immediate adjustment of the patient's hemodynamic management while the remainder of the IOE exam takes place.

To ensure that the examination is conducted efficiently, the methods that are used in assessing the severity of MV dysfunction are those that are more easily performed in a multitasking environment. As recommended by the ASE Nomenclature and Standards Committee and Task Force on Valvular Regurgitation, the assessment of the severity of MV dysfunction and its secondary pathophysiology integrates both the structural and Doppler parameters of severity weighted by the quality of data obtained and quantitative reliability (35). Severity is graded as mild, moderate, and severe, using terms such as "mild-to-moderate" or "moderate-to-severe" to characterize intermediate levels of severity (35). The term *trace regurgitation* is used to describe that which is barely detected. For mitral stenosis (MS), the terms mild, moderate, and severe are also used.

Subdued lighting (reduced monitor glare) and periods without electrocautery interference during critical portions of the intraoperative exam contribute to collecting quality 2-D images and Doppler-derived hemodynamic data. Such an atmosphere permits the precise recognition of intricate structural abnormalities (vegetation, thrombi, right-to-left shunts) that may have potentially devastating consequences if missed. It also enables the acquisition of the quality of diagnostic information that may confidently guide the pivotal surgical and hemodynamic decisions.

For organization purposes, the examination may be structured into two distinct phases: precardiopulmonary bypass (pre-CPB) and postcardiopulmonary bypass (post-CPB). The post-CPB incorporates an abbreviated preseparation bypass (pre-sep CPB) exam. Each of the phases has critical issues that are addressed during the progression of the procedure (Tables 28.5 and 28.6). For patients undergoing MV surgery, a priority directed exam may be performed at each of these phases of the surgical procedure. If the patient encounters hemodynamic instability at any point during the course of the procedure, an abbreviated overview exam is performed followed by a more focused diagnostic exam directed by the clinical course or as revealed during the abbreviated overview exam. If the patient's course is not entirely smooth, an examination following chest closure may direct clinical intervention or provide assurance.

For each stage of the surgical procedure, the abbreviated overview exam is followed by the focused diagnostic exam in addressing those issues that pertain to that stage of the surgery (Table 28.4). When the critical issues have been resolved and corresponding images stored digitally,

▶ **TABLE 28.5. The Precardiopulmonary Bypass (Pre-CPB) Exam**

1. **Confirm and Refine Preoperative Assessment**
   - Confirm MV dysfunction and severity
   - Determine repairability of valve
     - Refine pathoanatomy and mechanism
     - Explain variances
2. **Determine the Need for Unplanned Surgical Intervention**
   - Secondary pathophysiology
     - LV dysfunction
     - Increased LA or LAA thrombi
     - Pulmonary hypertension
     - RV dysfunction
     - Tricuspid regurgitation
     - Right to left shunt (PFO, ASD)
     - Hepatic congestion
   - Associated abnormality
     - Associated congenital anomalies
       - Cleft MV and primum ASD
     - Similar pathologic process
       - Ventricular dysfunction
       - Valve dysfunction
         - Acquired: rheumatic valve
         - Degenerative: myxomatous or calcific disease
         - Endocarditis
       - Vascular disorder
   - Unrelated process
     - Primary aortic valve stenosis or regurgitation
3. **Cannulation and Perfusion Strategy**
4. **Addresses Surgical Procedure-Specific Issues**
5. **Predict Complications**
   - Inability to repair
     - Documented risks
       - SAM and LVOTO: PMVL height, C-sept distance
       - Dilated annulus, MACa$^{++}$, >3 segments
       - Central MR jet
       - Rheumatic
       - Multiple mechanisms of valve dysfunction
       - Myxomatous and ischemic
       - Mitral stenosis
       - Endocarditis involving fibrous skeleton or annulus
   - Endocarditis
   - LVOT obstruction (MVRep or MVR)
   - Mitral annular calcification
     - Pseudoaneurysm
     - Perivalvular regurgitation
   - Ventricular dysfucntion
   - Coagulopathy (hepatic congestion)

the general comprehensive examination is completed by filling in any portions that were not performed during the focused diagnostic portion of the exam.

The conclusions of the systematic examination at the pre-CPB and post-CPB are communicated directly with the surgical team in addition to being documented in the patient's permanent medical record. The digital loops and images, which support the diagnostic conclusions and

▶ **TABLE 28.6A.** **Preseparation (Pre-Sep) CPB Examination**

| *Abbreviated Preseparation Exam* |
|---|
| • Abbreviated assessment of cardiovascular function<br>  • Cardiac performance<br>  • Initial screen for complications<br>    • Cannulation and perfusion-related<br>      • Check for dissection or intramural hematoma<br>    • Pre-CPB protruding plaques still present?<br>    • Procedure-related complications<br>    • New or secondary pathophysiology<br>• Initial assessment of MV surgery<br>  • Persistent MR or residual or new MS<br>  • Significant procedure-related complications<br>    (not improved by time)<br>    • Suture dehiscence<br>    • Leaflet damage<br>    • Pseudoaneurysm (slide-related)<br>    • MV stenosis<br>    • Pseudoaneurysm<br>    • Left circumflex obstruction<br>    • Latrogenic Shunt: ASD, aorta to LA fistula<br>    • SAM and LVOT obstruction<br>    • Significant perivalvular regurgitation<br>    • Mechanical leaflet malfunction<br>    • LVOT strut obstruction<br>    • Midventricular disruption<br>    • Ring dehiscence<br>    • Significant perivalvular fistula<br>    • LA avulsion<br>• Monitor micro-air clearance<br>• Assess ventricular function and optimal<br>  • Time for separation CPB<br>• Secondary pathophysiology<br>  • Pulmonary hypertension<br>  • RV dysfunction or TR<br>• Complications of cannulation and perfusion<br>  • Aortic dissection or intramural hematoma<br>  • Micro-air or atheromatous emboli<br>    • Myocardial ischemia |

▶ **TABLE 28.6B.** **Postseparation (Post-Sep) CPB Examination**

| |
|---|
| • Assess cardiovascular function<br>• Diagnose complications and mechanisms<br>  • MV repair<br>    • Incomplete repair<br>      • Primary mechanism<br>        • Residual prolapse<br>        • Residual annular dilatation<br>      • Secondary mechanisms<br>        • Repaired P2 with type IIIb (asymmetric)<br>        • New ischemic MR<br>        • Commissural regurgitation<br>  • Technique-related<br>    • Suture dehiscence<br>    • Interscallop malcoaptation<br>    • Overshortening leaflet<br>    • Leaflet damage<br>    • Pseudoaneurysm (slide-related)<br>    • MV stenosis<br>    • Pseudoaneurysm<br>    • Aortic valve incompetence<br>    • Circumflex coronary obstruction<br>    • Iatrogenic shunt: ASD, aorta to LA fistula<br>    • SAM and LVOT obstruction<br>  • MV replacement<br>    • Perivalvular regurgitation<br>    • Mechanical leaflet malfunction<br>    • LVOT strut obstruction<br>    • Midventricular disruption<br>    • Ring dehiscence<br>      Both MVRep and MVR<br>    • Perivalvular fistula<br>    • Pseudoaneurysm<br>    • LA avulsion<br>• Assess ventricular function<br>• Secondary pathophysiology<br>  • Pulmonary hypertension<br>  • RV dysfunction<br>• Complications of cannulation and perfusion<br>  • Aortic dissection or intramural hematoma<br>  • Micro-air emboli<br>    • Segmental ischemia<br>    • CNS dysfunction<br>  • Emboli (atheroma-related)<br>    • Infarcted or ischemic intestine<br>    • Stroke<br>    • Renal infarct |

constitute the complete systematic examination, are achieved for future retrieval for comparison and reviewed under an organized CQI process as recommended by the Intraoperative Council of the American Society of Echocardiography (29).

## Intraoperative Echocardiography (IOE) Examination and Outcomes

### *Precardiopulmonary Bypass (Pre-CPB IOE)*

#### *Critical Issues of the Pre-CPB Exam (Table 28.5)*

For patients with MV dysfunction, a decision to proceed with surgical intervention is one that has been established on the progression of the patient's clinical sympto-

matology and objective assessment of the severity of primary MV dysfunction and its secondary effects (20). Consequently, the pre-CPB exam is to verify the need for surgery and to focus on better understanding the underlying pathologic changes of the structural anatomy of the MVAp and the mechanism of MV dysfunction in addition to resolving other critical issues that are addressed in this phase.

Determining the severity of MV dysfunction is accomplished by the weighted integration methods of determining severity of valve dysfunction, incorporating the two-dimensional echocardiographic and Doppler exams (35,55,56). Detection of the severity of MR relies on established Doppler parameters, including color flow (CF) Doppler maximum jet area (CF Doppler MJA) mapping, CF Doppler vena contracta (VC) diameter (57–59), pulsed wave (PW) Doppler interrogation of the pulmonary veins (57,60–62), and proximal flow convergence (PFC) determination of the "peak" regurgitant orifice area (ROA) (63–66). Should there be significant discrepancies, more extensive volumetric quantitative techniques are used. Following surgical repair of the MV, the initial post-CPB exam is pivotal for long-term patient outcome. An incorrect assessment may unnecessarily return the patient to CPB for further repair or an unnecessary MVR exposing the patient to a lifetime of anticoagulation and all the risks associated with prosthetic valves. Inaccuracy may be introduced into this crucial decision-making period by suboptimal technical settings (CF Doppler gain, scale, wall filter, power, depth with lowered pulse repetition frequency, and frequency) or relying on CF Doppler alone for determining the severity of MR. Given the potential eccentricity of regurgitant jets following attempted valve repair, the potential for inherent inaccuracies with the various techniques come into focus. Utilizing more quantitative assessment methods (vena contracta, PFC, ROA), which are specifically suited for the character of the regurgitant jet (Table 28.12), provides a solid foundation for important decisions that may - significantly impact the patient's outcome and daily routine. A mutual understanding of these essential issues occurs outside of the operating room and permits time for hemodynamic equilibration and the efficient assessment of the surgical results using simplified quantitative parameters. MR jets, which are brief but of a significant size (by CF Doppler MJA), should be weighted for their duration. CF Doppler M-mode (color m-mode) enables an accurate visualization of the jet duration and depth of penetration (Fig. 28.39). If the severe jet is short-lived despite having a MJA of $> 6$ cm$^2$ (Nyquist 50 cm/sec–60 cm/sec), it may not be indicative of significant mitral regurgitant (67). Before returning to CPB and re-repair or MVR with greater than mild to moderate MR, a quantitative method of severity assessment (ROA, vena contracta) will improve the patient's long-term management (Fig. 28.39).

Assessment of MS similarly incorporates two-dimensional imaging and Doppler. The 2-D qualitative assessment incorporates a functional assessment of the MV apparatus utilizing the splitability index planimetery from the basal TG SAX imaging plane and (55, 68–70). As with the assessment of MR, CF Doppler provides a reliable screening assessment (71). Visualizing transmitral dia-stolic proximal flow convergence directs the exam to more quantitative methods of assessment. Use of PISA proximal flow convergence has been validated for determining the severity of MS. If the stenosis is subvalvular, it is inherently inaccurate. MVA in Doppler assessment of MS incorporates aspects of both CW and PW Doppler in providing a semiquantitative and quantitative assessment of the MV area. By measuring how rapidly the transvalvular pressure equilibrates between the LA and LV, the MV area may be determined using the pressure half-time and decelerating time methods (68–71). Except for circumstances of aortic regurgitation and issues of variance in assumptions for LA and LV compliance, these methods have proven reliable. The continuity equation incorporates both PW and CW Doppler techniques and is reasonably reliable as long as the reference valve is not regurgitant (55).

Determination of the mechanism of MV dysfunction for both MR and MS is assessed using a combination of 2-D echocardiography (annular size, segmental systolic and diastolic valve leaflet motion, and leaflet coaptation) and correlation with the corresponding color flow Doppler characterization of systolic regurgitant jet direction and/or diastolic flow disturbance visualized in the same imaging plane (29). In determining the mechanism of MR or MS, color flow Doppler is an essential component of the evaluation. With the surgical team understanding the etiology and mechanism of dysfunction, the feasibility of a successful valve repair or alternative replacement is better understood. The mechanism and underlying pathologic process directly affect the patient's long-term prognosis (29,53,55,56,74).

Other issues resolved by the pre-CPB exam include:

1. Evaluating the presence and severity of significant secondary or coexisting cardiovascular disease that would alter the patient's surgical management
2. Establishing the optimal cannulation-perfusion and myocardial protection strategy
3. Assessing cardiac function in determining the optimal intraoperative hemodynamic management of the patient
4. Assessing the probability for potential post-CPB complications related to the patient's MV surgery or use of cardiopulmonary bypass (aortic regurgitation, aortic dissection, and intramural hematoma).

The assessment of secondary physiology focuses on determining the presence of an increased LA pressure, pulmonary hypertension, secondary RV dysfunction with dilatation, and/or lateral enlargement of the tricuspid annulus. With MV dysfunction there may be increased left atrial pressure with chronic dilatation of the chamber. In acute MR, the LA does not dilate and the LA pressures are elevated more acutely with the onset of pulmonary congestion and hypertension. Utilizing PWD interrogation of

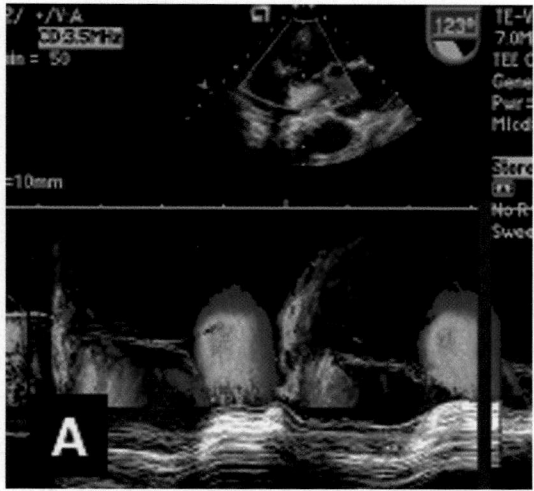

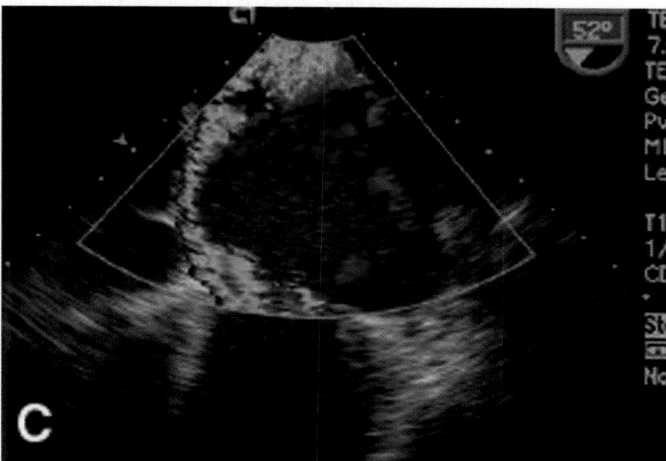

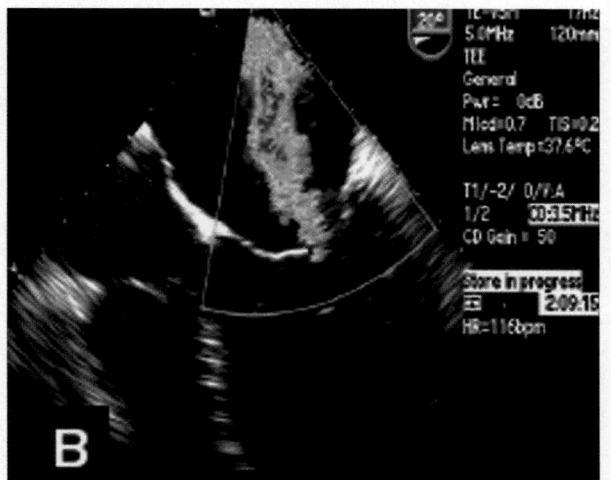

FIGURE 28.39A, B, C, and D. **A:** The post-CPB TEE exam following MVRep may reveal short duration MR jets with a significant maximum jet area. The color m-mode clarifies the duration of the jet. **B:** Color flow Doppler is a good screening technique to distinguish the presence of severe or mild MR. Eccentric jets will lead to an underestimation of MV severity due to the wall hugging (Coanda effect). **C:** In a patient with an A3 flail (ME Com$_R$ imaging plane), an eccentric posteriorly directed jet will lead to an underestimation of the severity of MR by CFD MJA due to the wall hugging (Coanda) effect. **D:** Due to the many factors influencing the jet area size (frequency, wall filter, gain, Nyquist limit, PRF, sector depth, and loading conditions), quantitative methods (including PISA ROA, and vena contracta) should be used to distinguish intermediate grades (mild to moderate, moderate, and moderate to severe). However, color flow Doppler is an essential component of the exam in determining mechanism of MR.

the pulmonary vein, the LAP may be estimated. If there is blunting of the S wave in all pulmonary veins, an elevation of LAP (> 15 mm Hg) is usually present (55–57). In chronic MR, the left atrium may dilate to greater than 70 mm (56,57). With persistent elevations of LAP, the patient may develop fixed pulmonary hypertension with RV dysfunction, eventually causing RV dilatation, and lateral enlargement of the tricuspid annulus, leading to tricuspid regurgitation in up to 25% of patients having MV surgery (75). The RAP may be elevated leading to chronic hepatic

congestion (diagnosed by a lack of respiratory variation in hepatic vein diameter) and in the present right-to-left shunting patent foramen ovale.

Notwithstanding the many valuable and recognized contributions that IOE has made to the patient undergoing valvular heart surgery, the ability to identify patients who are at a higher risk for postoperative stroke and neurocognitive dysfunction continues to have a daily impact on the management of these patients. This is not only a devastating complication that impacts patient morbidity and mortality, but it significantly increases the costs associated with valvular heart surgery. The cannulation and perfusion strategy is directed by the IOE assessment of the proximal ascending and descending aorta. Epiaortic scanning is performed if

1. Protruding plaques are seen in the descending aorta
2. Plaques are palpated at the anticipated site of cannulation or cross clamping
3. The patient has significant risk factors for aortic atheroma (103)

Significant aortic regurgitation may identify patients at risk for ventricular distension or ineffective antegrade cardioplegia administration, which may direct an alternative protection strategy, such as direct interostial administration of antegrade cardioplegia or more heavily weighted dependence on retrograde cardioplegia administration. As the cross clamp is released prior to reinstitution of a rhythm, cardiac distension may indicate the need for an AV vent through the pulmonary vein (76).

### The Pre-CPB IOE Exam and Outcome Studies (Table 28.5)

Intraoperative echocardiography (IOE) has been effectively utilized in guiding MVRep surgery since it was initially reported in 1986, using epicardial imaging with color flow Doppler determination of the mechanism of dysfunction (8). Not only has the IOE exam helped the individual patient, but it has also shortened the learning curves of cardiac surgeons and served as a catalyst to hasten the evolutionary development of MVRep. In 1998, Gillinov and colleagues reported on 1,072 patients who had successful MVRep surgery performed between 1985 and 1997 (77). The study included a subset of patients who had not received IOE guidance. In comparing those patients who received IOE compared with those who did not, the long-term durability was 98% compared to 92% (77). Following the initial surgical procedure, there was a preponderance of late failures that occurred within the first year (Figs. 28.40 and 28.41).

The potential repairability of the valve is an issue that affects the immediate management of the patient and impacts long-term outcome. Understanding the importance of the technical capabilities and experience of the surgeon and the perioperative team, the feasibility of MV repair is determined by the pathologic process and the mechanism and severity of dysfunction. It is the correlation of the direct surgical examination of the components of the valve apparatus with the real-time pre-CPB IOE exam of the same structures and determination of mechanisms of dysfunction, which yields a coordinated surgical strategy that will effectively navigate through those issues impacting the immediate and long-term outcome of the patient (Table 28.5).

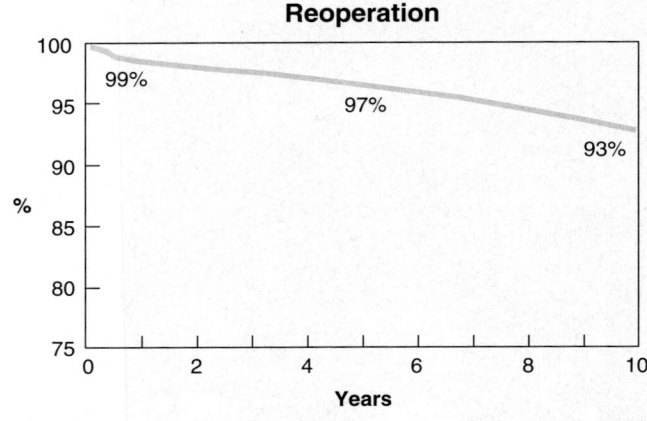

**FIGURE 28.40A.** Of 1,072 patients undergoing successful MV repair between 1985 and 1997, the long-term durability at 10 years was 93%.

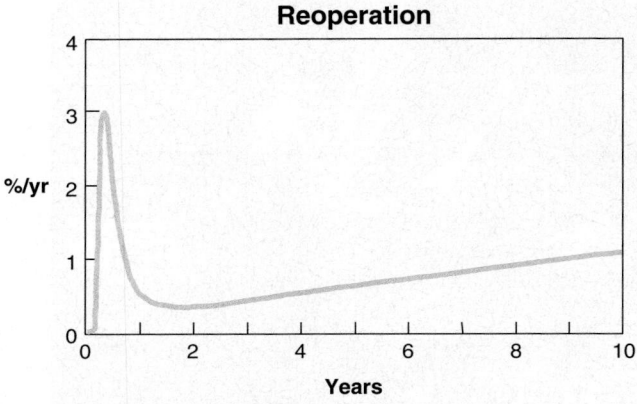

**FIGURE 28.40B.** Hazard curves for reoperation following successful MV repair. Though reoperations are an infrequent event, the first year is time of highest incidence.

### New Clinical Information

The pre-CPB IOE exam provides incremental information that impacts the surgical management of patients undergoing MV surgery. Michel-Cherqui et al. reported the results of 203 consecutive cardiac surgery patients and found a 17% incidence of IOE changing the preoperative diagnosis (78). Chaliki et al. found a 12% incidence of new findings influencing the intraoperative management of their patients (38). Lytle et al. reported that IOE discovered previously undiagnosed MV dysfunction requiring MVRep in 5% of 82 consecutive higher risk patients undergoing myocardial revascularization (18).

### Determine Mechanism and Probability of Repair

The IOE exam provides the surgeon with information that enables a more directed inspection of the mitral ap-

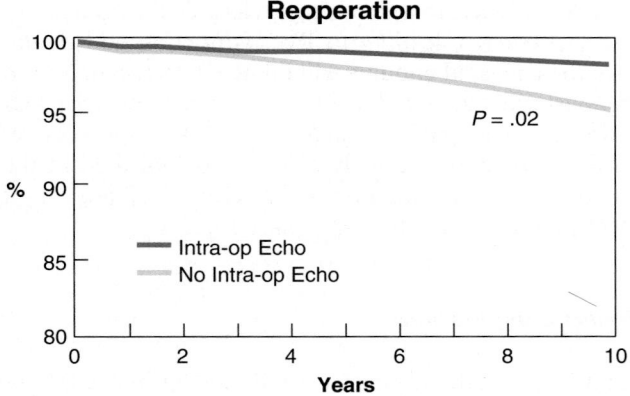

**FIGURE 28.41.** The patients who did not have intraoperative echo had a trend for lower long-term durability (92%) compared to those who received intraoperative guidance with TEE and /or epicardial echo (98%, p < 0.02) (77).

paratus. In 1992, Stewart et al. reported the Cleveland Clinic's initial experience with 286 patients undergoing MVRep (79). In those patients who received IOE guidance, the surgical diagnosis of mechanism and location was compared with the results of the pre-CPB exam. The IOE exam diagnosed the localized mechanisms most accurately with posterior-leaflet prolapse or flail (93%), anterior-leaflet prolapse or flail (94%), and restricted leaflet motion or rheumatic thickening (91%). It correctly diagnosed papillary muscle elongation or rupture in 75%, ventricular and annular dilatation in 72%, leaflet perforation in 62%, and bileaflet prolapse or flail in 44%. Of the 5% of patients who had more than one mechanism, the IOE was only able to diagnose both mechanisms in 38%, and one of the two mechanisms in 92%. Overall, the accuracy for diagnosing mechanisms was 85% (33). In a similar study, Foster et al. reported the high accuracy of utilizing a more regimented systematic IOE exam, reporting agreement between the TEE and surgical localizations of mechanisms in 96% of native MV segments or scallops (224 of 234 segments or scallops, p < 0.0001) and 88% of perivalvular prosthetic regurgitant segments (p < 0.001) (80). Lambert et al. reported on the ability of a consistent systematic examination to accurately determine the location and mechanism of MV dysfunction (compared with surgical inspection) in 96% compared with 70% in an IOE exam that was not systematically performed (81). Omran et al. prospectively evaluated 170 consecutive patients undergoing MVRep with a systematic segmental examination of the MVAp. They found that IOE accurately identified abnormal segments in 90 to 97% of patients (82). Segments that were most accurately identified as abnormal were P2 (97%) and least accurately identified were A3 (90%). The accuracy of correctly localizing to AMVL and PMVL was 95% and 100%, respectively

(82). In 1999, Caldarera et al. discovered that IOE provided accurate anatomic measurements of the anteroposterior diameter of the mitral annulus compared with surgical inspection (83). A measured diameter > 35 mm in the ME 4 Chr imaging plane was indicative of annular dilatation at the time of surgery requiring annuloplasty. In 1999, Enriquez-Sarano et al. compared the ability of IOE to accurately diagnose the etiology and mechanism of MV dysfunction in patients undergoing MVRep surgery with TTE (29). They found that IOE provided a superior ability to diagnose the correct etiology (99% vs. 95%) and mechanism of dysfunction (99% vs. 94%). The IOE exam was also more accurate in diagnosing MV prolapse (99% vs. 95%) and flail segments (99% vs. 83%, p < 0.001). The IOE exam was able to predict, on the basis of accurately diagnosing etiology and mechanism, those patients who were most likely to have a successful MVRep (p < 0.001) and a higher 5-year survival (p < .001) (29). Similar studies have consistently demonstrated the diagnostic capabilities of the IOE exam to accurately provide the surgical team with the information that will enable them to correlate their surgical findings in determining the optimal surgical strategy for repair or replacement of the valve.

### Variances with Preoperative Severity MV Dysfunction

Despite numerous reports demonstrating the ability to accurately determine the underlying anatomy and mechanism of dysfunction, there have been recognized discrepancies between the preoperative (both TEE and TTE) and intraoperative assessment of severity in some patients. Grewal et al. compared preoperative TEE with the IOE exam performed under general anesthesia to determine the unloading effect on the severity of MR. The severity of MR was assessed using color flow Doppler (CFD), maximal jet area (MJA), and vena contracta jet diameter (VCJD) (84). They found 22 of the 43 patients (51%) improved by at least one MR severity grade when assessed under general anesthesia. They found the most significant changes occurred in patients with functional MR, with normal MV leaflets (84). However, patients with structural leaflet dysfunction (flail) demonstrated little if any change in the MR severity. Bach et al. also compared the severity of preoperative TEE with the IOE using similar parameters of severity assessment (85). They determined that patients with structural valve leaflet abnormalities (flail) did not have a significant change in their severity assessment whereas those with functional MR decrease showed a significant MR (p < 0.001) (85).

In a report of 1,265 patients undergoing MV surgery in 1999, Chaliki et al. reported a total of 96 patients in whom the pre-CPB found no significant structural or functional abnormality of the mitral apparatus (38).

Based on this finding the decision was made not to surgically inspect the valve in 95 of these patients. In patients with ischemic MR undergoing myocardial revascularization, Cohn et al. reported on patients undergoing myocardial revascularization with moderate preoperative MR; 90% of these patients were downgraded to 0–2$^+$ by the IOE exam (19). Seven of the patients went from moderate MR to no MR intraoperatively and did not receive a MVRep or MVR. Postoperatively, 3 out of 7 patients returned to their original 3$^+$ MR, and 4 returned to 2$^+$ MR on their postoperative TTE (19).

All of these studies have made remarkable contributions to our understanding of the variances that we have observed in patients with "nonstructural" functional MR. Clearly, when MR is recorded an accompanying BP or other relevant information would enable a clearer understanding of the issue as it presents.

When explaining variances between the preoperative assessment and the intraoperative exam, as Thomas and many others have taught us, there are physical principles of ultrasound which we use daily that contribute to the variance in our intraoperative assessment (29,57). As explained in Chapter 1, the size of the maximum CF Doppler jet area (MJA) is determined by a number of considerations, including the regurgitant orifice area and the systolic LV-LA gradient accelerating the velocity and producing momentum (a product of velocity × flow rate and the most significant determinate of jet size), which is related to momentum (flow rate × velocity). Other factors include the eccentricity of the regurgitant jet (leads to wall constraint), and settings used on the ultrasound platform (power, transducer receiver gain, frequency of transducer—higher frequency transducer causes greater Doppler shift, wall filter, PRF, color scale or Nyquist limit, and size of scan sector—affecting pulse repetition frequency). Because of the closer proximity of the TEE transducer to the heart, higher frequencies can be used, causing a more pronounced jet area because of the relative lack of tissue attenuation at the imaging distance for TEE. By having the CF Doppler scale higher than what may have been used in the preoperative assessment, the MJA will be comparatively reduced.

From a clinical perspective, if the variance in the OR is more than two grades less, the possibility always exists that the patient may have had indolent ischemia at the time of the original exam. In these circumstances, if canceling the MV procedure is a consideration, altering the loading conditions with neosynephrine or challenging with a bolus of intravenous fluid may duplicate the MV dysfunction seen preoperatively. It is always a good idea to consult other colleagues who may provide insight into the patient's clinical course or more quantitative methods that may not be utilized on a routine basis in an intraoperative practice (18,62,63).

In MV disease that chronically elevates the pulmonary artery pressures, leading to RV dysfunction and dilatation, the tricuspid annulus will dilate laterally adjacent to the posterior tricuspid leaflet. The need for tricuspid valve repair in patients undergoing MV surgery is reported to be approximately 25% and is indicated in the presence of greater than moderate TR (75). Almost all of these procedures are tricuspid valve repairs.

### Predict Complications

In an era of minimally invasive and other cutting edge approaches to MV disease, the potential for difficulties keeps everyone vigilant. Such challenges do not become complications unless they remain undetected and adversely affect the patient. IOE clearly provides a safety net mechanism, enabling us to identify problems at a time when they may be more readily corrected. The pre-CPB has also been used to anticipate complications following MVRep and MVR (Table 28.5). Such complications are directly related to the surgical procedure, the patient's underlying disease process, or the use of cardiopulmonary bypass. Unsuccessful MVRep is classified as either immediate or late. Late failures occur after the patient's initial OR experience. Causes of immediate failure may be secondary to an extensively diseased valve, calcification, segmental involvement making the valve more difficult to repair, systolic anterior motion (SAM) of the MV with associated LVOT obstruction (LVOTO), suture dehiscence, development of ischemic MR, and incomplete repair second mechanism. Many of these causes may be detected by the pre-CPB IOE with a prediction of the difficulty of repair, raising the index of suspicion during the post pump evaluation. Marwick et al. reported on the factors associated with immediate failure during the initial MVRep procedure (86). Of 26 patients requiring second CPB runs for persistent MV, the causes were determined to be LVOT obstruction (38%), suture dehiscence (23%), and "incomplete repair" (38%) (86). Agricola et al. reported on 255 consecutive patients undergoing MVRep for MR receiving a quadrilateral resection (87). Twenty-one patients had significant residual MR related to:

1. Residual cleft, provoking interscallop malcoaptation
2. Residual prolapse of the anterior or posterior leaflets
3. Residual annular dilation
4. Left ventricular outflow obstruction
5. Suture dehiscence (64)

Omran et al. evaluated 170 consecutive patients undergoing MV repair, with 9% of patients receiving an MVR due to persistent significant MR (82). Using univariant and multivariant analysis, predictors of unsuccessful repair (or predicting the need for MV replacement) were:

1. MV annulus > 5.0 cm
2. MAC
3. Central MR jet
4. ≥ 3 segments/scallops with prolapse or flail

By allocating one point for each of these factors, if the score was 0, 1, or > 1 the observed risk was 0%, 10%, and 36% (82).

### Systolic Anterior Motion (SAM) with LVOT Obstruction (LVOTO)

Systolic anterior motion (SAM) with LVOT obstruction (LVOTO) and an associated posteriorly directed jet has been reported in up to 16% of patients undergoing MVRep for myxomatous MV dysfunction (86,88,89). More recent experiences place the incidence under 1%–2% of MVReps (37). When SAM with LVOTO occurs, inotropic agents and vasodilators (including vasodilating inhalation agents) should be discontinued to evaluate unprovoked mechanism of MR. If the administration of volume and pressor agents does not reverse the process, further repair may be required with a sliding annuloplasty, which reduces the height of the PMVL. In 1988, Schiavone et al. reported a small series of 12 patients with postrepair SAM and LVOT obstruction with a rigid ring (88). Of those patients who left the OR with persistent SAM and LVOTO, the severity of LVOTO had, in fact, diminished in follow-up at 27 months. However, when provoked with amyl nitrate, a significant gradient returned and was associated with significant MR (88). Lee et al. reported on a similar group of 14 patients, developing postrepair SAM and LVOT obstruction (89). They determined that these patients had common features of reduced pre-CPB coaptation to septal (C-sept) distances (2.65 cm) and PMVL systolic heights of 1.9 cm (Figs. 28.41A and 28.41B) (Fig. 28.43) (89). By effectively moving the coaptation line away from the interventricular septum, Carpentier developed the sliding annuloplasty in 1988 as a potential solution to these issues (90). Cosgrove et al. reported that sliding annuloplasty is performed on patients with a PMVL height of > 1.5 cm (Fig. 28.44) (91,92). Maslow et al. evaluated patients undergoing MV repair for myxomatous MV disease in attempting to identify echocardiographic predictors of LVOTO associated with SAM of the MV (93). Using intraoperative TEE and the ME 4 Chr imaging plane, the lengths of the coapted AMVL and PMVL leaflets, the distance from the coaptation point to the septum (C-Sept), annular diameters, and left ventricular internal diameter (LVID) at end systole were measured in 33 patients undergoing MV repair. Eleven patients developed significant SAM with LVOT obstruction and had smaller AL/PL ratios (0.99 vs. 1.95, p < 0.0001) and C-Sept distances (2.53 vs. 3.01 cm,

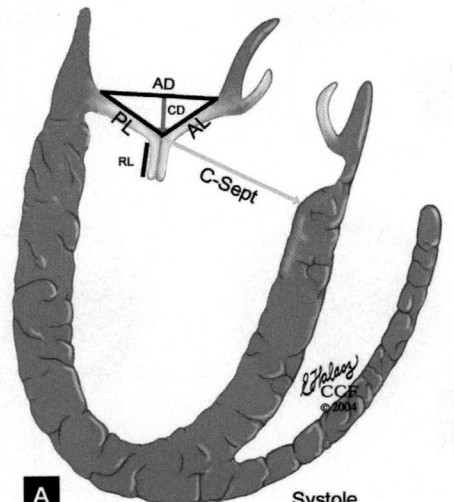 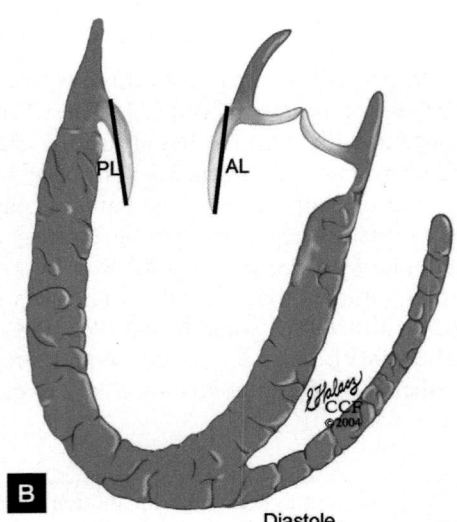

**FIGURE 28.42 A and B.** Lee et al. (89) and Maslow et al. (93) have demonstrated in two separate studies that SAM with LVOTO may be predicted by a tall PMVL (> 1.5) (89), AMVL/PMVL height < 1.0, (93), a cooaptation point to septal distance (C-sept) of < 2.53 (89) - 2.65 cm (93). Others have suggested an AMVL height of > 3.0 with reduced C-sept and an anteriorly displaced AL papillary muscle as other predictors. Measurements obtained in patients undergoing MV repair from the ME 4 Chr MV and ME LAX MV include the height of the PMVL (PL) and AMVL (AL), residual coaptated leaflet (RL), distance between superior plane of the annulus and coaptation point, the diastolic length of the AMVL and PMVL, and septal thickness in diastole.

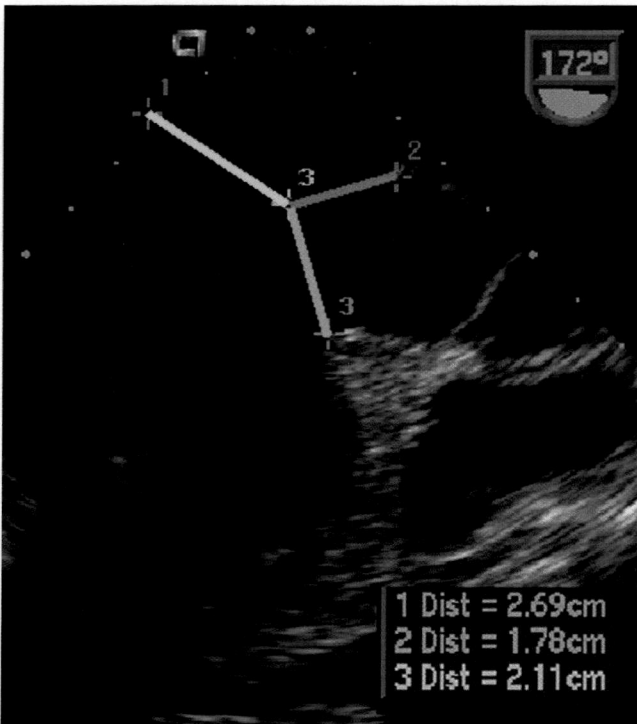

**FIGURE 28.43** Predictors of Post-MVRep SAM and LVOTO. AMVL:PMVL ratio less than 1.0, PMVL height > 1.5 cm, and a small systolic LVOT diameter (C-septal distance < 2.6 cm) would indicate a higher risk MVRep patient population for developing post-CPB SAM and LVOT obstruction (90–92).

p = 0.012) prior to pre-CPB compared to those who did not develop LVOT obstruction with SAM (93). These findings were consistent with studies demonstrating that SAM with LVOT obstruction following MVRep surgery is associated with anterior malposition of the point of coaptation. This study lends further support to the strategy of the sliding annuloplasty to prevent post-MVRep LVOTO (90–92). From these studies the predictive indicators of post-MVRep SAM with LVOTO would be a AMVL: PMVL ratio less than 1.0, PMVL height > 1.5 cm, and a small systolic LVOT diameter (C-septal distance < 2.6 cm)

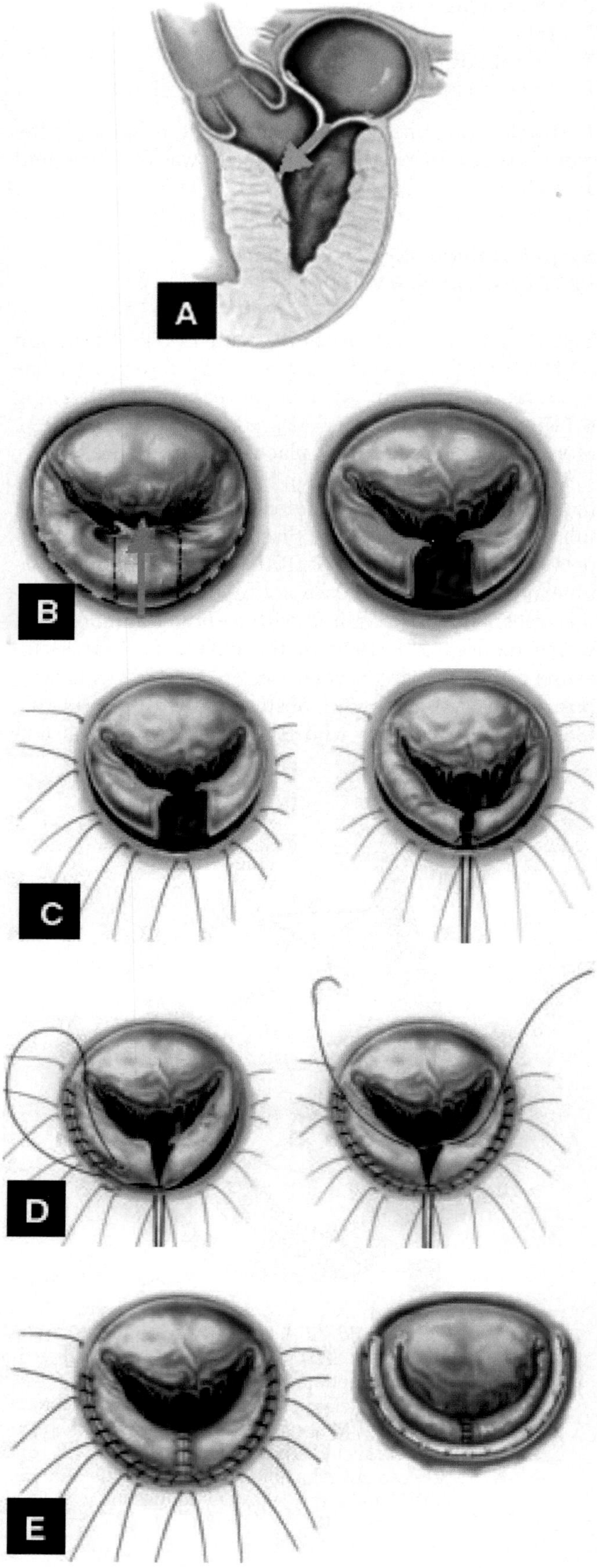

**FIGURE 28.44.** **A**: To prevent systolic anterior motion (SAM) of the MV with LV outflow tract obstruction (LVOTO), a sliding annuloplasty is performed. **B:** A quadrilateral resection of the P2 scallop with detachment of the PMVL from the annulus is performed. **C:** The posterior free edge of the respected P1 and P2 interface are anchored to the posterior annulus. **D:** The PMVL is reattached to the MV annulus posteriorly. **E:** A Cosgrove ring is used to reinforce the annuloplasty and prevent future annular dilatation. The procedure effectively increases the coaptation-septal distance (C-sept) (blue →). The coaptation distance is moved posteriorly, the height of the PMVL is reduced, and the distance between the septum and the coaptation point is increased.

would indicate a higher risk MVRep patient population for developing post-CPB SAM and LVOT obstruction and the potential need for a posterior MV complete or modified sliding annuloplasty.

### Periannular Annular Disruption

Other complications of MV surgery that may be predicted by the pre-CPB exam include post-CPB pseudoaneurysms (94,95). Patients with severe MAC in whom posterior annular debridement is required are at an increased risk. Demonstrating MAC prepump and consulting with the surgeon regarding the extent of resection alerts the team to the potential of pseudoaneurysm or annular disruption. Feindel reported a series of 54 patients with extensive mitral annular calcification. When calcium was debrided and a new mitral annulus was created by suturing a strip of pericardium onto the endocardium with annular reconstruction, the 5-year survival was 73% (94).

### LV Dysfunction

Post-CPB LV dysfunction may accompany MVRep. The greatest predictor of post-CPB LV dysfunction is preexisting LV function (96,97). The pre-CPB may also provide a quantitative indication for the need of post-CPB inotropic support. Patients with a pattern of restrictive diastolic dysfunction are at an increased risk for post-CPB dysfunction. Isada et al. reported the use of the CW Doppler interrogation of the MR jet and estimation of LV and RV dP/dt (Fig. 28.45). A dP/dt less than 800 was found to be predictive of the need for post-CPB support (97).

### Cannulation-Perfusion and Myocardial Protection Strategy

Davila-Roman et al. evaluated the relationship between the incidence of perioperative stroke and the presence of ascending aortic atheroma by examining 1,200 consecutive patients over the age of 50 with epiaortic echocardiography scanning (98). They determined that the incidence of stroke was almost 8 times greater in patients with greater than 3 mm to 5 mm plaques in the ascending aorta. They demonstrated in a subsequent study, in an older group of patients, that the incidence of stroke was 33% in those patients with plaques in the ascending aorta > 4 mm (99). Wareing et al. also demonstrated that the surgical practice of performing epiaortic echocardiography scanning only when plaques were palpated missed 38% of plaques at the site of aortic cannulation or cross clamp (100). Roach et al., in a large multicentered study involving over 2,100 patients, demonstrated a similar incidence of palpated atheroma documented by epivascular echocardiography, in addition to a strong association between atheromatous disease in the ascending aorta and postoperative focal neurological deficits (101). Subse-

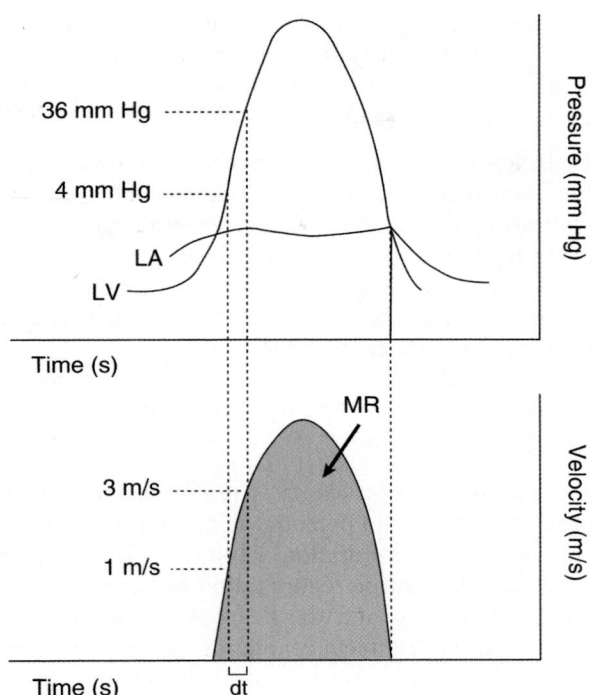

**FIGURE 28.45.** CW Doppler interrogation of the MR jet and estimation of LV and LV dP/dt is calculated by determining the time required for the spectral envelope velocity to increase from 1m/sec to 3m/sec, corresponding to a increase in the systolic LV-LA gradient from 4 mm Hg to 36 mm HG (gradient = $4V^2$). Isada et al. reported that a dP/dt < 800 was associated with the need for post-CPB support (97).

quent studies by Konstadt et al. have demonstrated a similar incidence of missed or underestimated plaques by palpation techniques (102). They demonstrated that TEE demonstration of the absence of significant descending aortic atheromatous disease in patients without significant risks for atheromatous disease. Patients with identified risk factors—age over 65 years, diabetes, neurologic history, previous CABG, and pulmonary disease—for atheromatous disease or demonstrable protruding plaques should receive epiaortic scanning to identify uncompromised areas for cannulation and cross clamping (103).

### Post-CPB Exam and Outcomes

#### Preseparation CPB Abbreviated Exam

For purposes of this discussion, the abbreviated exam prior to separation from CPB is included as part of the post-CPB exam, because it is functionally contiguous. This abbreviated exam serves as a safety net to immediately detect any significant complications that could adversely affect patients if they are prematurely weaned from CPB. A rapidly performed abbreviated overview exam is followed by a more complete evaluation of the surgical intervention and potential complications associated with the procedure and use of cardiopulmonary bypass. Important issues that are clarified by the IOE exam prior to separation from cardiopulmonary bypass include:

1. Detection of significant complications (aortic dissection, new segmental wall motion abnormality)
2. Optimizing the patient's cardiac performance
3. Assessing the function of other valves
4. Guidance of the de-airing process (microbubbles may be entrapped in the pulmonary circulation during an open cardiac surgical procedure)
5. Identifying the optimal time to separate from cardiopulmonary bypass (the heart is completely de-aired and ejecting effectively)

As soon as the cross-clamp is removed, IOE may be utilized to evaluate the potential distensibility of the LV caused by aortic regurgitation. Even though the patient may not have had aortic regurgitation pre-CPB, until the LVOT is pressurized and the heart is actively ejecting, there may not be complete coaptation of the aortic valve leaflets. If the heart is slow to initiate an intrinsic rhythm and eject on its own, placement of an LV vent may be warranted.

As the heart starts to eject, it is always tempting to diagnose the results of the valve repair or replacement. However, unless there is an obvious structural problem, the final verdict should wait until the heart has recovered and hemodynamics are optimized. Initial significant regurgitant jets may resolve following MV repair, and perivalvular regurgitation may be absent post-CPB after protamine has been administered in patients undergoing MV replacement (104–106). A rapid abbreviated examination may be performed to initially evaluate left ventricular function, TR, MR, aortic regurgitation, and the descending aorta for evidence of complications related to cannulation and perfusion while on CPB.

The passage of micro-air bubbles may also be visualized (Fig. 28.46). The IOE is a reliable monitor for micro-air that may be distributed to the cerebral circulation. When simultaneous recordings of intracranial Doppler and TEE visualizing the descending aorta are performed, detection of micro-air emboli in the cerebral circulation is simultaneous with micro-air visualization in the descending thoracic aorta (107). Strategies to prevent further embolization to the coronary arteries or cerebral circulation include:

1. Having the perfusionist increase aortic vent flow accordingly
2. Emptying the heart
3. Increasing pump flow and lowering the head with Trendelenburg positioning so that micro-air will accumulate at the ventricular apex and can be aspirated

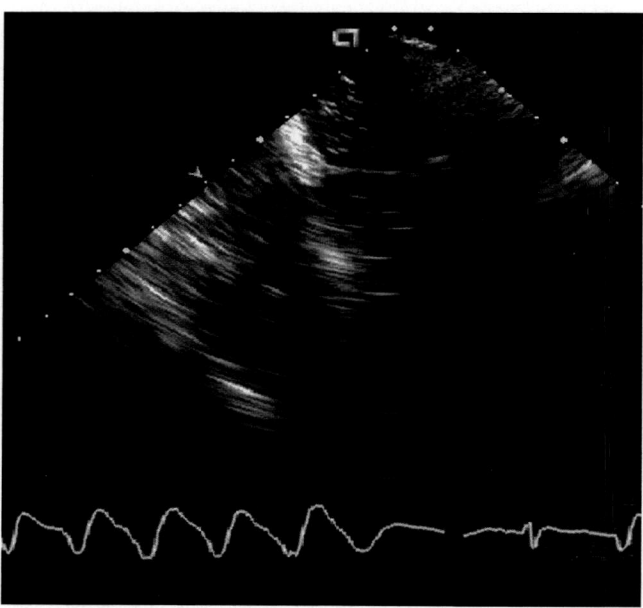

**FIGURE 28.46.** Micro-air detection. TEE detects the presence of significant amounts of micro-air bubbles that normally collect at the apex, LAA, and dome of the LA. Air emboli are more frequently seen in open cardiac procedures such as mitral valve surgery.

If waves of air are noticed that cycle with the ventilator, ventilation may be transiently interrupted until the micro air clears. Air may also collect at the dome of the LA adjacent to the aortic sinotubular junction or in the left atrial appendage. Micro air may be visualized in the proximal right or left main coronary arteries. If this occurs, the perfusion pressure may be increased to hasten passage of the micro-air through the circulation.

As the heart starts to more actively contract and the hemodynamics are optimized, assessment of the MV surgical intervention takes on more meaningful long-term significance. However, in addition to focusing on the surgical results, abbreviated IOE exams may avert the full effects of unfortunate complications. A rapidly performed abbreviated exam will detect complications, such as cannulation-related aortic dissections (Fig. 28.47). Functional assessments of left and right ventricle, tricuspid and aortic valves, the aorta proximal and distal to the cannulation site, and the interatrial septum (if a minimally invasive approach to the MV was utilized) will provide guidance for the optimal time of weaning from cardiopulmonary bypass.

### Post-CPB Clinical Issues (Tables 28.6, 28.13, and 28.14)

The post-CPB is an extension of the evaluation prior to separation from CPB. Following separation from CPB,

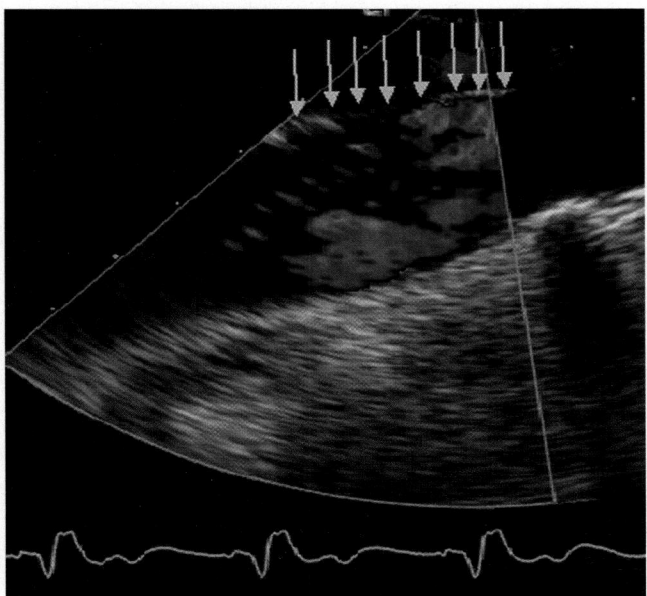

**FIGURE 28.47.** Post-CPB aortic dissection. A rapidly performed abbreviated exam will detect complications such as cannulation-related aortic dissections. To make certain that the finding is not an artifact, the pre-CPB documentation of the aortic anatomy is helpful for comparison.

overall cardiac performance may be assessed by an abbreviated overview examination (cardiac function and evaluation of cannulation-related complications) followed by an evaluation of the MV surgical procedure. In determining the success of the MVRep or MVR, a rapid 3-D screening for MR or MS is easily performed with CF Doppler (aliasing velocity set at 50 cm/sec to 60 cm/sec). Because of the MVRep technique, persistent MR is in a different location and requires a complete 3-D exam of the MV annulus. If significant (> mild) MR is seen by the initial CF Doppler screen (using MJA), a more quantitative method, such as simplified PISA estimate of peak ROA (scale set to 40 cm/sec, ROA = $r^2/2$ assessment), or vena contracta is performed (Fig. 28.48), use of CF Doppler maximal jet area may be misleading. While the MJA may appear to be significant, color m-mode may indicate a brief duration (< 50% systole) and MR of less significance. The duration of the color flow jet by color m-mode (CMM) or evaluating the severity of MR using more quantitative parameters, such as PISA (peak) ROA or vena contracta, may clarify the significance of the jet. As previously discussed, permitting a period for the heart to fully recover, before making a final decision of MR severity, will filter out those patients who may develop transient ischemic MR post-MVRep-related to myocardial ischemia encountered to some degree in all patients on CPB. If significant diastolic proximal flow convergence is found, a transvalvular gradient is performed using con-

tinuous wave (CW) Doppler. If the mean gradient is > 6 mm Hg to 8 mm Hg at a heart rate of 80 + 10 BPM consideration should be given to a second pump run and further repair or MVR.

### Post-CPB Complications

*MV Repair* Complications following MV repair or replacement, though infrequently encountered, include:

1. Residual MR
2. Residual or new MS
3. SAM or prosthetic strut protrusion with LVOT obstruction
4. Left or right ventricular dysfunction
5. Circumflex coronary "kinking" or occlusion from annuloplasty or valve ring suture
6. Pseudoaneurysm formation at site of debridement of mitral annular calcification
7. Shunts related endocarditis
8. Various shunts related to exposure
9. Air embolism
10. Aortic regurgitation secondary to suture placement or annular distortion
11. Complications related to cannulation and perfusion

Some of these complications could be potentially devastating. However, if recognized while the patient is in the operating room with the chest open, surgical intervention may prevent adverse impact on the patient's long-term course.

Mechanisms of persistent dysfunction following MVRep include SAM with LVOTO and a posterior jet of MR (Fig. 28.49), new or residual stenosis (Fig. 28.50), persistent primary mechanisms of MR, leaflet cleft or overshortening associated with PMVL resection (Fig. 28.70), anterior-leaflet override after a quadralateral resection of the PMVL, suture dehiscence, perivalvular MR following MVRep or MVR for endocarditis (Fig. 28.71), and new ischemic MR associated with transient postbypass ischemia. In patients receiving prosthetic valves, perivalvular MR is more frequent in patients with annular calcification and has been associated with reoperations. In each of these circumstances, the post-CPB IOE exam provided crucial identification of the mechanisms for the failed repair and directed their successful correction. In addition, with complete or incomplete chordal sparing techniques of MVR, the subvalvular apparatus may become entangled in the mechanical prosthesis apparatus, preventing complete leaflet closure (108).

Factors that may accentuate SAM and LVOTO with associated posteriorly directed MR include hypovolemia, excessive afterload reduction (vasodilators or anesthetic agents), and hyperdynamic ventricular function (increased sympathetic tone or inotropic agents). If the SAM persists following hemodynamic intervention with presors

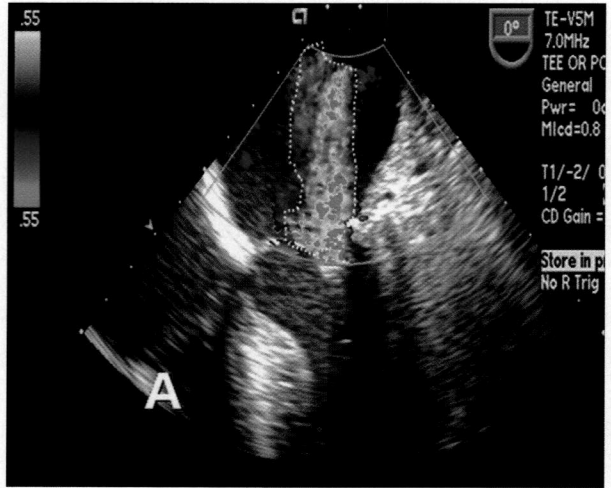

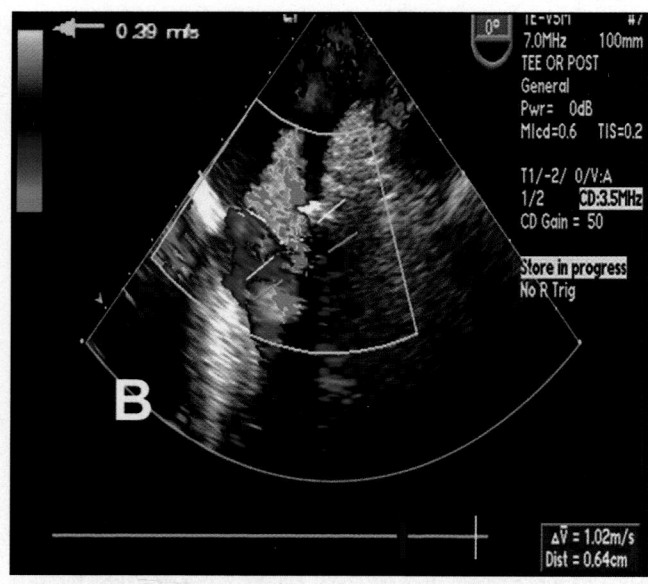

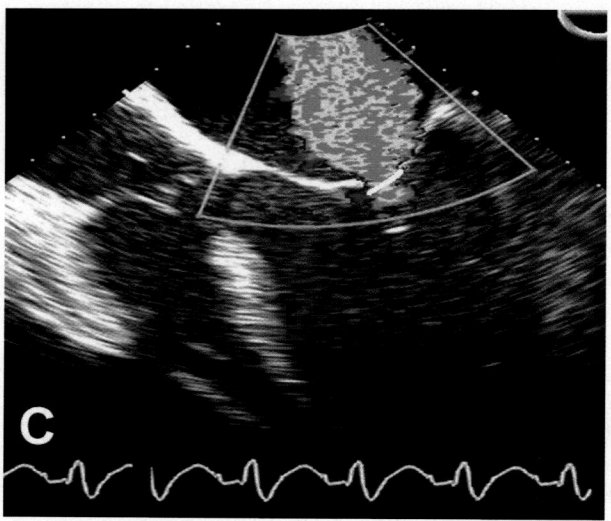

**FIGURE 28.48 A, B, and C.** Regurgitation following MVRep is initially detected using CF Doppler. However, more quantitative methods, (simplified PISA, vena contracta, systolic reversal PV) are recommended for determining the grade of severity.

and volume loading, the surgeon may elect to raise the height of coaptation by performing an annular slide (Figs. 28.44A and 28.44B) procedure. This effectively moves the mitral coaptation point further from the interventricular septum, thereby increasing the effective systolic diameter of the LVOT. In some circumstances, further attempts at valve repair are unsuccessful and valve replacement is necessary.

Other rare complications related to the MV procedure include ventricular septal defects following septal myectomy for correction of MR associated with SAM and myxomatous disease (Fig. 28.72), circumflex coronary occlusion with suture ligation or kinking during the placement of the prosthetic valve or annuloplasty ring (Figs. 28.54A and 28.54B), pseudoaneurysm following debridement of annular calcium (Figs. 28.55A–E), aortic regurgitation due to the anchoring trigonal suture for the annuloplasty

ring engaging the left coronary cusp or distorting the aortic valve annulus, and aortic dissections related to aortic decannulation. Various post-CPB shunts have been detected by IOE at the site of the atrial septal surgical approach, as well as between the LA and aorta (Figs. 28.56A and 28.56B). All of these complications may be diagnosed by intraoperative echocardiography while the chest is still open, if the index of suspicion is raised to a level where these concerns are routinely incorporated into the post-CPB examination.

### Post-CPB Outcomes

Post-CPB complications following MV surgery include those related to the MV procedure and those related to cardiac surgery with CPB in general. The need for second pump runs following MVRep varies widely from 2% to

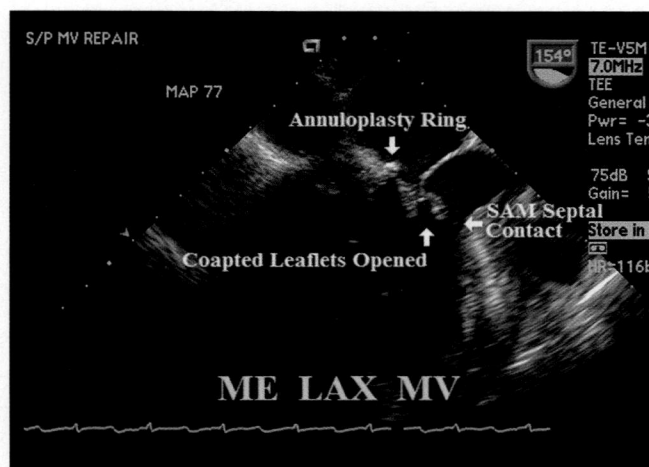

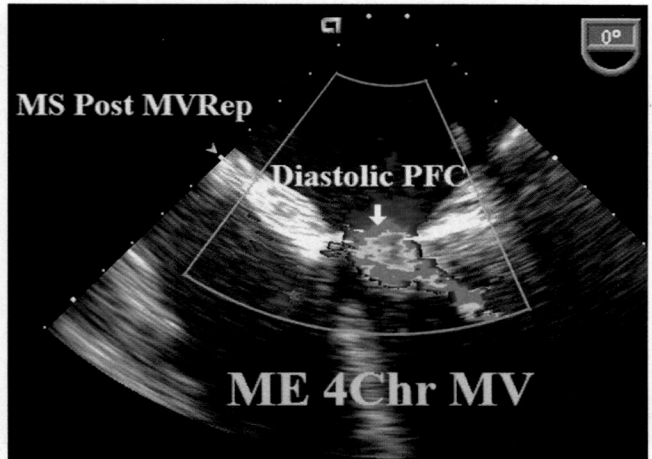

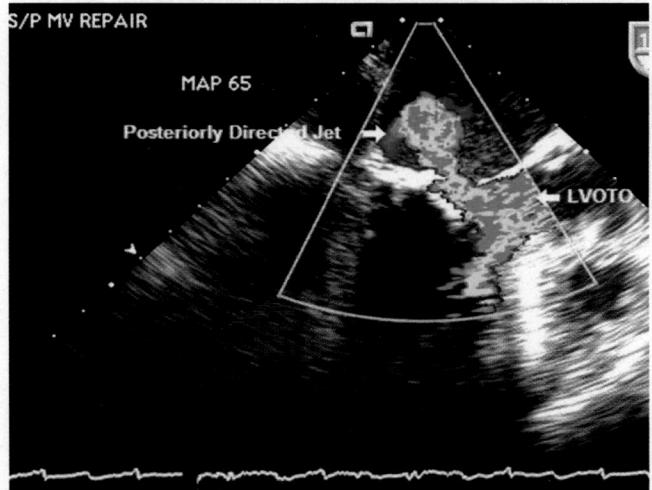

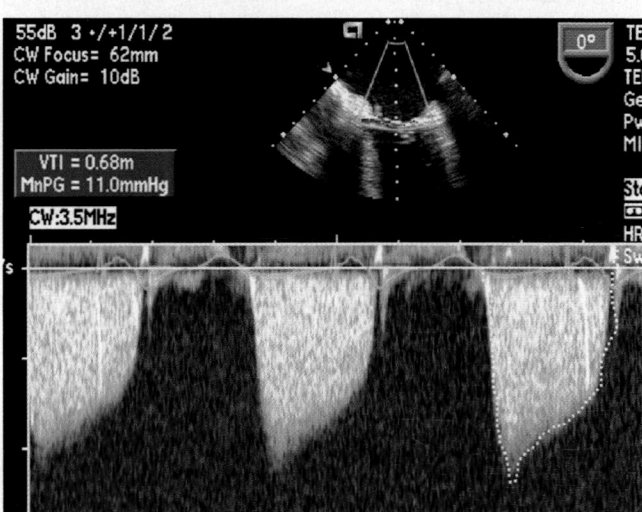

**FIGURE 28.49.** Post-MVRep SAM with LVOTO. Turbulence in the LVOT is a posteriorly directed MR jet characteristic for systolic anterior motion with LVOT obstruction.

**FIGURE 28.50.** Post-MVRep stenosis. Usually stenosis following MV reconstruction is associated with attempts to repair rheumatic disease with pure MS or combined MS and MR. However, cases of stenosis have been associated with repair of myxomatous MV disease using a smaller sized annuloplasty ring. **B:** CW Doppler will provide an estimation of the transvalvular gradient. the first sign of stenosis. Gradients are heart rate dependent, so a significant gradient should take the patient's heart rate into account. The presence of proximal flow convergence is usually the first indication of a significant gradient. PT½ is not a reliable method of assessing MV area post valvuloplasty due to compliance alterations changing the constant used in the calculation. MVA using the continuity equation (using TVI), the Gorlin calculation, is more reliable.

8%, and is dependent on the underlying etiology and mechanism of dysfunction in addition to the aggressiveness of attempted repairs (54,109). Fix et al. reported that patients requiring a second pump run do not incur additional morbidity or mortality, including increased inotrope use, prolonged ventilation, bleeding, and intensive care/hospital length of stay (110).

*Evaluation of Complications* The success rate for mitral repair is dependent upon the underlying pathoanatomy and mechanism of dysfunction. In patients at the Cleveland Clinic with myxomatous disease, second pump runs are required in less than 3% to 5% of patients (54,86,109). In this circumstance, IOE provides crucial information regarding the mechanisms for the failed repair. There have been a number of studies that have evaluated the causes of unsuccessful MVRep. Agri-

cola et al. reported on the mechanisms of failed MV repair in 255 consecutive patients undergoing MVRep who received a quadrilateral resection of the PMVL (87). Mechanisms of failed MVRep were detected by IOE in 21 patients requiring re-repair. Post-CPB determined the exact mechanism of immediate failure determined using IOE; the mechanisms included.

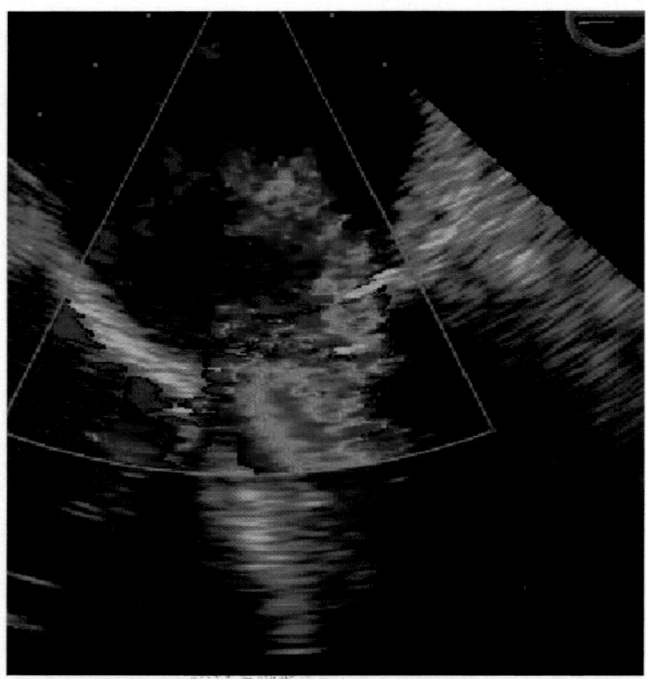

**FIGURE 28.51.** A leaflet cleft at the site of the quadralateral resection or overshortening of the PMVL may incomplete apposition and a posteriorly directed regurgitant jet.

1. Residual cleft provoking interscallop malcoaptation (9 patients)
2. Residual prolapse of the anterior (1 patient) or posterior leaflets (4 patients)
3. Residual annular dilation (3 patients)
4. Left ventricular outflow obstruction (2 patients)
5. Suture dehiscence (2 patients)

In 20 of 21 patients, IOE guided the repair with resolution of the residual MR. The one patient who required MVR had persistent SAM with LVOTO despite the performance of a sliding annuloplasty. SAM occurs most commonly in patients with extremely redundant myxomatous valves with tall PMVL and AMVL as well as hypertrophied ventricles with hyperdynamic function. SAM with LVOTO has occurred more frequently with rigid annuloplasty systems (87). Understanding the factors associated with SAM and LVOTO has provided for a more aggressive approach to this potential complication with the more frequent use of a sliding annuloplasty during the initial repair with a lowered 1% to 2% incidence of post-MVRep SAM and LVOTO (54,109,111). Gillinov et al. have reported that even with predictors of LVOTO, more than 90% of degenerative MVs can be repaired successfully by employing a sliding repair to reduce the risk of systolic anterior motion when the leaflet is > 1.5 cm long (92,93). If patients have a sigmoid-shaped superior septum, as is commonly seen in elderly

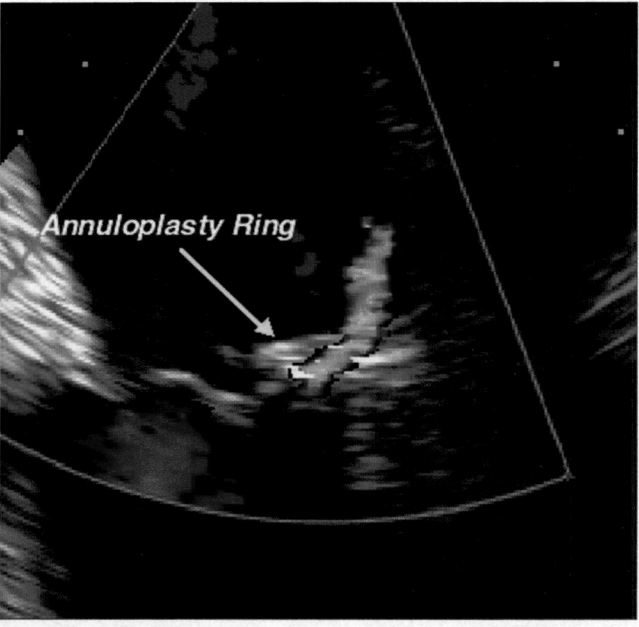

**FIGURE 28.52.** Fistula tract post-MV repair for endocarditis. Once identified, this was repaired with a pericarcial patch during a brief second pump run. The patient left the OR with no MR and had an uneventful postoperative course.

patients, a septal myectomy or MV replacement may be required (91). Close evaluation for a post-CPB VSD is warranted. Understanding those factors precipitating SAM with LVOTO also enables the hemodynamic man-

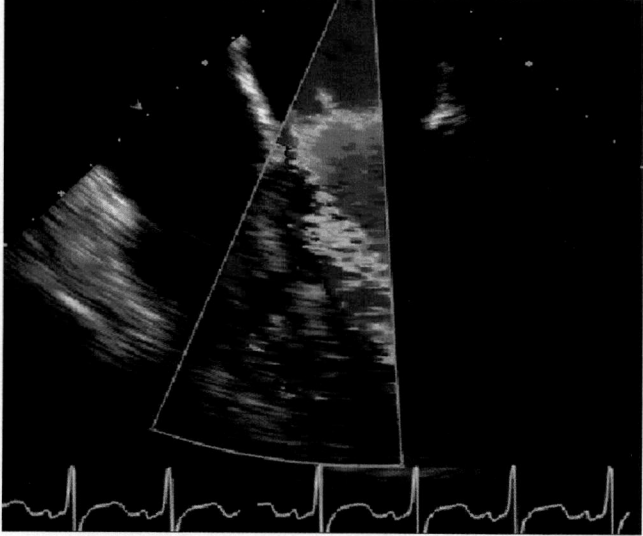

**FIGURE 28.53.** A VSD is an extremely rare complication of MV repair and is associated with the need to perform a septal myectomy in addition to primary reconstruction of the MV apparatus. Whenever a septal myectomy has been performed, great care is taken to closely interrogate the interventricular septum for a possible septal defect.

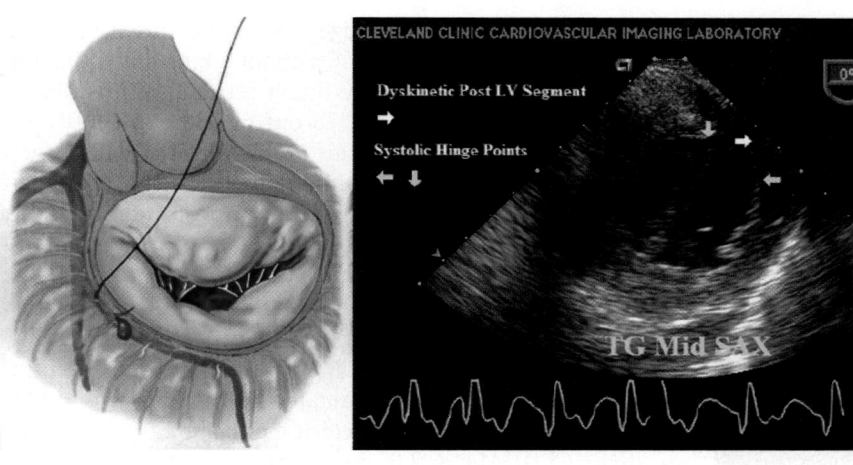

**FIGURE 28.54 A and B.** Occlusion of the left circumflex coronary artery (adjacent to the P1-P2 interface) by suture ligation or kinking of the vessel with placement of the annuloplasty ring or prosthetic mitral valve. This occlusion results in the development of a new or significantly more severe wall motion abnormality. With kinking of the vessel, the wall motion abnormality may be intermittent.

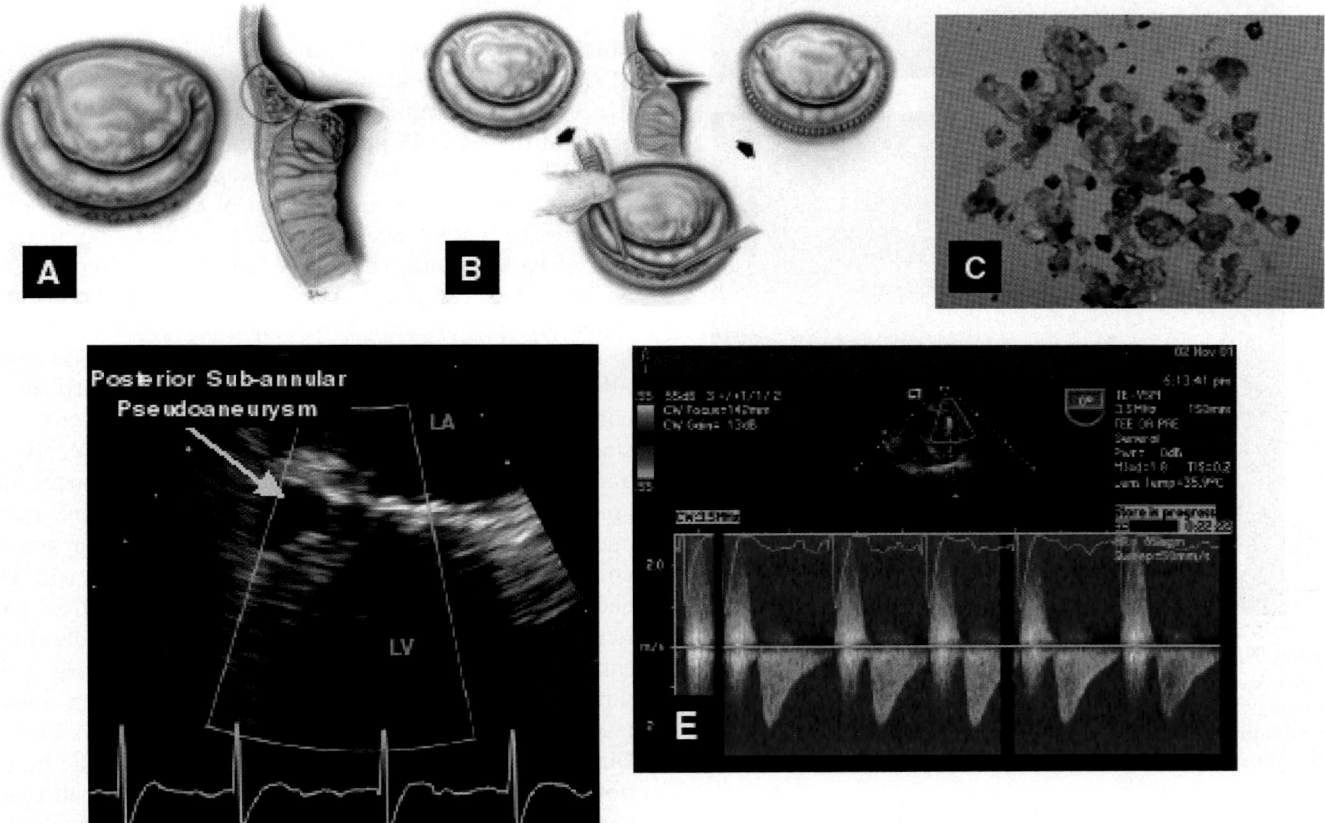

**FIGURE 28.55 A-E. A:** Mitral annular calcification limits annular mobility during systole thereby contributing to MR. **B** and **C:** Extensive debridement may be necessary and is associated with subannular aneurysms and pseudoaneurysm. Because the posterior annulus region is difficult to visualize in the open chest, intraoperative echo is important in establishing the diagnosis during the initial procedure. This patient required extensive debridement due to MAC while undergoing a MVRep. **D:** A subannular pouch was detected 20 minutes later and normal images of this area were visualized. **E:** PW Doppler documented the timing of the flow in and out of the pseudoaneurysm. The patient's subannular region was reinforced with pericardium, and he was weaned from CPB uneventfully and successfully discharged from the hospital.

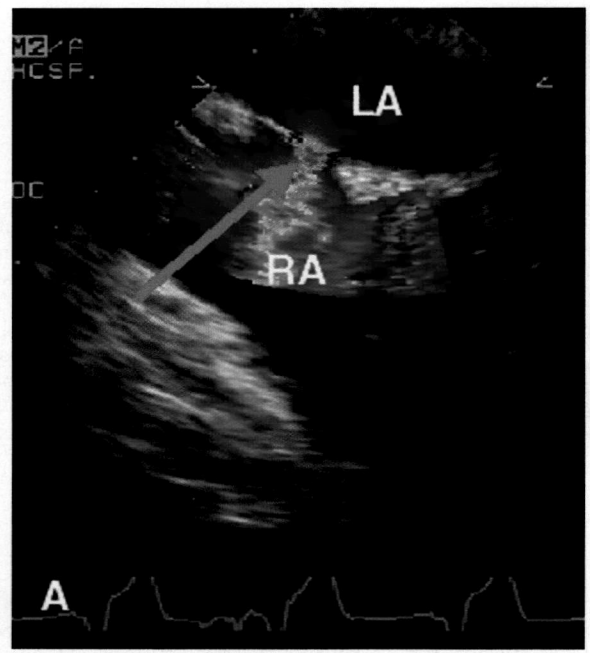

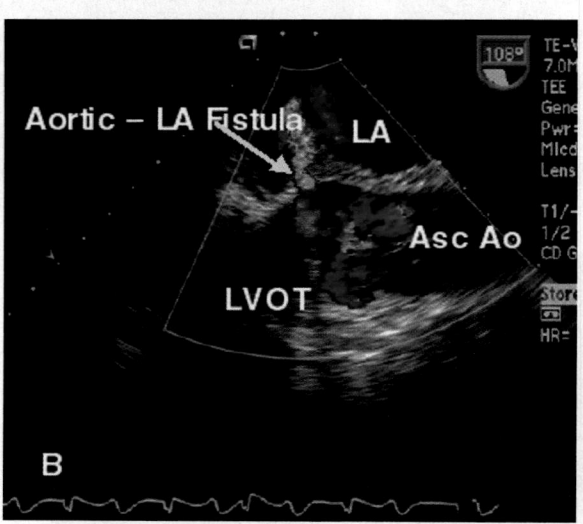

**FIGURE 28.56 A and B.** With the less invasive approaches to valve surgery, exposure is one of the determining factors influencing the success of the surgical procedure. The post-CPB examination closely examines for potential complications related to exposure.

agement of these patients to be anticipated and weaning the patient from CPB with adequate volume in the heart-lung machine to better ensure the ability to reverse mild LVOTO should it occur. Milas et al. have reported on the successful use of A-V sequential pacing in the successful management of SAM with LVOTO (111b).

Gatti et al. performed IOE on 108 consecutive patients who underwent MVRep for degenerative MV dysfunction with MR. Eleven patients had residual MR with a CFD MJA of $\geq 2.0$ cm$^2$ (112). They reported the successful use

of the Alferi edge-to-edge technique improving the amount of MR to $\leq 2.0$ cm$^2$ without taking down the original MVRep. Exactly how much residual MR is acceptable? Fix et al. evaluated 76 out of 530 consecutive patients undergoing MV repair (1987–1989) in whom there was persistent 1$^+$ or 2$^+$ MR and discovered that there were no significant differences in post-hospital mortality, thromboembolic events, hospitalizations for heart failure, or functional class (110). Kawano et al. used IOE in MVRep of 72 patients. They found residual MR with a grade of > 1$^+$ in 5 patients. One required immediate MVR and rapid progression of MR was required in the other three (15). Saiki et al. evaluated 42 patients who underwent MVRep for MR to determine the ability of post-CPB IOE (CFD MJA $\leq 2.0$ cm$^2$) to predict late outcome. Patients with trivial MR, continued to have trivial MR with no progression (p < 0.001) (113).

### Mitral Stenosis (MS)

Muratori et al. reported on 119 patients undergoing MVRep for predominant MR and reported a 0.8% incidence of newly acquired MS determined by transmitral gradient (88). CW Doppler is a routine part of the post-CPB echocardiography in MVRep and MVR in order to provide a baseline documentation of the patient's gradient. Post-CPB MS is usually associated with attempted repair of patients with rheumatic MV disease. New MS is an infrequent complication following MVRep. Following repair for nonrheumatic MR, a significant mean gradient (> 4 mm Hg to 6 mm Hg) is rare unless an edge-to-edge Alferi repair or commissural oversew is performed for a commissural prolapse or flail (109). In these circumstances, the mean gradient and heart rate are recorded and the valve area is planimetered using transgastric or epicardial imaging for accuracy (Fig. 28.57). Umana et al. and Privitera et al. reported on the transvalvular gradients following Alferi "bow-tie" repairs in patients with ischemic MR (116,117). Similar to prosthetic valves, patients following MVRep may have mildly elevated transvalvular mean gradients (less than 4 mm Hg to 6 mm Hg). Significant gradients following MVRep, however, have been reported in nonrheumatic valves (118). Due to differences in immediate post-CPB diastolic function of the left-sided chambers, the pressure half-time method for determining MV area cannot be accurately relied upon.

### Micro-Air and LV Function

In open cardiotomy procedures involving the MV, air is always an issue. Accepting the eventuality of such issues, despite the best attempts of de-airing, many surgical teams will flood the surgical mediastinal wound with CO$_2$ diffused through a surgical sponge to prevent a "jet wash" effect. Tingleff et al. evaluated 15 patients undergoing

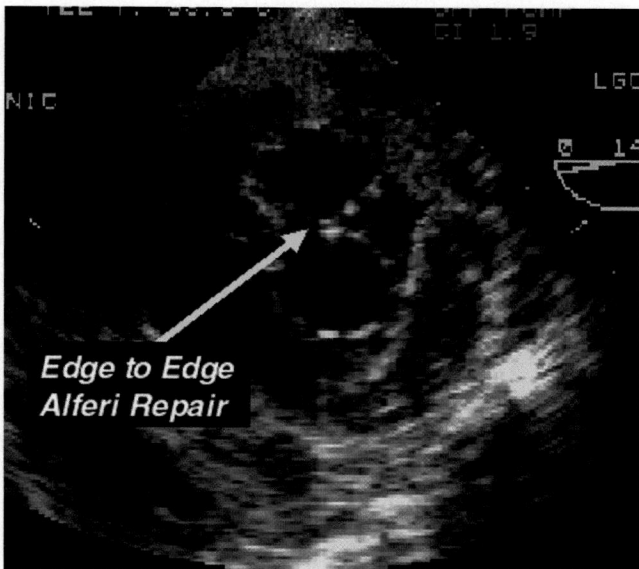

**FIGURE 28.57.** Following a MV repair utilizing an edge-to-edge "Alferi" repair technique, the transvalvular gradient and area of the double orifice are obtained to confirm that there is no significant stenosis (mean gradient > 6-8 mm Hg at a heart rate of 80 bpm, planimetered area > 2.5 cm²).

true open cardiotomy operations (119). All had micro-air originating in the pulmonary veins. Twelve of the 15 patients had new episodes of micro-air up to 28 minutes after termination of cardiopulmonary bypass (119). Secknus et al. evaluated the use of IOE in minimally invasive MV surgery in 52 patients. Intracardiac air was seen transiently in all patients and was associated with new LV dysfunction in 22 (20%) patients. A statistically significant difference (p < 0.001) was noted with a decreased incidence of LV dysfunction in those patients who had no micro-air boluses after weaning from CPB (120).

### Aortic Dissection

Varghese et al. reported on the IOE detection of an aortic dissection by the post-CPB IOE on a patient undergoing MVR (121). While most cannulation-related dissections are self-limiting, if not detected intraoperatively they can present catastrophic challenges. Significant ulcerated plaques or ascending aortic disease may lead to the use of alternative cannulation sites.

### Post-CPB LV Dysfunction

LV dysfunction following MV repair is usually associated with pre-CPB LV dysfunction, while the poor LV function post-CPB may be predicted by the pre-CPB IOE exam's assessment of diastolic and systolic parameters of LV function. LV dysfunction, however, may also be related to

the repair procedure with an open cardiac chamber. Procedure-related LV dysfunction post-CPB may be caused by micro-air embolization to the coronary perfusion bed, the effects of the CPB duration and adequacy of myocardial protection, or related to left circumflex coronary artery obstruction. Ischemia in the perfusion bed of the circumflex coronary artery may be caused by complete obstruction due to suture ensnarement near the lateral scallop of the PMVL as the annuloplasty or prosthetic valve ring is sutured in place (Figs. 28.54A and 28.54B). Kinking of the circumflex has also been reported when extensive resection of a redundant PMVL and sliding annuloplasty distorts the contour of the annular ring. Tavilla et al. reported a case of a damaged circumflex coronary artery associated with a sliding annuloplasty repair, emphasizing the ability of a routine post-CPB assessment to rapidly detect new wall motion abnormalities (122). While compromise of the coronary circulation is a rare complication of MVRep, three such encounters at our institution over the last twelve years have been recognized by abbreviated overview assessments during the pre-SEP CPB exam or shortly after weaning from CPB. In all patients the left circumflex has grafted with recovery of regional function without electrocardiographic or enzyme changes, suggesting a nontransmural or transmural infarct. Micro-air bubbles can cause regional wall motion abnormalities, usually in the more anterior originating right coronary artery. In 1990, Obarski et al. reviewed 224 patients undergoing either MV repair or replacement over a 24-month period and determined that 5.4% may have postoperative regional dysfunction related to micro-air embolization (123). Care is taken to adequately de-air the pulmonary circulation and pockets where air accumulates (ventricular apex, LAA, and dome of the LA).

### Annular Disruption Following Surgical Debridement

Patients who present with extensive posterior mitral annular calcification or periannular abscess requiring extensive debridement are at increased risk of periprosthetic or periannuloplasty ring fistula or pseudoaneurysm formation. With extensive subvalvular debridement, surgical reinforcement with pericardium is sometimes used. Fistulas or pseudoaneurysms between the LV and LA may also develop in patients with periannular abscesses (95,124) (Figs. 28.55A–28.55E). In 1998, Genoni et al. reported on two dissections of the left atrium during MVRep. The dissections were intraoperatively detected by TEE imaging and successfully managed without perioperative morbidity (124).

### Iatrogenic Shunts and Fistulas

Surgical exposure for minimally invasive MV surgery is an important determinant of successful exposure and the repair of the valve. In the initial experience with such devices, iatrogenic complications were encountered that were recognized by the IOE exam prior to separation from CPB. With recognition of these unusual findings, surgical intervention—while the patient was still cannulated, permitted their immediate resolution as potential issues in the postoperative course.

### Perivalvular MR following MVR

Perivalvular MR has an increased incidence in patients with mitral annular calcification and reoperation, and is associated with postoperative hemolysis. Though hemolysis is significantly decreased by comparison in MVRep, it can occur (58b). Morehead et al. reported the results of IOE in 27 patients undergoing MVR with IOE, utilizing CFD to detect intra- and perivalvular MR. Before the administration of protamine, a total of 55 jets were detected (104). The CF Doppler regurgitation by maximum jet area (MJA) decreased an average of 70% (p < 0.0001) by quantitative methods of assessment. Mitral and mechanical valves each had more jets and overall greater MJA when compared to aortic and tissue valves. With certain bioprosthetic MV prostheses, it is not unusual to see mild (1–2$^+$) central MR initially (Fig. 28.58). Ionescu et al. evaluated IOE in 300 patients undergoing MVR. With projections of cost savings from the complications that IOE diagnosed, they determined that extending routine

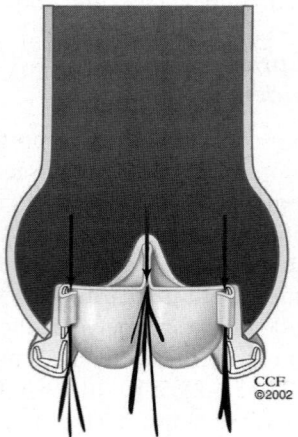

---

**FIGURE 28.58** All bioprosthetic valves have insignificant amounts of regurgitation up to mild (1+) within the sewing ring, and are usually central in origin and direction.

IOE use to patients undergoing MVR provided a cost savings of $109 per patient (125).

### Assessment of TV Repair

IOE evaluation of new TR or TVRep utilizes the ME 4 Chr TV focused image plane with 2 dimensional imaging and CFD MJA, vena contracta, and PISA PFC to determine the significance of TR post-CPB (35). In patients with significant metabolic derangements caused by hepatic congestion, correction of moderate TR which persists following attempted TVRep may be indicated. 5.3% of patients undergoing TVRep have required second pump runs (54). Similar to MVRep, the TV should be evaluated following hemodynamic equilibration. In a report of 401 patients undergoing cardiac surgery, the IOE altered the management of TVRep in 10% of patients; however, it was found that despite trivial TR with the post-CPB IOE, many patients will develop significant TR postoperatively as a reflection of poor RV dysfunction.

### Systematic IOE Examination in MV Surgery

#### Priority Directed Exam

The systematic examination in MV surgery is performed in an efficiently organized manner that will resolve those issues that guide intraoperative anesthetic-hemodynamic and surgical management of the patient, as well as document a comprehensive examination for future reference. As previously discussed, the systematic IOE examination in MV surgery is structured into a "priority directed exam" (abbreviated overview and focused diagnostic exam) and the more general comprehensive exam. Most pre-CPB exams are possible within a 10 to 15 minute period. Regardless of what name we attach to a portion of the exam, experienced intraoperative echocardiographers develop an organized sequence with which they are comfortable that enables them to:

1. Overview the cardiovascular anatomy and function and organize the patient's exam
2. Resolve these critical issues in the sequence of the examination and
3. Document a comprehensive TEE examination for future comparison

While it is always tempting to jump directly to the most impressive findings from the patient's preoperative evaluation, the previously mentioned studies provide evidence suggesting that there are instances where all current significant findings where not included in the results of the patient's preoperative evaluation. It is the abbreviated examination that permits the focused examination to proceed unimpeded, without the concern of last-minute revelations just before or after proceeding onto CPB. The abbreviated exam is followed by a focused and subsequent comprehensive IOE exam that is digitally stored for documentation and future reference (Table 28.4).

### Abbreviated Overview Exam (Table 28.7A, Fig. 28.24) (II)

The purpose of the abbreviated overview exam in patients undergoing MV surgery is to develop a complete understanding of the likely significant findings of the final exam from the outset. Because of the anatomic relation between the TEE probe position in the stomach and esophagus, every cardiac structure may be assessed utilizing 0° to 15° transducer angulation for transverse imaging. If abnormalities, such as mobile protruding atheroma or significant aortic regurgitation, are discovered it is possible to mobilize equipment and personnel for an epiaortic examination and include a more thorough examination of the aortic valve as discussed in Chapter 30. Once the TEE probe has been inserted, the following one-minute exam sequence may be performed in which 2-D and color Doppler assessment of the anatomy and function of all chambers, valves, and major thoracic vascular structures is obtained and digitally stored:

1. The TEE probe is advanced to the TG SAX$_{mid}$ imaging plane at a depth of approximately 40 cm. Using 2-D imaging and storage of a representative digital loop, the global LV and RV function are assessed.
2. For screening purposes only, color flow Doppler is initiated in a wide sector scan with an aliasing velocity at approximately 55 cm/sec. This will result in a PRF of 10 to 20 Hz, which is not reliable for detailed diagnostic evaluation. The TEE probe is slowly withdrawn with slight clockwise turning. By slightly advancing and withdrawing the TEE probe (2 cm) back and forth over the coaptation plane of the tricuspid valve, the valve structure and presence of abnormal regurgitation or turbulent transvalvular flow are noted and a representative digital loop is stored.
3. The TEE probe is slowly turned counterclockwise to the left and withdrawn to obtain a focused color Doppler view of the ME 4 Chr. Again, by slowly advancing and withdrawing the TEE probe (2 cm) back and forth over the coaptation plane of the MV, the structure and presence of abnormal regurgitation or stenosis is noted and a representative digital loop is stored.
4. The TEE probe is turned slightly clockwise and withdrawn until the ME 5 Chr is obtained with visualization of the LVOT and aortic valve Chr. Again, by slowly advancing and withdrawing the TEE probe (2 cm–3 cm) back and forth over the coaptation plane of the aortic valve and LVOT, the presence of abnormal regurgitation or turbulent systolic flow are noted and a representative digital loop is stored.
5. The TEE probe is slightly withdrawn (2 cm) from the ME 5 Chr to visualize the aortic root and presence of atheroma or pathology. A representative digital loop is stored in the ME asc aortic SAX.
6. The TEE probe is turned counterclockwise and the desc aorta SAX and LAX imaging plane is obtained. The entire descending aorta from the celiac axis to the arch and origins of the left subclavian, common carotid, and innominate may be visualized with 2-D and color. "Running" the descending thoracic aorta pre-CPB has proven valuable for detecting persistent patent ductus arteriosus in adults (Fig. 28.59). A representative digital loop of any significant atheroma is stored. If the atheroma is greater than 3 mm, epiaortic imaging is routinely performed (Figs. 28.60A–28.60D).

▶ **TABLE 28.7A.  Priority-Ordered Intraoperative Exam: Abbreviated Overview TEE Examination in Mitral Valve Surgery**

| Standard Imaging Plane | Probe Turn | Depth | CF Doppler Screen | Structures Examined |
|---|---|---|---|---|
| Transgastric SAX 2-D | | 40 cm | | LV & RV Fx |
| ME 4 Chr TV | Right | 35 cm | X | RV Fx<br>TR |
| ME 4 Chr MV | Left | 30 cm | X | LV Fx<br>MR MS |
| UE 5 Chr AoV | Central | 28 cm | X | LV Fx |
| UE LAX | Central | 26 cm | | Aortic root |
| Desc Th Ao SAX | Left | 40–20 cm | | Desc thoracic aorta |

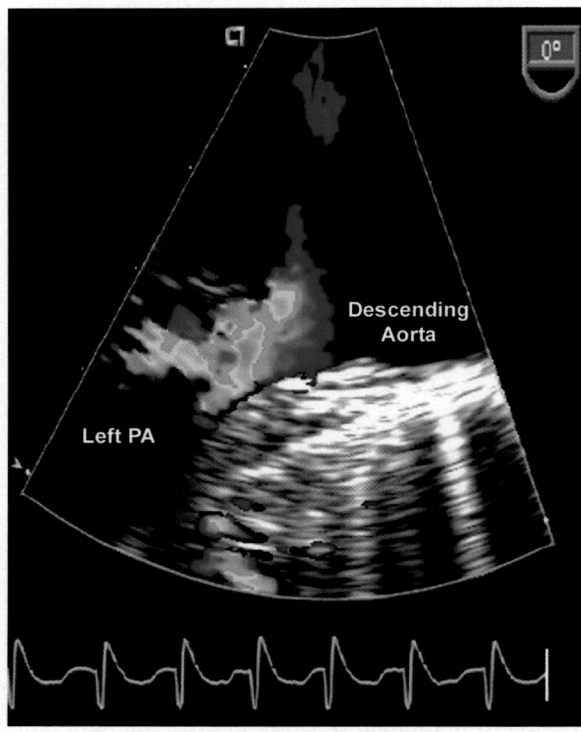

**FIGURE 28.59.** Evaluating the aorta for the rare patent ductus arteriosus may prevent interruption of strategies for cannulation and perfusion.

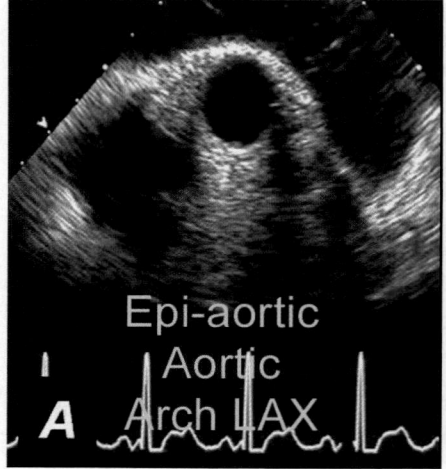

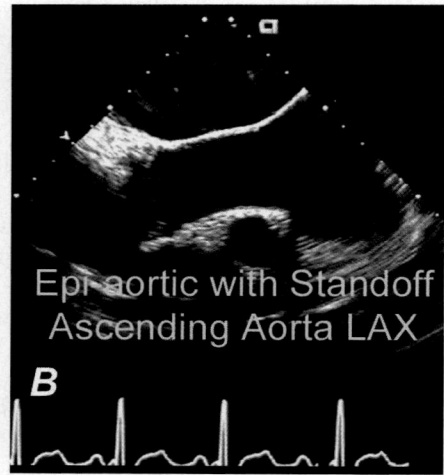

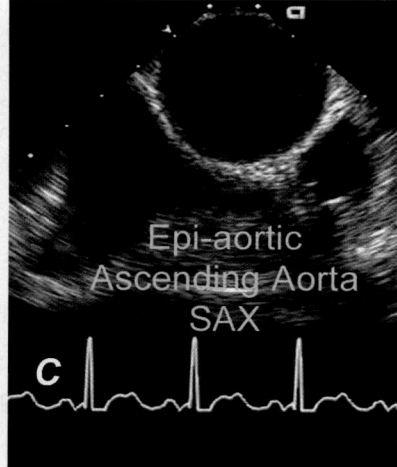

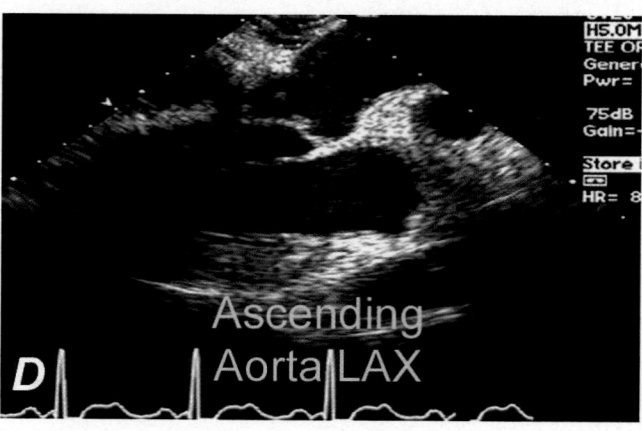

**FIGURE 28.60.** Epicardial scanning in patients with significant risk factors of developing atheroma or the finding of protruding plaques in the descending thoracic aorta warrants epiaortic scanning of the cannulation and cross-clamp sites.

In each of these rapid succession of imaging planes, the probe is advanced and withdrawn looking for evidence of valve regurgitation or transvalvular turbulence suggestive of stenosis. The ascending and descending thoracic aortas are evaluated for atheroma that would suggest the need for epicardial imaging. The results of this brief overview examination will serve as a guide for the organization of the remainder or the intraoperative examination.

### Focused Diagnostic IOE Exam in MV Surgery (Table 28.7B)

Experienced echocardiographers develop a natural sequence with which they feel most comfortable over time. The focused diagnostic exam sequence suggested here is guided by the rare necessity to initiate CPB sooner than anticipated or to return to CPB during the post-CPB exam. The posterior and superior location of the midesophagus in relation to the MV annulus and the central rotational axis of the transducer, which may be positioned in the center of the anterior mitral valve leaflet (AMVL), enable ideal imaging of the MVAp. With the possibility of 360° imaging of the MVAp at any depth with the multiplane transducer, it is possible to understand the 3-D anatomy of the MV anatomy and mechanism(s) of dysfunction. The anatomic progression of the depth of TEE probe insertion and transducer angulation permit an efficient and orderly progression with minimal probe or transducer manipulation.

As illustrated in Table 28.2, the MV apparatus is - examined utilizing up to 12 or more variations of the 6 recommended ASE/SCA cross-section imaging views at the midesophageal (ME 4 chamber MV, ME commissural MV, ME 2 chamber MV, and ME LAX MV) and transgastric imaging (TG basal SAX MV and TG 2 Chr MV) probe depths. A 3-D "feel" for the mitral apparatus anatomy is developed by advancing or withdrawing the TEE probe 2 cm to 3 cm (subtle anteflexing or retroflexing produces similar images) or by turning the TEE probe left (counterclockwise) and right (clockwise) from the standard midesophageal imaging planes. At every image plane 2-D, CFD, CWD, and PWD is performed. To orient the imaging field and to permit more efficient digital storage for the comprehensive examination, 2-D and CFD digital images are stored at initial depths that permit the visualization of the apex (in ME image planes) and the entire LV and RV in the TG SAX image planes. Should the need arise to initiate CPB, global and regional ventricular may be examined from the stored images and for future reference. Valve structures are examined in detail during the focused diagnostic exam by using the focusing or zoom option. This permits the visualization and storage of 2-D and CFD images with better image and color flow detail due to the increased magnification, as well as resolution and Doppler interrogation advantages related to increased pulse repetition frequency. 2-D and Doppler (CFD, CWD, and PWD) interrogation of the MV and adjacent structures (pulmonary veins, tricuspid valve, and hepatic veins) are digitally stored at each image plane prior to advancing in the sequence to the next imaging plane.

### Sequence of Focused Diagnostic IOE Exam in MV Surgery (Table 28.7B)

The approximate transducer angulation, probe manipulation (withdrawal or turning), and probe depth are included for each imaging plane. As previously noted, these approximations may vary from patient to patient due to individual variations as previously discussed (Fig. 28.12).

### Midesophageal Four-Chamber MV and Variations (Table 28.2, Figs. 28.25A and 28.27)

### Midesophageal Five-Chamber MV (Figs. 28.3B and 28.26)

### Lower-esophageal Four-Chamber MV (Figs. 28.3C and 28.27)

**TEE Probe Manipulation:** Following the brief abbreviated overview examination, the TEE probe is positioned at the ME 4 Chr at a probe depth of approximately 30 cm from the mouth with a transducer rotation of 0°–15°. Once this image plane is established the entire AMVL (A1, A2, A3) and PMVL (P1, P2, P3) may be evaluated by gradually withdrawing the probe 2 cm to 3 cm toward the head (or anteflexing) to the more superior ME 5 Chr imaging plane with visualization of the LVOT. This is followed by a slow advancement of the TEE probe toward the stomach 3 cm to 4 cm (or retroflexion). This maneuver permits the transducer imaging plane to diagonally travel over the entire mitral leaflet line of coaptation from the more superior anterolateral commissure to the more inferior posteromedial commissure (Fig. 28.25A). This maneuver is performed with 2-D and then with color flow Doppler, looking for regions of regurgitation or diastolic turbulence with stenosis.

In addition, the LV and RV global function may be assessed. The LV septum and lateral walls (base, mid, and apex) may be evaluated for regional wall motion. The RV septum and free wall may be evaluated.

### 1. Midesophageal Four-Chamber MV (Figs. 28.3A, 28.25A, and 28.25B)

**Transducer Depth:** 30 cm
**Transducer Rotation:** 0°–15°
**MV Structures:** A2, midcommissure, and P2 and/or P1
**Tricuspid Valve:** Septal, anterior, or posterior leaflet

TABLE 28.7B. Priority Ordered Intraoperative Exam Focused Diagnostic Exam

| ASE/SCA Standard Imaging Plane *Variation | Probe Turn Right = Clockwise Left = Counterclockwise | Angle Rotation (in degrees) | Probe Depth (in cm) | Chambers LV Segments | Valve Segments | Color Flow Doppler | CW Doppler | Pulse Wave Doppler |
|---|---|---|---|---|---|---|---|---|
| 1 ME 4 Chr | Midline | 0–15 | 30 | RA RV LA LV Septal & Lateral | A2 P1-2 | MR MS AR LVOT Obstruction | MR TVI MS PT$_{1/2}$ MS DT MS gradient (Peak & mean) | |
| 2 ME 5 Chr* | Midline | 0–15 | 28 | RA RV LA LV, LVOT, Anteroseptal & Post | A1 P1 ALC | MR MS AR LVOT Obstruction | MR TVI MS PT$_{1/2}$ MS DT MS gradient (Peak & Mean) *LVOTO* *AR/AS* | LUPV LLPV PW Doppler AR |
| 3 LE 4 Chr* | Midline | 0–15 | 30 | RA, RV, LA, LV Inferior-Septal Posterolateral | A3 P3 PMC | MR MS | MR TVI MS PT$_{1/2}$ MS DT MS gradient (Peak & mean) | |
| 4 ME Comm | Midline | 45–70 | 30 | LA LV Anterolateral & Inferior-Septal | P1 ALC A2 PMC P3 | MR MS | MR TVI MS PT$_{1/2}$ MS DT MS gradient (Peak & mean) | |
| 5 ME Comm Right* | Right | 45–70 | 30 | LA LV Aortic Valve Inferior-Septal Anterior-Anteroseptal | A1 A2 A3 | MR MS | MR TVI MS PT$_{1/2}$ MS DT MS gradient (Peak & mean) | |
| 6 ME Comm Left* | Left | 45–70 | 30 | LA LV Inferior-Lateral | P1-2 P2 P2-3 | MR MS | MR TVI MS PT$_{1/2}$ MS DT MS gradient (Peak & mean) | |

| # View | Orientation | Angle | Angle | Structures | Segments | Pathology | Measurements | Notes |
|---|---|---|---|---|---|---|---|---|
| 7 ME 2 Chr | Midline | 90 | 30 | LA<br>LV<br>Inferior and Septal<br>Anterolateral | A1A2A3<br>P3<br>PMC | MR MS | MR TVI<br>MS PT$_{1/2}$<br>MS DT<br>MS gradient<br>(Peak & mean) | |
| 8 ME 2 Chr Right | Right | 90 | 30 | LA<br>LV<br>Inferior-Anteroseptal<br>LVOT | A1A2A3<br>PMC<br>P3 | MR MS<br>AR AS<br>LVOT Obst | N/A | |
| 9 ME 2 Chr Left | Left | 90 | 30 | LA<br>LV<br>Inferior-Lateral | P3<br>P2 | MR MS | N/A | |
| 10 ME LAX | Midline | 130 | 30 | LA<br>LV<br>Anteroseptal Posterior<br>LVOT<br>Aorta | A2<br>P2<br>MidCom | MR MS<br>AR AS<br>LVOT Obst | MR TVI<br>MS PT$_{1/2}$<br>MS DT<br>MS gradient<br>(Peak & mean) | |
| 11 ME LAX Right* | Right | 130 | 30 | LA<br>LV<br>Anterior<br>Posterior-Lateral | P3<br>PMC<br>P2-3 | MR MS | MR TVI<br>MS PT$_{1/2}$<br>MS DT<br>MS gradient<br>(Peak & mean) | |
| 12 ME LAX Left* | Left | 130 | 30 | LA<br>LV<br>Posterior<br>Inferior-Septal | A1-2<br>ALC<br>P1-2 | MR MS | MR TVI<br>MS PT$_{1/2}$<br>MS DT<br>MS gradient<br>(Peak & mean) | |
| 13 Bicaval | Right from MELAX | 130 | 28 | LA, RA, IAS<br>Fossa Ovalis<br>PFO<br>SVC, IVC, Cor Sinus, | N/A | PFO<br>Cor Sinus | N/A | PW Doppler |
| 14 RUPV & RLPV (Bicaval) | Right | 135 | 135–28 | LA, RA, IAS<br>RUPV, RLPV<br>SVC, IVC, Cor Sinus | N/A | RUPV<br>RLPV | PV gradient in lung TP | Severe MR has systolic reversal |
| 15 TG SAX Basal | Midline | 0 | 32–35 | LV (anterior, lateral, posterior, inferior, septal segments)<br>RV | A1-2-3<br>ALC<br>P1-2-3<br>PLC | N/A | N/A | |
| 16 TG 2 Chr | Midline | 70–90 | 85 | LV anterior and inferior wall<br>Subvalvular apparatus | A2 P1-2 | MS MR<br>Subvalvular MS identification | N/A | |

**LV Structures:** (Infero) septum (base, mid, apex)

**RV Structure:** Septum and RV free wall

**CFD:** Interrogation for MR and severity assessment using MJA, vena contracta, PISA

**CWD:**

**MR:** CW intensity, peak transmitral velocity dP/dt, PISA peak $V_{MR}$

**MS:** Transmitral gradient, $PT_{1/2}$, DT, PISA peak $V_{MS}$

**PWD:**

**MR:** E or A dominance, volumetric calculations

**CMM:**

**MR:** Systolic PISA PCF radius calculation

Depending on the orientation of the MV commissure and transducer rotation angle, the 2-D plane may cut through the A2 and P2 and/or P1 segments of the MV. On the monitor in this imaging plane, the anterior leaflet is displayed on the right and the posterior leaflets on the left. Proceeding from left to right are A2, midcommissure, and P2 and/or P1.

### 2. Midesophageal Five-Chamber MV (ME 5 Chr MV) (Figs. 28.3B, 28.25A, and 28.26)

**Variation of ME 4 Chr MV**

**Transducer Depth:** 30 cm

**Probe Manipulation:** Withdraw from ME 4 Chr

**MV Structures:** A1, anterolateral commissure, and P1

**LV Structures:** LVOT, anterior septum (B, M, A), Lat-Post (B, M, A)

**LA:** Diameter

**RV Structure:** Anterior septum and anterior RV free wall

**Tricuspid Valve:** Septal and anterior leaflet

This imaging plane cuts through the left ventricular outflow track. Depending on the orientation of the MV commissure and transducer rotation angle, the 2-D plane may cut through the A1 segment, anterolateral commissure, and P1 segments of the MV. On the monitor in this imaging plane, the anterior leaflet is displayed on the right and the posterior leaflet on the left. Proceeding from left to right are A1, anterolateral commissure, and P1.

### 3. Lower-Esophageal Four-Chamber MV (LE Four Chr MV) (Figs. 28.3B, 28.25A, and 28.27)

**Variation of ME 4 Chr**

**Transducer Depth:** 32 cm

**Probe Manipulation:** Advance

**MV Structures:** A3 posteromedial commissure and P3

**LV Structures:** LVOT, anterior septum (B, M, A), Lat-Post (B, M, A)

**Tricuspid Valve:** Annular diameter, septal, and posterior leaflets

**RV Structure:** Inferior septum and inferior RV free wall, coronary sinus

Depending on the orientation of the MV commissure and transducer rotation angle, the 2-D plane may cut through

the A3 segment, posteromedial commissure, and the P3 scallop of the MV. On the monitor in this imaging plane, the anterior leaflet is displayed on the right and the posterior leaflet on the left. Proceeding from left to right are A3, posteromedial commissure, and P3.

**Diagnostic Capability:** Withdrawing the probe between the ME 4 Chr to the ME 5 Chr and then to the ME 4 Chr with 2-D and CFD imaging (aliasing velocity set at 50 cm/sec–55 cm/sec) every segment of the AMVL and PMVL may be evaluated for degree of thickness, characterization of systolic and diastolic leaflet motion (excessive, normal, or restricted), and the integrity of the chordae (primary and secondary), exact point of origin of regurgitant flow (proximal flow convergence visualized below plane of valve connecting to the vena contracta zone), or restricted stenotic antegrade flow (proximal flow convergence initiating above the annular plane and continuing through a funnel-shaped valve). If there is excessive regurgitant flow, for purposes of mechanism determination, the aliasing velocity scale is increased toward 70 cm/sec. If there are central and parallel regurgitant jets noted in adjacent imaging planes, where the PFC and vena contracta of only one are visualized, it is likely that these jets result from a similar mechanism, such as bileaflet tethering or symmetrical bileaflet prolapse. If two distinct jets are identified in the same or adjacent imaging planes and are crossing or directed in different directions, it is likely that these regurgitant jets represent two separate and distinct mechanisms of MR.

CW Doppler through the mitral inflow or regurgitant orifice may be utilized to interrogate for either a diastolic flow gradient or systolic regurgitation, utilizing the strength of the spectral envelope as indirect evidence of severity of MR. If the continuity equation is to be used for determination of MVA in the setting of MS, CW Doppler interrogation is performed using five or more cycles if the patient is in atrial fibrillation. The MV inflow TVI is measured using planimetry and entered.

### Left Upper and/or Lower Pulmonary Vein (Fig. 28.60.1A, B)

The left upper pulmonary is located adjacent to the aorta (laterally) and coumadin ridge (medially). Color flow Doppler is initiated and in the presence of significant MR, systolic color reversal may be seen. A Doppler cursor (line of interrogation) is placed parallel to the direction of pulmonary vein flow. With PWD, the pulmonary venous flow pattern is interrogated.

**TEE Probe Manipulation:** From the ME 4 Chr imaging plane, the TEE probe is slowly withdrawn and turned to the left (as the imaging plane passes through the ME 5 Chr, left atrium, and left atrial appendage).

**Diagnostic Value:** If there is severe MR, there will be systolic reversal of flow in the pulmonary vein as demon-

## Pulmonary Vein Doppler
### *Determinants of Waves*

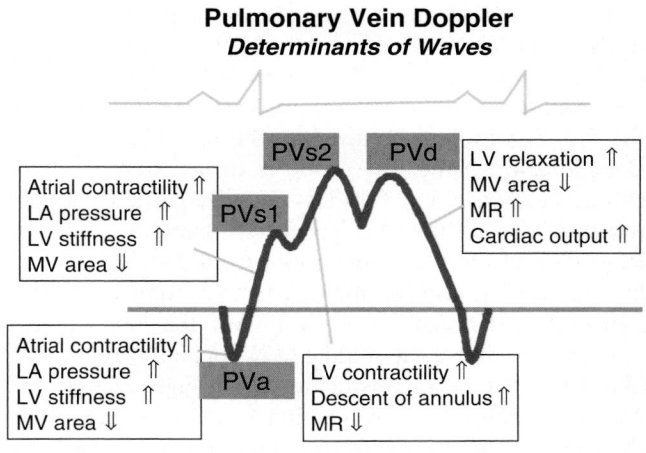

**FIGURE 28.60.1A.** Pulmonary vein doppler determinants of waves.

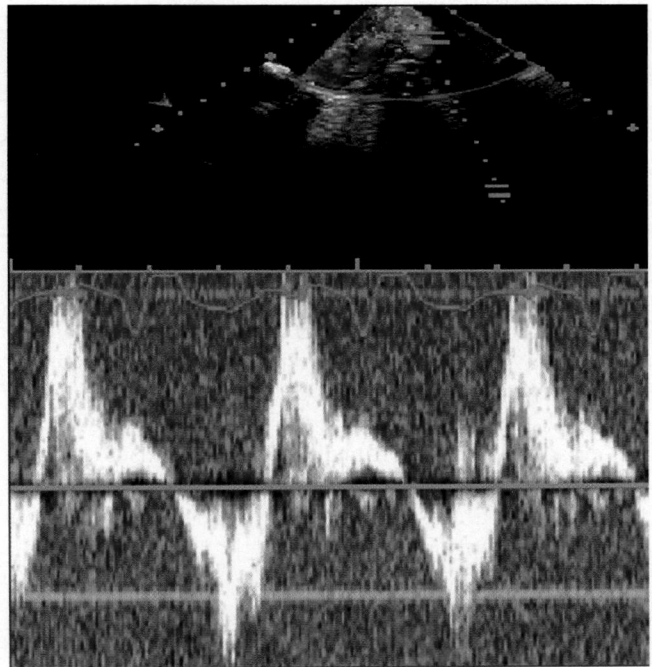

**FIGURE 28.60.1B.** PW Doppler left upper pulmonary vein.

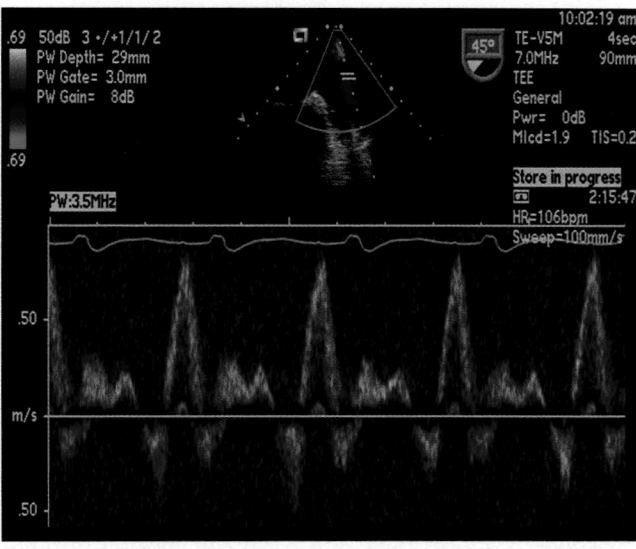

**FIGURE 28.61.** LUPV late systolic reversal is indicative of more severe MR. Finding systolic reversal in more than one pulmonary vein or the PV opposite the jet direction is more significant.

strated by the PW Doppler spectral envelope and timed by the onset of or following the ECG R wave (Fig. 28.61). If LA pressures are elevated above 15 mm Hg, there will be a blunting of the systolic wave. Advancing the probe with color flow Doppler may engage the left lower pulmonary vein.

### *Midesophageal Commissural MV and Variations (Figs. 28.3D and 28.28)*

**TEE Probe Manipulation:** From the midline ME 4 Chr imaging plane, the transducer angle is rotated forward to

45°–70° to obtain the ME Com imaging plane. 2-D imaging at this imaging plane and its associated right (clockwise) probe turn followed by a left (counterclockwise) turn enable visualization of every segment of the AMVL and PMVL in addition to color Doppler interrogation of the posteromedial, midcommissure, and posteromedial commissure.

### *4. Midesophageal Commissural MV (ME Com MV) (Table 28.2 and Fig. 28.28)*

**Transducer Depth:** 30 cm
**Probe Manipulation:** Midline
**Transducer Rotation:** 45°–70°
**MV Structures:** P3, posteromedial commissure, A2, anterolateral commissure, A1
May see flail P2 in center screen over A2 in systole
    **MV Annulus:** Major axis
**LV Structures:** Septal-inferior (B, M, A), anterolateral (B, M, A), LA: diameter
**CFD:** Visualize MR from posteromedial commissure, A2, anterolateral commissure, and A1
Depending on the orientation of the MV commissure and transducer rotation angle, the 2-D plane may cut through the P3 scallop, the posteromedial commissure, tip of A2, anterolateral commissure, and the P1 segments of the MV. On the monitor (proceeding from left to right) are P3, posteromedial commissure, A2, anterolateral commissure, and P1. The annular plane drawn between the MV annulus to the left on the screen and to the right usually represents the most inferior (closest to the apex) as-

pects of the saddle-shaped annulus. A plane drawn between these points consequently may overcall MV prolapse.

### 5. Midesophageal Commissural MV (Probe Turned Right) (ME Com$_R$ MV) (Table 28.2 and Fig. 28.29)

**Variation of ME Com MV**
**Transducer Depth:** 30 cm
**Transducer Rotation:** 45°–70°
**Probe Manipulation:** Turn right or clockwise
**MV Structures:** P3, posteromedial commissure, A3, A2, A1
**LV Structures:** Septal-inferior (B, M, A), anterior (B, M, ALA: diameter)
**CFD:** Visualize MR from posteromedial commissure, A3 or P3 flail

Depending on the orientation of the MV commissure and transducer rotation angle, the 2-D plane may cut through the P3 scallop, the posteromedial commissure, the A3 segment, A2 segment, and the A1 segment. On the monitor (proceeding from left to right) are P3, the posteromedial commissure, A3, A2, and A1.

### 6. Midesophageal Commissural MV (Probe Turned Left) (ME Com$_L$ MV) (Table 28.3F and Fig. 28.28A)

**Variation of ME Com**
**Transducer Depth:** 30 cm
**Probe Manipulation:** Turn left or counterclockwise
**Transducer Rotation:** 45°–70°
**MV Structures:** P3, P2, P1
**LV Structures:** Inferior (B, M, A), anterolateral (B, M, A)
**CFD:** Visualize MR from AMVL flail directed over P3, P2, or P1

Depending on the orientation of the MV commissure and transducer rotation angle, the 2-D plane may cut through the P3, P2, and P1 scallops. The commissure may not be visualized, except during diastole. On the monitor (proceeding from left to right) are P3, P2, and P1.

**Diagnostic Value:** Two-dimensional imaging at this imaging plane and its associated right (clockwise) probe turn followed by a left (counterclockwise) turn enable visualization of every segment of the AMVL and PMVL in addition to color Doppler interrogation of the posteromedial, midcommissure, and posteromedial commissure. The P1 scallop of the PMVL is on the right and protrudes from the anterolateral mitral annulus. The P3 scallop protrudes from the inferoposterior mitral annulus. The center of the AMVL (tip of A2) is seen centrally between P1 and P3 during cardiac cycle.

The ME Com imaging plane represents the long axis of the elliptically shaped MV annulus. Because the inferoseptal and anterolateral annulus in the ME Com imaging plane represents the lowest (closest to the apex) points of the saddle-shaped annulus, caution is taken in diagnosing excessive leaflet excursion above the plane of the annulus.

From the ME Com imaging plane, the probe is turned to the right (clockwise) and the AMVL is visualized proceeding A3-A2-A1 in a left-to-right order. Depending on the orientation of the MV commissure, the P3 scallop of the PMVL may be visualized to the left. From the ME Com imaging plane, the probe is turned to the left or counterclockwise. The PMVL is visualized. The P3 scallop protrudes from the left inferoposterior annulus and the P1 scallop of the PMVL protrudes from the right anterolateral annulus. The commissure is not visualized. With a flail middle (P2) scallop of the PMVL, the flail segment may be seen above the middle (A2) portion of the AMVL like a hooded cobra raising its head (Figs. 28.62A and 28.62B). When color flow imaging is utilized to determine the mechanism, the regurgitant jet appeared to be "confined" by the cobra's head. In the standard ME Com plane, the major axis of the MV annulus may be measured. A prolapsing or flail P1 or P3 segments may also be visualized in this imaging plane. As the probe is rotated to the right (clockwise) the imaging plane cuts through the A1-A2-A3 AMVL segments. This plane may also pass through the apex of the posteromedial commissure. If there is an isolated P3 segmental flail, it will be visualized in this plane with the regurgitant jet directed anteriorly away from the flail segment. In addition if there is a perforation or congenital cleft of the AMVL, with color flow Doppler, this maneuver will reveal the unusual regurgitant jet.

In addition the anterolateral and inferoseptal walls of the LV may be visualized. Scarring of these regions of the left ventricle may result in annular retraction or leaflet restriction. This imaging plane may demonstrate both the anterolateral and posteromedial papillary muscles. In addition, this plane permits evaluation of the LV portion of the tensor apparatus associated with the papillary muscle and annular continuity.

### Midesophageal Two-Chamber MV and Variations (ME 2 Chr MV) (Table 28.2 and Figs. 28.31–28.33)

**TEE Probe Manipulation:** From the ME Com imaging plane, the transducer is rotated forward to 80°–110°. In this view the AMVL protrudes from the anterolateral mitral annulus on the right. The AMVL segments A3-A2-A1 are visualized in left-to-right order. Again, depending on the orientation of the MV commissure, the P3 scallop of the PMVL may be visualized to the left protruding from the inferior mitral annulus. From the ME 2 Chr imaging plane, the TEE probe is turned to the right (clockwise), the plane is directed toward the posteromedial commissure. Again, depending on the orientation of the mitral commissure, it will initially pass through the A2 and A3 segments of the AMVL, the posteromedial commissure, and the P3 scallop. The visualized image (from left to right) will show the P3 scallop, the postero-

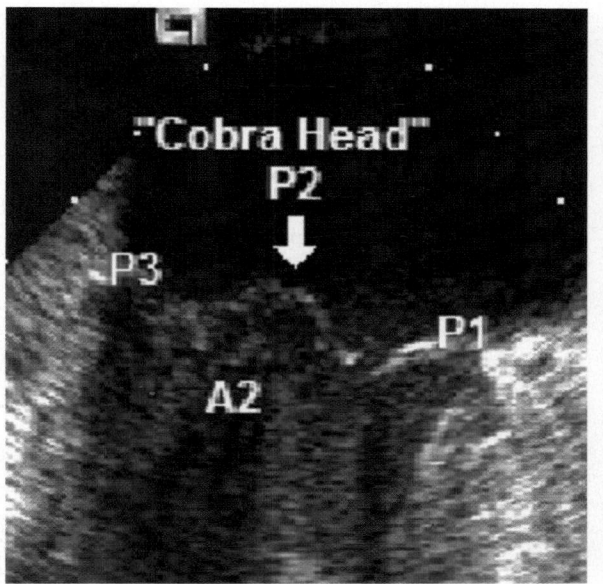 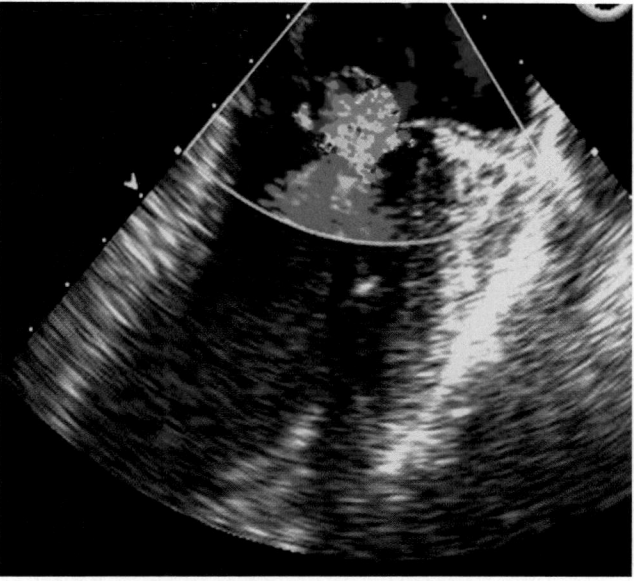

**FIGURE 28.62.** With a flail middle (P2) scallop of the PMVL, the flail segment may be seen rising above the middle (A2) portion of the AMVL like a hooded cobra raising its head. The anteriorly directed jet may be well confined by the P2 flail or prolapse.

medial commissure, and the A3 and A2 segments. From the ME 2 Chr imaging plane, the TEE probe is turned to the left (counterclockwise). This manipulation of the probe passes the imaging plane toward the middle of the posterior mitral annulus. As the imaging plane passes toward the posterior mitral annulus, only the PMVL will be visualized. Similar to the ME Com Left (counterclockwise), the P3, P2, and P1 scallops may be visualized going left to right.

### 7. Midesophageal Two-Chamber MV (ME 2 Chr MV) (Fig. 28.31)

**Transducer Depth:** 30 cm
**Probe Manipulation:** Midline
**Transducer Rotation:** 80°–110°
Depending on the orientation of the MV commissure and transducer rotation angle, the 2-D plane may cut through the P3 scallop, the posteromedial commissure, and the A3, A2, A1 segments. On the monitor (proceeding from left to right) are P3, posteromedial commissure, A3, A2, and A1.

### 8. Midesophageal Two-Chamber (Turned Right) (ME 2 Chr_R MV)

**Variation of ME 2 Chr MV**
**Transducer Depth:** 30 cm
**Transducer Rotation:** 80°–110°
**Probe Manipulation:** Turn right (clockwise)
**MV Structures:** P3, posteromedial commissure, A3, A2, and A1

**AoV:** NCC may be visualized
**LV Structures:** (Infero) septum (base, mid, apex)
**RV Structures:** Septum and RV free wall
**CFD:** Interrogation of entire commissure possible for maximum MR jet
Depending on the orientation of the MV commissure and transducer rotation angle, the 2-D plane may cut through the P3 scallop, the apex of the posteromedial commissure, the A3 segment, and the base of the A2 segment. On the monitor (proceeding from left to right) are P3, posteromedial commissure, A3, and A2.

### 9. Midesophageal Two-Chamber (Turned Left) (ME 2 ChrL MV) (Figs. 28.31A and 28.33)

**Variation of ME 2 Chr MV**
**Transducer Depth:** 30 cm
**Probe Manipulation:** Turn left or counterclockwise
**Transducer Rotation:** 80°–110°
**MV Structures:** P3, P2, and P1 scallops
**AoV:** NCC may be visualized
**LV Structures:** (Infero) septum (base, mid, apex)
**RV Structures:** Septum and RV free wall
**CFD:** Interrogation of entire commissure possible for maximum MR jet
Depending on the orientation of the MV commissure and transducer rotation angle, the 2-D plane may cut through the P3, P2, and P1 scallops. The commissure may not be visualized, except during diastole. On the monitor (proceeding from left to right) are P3, P2, and P1.
**Diagnostic Value:** This imaging plane is utilized for evaluating excessive motion of the P3 segment (flail or pro-

lapse). With color flow interrogation, it will demonstrate a regurgitant jet directed anteriorly. With an A3 flail, an inferoposteriorly directed jet will be visualized (Fig. 28.63). The left atrial appendage is consistently visualized in this plane where LAA appendage thrombi or spontaneous contrast may be visualized. Because of the parallel orientation of LAA flow with PW Doppler cursor, this is an ideal plane for interrogating the velocity of LAA systolic flow. In patients with LAA velocities below 50 cm/sec, there is a propensity to form thrombi in the appendage. The posteromedial papillary muscle and inferior wall of the LV may be evaluated in this imaging plane for infarcted scar with retraction of the inferior wall and annular retraction, which may result in an "override" of the A3 segment. Examination of the posteromedial papillary muscle may demonstrate calcification or scarring, which is usually associated with coronary disease. Such scarring may lead to a restriction of the medial segments of the AMVL or PMVL. Occasionally an infarcted papillary muscle may lead to elongation of the chordal attachment to the papillary muscle and associated segmental leaflet prolapse of one of the medial segments. The posteromedial papillary muscle is usually perfused by a single branch from the left circumflex or RCA.

### Midesophageal Long-Axis MV (Table 28.2 and Figs. 28.34–28.36)

**TEE Probe Manipulation:** From the ME 2 Chr imaging plane, the transducer plane is rotated forward to 110°–150°. This imaging plane passes through the minor

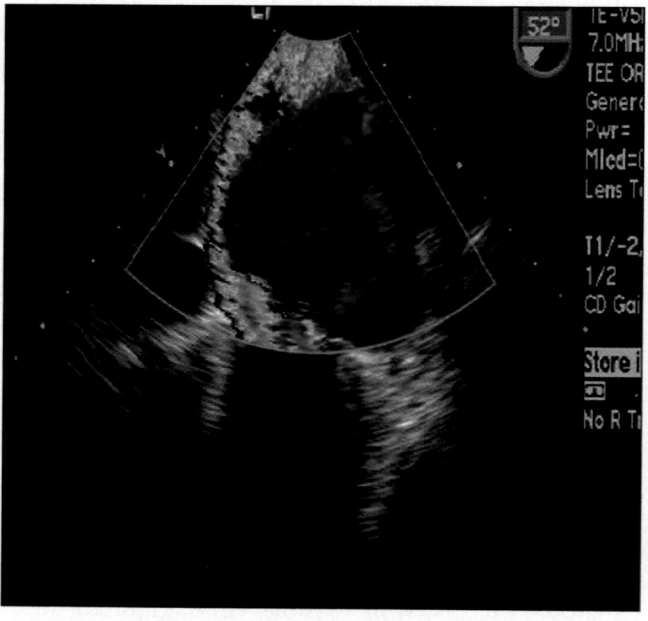

**FIGURE 28.63.** With an A3 flail, a inferoposteriorly directed jet will be visualized.

axis of the MV with a long-axis image of the aortic valve on the right. Moving from left to right, the base and edge of the P2 scallop of the PMVL is visualized and the A2 segment of the AMVL is visualized to the right.

### 10. Midesophageal Long-Axis MV (ME LAX MV)

**Transducer Depth:** 30 cm
**Transducer Rotation:** 110°–150°
**MV Structures:** P2, midcommissure and A2
   **MV Annulus:** Minor axis
**Aortic Valve:** (Left to right) NCC or LCC then RCC
**LV Structures:** Anteroseptum (B, M, A), posterior (B, M, A)
**RV Structure:** Septum and mid RV free wall
**CFD:** Interrogation for MR and severity assessment using maximum jet area, vena contracta, PISA (proximal flow convergence radius)
**CWD:**
   **MR:** CW intensity, peak transmitral velocity, dP/dt, PISA peak $V_{MR}$
   **MS:** Transmitral gradient, $PT_{1/2}$, DT, PISA peak $V_{MS}$
**PWD:**
   **MR:** E or dominance, volumetric calculations
**CMM:**
   **MR:** Systolic PISA radius calculation

Depending on the orientation of the MV commissure and transducer rotation angle, the 2-D plane passes through the minor axis of the MV annulus and aortic valve. The 2-D plane may cut through the P2 scallop, the midcommissure, and the A2 segment. On the monitor (proceeding from left to right) are P2, midcommissure, and the A2 segment of the MV. The aortic valve is seen on the right of the screen. The MV annulus to the left of the screen and to the right (adjacent to the aortic valve) are the most superior (farthest from the apex) aspects of the annulus. A plane drawn between these points, therefore, provides a more specific reference for diagnosing MV prolapse.

### 11. Midesophageal Long-Axis (Probe Turned Right) MV ME LAX$_R$ MV

**Variation ME LAX MV**
**Transducer Depth:** 30 cm
**Probe Manipulation:** Turn right clockwise
**Transducer Rotation:** 110°–150°
**MV Structures:** P2, posteromedial commissure with A3 possible, and P3
**LV Structures:** Posterior wall and septum (inferior) (base, mid, apex)
**RV Structure:** Septum (inf) and inferior RV free wall
**CFD:** Interrogation of entire posteromedial commissure possible

Depending on the orientation of the MV commissure, transducer rotation angle, and extent of probe manipulation, the 2-D plane may cut through the P2 scallop, the posteromedial commissure, and the P3 scallop. The commissure may not be visualized except during diastole. On the monitor (proceeding from left to right) are P2, possibly the posteromedial commissure, and P1.

### 12. Midesophageal Long-Axis Left MV (ME LAX$_L$ MV) (Fig. 28.36)

**Variation ME LAX MV**
**Transducer Depth:** 30 cm
**Probe Manipulation:** Left turn or counterclockwise
**Transducer Rotation:** 110°–150°
**MV Structures:** P2, anterolateral commissure with A1 possible, and P1
**LV Structures:** Posterolateral and anterior wall (base, mid, apex)
**AoV:** Will pass through AoV and LVOT transitioning from ME LAX$_R$ MV to ME LAX$_L$ MV
**CFD:** Interrogation of entire posteromedial commissure possible
Depending on the orientation of the MV commissure, transducer rotation angle, and extent of probe manipulation, the 2-D plane may cut through the P2 scallop, the anterolateral commissure, and P1 scallop. The commissure may not be visualized except during diastole. On the monitor (proceeding from left to right) are P2, possibly the anterolateral commissure, and P1.
**Diagnostic Value:** Because P2 is the most frequent flail or prolapsing segment of all the valve segments/scallops, this imaging plane will commonly demonstrate a flail P2 scallop with its characteristic anteriorly directed jet. In addition, measurements of the height of the PMVL, AMVL, C-sept distance, and minor MV annular diameter may be made in this view. With rightward (clockwise) turning of the probe from the ME LAX imaging plane, the imaging plane is directed toward the posteromedial commissure. MR from the posteromedial commissure may be visualized at this point. Again, depending on the orientation of the mitral commissure, as the probe is rotated toward the posteromedial commissure, it will initially pass through the medial aspect of the P2 scallop, the posteromedial commissure, and the A3 segment of the AMVL. The visualized image (from left to right) will show the medial portion of the P2 scallop, the posteromedial commissure, and the A3 segment of the AMVL. As the imaging plane passes through the apex of the posteromedial commissure, the medial aspect of the P2 and P3 scallops will be visualized from left to right on the monitor screen. If there is a flail segment of the A3 or the P3 scallop, it will be visualized by this maneuver.

From the ME LAX imaging plane, the TEE probe is turned to the left (counterclockwise). This manipulation of the probe passes the imaging plane toward the anterolateral commissure. If there is an anterolateral commissural regurgitant jet, it will be visualized at this point. De-

pending on the orientation of the mitral commissure, as the probe is rotated toward the anterolateral commissure, it will initially pass through the lateral aspect of the P2 scallop, the anterolateral commissure, and the A1 segment of the AMVL. The visualized image (from left to right) will show the lateral P2 scallop, the anterolateral commissure, the A1 segment, and the LVOT or aortic valve. As the imaging plane passes through the apex of the anterolateral commissure, the lateral aspect of the P2 scallop and the P1 scallop will be visualized going left to right on the monitor screen.

### 13. Bicaval Imaging Plane (Fig. 28.64)

**Transducer Depth:** 30 cm
**Probe Manipulation:** Turn left or counterclockwise
**Transducer Rotation:** 110°–150°
**TEE Probe Manipulation:** From the ME LAX imaging plane, the probe is turned clockwise to the right with the visualization of the bicaval imaging plane, with the SVC entering the atria from the right screen (Fig. 28.64). In addition the IVC and coronary sinus may be visualized as well as the cristae terminalis and right atrial appendage.
**Diagnostic Valve:** Color flow Doppler interrogation of the interatrial septum in the region of the fossa ovalis may demonstrate a patent foramen ovale. An injected contrast agent, such as 3 cc blood, 5 cc saline, and 2 cc air, which is dissolved between 2 syringes connected by a stopcock will reliably demonstrate the presence of an interatrial shunt if injected immediately upon release of then positive pressure Valsalva.

### 14. Right Upper Pulmonary Vein (Fig. 28.64)

**Transducer Depth:** 30 cm
**Probe Manipulation:** Turn right or clockwise
**Transducer Rotation:** 120°–140°
**TEE Probe Manipulation:** Rotation of the transducer forward to 130° and rightward turning (clockwise) of the TEE probe usually reveals the RUPV.
**Diagnostic Value:** If the regurgitant jet is directed laterally away from the RUPV, the PW Doppler interrogation of the RUPV may not be demonstrated equally on both sides. PMVL flails associated with significant regurgitation usually produce systolic reversal in the RUPV.

### RV Inflow-Outflow Imaging Plane (Fig. 28.65)

In this imaging plane, the anterior and septal leaflets are usually visualized. If the coronary sinus is visualized, the TV leaflet of the left lower portion of the screen is probably the posterior leaflet. The TV may be interrogated for regurgitation or stenosis.

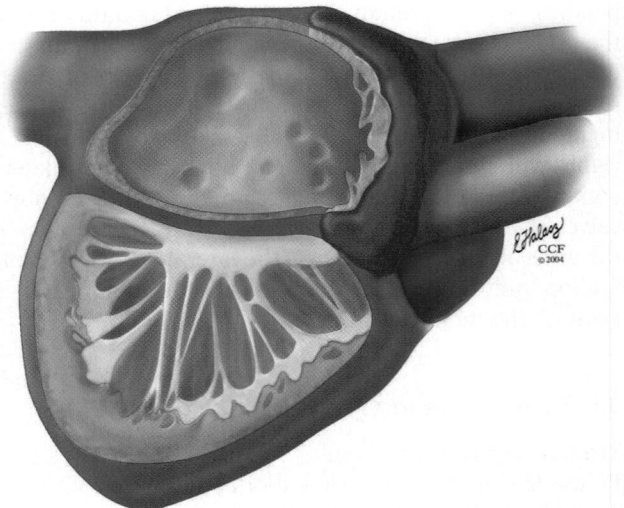

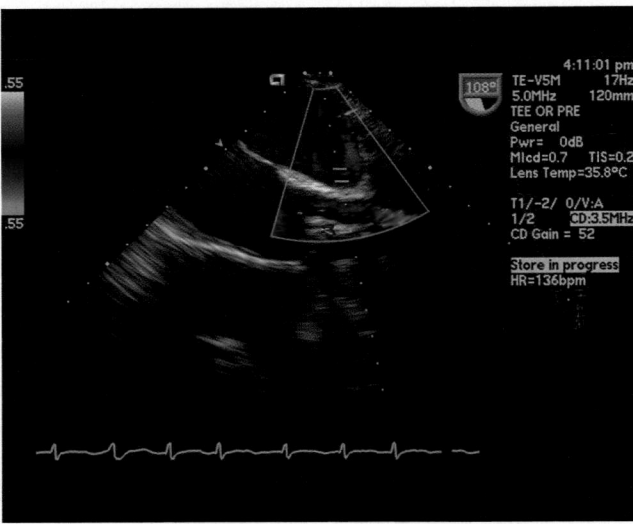

**FIGURE 28.64.** The bicaval imaging plane. By turning the probe to the right and/or rotating the transducer forward, the right upper pulmonary vein (RUPV) is visualized. PW Doppler is used to determine severe MR with systolic reversal.

**TEE Probe Manipulation:** From the bicaval view, the transducer is rotated back to between 30° and 45° where the ME aortic valve short axis (ME SAX AoV) is obtained. (If there was significant AS or AR the valve may be evaluated with 2-D using planimetry or CFD.) From the ME SAX AoV, the probe is slightly advanced until both the tricuspid and pulmonic valves are visualized.

**Diagnostic Valve:** If tricuspid regurgitation was visualized by the preoperative examination or the abbreviated overview examination, the tricuspid valve is evaluated at this point. From the RV inflow and outflow view, the significance of tricuspid regurgitation may be evaluated, as well as the degree of RV dysfunction and pulmonic valve regurgitation. With significant TR indicating the potential requirement of surgical repair, the hepatic veins may be interrogated for significance of systolic reversal of hepatic vein flow, which is an indication of 4+ TR.

### 15. Transgastric Basal Short Axis (TG SAX_B) (Table 28.2, Fig. 28.37)

**Transducer Depth:** 35 cm
**Transducer Rotation:** 0°–5°
In this imaging plane, the AMVL (A1-2-3, bottom to top) is visualized on the left and the PMVL (P1-2-3, bottom to top) is visualized on the right. The clear space to the left of the AMVL edge toward the bottom of the screen is the left ventricular outflow track (LVOT).
**TEE Probe Manipulation:** From the RV inflow-outflow or bicaval view, the transducer is rotated back to 0° and

the probe is advanced into the stomach at a depth of approximately 35 cm, with slight leftward flexion (counterclockwise rotation) of the smaller radial knob on the handle of the TEE probe.
**Diagnostic Value:** From the TG basal SAX, the competency of the MV may be evaluated for localization and determination of potential mechanism. With prolapsing

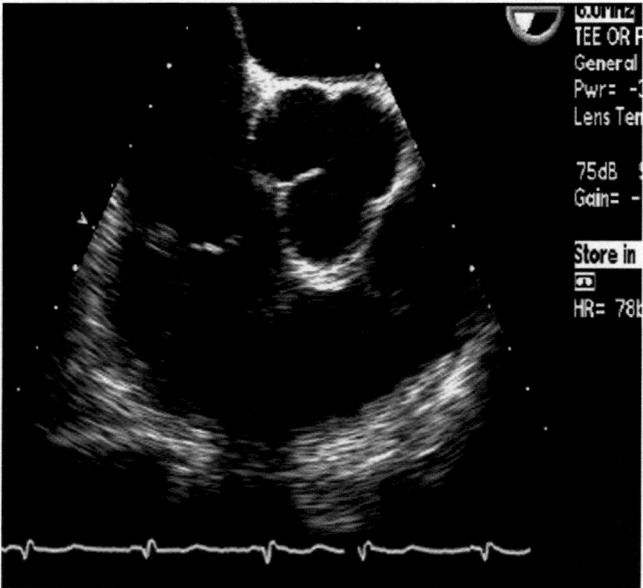

**FIGURE 28.65** In this image plane, the anterior and septal leaflets are usually visualized. If the coronary sinus is visualized, the TV leaflet of the left lower portion of the screen is probably the posterior leaflet.

segments, the may be an "echo-free" space adjacent to the line of coaptation with subsequent MR originating from the site of redundant leaflets. With MS, this imaging may be used to planimeter the valve or subvalvular apparatus. Because there may be more subvalvular stenosis in rheumatic MS, care should be taken to determine the level of most significant stenosis.

### 16. Transgastric Two-Chamber (TG 2 Chr) (Table 28.2, Fig. 28.38)

**Transducer Depth:** 35 cm
**Transducer Rotation:** 70°–90°
This image is similar to the ME 2 Chr imaging plane except that the ventricle is horizontally oriented. The AMVL (A1-2-3, bottom to top) is visualized at the bottom of the screen and the PMVL P2-3 is visualized at the top.

**TEE Probe Manipulation:** From the TG SAX imaging plane, the transducer is rotated forward to 70°–90° with the MV commissure positioned in the center of the imaging screen, and the transducer angle is rotated forward to obtain the TG 2 Chr imaging plane. Color Doppler may visualize regurgitation at this level. Clockwise turning of the probe may pass the imaging plane toward P1 and the anterolateral commissure. With color Doppler, isolation of the origin of a regurgitant jet near P1 or the anterolateral commissure may be confirmed.

**Diagnostic Value:** The TG 2 Chr is a useful imaging plane for evaluating the subvalvular apparatus in patients with rheumatic MS or MR. Looking for the associated anatomic findings of chordal fusion, loss of interchordal spaces, degree of calcification, and leaflet motion with color may demonstrate more significant subvalvular stenosis than valvular.

### General Comprehensive Exam

At the conclusion of the more focused diagnostic IOE exam, an account is taken with regard to the important diagnostic issues that need to be addressed, as well as the review of the cardiac valves, chambers, and aorta that are an important part of the comprehensive evaluation. Depending on which of the recommended standard imaging planes were omitted from the abbreviated focused diagnostic IOE exam, upon its completion the missing cross-sectional image views are obtained to complete the study. If the imaging planes that were discussed above had been the image sequence and interrogation utilized in an actual IOE exam, we would only require the TG SAX$_{MID}$ and deep TG LAX to document the comprehensive intraoperative multiplane TEE exam as recommended and endorsed by the ASE-SCA and these would be extremely valuable to have for future clinical reference.

## PATHOLOGY

Consistent with the principles of the intraoperative echocardiographic examination, evaluation of the patient undergoing MV surgery is to refine the understanding of the underlying etiology, pathologic changes in the anatomic structure of the apparatus, and mechanism of dysfunction. Compared to transthoracic echocardiography, the intraoperative TEE has an improved imaging capability to accomplish this and more accurately determines the functional anatomy and mechanism of dysfunction (92).

### Mitral Regurgitation (MR)

#### Etiology and Mechanisms of Mitral Regurgitation (Tables 28.8–28.10)

##### Etiologies

The etiologies of MR may be classified by either their acuity of onset or underlying etiology. The former classifies the etiology as being either acute or chronic. The latter classifies MR according to the acute or chronic pathologic process. Due to the reduced incidence of rheumatic MV disease in the United States and the increasing age of the patient population, the most common cause of both acute and chronic MR is myxomatous degeneration (126–130). In fact degenerative MR has become the predominant valvular abnormality involving the MV. Acute causes of MR are more commonly related to acute or chronic diseases, including myxomatous degeneration of the MV with associated chordal rupture. Other more common causes include endocarditis, ischemic heart disease (with or without PM rupture), and traumatic disruption of the MV apparatus.

The chronic causes of MR include myxomatous degeneration of the MV, mitral annular calcification, rheumatic valve disease, endocarditis, global LV dysfunction, hypertrophic obstructive cardiomyopathy (HOCM), radiation induced fibrosis and scarring, degenerative connective tissue disorders, and congenital abnormalities (cleft MV, parachute MV) (128). Some patients simply have a normal sized MV in a small heart and resulting mismatch.

##### Myxomatous Degeneration

Myxomatous degeneration is the most frequent cause of MR in the United States, occurring in 4%–5% of the population. It has also been referred to as "floppy MV," billowing mitral leaflet syndrome, MV prolapse, and fibro-elastic disorder. Of those patients with MV prolapse, only 10% to 15% develop progressive MR (126). A very small number of patients progress to surgical MR.

▶ TABLE 28.8. **Acute and Chronic Mitral Regurgitation:**
                **Etiology and Pathology**

| Chronicity | Etiology | Pathologic Anatomy |
|---|---|---|
| **Acute** | | |
| | Myxomatous | Ruptured chordae with segmental flail, endocarditis |
| Ischemia | Ischemic | Acute infarct of papillary muscle |
| | | PM tethering or rupture |
| | | Transient global dysfunction tethering |
| Inflammatory | Endocarditis | Leaflet perforation, vegetation obstructing closure, ruptured chordae, destruction of fibrous skeleton and annulus, associated with previous MV or AoV dysfunction or endocarditis |
| | Rheumatic fever | Thickening of leaflets, chordal elongation and prolapse of AMVL, enlarged annulus, active myocarditis with CHF |
| Other | Trauma | Ruptured papillary muscle, ruptured chordae, leaflet tear annular distortion |
| | Prosthetic | Sewing ring dehiscence, mechanical leaflet stuck open, endocarditis and bioprosthetic leaflet destruction |
| **Chronic** | | |
| Degenerative | Myxomatous | Annular enlargement eventually in all redundant leaflets with abnormal connective tissue thinning of chordae |
| | Mitral Annular Ca$^{++}$ | Posterior annulus Ca$^{++}$ deposition in granular or coalesced form creating subannular Ca$^{++}$ bars; extends into base of leaflets, causing immobilization; also deposited in annulus, decreasing mobility and systolic coaptation area |
| | Osteogenesis imperfecta | Chordal elongation and rupture |
| Ischemia | Dilated ischemic CM | Spherical remodeling with apical tethering of MVAp tethering |
| | Segmental infarct | PM infarct with tip elongation and segmental medial prolapse, inf-post infarct and restricted PM with decreased systolic annular motion |
| | Acute or chronic | Chronic LV remodeling and restrictive physiology; rapid development CHF and central and/or posterior MR due to restriction PMVL and apical tethering |
| Inflammatory | Rheumatic | Chronic fibrosis and Ca$^{++}$ of leaflets, chordae, PM, and annulus; commissural fusion with fish-mouth deformity (Type IIIa mechanism MR) |
| | Postradiation | Fibrosis of leaflets, annulus, and subvalvular apparatus with calcific degeneration leads to incomplete coaptation; accociated constrictive disease |
| | Rheumatoid arthritis | Rheumatic nodules on leaflets |
| | Systemic lupus | Liebman Sacks endocarditis at base valve and into subvalvular apparatus |
| | Atrial myxoma | Large myxoma may obstruct MV inflow |
| | Sarcoidosis | Papillary muscle granulomas may cause retraction |
| Congenital | Cleft MV leaflet | Usually AMVL associated with endocardial cushion defects, endocardial fibroelastosis, anomalous origin of coronary artery |
| | Parachute MV | Absence of papillary muscle, endocardial fibroelastosis |
| | Disproportional LV | LV cavity small for body size with resulting redundancy of MVAp structures |

Carpentier distinguishes Barlow's syndrome (MV prolapse) from the entity fibroelastic deficiency. Barlow's syndrome is characterized as occurring in middle-aged individuals and associated with excess tissue with myxoid degeneration. Fibroelastic deficiency is characterized as occurring more frequently in the elderly and is associated with leaflet thickening in the region of prolapse, with the remaining tissue being translucent and thinner than normal. Moderate annular dilatation is associated with fibroelastic deficiency (132).

In patients with myxomatous degeneration, there is annular thickening and dilatation, which is associated with infiltration of acid mucopolysaccharide material and architectural disorganization of elastin and collagen.

The clinical presentation of MV dysfunction in these patients is usually associated with annular dilatation and elongation of the primary chordae with associated chordal rupture. Patients with myxomatous degeneration may present with endocarditis, which leads to the potential for multiple mechanisms of valve dysfunction.

Eight hundred and thirty-three Omstead county residents, who were diagnosed with MV prolapse between 1989 and 1998, were followed for a 10-year period (133). The most frequent risk factors for cardiac death were moderate to severe MR and lowered ejection fraction. Secondary risk factors included left atrial enlargement, atrial fibrillation, and age $\geq$ 50. In patients with greater than moderate MR and decreased ejection fraction, < 50%

experienced a 10-year mortality of 45% with a yearly cardiovascular morbidity of over 6% per year. Mills et al. examined the mechanical properties of myxomatous MV leaflets and chordae and found they were more extensible than normal.

### Ischemic Mitral Regurgitation

By definition, ischemic MR is caused by coronary artery disease and may be transient or due to a previous myocardial infarction. Transient ischemia results in global or regional dysfunction with the potential of either apical tethering with the production of a central jet of MR. A regional abnormality (such as posterolateral dyskinesia) may result in dysfunction of the myocardium and papillary muscle subtending the posteromedial scallop (P3). This may result in uncoordinated coaptation with the opposing AMVL and transiently result in a posterior directed jet or central jet related to apical tethering (134).

### Endocarditis

Endocarditis involving the left-sided valve structures usually involves the aortic valve. If endocarditis involves the MV, it usually implies the coexistence of underlying degenerative or rheumatic valve disease. The most common organisms involved in MV endocarditis are *Streptococcus* (viridans and bovis) and *Staphylococcus* (aureus or epidermis) (135). Muehrcke et al. characterized pathologic abnormalities, including the presence of vegetations, leaflet perforation, chordal rupture, and abscess formation (136). In MV endocarditis the mechanism is usually associated with a preexisting underlying mechanism. Typical MV pathology associated with endocarditis includes leaflet perforation and obstructing vegetations that may interfere with antegrade flow into the left ventricle. Compared with TTE, TEE has a much higher resolution and is therefore usually performed when endocarditis is suspected. Karp reported that up to 18% of cases with multiple valve endocarditis involve the aortic and mitral valves (135). The lesion on the MV may be secondary to an aortic regurgitant jet lesion of the AMVL with the appearance of a wind sock.

### Rheumatic Mitral Regurgitation

Rheumatic MV disease with predominant regurgitation has many features that distinguish it from those associated with pure rheumatic stenosis. The regurgitant form is associated with less calcification of the valve leaflets and subvalvular apparatus. There is diffuse thickening and fibrosis of the leaflets, resulting in restriction in systole and diastole (Carpentier type IIIa). Acute rheumatic valvulitis is infrequently seen in the United States. It is associated with fibrosis of the valve leaflets with prolapse of the AMVL

causing predominant regurgitation (137). Other forms of the disease are amenable to surgical repair (138–141).

### Primary Pathophysiology

*Acute MR* Acute MR results in a sudden volume overload of the LV. Due to the increased preload, the LV may actually become hypercontractile with much of the stroke volume proceeding into a noncompliant LA during systole. Because both the LA and LV are not as compliant as in chronic disease process, patients rapidly develop pulmonary congestion, pulmonary hypertension, and eventually RV dysfunction with dilatation and tricuspid regurgitation. The secondary pathophysiology of acute and chronic MR differs significantly due to the stiff LA. The amount of volume that is ejected into the left atrium is dependent upon the size of the systolic regurgitant orifice, the systolic pressure gradient between the LV and LA, and the systolic ejection time (inversely proportional to heart rate dependent). With severe MR or a noncompliant left atrium, as the LAP progressively increases, the pressure differential between the LV and LA rapidly tapers at the end of systole, resulting in a "v wave cutoff sign" on CW Doppler (Fig. 28.66).

*Chronic MR* In chronic MR, the LA has time to become more compliant, resulting in extremely large LA chamber sizes. Because the amount of regurgitant vol-

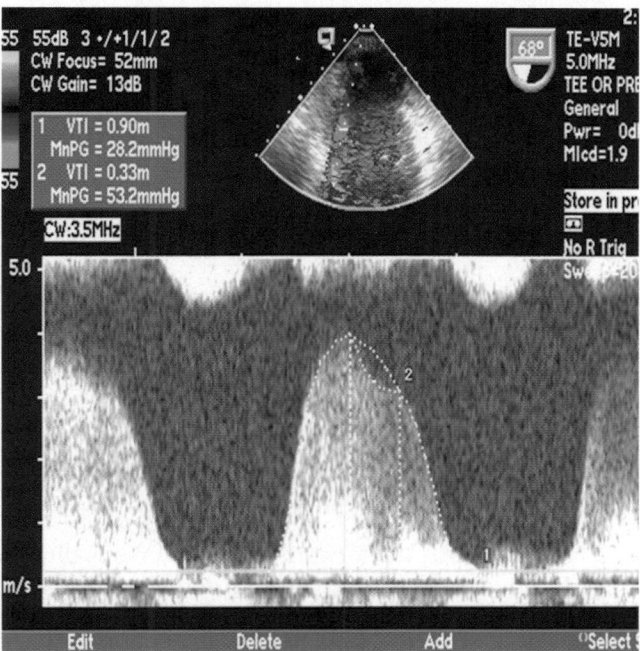

**FIGURE 28.66.** With severe MR or a noncompliant left atrium, as the LAP progressively increases, the pressure differential between the LV and LA rapidly tapers at the end of systole resulting in a "v wave cutoff sign" on CW Doppler.

▶ TABLE 28.9. **Etiology and Structural Alteration in the MVAp**

| Etiology | Annulus | MV Leaflets | Chordae | Papillary Muscles | Inf-Post and Antero-Lat LV |
|---|---|---|---|---|---|
| Myxomatous Degeneration | Enlargement | Redundant, thickened, prolapse | Elongated: propensity to rupture | Chordal attachment: tendency to rupture | Minimal effect |
| Ischemic MR | Retracted with scarring with decreased systolic narrowing and decreased apposition | Spherical LV causes tethering of both leaflets and tetted AMVL by secondary chordae | Attachment to papillary muscle head vulnerable with PM infarct | Solitary blood supply PMPM rupture or infarct with elongation or retraction | Scarred infarct leads to retraction of PMPM with asymmetrical restricted PMVL/ AMVL override Ischemic CM apical tethering |
| Rheumatic valve disease | Acute annular dilatation Chronic fibrosis with Ca$^{++}$ decreases systolic narrowing of MV commissure and malcoaptation of MV leaflets | Acute AMVL prolapse in children Chronic fibrosis and Ca$^{++}$ from leaflet edges toward base, comm fusion | Acute elongation and rupture | Inflammation with attachment elongation | Acute myocarditis with CHF and tethering Chronic myocarditis and underfilling with decreased systolic fx and restrictive physiology |
| Dilated cardiomyopathy | Annular dilatation associated with acute or chronic myocarditis post ant Diminished systolic mobility and malcoaptation | Tenting of AMVL by secondary chordal tethering and bileaflet tethering | Eccentric remodeling increases tension middle post annulus leads to ruptured primary chordae to middle scallop | Spherical ventricle causes tensor apparatus to tether leaflet closure | Diminished LV function increases systolic area or MV annulus with apical tethering |
| Endocarditis | Abcess invading fibrous skeleton and annulus | Leaflet perforations and vegetations | Destruction of chordae with rupture | Active infection of PM and myocardium leads to PM scarring | Active myocarditis |
| Mitral annular calcification | Ca$^{++}$ of annulus with reduced systolic narrowing of MV annula and malcoaptation of MV leaflets | Ca$^{++}$ from leaflet bases toward tips | Calcific degeneration with rupture | Calcific degeneration of PM tips leads to rupture of chordal attachment | Ca$^{++}$ extends into sub-annular tissue; may have Ca$^{++}$ bars interfering with coaptation or MV inflow |
| Postradiation | Accelerated degeneration with fibrosis, retraction, and diminished mobility, malcoaptation of leaflets | Thickening and fibrosis with accelerated degeneration and Ca$^{++}$; decreased apposition | Fibrosis and decreased structural integrity prone to rupture | Fibrosis of PM tips with scarring causes retraction MV leaflets in systole with variable tethering | Diastolic dysfunction with constrictive pericarditis; direct and indirect systolic dysfunction |

ume may be > 50%, the forward stroke volume is diminished. Eventually the LV may fail with end-diastolic diameters (EDD) greater than 70 mm (55). With chronic MR, the left ventricle may initially compensate for the added diastolic loading and ejection into a compliance chamber with hyperdynamic performance. However, if the loading conditions continue the ventricle will eventually fail. In

chronic MR, the effects of persistent volume overload of the left ventricle may be tolerated for years; however, the ventricle eventually begins to develop eccentric hypertrophy with the development of a spherically shaped and dilated ventricle, with an increased annular-apical distance, resulting in apical tethering of the mitral leaflets and a secondary mechanism of additional MR.

*(text continues on page 506)*

▶ TABLE 28.10. MV Apparatus: Pathology, Mechanism, and Surgical Technique

| Leaflet Motion and Carpentier Classification | MV Leaflets Motion | Annulus | PMVL Height ≥ 1.5 | MR Jet Origin | MR Jet Direction | Leaflet Surgery | Annular Surgery |
|---|---|---|---|---|---|---|---|
| Type 1 (associated with IIIb) | AMVL Normal PMVL Normal Symetric | Dilated | 1.6 | Length of commissure | Central origin | None | Ring annuloplasty |
| | AMVL Normal PMVL Normal Symetric | Normal | 1.3 | Leaflet body | Eccentric | Pericardial patch | Ring annuloplasty |
| Type II Excessive | Bileaflet prolapse Symmetric | Dilated | 2.2 | Point of incomplete coaptation | Central | PMVL quad resect | Ring annuloplasty slide |
| | Prolapse/Flail PMVL Asymmetric | Dilated | 2.0 | P2 | Anterior | P2 quad resect | Ring annuloplasty slide |
| | Prolapse Asymmetric/ Flail A2 | Dilated | 1.4 | A2 | Posterior | Chordal transfer PMVL quad resection | Ring annuloplasty |
| | Commissural Prolapse Asymmetric | Dilated | 1.4 | A3, P3 | Commissural | Suture commissure | Ring annuloplasty |
| Type IIIa Systolic/Diastolic Restricted Type IIIb | Rheumatic Symmetrical Bileaflet Restriction | Retracted, Ca++ | 1.0 | Entire commissure | Central | Open commissurotomy debridement | Ring annuloplasty |
| Type IIIb Systolic Restriction | PMVL Restriction Inf-Post Infarct Asymmetric | Retracted Inf-Post | 1.5 | P2-P3 | Posterior (AMVL Override) | None | Ring annuloplasty |
| Type IIIb (associated with Type I spherical ventricle apical tethering) | AMVL and PMVL Restriction Symmetric | Dilated | 1.4 | Along entire commissure | Central | None | Ring annuloplasty |

The surgical strategy is developed by the surgeon's correlation of their direct inspection of the anatomic components of the mitral valve apparatus with the findings of the intraoperative examination. The real-time assessment of the mechanism of dysfunction directs the surgeon to a closer inspection of segmental anatomy.
*Adapted from Stewart WJ. Intraoperative echocardiography in Topol's Textbook of cardiovascular medicine. Topol E, ed. Baltimore: Lippincott 2002.*

TABLE 28.11. MV Apparatus: Pathology, Mechanism, and Choice of Surgical Technique

| | 1 | 2 | 3 | 4 | 5 | 6 | 7 | 8 | 9 | 10 |
|---|---|---|---|---|---|---|---|---|---|---|
| | Myx Deg | | | | | Ischemic MR | Ischemic CM | Ruptured Postero-medial | Mitral Annular Ca++ | Endocarditis |
| | Bileaflet Pro P3A3 | Flail P3 | Flail A2 | Flail P2-Pro A1-2-3 P1+3 | Flail P2 Bileaflet Pro | Infarcted Inf-Post PM Seg and PMPM | | | Mild PMVL Restriction | Perforated AMVL A2 |
| **Annulus** | Dil | Dil | Dil | No | Dil | No | Yes | No | Sev Ca++ | No |
| P1 | NI | NI | NI | Pro | Pro | NI | Rest | NI | Rest | NI |
| P2 Lat | NI | NI | NI | FI | FI | Rest | Rest | NI | Rest | NI |
| P2 Med | NI | NI | NI | FI | FI | Rest | Rest | FI | Rest | NI |
| P3 | Pro | FI | NI | Pro | Pro | Rest | Rest | FI | Rest | NI |
| A1 | NI | NI | NI | Pro | Pro | NI | Rest | NI | NI | NI |
| A2 Lat | NI | NI | FI | Pro | Pro | NI | Rest | NI | NI | NI |
| A2 Med | NI | NI | FI | Pro | Pro | NI | Rest | FI | NI | NI |
| A3 | Pro | NI | NI | Pro | Pro | Pro | Rest | FI | NI | NI |
| PMVL Height | 2.2 | 2.2 | 1.3 | 2.0 | 1.2 | 1.4 | 1.1 | 1.2 | 1.0 | 1.3 |
| **Chordae** | | | | | | | | | | |
| P1 | NI | NI | NI | EI | EI | NI | Rest | NI | NI | NI |
| P2 Lat | NI | NI | NI | Rupt | Rupt | NI | Rest | NI | NI | NI |
| P2 Med | NI | NI | NI | Rupt | Rupt | NI | Rest | PM Rupt | NI | NI |
| P3 | EI | EI | NI | EI | EI | EI | Rest | PM Rupt | NI | NI |
| A1 | NI | NI | NI | EI | EI | NI | Rest | NI | NI | NI |
| A2 Lat | NI | NI | FI | EI | EI | NI | Rest | NI | NI | NI |
| A2 Med | NI | NI | FI | EI | EI | Ovr | Rest | PM Rupt | NI | NI |
| A3 | EI | NI | NI | EI | EI | Exc | Rest | PM Rupt | NI | NI |
| ALPM | NI | NI | NI | NI | NI | NI | Teth | NI | NI | NI |
| PMPM | NI | NI | NI | NI | NI | Ret | Teth | Rupt Head | NI | NI |
| Global LV | NI | NI | NI | NI | NI | ±Dil | Sph | Hyperdyn | NI | NI |

| | | | | | | | | | | |
|---|---|---|---|---|---|---|---|---|---|---|
| Inf-Post LV | NI | NI | NI | NI | NI | Akin | Hypo | NI | NI | NI |
| Scar | Hypo | Akin | NI | NI | NI | NI | Restr | Exc | Restr | NI |
| Ant-Lat LV | NI | NI | NI | NI | NI | NI | NI | NI | NI | NI |
| Leaflet Motion | Exc | Exc | Exc | Exc | Exc | Restr | Restr | Exc | Restr | Restr |
| MR Origin | PMC | P3 | PMC | P2 | P2 | P2-3 | ALC to PMC | Medial Half | A1-2-3 | A2 |
| MR Direction | Cen Com | Ant Lat | Ant | Ant | 1. Ant 2. Cen | Post | Cent | DiffusLat | Post | Ant |
| Motion Symmetrical | Sym | Asy | Asy | Asy | Asy | Asy | Sym | Asy | Asy | Sym |
| AnnPlast Ring | Yes | Yes | Yes | Yes | Yes | Yes | Yes | Yes | Yes | No |
| Slide | Yes Mod | Yes Mod | Yes Mod | Yes | No | No | No | No | No | No |
| Quad | No | Mod | Mod | Yes | Yes | No | No | ± | No | No |
| Com Sut | Yes | ± | Yes | No | No | No | No | No | No | No |
| Chor Transfer | ± | Yes | No | No | No | Yes | No | No | No | No |
| Patch | No | No | No | No | No | No | No | No | No | Yes |
| Other | | GortxCh | | | | | Alferi Repair | PM Rea or MVR | AnnDeb | |

The intraoperative exam of the MV involves a detailed assessment of the individual components of the MVAp including the annulus (dilation, Ca++, fibrosis), MV leaflets (thickness and motion), chordae (lengthy, thickness, fusion, and rupture), the papillary muscles (scarring, Ca++, elongation, retraction, rupture), and the LV complex (global function, inferoposterior and anterolateral segmental function). CF Doppler is used to characterize the mechanism. Regurgitant jets are characterized by their severity, origin, and direction of the jet. Excessive motion of a segment, produces a MR jet directed opposite the leaflet (unless the opposing leaflet has a similar degree of excessive motion). Symmetrical excessive or restricted leaflet motion produces a central jet. An asymmetrical segmental restriction is characterized by the MR jet being directed toward that segment from a "relative override" of the opposing leaflet segment. The surgical technique and probability of repair are determined by the etiology and the mechanism(s) of MR. Flail or prolapse of P2 is the most common presentation of myxomatous disease due to thinning of the fibrous annulus and localized annular dilitation.

In the examples above, every component of the MVAp has been evaluated. Surgical options for are included to illustrate how the IOE exam is incorporated into the decision-making process. All valve repairs usually incorporate an annuloplasty ring for additional support to prevent future annular dilitation seen in myxomatous degeneration and LV dysfunction. The five surgical techniques most commonly used in MVRep include: 1) an annuloplasty ring, 2) quadralateral resection, 3) sliding annuloplasty, 4) chordal transfer, or 5) commissural suture. Other techniques include the Alferi edge-to-edge suture, gortex chordae, and AMVL resection or plication.

Flail = Fl
Prolapse = Pro
Asymetrical= Asy
Symetrical Motion=Sym
Papillary Muscle Rupture = PM Rupt
PM Reattachment= PM Rea
Gortex Chordae= Gotx Ch
Severe Ca++ = Sec Ca++
Normal = NI
Excessive Leaflet Motion = Exc
Restricted Leaflet Motion = Restr
Hyperdynamic = Hyperdyn
Akinetic Segment = Akin

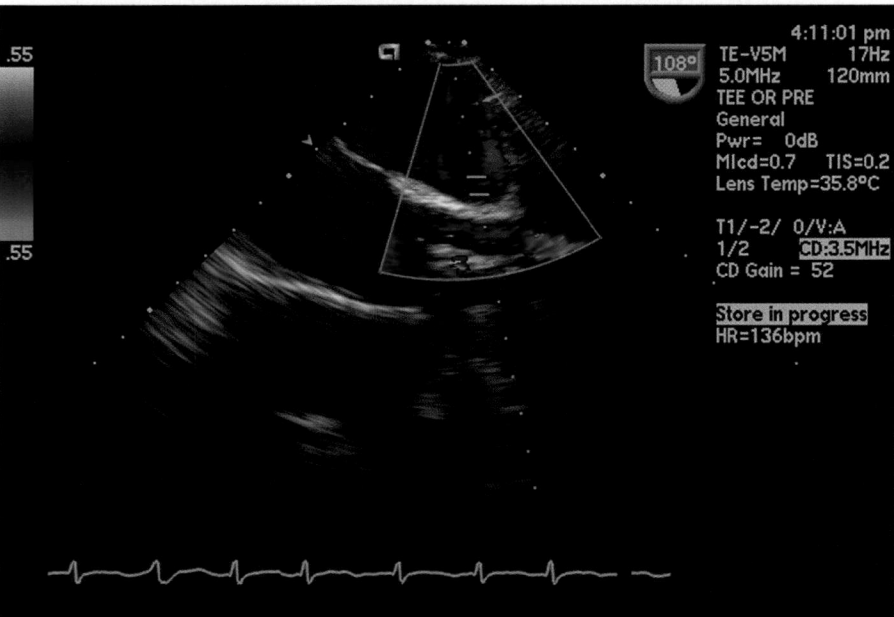

**FIGURE 28.67.** Right upper pulmonary vein (RUPV). By turning the probe to the right (clockwise) and/or rotating the transducer forward, the RUPV is visualized. PW Doppler is used to determine severe MR with systolic reversal.

## Mechanisms of Mitral Regurgitation (Fig. 28.68, Tables 28.9–28.11)

### MV Apparatus and Mechanism of Mitral Regurgitation (Table 28.9)

As previously discussed, the MVAp consists of five unique anatomic structures that work in concert as they function to prevent the retrograde flow of blood into the left atrium in systole, permit the antegrade flow into the LV during diastole, and maintain the functional integrity of the ventricle throughout the cardiac cycle. The range of etiologies of MV dysfunction produce pathognomonic changes in the structural integrity of one or more of the components of the MVAp (42,137,138). Each of the anatomic components of the MVAp may be structurally altered in a limited number of ways by the various pathologic processes. Apposition of the valve leaflets is an intricately choreographed process requiring each of the structures to work in concert to get the valve leaflets to the precise plane of apposition at the same time in the cardiac cycle. Significant regurgitation signals a failure of this integrated process. While on the surface, this would appear to occur because of excessive or restricted leaflet motion or annular dilatation, it is ultimately an expression of the abnormal structure and function of one or more of the components of the MVAp. The structural distortions include:

1. Annular dilatation or lack of mobility
2. Leaflet redundancy or retraction (fibrosis with calcification)
3. Chordal shortening, elongation, and rupture
4. Papillary muscle shortening, elongation, and rupture

5. Ventricular dilatation (apical tethering) or segmental abnormalities (transient dysfunction or scarring) (42,44,131)

In 1971, Carpentier characterized the mechanisms of MV dysfunction established on the principle that "function follows form." He recognized leaflet coaptation as the final manifestation of the structural integrity and function of the individual components. This led to the physiologic classification of MR based on the extent of systolic and diastolic excursion of the valve leaflets (129).

### Type I: Normal Leaflet Motion (Fig. 28.68)

MR that involves a type I mechanism (normal leaflet motion) may be associated with a dilated annulus frequently caused by myxomatous degeneration or the posterior annular dilatation associated with chronic congestive heart failure. A type I mechanism of MR may be seen in patients having endocarditis with leaflet perforations or a congenital cleft. The congenital cleft is frequently associated with endocardial cushion defects (142).

### Type II: Excessive Leaflet Motion (Fig. 28.68)

Because the annulosa fibrosa thins out in the region adjacent to the base of the P2 scallop, dilatation is frequently seen in this location with increasing tension being applied to the chordae at that point. With myxomatous degeneration, these chordae are abnormal and frequently rupture, resulting in a flail P2 segment that is the most

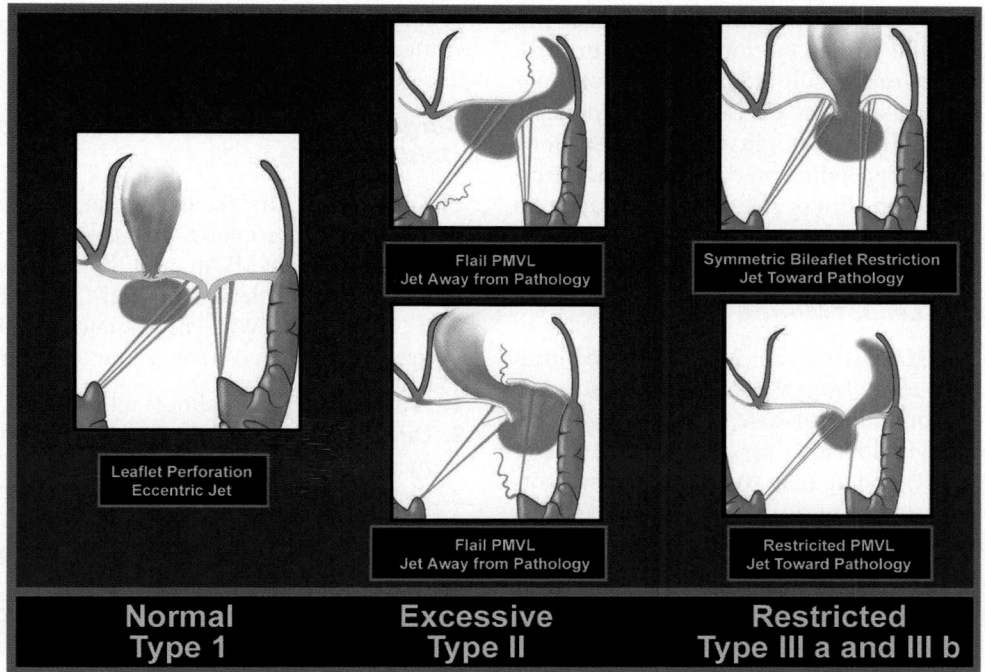

**FIGURE 28.68.** Mechanisms of MV dysfunction. Mitral regurgitation is produced by pathologic changes in the structural integrity of the one or more of the components of the MVAp that ultimately interferes with apposition of the valve leaflets. Normal apposition is prevented by mechanisms of dysfunction that are related to 1) normal leaflet motion (type I) with annular dilatation or a cleft or perforated leaflet, 2) excessive leaflet motion (type II), and 3) restricted leaflet motion in systole and diastole (IIIa) and restricted in just systole (IIIb) perforation.

frequent of all segmental leaflet abnormalities and the easiest to repair. Elongated chordae may lead to prolapse of the MV leaflet or a flail leaflet with the leaflet tip pointing toward the top of the atrium (47).

## Type III: Restricted Leaflet Motion (Fig. 28.68)

Type III is divided into IIIa (systolic and diastolic restriction) and IIIb (systolic restriction). Type IIIa is usually seen with rheumatic valve disease or extensive mitral annular calcification, which extends into the leaflet tips with restricted excursion both systole and diastole. Type IIIb is seen clinically in patients with eccentric hypertrophy with spherically shaped ventricles with associated apical tethering of the mitral apparatus. IIIb abnormalities may or may not be associated with annular dilatation. Because of incomplete coaptation, the jet originates centrally and, if there is symmetrical tethering, is centrally directed. With rheumatic disease, the feasibility of repair is the lowest of all etiologies (140).

## Intraoperative Echocardiography (IOE) and Mechanisms of MVAp Dysfunction

In patients with MR, the 2-D intraoperative exam is used to characterize the individual components of the MVAp (with a segment-by-segment analysis) and to evaluate how they function in concert with other related components. Added to the 2-D echocardiographic exam is the evaluation of the regurgitant jet, which is characterized by some of the following properties: location of origin, direction, and severity.

The direction of the regurgitant jet and its eccentricity may be predicted on the basis of leaflet excursion and the symmetrical excursion of the opposing leaflet segment. The presence of asymmetrical (unopposed) leaflet excursion (i.e., flail PMVL) results in a regurgitant jet away from the anatomic defect. Whereas symmetrical opposing leaflet excursion (i.e., bileaflet prolapse) produces a central regurgitant jet. If both leaflets have similar "normal" motion (type I as with annular dilatation), excessive motion (type II as with bileaflet prolapse), or restricted motion (type IIIa rheumatic or IIIb apical tethering) the MR jet will be central. If there is bileaflet prolapse, restriction, or normal motion associated with a dilated annulus, the resulting MR jet direction is central.

### Type I: Normal Leaflet Motion (Fig. 28.68)

Annular dilatation alone results in a lack of leaflet coaptation. Depending on the symmetry of the leaflet motion, the jet may either be central (symmetrical leaflet motion) or slightly posteriorly directed (mild PMVL restriction). With endocarditis, the leaflet motion remains normal; however, endocarditis may result in leaflet perforation or invasion of the cardiac skeleton. CF Doppler will detect a central or slightly posterior jet originating centrally along the line of coaptation, depending on the extent and severity of annular dilatation. Endocarditis may produce an eccentrically directed jet.

### Type II: Excessive Leaflet Motion (Fig. 28.68)

With asymmetrical excessive leaflet motion, the regurgitant flow is directed away from the leaflet with excessive motion. With myxomatous disease, patients will frequently have underlying bileaflet prolapse (with an associated central MR jet) and acutely rupture primary chordae to the PMVL, producing an anteriorly directed jet. The patient may have two distinct jet directions, including a central jet associated with the underlying bileaflet prolapse and an anterior jet associated with the flail segment.

### Type III Restricted Leaflet Motion (Fig. 28.68)

Because of incomplete coaptation, the regurgitant jet originates centrally and if there is symmetrical tethering, is centrally directed. With asymmetric restricted leaflet motion there may be an "override" of the opposing leaflet, and the jet is directed toward the abnormal leaflet. This is seen in posterior wall infarcts with unilateral retraction of the leaflet by a scarred papillary muscle or ventricular wall segment (136).

### Comparison of IOE Exam and Direct Surgical Inspection (Tables 28.10 and 28.11)

The surgical examination includes a direct inspection and determination of the passive mobility of the individual MVAp components. The characterization of leaflet motion by the surgeon and echocardiographer is similar but functionally distinct. The surgeon utilizes nerve hooks and passive extent of motion of the leaflet edge, whereas the echocardiographer characterizes the motion of the entire leaflet throughout the cardiac cycle. The echocardiographer is able to evaluate excursion of any portion of the leaflet above the annular plane. The surgeon evaluates the structure of the components of the MVAp and the range of motion of the valve leaflets. The surgeon may "fill up the heart" to demonstrate regions of the valve that do not passively coapt. The correlation of both evaluations results in a more accurate assessment of the mechanism. In the end, it is the merging of the perspectives that each provides that leads to the final understanding of the mechanism or mechanisms or dysfunction and the choice

of surgical techniques to be incorporated into the surgical strategy (30).

### Surgical Technique and IOE Characterization (Tables 28.10 and 28.11)

The choice of surgical technique and repair strategy is based upon the etiology, the structural integrity of each component of the MVAp, and the underlying mechanism of inadequate leaflet coaptation (Table 28.10) (36,37,54, 56,77,80,91,107). With myxomatous disease, there are five repair techniques that are most commonly employed:

1. Annuloplasty ring (almost all repairs) (77)
2. Quadrilateral resection (central or modified with segmental prolapse or flail PMVL)
3. Sliding annuloplasty (excessive length of PMVL > 1.5 cm)
4. Commissural suture (commissural flail or prolapse)
5. Chordal transfer (flip-over technique)

Other techniques used for this and other processes include:

1. The Alferi edge-to-edge
2. Gortex chordae
3. Chordal shortening (decreased freedom from reoperation)
4. Resection or plication (excessively long AMVL)
5. AMVL extension (for tenting due to apical tethering of secondary chordae)
6. Leaflet debridement (rheumatic or endocarditis)
7. External posterior wall patching between the lower segments and annulus (143)
8. Posterior inflatable baffle to offset tethering of dilated heart (144)
9. Cutting of secondary chordae for apical tethering with tenting of AMVL (145)

If there is excessive leaflet motion of the center P2 scallop of the posterior leaflet, a quadrilateral resection will likely be performed. If, however, there is excessive leaflet motion of the center of the AMVL with a posteriorly directed jet, a chordal transfer will likely be performed. Degenerative disease is associated with eventual annular dilatation. Gillinov et al. reported that long-term durability was diminished in those patients with a repair involving a stabilizing annuloplasty ring (30,77).

### IOE Assessment of MR Severity (Tables 28.13 and 28.14)

The intraoperative evaluation of patients presenting with known severe MR is focused on determining the repairability and determining the necessity of performing other surgical procedures. However, there are circumstances where severity assessment is critical to the management of a patient. Assessing the severity of any valve disease integrates multiple parameters of severity with weighting of the parameter used, according to the quality of the data, the ability to more accurately quantify, and the limitations of the technique for particular types of regurgitant jets. The methods of severity assessment in MR are organized as 2-D and Doppler-derived parameters of severity assessment (35,57).

Regurgitant jet timing is a factor that must be considered, especially if a short-lived regurgitant jet with a large spatial area is being used to determine if a patient should be returned to CPB for further repair surgery (67). Other parameters will provide the integrated guidance indicating the significance of MR of short duration. The parameters used to assess regurgitant valves are either 2-D and

Doppler-derived parameters, demonstrating the direct and indirect cause and the effects of acute and chronic regurgitation. The post-CPB assessment of MR utilizes CF Doppler as an initial screen for significant MR and, if found, is relied upon in conjunction with 2-D imaging to provide an understanding of mechanism(s) of unsuccessful MVRep and MVR.

### Two-Dimensional (2-D) IOE

Two-dimensional imaging provides direct indications of the severity of MV dysfunction, evaluating the indirect effect of regurgitation on the receiving chamber and valve structure. Patients with significant chronic MR have enlarged left atria. Significant MR is rarely associated with

▶ **TABLE 28.12A.** **Intraoperative Assessment of MR Severity: Qualitative and Semiquantitative Assessment**

| Parameter Two-Dimensional Imaging | Utility/Advantages | Limitations | Mild | Moderate | Severe |
|---|---|---|---|---|---|
| LA size | LAE with chronic MR NI LA size excludes significant chronic MR | Enlarged other conditions Severe acute MR may be normal | Normal | Normal or dilated | LAE |
| LV size | | | Normal | Normal or dilated | Dilated enlarged |
| MV apparatus | Flail or ruptured PM; severe MR | Limited to Flail and Ruptured PM | Normal or abnormal | Normal or abnormal | Flail leaflet/ rupt PM |
| **Doppler** | | | | | |
| CF Doppler maximum jet area (MJA) | Efficient screen for mild or severe MR | Technical: wall filter, power, aliasing velocity, color gain, frequency | MJA $< 4cm^2$ | Variable | MJA $> 8 cm^2$ PFC present Wall jet Circumferential |
| Aliasing velocity 50-60 cm/sec | Mechanism evaluation | Load dependent Wall impingement underestimates by 60% | | jet in LA | |
| PW Doppler | A wave dominance excludes severe MR | Dependent on load, diastolic fx, MVA, a fib Indirect inication | Dominant A wave | Variable | Dominant E wave E $> 1.2$ m/sec |
| PW Doppler PV flow | Systolic flow reversal indicates severe MR | Increased LAP, a fib, need R and L PV to call severe | Systolic dominance | Diastolic dominance | Systolic flow reversal |
| CW Doppler spectral density | Easy to perform | Qualitative | Faint envelope | Dense | "v" wave cut off sign |
| CW Doppler contour | Simple | Qualitative | Parabolic | Variable | Early peaking –triangular |

In the assessment of patients undergoing MV surgery, the purpose is to confirm the presence of MV dysfunction and focus on better understanding the underlying etiology and mechanism(s) of dysfunction. MR severity assessment becomes critical when previously undiagnosed MR is discovered or during the post-CPB exam when assessing the results of MV surgery. CF Doppler serves as a useful severity screening method capable of distinguishing mild from severe MR. However, intraoperative decisions based on the severity of MR (i.e., returning to cardiopulmonary bypass for further repair of the MV) should be founded on quantitative data such as regurgitant orifice area and vena contracta diameter with PW Doppler of the MV inflow and pulmonary veins serving as supporting information. The data is weighted according to its quality and its ability to reliably quantify the severity of regurgitation. Zoghbi WA, Enriquez-Sarano M, Foster E. et al. Recommendations for evaluation of the severity of native valvular regurgitation with two-dimensional and Doppler echocardiography. J Am Soc Echocardiogr 2003;16(7):777–802.

▶ TABLE 28.12B.   Quantitative Assessment

| | *Utilities/ Advantages* | *Limitations* | *Mild* | *Moderate* | *Severe* |
|---|---|---|---|---|---|
| **Vena Contracta width (cm)** | Good eccentric jets Efficient | Not useful for multiple MR jets Cannot add diameters | < 0.3 cm | 0.3–0.69 cm | Vena contracta width ≥ 0.7cm |

| **PISA Proximal Flow Convergence (PFC)** | *Utilities/ Advantages* | *Limitations* | *Mild* | *Mild to Moderate* | *Moderate to Severe* | *Severe* | |
|---|---|---|---|---|---|---|---|
| **Regurgitant volume (cc)** | | | | < 30 | 30–44 | 45–59 | ≥ 60 |
| **Regurgitant fractions (%)** | | | | < 30 | 30–39 | 40–49 | ≥ 50 |
| **ROA (cm²)** | PFC at aliasing velocity of 50-60 cm/sec sign MR | Eccentric jets Peak ROA only estimates mean ROA | < 0.20 | 0.20–0.29 | 0.30–0.39 | | ≥ 0.40 |

In the assessment of patients undergoing MV surgery, the purpose is to confirm the presence of MV dysfunction and focus on better understanding the underlying etiology and mechanism(s) of dysfunction. MR severity assessment becomes critical when previously undiagnosed MR is discovered or during the post-CPB exam when assessing the results of MV surgery. CF Doppler serves as a useful severity screening method capable of distinguishing mild from severe MR. However, intraoperative decisions based on the severity of MR (i.e., returning to cardiopulmonary bypass for further repair of the MV) should be founded on quantitative data such as regurgitant orifice area and vena contracta diameter with PW Doppler of the MV inflow and pulmonary veins serving as supporting information. The data is weighted according to its quality and its ability to reliably quantify the severity of regurgitation. Zoghbi WA, Enriquez-Sarano M, Foster E. et al. Recommendations for evaluation of the severity of native valvular regurgitation with two-dimensional and Doppler echocardiography. J Am Soc Echocardiogr 2003;16(7):777–802.

normal MV structure. Patients with a flail segment usually have severe MR. This holds true even if the CF Doppler demonstrates a small regurgitant jet area (RJA), such as that seen with an eccentric wall hugging jet or one associated with acute MR that is directed into a noncompliant LA. TEE imaging does not lend itself to see the entire LA, but massively enlarged atria associated with chronic MR are apparent (57).

### Doppler Assessment of MR

The regurgitant jet that is detected by CFD consists of a subvalvular zone of proximal flow convergence, the narrowest portion of the jet (at or just distal to the valve orifice on the LA side), and the spatial jet area in the LA. All components may yield distinct information, which, when

▶ TABLE 28.13.   Proximal Isovelocity Surface Area

**Proximal Flow Convergence Radius and Severity of MR**
$V_{aliasing}$ = 40 cm/sec or 1/12th (0.8) peak $V_{MR}$

| Grade | PISA Radius | ROA r²/2 (peak) | Regurgitant Volume (peak) |
|---|---|---|---|
| Mild | > 18.9 mm | 0.02 cm² | < 30 cc |
| Mod | 7.7–8.8 mm | 0.02–0.29 cm² | 30–40 cc |
| Mod Sev | 6.3–7.6 mm | 0.3–0.39 cm² | 45–59 cc |
| Sev | < 6.2 mm | ≥ 0.40 cm² | ≥ 60 cc |

integrated, provides a clearer understanding of the significance of the MV dysfunction. Doppler methods of severity assessment of MR have relied heavily on color flow determination of the maximal jet area (MJA).

### Color Flow Doppler Maximal Jet Area (MJA)

MJA may be utilized as an effective means for screening patients with severe or trivial MR and to characterize the mechanism of MR. However, MJA is not able to distinguish subtle differences of severity grade (35,57). MJA may not reflect the severity of valve dysfunction in acute MR or with eccentric MR (57). In addition, there are a host of settings that impact the MJA. While the MJA (utilizing an aliasing velocity near 50 to 60 m/s) is generally predictive of the severity of MR, it may underestimate the severity if it is eccentric or acute in etiology (Fig. 28.63) (35,57). If the absolute jet area is > 8 cm² there is severe MR, if < 4 cm² it is mild. All grades in between are not reliable as a stand-alone assessment of severity. The jet direction, however, is valuable in determining structural mechanisms.

### Vena Contracta Diameter (VCD)

Measuring the narrowest diameter of the regurgitant orifice at or distal to the anatomic orifice provides a more quantitatively and accurate method of assessment. The VCD should be from an image plane that is perpendicular to the commissural line of MR. The VCD is not dependent

▶ **TABLE 28.14.   Severity Assessment in MV Repair**

1. **CF Doppler Screening of Entire MV Coaptation Plane**
   - ME 4 Chr MV
   - ME 5 Chr MV (Ant-Lat Comm)
   - ME lower 4 Chr MV (Post-Med Comm)
     (aliasing velocity 50–60 cm/sec)
2. **If CF Doppler Detects MR Jet**
   - Use 2-D imaging to detect structural defect
   - Quantify amount
   - Use simplified PISA
     - Peak ROA > 0.3 cm$^2$ is moderately severe
   - Vena contracta diameter (VC > 0.3 cm is moderate)
     - Color m-mode may clarify closing regurgitation jet
       - Short lived < 40% systolic time interval
   - If moderate, integrate multiple methods
     - Weight toward quality of data obtained and quatitative reliability of parameter
   - Use other quantitative methods
     - PW Doppler PV: systolic reversal is severe
     - CW intensity of spectral envelope
     - MV inflow e > a more severe; e > 1.2 m/sec
     - Other volumetric methods
3. **When to Return to CPB for Further Repair**
   - Identified structural defect that will not
     - improve though less than moderate
     - SAM with LVOTO and MR
     - perforation, suture dehiscence identified mechanism
   - Greater than mild to moderate MR
     - ROA > 0.3 cm$^2$, regurgitant volume > 40–45 cc/beat
     - VC > 0.3 cm
   - If additional CPB time would jeopardize patient modify indications for return to CPB

on the flow rate, the LA-LV gradient, or the eccentricity of the MR jet. It does change throughout the cardiac cycle. Because of the small size of the VCD, focused zoom should be used to diminish the percentage of error. A VCD of < .3 cm$^2$ is consistent with mild MR whereas > 0.6 cm$^2$–0.8 cm$^2$ is severe (35,57). The presence of PFC and a width > 0.6 confirm the severity of the MR. Multiple small jets are not additive by diameter.

### *Proximal Flow Convergence (PFC)*

PFC (proximal flow convergence) is based on the principle that blood increases in velocity as it approaches a regurgitant orifice, resulting in hemispheric velocity shells (66). The presence of PISA (proximal isovelocity surface areas) with MR at an aliasing velocity of 50 cm/sec to 60 cm/sec is an indicator of clinically significant MR (35,57). When one does not see a flow convergence larger than 3 mm–4 mm at < 30 cm/sec, the MR would be trivial or at most mild. However, when the flow convergence is larger than 7 mm to 8 mm at the aliasing velocity > 50 cm/sec–60 cm/sec, the MR is severe (35). The size of the radius is strictly dependent on the aliasing velocity and alignment of the CFD parallel to the PISA. Not doing so will underestimate the severity of MR. The aliasing velocity must be adjusted down to obtain a hemispheric PFC. Assuming that the peak flow rate occurs simultaneously with the peak radius and peak regurgitant velocity, the (peak) regurgitant orifice area (ROA) may be determined with the following formula:

$$\text{(peak) ROA} = (6.28 \; r^2 \times V_a) \; / \; \text{peak } V_{MR}$$

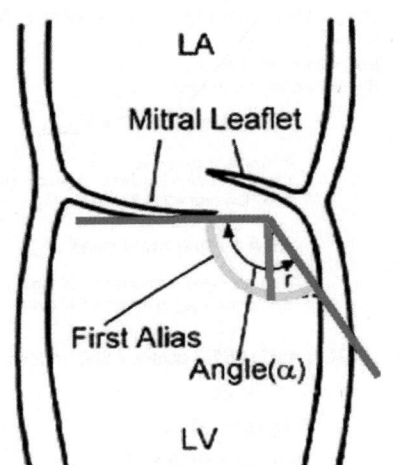
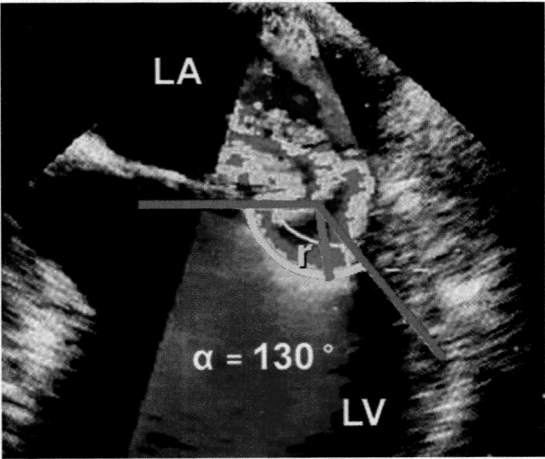

**FIGURE 28.69.** Peak ROA. Assuming that the peak flow rate is simultaneous with peak radius regurgitant velocity, the regurgitant orifice area (ROA) (at peak flow rate) may be determined with the formula above. (Where r is the aliasing radius between the orifice and interface, Va is the aliasing velocity, and $V_{MR}$ is the *peak* regurgitant velocity). Using aliasing velocity for ROA is most reliable with a hemispheric proximal flow convergence zone (adjust Nyquist limit down and/or baseline shift in direction of jet) and with absence of wall impingement. If there is wall impingement at the aliasing radius *r*, a reliable correction may be provided with the formula: ROA = (6.28 $r^2$ × Va) / peak $V_{MR}$ × angle/180° (66).

Where $r^2$ is the aliasing radium between the orifice and interface, $V_a$ represents the aliasing velocity and $V_{MR}$ is the peak regurgitant velocity. If there is wall impingement at the aliasing radius r, the wall constraint angle / 180° is multiplied by the ROA as a correction (Fig. 28.69) (65,66). An aliasing velocity must be hemispherical (decrease Nyquist limit or baseline shift in direction of jet) with the absence of wall impingement. Limitations apply to eccentric jets, nonhemispheric PFC, and variance of results using nonhemispheric aliasing velocities. Nonparallel alignment of the CW peak $V_{MR}$ results in an underestimation of the velocity peak and an overestimation of the (peak) ROA. If the ROA is > 0.4 cm², there is severe MR, if it is < 0.2 cm² it is mild. By multiplying the ROA by the MR TVI, the regurgitant volume may be determined (35).

### Simplified PISA Method (Fig. 28.70 and Table 28.14)

This shorthand method for effective regurgitant orifice area is consistent with the intraoperative requirement for efficiency and simplicity of quantitative measurement in a multitasking environment. There are two simplified PISA methods (57,66).

If we assume that the systolic pressure gradient between the LV and LA is 100 mm Hg (120 − 20 mm Hg) then we understand from the Bernoulli equation that the gradient 100 mm Hg = 4 peak $V^2$; and therefore peak V = 5 m/s.

Method One:
Aliasing Velocity set to 40 cm/sec

$$(\text{PEAK}) \ ROA = 2 \ \Pi \ r^2 \times V_a/V_P$$

$$(\text{peak}) \ ROA = \frac{6.28 \times 40 \ \text{cm/sec} \ r^2}{500 \ \text{cm/sec}} = \frac{251 \ r^2}{500}$$

$$(\text{peak}) \ ROA = \frac{1}{2} r^2$$

Method Two:
Aliasing Velocity set to 32 cm/sec

Because any ROA > 0.40 cm² is severe MR, if $V_P$ is also assumed to be 500 cm/sec then the Va must be 30 cm/sec for the ROA to equal 0.4 cm²

$$Va = \frac{0.4 \ \text{cm}^2 \times 500 \ \text{cm/sec}}{6.28 \times r^2 \ (1)}$$

$$Va = \frac{200 \ \text{cm}^3/\text{sec}}{6.28 \ \text{cm}^2} = 32 \ \text{cm/sec}$$

Therefore if the Va is set at 30 cm/sec and r is greater than 1 cm, the ROA is always > 0.4 cm².

The major advantages of the PISA method over the MJA method are that PISA is not influenced by color gain or affected by jet eccentricity.

### Continuous Wave Doppler (CWD)

The intensity of the spectral envelope signal is indicative of the severity of the MR. If the signal density is equiva-

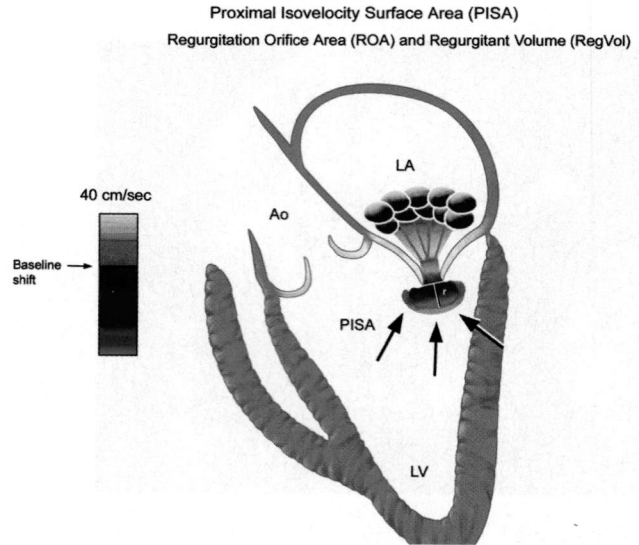

**FIGURE 28.70.** This shorthand method for regurgitant orifice area is consistent with the intraoperative need for efficiency and reliability of quantitative measurement. Assuming that the systolic pressure gradient between the LV and LA is 100 mm Hg (120 − 20 mm Hg), via the Bernoulli equation the peak velocity is 5 m/s. (LV-LA gradient = 100 mm Hg = 4 peak $V^2$ and therefore peak V = 5 m/s.) ROA = (2 $\pi r^2$ × Va) / peak VMR or ROA = $r^2$ (251/500) or $r^2$/2.

lent to the antegrade flow, the MR is significant. With more MR, the LA-LV gradient equilibrates and there is a V wave cutoff (Fig. 28.66). CWD of the TR jet may suggest pulmonary hypertension (PAS = CVP + 4 VTR$^2$) (35,57,146).

### Pulse Wave Doppler (PWD)

#### Transmitral Flow

PWD at the leaflet tips may be used as an indirect indication of the additional regurgitant flow. If the peak E wave velocity is > 1.2 m/sec, it is consistent with severe MR (assuming no MS). PWD may also be used to calculate regurgitant fraction; however, in the cardiac operating room it is rarely performed and only for guidance in borderline decisions. Borderline MR should not alter plans for MV surgery unless other complicating factors are present, placing the patient at extremely high risk for cannulation and CPB (35).

#### Pulmonary Venous Flow

PWD of the pulmonary vein inflow is an indirect method of assessing elevated LAP and is used to determine the presence of retrograde (reversal) of systolic pulmonary venous flow. Systolic reversal in more than two pulmonary veins is indicative of severe MR. Placing the cursor parallel to left upper PV flow into the LA at a PW depth of at least 2 cm into the pulmonary results in optimal spectral tracings (57,60–62). Blunting of the systolic waves is indicative of increased LAP and not specific for MR.

▶ **TABLE 28.15B. Etiology of Mitral Stenosis and Pathologic Anatomy: Less Frequent Causes of Mitral Stenosis**

| Etiology | Pathologic Changes Involving MV |
|---|---|
| Malignant Carcinoid | Rare but may lead to thickening and immobility of valves |
| Systemic Lupus | Inflammatory nodules (Libman-Sacks endocarditis resulting in inflammation and fusion of cusps) |
| Rheumatoid Arthritis | Rheumatoid nodules and secondary inflammation |
| Hunter-Hurley | Mucopolysaccharide deposition in valve leaflets |
| Cortriatriatum | Membrane in LA |
| Amyloid Deposits on Rheumatoid Valves | Rare presentation of amyloid, with amyloid deposition on rheumatic leaflets further decreasing mobility |

### Mitral Stenosis

#### Etiology and Mechanisms of Mitral Stenosis

*Etiology (Table 28.15)* Mitral stenosis (MS) most commonly results from longstanding rheumatic heart disease secondary to acute rheumatic fever. However, there are other potential causes of MS, including congenital, mitral annular calcification (extending onto leaflets),

▶ **TABLE 28.15A. Acute and Chronic Mitral Regurgitation: Etiology and Pathology**

| Etiology | Pathologic Anatomy | IOE Assessment |
|---|---|---|
| **Rheumatic** | 1) Thickened fibrotic Ca$^{++}$ leaflets with basal commissural fusion, and retraction with "fish-mouth" deformity and reduced mobility<br>2) Fibrotic Ca$^{++}$ of annulus with diminished mobility resulting in poor coaptation and MR<br>3) Subvalvular chordal fusion and obliteration of the effective interchordal orifice and subvalvular stenosis | 1) 2-D imaging demonstartes decreased mobility, leaflet thickening, subvalvular chordal fusion, and stenosis<br>2) Planimetry of MV area in transgastric after TG 2Chr CF Doppler confirms that subvalvular apparatus is not the most stenotic level; planimetry of the mitral valve area TG SAX<br>3) Annulus is fibrotic and frequently calcified with reduced mobility |
| **Mitral annular calcification** | 1) MAC$^{++}$ extends from posterior annulus into leaflet tips<br>2) Subannular and valvular fibrosis with Ca$^{++}$ bars impeding LV inflow | 1) 2-D imaging shows Ca$^{++}$ in PMVL and annulus<br>2) Leaflet Ca$^{++}$ reduces mobility with incomplete coaptation<br>3) Annular Ca$^{++}$ reduces mobility and contribution to coaptation<br>4) Subannular Ca$^{++}$ for bars which impede LV inflow. |
| **LA thrombus** | Associated with atrial fibrillation and associated with intermittent ball-valve occlusion of MV orifice | 2-D imaging demonstartes thrombus and spontaneous contrast with diminished LAA velocities under 0.5/sec |
| **LA Myxoma** | Attached to interatrial septum and, like thrombus, causes ball-valve type of abrupt obstruction of LV inflow. | 2-D imaging demonstrates myxoma with stalk attachment to IAS. |

parachute MV, obstructing masses (large atrial myxomas, thrombi), or endocarditis vegetations. Rarer causes of stenosis include valve abnormalities associated with inborn errors of metabolism, malignant carcinoid syndrome, systemic lupus, cardiac amyloid, and rheumatoid arthritis (41,42,44,46). The pathologic features of rheumatic valvular disease involving the MV include diffuse thickening, fibrosis, calcification of the valve leaflets, commissures, and subvalvular chordae. This results in thickened rigid valves, commissural fusion, and shortened fused chordae producing a "fish-mouth" shaped valve with both valvular and subvalvular stenosis. In addition rheumatic nodules are deposited in the myocardium (Aschoff bodies), which may produce underlying myocarditis. The MS ultimately leads to elevated LA pressures, pulmonary artery hypertension, RV dysfunction, and TR (with or without rheumatic involvement). The chronic elevation of LA pressure may result in atrial enlargement, stagnant blood flow (detected as spontaneous contrast), and thrombus formation.

### Mechanisms

Mechanisms of MS may be classified as those that are predominantly supravalvular (obstructing atrial myxoma, thrombus, or large obstructing vegetation), valvular (rheumatic, degenerative calcification), and subvalvular (rheumatic, parachute MV). Determining the mechanism of MS is essential for the purposes of MV repair. If there is significant subvalvular stenosis, repairing the valve apparatus may contribute to increased mobility, but the gradient will probably remain significantly elevated.

Rheumatic MV disease most commonly results from longstanding rheumatic heart disease secondary to acute rheumatic fever. Rheumatic valvular disease involving the MV is characterized pathologically by diffuse thickening, fibrosis, calcification of the valve leaflets, commissures, and subvalvular apparatus, including the chordae and heads of the papillary muscle. Significant disease usually appears after a latent period of 20–25 years, but may occur earlier with repeated exposures to rheumatic fever or active rheumatic myocarditis. The inflammatory process results in thickened and rigid valves, commissural fusion, and shortened fused chordae producing a "fish-mouth" shaped valve with potential for valvular and subvalvular stenosis. If there is restricted leaflet motion of the leaflet edges, it may result in a classic "hockey stick" deformity of the AMVL. Chronic rheumatic inflammation produces stenosis, or a combination of MS and MR. Isolated rheumatic MR is rare.

Mitral annular calcification (MAC) is a degenerative disease associated with aging and is found in 54% of males over the age of 60 (56). It is associated with arteriosclerosis of the aorta and coronary arteries. It is usually seen at the base of the posterior PMVL and extends

into the posterior LV wall. It may cause rigidity of the PMVL and calcific stenosis. The calcification and valve thickening progresses from the annulus toward the edge of the leaflets. There is reduced mobility of the saddle-shaped annulus with MAC and this may be associated with subvalvular calcific stenosis. The presence of annular calcification may require annular debridement and reconstruction for performance of either an annuloplasty or MV prosthesis, increasing the risk for pseudoaneurysms or annular disruption.

### Pathophysiology

Rheumatic MS results in the development of early diastolic gradient between the LA and LV. As the process continues, the gradient becomes elevated throughout late diastole. If there is coexisting MR, this may produce symptoms of pulmonary congestion earlier. The left atrium gradually dilates with MS, depending on the compliance changes in the atria. With enlarged LA, there is a propensity to develop atrial fibrillation, which, in the face of significant MS, may markedly reduce LV filling and overall forward cardiac output.

As the size of the MV decreases from 4.0 cm$^2$ to 1.0 cm$^2$, the gradient between the LV and LA may increase to 25 mm Hg with a mean > 10 mm Hg (56). This is manifest as a decreased e to f slope on m-mode or e to a slope on CWD. While the peak transvalvular gradient may be over 20 mm Hg at rest with a mean gradient > 8 mm Hg (55,56). Chronically, patients with greater than moderate MS have elevated LA pressures up to 30 mm Hg and associated pulmonary hypertension with RV dysfunction. The RV will chronically dilate, resulting in TV annular enlargement (> 3.5 cm), a lack of coaptation, and significant tricuspid regurgitation and hepatic congestion (55,56).

### Severity Assessment (Table 28.16)

As with MR, MS is best assessed using a weighted and integrated IOE approach of 2-D assessment (splitability score and planimetry) and Doppler (CFD, PISA, MVA calculation, CW and PWD determination of MVA) using the continuity equation and mean gradient, pressure half-time, and deceleration time.

### IOE Two-Dimensional Assessment of Severity of MS (Table 28.16)

Examination of the MVAp permits an identification of the underlying etiology. With more advanced rheumatic MS, features are pathognemonic. Unlike MS resulting from MAC, which extends from the base of the leaflets, rheumatic MS progresses from the leaflet tips toward the leaflet base. The TG basal SAX view aligned parallel to the annulus may demonstrate commissural fusion and re-

▶ TABLE 28.16.  Echocardiographic Splitability Index Based on MV Morphology

| Grade | Mobility | Leaflet Thickening | Subvalvular | Calcification |
|-------|----------|--------------------|-------------|---------------|
| 1 | Tips restricted | Normal 4-5 mm | < 1/3 below leaflet | Area |
| 2 | Base to mid-normal | Mid normal | 1/3 of chordae | Scattered areas on leaflet margins |
| 3 | Base normal | Throughout leaflet | 2/3 of chordae | Bright to mid leaflet portion |
| 4 | No movement | Marked throughout > 8–10 mm | No movement | $Ca^{++}$ throughout > 8–10 mm |

Wilkins GT, Weyman AE, Abascal VM, et al. Percutaneous balloon dilatation of the mitral valve: an analysis of echocardiographic variables related to outcome and the mechanism of dilatation. Br Heart J 1988;60:299–308.

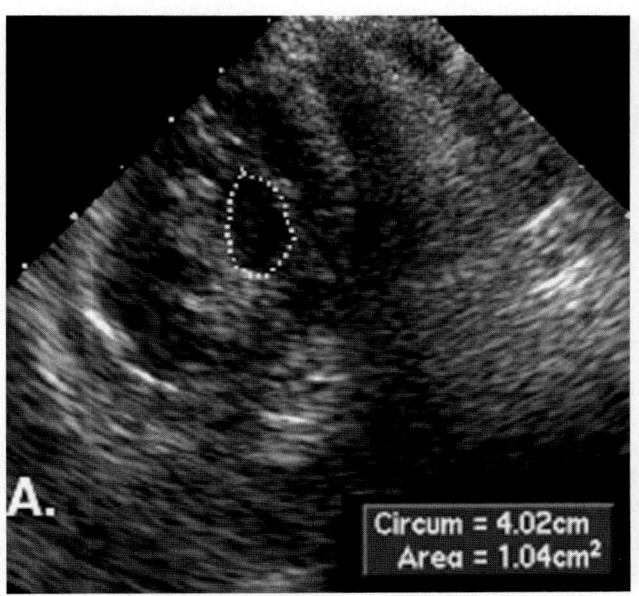

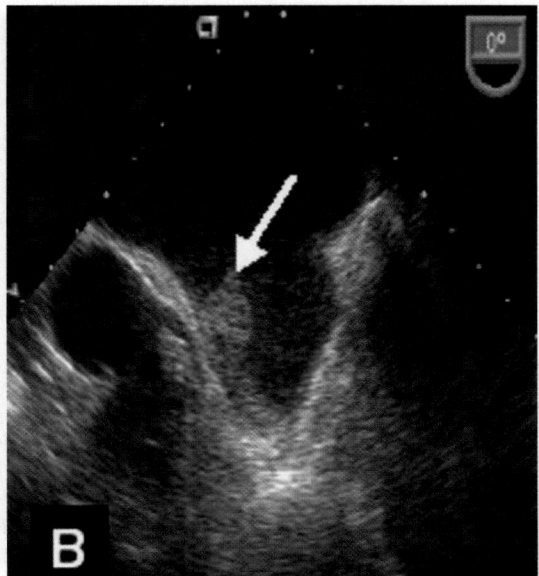

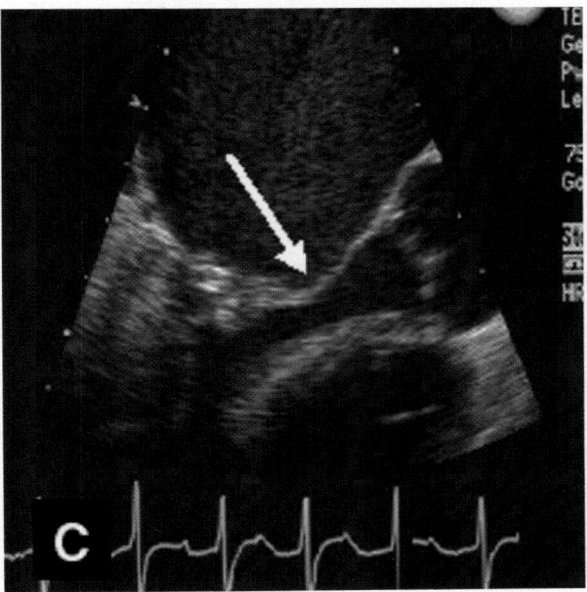

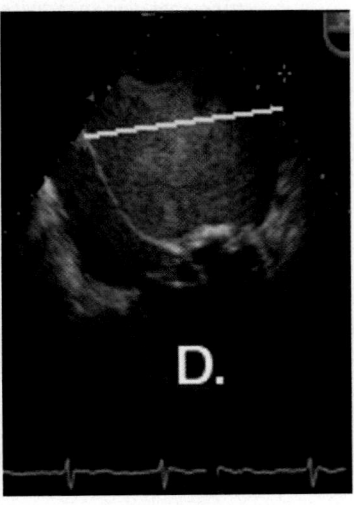

FIGURE 28.71 A, B, C, and D. **A:** Rheumatic MV stenosis may be valvular or subvalvular. Using CF Doppler in the TF 2Chr demonstrates PVC at the level of maximal stenosis. Using the TG basal SAX, the MV may be planimetered. Planimetry provides a reliable estimate of MVA if it is done at the level of the stenosis. **B-D:** Other findings in rheumatic valve disease include LAA thrombus **(B),** fusion of leaflet edges and a hockey stick deformity **(C),** and LA enlargement which must be estimated using TEE **(D).**

stricted valve motion. However, the TG 2 Chr MV image plane with color determines the level of the most significant stenosis. From the TG basal SAX, at the level of the most significant narrowing, a digital image loop is captured and advanced to the frame demonstrating maximal opening. Planimetering the MVA electronically provides a reliable estimation of the true valve area (Fig. 28.71). Planimetry may underestimate the severity due to echogenic shielding from the presence of $Ca^{++}$ in the valve annulus and the subvalvular degree of flow obstruction.

In 1988, Wilkins et al. evaluated patients over a 6-month period, who had balloon valvuloplasty for rheumatic MS. As discussed previously, they developed an echo score correlating with a propensity to restenose (68). This score was subsequently applied to 100 consecutive patients who underwent a similar procedure—valvotomy—and discovered that only one patient with a score > 8 restenosed (Table 28.17). To validate the ability to utilize TEE imaging to reliably determine a patient's splitability score, Marwick et al. compared the TTE and

TEE of 45 patients undergoing balloon valvuloplasty over two years. TEE was useful in MS, but there were significant differences between the TTE and TEE scores, with the TTE score 7.2 compared to TEE 5.9 (p < 0.001). The difference was thought to be subvalvular shielding by thickened and dense MV leaflets and a shielded transducer position on the LA side during esophageal imaging (147).

### Doppler Methods of Severity Assessment

A semiquantitative method of estimating MVA is to measure the pressure gradient, using CW Doppler interrogation across the MV inflow. A mean pressure gradient (from tracing the CW envelope) > 12 mm Hg severe MS, and < 5 mm Hg indicates less than moderate MS. Gradient is flow related, but if properly aligned, has less probability of inducible human error (55,56).

Quantitative methods of MS assessment are pressure half-time ($PT_{1/2}$), deceleration time (DT), continuity equa-

▶ **TABLE 28.17. MV Stenosis Severity Assessment**

| Left Atrial Size | LAE > 45 mm AP diameter |
| | *Exclude LAA thrombi* |
| PA Pressure | $PASP = 4(V_{TR})^2 + CVP*$ |
| | $PAM = (-0.45) AT + 79$ |
| Planimeter Valve Area | Difficult with heavy $Ca^{++}$, previous commissurotomy |
| Mean Gradient | Integrated Area of $MV_{Diastolic}$ Spectral Envelope |
| | *With atrial fibrillation, average 5 consecutive diastoles* |
| | *Gradient $\alpha$ flow across MV and MVA, therefore* |
| | *Severe MR produces larger than expected gradient* |
| Continuity Equation | $MVA = (D^2_{LVOT} \times 0.785) (TVI_{LVOT}) / TVI_{MV}$ |
| | *No AR, LVOT obstruction, or MR* |
| Deceleration Time | $MVA = 759 / DT$ |
| | $PT_{1/2} = 0.29 \times DT$ |
| | *Altered by diastolic dysfunction* |
| Pressure Half Time | $MVA = 220 / PT_{1/2}$ |
| | *Inaccurate with abnormal compliance (LA, LV), significant AR, or post valvuloplasty* |
| | *(AR reduces $PT_{1/2}$ and overestimates valve area)* |
| PISA | $MVA = 2 \pi R^2 \times V_{Aliasing} / Peak\ V_{MS} \times \alpha° / 180°$ |
| (Proximal Isovelocity Surface Area) | |
| | $V_{Aliasing}$ = Aliasing Velocity of Color Doppler |
| | R = radius from orifice to PISA interface |
| | Peak $V_{MS}$ = Peak CW Diastolic Doppler Velocity |

| *Normal = 4 – 6 cm²* | *Mild* | *Moderate* | *Severe* |
| --- | --- | --- | --- |
| Planimetered Area | 1.5 – 2.0 cm² | 1.0 – 1.5 cm² | ≤ 0.9 cm² |
| Mean Gradient ₍Diastolic₎ | < 6 mm Hg* | 6 – 12 mm Hg* | > 12 mm Hg* |
| Deceleration Time | < 517 m/sec | 517 – 690 m/sec | > 759 m/sec |
| Pressure Half Time | < 150 m/sec | 150 – 200 m/sec | > 220 m/sec |

Note: Symptoms = Gradient = MVA
  if not, must explain (rest vs. exercise, other etiology)
*Measured or estimated

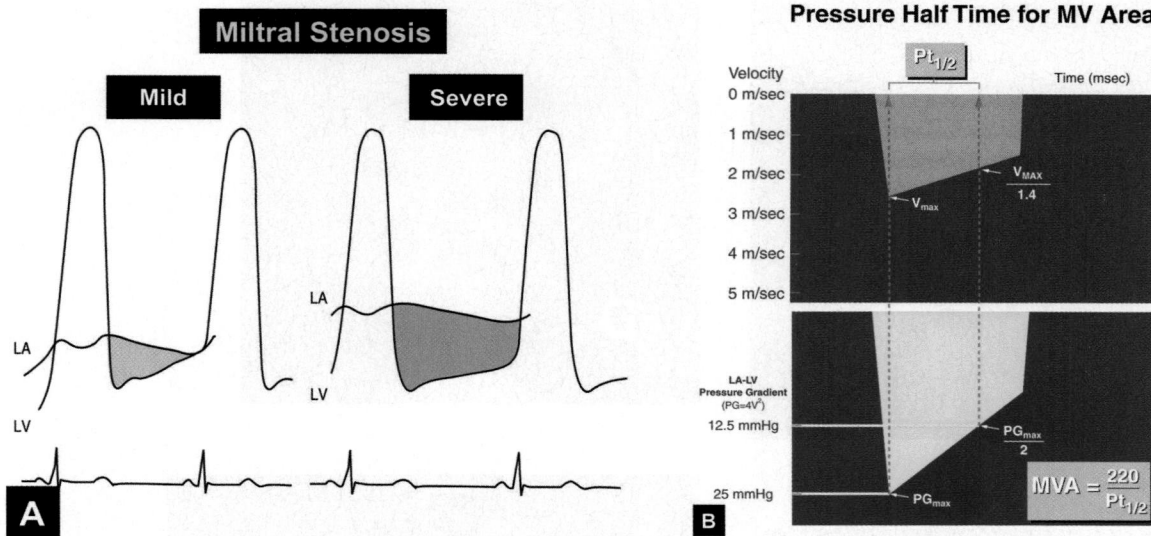

**FIGURE 28.72 A and B.** The peak instantaneous gradient (using the simplified Bernoulli equation), where V is the initial peak instantaneous velocity. Determining the time it requires for the gradient to drop by 50%. The MVA is calculated by dividing 220 by $PT_{1/2}$. The constant 220 is based on the relative diastolic properties of the LA and LV. Since severe MS is classified as a MVA < 1.0 cm$^2$, whenever $PT_{1/2}$ is > 220 msec, there is severe MS. There are circumstances that may lead to miscalculation including: 1) the presence of AR leading to a reduced $PT_{1/2}$ and overestimation of MVA due to more rapid equilibration of LA and LV pressure gradient, and 2) aging reduces the compliance of the LV, and the LA-LV gradient LV diastolic pressure rises faster than in normal complaint ventricles, hence a shorter $PT_{1/2}$ with and overestimation of MVA (55,56).

tion, or proximal isovelocity surface area (PISA). The CW spectral envelope demonstrates increased flow velocity across the valve, which corresponds to the increased valve gradient demonstrating a flattened slope of a slower reduction in LA and LV gradient. $PT_{1/2}$ is the time it takes for the initial peak instantaneous pressure gradient (4 × peak V$^2$) to drop by 50% (Fig. 28.72). Using standard calculation programs available on most platforms, these calculations are automatically calculated based on relative diastolic properties of the LA and LV dividing the constant 220 by the $PT_{1/2}$. Whenever $PT_{1/2}$ is ≥ 220 msec, there is severe MS with an estimated MVA < 1.0 cm$^2$. There are circumstances that lead to miscalculation, including the fact that AR reduces $PT_{1/2}$ and overestimates MVA (more rapid equilibration of LA-LV gradient), which leads to overestimation of MVA, or aging, which reduces the compliance of the LV with the LA-LV gradient causing a shorter and faster $PT_{1/2}$ and overestimation of MVA (55,56).

The deceleration time, or time it takes the peak velocity to reach 0 m/sec along the interpolated slope, may be used to calculate the MVA. The relation is characterized by the formula MVA = 759/DT. $PT_{1/2}$ may be calculated from the DT ($PT_{1/2}$ = 0.29 × DT). Therefore a DT greater than 760 msec is also suggestive of severe stenosis (55,56,71).

Another alternative for calculation of the MVA is utilizing the continuity equation based upon the principle that flow across one valve must equal flow across another (in the absence of regurgitation of either valve).

MV Flow = LVOT Flow and ($MV_A$ × $TVI_{MV}$ = Area $_{LVOT}$ × TVI $_{LVOT}$) therefore
MVA = (Area $_{LVOT}$) × (TVI $_{LVOT}$)/ TVI $_{MV}$

This technique involves obtaining the LVOT diameter at the aortic valve annulus in the ME LAX imaging plane, the PW Doppler VTI $_{LVOT}$ and the CW Doppler VTI across the MV. PISA (proximal isovelocity surface area) can also be used to calculate MVA (Figs. 28.73A–28.73D). Using the ME 4 Chr, CF Doppler interrogation of the MV is performed with a baseline shift to reduce the aliasing velocity away from the transducer. A digital loop is captured and the image is frozen in diastole to optimize the radius measurement of the first PISA interface zone. The atrial MV angle is then determined (Fig. 28.74). Rodriguez et al. validated a method for determining MV area, using the proximal flow convergence method of calculating flow rate (spherical area × aliasing velocity) (72). With the convergence funnel not being spherical, an adjustment was made for the typical funnel angle by the formula:

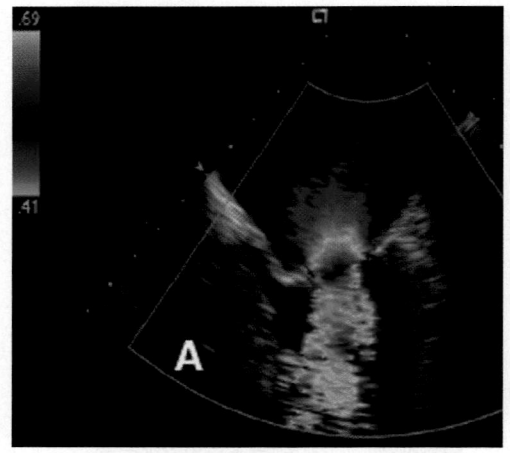

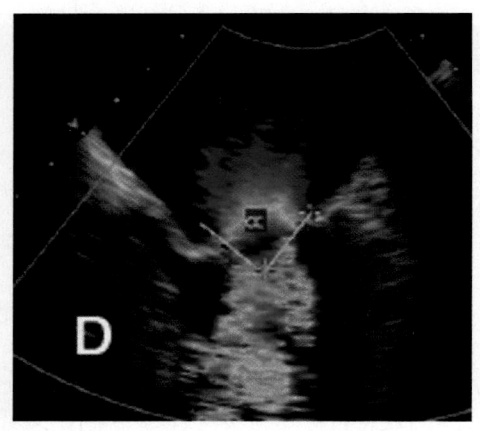

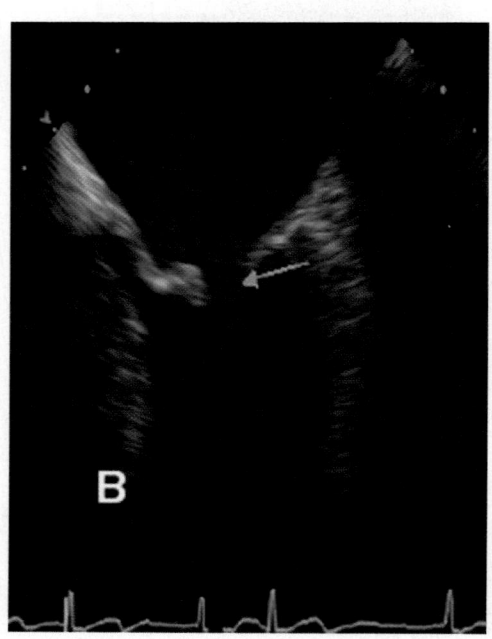

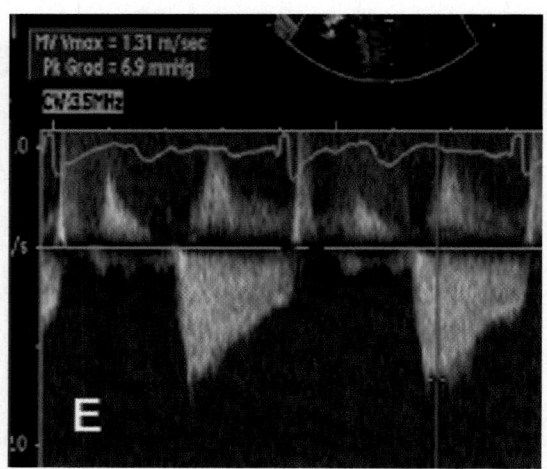

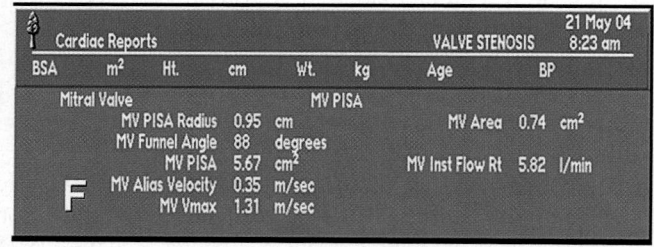

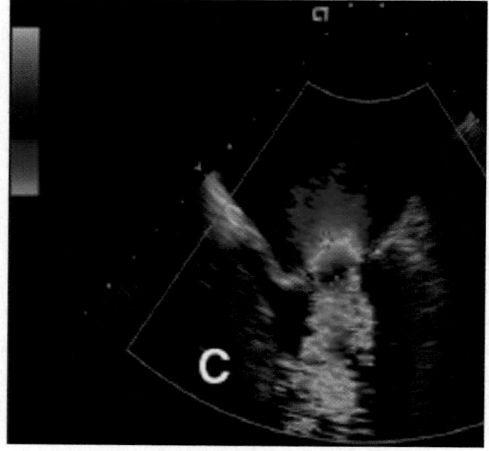

**FIGURE 28.73 A, B, C, D, E, and F.** PISA proximal flow convergence (PFC) is also used to calculate MVA. Using the ME four 4 Chr view, CF Doppler interrogation of the MV steno tic jet is performed with the zero baseline shifted upward to reduce the aliasing velocity away from the transducer. A digital loop is captured as the image is frozen in diastole to optimize the radius measurement of the first PISA interface zone. The atrial MV angle is then determined. Rodriguez et al. validated a method for determining MV area using the PVC velocity. Since the convergence funnel is not spherical, an adjustment is made for the funnel angle using the following:

$$\text{MV Flow Rate} = \text{Spherical Area} \times \text{Velocity Aliasing (angle/180°)}$$
$$\text{MV Flow Rate} = \text{Spherical Area} \times \text{Velocity Aliasing} \times (\text{angle}/180°)$$
$$\text{MV Flow Rate} = 2\,\pi r^2\,(V_{\text{Aliasing}}) \times (\text{angle}/180°)$$
$$\text{MVA} = \text{Flow Rate/Peak (CW Doppler)}\ V_{\text{MS}}$$

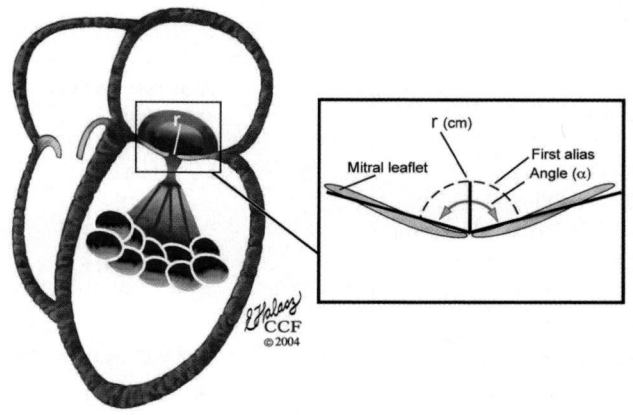

**FIGURE 28.74.** Rodriguez et al. validated a method for determining MV area using the proximal flow convergence method of calculating flow rate (*MV Flow Rate = Spherical Area × V$_A$*). When the convergence funnel is not spherical, an adjustment was made based on the funnel angle by the formula:

$$MV\ Flow\ Rate = Spherical\ Area × VA\ (angle\ \alpha /180°)$$
$$= 2\ \pi r^2\ V_A\ (angle\ \alpha /180°)$$
$$MVA = Flow\ Rate\ /\ Peak\ (CW\ Doppler)$$

$$MV\ Flow\ Rate = Spherical\ Area × Velocity_{Aliasing}\ (angle\ \alpha /180°)$$

$$MV\ Flow\ Rate = Spherical\ Area × Velocity_{Aliasing} × (angle\ /180°)$$
$$= 2\ \pi r^2\ (V_{Aliasing})\ × (angle\ /180°)$$

$$MVA = Flow\ Rate\ /\ Peak\ (CW\ Doppler)\ V_{MS}$$

Flow Convergence Method or PISA Method (Fig. 28.74)

## IOE Findings Associated with MV Dysfunction

### Secondary Pathophysiology in Mitral Valve Disease

*LA and LAA* In acute MR, blunting of the S wave is usually present in all pulmonary veins with a LAP > 15 mm Hg. Whereas in chronic MR, the left atrium may dilate to 70 mm (55,56). These patients may develop stagnant blood flow in the left atrial appendage. Because of the regurgitant jet, left atrial appendage thrombi are extremely rare except in instances of atrial fibrillation with combined rheumatic MS-MR, or low flow states due to severe ventricular dysfunction. With chronic MS, associated stagnant left atrial blood flow secondary has an increased risk for the development of thrombi in the left atrium and appendage. Predictors include the presence of atrial fibrillation, left atrial enlargement, spontaneous contrast, and PW Doppler peak LAA velocities under 0.5 m/sec (68). The presence of any of these risks is used as an indication for closure of the left atrial appendage. 2-D imaging may demonstrate spontaneous contrast in the LA, and the PW Doppler of the LAA may demonstrate low velocity flows under 0.5 m/sec, indicating that the patient is at an increased risk for developing LAA thrombi (75).

*Atrial Fibrillation* Up to 50% of patients undergoing MV surgery will have history of atrial fibrillation. Patients with transient paroxysmal atrial fibrillation often will have their inciting reentry focus at the junction of the pulmonary veins with the left atrium. In these patients, pulmonary vein isolation techniques achieve encouraging results when the LA is markedly enlarged. LA enlargement, as seen with chronic MR or MS, large areas of atrial tissue, which facilitate local macro reentry circuits. In patients who present to the OR in atrial fibrillation > 1 year duration, MV surgery is unlikely to remodel the LA enough to convert the patient back to normal sinus rhythm. The IOE exam in patients who have enlarged left atrium should document the LA dimensions in the 2-chamber imaging plane and ME LAX imaging planes. The finding of an enlarged left atrium (greater than 50 mm) indicates the potential for sustainable chronic atrial fibrillation (55,56). Patients who have undergone pulmonary vein isolation using percutaneous catheter ablation have demonstrated up to 23%–39% pulmonary vein stenosis within three days of their procedure. While this is not commonly reported with pulmonary vein isolation, documentation of pulmonary vein PW Doppler flows for future reference may prove useful.

*Pulmonary Hypertension* Persisting elevations of left atrial pressure may eventually result in proliferation of the intramural musculature of the pulmonary resistance vessels. Estimations of the PA systolic, mean, and diastolic pressures are possible using CW Doppler (Table 28.18) (33,56).

*RV Dysfunction* RV function is afterload-dependent, and the presence of persistently increased RV afterload leads to RV failure with tricuspid annulus dilatation, with resulting tricuspid regurgitation and passive congestion of the liver. RV failure causes dilation, ischemia, and decreased RV contractility. The 2-D IOE exam may demonstrate a septum that is flattened (D-shaped LV) and shifted toward the LV in systole with RV pressure overload, whereas, with RV volume overload associated with chronic TR, the septum is shifted in both systole and diastole.

*Tricuspid Valve Dysfunction (Table 28.19)* Chronically, patients with significant MS or MR have elevated LA pressures (up to 30 mm Hg). These pressures are associated with pulmonary systolic pressures of 60 or greater. Eighty-nine percent of patients undergoing tricuspid valve repair do so as a result of secondary pathophysiologic changes associated with primary MV disease and surgery (56). Up to 67% of patients undergoing MV surgery for rheumatic MS and/or MR are discovered to

▶ **TABLE 28.18.   Secondary Pathophysiology in MV Disease:
Estimation of Hemodynamic Pressures**

| Pressure Estimated | Required Measurement | Formula | Normal Values (mm Hg) |
|---|---|---|---|
| Estimated CVP | Respiratory IVC collapse | $\geq 40\% = 5$ mm Hg <br> $< 40\%$, (Nl RV) $= 10$ mm Hg <br> 0% and RV Dysfx $= 15$ mm Hg | 5 – 10 mm Hg |
| RV Systolic (RVSP) | Peak velocity$_{TR}$ <br> CVP or measured | $RVSP = 4(V_{TR})^2 + CVP$ <br> (No PS) | 16 – 30 mm Hg |
| RV Systolic (with VSD) | Systemic systolic BP <br> Peak V $_{LV-RV}$ | $RVSP = SBP - 4(V_{LV-RV})^2$ <br> *(No LVOT obstruction)* | with VSD usually > 50 |
| PA Systolic (PASP) | Peak velocity$_{TR}$ <br> CVP estimated or measured | $PASP = 4(V_{TR})^2 + CVP$ <br> (No PS; use estimated or measured CVP) | 16 – 30 mm Hg |
| PA Diastolic (PAD) | End Diastolic Velocity$_{PR}$ <br> CVP estimated or measured | $PAEDP = 4(V_{PR\ ED})^2 + CVP$ | 0 – 8 mm Hg |
| PA Mean (PAM) | Acceleration time (AT) to peak V$_{PA}$ | $PAM = (-0.45)\ AT + 79$ | 10 – 16 mm Hg |
| RV dP/dt | TR Spectral Envelope <br> T $_{TR(2m/sec)}$ – T $_{TR(1\ m/sec)}$ | $RV\ dP = 4V^2_{TR(2\ m/sec)} - 4V^2_{TR(2m/sec)}$ <br> $RV\ dP/dt = dP\ /\ T_{TR(2\ m/sec)} - T_{TR(1\ m/sec)}$ | > 150 mm Hg/ms |
| LA Systolic (LASP) | Peak V$_{MR}$ <br> Systolic BP (SBP) | $LASP = SBP - 4(V_{MR})^2$ <br> No LVOT gradient | 100–140 mm Hg |
| LA (PFO) | Velocity$_{PFO}$ <br> CVP estimated or measured | $LAP = 4(V_{PFO})^2 + CVP$ | 3–15 mm Hg |
| LV Diastolic (LVEDP) | End diastolic Velocity$_{AR}$ <br> Diastolic BP (DBP) | $LVEDP = DBP - 4(V_{AR})^2$ | 3–12 mm Hg |
| LV dP/dt | MR spectral envelope <br> T $_{MR(2\ m/sec)}$ – T $_{MR\ (1\ m/sec)}$ | $LV\ dP = 4V^2_{MR(2m/sec)} - 4V^2_{TR(2m/sec)}$ <br> $LV\ dP/dt = dP\ /\ T_{MR\ (2\ m/sec)} - T_{MR\ (1\ m/sec)}$ | > 800 mm Hg/ms |

have moderate or severe tricuspid regurgitation (75). In the presence of pulmonary hypertension with RV dilatation, the TV annulus dilates predominately at the bases of the anterior and posterior leaflets due to the basal septal leaflet incorporation into the central fibrous skeleton of the heart. Consequently, the regurgitant is frequently diffuse and directed septally and centrally. Klein et al. determined that tricuspid valve repair in MV surgery was associated with the most favorable outcome when both the mitral and tricuspid have greater than moderate TR (75). Other findings of severe TR are indicated by a TR jet area greater than 30% of the RA area or $\geq 6$ cm, dense CW spectral envelope of the TR jet, hepatic plethora, vena contracta > 0.7 cm, MJA, PISA > 0.6 cm to 0.9 cm with Nyquist at 28 cm/s, > 7 cm$^2$–10 cm$^2$, and hepatic vein systolic reversal (Table 28.19) (75). Duran et al. have also reported that tricuspid regurgitation that is moderate or severe should be repaired (140,150).

*Elevated RAP and PFO*   With elevated RAP, the fossa ovalis may become distended, revealing a patent foramen ovale. In the presence of severe pulmonary hypertension, a right-to-left shunt may occur leading to hypoxemia.

*Hepatic Congestion*   Patients with chronically elevated RA pressures or significant TR may develop chronic congestion of the liver. Hepatic plethora is diagnosed by having a lack of respiratory change in the diameter of the hepatic veins by M-mode echocardiography. PW Doppler may indicate severe TR by demonstrating systolic flow reversal or a systolic directional change as demonstrated by color flow Doppler.

### Associated Valvular or Coexisting Cardiac Pathology

*Associated Congenital Abnormalities*   Cleft MV leaflet abnormalities are commonly associated with specific congenital abnormalities. Endocardial cushion defects. Ostium primum ASD have been reported to be associated with cleft MV leaflets in 87% of cases (Fig. 28.75) and secundum ASD in 13%.

▶ **TABLE 28.19.**  **Intraoperative Assessment of TR Severity**

| Parameter 2-Dimensional Imaging | Utility/Advantages | Limitations | Mild | Moderate | Severe |
|---|---|---|---|---|---|
| **RA/RV/IVC size** *RA diameter < 4.6 cm* | RAE and RVE indicate chronic TR Normal RA and RV | RAE not specific RA normal in severe acute TR | Normal | Normal or dilated | Usually dilated |
| *RV diameter < 4.3 cm* Tricuspid valve | exclude signs of chronic TR Flail and poor coaptation with significant TR | Other findings not specific for significant TR | Normal | Normal or abnormal | Flail and Poor coaptation |
| **Doppler** | | | | | |
| **CF Doppler Max Jet Area (MJA) cm$^2$** *Nyquist limit 50–60 cm/ Not valid eccentric jets* | Efficient screen for TR | Note: tech factors and load conditions Underestimates eccentric jets | < 5 | 5–10 | > 10 |
| **PW Doppler Hepatic vein flow** | Simple | Blunting multiple causes | Systolic dominance | Systolic blunting | Systolic reversal |
| **CW Doppler Jet density—contour** | Simple Readily available | Qualitative Complementary data | Soft Parabolic | Dense Variable contour | Dense Triangular with early peaking |
| **Quantitative** | | | | | |
| **CF Dopppler Vena contracta diameter VCD (cm)** | Efficient Quantitative distinguishes mild from severe TR | Intermediates direct need of other parameters confirmation | Not defined | < 0.7 | > 0.7 |
| **PISA radius (cm)** *Baseline shift with Nyquist 28 cm/sec* | Quantitative | Validated in only a few studies | < 0.5 | 0.6 – 0.9 | > 0.9 |

In the assessment of patients undergoing MV surgery, the purpose of assessing the severity of tricuspid regurgitation is to determine the necessity of performing a TV repair. If the preoperative assessment of TR suggested the need for replacement, finding less TR should not be the determining factor in deciding to not proceed with TV repair.

*Rheumatic Valvular Heart Disease*  In patients presenting with rheumatic MV disease, 47% have some combination of rheumatic disease in other valves. Based on autopsy studies, the most frequent is aortic valve disease (32%), followed by mitral-aortic-tricuspid combination (9%), and mitral-tricuspid (4%) (135). Consequently, the aortic and tricuspid valves should be carefully interrogated for evidence of leaflet thickening and restricted aortic valve opening with commissural fusion when patients present for rheumatic MV surgery. If the degree of aortic stenosis is greater than mild to moderate, consideration is often given for replacement at the time of MV surgery because of the potential for progression to moderate or severe stenosis over a 15-year period (151). Patients with recurrent episodes of rheumatic fever may develop an active rheumatic myocarditis, leading to LV dysfunction and eccentric dilatation as demonstrated by 2-D IOE.

*Coexisting Myxomatous Disease*  Myxomatous MV disease is the etiology of MR in over 50% of cases (30). Similarly, myxomatous prolapse of the aortic valve is the most frequent cause of aortic regurgitation. While primary myxomatous degeneration of either of these valves is not associated with the other, prolapse of the mitral and aortic valves is seen in combination in patients with connective tissue disorders, such as Ehlers Danlos, Marfans, and osteogenesis imperfecta. In these patients, if the severity of the AR is greater than moderate, consideration is given to repair of the aortic valve unless there is architectural dilatation or distortion of the aortic root. Myxomatous tricuspid prolapse with TR has been reported in more than half of patients with MV prolapse. Because of the ability to reliably repair significant TR, TV repair is frequently performed in these patients.

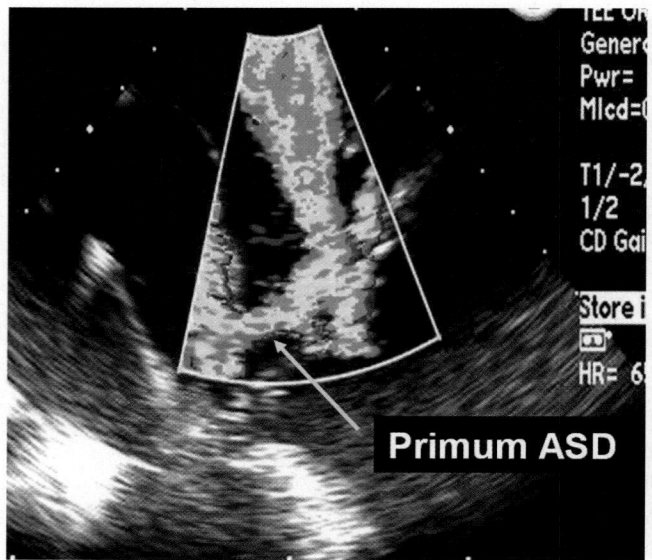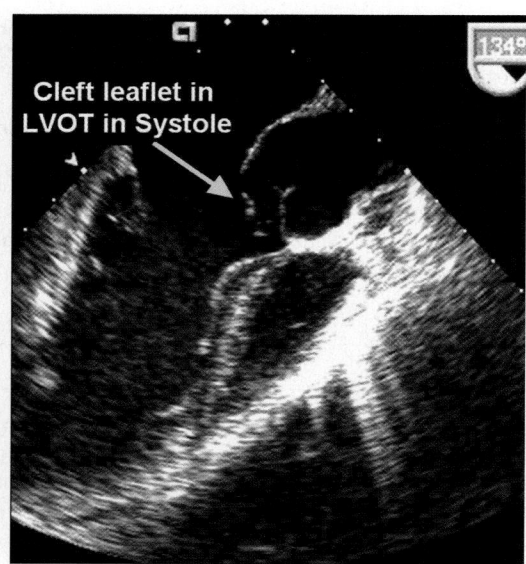

**FIGURE 28.75.** Cleft MV leaflet abnormalities are commonly associated with specific congenital abnormalities. Endocardial cushion defects (ostium primum ASD) has been reported to be associated with cleft MV leaflets in 87% of cases and secundum ASD in 13%.

*Coexisting Calcific Aortic Stenosis and MV Dysfunction* Calcific mitral and aortic valve disease are closely associated with aging. Calcific aortic stenosis is a frequent etiology of significant aortic stenosis in the elderly. Aronow et al. determined that calcific aortic stenosis may be present in 15% to 20% of elderly individuals over the age of 65 (25). In comparison, significant MR in the elderly is present in over 30% of the same population with MAC. In patients > 75 years old, more than one-quarter of patients with calcific aortic stenosis may have coexisting MAC with varying degrees of stenosis. While there is no close association between MAC, both are encountered in the same population.

### Aortic Stenosis or Regurgitation in Patient for MV Surgery

Coexistence of significant MR in the presence of AS or AR more frequently occurs in patients presenting for aortic valve surgery (see discussion below regarding moderate MR in patients with aortic valve stenosis). However, when significant AS or AR is found in the patient presenting for MV repair it may be with an incorrect assumption that the MR is secondary to coexisting ischemic heart disease. If there is greater than moderate aortic stenosis and dilatation of the LV, the replacement of the aortic valve is often considered in addition to MV repair. If, however, there is hypertrophy of the ventricle associated with the aortic valve disease, aortic valve replacement alone may correct the MR. If there is significant AR with ventricular dilatation, consideration is given to surgically correcting the aortic valve in addition to the MVRep. With the dilata-

tion, it is probable that the MR is secondary to apical tethering of the MV leaflets with an associated central jet of MR.

### Endocarditis of the Mitral and Aortic Valves

As previously discussed with MV endocarditis, it is unusual to have primary MV endocarditis with underlying MV disease or aortic valve endocarditis. Endocarditis involving multiple valves has been reported in more than 15% of cases, usually involving the aortic and mitral valves (135).

## MITRAL VALVE PROCEDURES

### Introduction

When surgical intervention is indicated for the optimal long-term management of a patient's MV dysfunction, valve repair is always the procedure of choice (36, 77,92,160,162). This is founded upon scientific evidence that, in comparison to MVR, MVRep offers lower operative mortality, improved long-term ventricular function, and greater freedom from thromboembolism, anticoagulant complications, endocarditis, and reoperation (77,92,160,162). While the repair of the MVAp is influenced by the underlying valve pathology and mechanism(s) of dysfunction, the precise application of repair techniques and the intraoperative assessment of the result of the surgical repair is guided by intraoperative echo. For patients undergoing MV surgery, there are issues related to the specific surgical intervention, which are addressed by the intraoperative examination. Those related to MVRep and MVR have been previously discussed.

## Mitral Valve Repair (MVRep)

### Historical Perspective

Though MVRep was first suggested in 1902 by Sir Thomas Brunton for patients with rheumatic MS (155), it was not until the early 1920s when Allen, Cutler, and Souttar, working independently, first developed such techniques. Due to the nonexistence of antimicrobials and methods for dealing with blood loss, further progress was limited (155,156). The surgical treatment of MR was limited to a diversion of the regurgitant jet until the idea of circumferentially reshaping the mitral annulus was advanced by Glover and Davila in 1938. However, it was not until the Gibbons introduction of the heart-lung machine in 1953 that Lillehei first attempted the correction of pure MR by reconstruction of the annulus in 1957 (158). Further clinical development of this radical concept, however, was postponed by the enthusiasm surrounding the introduction of the mechanical valve by Starr and Edwards in 1961. It was not until 1971 that Carpentier et al. presented their revolutionary new concept of a physiologic classification of mechanisms of MR and resulting clinical success (129). Duran advanced the development of repair techniques for the patients with combined stenotic and regurgitant rheumatic MV disease (159). These developments revolutionized the world of cardiac surgery and the era of modern valve repair began. Surgeons in the United States envisioned potential benefits for older patient populations with degenerative and ischemic regurgitation (159). Over the ensuing 20 years, a number of contributions have been made by various surgeons and cardiac centers and have established MVRep as the procedure of choice for the management of all etiologies of MR.

## MV Repair Compared to MV Replacement (Outcomes)

In 1987, Sand, Naftel, Blackstone, et al. first reported their remarkable results comparing MVRep with MVR (161). When they examined the outcome of 490 patients undergoing MVRep (101) and MVR (389) for MR, the 5-year survival was superior for MVRep (76% vs. 56%, p = 0.005) and superior for protection from endocarditis (0/101 vs. 11/389, p = 0.08). Because of this, a radical shift has occurred in the management of patients with MV dysfunction caused by all etiologies (77).

### MV Repair for Rheumatic Disease

The number of patients presenting for cardiac surgery with pure rheumatic MS has declined due to a decreased incidence of the disease and the number of patients receiving balloon valvuloplasty for its treatment (162,163). Rheumatic MV disease may produce a range of anatomic presentations, including MV prolapse associated with acute rheumatic valvulitis (rarely seen in United States) to the more chronic presentations of mixed MR and stenosis caused by the subvalvular thickening and fusion of the chordae, commissural fusion, and a fixed "fish-mouth" deformity with the Type IIIa systolic and diastolic restriction. Current indications for surgical intervention in patients with MS and/or MR include onset of congestive symptoms and new onset atrial fibrillation. If patients have atrial fibrillation, they are frequently referred for surgery irrespective of their echocardiographic splitability score. Patients with rheumatic MV disease usually present with restricted leaflet motion, causing either pure MS or a combination of both. Patients with pure MS with high splitability scores (> 8) or those with atrial fibrillation or those with mixed MS and MR are referred for surgery. David et al. have demonstrated that even if patients have higher splitability scores (> 8), repair may be possible if their anterior leaflets are pliable with a subvalvular structure that is not fused (141). In 2001, Carpenter et al. published their 20-year results of MV repair in degenerative MR (31). Between 1970 and 1994, they performed 951 reconstructive procedures (7% type I, 33% type II prolapse, 36% type III, and 24% combined type II AMVL and type III PMVL). Overall, they demonstrated a 10- and 20-year freedom of death (89% and 82%), freedom from reoperation (82% and 55%), and freedom from cardiac morbidity. Freedom from reoperation at 20 years was highest in type IIa/IIIp (65%), followed by type II (63%), and type III (46%). The main cause of reoperation was progression of MV fibrosis (31).

### MV Repair for Endocarditis

Endocarditis involving the left-sided valve structures usually involves the aortic valve. If endocarditis involves the MV, it implies coexistence of degenerative or rheumatic valve disease or it is secondary to a jet lesion from a posteriorly directed regurgitant jet associated with aortic valve endocarditis. In MV endocarditis the associated mechanism of regurgitation may be multiple mechanisms and includes the underlying valve abnormality, such as combined rheumatic MS-MR valve dysfunction or previously existing myxomatous degeneration of the MV. Endocarditis involving the MV produces a range of MV apparatus pathology, including isolated leaflet perforations (Type I) or secondary windsock defect from AR jet, vegetations attached to leaflets, ruptured chordae, and abscess cavities with erosion into the central intervalvular fibrosa (135). Repair of the MV in endocarditis involves patching of perforations, wide debridement and pericardial exclusion, and more aggressive reconstructive surgery where there is combined involvement of the aortic valve and intervalvular fibrosa. Muehrke et al. have reported an 80% success rate in repair of infected mitral valves (136).

### MV Repair for Ischemic Heart Disease

Ischemic MR is classified as either transient or chronic. The chronic form involves an infarction and may result in a ruptured papillary muscle (type II), elongation of the papillary muscle head with leaflet prolapse (type II), or functional regurgitation associated with ventricular remodeling and apical tethering (type IIIb with or without type I annular dilatation) or a posterior and/or lateral infarct impacting the mitral apparatus in that region (IIIb). While all three are approachable by reconstructive technique, the decision to proceed with repair or replacement is patient dependent. Due to the potential catastrophic nature of the effects of an acute failure of a reattached papillary muscle head, MV replacement is usually performed. Papillary muscle infarction, which results in chordal elongation, causes a focal prolapse of a segment of the AMVL or PMVL scallop. Often these patients are referred for surgical management of coexisting myxomatous and coronary disease. Recently, Reece et al. compared 110 CABG patients, with type IIIb with or without type I annular dilatation, who either had MV repair (54 undersized annuloplasty ring with or without a posterior patch) or MV replacement (subvalvular sparring technique) (143). Comparing the MV repair with the MV replacement group they demonstrated a superior in-hospital mortality (1.9% vs. 10.7%), shorter length of stay (9.7 days vs. 13.1 days), lower infection rate (9% vs. 13%), shorter CPB times (112 min vs. 132 min), and shorter cross-clamp times (152 min vs. 171 min) (140). They concluded that MV repair was superior to MV replacement with regard to perioperative mortality and morbidity. In 2001, Gillinov et al. reported on 482 patients with ischemic MR who underwent either MV repair or replacement and were propensity matched into a better-risk and poor-risk group (36). They found that MV repair compared to MV replacement in the better-risk group demonstrated superior survivals at 30 days, 1 year, and 5 years (94% vs. 81%, 82% vs. 56%, 58% vs. 36%; p = .08) (36). There was no significant difference in the poor-risk group. Ischemic MR patients with papillary muscle rupture have a better long-term survival compared with those patients with chronic failure and apical tethering (36).

### MV Repair for Myxomatous MV Disease

Myxomatous degeneration is the most common indication for MVRep, with 90% of such valves being repairable. In the general population, 4% to 5% of individuals may have mitral valve prolapse potentially leading to surgical intervention in up to 5% (164). The surgical approaches that have been developed are directed at the underlying pathology of redundant myxomatous leaflets, thinned and elongated chordae—which are prone to rupture—and annular dilatation. Patients with significant MR secondary to structural abnormalities of the apparatus eventually require surgical intervention. If untreated, the natural history indicates that patients will develop progressive heart failure and many will develop atrial fibrillation. Valve repair for myxomatous is accomplished in the majority of patients, using five surgical techniques, including a central or modified quadrilateral resection of the PMVL, chordal transfer, annuloplasty, commissural closure, and a sliding annuloplasty. Other surgical techniques include addition of gortex chords, chordal shortening, anterior leaf resection (Pomeroy procedure), and anterior leaflet plication.

Gillinov et al. reported on the long-term durability of MV repair at the Cleveland Clinic in 1,072 patients who underwent primary isolated MVRep for valvular regurgitation caused by degenerative disease between 1985 and 1997. In this study 1-, 5-, and 10-year freedom from reoperation were reported as 98.7%, 96.9%, and 92.9%, respectively. Freedom from reoperation was highest in those patients with PMVL prolapse or flail (98%, type II), and those who received an intraoperative assessment by transesophageal or epicardial echocardiography and annuloplasty with leaflet resection (77). Using multivariant analysis, they found that the risks of reoperation were decreased by use of IOE and use of an annuloplasty ring, and were increased by use of chordal shortening and non-PMVL pathology. Of the 30 patients with late MV dysfunction, the repair failed in 16 (53%) as a result of progressive degenerative disease. Death before reoperation was increased in patients having isolated anterior leaflet prolapse, annular calcification, and by use of chordal shortening or annuloplasty alone.

Carpentier and Deloche reported their long-term, 20-year results in the first 162 consecutive patients who underwent nonrheumatic MV repair for degenerative MV regurgitation between 1970 and 1984 (31). The Carpentier mechanism was type II in 152 (PMVL 93, AMVL 28, bileaflet in 31). There were three postoperative deaths and three reoperations in the first month. The remaining patients with MV repair were followed for a median of 17 years. The survival was 48% for 20 years, which is similar to a normal population. The cardiac death and cardiac morbidity were 19% and 26%, respectively. For patients with PMVL involvement, the 10- and 20-year freedom from reoperation was 98.5% and 93%, whereas AMVL was 86.2% and bileaflet involvement was 88.1% and 82.6% (31).

## Clinical Guidelines for MV Repair

In 1996, Ling et al. reported a study that evaluated the optimal timing of surgical intervention for 221 patients with severe MR caused by a myxomatous Carpentier type II flail or prolapse mechanism (28). These patients were separated into two groups that were designated as Group 1 (early surgery < 1 month) and Group 2 (those patients who had surgery after 1 month or not at all). Both groups had similar comorbidities and no significant incidence of coronary disease by angiography in small subsets of either group. It was found that those patients who had earlier surgery (within 1 month of being diagnosed with clinically significant MR) had improved survival at 5 and 10 years ($p = 0.28$). In addition, the early surgery patients demonstrated decreased operative mortality ($p = 0.17$), a decreased likelihood of progressive congestive heart failure, and better long-term survival with diminished cardiovascular mortality ($p = .002$). The authors concluded by suggesting a strategy of earlier surgery in acceptable candidates, with severe MR, with a high probability of successful MV repair (28).

Because of this and similar studies, in 1998 the American College of Cardiology and American Heart Association Task Force on Guidelines in Valvular Heart Disease recommended the following as indications for MVRep surgery in patients with MR:

1. ≥ Functional Class II symptoms and severe MR
2. Asymptomatic patients with severe MR and LV dysfunction (LVESD > 45 mm) and MS
3. > Functional Class III with MVA < 1.5 cm$^2$
4. With an echocardiography score < 8, balloon valvuloplasty optional (33)

## Moderate MR in Patients for Aortic Valve Surgery

When patients are discovered to have coexisting functional MR in the presence of significant aortic valve dysfunction, it is usually in the setting of primary aortic valve surgery Christenson et al. evaluated 60 consecutive patients with aortic stenosis and MR to determine the effect of aortic valve replacement on the severity of MR. They found that unless there was irreversible eccentric remodeling, the repair or correction of the aortic valve dysfunction resulted in an improvement of the severity of MR (153). Conversely, if there is moderate MR and spherical remodeling, they found that it was unlikely that the MR would be diminished. Gillinov et al. reported a study evaluating 813 patients undergoing AVR in addition to either MVRep (295) or MVR (518) from 1975 to 1998. MVR was more common in patients with severe MS ($p = 0.0009$), atrial fibrillation ($p = 0.0006$), and in patients receiving a mechanical aortic prosthesis ($p = 0.0002$). Hospital mor-

tality rate for MVR was 5.4% ($p = 0.4$). Survivals at 5, 10, and 15 years were 79%, 63%, and 46%, after MVRep compared to 72%, 52%, and 34%, after replacement ($p = 0.01$). Late survival was increased by MVRep rather than replacement ($p = 0.03$) in all subsets of patients, including those with severe MS. In many patients with double valve disease, aortic valve replacement and MVRep may improve late survival rates and is the preferred strategy when MVRep is possible (154).

## Mitral Valve Replacement (MVR)

In MV replacement, the post-CPB echocardiographic evaluation focuses on the integrity of the valve, presence of perivalvular regurgitation, underlying LV function, and potential for valve strut interference with LVOT blood flow. Because of the left-sided systolic pressures, small spaces between the valvular sewing ring and mitral annulus may result in small, but high velocity, perivalvular regurgitation. Such high velocity has a propensity to cause hemolysis and requires further evaluation or repair of the sewing ring leak. It is imperative that regurgitant jets associated with valve replacement be localized as either originating from within the sewing ring or as perivalvular. Localization and quantification of the regurgitant jet associated with prosthetic valves is one of the most difficult challenges in IOE due to the artifacts associated with an echo-dense valve ring or mechanical leaflets. Use of multiple imaging views and/or epicardial imaging is often necessary to achieve a confident conclusion. Helpful clues in this dilemma include the almost universal presence of small regurgitant jets with bioprosthetic valves and the characteristic regurgitant patterns of the various mechanical valves. In addition, the application of gentle manual pressure posteriorly on the sewing ring, may obliterate some perivalvular leaks, confirming the diagnosis. In patients receiving a bileaflet (St. Jude, Carbomedics) or a tilting disc, it is important to visualize an appropriate range of motion of the individual leaflets or disc.

In nonchordal sparring, MVR is associated with reduced ventricular function due to disruption of the mitral tensor apparatus. This is especially prevalent in those circumstances when the surgeon was not able to maintain the continuity of the mitral tensor apparatus. In addition, the propensity for disruption of the posterior LV or annulus is increased in such circumstances. Such disruption is preceded by identifiable intramyocardial areas of turbulence permitting the echocardiographer to alert the surgeon prior to a catastrophic myocardial rupture.

With the implantation of higher profile valves in the mitral position, the valve struts may protrude into the LVOT if not appropriately aligned. While some prosthetic valve models permit an in situ rotation of the valve, significant obstruction to LVOT flow may require reimplantation of the prosthetic valve.

## Mitral Valve Homograft

Acar et al. reported on the use of MV homografts for patients who had MV dysfunction that was too extensive for successful repair (166). Forty-three patients underwent MVR with a cryopreserved mitral homograft in patients with acute endocarditis (14), rheumatic stenosis (26), systemic lupus endocarditis (2), and marasmic endocarditis (1). Partial homograft was performed in 21 and total in 22. Follow-up at 14 months demonstrated 1 reoperation for restenosis and 1 death (pulmonary neoplasm). Thirty-three patients were in sinus rhythm, no to minimal MR in 33, and mild MR in 5 with an average MVA of 2.4 cm$^2$. Since the initial experience this procedure has been performed in selected institutions (166,167).

### Pre-CPB IOE Exam

The IOE exam has unique requirements for confirming that the mechanism of dysfunction is irreparable. The homograft was matched to measurements provided by the pre-CPB or pre-OR TEE. Using the ME 4 Chr imaging plane, the diastolic "height" was measured from the hinge point to the distal edge. In systole, the anteroposterior diameter of the annulus was measured, as well as the distance between the annular planes in the image to the tip of the anterolateral papillary muscle. These measured parameters (plus 3 mm) were matched with harvested mitral homographs.

### Post-CPB IOE Exam

The post-CPB assessment of the homograft includes a determination of the presence of MR, MV area by planimetry, and the transvalvular gradient. MR was minimal in 15

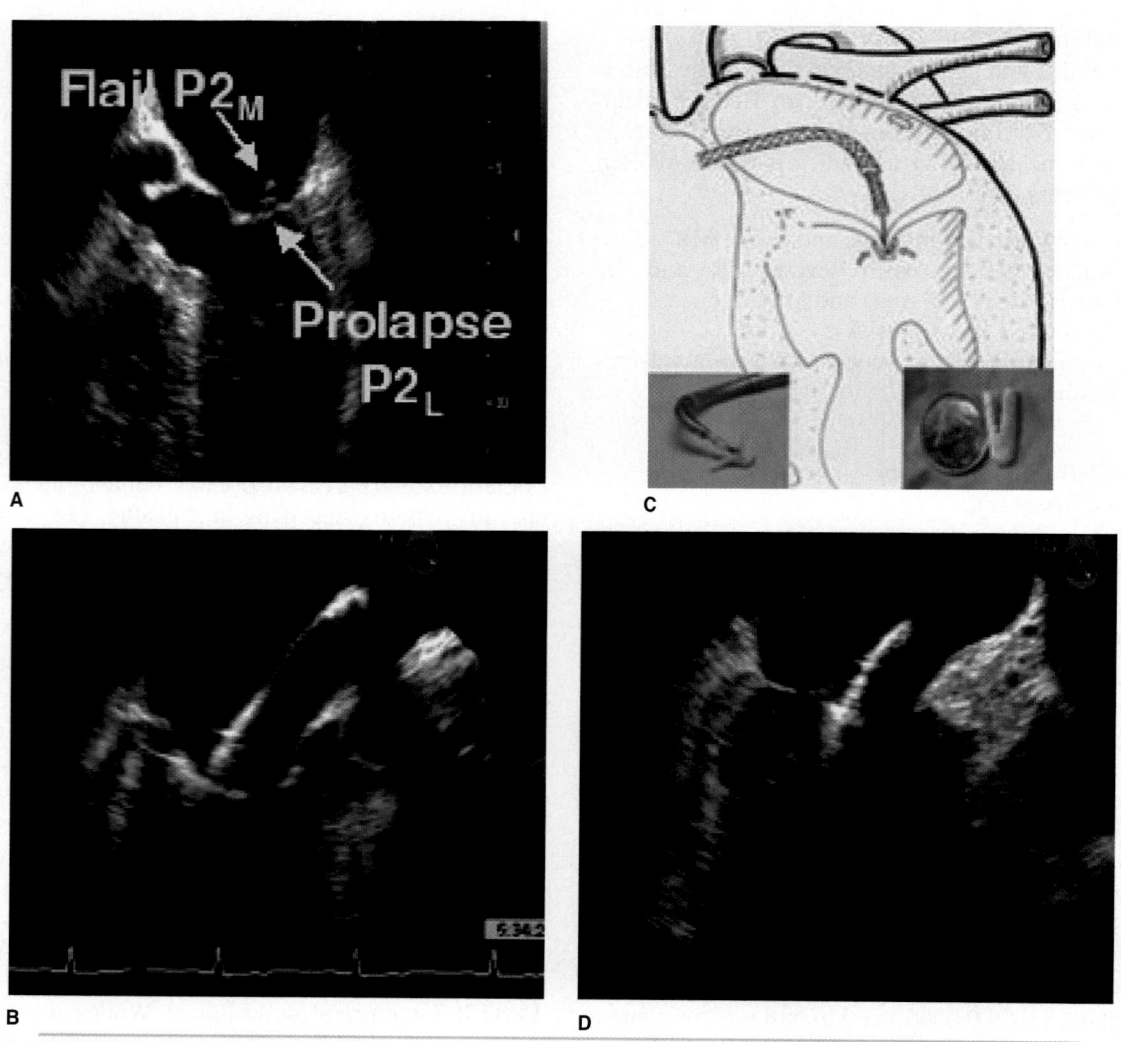

**FIGURE 28.76 A,B,C, and D.** Percutaneous mitral valve repair utilizing an "Alferi" clip of a segmental flail P2 (medial half). Device was positioned and deployed under TEE and fluoro guidance (168).

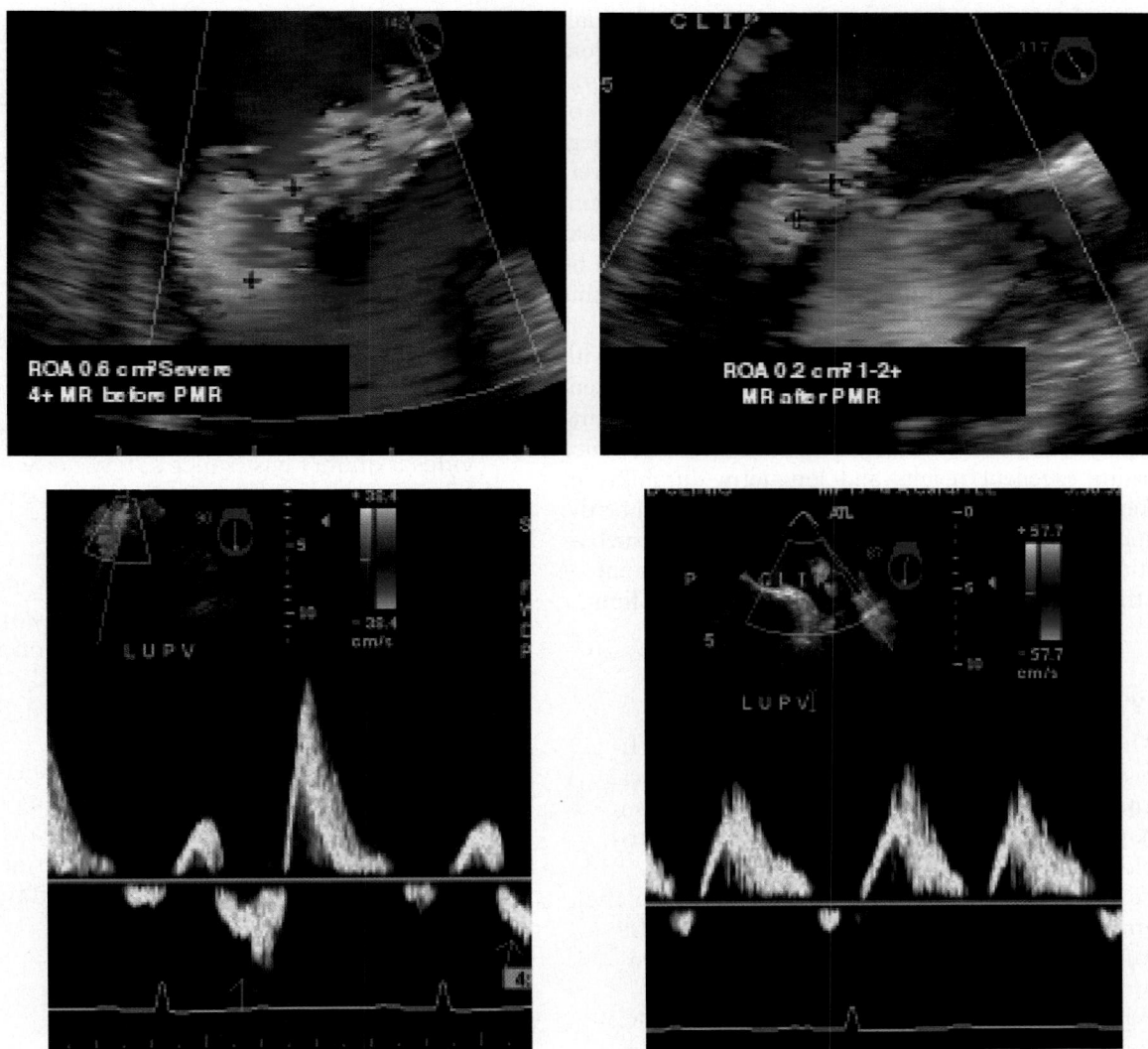

**FIGURE 28.77 A,B,C, and D.** Severity of MR was reduced from a ROA of 0.6 cm² (severe) to 0.2 cm² (mild). Pulmonary vein systolic reversal reverted to normal S:D.

patients and mild in 6. The mean transvalvular gradient was 3 ± 2 mm Hg and the valve area measured 2.5 cm² by planimetry (166).

## FUTURE OF MV SURGERY AND IOE

Some of the most exciting developments in MV surgery are the evolving percutaneous approaches to myxomatous as well as ischemic MR and the rapid progress being made toward real-time 3-D imaging with CF Doppler. Just as intraoperative echo has enabled new approaches to MV disease, such as advanced MVRep to more safely and rapidly evolve into their full potential; innovations will continue to challenge the intraoperative echocardiographer using ultra-

sound technology. Today, patients with segmental flail myxomatous mitral valves are undergoing percutaneous placement of edge-to-edge Alferi clipping devices (Figs. 28.76 and 28.77). Initial experiences at the Cleveland Clinic have demonstrated an immediate reduction of severe MR to trivial-to-mild MR with simultaneous reductions in elevated pulmonary artery pressures. However, in pushing the frontier, difficulties are encountered. Intraoperative echocardiography enables the surgical intervention team to correct these issues before an adverse effect occurs, thereby ensuring not only the safety of the patient but the ability to realize the full potential of innovative medical approaches to cardiovascular disease.

Three-dimensional imaging with CF Doppler echo is reconstructed within 90 seconds of obtaining 30-second period of data acquisition, permitting the "virtual" visualization in intricate detail of MVAp anatomy and function. The digital viewing capability enables the echocardiographer to guide the cardiac surgeon to the exact site(s) of dysfunction using 3-D identification of prolapsing segments with CF Doppler identification of flow convergence. Three-dimensional IOE will enable us to better understand the mechanisms of unsuccessful repair so that patients with remote chances of successful repair will be more likely to benefit from the many advantages of this procedure.

As our population continues to age, patients with milder forms of myxomatous degeneration will present with complex mechanisms of MV dysfunction, involving multiple etiologies. If we are to continue to experience the same excellent results and long-term durability of MVRep in these more complicated patients, it will be the advanced diagnostic capabilities that innovations such as real-time three-dimensional IOE bring to the point of care that will enable us to push the envelope to its limit.

### KEY POINTS

- The mitral valve apparatus consists of the fibrous cardiac skeleton, saddle-shaped mitral annulus, mitral valve (MV) leaflets, chordae, papillary muscles, and ventricular wall complex.
- Pathologic processes may structurally alter the anatomic integrity of the components of the mitral valve apparatus (MVAp), resulting in mitral valve dysfunction.
- While the intraoperative echocardiographic exam confirms the presence of MV dysfunction and its (intraoperative) severity, its most significant role is refining the understanding of the structure and mechanism(s) of MV dysfunction.
- Mitral valve repair is the treatment of choice for mitral valve (MV) dysfunction resulting from all etiologies.
- In MV surgery, the most significant surgical issues that the IOE exam resolves are the repairability of the MV apparatus, the necessity to perform other surgical interventions, and the postcardiopulmonary bypass (post-CPB) assessment of the surgical procedure and complications.
- In addition to the expertise and experience of the surgical team, the probability of mitral valve repair is dictated by etiology apparatus and mechanism of dysfunction. These are determined by the intraoperative echocardiographic exam in conjunction with the sur-

geon's direct inspection of the mitral valve apparatus.
- The intraoperative echocardiography exam may be organized by priority to insure that critical issues are addressed should the patient require the initiation of cardiopulmonary bypass.
- The precardiopulmonary bypass also determines the secondary or associated pathophysiology, cannulation-perfusion strategy, the potential for post-CPB complications, and provides an ongoing assessment of cardiac function.
- The postcardiopulmonary bypass exam provides a quality assurance safety net with the assessment of the surgical procedure and diagnosis of complications.
- Consistent with the recommendations of the ASE Standards Committee and Task Force on Native Valve Regurgitation, the intraoperative exam relies on a weighted-integration method of severity assessment for all valve dysfunction. This may be efficiently performed in a multitasking environment.
- Color flow Doppler (maximal jet area) is a useful screening method for determining the presence of ≥ severe or ≤ trivial mitral valve regurgitation. More quantitative methods are recommended in addition to color flow Doppler (maximal jet area).

### REFERENCES

1. Johnson ML, Holmes JH, Spangler RD, et al. Usefulness of echocardiography in patients undergoing MV surgery. J Thorac Cardiovasc Surg 1972;64:922–28.
2. Frazin L, Talano JV, Stephanides L. Esophageal echocardiography. Circulation 1975;54:102–04.
3. Hisanga K, Hisanaga A, Nagata K, et al. A new transesophageal real-time two-dimensional echocardiographic system using a flexible tube and its clinical application. Proc Jpn Soc Ultrason Med 1977;32:43–5.
4. Hanrath P, Kremer P, Langenstein BA. Transosophageal echokardiographie: ein neues verfahren zur dynamischen ventrikelfunktionsanalyse. Dtsch Med Wochenschr 1981;106:533.
5. Kremer P, Roizen MT, Gutman J, et al. Cardiac monitoring by transesophageal 2-D echocardiography during abdominal aortic aneurysmectomy. Circulation 1982;66:II-179(abst).
6. Goldman ME, Mindich BP, Teichholz LE, et al. Intraoperative contrast echocardiography to evaluate MV operations. J Am Coll Cardiol 1984;4:1035–40.
7. Takamoto S, Kyo S, Adachi H, et al. Intraoperative color flow mapping by real-time two-dimensional Doppler echocardiography for evaluation of valvular and congenital heart disease and vascular disease. J Thorac Cardiovasc Surg 1985;90:802–12.
8. Stewart WJ, Salcedo EE, Schiavone WA, et al. Intraoperative Doppler color flow mapping in valve conservation

surgery. Proc Tenth World Congress Cardiology 1986:247 (abst).

9. Stewart WJ, Currie PJ, Agler DA, et al. Intraoperative epicardial echocardiography: technique, imaging planes, and use in valve repair for mitral regurgitation. Dynamic Cardiovasc Imaging 1987;1:179–84.

10. Kyo S, Takamoto S, Matsumura M, et al. Immediate and early postoperative evaluation of results of cardiac surgery by transesophageal two-dimensional Doppler echocardiography. Circulation 1987;76:113–21.

11. Rankin JS, Livesey SA, Smith LR, et al. Trends in the surgical treatment of ischemic mitral regurgitation: effects of mitral valve repair on hospital mortality. Semin Thorac Cardiovasc Surg 1989;1:149–63.

12. Mishra M, Chauhan R, Sharma KK, et al. Real-time intraoperative transesophageal echocardiography——how useful? Experience of 5,016 cases. J Cardiothorac Vasc Anesth 1998;12:625–32.

13. Sutton DC, Kluger R. Intraoperative transesophageal echocardiography: impact on adult cardiac surgery. Anesth Intensive Care 1998;26:287–93.

14. Stewart WJ, Currie PJ, Salcedo EE, et al. Intraoperative Doppler color flow mapping for decision-making in valve repair for mitral regurgitation. Technique and results in 100 patients. Circulation 1990;81:556–66.

15. Kawano H, Mizoguchi T, Aoyagi S. Intraoperative transesophageal echocardiography for evaluation of mitral valve repair. J Heart Valve Dis 1999;8(3):287–93.

16. Abraham TP, Warner JG, Kon ND, et al. Feasibility, accuracy, and incremental value of intraoperative three-dimensional echocardiography in valve surgery. Am J Cardiol 1997;80(12):1577–82.

17. Aklog L, Filsoufi F, Flores KQ, et al. Does coronary artery bypass grafting alone correct moderate ischemic mitral regurgitation? Circulation 2001;104[12 Suppl 1]:I68–75.

18. Savage RM, Lytle BW, Aronson S, et al. Intraoperative echocardiography is indicated in high-risk coronary artery bypass grafting. Ann Thorac Surg 1997;64:368–73.

19. Cohn LH, Rizzo RJ, Adams DH, et al. The effect of pathophysiology on the surgical treatment of ischemic mitral regurgitation: operative and late risks of repair versus replacement. Eur J Cardiothorac Surg 1995;9:568–74.

20. Cheitlin MD, Armstrong WF, Aurigemma GP, et al. ACC/AHA/ASE 2003 guideline update for the clinical application of echocardiography—summary article: a report of the American College of Cardiology/American Heart Association Task Force on Practice guidelines (ACC/AHA/ASE Committee to Update the 1997 Guidelines for the Clinical Application of Echocardiography). J Am Coll Cardiol 2003; 42(5):954–70.

21. Bonow RO, Smith SC Jr. Cardiovascular manpower: the looming crisis. Circulation 2004;109(7):817–20.

22. National Center for Health Statistics, Owings MF, Lawrence L. Detailed diagnosis and procedures: National Hospital Discharge Survey, 1997. Vital and health statistics. Series 13. No. 145. Washington, D.C.: Government Printing Office, December 1999.

23. 2003 United States Census Bureau Statistics.

24. Singh JP, Evans JC, Levy D, et al. Prevalence and clinical determinants of mitral, tricuspid, and aortic regurgitation (the Framingham Study). Am J Cardiol 1999;83:897–902.

25. Aronow WS, Ahn C, Kronzon I. Echocardiographic abnormalities in African-American, Hispanic, and white men and women aged > 60 years. Am J Cardiol 2001;87(9):1131–33.

26. Horstkotte D. Pathomorphological aspects, etiology and natural history of acquired mitral valve stenosis. Eur Heart J 1991;12[Suppl B]:55–60.

27. Supino PG, Borer JS, Yin A. The epidemiology of valvular heart disease: an emerging public health problem. Adv Cardiol 2002;39:1–6.

28. Ling LH, Sarano ME, Seward JB, et al. Clinical outcome of mitral regurgitation due to flail leaflet. N Engl J Med 1996;335:1417–23.

29. Enriquez-Sarano M, Basmadjian AJ, Rossi A, et al. Progression of mitral regurgitation: a prospective Doppler echocardiographic study. J Am Coll Cardiol 1999;34(4):1137–44.

30. Gillinov AM, Cosgrove DM. Mitral valve repair for degenerative disease. J Heart Valve Dis 2002;11[Suppl 1]:S15–S20.

31. Braunberger E, Deloche A, Berrebi A, et al. Very long-term results (more than 20 years) of valve repair with Carpentier's techniques in nonrheumatic mitral valve insufficiency. Circulation 2001;104[Suppl I]:I-8–I-11.

32. Enriquez-Sarano M. Timing of mitral valve surgery. Heart 2002;87(1):79–85.

33. Bonow RO, Carabello B, de Leon AC, et al. ACC/AHA guidelines for the management of patients with valvular heart disease. Executive Summary. A report of the American College of Cardiology/American Heart Association Task Force on Practice Guidelines (Committee on Management of Patients with Valvular Heart Disease). Circulation 1998;98:1949–84.

34. The Society of Thoracic Surgeons National Cardiac Surgery Database: Executive Summary 2003. December 2003. Chicago: The Society of Thoracic Surgeons.

35. Zoghbi WA, Enriquez-Sarano M, Foster E, et al. Recommendations for evaluation of the severity of native valvular regurgitation with two-dimensional and Doppler echocardiography. J Am Soc Echocardiogr 2003;16(7):777–802.

36. Gillinov AM, Cosgrove DM, Lytle BW, et al. Surgery for acquired heart disease: reoperation for failure of mitral valve repair. J Thorac Cardiovasc Surg 1997;113:467–75.

37. Enriquez-Sarano M, Nkomo V, Mohty D, et al. Mitral regurgitation: predictors of outcome and natural history. Adv Cardiol 2002;39:133–43.

38. Chaliki HP, Click RL, Abel MD. Comparison of intraoperative transesophageal echocardiographic examinations with the operative findings: prospective review of 1918 cases. J Am Soc Echocardiogr 1999;12:237–40.

39. Sheikh KH, de Bruijn NP, Rankin JS, et al. The utility of transesophageal echocardiography and Doppler color flow imaging in patients undergoing cardiac valve surgery. J Am Coll Cardiol 1990;15:363–72.

40. Shah PM, Raney AA, Duran CM, et al. Multiplane transesophageal echocardiography: a roadmap for mitral valve repair. J Heart Valve Dis 1999;8:625–29.

41. Perloff JK, Roberts WC. The mitral apparatus: functional anatomy of mitral regurgitation. Circulation 1972;46:227.

42. Becker AE, de Wit APM. The mitral valve apparatus: a spectrum of normality relevant to mitral valve prolapse. Br Heart J 1980;42:680–89.

43. DePlessis LA, Marchand P. The anatomy of the mitral valve and its associated structures. Thorax 1964;19:221–27.

44. Rusted IE, Schiefley CH, Edwards JE. Studies of the mitral valve. I. Anatomic features of the normal mitral valve and associated structures. Circulation 1952;6:825–31.

45. Brock RC. The surgical and pathological anatomy of the mitral valve. Br Heart J 1952;14:489–513.

46. Zimmerman J, Bailey CP. The surgical significance of the fibrous skeleton of the heart. J Thorac Cardiovasc Surg 1962;44:701–12.

47. Kunzelman KS, Reimink MS, Cochran RP. Annular dilation increases stress in the mitral valve and delays coaptation: a finite element computer model. Cardiovasc Surg 1997;5(4):427–34.

48. Flashskampf FA, Chandra S, Gaddipatti A, et al. Analysis of shape and motion of the mitral annulus in subjects with and without cardiomyopathy by echocardiographic 3-dimensional reconstruction. J Am Soc Echocardiogr 2000;13(4):277–87.

49. Lam JHC, Ranganathan N, Wigle ED, et al. Morphology of the human mitral valve. I. Chordae tendineae: a new classification. Circulation 1970;41:449–58.

50. Stümper O, Fraser AG, Ho SY, et al. Transesophageal echocardiography in the longitudinal axis: correlation between anatomy and images and its clinical implications. Br Heart J 1990;64:282–88.

51. Voci P, Bilotta F, Caretta Q, et al. Papillary muscle perfusion pattern: a hypothesis for ischemic papillary muscle dysfunction. Circulation 1995;91:1714–18.
52. Shanewise JS, Cheung AT, Aronson S, et al. ASE/SCA guidelines for performing a comprehensive intraoperative multiplane transesophageal echocardiography examination: recommendations of the American Society of Echocardiography Council for Intraoperative Echocardiography and the Society of Cardiovascular Anesthesiologists Task Force for Certification in Perioperative Transesophageal Echocardiography. J Am Soc Echocardiogr 1999;12(10): 884–900.
53. Kumar N, Kumar M, Duran CMG. A revised terminology for recording surgical findings of the mitral valve. J Heart Valve Dis 1995;4:70–5.
54. Stewart WJ. Intraoperative echocardiography. In: Topol E, ed. Textbook of cardiovascular medicine. Baltimore: Lippincott, 2003.
55. Otto C. Valvular stenosis: diagnosis, quantitation, and clinical approach. In: Otto C, ed. Textbook of clinical echocardiography, 2nd ed. Philadelphia: WB Saunders, 2000: 229–64.
55b. Echocardiographic measurements and normal values. In: Feigenbaum H, ed. Echocardiography. Philadelphia: Lea & Febiger, 1994:658–83.
55c. Hemodynamic assessment. In: Oh J, Seward JB, Tajik AJ, eds. The Echo Manual. Philadelphia: Lippincott-Raven, 59–72.
56. Carabello BA. Timing of surgery for mitral and aortic stenosis. Cardiol Clin 1991;9:229–38.
56b. Valvular heart disease. In: Oh J, Seward JB, Tajik AJ, eds. The Echo Manual. Philadelphia: Lippincott-Raven, 103–32.
57. Thomas JD. Doppler echocardiographic assessment of valvar regurgitation. Heart (British Cardiac Society) 2002;88 (6):651–57.
58. Grayburn P, Fehske W, Omran H, et al. Multiplane transesophageal echocardiographic assessment of mitral regurgitation by Doppler color flow mapping of the vena contracta. Am J Cardiol 1994;74:912–17.
59. Hall SA, Brickner ME, Willett DL, et al. Assessment of mitral regurgitant severity by Doppler color flow mapping of the vena contracta. Circulation 1997;95:636–42.
60. Klein AL, Stewart WJ, Bartlett J, et al. Effects of mitral regurgitation on pulmonary venous flow and left atrial pressure: an intraoperative transesophageal echocardiographic study. J Am Coll Cardiol 1992;20:1345–52.
61. Pu M, Griffin BP, Vandervoort PM, et al. The value of assessing pulmonary venous flow velocity for predicting severity of mitral regurgitation: a quantitative assessment integrating left ventricular function. J Am Soc Echocardiogr 1999; 12: 736–43.
62. Klein AL, Savage RM, Kahan F, et al. Experimental and numerically modeled effects of convergence altered loading conditions on pulmonary venous flow and left atrial pressure in patients with mitral regurgitation. J Am Soc Echocardiogr 1997;10(1):41–51.
63. Pu M, Vandervoort PM, Griffin BP, et al. Quantification of mitral regurgitation by the proximal convergence method using transesophageal echocardiography. Clinical validation of a geometric correction for proximal flow constraint. Circulation 1995;92:2169–77.
64. Rivera JM, Vandervoort PM, Thoreau DH, et al. Quantification of mitral regurgitation using the proximal flow convergence method: a clinical study. Am Heart J 1992;124: 1289–96.
65. Rodriguez L, Anconina J, Flachskampf FA, et al. Impact of finite orifice on proximal flow convergence: implications for Doppler quantification of valvular regurgitation. Circ Res 1992;70:923–30.
66. Pu M, Prior DL, Fan X, et al. Calculation of mitral regurgitant orifice area with use of a simplified proximal convergence method: initial clinical application. J Am Soc Echocardiogr 2001;14:180–85.
67. Schwammenthal E, Chen C, Giesler M, et al. New method for accurate calculation of regurgitant flow rate based on
68. Wilkins GT, Weyman AE, Abascal VM, et al. Percutaneous balloon dilatation of the mitral valve: an analysis of echocardiographic variables related to outcome and the mechanism of dilatation. Br Heart J 1988;60:299–308.
69. Martin RP, Rakowski H, Kleiman JH, et al. Reliability and reproducibility of two dimensional echocardiograph measurement of the stenotic mitral valve orifice area. Am J Cardiol 1979;43:560–68.
70. Carabello BA, Crawford FA Jr. Valvular heart disease. N Engl J Med 1997;337(1):32–41; Erratum in: N Engl J Med 1997; 337(7):507.
71. Hatle L, Brubakk A, Tromsdal A, Angelsen B. Noninvasive assessment of pressure drop in MS by Doppler ultrasound. Br Heart J 1978;40:131–40.
72. Rodriguez L, Thomas JD, Monterosso V, et al. Validation of the proximal flow convergence method. Calculation of orifice area in patients with mitral stenosis. Circulation 1993;88: 1157–65.
73. Kulas A, Enriquez-Sarano L, Troley C, Acar J. Value of correction by receiving gains in the determination of mitral valve surface area by two-dimensional echocardiography. Arch Mal Coeur Vaiss 1982;75:757–66.
74. Enriquez-Sarano M, Freeman WK, Tribouilloy CM, et al. Functional anatomy of mitral regurgitation: accuracy and outcome implications of transesophageal echocardiography. J Am Coll Cardiol 1999;34:1129–36.
75. Bajzer CT, Stewart WJ, Cosgrove DM, et al. Tricuspid valve surgery and intraoperative echocardiography: factors affecting survival, clinical outcome, and echocardiographic success. J Am Coll Cardiol 1998;32(4):1023–31.
76. Moisa RB, Zeldis SM, Alper SA, et al. Aortic regurgitation in coronary artery bypass grafting: implications for cardioplegia administration. Ann Thorac Surg 1995;60:665–68.
77. Gillinov AM, Cosgrove DM, Blackstone EH, et al. Durability of mitral valve repair for degenerative disease. J Thorac Cardiovasc Surg 1998;116:734–43.
78. Michel-Cherqui M, Ceddaha A, Liu N, et al. Assessment of systematic use of intraoperative transesophageal echocardiography during cardiac surgery in adults: a prospective study of 203 patients. J Cardiothorac Vasc Anesth 2000; 14:45–50.
79. Stewart WJ, Currie PJ, Salcedo EE, et al. Evaluation of mitral leaflet motion by echocardiography and jet direction by Doppler color flow mapping to determine the mechanisms of mitral regurgitation. J Am Coll Cardiol 1992;20:1353–61.
80. Foster GP, Isselbacher EM, Rose GA, et al. Accurate localization of mitral regurgitant defects using multiplane transesophageal echocardiography. Ann Thorac Surg 1998;65(4): 1025–31.
81. Lambert AS, Miller JP, Merrick SH, et al. Improved evaluation of the location and mechanism of mitral valve regurgitation with a systematic transesophageal echocardiography examination Anesth Analg 1999;88(6):1205–12.
82. Omran AS, Woo A, David TE, et al. Intraoperative transesophageal echocardiography accurately predicts mitral valve anatomy and suitability for repair. J Am Soc Echocardiogr 2002;15(9):950–57.
83. Caldarera I, Van Herwerden LA, Taams MA, et al. Multiplane transesophageal echocardiography and morphology of regurgitant mitral valves in surgical repair. Eur Heart J 1995; 16(7):999–1006.
84. Grewal KS, Malkowski MJ, Kramer CM, et al. Multiplane transesophageal echocardiographic identification of the involved scallop in patients with flail mitral valve leaflet: intraoperative correlation. J Am Soc Echocardiogr 1998;11: 966–71.
85. Bach DS, Deeb GM, Bolling SF. Accuracy of intraoperative transesophageal echocardiography for estimating the severity of functional mitral regurgitation. Am J Cardiol 1995; 76(7):508–12.
86. Marwick TH, Stewart WJ, Currie PJ, et al. Mechanisms of failure of mitral valve repair: an echocardiographic study. Am Heart J 1991;122(1 Pt 1):149–56.

87. Agricola E, Oppizzi M, Maisano F, et al. Detection of mechanisms of immediate failure by transesophageal echocardiography in quadrangular resection mitral valve repair technique for severe mitral regurgitation. Am J Cardiol 2003; 91(2):175–79.
88. Schiavone WA, Cosgrove DM, Lever HM, et al. Follow-up of patients with left ventricular outflow tract obstruction after Carpentier ring mitral valvuloplasty. Circulation 1988;78(3 Pt 2):I60–5.
89. Lee KS, Stewart WJ, Lever HM, et al. Mechanism of outflow tract obstruction causing failed mitral valve repair. Anterior displacement of leaflet coaptation. Circulation 1993;88:II-24–II-29.
90. Carpentier A. The sliding leaflet technique. Le Club Mitrale Newsletter 1988 Aug.
91. Gillinov AM, Cosgrove DM 3rd. Modified sliding leaflet technique for repair of the mitral valve. Ann Thorac Surg 1999;68(6):2356–57.
92. Gillinov AM, Wierup PN, Blackstone EH, et al. Is repair preferable to replacement for ischemic mitral regurgitation J Thorac Cardiovasc Surg 2001;122(6):1125–41.
93. Maslow AD, Regan MM, Haering JM, et al. Echocardiographic predictors of left ventricular outflow tract obstruction and systolic anterior motion of the mitral valve after mitral valve reconstruction for myxomatous valve disease. J Am Coll Cardiol 1999;34(7):2096–104.
94. Feindel CM, Tufail Z, David TE. Mitral valve surgery in patients with extensive calcification of the mitral annulus. J Thorac Cardiovasc Surg 2003;126(3):777–82.
95. David TE, Feindel CM, Armstrong S, Sun Z. Reconstruction of the mitral anulus. A ten-year experience. J Thorac Cardiovasc Surg 1995;110(5):1323–32.
96. David TE, Armstrong S, Sun Z. Left ventricular function after mitral valve surgery. J Heart Valve Dis 1995;4 [Suppl 2]:S175–80.
97. Savage RM, Isada LR, Torelli J, et al. Echo-Doppler derived dP/dt predicts perioperative course of patients following mitral valve repair. Anesth Analg 1993;(Abst)Apr.
98. Davila-Roman VG, Barzilai B, Wareing TH, et al. Atherosclerosis of the ascending aorta. Prevalence and role as an independent predictor of cerebrovascular events in cardiac patients. Stroke 1994;25:2010.
99. Davila-Roman VG, Phillips KJ, Daily BB, et al. Intraoperative transesophageal echocardiography and epiaortic ultrasound for assessment of atherosclerosis of the thoracic aorta. J Am Coll Cardiol 1996;28:942–47.
100. Wareing TH, Davila-Roman VG, Barzilai B, et al. Management of the severely atherosclerotic ascending aorta during cardiac operations. A strategy for detection and treatment. J Thorac Cardiovasc Surg 1992;103:453–62.
101. Roach GW, Kacchuger M, Mangano C, et al. Adverse cerebral outcomes after coronary bypass surgery. N Engl J Med 1996;335:1857.
102. Konstadt SN, Reich DL, Quintana C, et al. The ascending aorta: how much does transesophageal echocardiography see? Anesth Analg 1994;78:240–44.
103. Newman MF, Wolman R, Kanchuger M, et al. Multicenter preoperative stroke risk index for patients undergoing coronary artery bypass graft surgery. Multicenter Study of Perioperative Ischemia (McSPI) Research Group. Circulation 1996;94[Suppl 9]:II-74–II-80.
104. Morehead AJ, Firstenberg MS, Shiota T, et al. Intraoperative echocardiographic detection of regurgitant jets after valve replacement. Ann Thorac Surg 2000;69:135–39.
105. Thomas JD, Vandervoort PM, Pu M, et al. Doppler/echocardiographic assessment of native and prosthetic heart valves: recent advances. J Heart Valve Dis 1995;4[Suppl 1]:S59–63.
106. Cohen GI, Davison MB, Klein AL, et al. A comparison of flow convergence with other transthoracic echocardiographic indexes of prosthetic mitral regurgitation. J Am Soc Echocardiogr 1992;5(6):620–27.
107. Intracranial Doppler
108. David TE. Dynamic left ventricular outflow tract obstruction when the anterior leaflet is retained at prosthetic mitral valve replacement. Ann Thorac Surg 1988;45(2):229.
109. Grimm RA, Stewart WJ. The role of intraoperative echocardiography in valve surgery. Cardiol Clin 1998;16:477–89.
110. Fix J, Isada L, Cosgrove D, et al. Do patients with less than "echo-perfect" results from mitral valve repair by intraoperative echocardiography have a different outcome? Circulation 1993;88:II-39–II-48.
111. Freeman WK, Schaff HV, Khandheria BK, et al. Intraoperative evaluation of mitral valve regurgitation and repair by transesophageal echocardiography: incidence and significance of systolic anterior motion. J Am Coll Cardiol 1992;20:599–609.
111b. Milas BL, Bavaria JE, Koch CG, Troianos CA. Case 8-2001. Resolution of systolic anterior motion after mitral valve repair with atrial pacing. J Cardiothorac Vasc Anesth 2001; 15(5):641–48.
112. Gatti G, Cardu G, Trane R, Pugliese P. The edge-to-edge technique as a trick to rescue an imperfect mitral valve repair. Eur J Cardiothorac Surg 2002;22(5):817–20.
113. Saiki Y, Kasegawa H, Kawase M, et al. Intraoperative TEE during mitral valve repair: does it predict early and late postoperative mitral valve dysfunction? Ann Thorac Surg 1998;66(4):1277–81.
114. Muratori M, Berti M, Doria E, et al. Transesophageal echocardiography as predictor of mitral valve repair. J Heart Valve Dis 2001;10:65–71.
115. Kaplan SR, Bashein G, Sheehan FH, et al. Three-dimensional echocardiographic assessment of annular shape changes in the normal and regurgitant mitral valve. Am Heart J 2000;139:378–87.
116. Umana JP, Salehizadeh B, et al. "Bow-tie" mitral valve repair: an adjuvant technique for ischemic mitral regurgitation. Ann Thorac Surg 1998;66(5):1640–46.
117. Privitera S, Butany J, Cusimano RJ, et al. Images in cardiovascular medicine. Alfieri mitral valve repair: clinical outcome and pathology. Circulation 2002;106(21): 173–74.
118. Ibrahim MF, David TE. Mitral stenosis after mitral valve repair for non-rheumatic mitral regurgitation. Ann Thorac Surg 2002;73(1):34–6.
119. Tingleff J, Joyce FS, Pettersson G. Intraoperative echocardiographic study of air embolism during cardiac operations. Ann Thorac Surg 1995;60:673–77.
120. Secknus MA, Asher CR, Scalia GM, et al. Intraoperative transesophageal echocardiography in minimally invasive cardiac valve surgery. J Am Soc Echocardiogr 1999;12(4): 231–36.
121. Varghese D, Riedel BJ, Fletchker SN, et al. Successful repair of intraoperative aortic dissection detected by transesophageal echocardiography. Ann Thorac Surg 2002;73(3): 953–55.
122. Tavilla G, Pacini D. Damage to the circumflex coronary artery during mitral valve repair with sliding leaflet technique. Ann Thorac Surg 1998;66(6):2091–93.
123. Obarski TP, Loop FD, Cosgrove DM, et al. Frequency of acute myocardial infarction in valve repairs versus valve replacement for pure mitral regurgitation. Am J Cardiol 1990;65(13):887–90.
124. Genoni M, Jenni R, Schmid ER, et al. Treatment of left atrial dissection after mitral valve repair: internal drainage. Ann Thorac Surg 1999;68(4):1394–96.
125. Ionescu AA, West RR, Proudman C, et al. Prospective study of routine perioperative transesophageal echocardiography for elective valve replacement: clinical impact and cost-saving implications. J Am Soc Echocardiogr 2001;14(7): 659–67.
126. Mills WR, Barber JE, Skiles JA, et al. Clinical, echocardiographic, and biomechanical differences in mitral valve prolapse affecting one or both leaflets. Am J Cardiol 2002; 89(12):1394–99.
127. Robert WC. Morphologic aspects of cardiac valve dysfunction. Am Heart J 1992;123:1610.

128. Braunwald E. Mitral regurgitation: physiologic, clinical, and surgical considerations. N Engl J Med 1969;281(8): 425–33.

129. Carpentier A, Deloche A, Dauptain J, et al. A new reconstructive operation for correction of mitral and tricuspid insufficiency. J Thorac Cardiovasc Surg 1971;61:1–13.

130. Waller BF, Morrow AG, Maron BJ, et al. Etiology of clinically isolated, severe, chronic, pure mitral regurgitation: analysis of 97 patients over 30 years of age having mitral valve replacement. Am Heart J 1982;104:276–88.

131. Hanson TP, Edwards BC, Edwards JE. Pathology of surgically excised mitral valves: one hundred cases. Arch Pathol Lab Med 1985;109:823.

132. Fornes P, Heudes D, Fuzellier J, et al. Correlation between clinical and histologic patterns of degenerative mitral valve insufficiency: a histomorphometric study of 130 excised segments. Cardiovasc Path 1999;8(2):81–92.

133. Rosen SE, Borer JS, Hochreiter C, et al. Natural history of the asymptomatic/minimally symptomatic patient with severe mitral regurgitation secondary to mitral valve prolapse and normal right and left ventricular performance. Am J Cardiol 1994;74:374–80.

134. Kwan J, Shiota T, Agler DA, et al. Geometric differences of the mitral apparatus between ischemic and dilated cardiomyopathy with significant mitral regurgitation: real-time three-dimensional echocardiography study. Circulation 2003;107(8):1135–40.

135. Karp RB. Role of surgery in infective endocarditis. Cardiovasc Clin 1987;17:141.

136. Muehrcke DD, Cosgrove DM, Lytle BW, et al. Is there an advantage to sparing infected mitral valves? Ann Thorac Surg 1997;63:1718.

137. Marcus RH, Sareli P, Pocock WA, Barlow JB. The spectrum of severe rheumatic mitral valve disease in a developing country: correlations among clinical presentation, surgical pathologic findings, and hemodynamic sequelae. Ann Intern Med 1994;120:177–83.

138. Olson LJ, Subramanian R, Ackermann DM, et al. Surgical pathology of the mitral valve: a study of 712 cases spanning 21 years. Mayo Clin Proc 1987;62:22–34.

138b. Carpentier A, Chauvaud S, Fabiani JN, et al. Reconstructive surgery of mitral valve incompetence, ten-year appraisal. J Thorac Cardiovasc Surg 1980;79:338–48.

139. Carpentier AF, Pellerin M, Fuzellier JF, Relland JY. Extensive calcification of the mitral valve anulus: pathology and surgical management. J Thorac Cardiovasc Surg 1996;111 (4):718–29; discussion, 729–30.

140. Duran CM, Gometza B, Balasundaram S, et al. A feasibility study of valve repair in rheumatic mitral regurgitation. Eur Heart J 1991;12:34–8.

141. David TE. The appropriateness of mitral valve repair for rheumatic mitral valve disease. J Heart Valve Dis 1997;6(4): 373–74.

142. Carpentier A. Cardiac valve surgery: the "French Connection." J Thorac Cardiovasc Surg 1983;86:323.

143. Reece TB, Tribble CG, Ellman PI. Mitral repair is superior to replacement when associated with coronary artery disease. Ann Surg 2004;239(5):671–75; discussion, 675–77.

144. Messas E, Pouzet B, Touchot B, et al. Efficacy of chordal cutting to relieve chronic persistent ischemic mitral regurgitation. Circulation 2003;108[Suppl 1]:II-111–5.

145. Levine RA, Hung J. Ischemic mitral regurgitation, the dynamic lesion: clues to the cure [comment]. J Am Coll Cardiol 2003;42(11):1929–32.

146. Enriquez-Sarano M, Bailey KR, Seward JB, et al. Quantitative Doppler assessment of valvular regurgitation. Circulation 1993;87:841–48.

147. Marwick TH, Torelli J, Obarski T, et al. Assessment of the mitral valve splitability score by transthoracic and transesophageal echocardiography. Am J Cardiol 1991;68: 1106–07.

148. Flachskampf FA, Weyman AE, Gillam L, et al. Aortic regurgitation shortens Doppler pressure half-time in mitral stenosis: clinical evidence, in vitro simulation and theoretic analysis. J Am Coll Cardiol 1990;16:396–404.

149. Nakatani S, Masuyama T, Kodama K, et al. Value and limitations of Doppler echocardiography in the quantification of stenotic mitral valve area: comparison of the pressure half-time and the continuity equation methods. Circulation 1988;77:78–85.

150. Duran CM. Tricuspid valve surgery revisited. J Cardiac Surg 1994;9:242–47.

151. Choudhary SK, Talwar S, Juneja R, et al. Fate of mild aortic valve disease after mitral intervention. J Thorac Cardiovasc Surg 2001;122:583.

152. Enriquez-Sarano M, Tajik AJ, Bailey KR, Seward JB. Color flow imaging compared with quantitative Doppler assessment of severity of mitral regurgitation: influence of eccentricity of jet and mechanism of regurgitation. J Am Coll Cardiol 1993;21:1211–29.

153. Christenson JT, Jordan B, Bloch A, et al. Should a regurgitant mitral valve be replaced simultaneously with a stenotic valve? Tex Heart Inst J 2000;27:350–55.

154. Gillinov AM, Blackstone EH, White J, et al. Durability of combined aortic and mitral valve repair. Ann Thorac Surg 2001;72(1):20–7.

155. Brunton T. Preliminary note on the possibility of treating mitral stenosis by surgical methods. Lancet 1902;1:352.

156. Cutler EE, Levine SA, Beck CS. The surgical treatment of mitral stenosis: experimental and clinical studies. Arch Surg 1924;9:689–821, 104–05.

157. Souttar HS. The surgical diagnosis of mitral stenosis. Brit Med J 1925;2:605.

158. Lillehei CW, Gott VL, DeWall RA, et al. Surgical correction of pure mitral insufficiency by annuloplasty under direct vision. Lancet 1957;77:446–49.

159. Duran CG, Pomar JL, Revuelta JM, et al. Conservative operation for mitral insufficiency. Critical analysis supported by postoperative hemodynamic studies in 72 patients. J Thorac Cardiovasc Surg 1980;79:326.

160. McGoon DC, et al. Repair of mitral insufficiency due to ruptured chordae tendineae. J Thorac Cardiovasc Surg 1960;39:357–62.

161. Sand ME, Naftel DC, Blackstone EH, et al. A comparison of repair and replacement for mitral valve incompetence J Thorac Cardiovasc Surg 1987;94(2):208–19.

162. Gillinov AM, Cosgrove DM 3rd, Shiota T, et al. Cosgrove-Edwards Annuloplasty System: midterm results. Ann Thorac Surg 2000;69(3):717–21.

163. Edwards JE. Pathology of mitral incompetence. In: Silver MD, ed. Cardiovascular pathology, vol. 1. New York: Churchill Livingstone, 1983:575.

164. Gordis L. The virtual disappearance of rheumatic fever in the United States: lessons in the rise and fall of disease. T. Duckett Jones Memorial Lecture, Circulation 1985;72:1155.

165. Appelblatt NH, Willis PW, Lenhart, et al. Ten to 40 year follow up of patients with systolic click with and without late systolic murmur. Am J Cardiol 1979;35:119.

166. Acar C, Farge A, Ramsheyi A. Mitral valve replacement using a cryopreserved mitral homograft. Ann Thorac Surg 1994;57(3):746–48.

167. Chauvaud S, Waldmann T, d'Attellis N, et al. Homograft replacement of the mitral valve in young recipients: mid-term results. Eur J Cardiothorac Surg 2003;23(4):560–66.

168. Block PC. Percutaneous mitral valve repair for mitral regurgitation. J Interv Cardiol 2003;16:93–96.

## TERMINOLOGY AND ABBREVIATIONS

**IOE exam**   **Intraoperative echocardiographic examination** consisting of transesophageal echocardiography and epicardial imaging as required in addressing the critical issues in mitral valve surgery

| | |
|---|---|
| MV | **Mitral valve** |
| MVAp | **Mitral valve apparatus** consisting of the fibrous skeleton and annulus, valve leaflets, chordae, papillary muscles, and left ventricular wall between the attached papillary muscles and annulus |
| PMVL | **Posterior mitral valve leaflet** |
| P1 | **Lateral scallop PMVL (both ASE/SCA and Duran nomenclature)** |
| P2 | **Middle scallop PMVL (ASE/SCA), medial scallop (Duran)** |
| P3 | **Medial scallop PMVL (ASE/SCA)** |
| PM1 | **Duran nomenclature, middle scallop lateral half** |
| PM2 | **Duran nomenclature, middle scallop medial half** |
| AMVL | **Anterior mitral valve leaflet** |
| A1 | **Lateral segment, AMVL** |
| A2 | **Middle segment, AMVL** |
| A3 | **Medial segment, AMVL** |
| PM | **Papillary muscle** |
| ALC | **Anterolateral commissure (Duran C1)** |
| PMC | **Posteromedial commissure (Duran C2)** |
| ALPM | **Anterolateral papillary muscle (Duran M1)** |
| PMPM | **Posteromedial papillary muscle (Duran M2)** |
| MVR | **Mitral valve replacement** in which the secondary and tertiary chordal attachments are left intact (chordal sparing) or they are removed (nonchordal sparing) and replaced with a mechanical, bioprosthetic MV prosthetic valve or homograft. |
| MVRep | **MV repair** |
| Pre-CPB | **Precardiopulmonary bypass period** |
| PreSep | The period prior to separating from cardiopulmonary bypass |
| CPB | **Cardiopulmonary bypass** |
| Post-CPB | **Period following separation from CPB** |
| MS | **Mitral stenosis** |
| MR | **Mitral regurgitation** |
| CF Doppler | **Color flow Doppler** |
| MJA | **Maximal jet area** |
| PCV | **Proximal flow convergence** |
| PISA | **Proximal isovelocity surface area** |
| $PT_{1/2}$ | **Pressure half time method of calculating MV area** |
| DT | **Deceleration time** |
| PW Doppler | **Pulse wave Doppler** |
| CW Doppler | **Continuous wave Doppler** |
| TEE | **Transesophageal echocardiography** |
| ECE | **Epicardial echocardiography** |
| ME 4 Chr | **Midesophageal 4 chamber** |
| ME 5 Chr | **Midesophageal 5 chamber** |
| ME Com | **Midesophageal commissural image plane** |
| ME ComR | **Midesophageal commissural image plane with probe turned right (clockwise)** |
| ME ComL | **Midesophageal commissural image plane with probe turned left (counterclockwise)** |
| ME 2 Chr | **Midesophageal 2 chamber** |
| ME 2 ChrR | **Midesophageal 2 chamber with probe turned right (clockwise)** |
| ME 2 ChrL | **Midesophageal 2 chamber with probe turned left (counterclockwise)** |
| ME LAX | **Midesophageal long axis** |
| ME LAXR | **Midesophageal long axis with probe turned right (clockwise)** |
| ME LAXL | **Midesophageal long axis with probe turned left (counterclockwise)** |
| TG SAXb | **Basal transgastric short axis** |
| TG 2 Chr | **Transgastric 2 chamber** |
| TR | **Tricuspid regurgitation** |
| AR | **Aortic regurgitation** |
| AS | **Aortic stenosis** |

## QUESTIONS

1. Which of the following are predictors of a successful MV repair for severe mitral insufficiency?
   A. MV annulus dimension of 51 mm
   B. Severe mitral annular calcification
   C. Splitability score of 12 in rheumatic MV disease
   D. AMVL prolapse
   E. PMVL flail

2. Which of the following best characterizes a post-CPB finding that would require a return to cardiopulmonary bypass for further reconstructive MV surgery (Nyquist limit of 55 cm/sec)?
   A. CF Doppler maximum jet area of 1 cm$^2$
   B. Color flow Doppler maximum jet area of 5 cm$^2$
   C. Vena contracta diameter 0.3 cm
   D. PISA "peak" ROA 0.3 cm$^2$
   E. None of the above

3. Which of the following are predictors of post-MVRep SAM and LVOTO?
   A. AMVL:PMVL ratio of > 1.3
   B. Coaptation to septal distance (C-Sept) of 3.2
   C. Septal thickness 2.3 cm$^2$
   D. PMVL height 2.1 cm
   E. PMVL flail

4. What percentage of patients with a myxomatous flail MV leaflet either have surgery or die within 10 years of their diagnosis?
   A. 10%
   B. 30%
   C. 60%
   D. 90%
   E. 100%

5. Which of the following patients with rheumatic MR and MS are most likely to have a successful MV repair?
   A. 38-year-old patient with MVA 1.2 cm$^2$ and splitability score 12
   B. 46-year-old patient with MVA 1.8 with subvalvular stenosis
   C. 15-year-old patient with mild MS and severe MR with AMVL prolapse
   D. 65-year-old patient with severe MAC and splitability score 6
   E. 69-year-old patient with MVA of 0.7 cm$^2$ and splitability score of 9

# Surgical Considerations in Aortic Valve Surgery

### *Cristiano N. Faber and Nicholas G. Smedira*

Aortic valve disease is the number one indication for valve replacement. At the Cleveland Clinic Foundation, the number of aortic valve operations has steadily increased over the last five years, with almost 1,000 patients having some type of aortic valve surgery between 1999 and 2000 (Fig. 29.1). With the increasing life expectancy of the American population (1), these numbers will continue to rise with an increasing prevalence of degenerative aortic disease among older patients.

The surgical treatment of aortic valve continues to evolve. The development of new valve prosthesis, surgical techniques, and intraoperative echocardiographic assessment of the anatomy and function of the aortic valve contributed to a more individualized approach to each patient. Intraoperative echocardiography, especially transesophageal echocardiography, offers the surgeon a more detailed and dynamic understanding of the aortic root, valve, and left ventricular outflow tract. In addition to its clinical benefits, routine intraoperative TEE has also been shown to have cost-saving implications in patients undergoing valve surgery (2).

Nowadays, intraoperative transesophageal echocardiogram is an important part of decision-making during valve surgery. Such evaluations can have a great impact on the selection of prosthesis size, type of prosthesis that would better fit patient's anatomy (3), and repair techniques used (4).

## ANATOMY/PATHOLOGY

There are two mechanisms of aortic valve failure: aortic stenosis and aortic insufficiency. A diseased aortic valve can present both abnormalities at the same time but most frequently one pattern will be dominant.

*Aortic stenosis* (AS) is caused by calcific aortic stenosis (congenital bicuspid valve), rheumatic disease, and atherosclerotic degenerative process. The manifestation of all forms is the same and represents a decrease in the effective valve orifice area and obstruction to the ejection of blood from the left ventricle (LV). This increased afterload

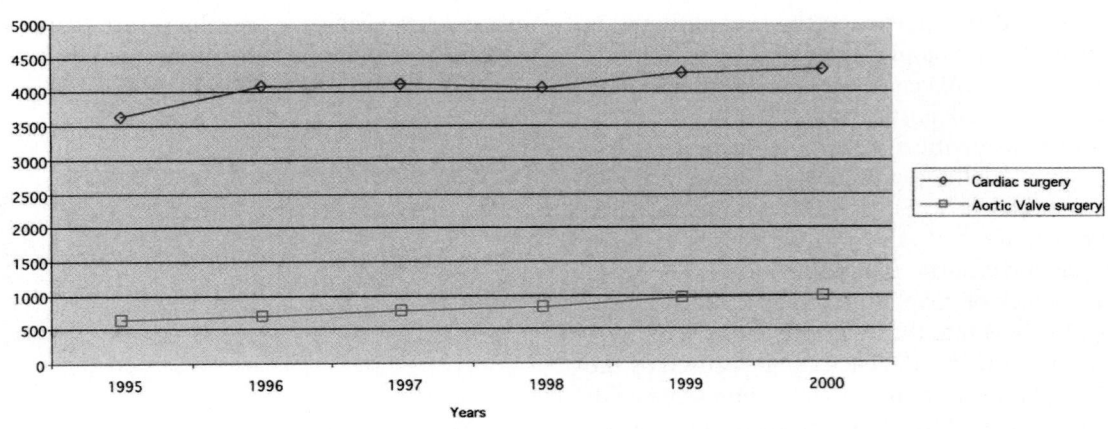

**FIGURE 29.1.** Aortic valve surgery at the Cleveland Clinic Foundation.

will lead to concentric ventricular hypertrophy and eventually LV dysfunction.

Congenital bicuspid valve abnormalities are characterized by unequal cusp size due to the fusion of right and left cusps, presence of a central raphe, and smooth cusp margins (5). The abnormal flow through the valve is associated with wear and tear of the cusps, which predisposes to calcifications that are more pronounced on the raphe of the conjoined cusp and at the commissures and adjacent aorta (6). Over time, the slow calcification results in significant stenosis during the fifth to sixth decades of life (the most common cause of AS in this age group) (6). Usually the stenosis is accompanied by trivial regurgitation.

Degenerative-calcific process is the most common cause of AS in the adult (7). Histological analysis of the early lesions of valvular aortic stenosis show displacement of the subendothelial elastic lamina; accumulation of a cellular infiltrate of macrophage and T lymphocytes; and deposition of protein, lipid, and calcium. The adjacent fibrosa is also abnormal, with accumulation of fibrous protein, lipid, and calcium minerals (8,9). It is postulated that the development of aortic stenosis is an active process, in part mediated by chronic inflammation, rather than a consequence of aging, and evidence suggests that this inflammatory process is fueled by atherosclerotic risk factors (6).

Apoptosis may also play a role in the mechanism of valvular disease (10). Apoptosis of fibroblasts and endothelial cells of the aortic valve, ranging from focal disruption of individual endothelial cells to extensive denudation of entire endothelium, leads to calcific deposits within the cellular fragments, and this programmed cellular death is increased by hypercholesterolemia (11).

The aortic valve is tricuspid and the calcification involves the cusps, commissures, annulus, sinuses of Valsalva and ascending aorta. It is often present in patients over 65 years of age and its prevalence increases with age. Associated rheumatic disease can accelerate this process, which, despite the low incidence in the United States, is still very prevalent in developing countries.

*Aortic insufficiency* (AI) can be caused by native valve endocarditis, congenital aortic valve disease, myxomatous aortic valve, rheumatic disease, and ascending aortic enlargement from multiple pathologies (please refer to Chapter 35, Assessment in Surgical Procedures for Congestive Heart Failure, for valve insufficiency associated with ascending aortic/aortic root pathologies). The main mechanism is a lack of coaptation of aortic cusps resulting in retrograde flow into the LV during diastole.

In endocarditis, the insufficiency can be caused by the presence of vegetations, injury of the commissure with prolapse of the cusp, perforation of the cusp, and destruction of the aortic annulus due to an abscess cavity.

AI caused by prolapse of the cusps of the aortic valve is more common in congenital bicuspid aortic valve and is caused by prolapse of the free edge of the conjoined leaflet (12), while in myxomatous degeneration of the aortic valve the prolapse is due to redundant and thickened cusps.

Predominant aortic valve insufficiency is not a common presentation of rheumatic disease, and when it happens it is due to shortening of the cusps caused by scar.

## SURGICAL CONSIDERATIONS: AORTIC VALVE REPAIR

When feasible, aortic valve repair is the surgical treatment of choice. In adults, stenotic valves are rarely amenable to repair as decalcification procedures were associated with early failure so that now most efforts at valve repair occur in patients with aortic insufficiency (13,14).

Repair of an insufficient aortic valve requires an understanding of the mechanisms of valve failure. The intraoperative echocardiogram provides the detailed information to help formulate repair plans and assess the results of the repair. Identification of the diseased cusp, mechanism of regurgitation, size of the annulus, and presence of calcification of the aortic annulus are paramount when choosing the repair technique.

In the insufficient tricuspid aortic valve the main cause of prolapse is elongation of the leaflet with prolapse or rupture of the free edge of the cusp at an area of fenestration. In those cases a triangular resection of the leaflet is performed (Fig. 29.2).

Frequently an annuloplasty needs to be added to the repair to reduce the circumference of the annulus and increase coaptation. This is accomplished by placing a horizontal mattress suture buttressed with Teflon felt at the commissure (Fig. 29.3). The amount of commissural plication is determined by the level of the suture. The lower into the left ventricular outflow tract the suture is the greater the annular plication performed (Fig. 29.4).

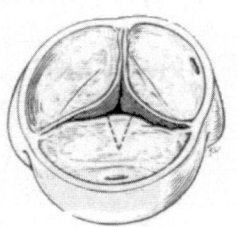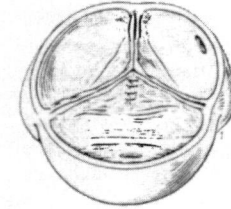

**FIGURE 29.2.** Triangular resection of the prolapsing free edge of the cusp.

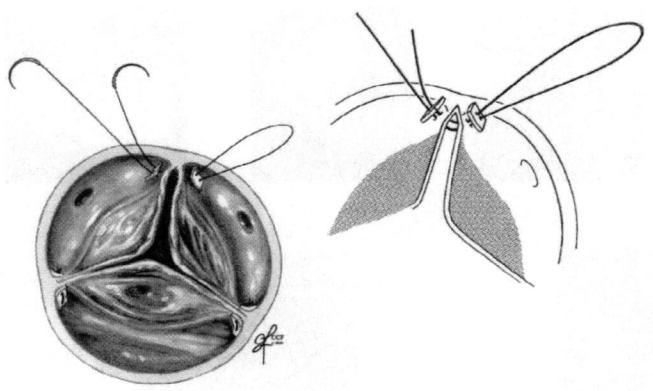

**FIGURE 29.3.** Aortic annuloplasty.

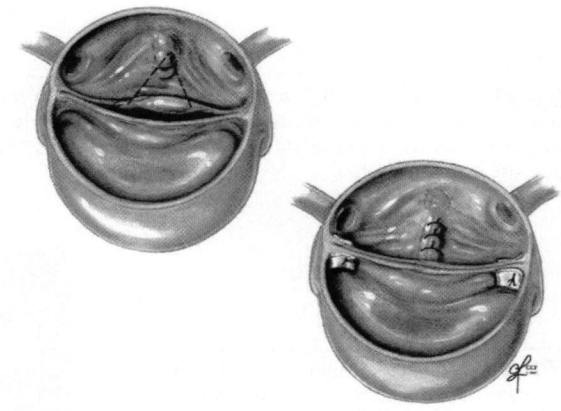

**FIGURE 29.5.** Triangular resection of the cojoined leaflet at the level of the raphe and aortic annuloplasty.

For repair of a bicuspid aortic valve the technique is very similar with the resection or plication of the redundant central portion of the prolapsing leaflet, at the site of the raphe, followed by annuloplasty (Fig. 29.5).

Those techniques are shown to effectively eliminate aortic insufficiency (15). To achieve good long-term results, at the end of the repair there should be minimal or no aortic insufficiency.

At the Cleveland Clinic, 94 bicuspid valves and 33 tricuspid valve repairs were analyzed. Tricuspid valve repair, most often involving the right coronary cusp (82% of the time), was less reproducible than bicuspid valve repair. Persistent intraoperative aortic regurgitation requiring valve replacement occurred in 15% of the tricuspid valve repairs versus 0% for bicuspid repairs. Overall freedom from reoperation if the patient left the operating room without AI was 93% for bicuspid repairs and 83% for tricuspid valve repairs at 5 years.

## SURGICAL CONSIDERATIONS: AORTIC VALVE REPLACEMENT

The implantation technique for a stented prosthesis is the same for mechanical as well biological valves and often consists of placement of non-everting braided polyester mattress sutures, with or without pledgets (Fig. 29.6). The native valve must be excised and the annulus carefully debrided to maintain left ventricular and aortic continuity. The sutures are passed through the sewing ring of the valve and the valve is seated (Fig. 29.7).

Although the technique is the same, for mechanical prosthesis, there are different positions in which the valve can be seated in the aortic annulus, depending on the type of valve utilized. The valve can be implanted in an intraannular or supraannular position depending on its design (Fig. 29.8).

The advantage of the supraannular position is that the valve itself sits above the annulus, because the sewing

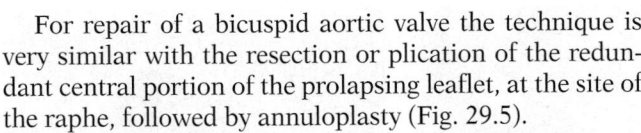

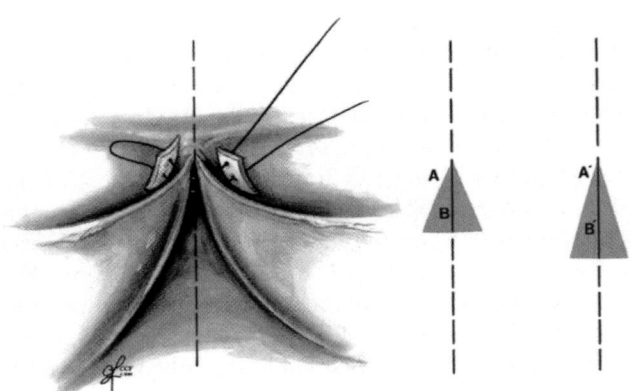

**FIGURE 29.4.** The amount of annular plication is determined by the level where the suture is placed. The lower the suture is placed the more annular plication is achieved (AB → A'B').

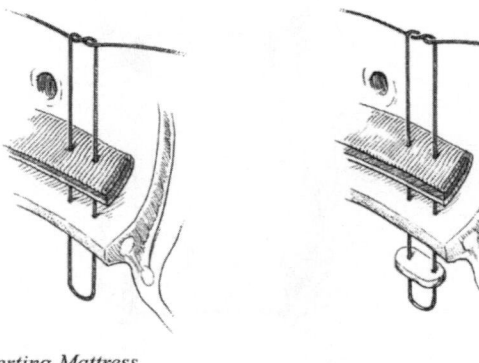

*Non-Everting Mattress*

**FIGURE 29.6.** Most common type of suture technique utilized for implantation of stented valves. (Courtesy of Sulzer Carbo-Medics, Inc.)

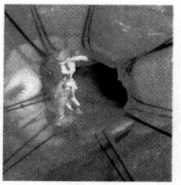 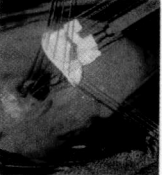 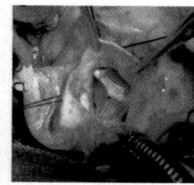

**FIGURE 29.7.** Implantation of a stented bioprosthesis in the intraannular position. The sutures are placed in the aortic annulus, then in the sewing ring of the valve and the prosthesis is finally seated in the aortic annulus.

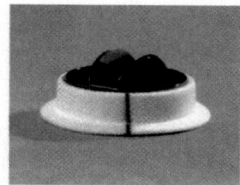 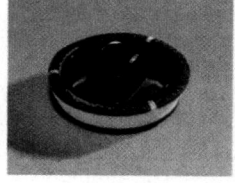

**FIGURE 29.8.** Supraannular and intraannular mechanical aortic valves. Note the inflow valve positioning if the sewing ring is in the supraannular (TopHat™) valve. (Courtesy of Sulzer CarboMedics, Inc.)

**SulzerCarbomedics TopHat™ valve**          **SulzerCarbomedics "R" Aortic valve**

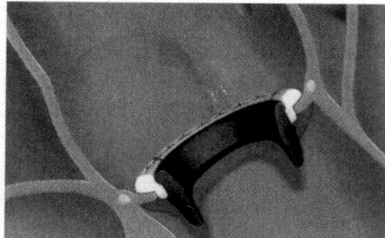 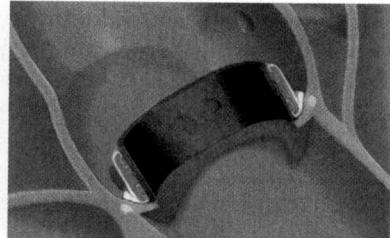

**FIGURE 29.9.** Position of the aortic valve in relation to the aortic annulus. (Courtesy of Sulzer CarboMedics, Inc.)

cuff is positioned at the inflow level of the valve, moving the housing of the valve to a supraannular position (Fig. 29.9). This theoretically allows one to place a larger valve in the same patient with lower pressure gradients than a smaller valve implanted in the intraannular position (Fig. 29.10).

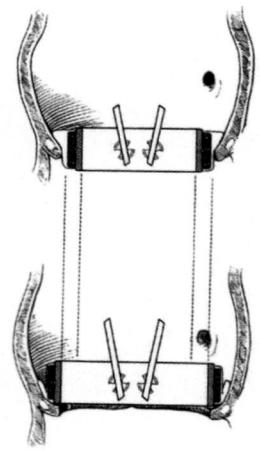

**FIGURE 29.10.** Intraannular and supraannular positioning of the aortic valve prosthesis. Note that in the supraannular position the structural components of the valve are above the annulus, providing an increased orifice area. (Courtesy of Sulzer CarboMedics, Inc.)

This would be beneficial in cases were the aortic root is small, avoiding the increased morbidity and mortality associated with aortic root enlargement (16). These valves have been used with low mortality and morbidity, but careful attention needs to be taken when sizing this type of valve. Forcing a large prosthesis into the annulus could cause obstruction of the coronaries, dehiscence of the prosthesis, or paravalvular aortic insufficiency (17).

Stentless tissue heterografts require a more demanding implantation technique than stented prosthesis, but offer better hemodynamics. Two stentless heterografts are currently available in the United States: the Toronto SPV® valve (St. Jude Medical; St. Paul, Minnesota) and the Freestyle® aortic root bioprosthesis (Medtronic Heart Valves; Minneapolis, Minnesota). The difference between the two valves is that the Toronto SPV has most of the porcine sinuses of Valsalva removed for subcoronary implantation, leaving a rim of aorta at the commissures and at the base of the sinuses for suture placement. The Freestyle® contains the porcine aortic valve and ascending aorta (Fig. 29.11).

Both valves can be implanted in the subcoronary position, using what is called the *freehand technique.* This is a two suture line technique where the proximal (inflow) suture is circular and located at the aortic annulus, and the distal (outflow) suture line follows the commissures and base of the sinuses of Valsalva (Fig. 29.12).

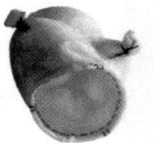
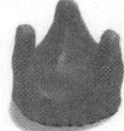

Freestyle® Medtronics        Toronto SPV® St Jude Medical

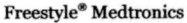

**FIGURE 29.11.** Stentless aortic xenografts. (Picture of Freestyle® valve courtesy of Medtronics, Inc.; picture of Toronto SPV® valve courtesy of St. Jude Medical, Inc.)

More commonly the Freestyle® valve is implanted using the full-root or the root-inclusion technique. For the full-root technique, the patient's proximal aorta is removed and the valve interposed between the left ventricle and ascending aorta with reimplantation of the coronary ostia.

When using a stentless valve and the subcoronary technique, it is very important to verify that the diameter of the patient's sinotubular junction is within normal limits otherwise there will be poor coaptation of the cusps and consequent aortic regurgitation. For this reason it is necessary that the aortic root is assessed carefully during the intraoperative echocardiogram. After the operation is completed the competence of the valve must be assessed; it is not uncommon to have a small paravalvular leak right after discontinuation of cardiopulmonary bypass, so the valve needs to be reassessed after heparin reversal. If the full-root technique is used, the evaluation of the patency of the proximal segments of the coronaries should be done to exclude kinking due to malpositioning.

Homografts, which are constituted of cadaveric aortic root (with a left ventricle muscle band, with or without the anterior leaflet of the mitral valve and ascending aorta) are very useful when extensive compromise of the aortic root is present (Fig. 29.13).

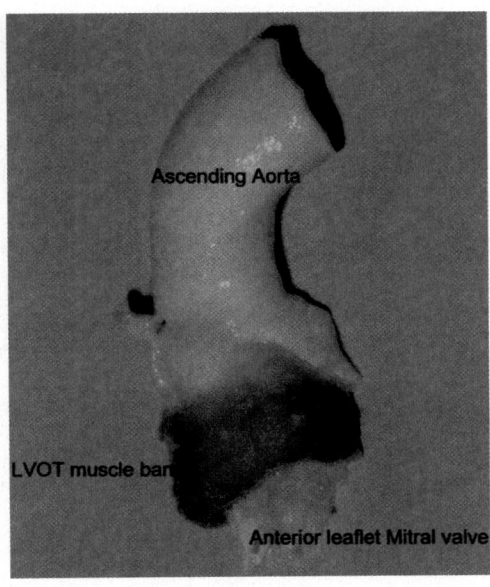

**FIGURE 29.13.** Cadaveric homograft. Composed of aortic root, ascending aorta, left ventricle outflow tract (LVOT) muscle band, and the anterior leaflet of the mitral valve.

Due to the pliability of human tissue and resistance to infection, these valves are used commonly to replace an infected aortic valve. They are implanted using the full-root technique and require the same intraoperative echocardiographic evaluation as a stentless valve (Fig. 29.14). Any distortion when suturing the valve to the aortic annulus can cause important aortic insufficiency and kinking of the coronary arteries.

Another alternative for aortic valve replacement, especially in young patients, is the Ross procedure, which consists of an aortic valve replacement with pulmonary autograft and reconstruction of the right ventricular outflow graft with a pulmonary homograft (Fig. 29.15).

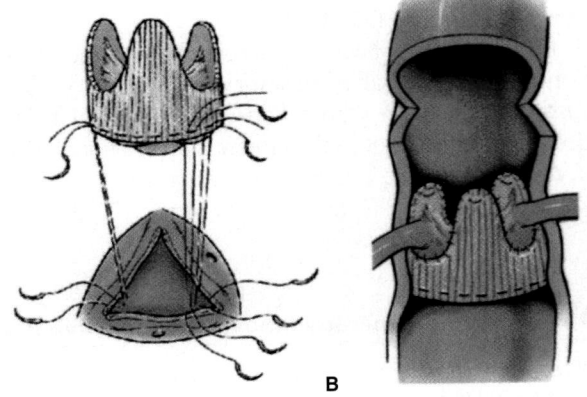

**FIGURE 29.12.** Stentless aortic valve implantation. The inflow suture line is placed in a single horizontal line on the fibrous tissue of the annulus **(A)**, while the outflow suture line follows the shape of the distal edge of the valve **(B)**. (Courtesy of St. Jude Medical, Inc.)

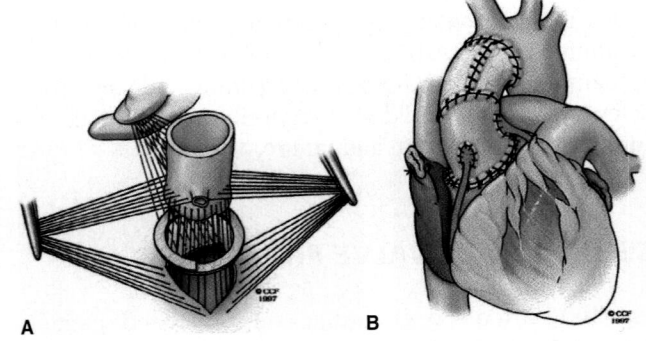

**FIGURE 29.14. A:** After removal of the aortic valve, the homograft is implanted using interrupted stitches placed into the aortic annulus (a strip of felt can be used to reinforce the annulus and also with hemostatic purposes). **B:** Final aspect of a cadaveric homograft implanted using the full-root technique.

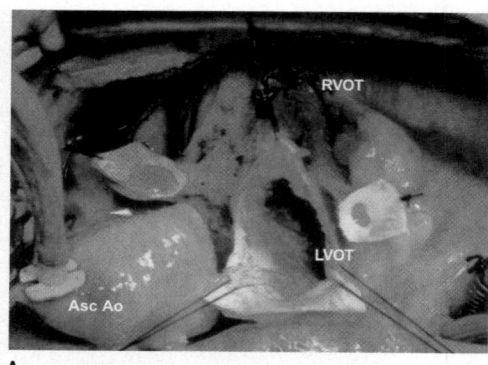 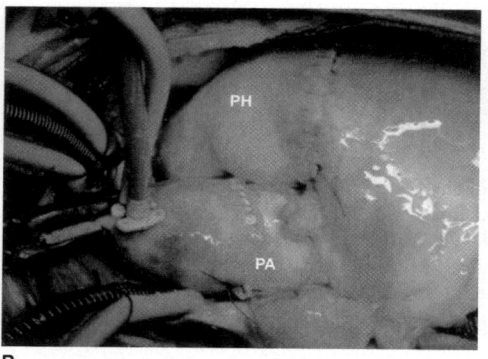

**FIGURE 29.15.** Ross procedure. **A:** Pulmonary autograft is harvested and the aortic valve is removed. **B:** Final aspect of the heart after implantation of the pulmonary autograft in the aortic position and a pulmonary homograft into the right ventricular outflow tract. *RVOT,* right ventricle outflow tract; *LVOT,* left ventricle outflow tract; *Asc. Ao,* ascending aorta; *PH,* pulmonary homograft; *PA,* pulmonary autograft.

The aortic anatomy is important: because the pulmonary autograft is a stentless valve, any abnormality of the aortic root and sinotubular junction could result in valvular regurgitation. The diameter of the aortic annulus should be measured, as well as the diameter of the ascending aorta and the sinotubular junction. Relative contraindications to a Ross procedure would be a bicuspid aortic valve with dilation of the aortic annulus beyond 30 mm. Extensive aortic dilatation can be seen as an indicator of a possible connective tissue disorder with increased risk of future autograft dilatation.

The evaluation of the pulmonary autograft is best done by transesophageal echocardiography. The pulmonary valve should be tricuspid without any degree of regurgitation. Another very important factor is the size of the pulmonary annulus and specifically the sinotubular junction; these structures should have normal diameters for the age of the patient. Pulmonary artery sinotubular junction size is the primary measure on which the matching (aortic annulus versus pulmonary sinotubular junction) is based. In case of size mismatch (i.e., aortic annulus 3 mm to 4 mm bigger than the pulmonary sinotubular junction) the aortic annulus is downsized. At the end of the procedure the autograft should be assessed for anatomy and valve competence. Persistent mild (1+) regurgitation will likely result in early progression and failure.

The ideal prosthesis for patients with aortic pathology not amenable to repair would be the one with a low structural deterioration rate, low rates of thromboembolic events without the necessity for anticoagulation, availability, high resistance to infection, and ease of implant. Such a device unfortunately is still not available, so when choosing the best prosthesis for the patient, one should balance the advantages and disadvantages of the different valves available.

Operative mortality is equivalent for all types of aortic valve replacements (AVR) (Table 29.1). With respect to bioprosthetic and allograft valves, the main advantage is that anticoagulation is not required, with thromboembolism rates and hemorrhage related to anticoagulation lower than that of mechanical valves (18–24). Another proposed advantage of the stentless valves (xenografts, homografts, and autografts) is superior hemodynamic performance (25–29). However, it is yet to be shown that lower postoperative transvalvular gradients translate into improved survival (27,30,31).

Biologic valves have an increased resistance to infection and are the valves of choice in patients with endocarditis. In patients with extensive aortic annular destruction, homograft root replacement is a very good option as it can exclude the abscess cavities from the circulation and reconstruct the left outflow tract (32–34). At the

## SELECTION OF VALVE PROSTHESIS

Ask 100 cardiologists, cardiac surgeons, and patients which valve is the most appropriate for a given situation and you will get 100 different answers. If possible, aortic valve repair should be considered the technique of choice for patients with isolated aortic regurgitation.

▶ **TABLE 29.1. Operative mortality and valve type**

| | |
|---|---|
| Stented xenografts | 2.5% to 8.0% |
| Stentless xenograft | 3.5% to 8.0% |
| Homografts | 3.0% to 6.0% |
| Mechanical prosthesis | 2.0% to 7.0% |
| Pulmonary autografts | 4.0% to 8.0% |

Cleveland Clinic Foundation, a homograft is the valve of choice for patients with native and prosthetic aortic valve endocarditis. Along with homografts, pulmonary autografts have also been demonstrated as a good alternative in endocarditis (34).

Limited durability is the major disadvantage of any bioprosthesis. The bulk of data shows that for patients over 65 years of age, a stented aortic bioprosthesis is a very good alternative. The follow-up is now extended for over 15 years and shows an 82% freedom from structural valve deterioration (18,21). Younger age and poor ventricular function (ejection fraction < 39%) were identified as independent predictors of structural valve deterioration (36). For children and young adults pulmonary autografts have become widely accepted as a good alternative for valve replacement, due to the potential for regeneration and growth (37,38).

Due to the excellent freedom from structural deterioration rate, mechanical valves are often considered a good choice when replacement is needed in patients between the ages of 30 and 60 (39–42). Unfortunately, due to the need for long-term anticoagulation, these valves are associated with more frequent bleeding and thromboembolic complications than biologic valves (Fig. 29.16) (20,40).

For patients under 30 years of age, a Ross procedure is probably the best operation. If performed by an experienced surgeon, this aortic valve replacement gives the patient the greatest chance of having a life without needing anticoagulation or another valve replacement. In addition the autograft has the potential to grow, which would be desirable in young patients (35).

Aortic homografts are a reasonable alternative in young patients, but there is data suggesting that younger patients are at increased risk for early structural valve deterioration (43–45). Bioprostheses have a similar problem in this age group, but reoperation for valve deterioration is much easier after a stented valve when compared to an autograft or an allograft.

Autografts, homografts, stented or stentless bioprostheses, and mechanical valves are all recommended by "experts" for patients between 40 and 60 years of age. A patient must weigh lifestyle considerations (skydiving, hunting, motor cross, etc.) against the risk of anticoagulation complications or the likelihood of structural valve deterioration and the need for reoperation.

The Cleveland Clinic Foundation favors aortic homografts in this age group and have lowered the age for using bioprosthesis AVR to patients younger than 60 years of age. The argument supporting this is that the mortality risk of a reoperation for bioprosthetic valve dysfunction is about 1%, which is better than the long-term risk of anticoagulation related hemorrhage and thromboembolism.

Over the age of 65 years old a stented bioprosthesis is the valve of choice for some. It is a quick and safe operation with the expectation of low morbidity and an infrequent need for replacement. However, controversy exists. Some surgeons feel that this valve is too small in larger patients and a transvalvular gradient is maintained, less left ventricular mass regression is obtained, and consequently lower survival when compared to stentless valve (22,27). Despite the knowledge that an increase in left ventricular mass predicts a higher incidence of death attributable to cardiovascular disease (46), and is associated with increased mortality in patients with AS and AI, it has not been shown conclusively that this lower gradient translates into better survival (47).

## CONCLUSION

In an effort to avoid the complications associated with mechanical valve prosthesis and long-term anticoagulation, valve repair, and valve replacement with biologic valves are the procedures of choice for aortic valve dysfunction. As such, a solid understanding of aortic valve and aortic root anatomy and function are required. A great deal of this understanding has come from echocardiographic analysis of aortic pathology after aortic replacement.

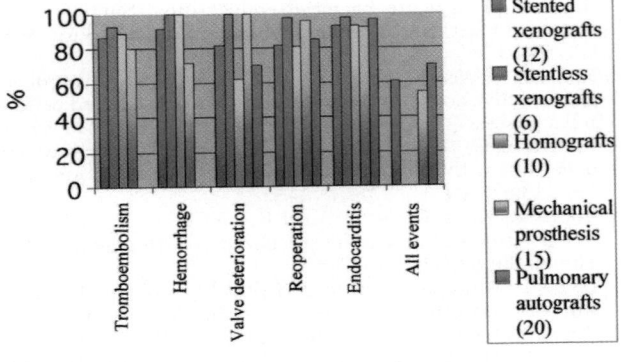

**( ) years of follow-up**

**FIGURE 29.16.** Freedom of events after aortic valve replacement.

### KEY POINTS

- Knowledge of aortic valve and root anatomy is critical to successful aortic valve repair and replacement.
- Valve repair techniques are applicable for prolapsing bicuspid and tricuspid leaflets and aortic root aneurysms.

- Sinotubular junction diameter is the most important measurement for the proper size selection of stentless valves.
- There is no perfect replacement valve.
- Biologic valves have the advantages of lower thromboembolism and anticoagulation related hemorrhage rates, but the disadvantage of decreased durability when compared to mechanical valves.

## REFERENCES

1. Hyatsville M. Monthly vital statistics report. National Center for Health Statistics. Report of final mortality statistics 1999;47(19).
2. Ionescu A, West R, Proudman C, Butchard E, Fraser A. Prospective study of routine perioperative transesophageal echocardiography for elective valve replacement: clinical impact and cost-saving implications. J Am Soc Echocardiogr 2001 Jul;14(7):659–67.
3. Guarracino F, Zussa C, Polesel E, Rigo F, Penzo D, De Cosmo D. Influence of transesophageal echocardiography on intraoperative decision making for Toronto stentless prosthetic valve implantation. J Heart Valve Dis 2001;10(1):31–4.
4. David T. Aortic valve repair for management of aortic insufficiency. Adv Card Surg 1999;11:19–59.
5. Ward C. Clinical significance of the bicuspid aortic valve. Heart 2000;83: 81–5.
6. Mohler E. Are atherosclerotic processes involved in aortic valve calcification? Lancet 2000;356(12):524–5.
7. Bonow R, Carabello B, de Leon A, et al. ACC/AHA guidelines for the management of patients with valvular heart disease: a report of the American College of Cardiology/American Heart Association Task Force on Practice Guidelines (Committee on Management of Patients with Valvular Heart Disease). J Am Coll Cardiol 1998;32:1486–588.
8. Leggett M, Otto C. Aortic valve disease. Curr Opin Cardiol 1996;11:120–25.
9. Otto C, Kuusisto J, Reichenbach D, Gown A, O'Brien K. Characterization of the early lesion of degenerative valvular aortic stenosis: histological and immunohistochemical studies. Circulation 1994;90:844–53.
10. Lee Y, Chou Y. Pathogenetic mechanism of senile calcific aortic stenosis: the role of apoptosis. Chin Med J 1998;111(10):934–9.
11. Rajamannan N, Sangiorgi G, Springett M, et al. Experimental hypercholesterolemia induces apoptosis in the aortic valve. J Heart Valve Dis 2001;10(3):371–74.
12. Roberts W, Morrow A, McIntosh C, Jone M, Epstein S. Congenitally bicuspid aortic valve causing severe, pure aortic regurgitation superimposed infective endocarditis. Analysis of 13 patients requiring aortic replacement. Am J Cardiol 1981;47(2):206–9.
13. Feindel C, David T. Heart valve surgery. Curr Opin Cardiol 1993;8(2):247–53.
14. Shapira N, Lemole G, Fernandez J, et al. Aortic valve repair for aortic stenosis in adults. Ann Thorac Surg 1990;50:110–20.
15. Cosgrove D, Rosenkranz E, Hendren W, Bartlett J, Stewart W. Valvuloplasty for aortic insufficiency. J Thorac Cardiovasc Surg 1991;102:571–7.
16. Sommers K, David T. Aortic valve replacement with patch enlargement of the aortic annulus. Ann Thorac Surg 1997;63(6):1608–12.
17. Bernal J, Martin-Duran R, Rabasa J, Revuelta J. The CarboMedics "Top Hat" supranuular prosthesis. Ann Thorac Surg 1999;67:1299–303.
18. Banbury M, Cosgrove D, Lytle B, Smedira N, Sabik J, Saunders C. Long-term results of the Carpentier-Edwards pericardial aortic valve: a 12-year follow-up. Ann Thorac Surg 1998;66:S73-6
19. Banbury M, Cosgrove D, White J, Blackstone E, Frater R, Okies J. Age and valve size effects on the long-term durability of the Carpentier-Edwards aortic pericardial bioprosthesis. Ann Thorac Surg 2001;72(3):753–7.
20. Hammermeister K, Gulshan K, Henderson W, Oprian C, Kim T, Rahimtoola S. A comparison of outcomes in men 11 years after heart valve replacement with mechanical valve or bioprosthesis. N Engl J Med 1993;328(18):1289–96.
21. Corbineau H, De La Tour B, Verhoye J, Langanay T, Lelong B, Leguerrier A. Carpentier-Edwards supraannular porcine bioprosthesis in aortic position: 16-year experience. Ann Thorac Surg 2001;71:S228-31.
22. David T. Aortic valve replacement with stentless porcine bioprosthesis. J Card Surg 1998;13(5):344–51.
23. Lytle B, Cosgrove D, Taylor P, et al. Primary isolated aortic valve replacement. Early and late results. J Thorac Cardiovasc Surg 1989;97:675–94.
24. Stein P, Alpert J, Dalen J, Horstkotte D, Turpie A. Antithrombotic therapy in patients with mechanical and biological prosthetic heart valves. Chest 1998;114(5 Suppl):602S– 10S.
25. Maselli D, Pizio R, DiBella I, De Gasperis C. Left ventricular mass reduction after aortic valve replacement: homografts, stentless and stented valves. Ann Thorac Surg 1999;67(4):966–71.
26. Pibarot P, Dumesnil J, Leblanc M, Cartier P, Metras J. Changes in left ventricular mass and function after aortic valve replacement: a comparison between stentless and stented bioprosthetic valves. J Am Soc Echocardiogr 1999;12(11):981–7.
27. Westaby S, Horton M, Jin X, et al. Survival advantages of stentless bioprosthesis. Ann Thorac Surg 2000;70:785–91.
28. Fries R, Wendler O, Schieffer H, Schafers H. Comparative rest and exercise hemodynamics of 23-mm stentless versus 23-mm stented aortic bioprosthesis. Ann Thorac Surg; 2000; 69:817–22.
29. Bah D, David T, Yacoub M, et al. Hemodynamics and left ventricular mass regression following implantation of the Toronto SPV stentless porcine valve. Am J Cardiol 1998;82(10):1214–19.
30. Park S, Reardon M. Current status of stentless aortic xenografts. Curr Opin Cardiol 2000;15(2):74–81.
31. Walther T, Falk V, Langebartels G, Kruger M, et al. Prospectively randomized evaluation of stentless versus conventional biological aortic valves. Impact on early regression of left ventricular hypertrophy. Circulation 1999;100(Suppl II):II6–II10.
32. Ergin M, Raissi S, Follis F, Lansman S, Griepp R. Annular destruction in acute bacterial endocarditis. Surgical techniques to meet the challenge. J Thorac Cardiovasc Surg 1989;97:755–63.
33. Knosalla C, Weng Y, Yankah A, et al. Surgical treatment of active infective aortic valve endocarditis with associated periannular abscess–11 year results. Eur Heart J 2000;21:490–97.
34. Pettersson G, Tingleff J, Joyce F. Treatment of aortic valve endocarditis with the Ross operation. Eur J Cardiothorac Surg 1998;13:678–84.
35. Elkins R, Knott-Craig C, Ward K, McCue C, Lane M. Pulmonary autograft in children: realized growth potential. Ann Thorac Surg 1994;57:1387–94.
36. David T, Ivanov J, Armstron S, Feindel C, Cohen G. Late results of heart valve replacement with the Hancock II bioprosthesis. J Thorac Cardiovasc Surg 2001;121(2): 268–78.
37. Elkins R. The Ross operation: a 12-year experience. Ann Thorac Surg 1999;68:S14–8.
38. Ross D, Jackson M, Davies J. Pulmonary autograft aortic valve replacement. Long-term results. J Cardiac Surg 1991;6 (Suppl 4):529–33.
39. Carrier M, Pellerin M, Perrault L, et al. Aortic valve replacement with mechanical and biological prosthesis in middle-aged patients. Ann Thorac Surg 2001;71:S253–6.

40. Peterseim D, Cen Y, Cheruvu S, et al. Long-term outcome after biologic versus mechanical aortic valve replacement in 841 patients. J Thorac Cardiovasc Surg 1999;117:890–7.
41. Li H, Hahn J, Urbanski P, Torka M, Grunkemeier G, Hacker R. Intermediate-term results with 1019 CarboMedics aortic valves. Ann Thorac Surg 2001;71:1181–87.
42. Zellner J, Kratz J, Crumbley A, et al. Long-term experience with the St. Jude Medical valve prosthesis. Ann Thorac Surg 1999;68:1210–8.
43. Yacoub M, Rasmi N, Sundt T, et al. Fourteen-year experience with homovital homografts for aortic valve replacement. J Thorac Cardiovasc Surg 1995;110:186–94.
44. Aklog L, Carr-White G, Birks E, Yacoub M. Pulmonary autograft versus aortic homograft for aortic valve replacement: interim results from a prospective randomized trial. J Heart Valve Dis 2000;9:176–89.
45. Lund O, Chandrasekaran V, Grocott-Mason R, et al. Primary aortic valve replacement with allografts over twenty-five years: valve-related and procedure-related determinants of outcome. J Thorac Cardiovasc Surg 1999;117(1):77–90; discussion 90–1.
46. Levy D, Garrison R, Savage D, Kannel W, Castelli W. Prognostic implications of echocardiographically determined left ventricular mass in the Framingham Heart Study. N Engl J Med 1990;322:1561–6.
47. Medalion B, Blackstone E, Lytle B, White J, Arnold J, Cosgrove D. Aortic valve replacement: is valve size important? J Thorac Cardiovasc Surg. 2000;119(5):963–74.

## QUESTIONS

1. What is the most common aortic valve lesion amenable to repair?
   A. Leaflet prolapse
   B. Ascending aortic enlargement
   C. Mixed regurgitation/stenosis
   D. Endocarditis

2. What is the advantage of the Ross operation (autograft) when compared to the aortic homograft (allograft)?
   A. Greater resistance to infection
   B. Shorter cross clamp times
   C. Ease of insertion
   D. Potential for growth

3. What is the most important measurement to select the proper size stentless valve?
   A. Aortic annulus
   B. Sinus of Valsalva
   C. Sinotubular junction
   D. Proximal ascending aorta

# Chapter 30

# Assessment in Aortic Valve Surgery

*Christopher A. Troianos*
*Questions and answers: Lori B. Heller*

Intraoperative echocardiography during aortic valve surgery provides critical information for surgical decision-making and hemodynamic management. Transesophageal echocardiography (TEE) provides high-resolution images of the aortic valve due to the close proximity of the valve to the esophagus. Evaluation of leaflet morphology and mobility, degree of calcification, aortic root disease, and etiology of valve dysfunction are important aspects of two-dimensional evaluation. Accurate determination of valve and aortic root dimensions is important for guiding therapy and choosing the type and size of a prosthesis to implant. Postoperative assessment identifies complications associated with repair or replacement, and prompts surgical intervention to correct inadequate valve repair and reoperation for complications. Clinical information provided by TEE permits appropriate hemodynamic management for patients with aortic valve disease, which is particularly important in patients with manifestation of chronic disease, whether they have stenosis, regurgitation, or both. The application of Doppler echocardiography (pulsed wave, continuous wave, and color), with two-dimensional imaging allows for the complete evaluation of stenotic and regurgitant lesions (discussed in detail in Chapter 15, Assessment of the Aortic Valve). This current chapter reviews the transesophageal echocardiographic anatomy, aortic valve disease pathophysiology, and echocardiographic evaluation of the aortic valve, with particular emphasis on critical issues that arise during aortic valve surgery. Indications for evaluation, implications for surgical intervention, and associated cardiovascular lesions are also discussed.

## CRITICAL ISSUES DURING AORTIC VALVE SURGERY

Echocardiography provides essential information in the evaluation of patients with aortic valve disease. Intraoperative echocardiography is used to confirm the pre-

operative diagnosis, determine the feasibility of repair versus replacement, measure the size of valve to be implanted, and evaluate the implanted or repaired valve for complications. Preoperative valve sizing is important when valves of limited availability, such as homografts, are to be implanted (1). For patients undergoing aortic valve replacement for aortic stenosis, intraoperative TEE has been shown to alter the surgical plan in 13% of patients (Table 30.1) (2). The patient with mild to moderate aortic valve disease scheduled for nonaortic valve cardiac surgery, as well as the patient with previously unsuspected aortic valve disease present clinical dilemmas. TEE assists with this intraoperative decision making. The size of the annulus must be considered when deciding whether a valve with only moderate stenosis should be replaced. Patients with small annular diameters may not derive as significant a benefit from aortic valve replacement as patients in whom a larger valve could be implanted. The issue of whether or not to intervene in patients with mild to moderate disease is more important

▶ TABLE 30.1. Impact of Intraoperative TEE during Aortic Valve Replacement in 383 Patients (2)

| New findings before bypass | Surgical impact |
| --- | --- |
| 7 PFO | 2 closed |
| 2 masses (TV fibroelastoma, LVOT accessory chordae) | 2 removed |
| 5 LAA thrombi | 5 removed |
| 10 homograft annular size measurements | 10 sized |

| New findings after bypass | Surgical impact |
| --- | --- |
| 1 new wall motion abnormality | No change |

*PFO*, patent foramen ovale; *LAA*, left atrial appendage; *TV*, tricuspid valve; *LVOT*, left ventricular outflow obstruction. From Nowrangi SK, et al. J Am Soc Echocardiogr 2001;14:863–6.

for patients with stenosis rather than regurgitation, because of the higher mortality associated with reoperation in patients with aortic stenosis who have had previous coronary artery bypass grafting (CABG) (3). Finally, intraoperative echocardiography is used to differentiate aortic valve disease from other causes that produce a gradient between the left ventricle and aorta, such as hypertrophic obstructive cardiomyopathy and supravalvular stenosis.

## Role of TEE in Surgical Decision-Making

Intraoperative TEE among patients with known aortic valve disease undergoing valve replacement is used to confirm the preoperative diagnosis and determine the etiology of valve dysfunction. High-resolution images, owing to the close proximity of the valve and the esophagus, permit accurate diagnosis of the mechanism of valve dysfunction, a key aspect for determining the feasibility of repair versus replacement. The vast majority of aortic valves suitable for repair have regurgitant lesions rather than stenotic lesions. Valve repair for patients with aortic dissection involves resuspension of the cusps, and is easily performed and highly successful in the absence of additional leaflet pathology.

Postoperatively, TEE is used to evaluate the success of repair or function of the prosthetic valve. The degree of residual aortic regurgitation is an important aspect of valve repair evaluation and determines the need for further surgery and possible valve replacement. The number and area of regurgitant jets present after aortic valve replacement are less than after mitral valve replacement, but there is a similar percentage decrease of regurgitant jet area after protamine administration (4a). Patients undergoing the Ross procedure for autograft replacement of their aortic valve also require evaluation of the prosthetic pulmonic valve.

TEE is important for guiding hemodynamic therapy during aortic valve surgery. An accurate evaluation of left ventricular function is important during the immediate postoperative period because of the inherently low ventricular compliance present among patients with left ventricular hypertrophy, due to long-standing aortic stenosis or chronic hypertension. Left ventricular volume is more accurately determined by two-dimensional echocardiographic assessment of LV cross-sectional area than by filling pressures measured with a pulmonary artery catheter (4b). Characteristically, patients with low LV compliance often require volume infusion despite high filling pressures in the postbypass period. Clinical information provided by TEE permits appropriate hemodynamic management for patients with aortic valve disease before, during, and after aortic valve surgery.

## APPROACH

### Focused Intraoperative Echocardiography Exam

A focused intraoperative echocardiography exam is a brief pointed assessment on the anatomy and function most pertinent to the surgeon. For patients in whom the preoperative diagnosis of aortic valve disease is confirmed and well established, this usually entails a verification of the preoperative findings including the elucidation of the etiology of valve dysfunction, an estimation of valve size, and an assessment of associated findings. For patients with severe aortic stenosis, the diagnosis is confirmed simply by a two-dimensional echocardiographic evaluation of the valve, utilizing the midesophageal aortic valve short-axis view (Fig. 30.1). The valve appears severely restricted and heavily calcified. This aortic valve short-axis view is developed at the midesophageal level by rotating the transducer forward 30° to 60° and anteflexing the probe. This view is important for tracing the aortic valve orifice area, using planimetry, and for identifying the site of aortic regurgitation using color flow Doppler. Rotating the multiplane angle forward to 110° to 150° develops the midesophageal aortic valve long-axis (ME AV LAX) view (Fig. 30.2). This view provides imaging of the left ventricular outflow tract, aortic valve, and aortic root and allows differentiation of valvular from subvalvular and supravalvular pathology.

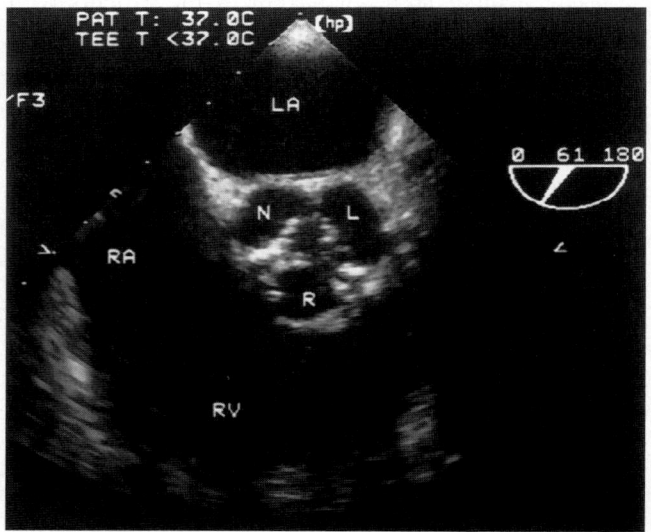

**FIGURE 30.1.** Transesophageal echocardiogram of the midesophageal aortic valve short-axis view during systole in a patient with aortic stenosis. *L, R,* and *N,* left, right, and noncoronary aortic valve cusps, respectively; *LA,* left atrium; *RA,* right atrium; *RV,* right ventricle.

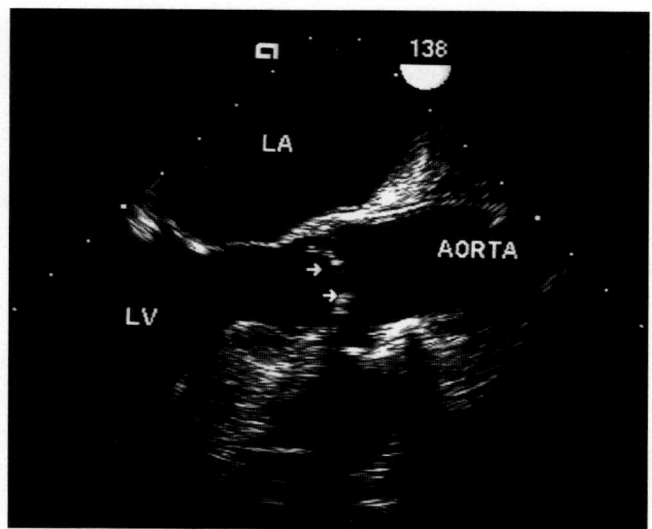

**FIGURE 30.2.** Transesophageal echocardiogram of the midesophageal aortic valve long-axis view during systole in a patient with aortic stenosis. A multiplane probe at 138° provided this view of an aortic valve with doming leaflets (*arrows*). Leaflet doming is a qualitative sign of stenosis. The proximal ascending aorta is also imaged in this view. *LA,* left atrium; *LV,* left ventricle.

Quantifying the severity of stenosis by either gradient or area determination is usually not necessary during the focused exam of a patient whose diagnosis of aortic stenosis was firmly established preoperatively, but is often included in a more comprehensive exam. Area determination by planimetry in patients with severe aortic stenosis may be difficult to perform due to shadowing of the valve by the heavy calcification. Area determination with the continuity equation in patients with severe stenosis is of benefit to the novice echocardiographer who requires practice in obtaining the transgastric views necessary for measuring aortic valve flow. A peak velocity measurement provides some indication of the severity of stenosis, but must be taken in the context of the left ventricular function.

A focused exam in patients with severe aortic regurgitation undergoing aortic valve surgery involves a two-dimensional echocardiographic evaluation to determine the etiology of the regurgitation (leaflets vs. aortic root) and a color flow Doppler interrogation of the left ventricular outflow tract to evaluate the severity of the regurgitation. The etiology directs the surgeon as to the feasibility of repair versus replacement, and the techniques to be employed for repair. The postoperative assessment is important for ascertaining the success of the repair. The degree of residual aortic regurgitation is an essential aspect of valve repair evaluation and determines the need for further revisions or possible valve replacement.

For patients undergoing valve replacement, another aspect of the focused exam is determination of valve size and suitability of the implantation of specific valve types. The midesophageal aortic valve long-axis view is used to measure annular diameter and size of the aortic root. A size discrepancy of greater than 10% between the diameters of the aortic annulus and sinotubular junction makes implantation of a stentless aortic valve unfeasible. The points at which the measurements are made are indicated in Fig. 30.3. The annular diameter measurement is the size used for implantation of mechanical and stented bioprosthetic valves, while the sinotubular junction diameter is the size used for implantation of stentless aortic valves.

## Comprehensive Intraoperative Echo Exam

An accurate, comprehensive intraoperative echocardiography examination is paramount to the surgical decision-making process, particularly in patients in whom the severity of disease is borderline or moderate. The intraoperative echocardiography exam in these situations should utilize the full diagnostic potential of this tool and be performed by echocardiographers with advanced training (5). More than one method should be employed to assess the severity of disease, because the assessment will be used to guide the surgical decision. The severity of aortic stenosis can be determined by two-dimensional echocardiography, gradient determination by measurement of transaortic velocity, and area determination by planimetry and the continuity equation.

Hemodynamic assessment of antegrade and retrograde aortic valve flow requires a parallel orientation of

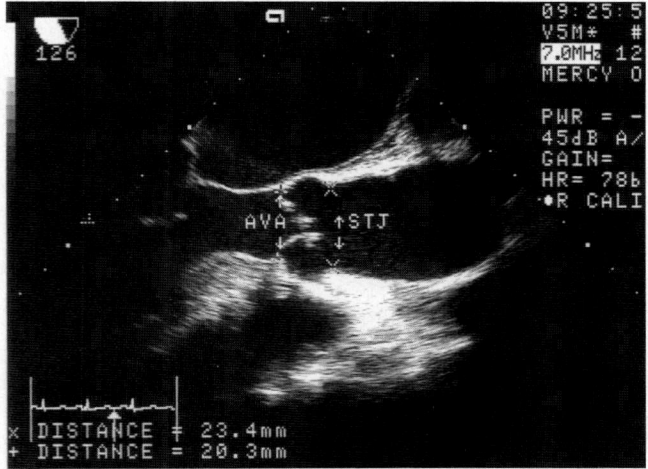

**FIGURE 30.3.** Transesophageal echocardiogram of the midesophageal aortic valve long-axis view indicating where measurements are made of the aortic valve annulus (*AVA*) and sinotubular junction (*STJ*) diameters.

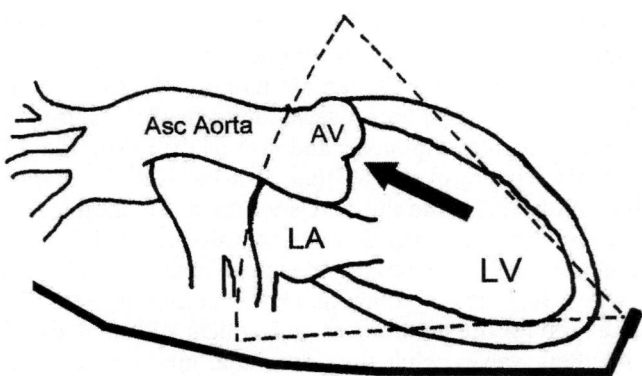

**FIGURE 30.4.** Illustration of the TEE probe position for the deep transgastric view of the aortic valve that allows a parallel orientation of blood flow through the aortic valve (*AV*) and left ventricular outflow tract (*arrow*). *LA*, left atrium; *LV*, left ventricle; *Asc*, ascending. From Troianos CA. Aortic valve. In: Konstadt SN, Shernan S, and Oka Y, eds. Clinical transesophageal echocardiography: a problem-oriented approach, 2nd ed., Philadelphia: Lippincott, Williams & Wilkins with permission.

blood flow and the Doppler beam (Fig. 30.4). The midesophageal views used for two-dimensional evaluation are inadequate for this assessment because blood flow in these windows is perpendicular to the Doppler beam. Conversely, the two transgastric views are more useful for interrogating flow across the aortic valve, but not as useful for detailed two-dimensional anatomic assessment due to the far field position of the aortic valve. The *deep* transgastric long-axis (deep TG LAX) view is developed from the transgastric midshort-axis view by advancing the probe past the midpapillary window, then gently withdrawing the probe with slight anteflexion and leftward flexion until the aortic valve is viewed in the middle or left side of the image in the far field (Fig. 30.5). The trans-

gastric long-axis (TG LAX) view is developed from the transgastric midshort-axis view by rotating the transducer forward from 0° to 90° to 120° until the aortic valve is viewed on the right side of the image in the far field (Fig. 30.6). Either one or both of the transgastric views can be used to measure the velocity of blood flow through the aortic valve and left ventricular outflow tract because of the parallel orientation of transaortic blood flow and the Doppler beam. It is important for the echocardiographer to become familiar with both approaches, because these views are often difficult to obtain and require considerable practice and expertise. Stoddard et al. demonstrated 56% feasibility among the first 43 patients studied as compared to 88% feasibility among the latter 43 patients studied, suggesting a significant learning curve in measuring aortic valve blood flow velocity via the transgastric approach (6). Data obtained intraoperatively is compared to preoperative assessment, and intraoperative surgical inspection of the valve can be used as a gauge of accuracy in aortic valve evaluation.

A common clinical dilemma facing clinicians who care for cardiac surgical patients is the patient with coronary artery disease (CAD) requiring coronary artery bypass grafting (CABG), who is found to have moderate aortic stenosis. Accepted practice for patients undergoing CABG with severe aortic stenosis (valve area < 1.0 cm$^2$ and gradient > 40 mm Hg) is for combined aortic valve replacement (AVR) and CABG. Conversely, the consensus is CABG only for patients with CAD and mild aortic stenosis [aortic valve area (AVA) > 1.5 cm$^2$ and aortic valve gradient (AVG) < 25 mm Hg]. Patients with moderate aortic stenosis (AVA of 1.0–1.5 cm$^2$ and AVG of 25–40 mm Hg) undergoing CABG present a clinical controversy. Should

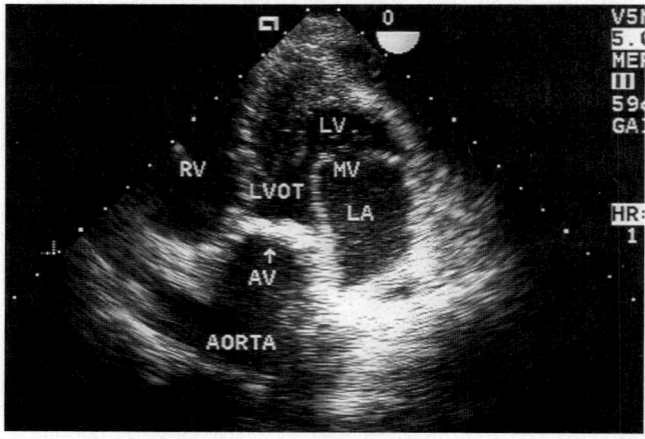

**FIGURE 30.5.** Transesophageal echocardiogram of the deep transgastric view. *AV*, aortic valve; *LA*, left atrium; *LV*, left ventricle; *LVOT*, left ventricular outflow tract; *AORTA*, ascending aorta; *MV*, mitral valve; *RV*, right ventricle.

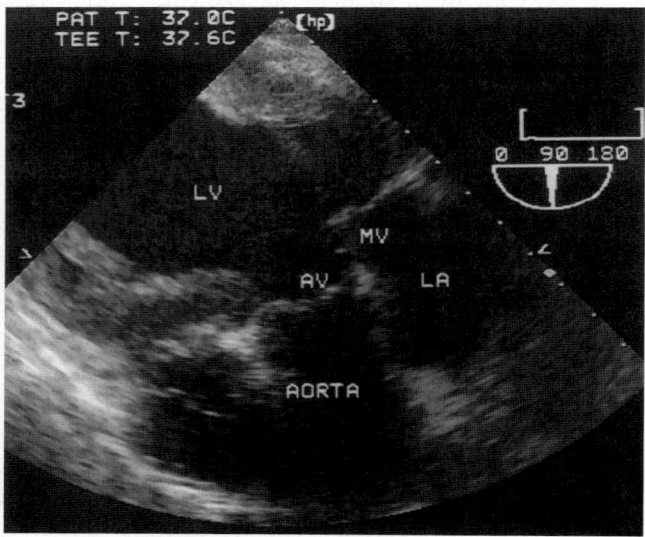

**FIGURE 30.6.** Transesophageal echocardiogram of the transgastric long-axis view. *AV*, aortic valve; *AORTA*, aortic root; *LA*, left atrium; *MV*, mitral valve; *LV*, left ventricle.

the patient with moderate aortic stenosis undergoing CABG have CABG alone or combined AVR and CABG?

The dilemma exists in patients with aortic stenosis that is not severe and often asymptomatic. These patients would not be candidates for AVR based on the severity of aortic stenosis alone, but because they are undergoing CABG surgery, consideration is made for concomitant aortic valve replacement. Aortic valve replacement after previous coronary artery bypass grafting is associated with higher mortality than combined aortic valve and coronary bypass surgery (7). It is therefore important to identify even moderate aortic stenosis during coronary bypass surgery and consider combination surgery to avoid the higher mortality associated with reoperation.

The degree of aortic stenosis is important for surgical management, because valves with a smaller valve area will progress more rapidly to cause symptoms related to aortic stenosis. The aortic valve short-axis view allows measurement of aortic valve orifice area by two-dimensional planimetry, which provides good correlation with other methods used for assessment of aortic stenosis (8). The probe is manipulated to provide the image with the smallest orifice to ensure that the cross section is of the leaflet tips. A cross section that is oblique or inferior to the leaflet tips overestimates the orifice size. The valve appears circular in a true short-axis cross section with all three cusps being viewed simultaneously and equal in shape. Multiplane TEE simplifies the location of the actual orifice by imaging the aortic valve, first in long axis to identify the smallest orifice at the leaflet tips. The orifice is centered on the image display screen and the trans-

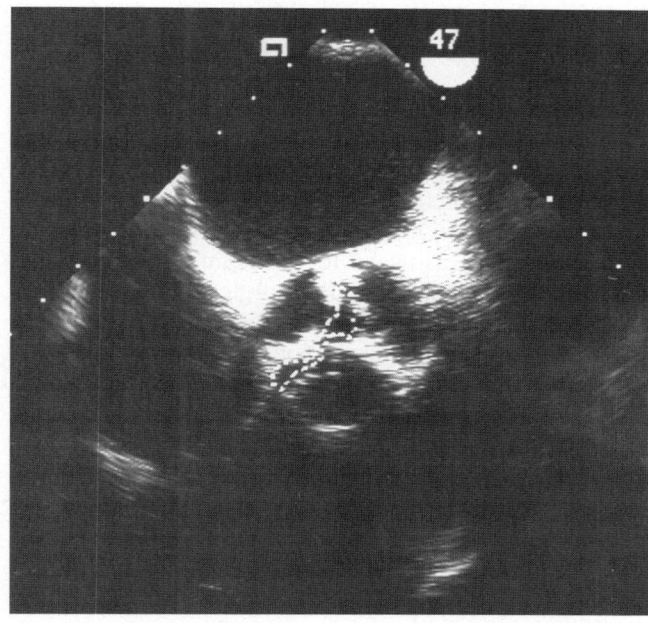

**FIGURE 30.8.** Transesophageal echocardiogram of the midesophageal aortic valve short-axis view during systole in a patient with aortic stenosis, using planimetry to measure aortic valve area.

ducer position is stabilized within the esophagus as the multiplane angle is rotated backward to the short-axis view. The smallest orifice is traced and the two-dimensional cross-sectional area is displayed (Fig. 30.8). Limitations to planimetry are:

1. Inability to obtain an adequate short-axis view
2. Heavy calcification (particularly posterior), which causes shadowing of the valve
3. The presence of "pinhole" aortic stenosis, in which the valve orifice cannot be identified

The presence of these elements suggests advanced disease or the likelihood of rapid progression of aortic stenosis, and favors a decision to replace the valve during concomitant CABG surgery.

Intraoperative echocardiography is not only critical in the evaluation of the aortic valve, but in the evaluation of cardiac and vascular structures that are affected by the techniques employed during aortic valve surgery. Evaluation of left ventricular function is important, because patients with aortic stenosis develop left ventricular hypertrophy, decreased left ventricular compliance, and are prone to myocardial ischemia. TEE provides early indication of myocardial ischemia through monitoring of regional wall motion, and a global assessment of overall contractility and volume loading. Patients with aortic stenosis have decreased left ventricular compliance; therefore assessment of preload using pulmonary artery catheter data often provides misleading information.

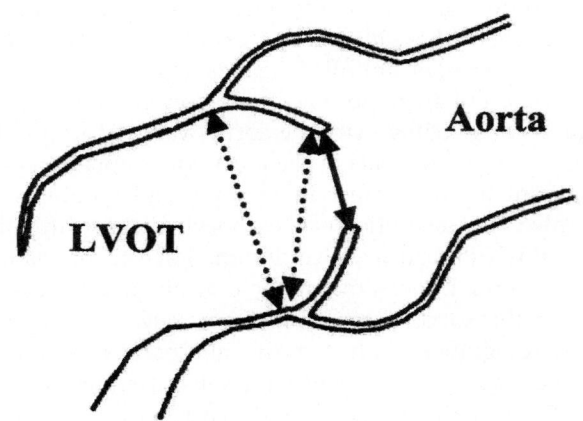

**FIGURE 30.7.** Illustration of various cross-sections that may be used to perform planimetry measurements of aortic valve orifice size. The *solid line* indicates the correct cross section at the tips of the aortic cusps. The two *dotted lines* indicate an oblique cross section and a cross section that is inferior to the leaflet tips. Both would result in an overestimation of aortic valve orifice size. From Troianos CA. Perioperative echocardiography. In Troianos CA, ed. Anesthesia for the cardiac patient. St. Louis: Mosby; 2002;155, with permission.

TEE provides a more accurate assessment of preload by thorough imaging of intracavitary volume and global contractility.

Patients with aortic valve disease develop diastolic dysfunction, which also can be evaluated and monitored with intraoperative echocardiography. Long-standing left ventricular dysfunction leads to mitral regurgitation, pulmonary hypertension, and ultimately right ventricular dysfunction. TEE is useful for managing these problems intraoperatively and for guiding surgical management decisions about the need for cardiac surgical intervention. For example, mitral regurgitation secondary to increased left ventricular systolic pressure from aortic stenosis will likely improve with aortic valve replacement. However, intrinsic mitral valve disease or mitral regurgitation due to hypertrophic obstructive cardiomyopathy may not improve after aortic valve replacement, and may in fact worsen.

Dilation of the ascending aorta may be a consequence of long-standing aortic stenosis due to the body's adaptive mechanism in promoting left ventricular ejection, or may be secondary to intrinsic disease within the aortic walls. The latter is more likely to require surgical intervention, while the former does not require surgical correction unless the dilation is severe. Evaluation of the aorta is also important for determining the cannulation site and for guiding perfusion strategies, in addition to identifying atheromatous disease in the proximal ascending aorta, implicated as a leading cause of neurologic injury.

Postoperatively, the comprehensive examination is focused on the function of the prosthetic valve, postimplant complications, and resolution of dynamic lesions not surgically addressed. Postbypass echocardiography is particularly important for patients undergoing valve repair to assess the success of repair. The presence of aortic regurgitation after aortic valve repair is a poor prognostic indicator, as these patients commonly require reoperation for definitive correction.

## AORTIC VALVE APPARATUS

Understanding the role of intraoperative echocardiography in aortic valve surgery requires knowledge of the anatomy and function of the aortic valve apparatus. The leaflets and the supporting and surrounding structures constitute the aortic valve apparatus (Fig. 30.9). Akin to the mitral valve apparatus being comprised of chordae tendineae, papillary muscles, and the annulus, the aortic valve apparatus is comprised of the valve cusps, the sinuses of Valsalva, the proximal ascending aorta, and the left ventricular outflow tract. Abnormalities involving any of these structures can lead to aortic valve dysfunction. Proximal to the aortic valve, the left ventricular outflow tract consists of the inferior surface of the anterior mitral

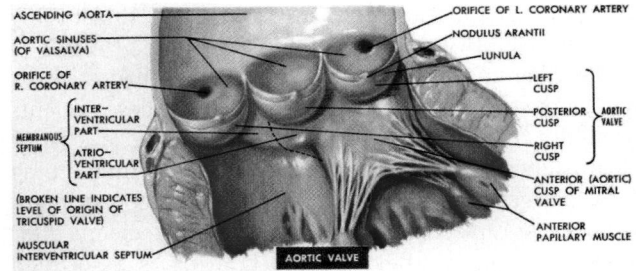

**FIGURE 30.9.** Illustration of the aortic valve apparatus consisting of three leaflets, left ventricular outflow tract, ascending aorta, and annulus. The lunula on each leaflet provides overlap during coaptation and serves to distribute stress from the leaflets to the commissures. From Netter FH. Heart (Vol. 5):12. In Netter FH. The Ciba collection of medical illustrations, New York: Ciba Pharmaceutical Company 1978, with permission.

leaflet, the ventricular septum, and the posterior left ventricular free wall.

The pressure drop across the aortic valve during diastole generates considerable stress within the leaflets. An intact apparatus allows distribution of this stress from the leaflets to the surrounding fibrous structure to which the leaflets are attached (9). The leaflets are also supported by one another along the region of coaptation on the leaflet called the lunula (Fig. 30.9). The stress is then distributed along the leaflet edges to corners of the commissures (9). Further stress reduction occurs through distribution of stress to the sinuses of Valsalva, which are three bulges or pouch-like dilations in the aortic wall associated with each leaflet (Fig. 30.9). The radius of curvature within these bulges in the aortic wall decreases between systole and diastole to accommodate the stress in accordance with LaPlace's law (9,10). The sinuses not only play an important role in leaflet closure by distributing stress, but their presence also prevents the leaflets from making contact with the aortic wall during systole. All of these components of the aortic valve apparatus are important for the proper functioning and durability of the valve. Any disruption of these mechanisms within the apparatus will lead to valve dysfunction and premature deterioration. Understanding these mechanisms is essential for the surgeon repairing these valves and to the echocardiographer who must interpret echocardiographic findings associated with valve dysfunction and communicate these findings to the surgeon.

A normal aortic valve appears as two thin lines that open parallel to the aortic walls in the midesophageal aortic valve long-axis (ME AV LAX) view. This view also provides imaging of the ascending aorta and LVOT (Fig. 30.10) and provides valuable insight into the function of the aortic valve apparatus. With atrial contraction and left ventricular filling during late diastole, a 12% expansion of the aortic root is observed 20 to 40 milliseconds prior to

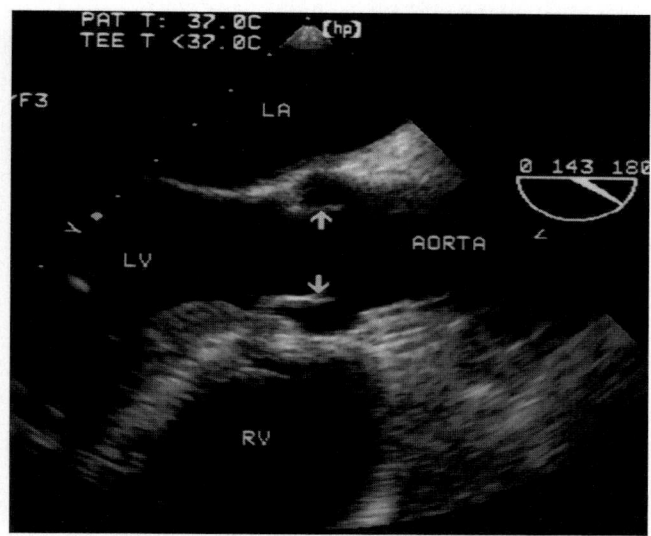

**FIGURE 30.10.** Transesophageal echocardiogram of the midesophageal aortic valve long-axis view during systole. A multiplane probe at 143° provided this view of a normal aortic valve with leaflets (*arrows*) that open parallel to the aortic walls. The proximal ascending aorta is also imaged in this view. *LA,* left atrium; *LV,* left ventricle; *RV,* right ventricle.

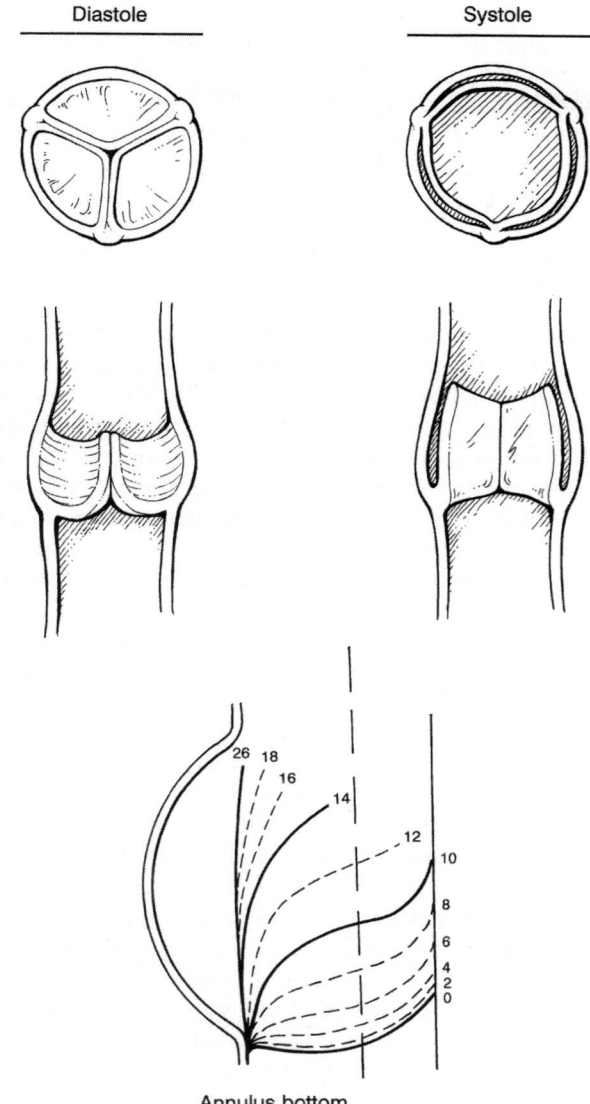

**FIGURE 30.11.** Positions of the aortic valve leaflets at end diastole and end systole and of a single leaflet in profile during ejection as the leaflet moves from the closed position (0) to fully opened (26). Note how the fully opened leaflet tends to produce a uniform diameter above the ventricular-arterial junction. From Mihaljevic T, Paul S, Cohn LH, Wechsler A. Pathophysiology of aortic valve disease. In Cohn LH, Edmunds LH Jr, eds. Cardiac surgery in the adult. New York: McGraw-Hill, 2003: 791–810, with permission.

aortic valve opening (9,11,12). Dilation of the aortic root alone contributes 20% to leaflet opening (9). The effect of this aortic root dilation actually causes the leaflets to open before any positive pressure from ventricular contraction is applied (9,13). As previously mentioned, leaflet stress during diastole is distributed along the leaflet edges, to the commissures, and to the aortic root. Just before the onset of systole, with no tension within the leaflets and the aortic root dilated, the leaflets open rapidly with the onset of ventricular contraction, offering minimal resistance to left ventricular ejection (9,14).

The sinuses of Valsalva play an important role during systole, allowing the leaflets to fully open without making contact with the aortic wall. In addition, because a space is maintained between the leaflets and the aortic wall, the leaflets rapidly close at the onset of diastole (Fig. 30.11). The sinuses provide a reservoir of blood for developing vortices that move toward the ventricular arterial junction as the velocity of blood flow declines during systole (9). These vortices within the sinuses of Valsalva prime the leaflets for closure, so that as soon as the pressure between the ventricle and aorta equalizes, the leaflets rapidly close.

## PATHOLOGY

### Pathophysiology of Aortic Stenosis

The most frequent causes of aortic stenosis are calcific stenosis in the elderly, rheumatic valvulitis, and congeni-

tal anomalies (bicuspid, rarely unicuspid) that lead to accelerated leaflet calcification and restriction. The mechanism of stenosis occurs from calcification of the leaflets (calcific, rheumatic, or congenital) or commissural fusion (usually rheumatic). Subaortic stenosis (subaortic membrane or ridge, and asymmetric septal hypertrophy) and supravalvular stenosis (narrowed aortic root) mimic aortic stenosis, but do not represent true valvular stenosis.

Many of the echocardiographic techniques used for hemodynamic assessment of the aortic valve, however, can also be used to evaluate the severity of subvalvular and supravalvular pathology. Asymmetric septal hypertrophy or hypertrophic obstructive cardiomyopathy is further discussed in Chapter 15.

## Echocardiographic Evaluation of Aortic Stenosis

An important sign of aortic stenosis is leaflet doming during systole observed in the midesophageal long-axis view with two-dimensional echocardiography (Fig. 30.2). The leaflets are curved toward the midline of the aorta instead of parallel to the aortic wall. Leaflet doming is such an important observation that this finding alone is sufficient for the qualitative diagnosis of aortic stenosis. Coincident with doming is reduced leaflet separation (< 15 mm), which is appreciated in both the short- and long-axis views of the aortic valve. The short-axis view of the aortic valve (Fig. 30.1) permits evaluation of leaflet motion and calcification, commissural fusion, and leaflet coaptation. This short-axis view (30° to 60°) is used for measuring the aortic valve orifice area by two-dimensional planimetry, which provides good correlation with other methods used for assessment of aortic stenosis (8). The probe is manipulated to provide the image with the smallest valvular cross-sectional area to ensure that the imaging plane is at the level of the leaflet tips or smallest orifice.

The two-dimensional evaluation of the aortic valve is usually sufficient to confirm the diagnosis of aortic stenosis. Patients with a diagnosis of moderate aortic stenosis, who are not predetermined to undergo an aortic valve replacement, require more sophisticated evaluation of their aortic valve disease. Doppler echocardiography is used to quantitate the severity of aortic stenosis by measuring transvalvular blood velocity. The peak pressure gradient is estimated from the peak velocity measurement using the modified Bernoulli equation:

$$\text{Aortic Valve Gradient} = 4 \times (\text{Aortic Valve Velocity})^2$$

The deep TG LAX view is used to direct the ultrasound beam in a parallel alignment with blood flow in the LVOT and through the aortic valve (Fig. 30.5). A parallel alignment of the ultrasound beam and aortic valve flow can also be obtained with the TG LAX view (Fig. 30.6).

The continuous wave Doppler cursor is aligned with the narrow, turbulent, high-velocity jet and the spectral Doppler display is activated. Accurate localization provides a distinctive audible sound and high-velocity (> 3 m/sec) spectral Doppler recording that exhibits a fine feathery appearance and a midsystolic peak (Fig. 30.12).

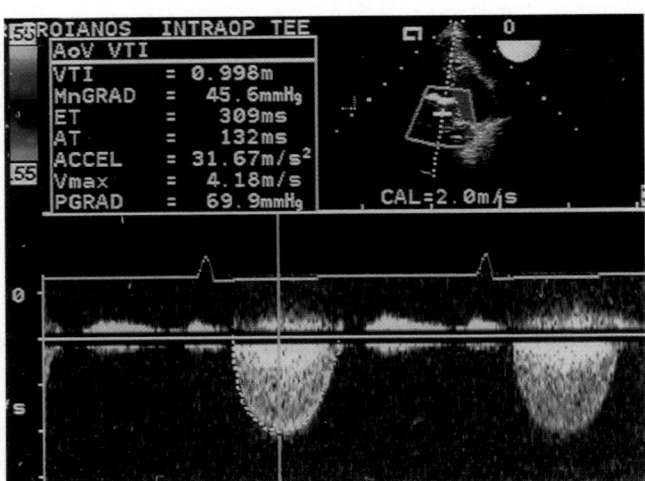

**FIGURE 30.12.** Continuous wave spectral Doppler velocities through a stenotic aortic valve. The fine, feathery appearance of the high (4.18 m/sec) velocities with a midsystolic peak indicates flow through a stenotic aortic valve. The denser lower velocities near the baseline indicate flow through the left ventricular outflow tract.

Planimetry of the velocity over time spectral Doppler analysis of transaortic blood flow yields the velocity time integral (VTI) and an estimate of mean aortic valve gradient.

A gradient across a stenotic orifice is dynamic because of its dependence on flow. As the flow (or cardiac output) through the valve decreases, the gradient also decreases. Conversely, as flow or the force of contraction increases, the gradient also increases. It is important to correctly identify the origin of the gradient between the left ventricle and aorta as either valvular, subvalvular, or supravalvular based upon two-dimensional imaging. The shape of the spectral Doppler display differs depending on the etiology of the outflow obstruction. Aortic stenosis produces a rounded pattern with a midsystolic peak (Fig. 30.12), while LVOT obstruction produces a "dagger-shaped" pattern. Limitations to assessing the severity of stenosis by transvalvular velocity measurement are listed in Table 30.2.

Valve area is considered a more constant and less dynamic assessment of aortic stenosis, but the more pliable (moderately stenotic, nonrheumatic) valves may open more with increased contractility (15). The continuity equation is used for calculation of valve area, based on the assumption that blood flowing through sequential areas of a continuous, intact, vascular system must be equal. Blood flowing through the LVOT is thus equated with blood flow through the aortic valve.

$$\text{Aortic Valve}_{\text{BLOOD FLOW}} = \text{LVOT}_{\text{BLOOD FLOW}}$$

▶ TABLE 30.2. **Limitations to Assessing the Severity of Aortic Stenosis by Transvalvular Velocity Measurement**

| Etiology of limitation | Consequence |
|---|---|
| Decreased transvalvular flow | |
|   Severe LV dysfunction | |
|   Severe mitral regurgitation | Decreased pressure gradient |
|   Left-to-right intracardiac shunt | |
|   Low cardiac output | |
| Increased transvalvular flow | |
|   Hyperdynamic LV function | |
|   Sepsis | Increased pressure gradient |
|   Hyperthyroidism | |

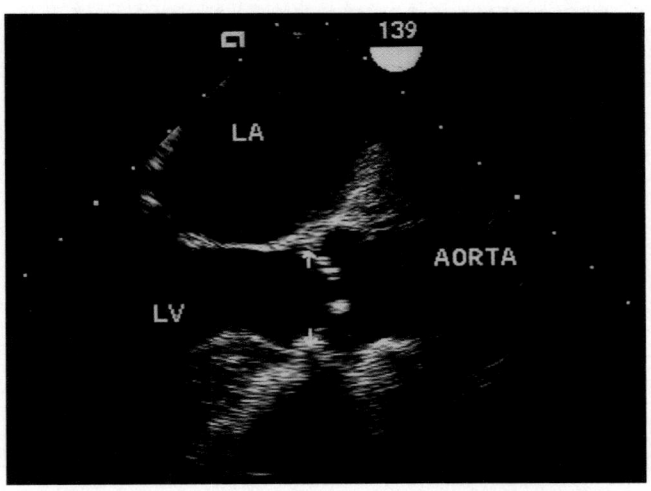

**FIGURE 30.13.** Transesophageal echocardiogram of the midesophageal aortic valve long-axis view during systole, indicating the site of measurement of the left ventricular outflow tract diameter (*arrows*). *LA*, left atrium; *LV*, left ventricle.

Substitution of blood flow with the product of velocity (VTI) and cross-sectional area yields:

$$\text{Aortic Valve Area} \times \text{Aortic Valve}_{VTI} = \text{LVOT}_{AREA} \times \text{LVOT}_{VTI}$$

Aortic valve area is then calculated as:

$$\text{Aortic Valve Area} = \frac{\text{LVOT}_{AREA} \times \text{LVOT}_{VTI}}{\text{Aortic Valve}_{VTI}}$$

$\text{LVOT}_{VTI}$ is measured by placing the pulsed wave Doppler sample volume in the LVOT just inferior to the aortic valve, and tracing the spectral Doppler velocity over time. $\text{LVOT}_{AREA}$ is determined by using the midesophageal aortic valve long-axis view and by measuring the LVOT diameter (d) near the aortic valve annulus (Fig. 30.13) to correspond to the same anatomic location as the pulsed wave Doppler recording of LVOT velocity. $\text{LVOT}_{AREA}$ is calculated by assuming the LVOT is circular. Using the formula

$$\text{AREA} = \pi \times (d/2)2. \ \text{LVOT}_{AREA}$$

provides the greatest source of error in the continuity equation because measurements of LVOT diameter are squared to calculate $\text{LVOT}_{AREA}$.

It is imperative to measure VTI for the aortic valve and LVOT using the same cardiac beat in patients with irregular cardiac rhythms. Instead of using pulsed wave Doppler to measure LVOT velocity, the $\text{LVOT}_{VTI}$ is traced from the aortic valve continuous wave spectral Doppler display. This "double envelope" technique (16) circumvents the problem of different stroke volumes for different beats, but can also be used for patients with a regular rhythm. An alternative to measuring aortic valve and LVOT VTI from the same cardiac beat in patients with an irregular rhythm is to measure aortic valve and LVOT VTI of several (seven or more) cardiac beats and taking the average VTI for each in calculation of aortic valve area.

Stroke volume affects the calculation of aortic valve area, even in patients with a regular sinus rhythm. Use of dobutamine to induce a larger stroke volume yields a slighter larger area that is related to the continuity equation rather than an actual change in valve area (17,18). Limitations to determination of aortic valve area by the continuity equation are summarized in Table 30.3.

▶ TABLE 30.3. **Limitations to Determination of Aortic Valve Area by the Continuity Equation**

| Limitation | Etiology | Consequence |
|---|---|---|
| Inadequate transgastric view | Patient anatomy | Inability to position Doppler beam parallel to high velocity jet for velocity measurements |
| Inability to identify high velocity jet | Pinhole aortic stenosis | Inability to measure transvalvular flow |
| Inability to measure an accurate LVOT diameter | Anatomic relation between LVOT and esophagus | Error in valve area calculations |

## Echocardiographic Findings Associated with Aortic Stenosis

Patients with aortic stenosis commonly have left ventricular hypertrophy, which is an adaptive mechanism in response to the chronic pressure overload. Increased wall thickness reduces wall stress by distributing the pressure overload over greater myocardial mass, as indicated by La Place's Law:

$$\text{Wall stress} = \frac{\text{Pressure} \times \text{Volume}}{\text{wall thickness}}$$

The major perioperative implication is that estimates of left ventricular filling pressure are not reliable indicators of volume loading because of the associated decreased left ventricular compliance. The second major concern is the development of systolic anterior motion of the mitral valve because of the septal hypertrophy after aortic valve replacement for aortic stenosis. Although this condition is well recognized with asymmetric septal hypertrophy, SAM can also occur in patients with *symmetric* septal hypertrophy after aortic valve replacement. This is usually a manifestation of the abrupt reduction in left ventricular afterload associated with an under-filled left ventricle in patients with septal or concentric hypertrophy. The condition usually resolves with administration of volume, phenylephrine, and discontinuation of inotropic and chronotropic medications.

Patients with long-standing aortic stenosis develop diastolic dysfunction. This is evaluated using mitral inflow velocities and pulmonary venous flow patterns as discussed earlier in this book. Systolic function is preserved until late in the disease progression when left ventricular dilation develops. Systolic dysfunction due to aortic stenosis is usually reversible with valve replacement; however, systolic dysfunction due to myocardial infarction may not improve. Underestimation of the severity of aortic stenosis by gradient determination occurs in patients with decreased systolic function.

Many patients with aortic stenosis also have aortic regurgitation (AR). The diastolic regurgitation of blood into the left ventricle increases transaortic blood flow during systole, yielding a higher gradient for a given aortic valve orifice. The presence of AR does not affect continuity equation area calculations because the increased systolic flow affects measurements in the LVOT and the aortic valve equally.

Patients with aortic valve disease may also have mitral valve disease, manifested as mitral stenosis, regurgitation, or both. The presence of mitral stenosis causes an underestimation of the severity of aortic stenosis by gradient determination because of decreased transaortic blood flow.

## Pathophysiology of Aortic Regurgitation

Aortic regurgitation (AR) is caused by either intrinsic disease of the aortic cusps or secondarily from diseases affecting the ascending aorta. Intrinsic valvular problems include rheumatic, calcific, and myxomatous valvular disease; endocarditis; traumatic injury; and congenital abnormalities. Conditions affecting the ascending aorta that lead to aortic regurgitation include annular dilatation and aortic dissection (secondary to blunt trauma or hypertension), mycotic aneurysm, cystic medial necrosis, Marfan's syndrome, and chronic hypertension. The most common cause of pure aortic regurgitation is no longer postinflammatory due to the decreasing prevalence of rheumatic heart disease among cardiac surgical patients (19). Aortic root dilation is now the most common etiologic factor, to the increased prevalence of degenerative disease, followed by postinflammatory disease and bicuspid valve disease.

## Echocardiographic Evaluation of Aortic Regurgitation

The aortic valve, ascending aorta, and LVOT are inspected using the ME AV LAX view. Normal leaflets are often not visible during diastole, because they are parallel to the Doppler beam when closed. Stenotic leaflets that dome during systole often do not completely coapt during diastole, leading to aortic regurgitation. The diagnosis of leaflet prolapse is made when aortic leaflet tissue is imaged in the LVOT below the annular plane during diastole (Fig. 30.14). An aortic dissection in the aortic root causes

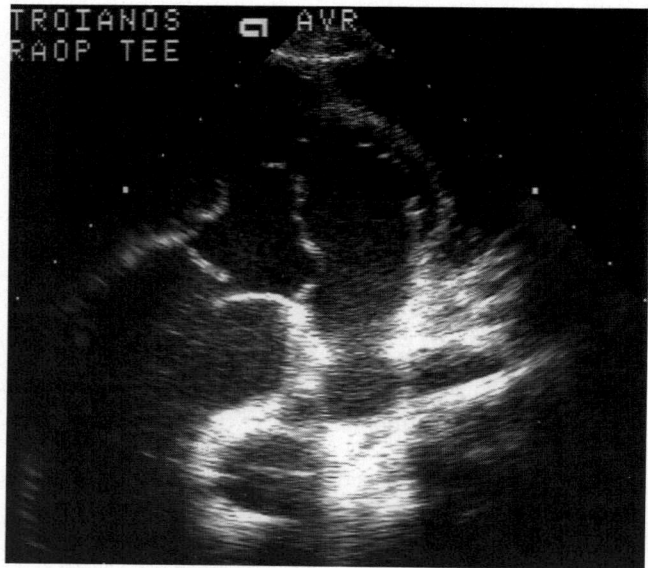

**FIGURE 30.14.** Transesophageal echocardiogram of the deep transgastric view of the aortic valve during diastole, indicating leaflet prolapse.

disruption of leaflets from the aortic annulus and may cause leaflet prolapse. Two-dimensional echocardiography is used to determine the etiology of the aortic regurgitation by identifying structural abnormalities of the leaflets or aortic root.

Although two-dimensional echocardiography is not useful for quantifying the severity of AR, there are several associated echocardiographic features. The left ventricle is dilated and more spherical in shape with chronic AR, but not necessarily with acute AR. The mitral valve exhibits premature closure and fluttering of the anterior mitral leaflet during diastole.

Doppler echocardiography is used to quantitate the severity of AR by several techniques that involve color, pulsed wave, and continuous wave Doppler. These techniques are sensitive and reliable, but all have limitations. Color Doppler applied to ME AV SAX (30° to 50° multiplane angle) is useful for localizing the site of regurgitation (Fig. 30.15). Despite the orthogonal relationship between the aortic valve flow and Doppler beam in this short-axis view, the regurgitant orifice is identifiable because the AR jet is usually not completely orthogonal to the Doppler beam, particularly if the jet is eccentric. The ME AV LAX view (120° to 150° multiplane angle) is the most useful for quantitating the severity of AR. Color

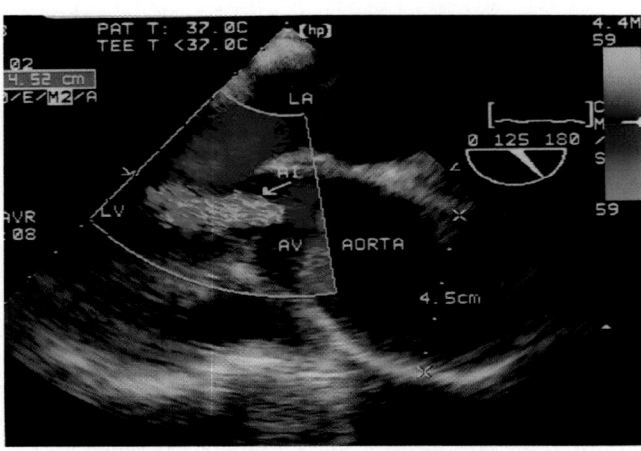

**FIGURE 30.16.** Transesophageal echocardiogram of the midesophageal aortic valve long-axis view with color flow Doppler in a patient with aortic insufficiency (*AI*). *LA*, left atrium; *LV*, left ventricle; *AV*, aortic valve.

Doppler reveals a flow disturbance in the left ventricular outflow tract originating from the aortic valve and directed into the left ventricle (Fig. 30.16). A central jet is usually caused by aortic root dilatation, whereas an eccentric jet often implies a leaflet abnormality. The width of the jet at the orifice compared to the width of the LVOT correlates with angiographic determinants of aortic regurgitation (Table 30.4) (20).

Although the jet width/LVOT width method is easy to use and provides sufficient information to make clinical decisions, other methods are sometimes necessary to evaluate patients with aortic regurgitation. Continuous wave Doppler is used to determine the severity of AR by measuring the deceleration slope of the regurgitant jet. A deep transgastric or transgastric long-axis view aligns the regurgitant jet with the Doppler beam. Color Doppler is useful for identifying the location and direction of the AR jet, while the Doppler cursor is placed within the jet to obtain the continuous wave spectral velocity profile (Fig. 30.17). The velocity of the regurgitant jet declines more rapidly in patients with severe AR because the larger regurgitant orifice allows a more rapid equilibration of the aortic and left ventricular pressures. The limitations of

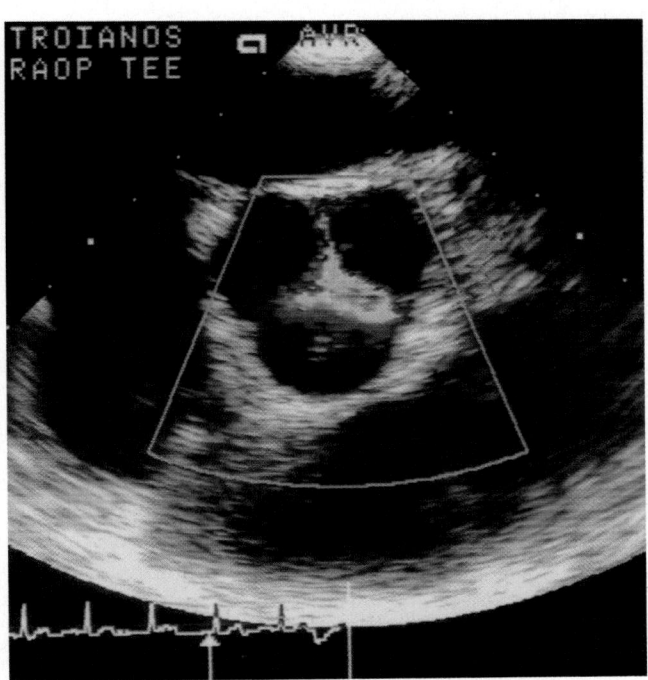

**FIGURE 30.15.** Transesophageal echocardiogram of the midesophageal aortic valve short-axis view with color flow Doppler in a patient with aortic insufficiency. The origin of the aortic insufficiency is predominantly between the right and left coronary cusps. From Troianos CA. Perioperative echocardiography. In Troianos CA, ed. Anesthesia for the cardiac patient. St. Louis: Mosby; 2002, with permission.

▶ **TABLE 30.4. Grading Aortic Insufficiency**

| Severity of aortic insufficiency | Jet width/LVOT width ratio (20) |
|---|---|
| 1+ | < 0.25 |
| 2+ | 0.25 to 0.46 |
| 3+ | 0.47 to 0.64 |
| 4+ | > 0.64 |

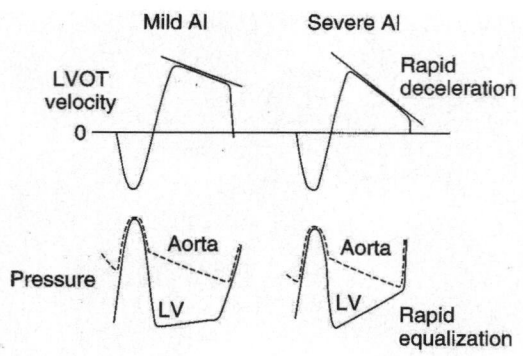

**FIGURE 30.17.** Illustration of the association between the left ventricular outflow tract (*LVOT*) deceleration slope and the pressure difference between the aorta and left ventricle (*LV*) during diastole. The deceleration slope is steeper and approaches zero velocity more rapidly with severe aortic insufficiency (*AI*) as the pressures in the aorta and left ventricle equalize more rapidly. From Troianos CA. Perioperative echocardiography. In Troianos CA, ed. Anesthesia for the cardiac patient. St. Louis, Mosby; 2002, with permission and adapted from Feigenbaum H. Echocardiography, 5th ed. Philadelphia: Lea & Febiger, 1994, 286, with permission.

this technique are discussed in Chapter 15, Assessment of the Aortic Valve.

Pulsed wave Doppler is used to detect retrograde flow in the aorta during diastole. Holodiastolic flow in the abdominal aorta is sensitive and specific for severe aortic insufficiency. Retrograde flow throughout diastole (holodiastolic) in the distal descending thoracic aorta (21) or the abdominal aorta (Fig. 30.18) (22) indicates severe aortic regurgitation.

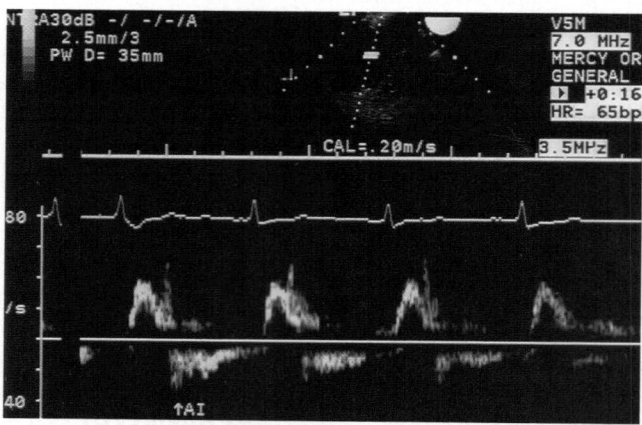

**FIGURE 30.18.** Pulsed wave Doppler spectral velocity of blood flow in the descending thoracic aorta. The retrograde flow throughout diastole (arrow) is termed holodiastolic and is associated with severe aortic insufficiency. From Troianos CA. Perioperative echocardiography. In Troianos CA, ed. Anesthesia for the cardiac patient. St. Louis: Mosby; 2002; 155, with permission.

## Echocardiographic Findings Associated with Aortic Regurgitation

Chronic left ventricular volume overload causes progressive left ventricular dilation over many years, while systolic function is preserved. Ejection fraction is initially normal while end-diastolic dimensions are increased. In contrast to aortic stenosis, the ventricle remains relatively compliant until systolic dysfunction ensues late in the course of the disease process. And, unlike aortic stenosis, the systolic dysfunction is not reversible. Acute aortic regurgitation is not associated with left ventricular dilation because the adaptive left ventricular dilation has not yet occurred. This lack of adaptation is associated with a decreased left ventricular compliance and a rapid onset of symptoms. Other echocardiographic findings include premature mitral valve closure and fluttering of the mitral valve leaflets. Depending on the etiology of the AR, aortic root abnormalities may also be present, including aortic dissection or aneurysm.

Aortic regurgitation causes an overestimation of mitral valve area by the pressure half-time (PHT) method of determining mitral orifice size. The PHT method utilizes the relationship between mitral inflow deceleration and mitral valve area. Deceleration is based on the equalization of pressure in the left atrium and the left ventricle and is prolonged as mitral orifice size decreases. In the absence of AR, left ventricular volume (and subsequently left ventricular pressure) increases via mitral inflow alone. In the presence of AR, left ventricular pressure increases by both mitral inflow and aortic regurgitation, and gives the impression that mitral inflow is better than actual, thus underestimating the severity of mitral stenosis.

## SPECIFIC AORTIC VALVE PROCEDURES

### Aortic Valve Replacement

The role of intraoperative echocardiography for aortic valve replacement is to confirm the diagnosis of aortic valve dysfunction and evaluate the left ventricular outflow tract, aortic annulus, and proximal ascending aorta for abnormalities that impact aortic valve replacement, as well as evaluate secondary and associated abnormalities. Providing the surgeon with an estimate of the size of the valve to be implanted allows the surgeon to consider prosthetic valve options and determine whether the annulus needs to be enlarged. The diameter of the annulus is measured trailing edge to leading edge at the point of leaflet attachment, using the midesophageal aortic valve long-axis view (Fig. 30.3). The question is often asked whether to make this measurement during systole or diastole. In reality, it likely does not matter because the annular size does not change significantly within the cardiac cycle. It certainly does not change by an entire valve size. It may be easier to make the measurement during systole, because the point of leaflet attachment to the annulus is more easily identified.

It is important to identify aortic regurgitation with intraoperative echocardiography because of the impact on cardioplegia administration for myocardial protection. Severe aortic regurgitation necessitates an altered myocardial perfusion strategy, such as retrograde cardioplegia administration via a coronary sinus catheter. TEE is useful for guiding and confirming cannulation of the coronary sinus. Severe calcification within the aortic annulus may affect the ease of valve seating and the presence of paravalvular leaks after implantation. Atheromatous disease in the aortic root may necessitate debridement or aortic root replacement. Aneurysmal dilation and dissection involving the ascending aorta contribute to aortic valve dysfunction. These conditions require replacement of the ascending aorta concomitant with the aortic valve. If coronary reimplantation is required, thorough evaluation of regional and global left ventricular contractility is crucial after separation from cardiopulmonary bypass.

As mentioned previously, aortic valve disease causes secondary abnormalities and necessitates a thorough intraoperative echocardiographic evaluation of associated structures. Inspection for mitral and tricuspic regurgitation, assessment of left ventricular diastolic and right ventricular systolic function, and calculation of pulmonary artery pressure are integral to the intraoperative evaluation of patients undergoing aortic valve surgery, regardless of what procedure will be employed to correct the aortic valve pathology.

After cardiopulmonary bypass, the prosthetic valve function is assessed by evaluating leaflet motion with two-dimensional echocardiography. It is important to know what type of prosthetic valve was implanted in order to make an accurate assessment of prosthetic valve function. Some echocardiographers routinely measure the gradient across the prosthetic aortic valve, during the postbypass period. Caution must be exercised in order to avoid unnecessary concern for valve dysfunction due to a higher than expected gradient determination immediately after cardiopulmonary bypass. The gradient is affected by flow and these patients are commonly in a "high output" state immediately after bypass. The systemic vascular resistance is usually low, inotropes are being infused, and the patient is usually anemic. All of these factors, in addition to the size of the valve relative to the size of the patient, contribute to a higher than expected gradient across an aortic valve after bypass. It is most important to evaluate leaflet mobility and observe the function of the prosthetic valve with two-dimensional echocardiography than to rely solely on a Doppler-derived estimate of the valve gradient. Large intravalvular leaks are not normal and require further investigation. Small in-

travalvular leaks are common, depending on the type of prosthetic valve implanted. Bioprosthetic valves may have no intravalvular leaks or a small central leak. Mechanical valves may have one or several small intravalvular leaks, depending on the type of valve. The presence of paravalvular leaks is usually a concern after aortic valve replacement, but the degree of concern depends on the size of the leak and whether or not the leak persists after protamine administration. For a more comprehensive review of prosthetic valve evaluation, see Chapter 18, Assessment of Prosthetic Valves.

## Stentless Aortic Valves

The ideal valve replacement for an aortic valve has a minimal transvalvular gradient, minimal risk of thromboembolism, and is durable for the life of the patient. Stentless valves and stented bioprosthetic valves do not require chronic anticoagulation therapy, but stentless valves offer a superior hemodynamic profile. The lack of a sewing ring and valve struts supporting the cusps makes implantation more time-consuming and sometimes more difficult, but their absence results in a better hemodynamic profile. The pliability of stentless valves and the lack of struts allow for a more laminar flow pattern, lower pressure gradients, and a larger effective orifice size compared to a similar size stented bioprosthesis. There is also, theoretically, less stress on the leaflets of a stentless valve than a stented bioprosthesis, because the stress is distributed to the commissures and aortic wall, similar to a native aortic valve (as previously described). Newer anticalcification treatments may reduce calcium deposit on these valves, prolonging their durability. The disadvantage of these valves is the risk of distortion during implantation, leading to valve dysfunction.

There are many valves classified as stentless that are suitable for implantation in the aortic position, including homografts, autografts, and manufactured or processed valves. Although there are several stentless manufactured or processed valves on the market, specific discussion in this chapter will be in reference to the most commonly used valves, the Toronto SPV® and the Medtronic Freestyle aortic root.

The Toronto SPV® is an excised porcine aortic valve that has been trimmed, cross-linked, sterilized, preserved in glutaraldehyde, and wrapped in polyester fabric. The valve has the advantage of the more superior hemodynamic profile, similar to a homograft. This manufactured valve is available in sizes 21 mm, 23 mm, 25 mm, 27 mm, and 29 mm and is more readily available than homografts. Proper valve sizing and implantation is crucial to the function of the valve. Measurements are made at the sinotubular junction and aortic valve annulus (Fig. 30.3) to determine proper sizing because the valve is sewn both to the annulus (inflow sutures) and aortic wall (outflow

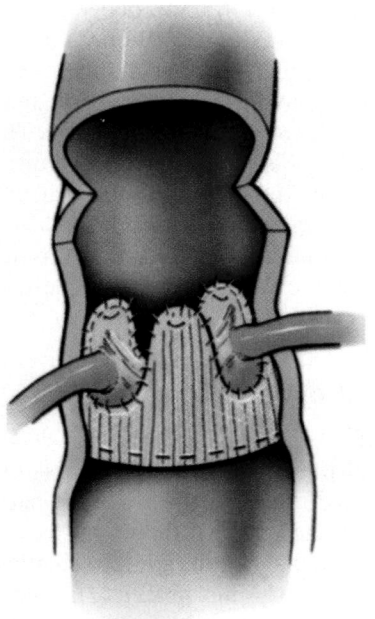

**FIGURE 30.19.** Illustration of the Toronto SPV® valve indicating its position within the aortic root and two suture lines (inflow and outflow). (From St. Jude Medical, with permission.)

▶ **TABLE 30.5.** Toronto SPV® Valve Sizing (all values are in mm)

| Sinotubular junction diameter | Annular diameter | Toronto SPV® valve size |
|---|---|---|
| 21 | 19–21 | 21 |
| 23 | 21–23 | 23 |
| 25 | 23–25 | 25 |
| 27 | 25–27 | 27 |
| 29 | 27–29 | 29 |

suture line) (Fig. 30.19). The diameter of the annulus is measured trailing edge to leading edge at the point of leaflet attachment using the midesophageal aortic valve long-axis view (Fig. 30.3). The sinotubular junction diameter is measured trailing edge to leading edge at the top of the sinuses of Valsalva (Fig. 30.3). The sinotubular junction diameter is used for the valve size and should not be more than 10% (or one valve size) greater than the annular diameter (Table 30.5). Implantation of a valve that "fits" the annulus, but is too small for the sinotubular junction, will result in valve distortion and intravalvular regurgitation due to the leaflets being "pulled apart" by the aortic wall. Oversizing may lead to leaflet buckling and asymmetric valve closure.

Similar to the Toronto SPV®, the Medtronic Freestyle aortic root is also obtained from the porcine aortic root and lacks rigid sewing and supporting struts. In contrast to the Toronto SPV®, the ascending aorta is intact with ligated coronary arteries on the Freestyle valve and sculpted by the surgeon to one of three possible configurations (Fig. 30.20) (23). Two suture lines are used to implant this valve. The inflow sutures are placed into the annulus, similar to the Toronto SPV®. The outflow sutures, however, vary according to the implantation technique chosen: full root, root-inclusion, complete subcoronary, or modified subcoronary. The variety of implantation options provided by this valve is an advantage that reduces the problems associated with implanting the Toronto SPV® in patients with > 10% annular-sinotubular junc-

tion diameter discrepancies. Some disadvantages of this valve are the expertise and sculpting required by the surgeon to implant it and greater implantation time.

Prebypass TEE provides a detailed assessment of native anatomic structures. Particular attention is directed to the annular and sinotubular junction diameters. Dilation of the aortic root at the sinotubular junction may result in significant valvular regurgitation. This condition must be communicated to the surgeon, so that repair of the aortic root accompanies the use of a stentless valve (23). In the absence of significant aortic root dilation, the Toronto SPV® valve size chosen is the sinotubular junction diameter. This diameter must not be more than 10% larger than the annular diameter, or the valve will not seat properly into the annulus. Either another valve option must be selected or the size of either the annulus or sinotubular ridge must be altered to accommodate the Toronto SPV®. A recent study utilizing the Sorin Pericarbon stentless valve demonstrated better valve competence and a better hemodynamic profile if the valve size chosen was between 3 mm and 4 mm greater than the annular diameter. Patients with aortic root dilation underwent surgical revision of the noncoronary sinus to maintain the

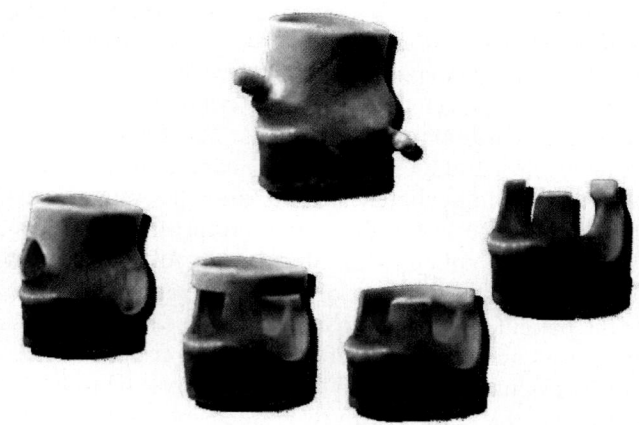

**FIGURE 30.20.** Illustration of the Medtronic Freestyle valve indicating various configurations used for implantation. (From Medtronic Corporation, with permission.)

sinotubular junction diameter within 115% of the aortic annulus diameter (24).

Postbypass TEE is used to evaluate leaflet mobility and detect any abnormal flow disturbance that may indicate valve malfunction. Two-dimensional echocardiography is used to evaluate the valve in its short and long axes. A multiplane probe is rotated to multiplane angles of 30°–60° and 120°–150°, respectively, to obtain these images and assess leaflet mobility. Leaflet prolapse or lack of leaflet coaptation may indicate problems with implantation, sizing, or malposition. Color flow Doppler is used to evaluate flow patterns across the valve and to detect intravalvular or paravalvular leaks. Prolapse of a single leaflet would most likely result in an eccentric jet, while lack of leaflet coaptation would result in a central regurgitant jet. A small central jet of AR is usually not cause for concern and most surgeons would not routinely reopen the aorta to evaluate a trace central jet of AR. Paravalvular leaks are generally uncommon with stentless valves because there are two suture lines. The outflow suture line is considered to be hemostatic. If the inflow suture line is not completely occlusive, systolic flow may be detected around the valve. If the outflow suture line is incompetent, one should expect to see diastolic flow around the valve. Small paravalvular leaks often resolve with protamine administration. However, larger (moderate to severe) paravalvular or intravalvular leaks are not likely to resolve after protamine administration. Provided that leaflet mobility is normal, routine measurement of stentless valve gradients immediately after bypass is not required. (See discussion earlier in this chapter.) These valves are easier to image with echocardiography than stented bioprosthetic valves and mechanical valves. The aortic wall appears thicker in the proximal ascending aorta due to the overlap of the native aortic wall and the aortic graft. An echolucent space may also be observed between the porcine and native aortic walls (23). This paravalvular space should be interrogated with color flow Doppler, particularly if the space varies in size during the cardiac cycle. Expansion of the space with color entry during systole implies communication of the space with the left ventricular outflow tract, which may be expected if the inflow suture line is not hemostatic. Expansion of the space with color entry during diastole implies communication with the ascending aorta. A diagnosis of partial valve dehiscence is made in patients with significant paraprosthetic diastolic regurgitation visualized through an echolucent space (23). A paraprosthetic echolucent space that does not vary in size and lacks color flow Doppler disturbance does not require surgical exploration if valve function is not affected. A persistent or expanding paraprosthetic echolucent space present for several weeks after implantation raises concerns for a paravalvular infection due to abscess formation (23).

## Aortic Valve Homograft

Homografts provide many desirable valve characteristics, such as an excellent hemodynamic profile and resistance to infection, and do not require long-term anticoagulation therapy. These valves have excellent durability, with a 10-year 92% freedom of reoperation from graft-related causes (25). These characteristics make homografts particularly suitable for younger patients and those with active endocarditis (26). Disadvantages are a shortage of supply and tissue failure (1). Recent advances have improved their durability and storage time, promoting a renewed interest in use of these valves (1).

Prebypass TEE provides a detailed assessment of native anatomic structures. Particular attention is directed to the annular and sinotubular junction diameters. The annular diameter is measured in a manner similar to that described above for mechanical and stentless valves. However, for patients in whom a homograft is planned, internal annular diameter must accommodate the external diameter of the homograft. For this reason, a valve size of 2 mm to 3 mm less than the measured native annulus (internal diameter) is selected as the homograft size. Transesophageal echocardiography is useful for measuring annular diameter and predicting the size of the homograft to be implanted (27). Accurate estimation of homograft size with intraoperative echocardiography reduces aortic cross-clamp and bypass times if the homograft is thawed before the surgeon directly measures the annular size after aortotomy. The difference between the aortic annular size measured with intraoperative echocardiography as compared with the size measured by the surgeon is less than 1 mm in 94% of patients and less than 2 mm in all patients, with an average difference of 0.6 mm (28). It is also important to measure the sinotubular junction diameter so that the implanted homograft is proportional to the size of the supravalvular ridge (29).

Postbypass TEE is used to evaluate leaflet mobility and detect any abnormal flow disturbance that may indicate valve malfunction. Two-dimensional echocardiography is used to evaluate the valve in its short and long axes. A multiplane probe is rotated to multiplane angles of between 30° and 60° and 120° and 150°, respectively, to obtain these images and assess leaflet mobility. The same issues previously discussed with stentless aortic valves apply to homografts. Namely, the valves are prone to distortion and malposition during implantation due to the absence of a sewing ring. Leaflet prolapse or lack of leaflet coaptation may indicate problems with implantation, sizing, or malposition. Color flow Doppler is used to evaluate flow patterns across the valve and to detect intravalvular leaks. Prolapse of a single leaflet would most likely result in an eccentric jet, while lack of leaflet coaptation would result in a central regurgitant jet. The frequency of problems with homograft implantation requiring a return to cardiopulmonary bypass may be higher (11.6% in one study) (28), compared with implantation of a prosthetic valve. Intraoperative echocardiography is valuable for identifying these problems, which are primarily aortic regurgitation and myocardial ischemia (with coronary reimplantation) (30). Homografts implanted using an inclusion technique have the same issues previously described in the section on stentless aortic valves: a thicker aortic wall and a potential space between the homograph and native aortic walls. Postbypass color flow Doppler interrogation and observation of the size of the space throughout the cardiac cycle are important for identifying valve dehiscence.

## Combined Aortic Valve-Aortic Root Replacement

Patients with aortic valve disease and aortic root disease (aneurysm, dissection) require a combined aortic valve-aortic root replacement. The role of intraoperative echocardiography is to evaluate the aortic valve for repair versus replacement and to identify the extent of disease in the aorta both proximally and distally. The pathophysiologic process affecting the aortic valve with both aneurysm and dissection is regurgitation. Otherwise normal leaflet anatomy allows for aortic valve repair by resuspension of the cusps in cases of dissection and annular placation in cases of aortic root dilation. Aortic valve repair is possible in 70% of patients with type A dissection (31,32). Patients with an abnormal aortic valve in the setting of dissection or aneurysm require a combined valve-conduit approach for replacement. Patients with significant aortic root pathology, due to cystic medial necrosis or a significantly dilated aortic root, require a valve conduit approach with coronary artery reimplantation into the graft. The graft is extended to replace the affected segment of diseased aorta.

In cases of aortic dissection, it is important to identify coronary artery involvement with proximal extension of the dissection, and involvement of the great vessels with extension of the dissection into the arch. Epiaortic ultrasound is a necessary adjunct to TEE for the intraoperative evaluation of the distal ascending aorta and proximal aortic arch because these areas cannot be imaged with TEE. The right main stem bronchus is interpositioned between these aortic segments and the esophagus, making these areas inaccessible for imaging by TEE. Aneurysmal involvement of these aortic segments can be appreciated by surgical inspection. The involvement of these aortic segments in the disease process has important implications in placement of the arterial perfusion and cardioplegia cannula, in addition to the surgical approach and the need for deep hypothermic circulatory arrest. It is important to confirm cannulation of the true lumen when a femoral cannulation site is chosen for arterial perfusion

during cardiopulmonary bypass. The true lumen is identified by systolic expansion, generally higher velocity flow, and absence of spontaneous echocontrast. True lumen cannulation is confirmed by observing a wire inserted into the femoral catheter threaded far enough to allow imaging of the wire in the thoracic aorta with TEE. The observation of fluid contrast with initiation of cardiopulmonary bypass provides further confirmation of true lumen cannulation via the femoral artery. Intraoperative echocardiography is also used for identifying pericardial and pleural fluid, evaluating global and regional myocardial contractility, estimating the valve size (if not repairable), and measuring the diameter of the various aortic segments.

Postbypass echocardiography is used to evaluate the repaired native or prosthetic aortic valve, the aortic anastomoses, and left ventricular wall motion. Persistent regurgitation, paraprosthetic regurgitation, and new persistent wall motion abnormalities may indicate complications of surgery that require a return to cardiopulmonary bypass for correction. The frequency of a return to cardiopulmonary bypass is 3.8% after aortic aneurysm surgery (33). The postbypass echocardiographic evaluation of patients undergoing surgery for aortic dissection should demonstrate reduced flow in the false lumen. Persistent flow and absence of thrombus in the false lumen are poor prognostic indicators and indicate a greater risk of the dissection extending within the aorta. These patients require more intensive observation postoperatively. (34).

## Aortic Valve Repair

The preoperative echocardiography examination plays a key role in identifying aortic valves suitable for repair. Stenotic valves and valves with regurgitation due to leaflet restriction (degenerative, calcific) or retraction (rheumatic) comprise the most common etiologies of aortic regurgitation, but unfortunately these valves are not amenable to repair. Repair is a suitable option among patients with aortic regurgitation due to single-leaflet prolapse of either a tricuspid or congenitally bicuspid valve. Although leaflet prolapse is observed in tricuspid aortic valves, this lesion most commonly affects bicuspid valves (35). The prolapsing area of the leaflet is resected and reapproximated with suture (Figs. 30.21 and 30.22). Annuloplasty is often performed in association with the triangular resection of the prolapsing leaflet. Calcification limits the potential for valve reconstruction and is usually included in the resected portion of the leaflet.

Regurgitant lesions with anatomically normal leaflets and mobility are commonly caused by aortic root dilation and have a characteristic central jet of regurgitation. Annular dilation secondary to aortic root dilation can be repaired if annular dilation is limited and the leaflets are

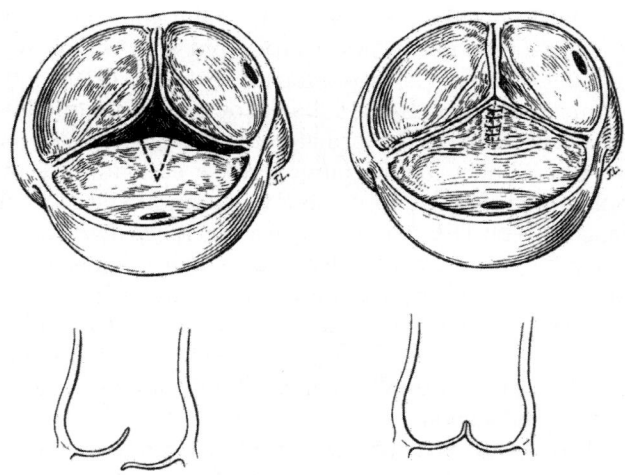

**FIGURE 30.21.** Aortic valve repair involving a tricuspid valve with a single-leaflet prolapse. Triangular resection of the free edge of the prolapsing cusp results in normal leaflet size and coaptation. From Cosgrove DM, Rosenkranz ER, Hendren WG, et al. Valvuloplasty for aortic insufficiency. J Thorac Cardiovasc Surg 1991;102:571–7, with permission.

otherwise anatomically normal. The size and morphology of the aortic root is determined with TEE. A normal aortic root consists of three sinuses of Valsalva that are symmetrical in shape and at most 2 mm to 3 mm larger than the valve annulus (33). Carpentier's technique of correcting annular dilation employs continuous circumferential horizontal mattress sutures placed through the annulus (35,36). Cosgrove's technique places sutures at the com-

missures to advance the sinotubular ridge inward and allow central coaptation (Fig. 30.23) (35). This method provides selected plication to the most affected areas of the valve (usually the commissures).

Valve repair for patients with aortic dissection involves resuspension of the cusps, and is easily performed and highly successful in the absence of additional leaflet pathology. Leaflet perforation caused by endocarditis can be repaired by patch or primary closure if destruction is limited to a small perforation of a single leaflet.

Intraoperative echocardiography after aortic valve repair identifies residual aortic regurgitation and the mechanism of valve dysfunction. The frequency of failed aortic valve repair is higher (14.4%) when compared to mitral valve repair (6.6%), owing to the increased technical difficulty associated with this procedure (33). Even with a perfect result in the course of repairing a prolapsing leaflet of a congenitally bicuspid valve, the leaflets appear thickened, bicuspid, and mildly stenotic (with leaflet doming) (33). The mechanism of valve dysfunction aids the surgeon to decide whether to attempt additional repair or to replace the valve.

## Ross Procedure

The pulmonary-aortic switch or Ross procedure involves excision of the patient's own pulmonic valve, implantation of the autograft into the aortic position, and implantation of a homograft or bioprosthetic valve into the pulmonic position (Fig. 30.24). This also results in an excellent hemodynamic profile, durability, and resistance to infection, and obviates the need for long-term anticoagulant therapy. There is also the potential for growth of this living tissue, making this an attractive option for younger patients (37). Disadvantages to this procedure

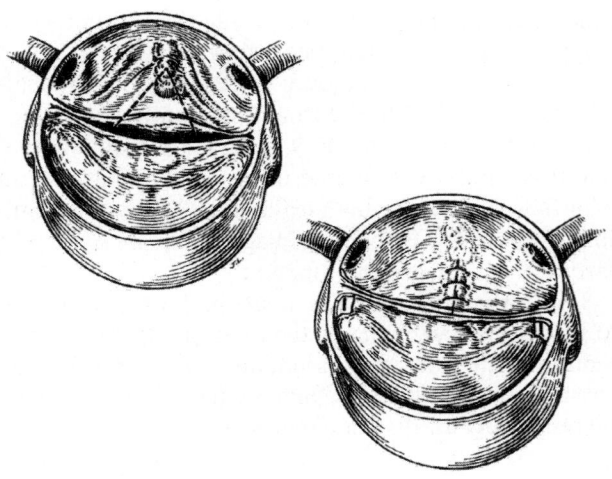

**FIGURE 30.22.** Aortic valve repair, involving a bicuspid valve with leaflet prolapse involves resection of the raphe when present, triangular resection of prolapsing cusp, and annuloplasty. From Cosgrove DM, Rosenkranz ER, Hendren WG, et al. Valvuloplasty for aortic insufficiency. J Thorac Cardiovasc Surg 1991;102:571–7, with permission.

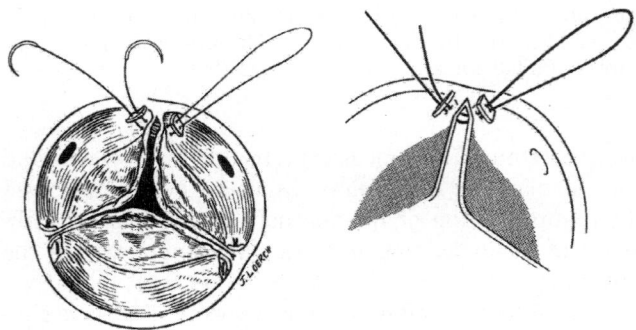

**FIGURE 30.23.** Aortic valve annuloplasty is performed by placing horizontal mattress sutures buttressed with Teflon felt at each commissure. Care is taken to avoid leaflet contact as the suture passes through the annulus, into the outflow tract, and back through the annulus. From Cosgrove DM, Rosenkranz ER, Hendren WG, et al. Valvuloplasty for aortic insufficiency. J Thorac Cardiovasc Surg 1991;102:571–7, with permission.

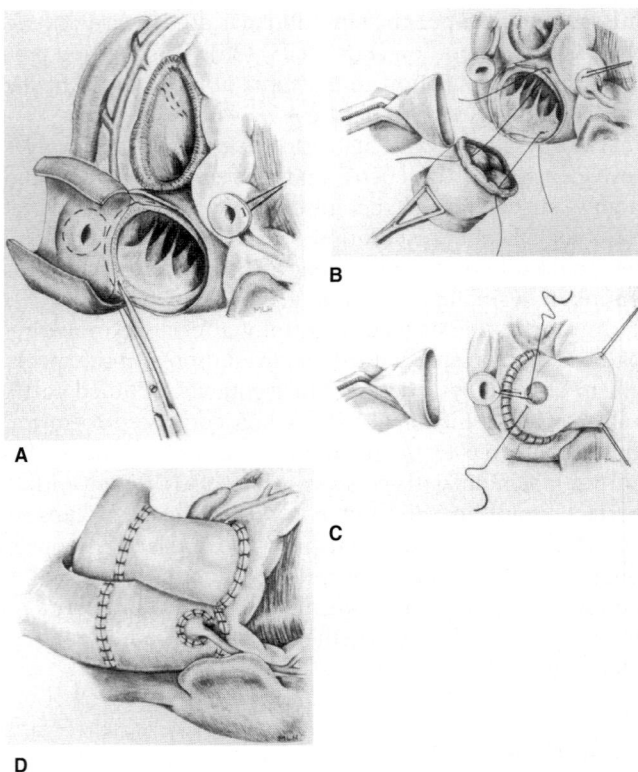

**FIGURE 30.24.** Ross Procedure root replacement technique. **A:** Generous cuffs of aorta are left attached to the right and left coronary ostia. Minimal mobilization of these arteries is performed. The remaining proximal aorta is excised, transecting the aorta below the aortic annulus in the interleaflet triangle. **B:** The pulmonary autograft is in an anatomic position with the posterior sinus of the autograft, becoming the new left coronary sinus (stay sutures omitted from drawing). The remaining sutures for orientation are placed to position the new right coronary sinus and to trifurcate the aortic annulus. **C:** Completion of the pulmonary autograft root implantation with selection of the site of implantation of the right coronary artery with the autograft distended. **D:** The pulmonary homograft reconstruction of the right ventricle outflow tract is done with two continuous suture lines. From Elkins RC. Aortic valve: Ross procedure. In Kaiser LR, Kron IL, Spray TL, eds. Mastery of cardiothoracic surgery. Philadelphia, Lippincott-Raven; 1998.

are the required technical expertise of the surgeon and the valvular size constraints discussed below. The need for reimplantation of the coronary arteries and the absence of a sewing ring increases the complexity of the procedure.

The presence of significant aortic valve disease is confirmed and the etiology of the valve disease is identified. Identification of etiology is important because progressive valvulitis is a cause of early postoperative valve dysfunction in patients with rheumatic valve disease (38). An important aspect of the intraoperative evaluation, besides confirming the presence of aortic valve disease, is the suitability of the pulmonic valve for transplantation into

the aortic position. Primarily, the pulmonic valve itself must be a functionally normal tricuspid valve without significant stenosis or regurgitation. The size of the pulmonic valve must also be suitable for transplantation into the aortic position. Epicardial echocardiography is an important adjunct for the intraoperative evaluation of the pulmonic valve due to its anterior location and difficult imaging with TEE. Patients with a difference in the aortic and pulmonic valve diameters of less than 3 mm have less postbypass and postoperative autograft regurgitation (39). Dilation of the aortic annulus or proximal ascending aorta may indicate unrecognized connective tissue disease that progresses after autograft implantation, leading to annular dilation.

The postbypass echocardiography examination focuses on the function of the autograft, the pulmonary allograft, and regional left ventricular contractility. The close proximity of the septal perforator branch of the left anterior descending coronary artery to the pulmonic valve makes compromise of the septal blood flow a potential complication during pulmonic valve harvesting. TEE is used to evaluate left ventricular contractility, particularly myocardial thickening and radial shortening in the basal anteroseptal segment to assess patency of the septal perforator. Regional contractility is assessed in other areas of the left and right ventricles as an indicator of coronary malperfusion due to problems that may arise from coronary reimplantation or bleeding.

The two-dimensional midesophageal short- and long-axis views are used to evaluate the function of the autograft. Particular attention is paid to leaflet coaptation—evaluating for leaflet prolapse, and restriction of leaflet mobility. Color flow Doppler to these views detects aortic regurgitation. The degree of regurgitation is best determined with the long-axis view, while the location of the coaptation defect is identified using the short-axis view. More than a minimal amount of regurgitation indicates possible valve distortion during implantation and a need to return to cardiopulmonary bypass. The pulmonary allograft is similarly evaluated using two-dimensional and color flow Doppler for both leaflet mobility and regurgitation, respectively. Epicardial imaging may be required to adequately evaluate valve function.

The aortic root and proximal pulmonary artery are evaluated for narrowing at the anastomotic site and for dilation of the proximal ascending aorta. Baseline measurements are important for long-term follow-up given the propensity for disease progression.

## Percutaneous Aortic Valve Surgery

Percutaneous aortic valve surgery is a new procedure in development that involves the placement of a prosthesis across the aortic valve, using an intravascular approach. The general principle utilizes a collapsible bioprosthetic valve mounted within an expandable stent. Lutter et al. described their experience with a porcine aortic valve mounted into a self-expandable nitinol stent by means of a suture technique (41). They implanted 6 valves in the descending aorta and 8 valves in a subcoronary position in the ascending aorta of 14 anesthetized pigs, via the left iliac artery or infrarenal aorta. One animal died of ventricular fibrillation, and technical failure (stent twisting) occurred in two animals. The remaining 11 valved stents demonstrated low transvalvular gradients, physiologic regurgitation in only 8 animals, and mild regurgitation in 3 animals (41).

Cribier et al. reported the first human implantation of a percutaneous aortic valve in a 57-year-old man with calcific aortic stenosis, cardiogenic shock, subacute leg ischemia, and other associated noncardiac medical problems (42). Valve replacement was declined for this patient. Although balloon valvuloplasty had been performed, the results were nonsustained. The investigators used an antegrade transseptal approach to successfully implant the percutaneous heart valve within the diseased aortic valve. Their valve was composed of three bovine pericardial leaflets mounted within a balloon-expandable stent. The placement was accurate and stable with no impingement of coronary artery blood flow or interference with mitral valve function. A mild degree of paravalvular regurgitation was present after implantation. Valvular function remained satisfactory for 4 months after the procedure, assessed with sequential transesophageal echocardiograms without the recurrence of heart failure. The patient died 17 weeks after implantation due to noncardiac complications from worsening leg ischemia, amputation, and infection (42).

Transesophageal echocardiography will play a critical role in percutaneous aortic valve implantation. In addition to determining feasibility of the procedure in the patient, TEE will assist with sizing, placement, and stabilization of the device. Postimplantation exams will be utilized to detect complications. These complications include displacement of the device, obstruction of coronary artery blood flow, and damage to the mitral valve. Patients with calcific disease face similar complications as with balloon valvuloplasty, such as embolic events associated with the procedure. Continued improvements in the device and implantation techniques may provide a viable option in the treatment of patients with aortic valve disease.

*The editors acknowledge Lori B. Heller for her editorial contributions to this chapter.*

## KEY POINTS

- Epiaortic, epicardial, and transesophageal echocardiography are valuable intraoperative tools used for the complete evaluation of the aortic valve and ascending aorta. Two-dimensional imaging combined with pulsed wave, continuous wave, and color Doppler allow quantitative evaluation of stenotic and regurgitant lesions.
- Focused and comprehensive echocardiographic examinations are performed during aortic valve surgery to confirm the preoperative diagnosis, evaluate the severity of aortic valve disease, determine the feasibility of aortic valve repair versus replacement, and evaluate the success of surgical correction.
- The aortic valve apparatus is comprised of the valve cusps, sinuses of Valsalva, proximal ascending aorta, and left ventricular outflow tract. Abnormalities involving any of these structures can lead to aortic valve dysfunction.
- Intraoperative echocardiography during aortic valve replacement is used to estimate the size of the valve to be implanted, assess the function of the prosthetic valve, assess de-airing maneuvers, evaluate ventricular function, and evaluate the thoracic aorta.
- Implantation of a stentless aortic valve requires measurements of both the aortic annulus and sinotubular junction.
- Preoperative TEE for patients undergoing homograft implantation is useful for determining homograft size before aortotomy, reducing cross clamp time, and ensuring availability of this limited-availability valve.
- Combined aortic root and aortic valve procedures are long, technically demanding, and associated with serious complications that can be diagnosed with intraoperative echocardiography.
- Aortic valve repair is a suitable option for patients with aortic regurgitation due to single-leaflet prolapse of either a tricuspid or congenitally bicuspid valve. Moderate-to-severe regurgitation is cause for concern after repair, and often necessitates return to cardiopulmonary bypass for further correction.
- The Ross procedure involves the use of the patient's own pulmonic valve as an autograft replacement of the aortic valve and an allograft replacement of the pulmonic valve. Echocardiography plays an important role in determining the suitability of the patient for this procedure, and to identify complications that may arise. These complications include valve dysfunction, aortic root dilation due to disease progression, proximal pulmonary artery stricture, and inadequate coronary perfusion.

- Percutaneous aortic valve surgery involves the placement of a bioprosthetic, collapsible aortic valve mounted on an expandable stent through a percutaneous approach. As this technology develops, TEE will play a critical role in the evaluation of patients suitable for percutaneous aortic valve implantation, sizing, placement, and stabilization of the device, and postimplantation evaluation for complications.

## REFERENCES

1. Oh CC, Click RL, Orszulak TA, et al. Role of intraoperative transesophageal echocardiography in determining aortic annulus diameter in homograft insertion. J Am Soc Echocardiogr 1998;11:638–42.
2. Nowrangi SK, Connolly HM, Freeman WK, Click RL. Impact of intraoperative transesophageal echocardiography among patients undergoing aortic valve replacement for aortic stenosis. J Am Soc Echocardiogr 2001;14:863–6.
3. Filsoufi F, Aklog L, Adams DH, Byrne JG. Management of mild to moderate aortic stenosis at the time of coronary artery bypass grafting. J Heart Valve Dis 2002;11(Suppl 1): S45–S49.
4a. Morehead AJ, Firstenberg MS, Shiota T, et al. Intraoperative echocardiographic detection of regurgitant jets after valve replacement. Ann Thorac Surg 2000;69:135–9.
4b. Kumar A, Anel R, Bunnell E. Pulmonary artery occlusion pressure and central venous pressure fail to predict ventricular filling volume, cardiac performance, or the response to volume infusion in normal subjects Critical Care Med 2004;32(3):691–9.
5. Cahalan MK, Abel M, Goldman M, et al. American Society of Echocardiography; Society of Cardiovascular Anesthesiologists. American Society of Echocardiography and Society of Cardiovascular Anesthesiologists task force guidelines for training in perioperative echocardiography. Anesth Analg 2002;94:1384–8.
6. Stoddard MF, Hammons RT, Longaker RA. Doppler transesophageal echocardiographic determination of aortic valve area in adults with aortic stenosis. Am Heart J 1996;132: 337–42.
7. Odell JA, Mullany CJ, Schaff HV, et al. Aortic valve replacement after previous coronary artery bypass grafting. Ann Thorac Surg 1996;62:1424–30.
8. Hoffmann R, Flachskampf FA, Hanrath P. Planimetry of orifice area in aortic stenosis using multiplane transesophageal echocardiography. J Am Coll Cardiol 1993;22:529–34.
9. Mihaljevic T, Paul S, Cohn LH, Wechsler A. Pathophysiology of aortic valve disease. In: Cohn LH, Edmunds LH Jr, eds. Cardiac surgery in the adult. New York: McGraw-Hill, 2003; 791–810.
10. Thubrikar MJ, Nolan SP, Aouad J, Deck JD. Stress sharing between the sinus and leaflets of canine aortic valve. Ann Thorac Surg 1986;42:434–40.
11. Deck JD, Thubrikar MJ, Schneider PJ, Nolan SP. Structure, stress, and tissue repair in aortic valve leaflets. Cardiovasc Res 1988;22:7–16.
12. Thubrikar M, Harry R, Nolan SP. Normal aortic valve function in dogs. Am J Cardiol 1977;40:563–68.
13. Gnyaneshwar R, Kumar RK, Komarakshi RB. Dynamic analysis of the aortic valve using a finite element model. Ann Thorac Surg 2002;73:1122–29.
14. Mercer JL. The movements of the dog's aortic valve studied by high speed cineangiography. Br J Radiol 1973;46:344.
15. Shively BK, Charlton GA, Crawford MH, et al. Flow dependence of valve area in aortic stenosis: Relation to valve morphology. J Am Coll Cardiol 1998;31:654–60.
16. Maslow AD, Mashikian J, Haering JM, et al. Transesophageal echocardiographic evaluation of native aortic valve area: Utility of the double-envelope technique. J Cardiothorac Vasc Anesth 2001;15:293–9.
17. Rask LP, Karp KH, Eriksson NP. Flow dependence of the aortic valve area in patients with aortic stenosis: assessment by application of the continuity equation. J Am Soc Echocardiogr 1996;9:295–9.
18. Lin SS, Roger VL, Pascoe R, et al. Dobutamine stress Doppler hemodynamics in patients with aortic stenosis: feasibility, safety, and surgical correlations. Am Heart J 1998; 136:1010–6.
19. Cosgrove DM, Rosenkranz ER, Hendren WG, et al. Valvuloplasty for aortic insufficiency. J Thorac Cardiovasc Surg 1991;102:571–7.
20. Perry GJ, Helmcke F, Nanda NC, et al. Evaluation of aortic insufficiency by Doppler color flow mapping. J Am Coll Cardiol 1987;9:952–9.
21. Sutton DC, Kluger R, Ahmed SU, et al. Flow reversal in the descending aorta: a guide to intraoperative assessment of aortic regurgitation with transesophageal echocardiography. J Thorac Cardiovasc Surg 1994;108:576–82.
22. Takenaka K, Sakamoto T, Dabestani A, et al. Pulsed Doppler echocardiographic detection of regurgitant blood flow in the ascending, descending and abdominal aorta of patients with aortic regurgitation. J Cardiol 1987;17:301–9.
23. Bach DS. Echocardiographic assessment of stentless aortic bioprosthetic valves. J Am Soc Echocardiogr 2000;13:941–8.
24. Bach DS. J Am Soc Echocardiogr 2000;13(10):941–8.
25. Jin XY. Semin Thorac Cardiovasc Surg 2001;13(4 Suppl 1):67–74.
26. Doty JR, Salazar JD, Liddicoat JR, et al. Aortic valve replacement with cryopreserved aortic allograft: ten-year experience. J Thorac Cardiovasc Surg 1998;115:371–9.
27. Petrou M, Wong K, Albertucci M, et al. Evaluation of unstented aortic homografts for the treatment of prosthetic aortic valve endocarditis. Circulation 1994;90:II-198–II-204.
28. Fan CM, Liu X, Panidis JP, et al. Prediction of homograft aortic valve size by transthoracic and transesophageal two-dimensional echocardiography. Echocardiography 1997;14: 345–48.
29. Stewart WJ, Gillam L, Morehead AJ, et al. Impact of intraoperative echocardiography on homograft aortic valve surgery. J Am Coll Cardiol 1993;21:17A.
30. Kunzelman KS, Grande KJ, David TE, et al. Aortic root and valve relationships. Impact on surgical repair. J Thorac Cardiovasc Surg 1994;107:162–70.
31. Reddy VM, Rajasinghe HA, Teitel DF, et al. Aortoventriculoplasty with the pulmonary autograft: the "Ross-Konno" procedure. J Thorac Cardiovasc Surg 1996;111:158–65.
32. Jex RK, Schaff HV, Piehler JM, et al. Repair of ascending aortic dissection: Influence of associated aortic valve insufficiency on early and late results. J Thorac Cardiovasc Surg 1987;93:375–84.
33. Mazzucotelli JP, Deleuze PH, Baufreton C, et al. Preservation of the aortic valve in acute aortic dissection: long-term echocardiographic assessment and clinical outcome. Ann Thorac Surg 1993 Jun;55(6):1513–17.
34. Grimm RA, Stewart WJ. The role of intraoperative echocardiography in valve surgery. Cardiol Clin 1998;16:477–89.
35. Erbel R, Oelert H, Meyer J, et al. Effect of medical and surgical therapy on aortic dissection evaluated by transesophageal echocardiography. Implications for prognosis and therapy. The European Cooperative Study Group on Echocardiography. Circulation 1993;87:1604–15.
36. Cosgrove DM, Rosenkranz ER, Hendren WG, et al. Valvuloplasty for aortic insufficiency. J Thorac Cardiovasc Surg 1991;102:571–7.
37. Carpentier A. Cardiac valve surgery—"the French correction." J Thorac Cardiovasc Surg 1983;86:323–37.

38. Walls JT, McDaniel WC, Pope ER, et al. Documented growth of autogenous pulmonary valve translocated to the aortic valve position. J Thorac Cardiovasc Surg 1994;107:1530–1.
39. al-Halees Z, Kumar N, Gallo R, et al. Pulmonary autograft for aortic valve replacement in rheumatic disease: a caveat. Ann Thorac Surg 1995;60(2 Suppl):S172–5.
40. Stewart WJ, Secknus MA, Thomas JD, et al. Intraoperative echocardiography in the Ross procedure. J Am Coll Cardiol 1996;27:190A.
41. Lutter G, Kuklinski D, Berg G, et al. Percutaneous aortic valve replacement: an experimental study. I. Studies on implantation. J Thorac Cardiovasc Surg 2002;123:768–76.
42. Cribier A, Eltchaninoff H, Bash A, et al. Percutaneous transcatheter implantation of an aortic valve prosthesis for calcific aortic stenosis: first human case description. Circulation 2002;106:3006–8.

## QUESTIONS*

1. Which valve would be least suitable for repair?
   A. Congenitally bicuspid valve that has a dilated annulus and moderate AI
   B. Perforated noncoronary cusp with severe AI and mild AS
   C. Rheumatic valve with moderate AI
   D. Moderate AI in the setting of mild aortic stenosis

2. After homograph placement, which of the following should be inspected?
   A. Valve leaflets for mobility and competence
   B. Paravalvular area for regurgitant leaks
   C. Mitral valve
   D. Distal anastomotic site for diastolic leaks

3. If the aortic root is dilated
   A. a stentless heterograph is not a viable option.
   B. a stentless valve can be placed, as long as the STJ diameter exceeds the annulus diameter by 10%.
   C. an aortoplasty must be performed.
   D. a stentless valve can be placed, but either a root replacement or an aortoplasty should be considered.

4. If _____ is seen postbypass, one should consider returning to bypass for intervention:
   A. mild paravalvular leak (2 mm) after replacement with a stentless aortic valve
   B. paravalvular thickening that leads to mild restriction of movement of a single leaflet of the aortic valve
   C. trace AI after homograph placement
   D. mild AI after stentless aortic valve placement

*Questions provied by Lori B. Heller.

# Surgical Decision Making in Major Vascular Disease

# Assessment of Surgery of the Aorta

*Marc Kanchuger and Ellise Delphin*

The first successful reparative surgery of the thoracic aorta occurred between 1949 and 1953, without the benefit of sophisticated diagnostic equipment, or high-tech surgical and anesthetic techniques. Dubost was the first to successfully remove an abdominal aortic aneurysm and replace it with a homograft in 1951 (1). Gross (2), Swan (3), Lam (4), and DeBakey (5) accomplished the successful treatment of both coarctation and aneurysms of the descending aorta. Although the origin of extracorporeal circulation is difficult to trace, it is most often attributed to Gibbon (6). This innovation permitted the first successful resection and graft placement in the ascending aorta, followed by successful resection and graft placement of the aortic arch. Over the past four decades, major advances in diagnostic modalities, such as anesthetic management of myocardial, cerebral, and spinal cord preservation and surgical tactics, have dramatically improved survival and quality of life after aortic surgery. The refinement and expanded use of transesophageal echocardiography as a diagnostic modality for aortic disease has refined perioperative care. Preoperative diagnosis of aortic disorders has become less invasive due to the unique sensitivity and specificity of transesophageal echocardiography. Intraoperative diagnosis of atheromatous disease has enabled improved outcomes in cardiac surgery because it serves as a guide to operative technique.

## CLASSIFICATION AND EPIDEMIOLOGY OF DISEASES OF THE AORTA

Diseases of the aorta are generally considered to fall into five major groups:

1. Aneurysms
2. Dissections
3. Traumatic lesions
4. Atherosclerotic disease, including penetrating atherosclerotic ulcer and intramural hematoma
5. Other disease

## Aneurysms

### Description

*Aneurysm* is defined as a localized or diffuse aortic dilatation of more than 50% normal diameter (7). Dilatation is progressive and develops from weakening of the aortic wall. Aneurysms may be congenital or acquired. The etiology of congenital aneurysms is often connective tissue disease, such as Marfan's syndrome or Ehlers Danlos syndrome. Acquired aneurysms are more common and are often due to atherosclerotic disease in combination with degenerative changes of the media. Advanced age, smoking, and hypertension are often associated with this type of acquired aneurysm. In addition to atherosclerotic disease and cystic medial necrosis, acquired aneurysms may be caused by trauma, infection, inflammation, or iatrogenic causes. Sixty-five percent of aneurysms only involve the abdominal aorta, while 11% involve the thoracoabdominal aorta, and 6% affect the distal thoracic aorta and arch (8).

### Epidemiology

The incidence and prevalence of thoracic aneurysms in the United States population are difficult to estimate. The best population-based study to date, by Bickerstaff et al. (9), reported the incidence of newly diagnosed thoracic aneurysms as 5.9 per 100,000 person-years. The lifetime probability of rupture is 75%–80%, with 5-year untreated survival rates in the range of 10 to 20%. In nondissecting abdominal aneurysms, size significantly influences median time to rupture with a 43% risk of rupture within one year for aneurysms greater than 6 cm, and an 80% risk with those greater than 8 cm (10). Juvonen described the natural history of thoracic and thoracoabdominal aneurysms in 114 patients. In this group, maximal diameter of greater than 5.8 cm was an independent risk factor for rupture as were advanced age, pain, and chronic obstructive pulmonary disease (11).

## Dissection

### Description

Aortic dissection is one of the most serious forms of aortic disease, often requiring emergency surgery and aggressive medical care. A tear in the intima allows blood to escape from the true lumen of the aorta, creating a separation of the intima from the media, resulting in a false lumen. By definition, the true lumen is surrounded by intima, and the false lumen lies between the dissected layers. The dissection may remain localized or may propagate longitudinally and distally.

Two classification systems have been used to describe aortic dissections: the DeBakey system and the Stanford system (12,13). DeBakey classifies dissections into three types: Type I, intimal tear in the ascending aorta with extension of the dissection to the descending aorta; Type II, intimal tear in the ascending aorta with dissection confined to the ascending aorta; and Type III, tear beginning in the descending aorta (Fig. 31.1). The Stanford classification system is simpler and uses two groups: Type A dissections that involve the ascending aorta and Type B dissections involving only the descending aorta. The Stanford classification has become more popular because it is related to both therapeutic approach and risk. Type A dissections carry a mortality of 90% to 95% without surgical intervention and account for approximately 65% to 70% of all aortic dissections. Type B dissections carry a 40% mortality and medical management is the preferred type of therapy.

### Epidemiology

The incidence of aortic dissection is approximately 5 per million population per year (14). Independent risk factors for aortic dissection include hypertension, advanced age, connective tissue disorders (Marfan's syndrome), congenital diseases such as coarctation of the aorta, trauma, and perhaps pregnancy. The disease predominantly affects men between 50 and 70 years of age.

## Traumatic Aortic Disease

### Description

Traumatic aortic injuries are the result of either blunt or penetrating trauma. Blunt (acceleration/deceleration) injuries occur from sheer forces that directly damage the arterial wall. The damage typically occurs at the transition point between the aortic arch, a fixed structure, and the more mobile descending aorta. These injuries are typical of motor vehicle accidents. Penetrating injuries occur secondary to stab and gunshot wounds.

### Epidemiology

Of the 100,000 blunt chest trauma hospital admissions per year, approximately 3,000 have aortic injuries requiring surgery (15). Patients with penetrating chest trauma have an incidence of aortic injury of approximately 4% (16). The survival of patients with either blunt or penetrating chest trauma is poor. Most of the patients die before reaching the emergency room. For those who reach the hospital, immediate diagnostic and surgical management are crucial.

## Atherosclerotic Disease

### Description

Atherosclerotic disease of the aorta is pathologically similar to this disease process in the other arteries of the body. Collections of macrophages laden with lipid develop into fibrous plaques that form focal lesions. Over time, they are covered by a layer of smooth muscle cells (17,18). Penetrating aortic ulcers (PAU) occur when an ulceration of an atherosclerotic plaque erodes into the media. This process may progress to the formation of aneurysm, dissection, aortic intramural hematoma (AIH), or aortic rupture. AIH has been defined as a localized separation of the layers of the aortic wall by partially or totally clotted blood, without an intimal tear. Due to their common clinical manifestations AIH, PAU, and aortic dissection have been called "acute aortic syndrome." The rapid progression of both AIH and PAU to life-threatening disease warrants the same urgent approach to diagnosis as in aortic dissection. Patients with any of the three disorders may present with excruciating back pain and may progress to aortic rupture.

Lesions of the ascending aorta and arch have been identified as risk factors for stroke, peripheral emboliza-

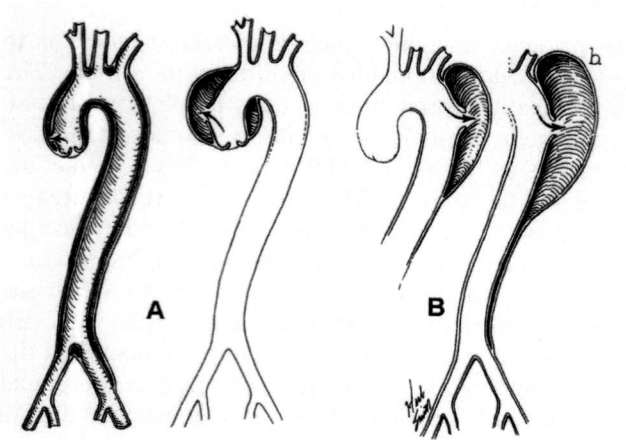

**FIGURE 31.1.** Stanford (A and B) and Debakey (Types 1, 2, 3) classification of aortic dissection. See text for details. Reprinted from Text Book of Surgery, Sabiston: 1998, with permission.

tion, perioperative stroke, as well as neuropsychological dysfunction after open heart surgery (19,20). Atheroemboli, thromboemboli, and plaque thickness > 4 mm correlate with embolic risk. Twelve percent of patients have recurrent strokes within a year, and 33% of patients have emboli. In addition, in patients undergoing cardiopulmonary bypass with identifiable aortic atheroma by transesophageal echocardiography, the risk of stoke is 12%, six times higher than the usual stroke rate.

### Epidemiology

Both aortic dissection and AIH seem to be widely distributed in all segments of the aorta. PAU tends to affect an older population with more cardiac risk factors and more widely spread disease. It occurs predominantly in the descending aorta. The natural history and management of AIH and PAU have not been defined.

The prevalence of aortic arch atheromas in patients with embolic disease has been identified to be approximately 30% in retrospective case-controlled studies, as compared to 4% to 13% in control subjects (21–23).

## OTHER DISEASE

### Congenital Anomalies

#### Description

Coarctation of the aorta, anomalies of the arch and great vessels, and patent ductus arteriosus are the most common adult congenital anomalies of the aorta. Coarctation of the aorta is the most common, and most likely to become problematic in adult life. It consists of a congenital narrowing of the aorta at the area of insertion of the ligamentum arteriosum. Diagnosis is made on physical examination. Hypertension is present in the upper extremities with weak or absent pulses in the lower extremities. Chronic increase in left ventricular afterload can result in hypertrophy or heart failure (24).

#### Epidemiology

Coarctation occurs in about 7% of all patients with congenital heart disease. It is twice as common in males as in females.

### Connective Tissue Disease

#### Description

Marfan's syndrome is an autosomal dominant connective tissue disorder that causes cystic medial necrosis of the aorta. Aortic dilatation and aneurysm result due to the weakened medial layer of elastin. The severe form of the disease is due to a mutation of a single allele of the fibrillin gene. Other connective tissue disorders, such as Ehlers-Danlos syndrome, often present in the same manner.

### Epidemiology

The incidence of Marfan's syndrome in the general population is 1 in 10,000. Ehlers-Danlos is more common, with an incidence of 1 in 5,000. Surgery is advised when the dilation reaches a size of 5.5 cm, due to the propensity of these aneurysms to rupture (25,26).

## TUMOR

Primary tumors of the aorta are rare. They are most often sarcomas or leiomyosarcomas that occur in the descending aorta. Sarcoma has been reported to develop at the site of Dacron grafts (27,28).

## TRANSESOPHAGEAL ECHOCARDIOGRAPHY OF THE AORTA

### Anatomy of the Aorta

Transesophageal echocardiographic evaluation, as well as anesthetic and surgical perioperative management depend not only upon the etiology of disease, but also upon the segment of the aorta involved. The aorta is divided into four parts:

1. Ascending aorta
2. Transverse aortic arch
3. Descending thoracic aorta
4. Thoracoabdominal aorta

The aortic root, the proximal third of the ascending aorta, begins at the aortic valve and houses the sinuses of Valsalva and the right and left coronary arteries. The root is particularly vulnerable in Marfan's syndrome. It courses posterior, superior, and rightward to the right ventricular infundibulum and the pulmonary valve. The middle third of the ascending aorta remains to the right of the main pulmonary artery, anterior to the right pulmonary artery and superior to the superior vena cava. The distal third of the ascending aorta lies anterior to the trachea and right main stem bronchus, courses superior to the pulmonary artery and posterior to the innominate vein. Sixty to 70% of aneurysm dissections occur in the ascending aorta (9).

The aortic arch curves upward between the ascending and descending aortas. Originating from the arch are the innominate (brachiocephalic) artery, the left common carotid artery, and the left subclavian artery, which carry blood to the brain. Both the innominate and left common carotid arteries lie close to the anterior aspect of the trachea. The left subclavian artery lies to the left of the trachea.

The descending thoracic aorta lies distal to the left subclavian artery and curves posteriorly to lie posterior to the esophagus at approximately intercostal space 12. The thoracoabdominal aorta is the descending thoracic and the abdominal aorta.

The wall of the aorta is composed of the intimal, medial, and adventitial layers. The intimal surface is composed of a confluent monolayer of endothelial cells. It is responsible for the regulation of vasomotor tone, inflammatory and immunologic reactions, and coagulation. Eighty percent of aortic wall thickness is comprised by the media, layers of smooth muscle cells intermeshed with connective tissue material. The adventitial layer contains the vasa vasorum, lymphatics, and collagen (29).

## TRANSESOPHAGEAL ECHO EXAMINATION OF THE THORACIC AORTA

Most segments of the thoracic aorta can be clearly imaged with multiplane transesophageal echocardiography (TEE) as the aorta descends along the esophagus. Two blind spots, the distal ascending aorta and the proximal aortic arch, occur due to the intervening trachea and left main stem bronchus. Epiaortic scanning may be useful during surgery in order to visualize these two areas.

Examination of the ascending aorta begins with the midesophageal aortic valve long-axis view at 120 degrees (Fig. 31.2). Slight withdrawal of the probe and rotation of the angle back to 45 degrees will allow further visualiza-

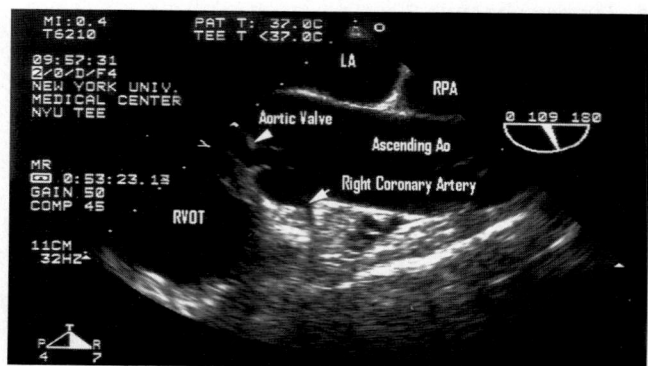

**FIGURE 31.2.** Longitudinal (109°) view of the ascending aorta (*Ascending Ao*) demonstrating an open aortic valve and the right coronary artery off the right coronary sinus. Note the relationships to the right pulmonary artery (*RPA*), left atrium (*LA*), and the right ventricular outflow tract (*RVOT*). Reprinted from Konstadt SN, Shernan S, Oka Y. *Clinical Transesophageal Echocardiography.* Philadelphia: Lippincott, Williams & Wilkins, 2003, with permission.

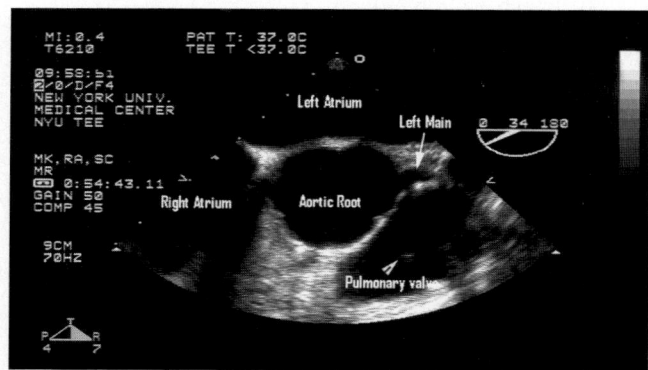

**FIGURE 31.3.** Slightly oblique transverse (34°) view of the base of the heart through the aortic root demonstrating the left main coronary artery (*Left Main*) arising from the left coronary sinus. The tip of the pulmonic valve is above the *arrow.* Reprinted from Konstadt SN, Shernan S, Oka Y. *Clinical Transesophageal Echocardiography.* Philadelphia: Lippincott, Williams & Wilkins, 2003, with permission.

tion of the ascending aorta. The midesophageal ascending aortic short-axis view appears simply by rotating the angle between 0 to 45 degrees (Figs. 31.3 and 31.4). This view displays the main and right pulmonary arteries as longitudinal structures and the aorta as a circular section. The diameter of the aorta may be measured in either the short- or long-axis views.

Examination of the descending thoracic aorta begins by turning the probe to the left from the midesophageal four-chamber view until a circular structure appears in the upper center of the echo image. This view is called the descending aorta short-axis view and is best viewed with an enlarged picture at a depth of 6 cm to 8 cm (Fig. 31.5). The rotation of the multiplane probe to 90 degrees will produce a horizontal long-axis view of the descending aorta (Fig. 31.6). The entire descending thoracic and upper abdominal aorta can be imaged in either long- or short-axis by slowly advancing and withdrawing the

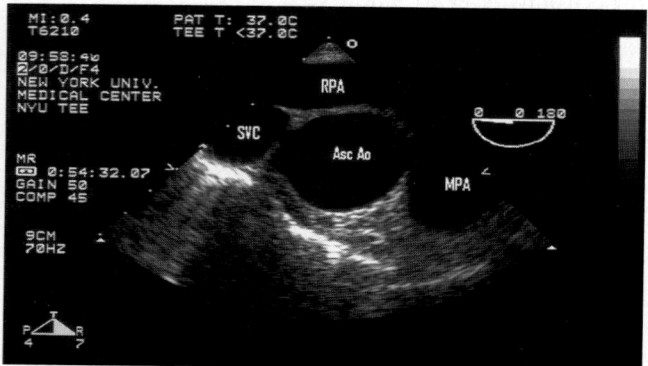

**FIGURE 31.4.** Transverse (0°) view of the ascending aorta (*Asc Ao*) at the base of the heart, just superior to the sinotubular ridge. Note the relationship of the right pulmonary artery (*RPA*), superior vena cava (*SVC*), and main pulmonary artery (*MPA*).

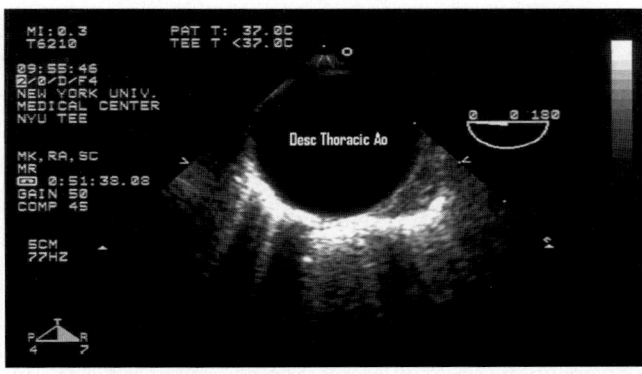

**FIGURE 31.5.** Transverse (0°) view of the descending thoracic aorta (*Desc Thoracic Ao*). Reprinted from Konstadt SN, Shernan S, Oka Y. *Clinical Transesophageal Echocardiography.* Philadelphia: Lippincott, Williams & Wilkins, 2003, with permission.

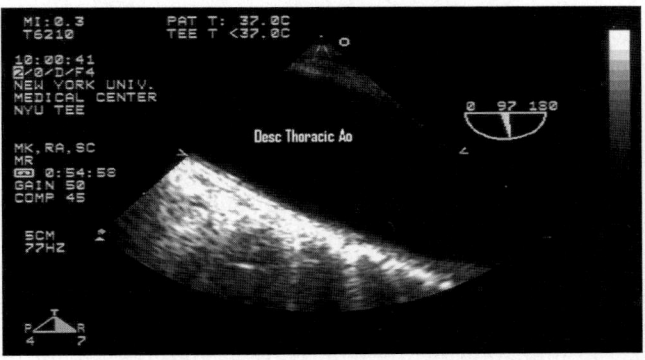

**FIGURE 31.6.** Longitudinal (97°) view of the descending thoracic aorta (*Desc Thoracic Ao*). Reprinted from Konstadt SN, Shernan S, Oka Y. *Clinical Transesophageal Echocardiography.* Philadelphia: Lippincott, Williams & Wilkins, 2003, with permission.

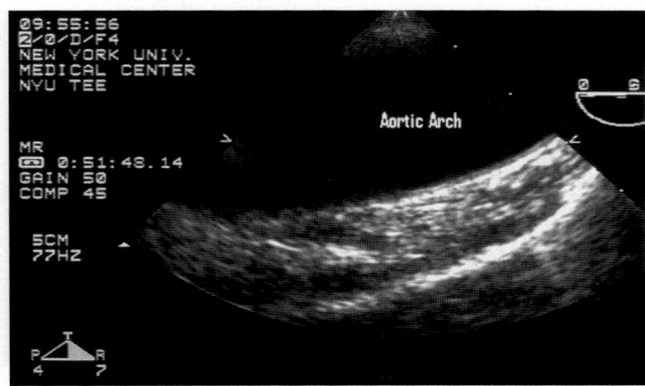

**FIGURE 31.7.** Transverse (0°) view of the distal aortic arch (*Aortic Arch*). Reprinted from Konstadt SN, Shernan S, Oka Y. *Clinical Transesophageal Echocardiography.* Philadelphia: Lippincott, Williams & Wilkins, 2003, with permission.

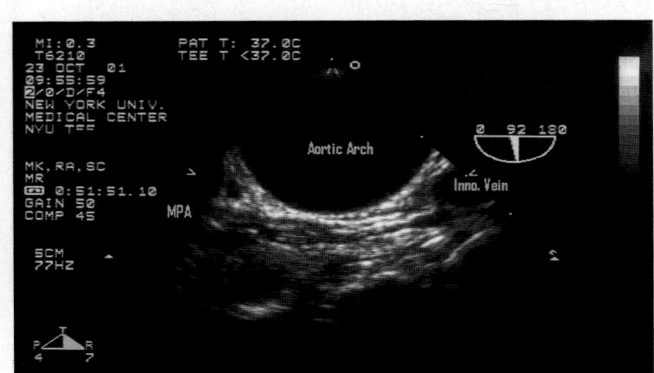

**FIGURE 31.8.** Longitudinal (92°) view of the midaortic arch, demonstrating its relationship to the main pulmonary artery (*MPA*) and the innominate vein (*Inno Vein*). Reprinted from Konstadt SN, Shernan S, Oka Y. *Clinical Transesophageal Echocardiography.* Philadelphia: Lippincott, Williams & Wilkins, 2003, with permission.

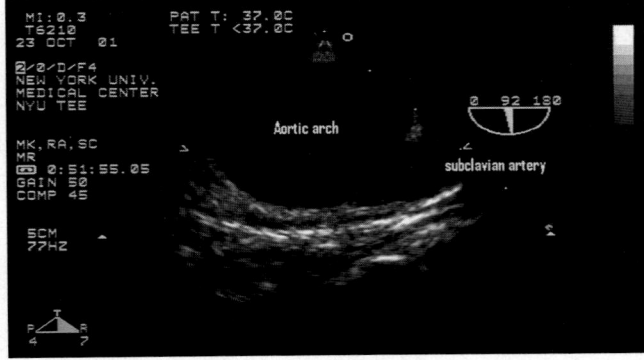

**FIGURE 31.9.** Longitudinal (92°) view of the midaortic arch, demonstrating the takeoff of the left subclavian artery (*subclavian artery*). Reprinted from Konstadt SN, Shernan S, Oka Y. *Clinical Transesophageal Echocardiography.* Philadelphia: Lippincott, Williams & Wilkins, 2003, with permission.

probe. It is often difficult to pinpoint the exact location of a descending aortic lesion due to the changing positional relationship of the esophagus and the aorta. Localization of aortic wall lesions is often marked in terms of their distance from the left subclavian artery.

As the probe is withdrawn at an angle of 0 degrees the circular descending aorta becomes an elliptical structure, the aortic arch. This view is called the upperesophageal aortic arch long-axis view (Fig. 31.7). The distal arch is to the right of the image and the proximal arch to the left, with the posterior wall at the top and the anterior wall below. Turning the probe to the right and the left will allow full visualization of the length of the arch. A short-axis aortic arch view may be obtained by rotating the multiplane angle to 90 degrees (Fig. 31.8).

The arch vessels are often difficult to image adequately. Beginning with the upperesophageal long-axis view, withdrawal of the probe superiorly, and rotation of the multiplane angle to 20 to 40 degrees may allow visualization of the proximal left subclavian and carotid arteries (Figs. 31.9–31.11). Visualization of one of these two

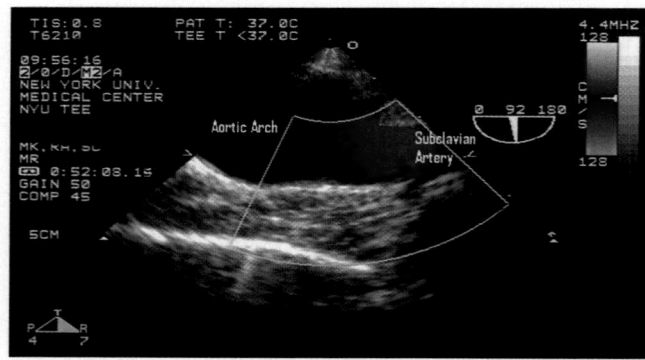

**FIGURE 31.10.** Color Flow Doppler in the longitudinal (92°) view of the midaortic arch, demonstrating nonturbulent normal blood flow in the left subclavian artery.

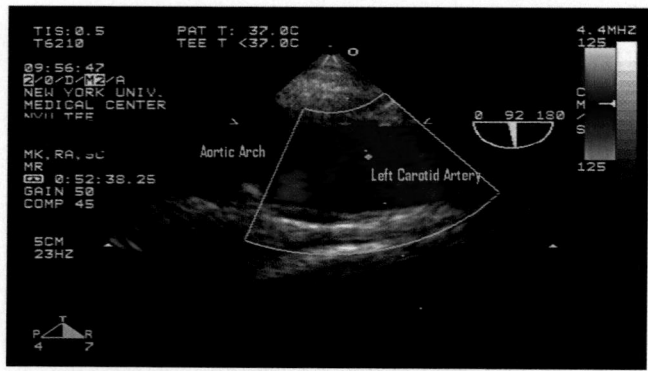

**FIGURE 31.11.** Color Flow Doppler in the longitudinal (92°) view of the midaortic arch, demonstrating nonturbulent normal blood flow in the left carotid artery takeoff.

structures is reported to occur approximately 60% of the time, while both are visualized 75% of the time. The innominate artery and the distal ascending aorta are obscured from view by the air-filled trachea (30,31).

## STRUCTURES

### TEE Sensitivity and Specificity by Disease Classification

#### Comparison to Other Diagnostic and Monitoring Modalities

Transesophageal echocardiography has become increasingly valuable as a diagnostic and monitoring modality in thoracic aortic disease. One unique advantage is its portability to all locations, allowing the unstable patient to remain in a monitored critical care setting. In addition, with advances in echo technology over the past 20 years, higher degrees of resolution of the normal and abnormal pathology of the three layers of the aortic wall and the aortic lumen may be obtained.

## Aneurysm

Thoracic aortic aneurysms are often detected in asymptomatic patients undergoing examination for other disease. Symptoms occur as the aneurysm ruptures or enlarges and compresses adjacent structures, which may include the esophagus, lung, and superior vena cava.

Chest x-ray often reveals larger aneurysms as an enlarged mediastinum, aortic knob, or tracheal deviation. Smaller aneurysms are often entirely missed by chest films. Angiography continues to be the gold standard for evaluation of size and location. Computed tomography and magnetic resonance imaging are replacing more invasive angiography as diagnostic tools. No studies have been performed to compare the accuracies of these techniques. TEE is becoming an alternative to these modalities, particularly if aortic dissection is suspected. The portability and rapidity of TEE diagnosis makes it the diagnostic modality of choice if the patient is unstable. Comparison to other diagnostic modalities has been more specific in aortic dissection and is described below.

## Dissection

Aortic dissection is catastrophic and has an extremely high mortality in the first 48 hours. Early diagnosis and treatment with either surgical or medical therapy can improve outcome. In the hemodynamically stable patient a thorough TEE exam should be performed, including (1) examination of the left ventricle and assessment of global function, (2) aortic valve examination to detect the presence and degree of regurgitation (Fig 31.12), and (3) examination for pericardial or pleural effusion or hemothorax. In the unstable patient the TEE exam should proceed directly to the examination of the aorta, as described above. The size of the aortic root, ascending aorta, and descending aorta should be measured and any increased

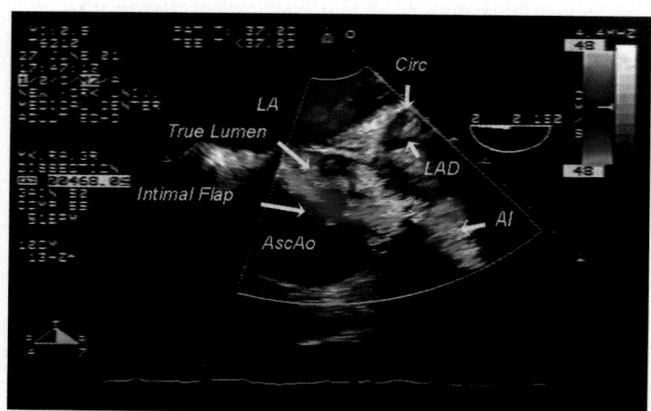

**FIGURE 31.12.** Color Flow Doppler exam of a patient with an acute aortic dissection and aortic insufficiency (*AI*). Note the flow in the circumflex coronary artery and the left anterior descending artery (*Circ, LAD*).

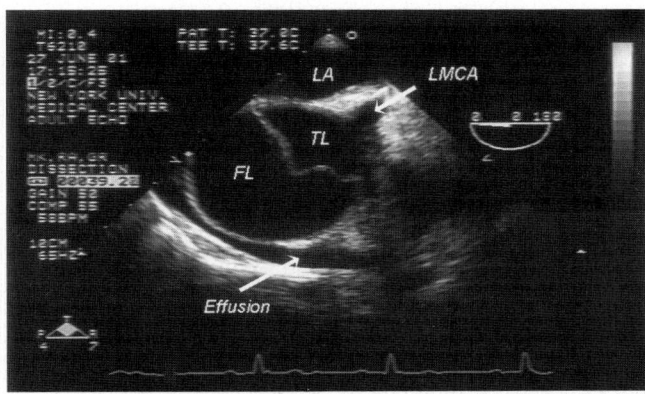

**FIGURE 31.13.** Transverse view of complete aortic dissection at the level of the left main coronary artery (*LMCA*). Note the pericardial effusion.

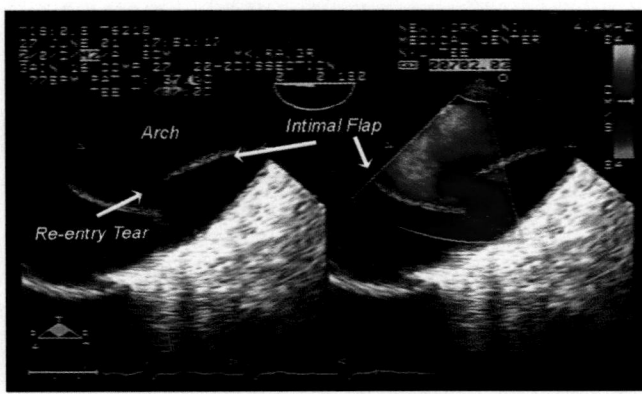

**FIGURE 31.16.** Transverse view of the aortic arch, demonstrating the entry point of an intimal flap.

diameter of the aorta is noted. High gain settings will allow better visualization of any thrombus or spontaneous echo contrast. The pathognomonic echocardiographic appearance of dissection is an undulating linear density (intimal flap) within the aortic lumen separating a true and false lumen, which have different Doppler flow patterns (Figs. 31.13–31.16). These criteria may be too restrictive, and dissection should be suspected whenever the single aortic wall appearance is replaced by two separate echo densities, one representing the intimal wall and the other the outer media and adventitia.

The previous gold standard for diagnosis of dissection was aortography. Other new technologies, including CT scans, MRI, transthoracic echocardiography (TTE), and TEE have been used for diagnosis. The portability, low cost, speed, and accuracy of TEE have made it an increasingly popular first choice for diagnosis. At least seven studies involving 50 to more than 100 patients have reported on the sensitivity and specificity of TEE in the diagnosis of dissection (32). The sensitivity was high, between 97% and 100%, and the specificity ranged from 77% to 100%. A series of 110 patients compared TTE, TEE, CT, and MRI (33). Sensitivities were low for TTE (59%) as compared to the other three imaging modalities: TEE (98%), CT (94%), and MRI (98%). The specificities were TTE (83%), TEE (77%), CT (87%), and MRI (98%). Due to the outstanding accuracy of MRI the authors of this study recommended MRI as the initial diagnostic procedure in stable patients and TEE in unstable patients. The low range of specificity of TEE may be attributed to difficulty of visualization of the ascending aorta with monoplane and biplane probes. Reverberation artifacts are common in dilated ascending aortas and may lead to false positive diagnosis of type II dissection. False negatives can occur when the dissection is in the upper ascending aorta or the proximal arch due to blind spots caused by the air-filled trachea (34). Recent studies have evaluated the diagnostic accuracy of multiplane TEE and have noted improved accuracy, with sensitivity between 98% and 100% and specificity between 94% and

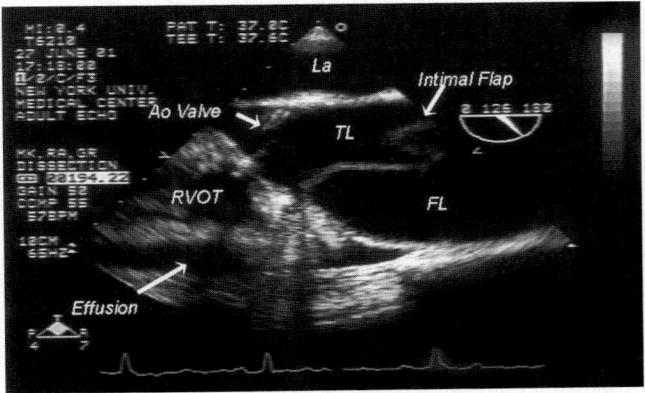

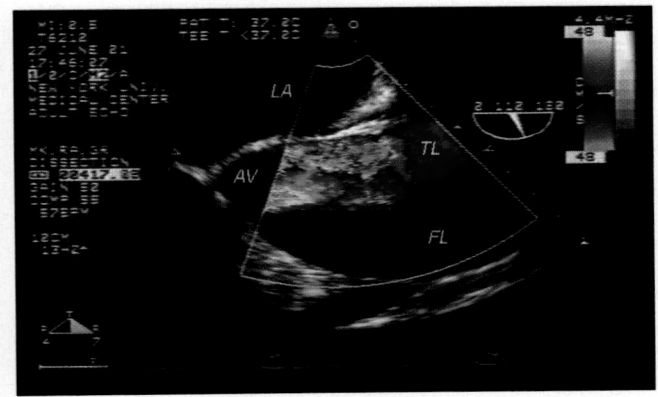

**FIGURES 31.14. and 31.15.** Longitudinal view of the ascending aorta of the same patient shown in Figure 31.13. Note the absence of flow in the false lumen (*FL*).

95% (35,36). Measures that have been used in order to increase accuracy have been the combination of TEE with M-mode echocardiography in order to recognize reverberation artifacts (37) and refinement of diagnostic criteria to state that patients with thickened aortic walls with an inner echo that was smooth and highly echo reflective were most likely to have intimal flaps (38).

In addition to accuracy, many factors have importance when choosing an initial diagnostic modality for suspected aortic dissection. TEE is completed quickly, is portable, is low cost, and is less invasive than CT and aortography. In addition, TEE can provide accurate information about the following factors that are relevant to surgical decision making: (1) the extent of the dissection, (2) the entry and exit points, (3) involvement of the aortic valve or other branches of the aorta, (4) left ventricular function, and (5) the presence of pericardial or pleural fluid. TEE may be used as the sole modality to evaluate these patients prior to surgery.

## Traumatic Disease of the Aorta

Trauma to the aorta, whether blunt or penetrating, carries a high early mortality. Accurate and immediate diagnosis and therapy are crucial to survival. Conventional management with aortography is limited by the risk of contrast, further vascular damage, and inconvenience. The speed and portability of TEE has increased its use in the diagnosis and management of traumatic disease. Goarin et al. described the various TEE findings in traumatic disease after studying 28 patients (39). These include thick stripes reflecting damage to the intima and media, intimal flaps, changes in the shape of the aorta with either fusiform dilatation or distortion of the circular shape, and less commonly intraluminal thrombus or medial hematoma (Fig. 31.17).

In 1995, Vignon et al. proposed an echocardiographic classification dividing aortic trauma into four types: trau-matic intimal tears, partial subadventitial aortic disruptions, subtotal subadventitial disruptions, and subadventitial disruption. Intimal tears appear as thin, linear echo densities; they can be managed medically and have a good prognosis. Subadventitial disruptions require urgent surgical treatment. Partial disruptions appear as deep breaks in the continuity of the aortic wall. Subtotal disruptions are characterized by a tear, involving at least two-thirds of the aortic wall, and total disruptions appear as a thick flap with the media completely separated from the adventitia (40).

Several studies involving relatively small numbers of patients have evaluated the sensitivity and specificity of TEE in aortic trauma. The sensitivity of TEE for diagnosing aortic trauma ranges from 57% to 100% and the specificity from 84% to 100%. The large range in these results may be attributed to whether trauma surgeons or cardiologists interpreted the echos, with surgical interpretation being less accurate (41–46). The ability to simultaneously evaluate cardiac function, volume status, effusions, and valvular abnormalities using TEE suggests that it may become a crucial part of the initial diagnostic evaluation of traumatic injury to the aorta.

## Atherosclerotic Disease of the Aorta

The development of aortic atheromas follows the natural history of atherosclerotic disease, increasing with age and insidiously progressing through the years. It correlates with the other risk factors for atherosclerosis: smoking, hypercholesterolemia, and hypertension. Thoracic aortic plaque is most often seen in the elderly (> 70 years). Embolization from aortic plaque is responsible for stroke and peripheral vasoocclusive disease, and is the most common cause of stroke during open heart surgery.

Intraoperative detection of aortic atheroma is feasible with both epiaortic and transesophageal echocardiography. The three-stage grading system devised by Tunick et al. is the simplest and most commonly used. Grade I (insignificant) plaque is < 2 mm (Fig. 31.18); Grade II (moderate disease) is plaque or intimal thickening of 2 mm to 5 mm (Figs. 31.19 and 31.20), and Grade III (severe disease) plaque > 5 mm or mobile (Figs. 31.21–31.24) (47,48). CT scanning, used to evaluate patients who also had TEE, was found to have a sensitivity of 87% and a specificity of 82%. Gated MRI studies found fewer Grade III plaques when compared to TEE. In comparison to epiaortic scanning, TEE has been found to be superior for plaque identification in the descending aorta and arch, but has a poor predictive value in detecting disease in the ascending aorta. A combination of both techniques is recommended in patients at high risk for disease in the distal ascending aorta (49–52).

The incidence of perioperative stroke correlates with the TEE grade of atherosclerotic plaque. Several studies have found a stroke rate of approximately 30% in patients

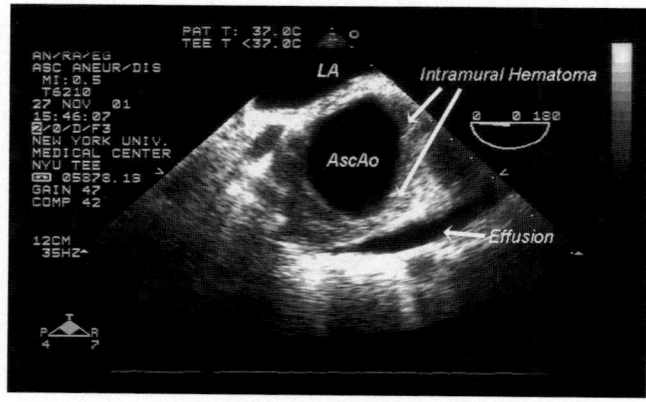

**FIGURE 31.17.** Intramural hematoma of the ascending aorta in a patient who suffered a rapid deceleration.

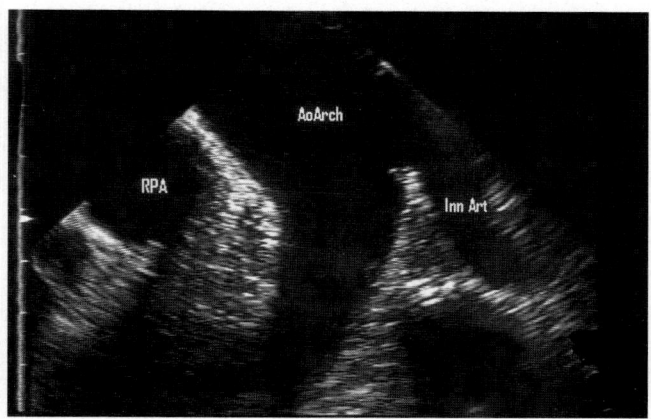

**FIGURE 31.18.** Epiaortic scan of the proximal aortic arch (*Ao Arch*), showing normal intima, Grade I. Note the innominate artery (*Inn Art*). Reprinted from Konstadt SN, Shernan S, Oka Y. *Clinical Transesophageal Echocardiography.* Philadelphia: Lippincott, Williams & Wilkins, 2003, with permission.

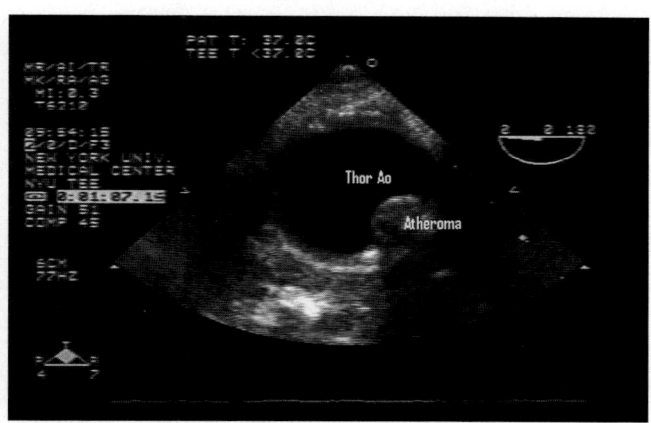

**FIGURE 31.21.** Transverse view of the thoracic aorta, showing severe protruding intimal atherosclerosis with ulcerations. Reprinted from Konstadt SN, Shernan S, Oka Y. *Clinical Transesophageal Echocardiography.* Philadelphia: Lippincott, Williams & Wilkins, 2003, with permission.

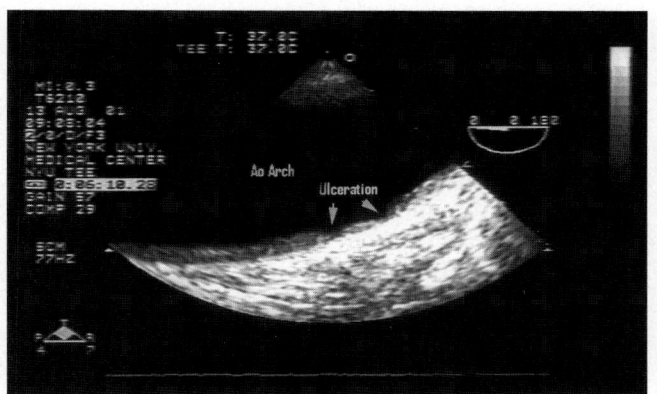

**FIGURE 31.19.** Transverse view of the aortic arch, showing mild intimal atherosclerosis with ulcerations.

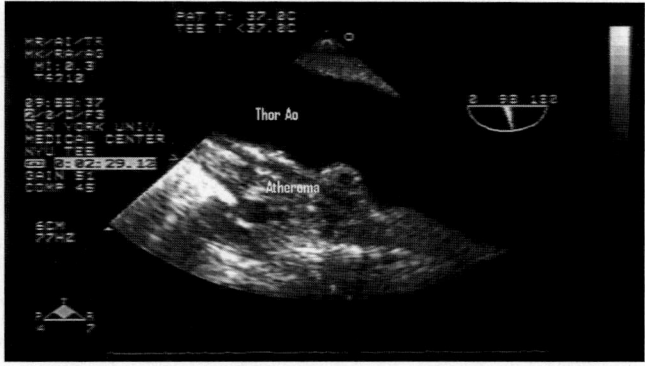

**FIGURE 31.22.** Longitudinal view of the thoracic aorta, showing severe protruding and ulcerated complex atheromatous disease. Reprinted from Konstadt SN, Shernan S, Oka Y. *Clinical Transesophageal Echocardiography.* Philadelphia: Lippincott, Williams & Wilkins, 2003, with permission.

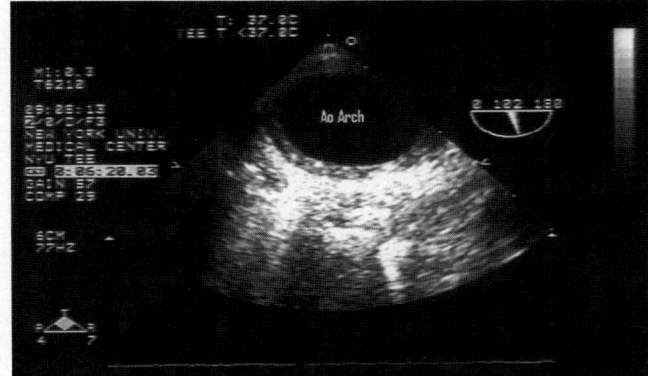

**FIGURE 31.20.** Longitudinal view of the aortic arch, showing mild intimal atherosclerosis.

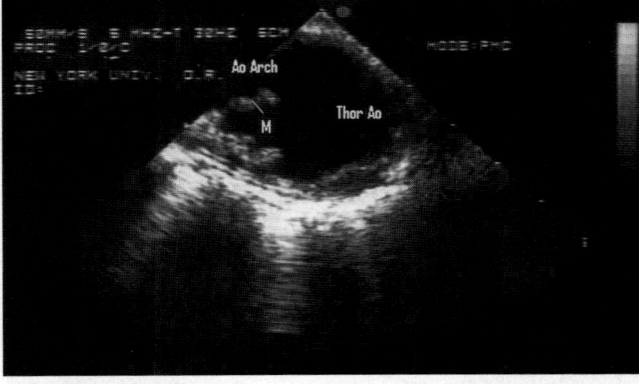

**FIGURE 31.23.** Transverse view of distal aortic arch (*Arch*) where it meets the thoracic aorta, showing a large mobile (*M*) atheroma.

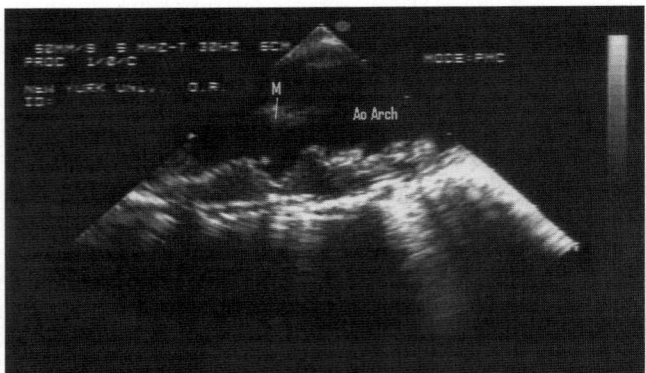

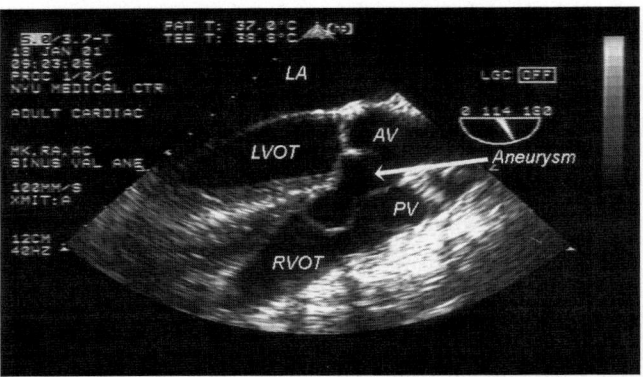

**FIGURE 31.24.** Transverse view of the aortic arch (*arch*) more proximally, showing a large mobile (*M*) atheroma.

**FIGURE 31.26.** Sinus of Valsava aneurysm, demonstrating protrusion into the right ventricular outflow tract (*RVOT*).

with Grade III plaque when surgical technique was not modified (53,54).

## Other Disease

### Coarctation of the Aorta

Two-dimensional echocardiography can identify the site and length of the coarctation. Doppler studies record and quantify the pressure gradient. Transesophageal echocardiography and magnetic resonance imaging or digital angiography allow visualization of the length and severity of the obstruction.

### Tumors

The position and extent of aortic tumors are discernable on TEE (Fig. 31.25).

### Sinus of Valsalva Aneurysms

The diagnosis of sinus of Valsalva aneurysms can be made by TEE (Figs. 31.26 and 31.27).

## PATHOPHYSIOLOGY OF AORTIC DISEASE

### Role of TEE in Anesthetic and Surgical Management

#### Disease of the Ascending Aorta and Arch

The surgical approach to disease of the ascending aorta and arch is median sternotomy, regardless of the disease process. The procedure depends upon the type and extent of the disease, ranging from insertion of a tubular graft to replace the diseased segment of the aorta to procedures that require the replacement of the aortic valve, reimplantation of the coronary arteries, and reimplantation of the arch vessels. These procedures invariably involve cardiopulmonary bypass. Surgical mortality for acute type A dissection remains high at 40%, while those undergoing elective repair for aneurysms and dissection have a mortality of 10%.

Patients presenting for ascending aorta and arch surgery often have coexisting medical conditions related

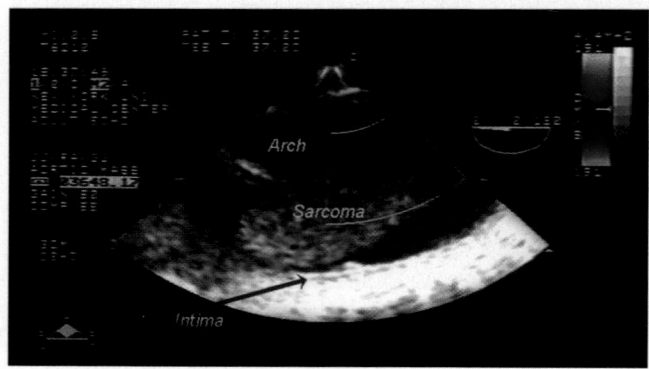

**FIGURE 31.25.** Large sarcoma of the aortic arch.

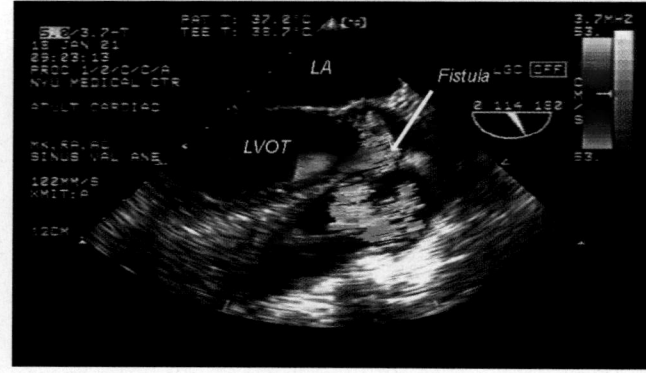

**FIGURE 31.27.** Sinus of Valsava aneurysm, demonstrating protrusion into the right ventricular outflow tract (*RVOT*). Note the AV fistula on color Doppler.

to atherosclerotic disease, including ischemic heart disease, peripheral vascular disease, and cerebral vascular disease. Careful evaluation of these conditions preoperatively will determine the nature of intraoperative monitoring and management. Standard monitors as well as arterial blood pressure, Swan-Ganz catheters, and TEE are routine for surgery on the ascending aorta and arch. Postinduction TEE evaluation of the heart can provide information about volume status, regional wall motion abnormalities, and aortic valve competence, as well as estimates of stroke volume and ejection fraction. Examination of the thoracic aorta will provide information of the extent of aortic disease, including size and extension of the aneurysm or dissection and grading and location of atheroma prior to the placement of cannulae for cardiopulmonary bypass. TEE-guided placement of femoral venous catheters and retrograde cardioplegia catheters occur prior to bypass. Surgery may be complicated by blood pressure lability due to intravascular volume shifts, surgical manipulation, effects of anesthetic agents, or rapid blood loss. In addition, many of these patients have myocardial disease that may result in intraoperative myocardial ischemia or heart failure. Continuous TEE monitoring during the procedure allows immediate detection and treatment of ischemic changes and differences in ventricular function and volume status. Examination of the aorta after cardiopulmonary bypass aids in determining the reestablishment of flow to the proper lumens and the safety of wraps of the graft (Fig. 31.28).

### Descending Thoracic Aortic Disease

Surgical repair of lesions of the descending aorta is performed in the right lateral decubitus position via a posterolateral thoracotomy. Cannulae are inserted for the perfusion of the distal aorta by partial left heart bypass or partial cardiopulmonary bypass. Vascular cross clamps are placed to isolate the diseased section of the aorta in order to allow anterograde flow to the coronary and brachiocephalic vessels and retrograde flow via the femoral arteries to vessels below the clamp.

Preoperative considerations for patients with descending aortic disease are similar to those described above for disease of the ascending aorta and arch. Appropriate monitoring during anesthesia consists of standard monitors, invasive blood pressure, pulmonary artery catheter monitoring, and TEE. A complete postinduction TEE examination provides information about concomitant cardiac disease and left ventricular dysfunction. Aortic pathology can be visualized and confirmed (Fig. 31.29). Cannula position in the femoral artery can be monitored with TEE in order to insure that the cannula is positioned in the true lumen. Surgical repair of descending aortic disease is always accompanied by rapid hemodynamic changes due to alterations in preload and afterload. Preload change can arise from aortic rupture or extensive bleeding during the procedure. Abrupt changes in afterload are caused by aortic clamping and unclamping and may result in myocardial dysfunction that can be diagnosed early with the use of TEE.

### Atherosclerotic Disease and Its Relationship to Cardiac Surgery

Embolic stroke and peripheral emboli are serious complications of open heart surgery performed with cardiopulmonary bypass (54–56). These events are particularly common in elderly patients (> 70 years). There are a variety of etiologies for these embolic phenomena, including air emboli, pump debris, aortic manipulation and dislodging of thrombi during cross clamping of the aorta, graft anastomosis, cannula placement, or a sandblasting effect from cannula flow. Ascending aorta and arch atheroma visualized by TEE have been correlated with a high risk of perioperative stroke in patients undergoing cardiopulmonary bypass. Identification of atheroma by

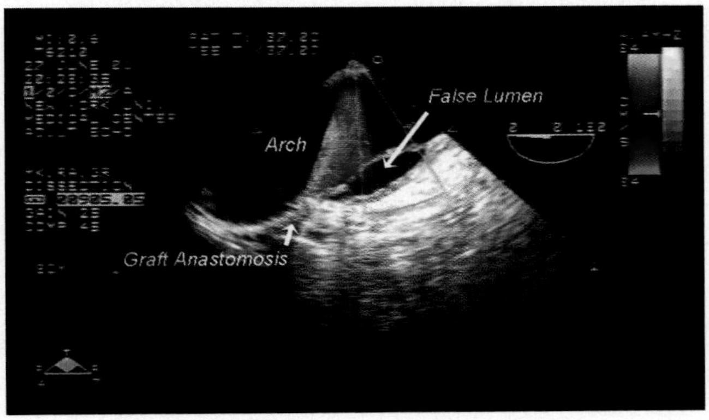

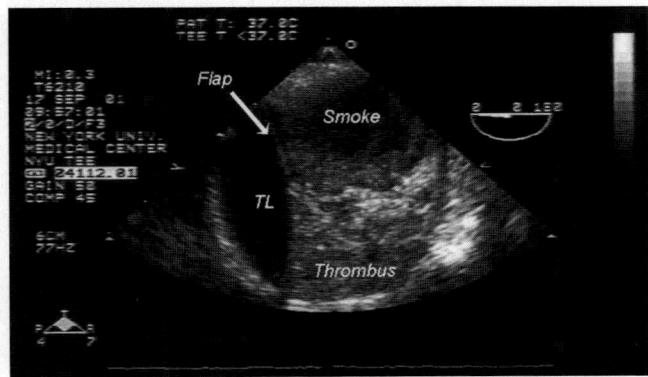

**FIGURE 31.28.** Postbypass examination of the aortic arch (*Arch*), demonstrating proper placement of an ascending aortic graft with reestablishment of flow to the true lumen.

**FIGURE 31.29.** Prebypass examination of a large descending thoracic aortic aneurysm. Dissection demonstrating thrombus formation and low flow in the false lumen.

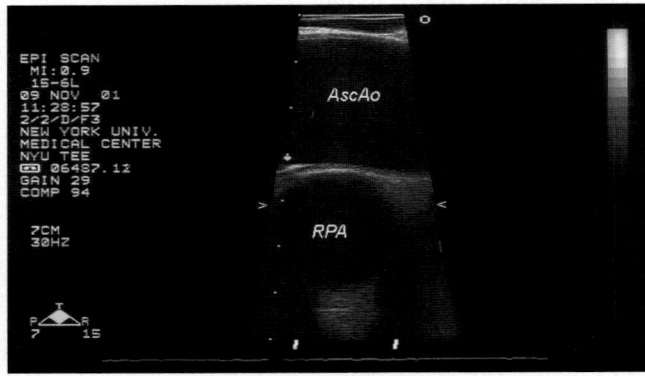

**FIGURE 31.30.** Longitudinal view of the ascending aorta using a 7.5 mghz epiaortic probe, demonstrating a normal aorta.

palpation is not as successful with 83% of plaques identified by TEE missed by palpation (57). Evaluation of the ascending aorta by epiaortic ultrasound has been found to be superior to TEE (Figs. 31.30 and 31.31). The most successful approach proves to be a combination of TEE and epiaortic scanning (Fig. 31.32) (58–60).

Aortic arch atheromas larger than 5 mm (Grade III) prove to be a highly significant risk factor for perioperative stroke, with an incidence of 11.6%. In a subgroup of patients who had atherectomy prior to either valve replacement or bypass grafting, the stroke incidence rose to 35%. These most often resulted in major neurologic events with an in-hospital mortality of 39% and significantly prolonged hospitalizations in the group that survived. Those who left the hospital often had major disability. In addition, the in-hospital mortality of all patients with arch atheroma with or without neurologic complications was close to 15% (61,62).

These patients represent a very high risk group. Arch atherectomy clearly increases the morbidity during open heart surgery and should not be performed. A complete

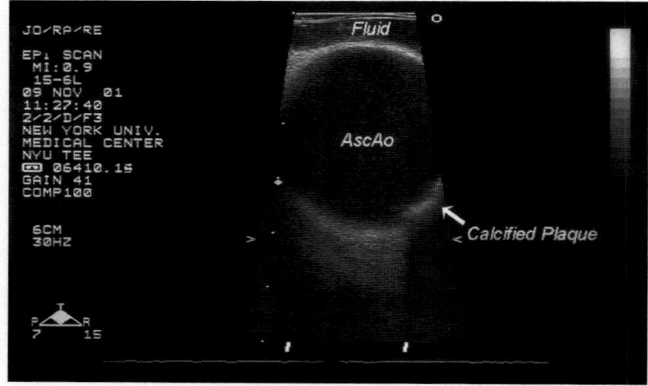

**FIGURE 31.31.** Transverse view of the ascending aorta using a 7.5 mghz epiaortic probe, demonstrating a small plaque posterior in the ascending aorta.

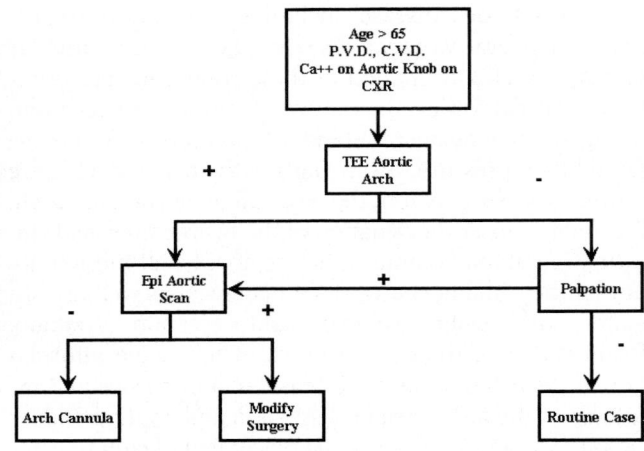

**FIGURE 31.32.** Flow chart of operative diagnosis and management of aortic atherosclerosis during cardiac surgery.

examination of the aorta after the induction of anesthesia and the use of the grading system for plaque will outline the extent of aortic disease. In coronary surgery, which may be performed off pump, the presence of severe atheromatous disease may influence the surgical decision to avoid cardiopulmonary bypass. If off-pump surgery is not an option, as in valvular or intracardiac surgery, location of atheromas can guide the placement of cross clamps, cardioplegia cannulae, and coronary grafts (63–69).

### KEY POINTS

- The refinement and expanded use of transesophageal echocardiography as a diagnostic modality for aortic disease has refined perioperative care.
- When compared to traditional and more invasive methods of diagnosis, such as angiography, MRI, and CT scanning, TEE demonstrates unique specificity and sensitivity.
- TEE is a portable, noninvasive rapid diagnostic tool that has improved patient safety by decreasing the time to diagnosis preoperatively.
- Intraoperative TEE is useful as a guide to reparative surgery of the aorta.
- Intraoperative diagnosis of atheromatous disease has enabled improved outcomes in cardiac surgery as it serves to guide operative technique.

### REFERENCES

1. Dubost C, Allary M, Oecanomos N. Resection of an aneurysm of the abdominal aorta: reestablishment of the continuity by a preserved human arterial graft, with the results after five months. Arch Surg 1952;64:405–9.

2. Gross RE, Bill AH Jr, Pierce EC. II: methods for the preservation and transplantation of arterial grafts. Observations on arterial grafts in dogs: report of transplantation of preserved arterial grafts in 9 human cases. Surg Gynecol Obstet 1949; 88:689–93.

3. Swan H, Maaske C, Johnson M, et al. Arterial homografts. II. Resection of the thoracic aortic aneurysm using a stored human arterial transplant. Arch Surg 1950;61:732–37.

4. Lam CR, Avram HH. Resection of the descending thoracic aorta for aneurysm. A report of the use of a homograft in a case and an experimental study. Ann Surg 1951;134: 734–39.

5. Debakey ME, Codey DA. Successful resection of aneurysm of the thoracic aorta and replacement by graft. JAMA 1953; 152:673–76.

6. Gibbon JH Jr. Application of mechanical heart lung apparatus to cardiac surgery. Minn Med 1954;37:171–75.

7. Johnston KW, Rutherford RB, Tilson MD, et al. Suggested standards for reporting on arterial aneurysms. Subcommittee on reporting standards for arterial aneurysms, Ad Hoc Committee on Reporting Standards, Society for Vascular Surgery, and North American Chapter, International Society for Cardiovascular Surgery. J Vasc Surg 1991;13:452–58.

8. Crawford ES. A prospective randomized study of cerebrospinal fluid drainage to prevent paraplegia after high risk surgery on the thoracoabdominal aorta. J Vasc Surg 1991; 13:36–45.

9. Bickerstaff LK, Pairoleto PC, Hollier LH, et al. Thoracic aortic aneurysms. A population based study. Surgery 1982; 92:1103–8.

10. Szilagyi DE, Elliot JP, Smith RF. Clinical fate of the patient with asymptomatic abdominal aneurysm and unfit for surgical treatment. Arch Surg 1972;104:600–4.

11. Juvonen T, Ergin MA, Galla JD, et al. Prospective study on the natural history of thoracic aortic aneurysm. Ann Thor Surg 1997;63:1533–45.

12. DeBakey ME, McCollum CH, Crawford ES, et al. Dissection and dissecting aneurysms of the aorta: twenty year follow up of 527 patients treated surgically. Surgery 1982;92:1118–34.

13. Daily PO, Trueblood HW, Stinson ED, et al. Management of acute aortic dissections. Ann Thorac Surg 1970;10:237–47.

14. Wheat MW Jr. Acute dissecting aneurysms of the aorta. Diagnosis and treatment. Am Heart 1980;99:373–87.

15. Von Kessler LK, Fischer A, Vogt P, et al. Diagnosis and management of blunt great vessel trauma. J Card Surg 1997;12: 181–92.

16. Demetriades D. Penetrating injuries to the thoracic great vessels. J Card Surg 1997;12:173–80.

17. Stary HC, Chandler AB, Glagov S, et al. A definition of initial, fatty streak, and intermediate lesions of atherosclerosis. A report from the Committee on Vascular Lesions of the Council on Arteriosclerosis, American Heart Association. Circulation 1994;89:2462–78.

18. Lindsay J Jr, Beall AC Jr, DeBakey ME. Diagnosis and treatment of diseases of the aorta, in Alexander RW, Schlant RC, Fuster V, eds. Hurst's The Heart, 9th edition. New York: McGraw-Hill, 1998:2170–75.

19. Roach GW, Kanchuger M, Mangano CM, et al. Adverse cerebral outcomes after coronary bypass surgery. Multicenter Study of Perioperative Ischemia Research Group and the Ischemia Research and Education Foundation Investigators. NEJM 1996;35:1857–63.

20. Marschall K, Kanchuger M, Kessler K, et al. Superiority of transesophageal echocardiography in detecting aortic arch atheromatous disease: Identification of patients at increased risk of stroke during cardiac surgery. J Cardiothorac Vasc Anesth 1994;8:5–13.

21. Karalis DG, Krishnaswamy C, Victor MF, et al. Recognition and embolic potential of intraaortic atherosclerotic debris. J Am Coll Cardiol 1991;17:73–8.

22. The French Study of Aortic Plaques in Strokes Group. Atherosclerotic disease of the aortic arch as a risk factor for recurrent ischemic stroke. NEJM 1996;334:1216–21.

23. Stone DH, Hawke MW, laMonte M, et al. Ulcerated atherosclerotic plaques in the thoracic aorta are associated with cryptogenic stroke. Am Heart J 1995;130:105–8.

24. Lindsay J Jr., DeBakey ME, Beall AC. Diagnosis and treatment of diseases of the aorta, in Schlant RC, Alexander RW, et al., eds. Hurst's The Heart, 8th ed. New York: McGraw-Hill, 1994:2170–75.

25. Isselbacher EM, Eagle KA, Desanctis RW. Diseases of the aorta, in Braunwald E, ed. Heart Disease, 5th ed. Philadelphia: Saunders 1997:1546.

26. Hollister DW, Godfrey M, Sakai LY, et al. Immunohistologic abnormalities of the microfibrillar-fiber system in Marfan syndrome. NEJM 1990;323:152–9.

27. Fyfe BS, Quintana CS, Kaneko M, et al. Aortic sarcoma four years after Dacron graft insertion. Ann Thorac Surg 1994;58: 1752–4.

28. Navarra G, Occhionorelli S, Mascoll F, et al. Primary leiomyosarcoma of the aorta. Report of a case and review of the literature. J Cardiovasc Surg 1994;35:333–6.

29. Pick TP, Howden R. The Aorta, in Gray's Anatomy. Philadelphia: Running Press, 1974:475–80.

30. Delphin E, Kanchuger M. Aortic atherosclerosis. In: Konstadt SN, ed. Clinical transesophageal echocardiography. Philadelphia: Lippincott Williams & Wilkins, in press.

31. Katz ES, Konecky N, Tunick, et al. Visualization and identification of the left common carotid and left subclavian arteries: A transesophageal echo approach. J Am Soc Echocardiog 1996;9:58–61.

32. Willens HJ, Kessler KM. Transesophageal echocardiography in the diagnosis of diseases of the thoracic aorta. Chest 1999;116:1772–9.

33. Nienaber CA, Kodolitsch YU, Nicholas V, et al. The diagnosis of thoracic aortic dissection by noninvasive imaging procedures. NEJM 1993;328:1–9.

34. Applebee AF, Walker PG, Yeoh JK, et al. Clinical significance and origin of artifacts in transesophageal echocardiography of the thoracic aorta. J Am Coll Cardiol 1993;21:754–60.

35. Koren A, Kim CB, Hu BS, et al. Accuracy of biplane and multiplane transesophageal echocardiography in diagnosis of typical acute aortic dissection and intramural hematoma. J Am Coll Cardiol 1996;28:627–36.

36. Sommer T, Fehske W, Holzkuecht N, et al. Aortic dissection: a comparative study of diagnosis with spiral CT, multiplanar transesophageal echocardiography and MR imaging. Radiology 1996;199:347–52.

37. Evangelista A, Garcia del Castillo H, Gonzalez-Alujas T, et al. Diagnosis of ascending aortic dissection by transesophageal echocardiography: utility of M mode in recognizing artifact. J Am Coll Cardiol 1996;27:102–7.

38. Nishino M, Tanouchi J, Tanaka K, et al. Transesophageal echocardiographic diagnosis of thoracic aortic dissection with the completely thrombosed false lumen. J Am Soc Echocardiogr 1996;9:79–85.

39. Goarin JP, Catoire P, Jacquens Y, et al. Use of transesophageal echocardiography for diagnosis and management of traumatic aortic injury. Chest 1997;112:71–80.

40. Vignon P, Gueret P, Vedrinnen JM, et al. Role of transesophageal echocardiography in the diagnosis and management of traumatic aortic disruption. Circulation 1995;92: 2959–68.

41. Smith MD, Cassidy JM, Souther S, et al. Transesophageal echocardiography in the diagnosis of traumatic rupture of the aorta. NEJM 1995;332:356–62.

42. Karalis DG, Victor MF, Davis GA, et al. The role of echocardiography in blunt chest trauma: a transthoracic and transesophageal echocardiographic study. J Trauma 1994;32: 53–8.

43. Minard G, Schurr MJ, Croce MA, et al. A prospective analysis of transesophageal echocardiography in the diagnosis of traumatic disruption of the aorta. J Trauma 1996;40:225–30.

44. Saletta S, Lederman E, Fein S, et al. Transesophageal echocardiography for the initial evaluation of the widened mediastinum in trauma patients. J Trauma 1995;39:137–42.

45. Catoire P, Orliaguet G, Liu N, et al. Systematic transesophageal echocardiography for the detection of mediastinal lesions in patients with multiple injuries. J Trauma 1995;38:96–102.
46. Shapiro MJ, Durham RM, Labovitz AJ. TEE: a niche not yet carved (editorial). J Trauma 1992;32:767.
47. Tunick PA, Perez JL, Kronzon I. Protruding atheromas in the thoracic aorta and systemic embolization. Ann Int Med 1991;115:423–7.
48. Tunick PA, Rosenzweig BP, Katz ES, et al. High risk for vascular events in patients with protruding atheroma: a prospective study. J Am Coll Cardiol 1994;23:1085–90.
49. Tenenbaum A, Garniek J, Shemesh, et al. Dual-helical CT for detecting aortic atheromas as a source of stroke: comparison with transesophageal echocardiography. Radiology 1998;208:153–7.
50. Seelos KC, Funari M, Higgins CB. Detection of aortic arch thrombus using MR imaging. J Comput Assist Tomogr 1991;15:224–47.
51. Krinsky G, Reuss PM. MR angiography of the thoracic aorta. Magn Reson Imaging Clin Am 1998;6:293–320.
52. Kutz SM, Lee VS, Tunick PA, et al. Atheromas of the thoracic aorta: comparison of TEE and MRA (abstr). J Am Coll Cardiol 1999;33:414A.
53. Tunick PA, Kronzon I. Atheromas of the thoracic aorta: clinical and therapeutic update. 2000;35:545–54.
54. Davila-Roman VG, Barzilai TH, Wareing TH, et al. Atherosclerosis of the ascending aorta: prevalence and role as an independent predictor of cerebrovascular events in cardiac patients. Stroke 1994;25:2010–16.
55. Barzilai TH, Marshall Jr WG, Saffitz JE, et al. Avoidance of embolic complications by ultrasonographic characterization of the ascending aorta. Circulation 1989;80:275–79.
56. Weinberger J, Azhar S, Danisi F, et al. A new noninvasive technique for imaging atherosclerotic plaque in the aortic arch of stroke patients by transcutaneous real time B mode ultrasonography: an initial report. Stroke 1998;29:673–76.
57. Konstadt SN, Reich DL, Quintana C, et al. The ascending aorta: how much does transesophageal echocardiography see? Anesth Analg 1994;78:240–44.
58. Davila-Roman VG, Murphy SF, Nickerson NJ, et al. Intraoperative transesophageal echocardiography and epiaortic ultrasound for assessment of atherosclerosis of the thoracic aorta. J Am Coll Cardiol 1996;28:944–7.
59. Marshall WG, Barzilai B, Kouchoukos NT, et al. Intraoperative ultrasound imaging of the ascending aorta. Ann Thorac Surg 1989;48:339–44.
60. Katz ES, Tunick PA, Rusinek H, et al. Protruding aortic atheromas predict stroke in elderly patients undergoing cardiopulmonary bypass: a review of our experience with intraoperative transesophageal echocardiography. J Am Coll Cardiol 1992;20:70–7.
61. Wareing TH, Davila-Roman VG, Barzilai AB, et al. Management of the severely atherosclerotic ascending aorta during cardiac operations: a strategy for detection and treatment. J Thorac Cardiovasc Surg 1992;103:453–62.
62. Stern A, Tunick PA, Culliford AT, et al. Protruding aortic arch atheromas: risk of stroke during heart surgery with and without aortic arch atherectomy. Am Heart J 1999;138:746–52.
63. Gardner TJ, Korneffer P, Manolio TA, et al. Stroke following coronary artery bypass grafting: a ten year study. Ann Thorac Surg 1985;40:574–81.
64. Salomon NW, Page US, Bigelow JC, et al. Coronary artery bypass grafting in elderly patients. J Thorac Cardiovasc Surg 1991;101:209–18.
65. Faro RS, Golden MD, Javid H, et al Coronary revascularization in septuagenarians. J Thorac Cardiovasc Surg 1983;86:616–20.
66. Katz ES, Tunick PA, Rusineck. Palpation vs. TEE
67. Wareing TH, Davila-Roman VG, Daily B, et al. Strategy for the reduction of stroke incidence in cardiac surgical patients. Ann Thorac Surg 1993;55:1400–8.
68. Applebaum RM, Cutler WM, Bhardwaj N, et al. Utility of transesophageal echocardiography during port-access minimally invasive cardiac surgery. Am J Cardiol 1998;82:183–88.
69. Trehan N, Mishra M, Dhole S, et al. Significantly reduced incidence of stroke during coronary artery bypass grafting using transesophageal echocardiography. Eur J Cardiothorac Surg 1997;11:234–42.
70. Trehan N, Mishra M, Kasliwal R, et al. Prevention of stroke during coronary bypass surgery in patients with protruding aortic atheromas identified by transesophageal echocardiography (abstr). J Am Soc Echocardiogr 1999;12:413.

## QUESTIONS

1. An aortic aneurysm is defined as containing adventitia, media, and intimae, and being dilated _____.
   A. 1.25 × normal
   B. 1.5 × normal
   C. 1.75 × normal
   D. > 2 × normal

2. Transesophageal echo is *not* useful for visualizing the _____.
   A. sinus of Valsalva
   B. transverse aortic arch
   C. distal ascending aorta
   D. thoracic aorta

3. What is the "gold standard" for diagnosing aortic aneurysms?
   A. Angiography
   B. CAT scan
   C. MRI scan
   D. TEE

4. What is the most rapid and reliable way to diagnose an intrathoracic aortic aneurysm?
   A. Angiography
   B. CAT scan
   C. MRI scan
   D. TEE

# Surgical Decision Making in Congestive Heart Failure

# Pathophysiology of Patients with Congestive Heart Failure

*James B. Young*

Though many clinicians believe they can easily describe a patient with heart failure, in fact, the definition of the syndrome is nebulous. Previously, congestive heart failure was thought of primarily as a dropsical or fluid retention state in a setting, generally, of hypertension, valvular heart disease, or chronic ischemic heart syndromes. Perhaps the best representation of this is the remarkable illustrations created by Dr. Frank Netter in *The Ciba Collection of Medical Illustrations* series (1). Figure 32.1 is a montage of his depiction of a patient with chronic congestive heart failure in comparison to an acute pulmonary edema patient. The fluid retention state is part of a syndrome where cardiomegaly is noted, pulmonary edema and mesenteric congestion is apparent, and the patient is symptomatic with profound weakness, fatigue, and dyspnea—both at exertion and at rest (orthopnea and paroxysmal nocturnal dyspnea). Acute heart failure is also often noted and generally seen in individuals with sudden pulmonary edema associated mostly with hypertensive crises, acute valvular insufficiency (sudden aortic or mitral insufficiency), or acute coronary syndromes (unstable angina and myocardial infarction). These disease states can also be blamed for subsequent ventricular hypertrophy and cardiac chamber dilation. Also displayed in the Fig. 32.1 montage is Netter's summary of the etiologic events leading up to, and the pathophysiology of, heart failure. Early definitions of heart failure focused on the concept that hemodynamic abnormalities were largely rooted in systolic and, to a lesser extent, diastolic dysfunction rather than detrimental cardiac remodeling. A quite commonly quoted definition of heart failure previously described the state as one in which the cardiac output was inadequate to meet the metabolic demands of the body. It was felt that this led to the circulatory, and particularly renal perfusion, aberrations that prompted fluid retention, leading to congestion. Of course, this definition of heart failure is correct, however, limited in scope. Heart failure is a vastly more complex syndrome,

and we now know that cardiac and circulatory failure can be seen in patients with more normal intracardiac hemodynamics and cardiac output. This has been summarized in many recent overviews (2–6).

Figure 32.2 attempts to put into context the many facets of the heart failure syndrome that, perhaps, better explain its pathophysiology and define the syndrome. Primarily, heart failure should take into context the broader definition of "failure," which is the inability to measure up to certain normal standards (Fig. 32.2). Thus, heart failure can be defined as failure of normal molecular biodynamic processes, failure of normal cellular responses to signaling hormones or other circulating substances, and failure of the heart with respect to proper filling and emptying. Failure, too, can be defined by circulatory flow perturbation, sometimes so subtle that it cannot be objectively measured or easily studied. As Fig. 32.2 suggests, one sort of injury or disease induction process is noted, with these changes then intertwining with one another. Molecular biodynamic alterations lead to differences in cellular membrane receptor expression (up and down regulation of beta-1 and beta-2 adrenergic receptors, for example) and a drive toward myocyte hypertrophy, which leads to anatomic or morphologic remodeling of the heart (cardiac muscle hypertrophy and chamber dilation). It is the anatomic and morphologic dilation that most commonly was associated with heart failure when studied previously. Thus, the myocyte and muscle enlargement noted in patients with dropsy and hypertension reflected this pathophysiologic change. Perhaps, today, the two most important characteristics of heart failure are the molecular biodynamic perturbations that lead to detrimental remodeling of the heart. Figure 32.3 characterizes this remodeling process, demonstrating a dilated and hypertrophied heart compared to a more normal shaped specimen, and also shows the myocyte hypertrophy, which is an important component of remodeling, with interstitial fibrosis that contributes to functional derangements.

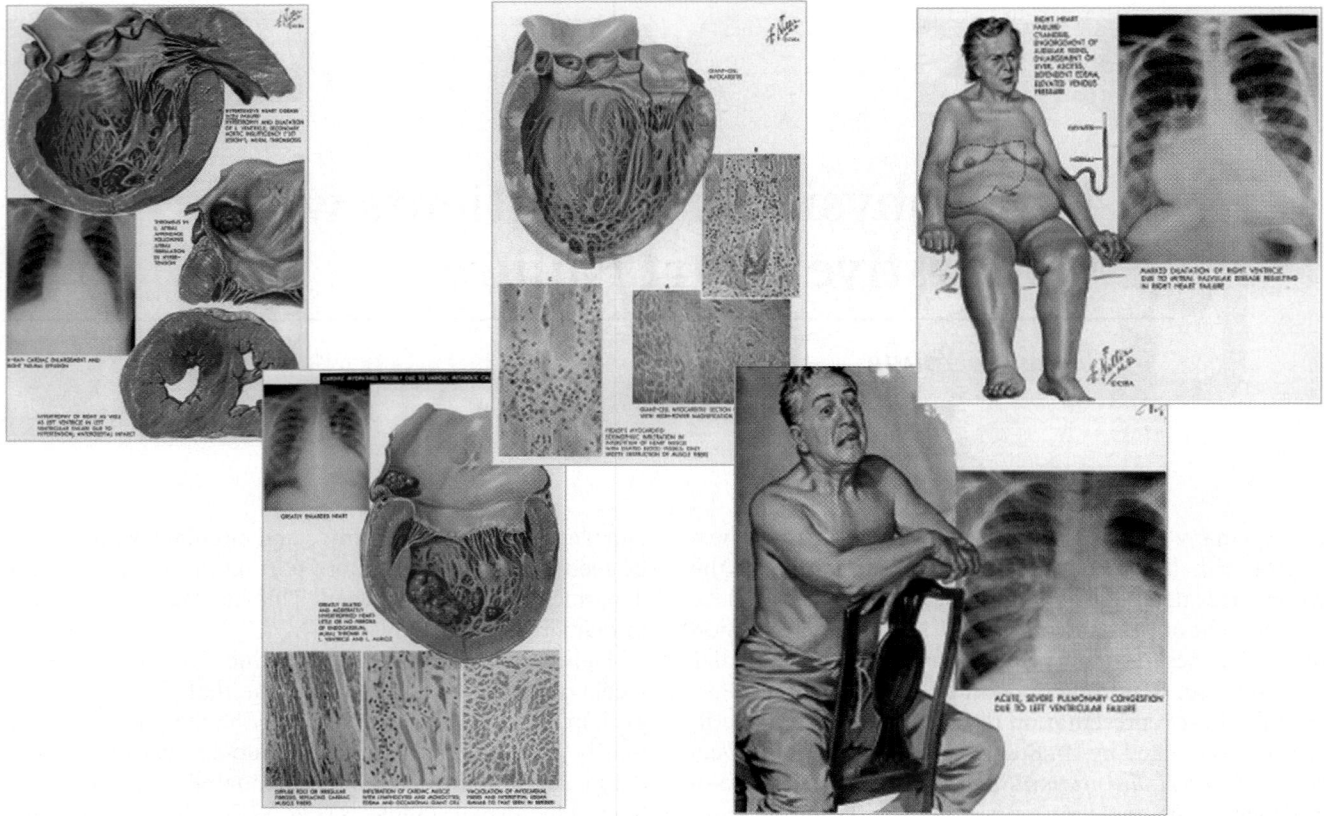

**FIGURE 32.1.** Dr. Frank Netter's Ciba collection montage of acute and chronic heart failure. Modified from Netter FH, Yonkman EF, eds. The heart. The Ciba collection of medical illustrations, vol. 5. A compilation of paintings on the normal and pathologic anatomy and physicology and embryology and disease of the heart. Ciba, 1969.

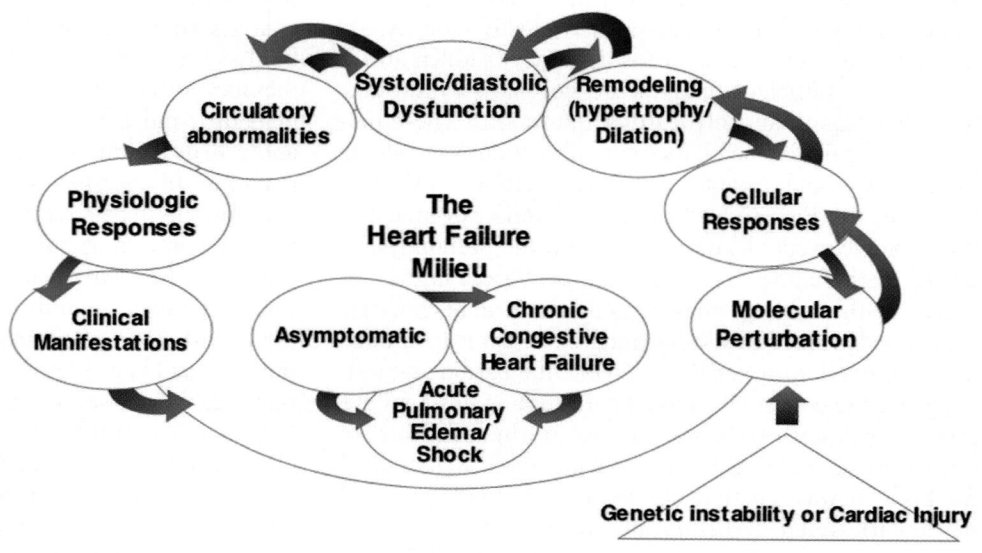

**FIGURE 32.2.** The facets of heart failure: Complexity of the syndrome. Modified from Kirklin JK, Young JB, McGiffin DC. Patho-physiology and clinical features of heart failure. In: Heart transplantation. Philadelphia: Churchill Livingstone, 2002.

"Failure is the inability to measure up to certain normal standards"
Webster's Dictionary

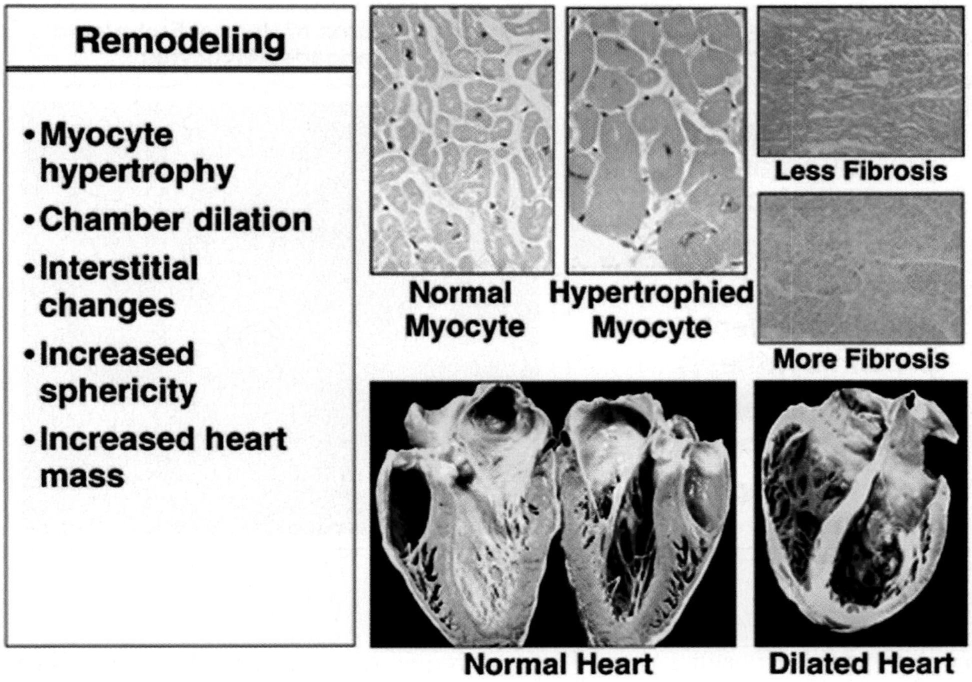

**Remodeling**

- **Myocyte hypertrophy**
- **Chamber dilation**
- **Interstitial changes**
- **Increased sphericity**
- **Increased heart mass**

Normal Myocyte    Hypertrophied Myocyte

Less Fibrosis

More Fibrosis

Normal Heart    Dilated Heart

FIGURE 32.3. Cardiac remodeling leading to heart failure. Modified from Kirklin JK, Young JB, McGiffin DC. Pathophysiology and clinical features of heart failure. In: Heart transplantation. Philadelphia: Churchill Livingstone, 2002.

A great deal of information has come to light recently regarding the molecular biodynamic abnormalities seen in heart failure. Interestingly, a common theme of many "over" and "under" gene expression knockout animal models has been the induction of cardiac hypertrophy. It is now known that several pathways exist that stimulate a variety of mitochondrial protooncogenes that regulate contractile protein production, causing increases in these important cellular elements such that individual myocytes enlarge in an attempt to augment contractility. Perhaps most important are the neuroadrenergic mediators, such as epinephrine and norepinephrine, angiotensin II, endothelin, and several proinflammatory cytokines, such as interleukin-6. Not to be discounted, however, is the importance of the stretch-mediated hypertrophy pathways. This explains the downward spiraling problems failing hearts demonstrate. As cells enlarge and as the cardiac chamber stretches even further, there is a self-promotion of growth that leads to further deleterious and detrimental cardiac remodeling. The intricacy and overlapping network of signal transduction pathways, which contributes to this vexatious problem, is brilliantly summarized by Katz and shown in Fig. 32.4 (3).

Obviously, cardiac injury and the subsequent remodeling lead to contractile and relaxation abnormalities. Figure 32.5 demonstrates classic pressure volume curves, which traditionally have been used to characterize, at the hemodynamic level, cardiac dysfunction. Traditionally, when heart failure is thought of, most have systolic left ventricular dysfunction in mind. We now know, however, that diastolic dysfunction or relaxation abnormalities can

be extraordinarily common in patients presenting with symptomatic heart failure. Systolic left ventricular dysfunction in the past has been primarily characterized by a low ejection fraction. Interestingly, today, epidemiologic studies suggest that between 30% and 50% of patients presenting and hospitalized with decompensated congestive heart failure have left ventricular ejection fractions in the normal range. It is likely that the vast majority of patients have a combination of both systolic and diastolic left ventricular dysfunction when heart failure is present. Again, it is important to understand that large degrees of variation are present with some patients having primarily systolic, and others primarily diastolic dysfunction, but some sort of combination is always present.

Systolic left ventricular dysfunction is defined as reduction in contractile capabilities, which translates into a decreased ejection fraction generally measured as a lower stroke volume. In an attempt to capitalize on the so-called Starling-Frank physiologic relationship, as the heart dilates and ventricular volume rises, contractility due to higher filling pressures ensues. Thus, end diastolic pressure and volume generally rise in heart failure, as can be seen in Fig. 32.5, but pressure generated during contraction often falls and ejection volume, overall, drops. Thus, at any given end-diastolic pressure, forward cardiac flow can be diminished. In pure forms of diastolic dysfunction, ejection volume and ejection fraction are generally maintained but, for any given cardiac volume, the intracardiac end-diastolic pressure is higher. The specific definition of diastolic dysfunction is, then, a higher left ventricular end diastolic pressure at normal or low left

## Molecular Biodynamics

- **Altered cellular protein/organelle repair-replacement**
- **Reversion to fetal phenotype**
- **Accelerated/enhanced protein synthesis**
- **Inefficient contractile elements produced**
- **Shift from repair to growth**

## Growth Patterns of Normal Embryonic & Overloaded Myocytes

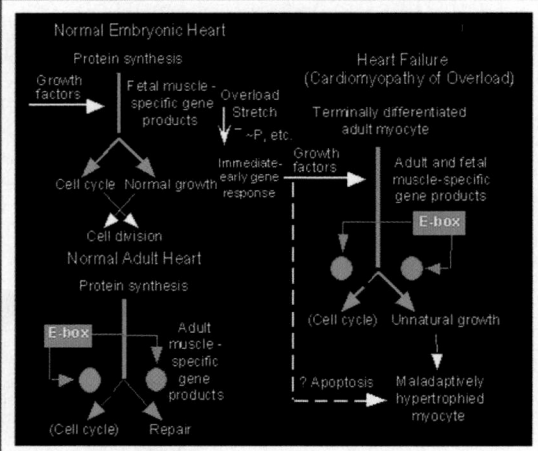

\* After Katz A.

**FIGURE 32.4.** Cardiac hypertrophy signal transduction pathways. Modified from Kirklin JK, Young JB, McGiffin DC. Pathophysiology and clinical features of heart failure. In: Heart transplantation. Philadelphia: Churchill Livingstone, 2002.

ventricular end diastolic volume. As mentioned, and demonstrated in Fig. 32.5, most patients with heart failure actually have a mixture of systolic and diastolic left ventricular myocardial failure with one aspect usually predominating over the other. The hemodynamics of heart failure should be considered a continuum. Less should be made of the distinction between systolic and diastolic left ventricular dysfunction, except when the left ventricular ejection fraction is normal or near normal. This is important from the pathophysiologic standpoint, but perhaps more important when we address therapeutic strategies.

Figure 32.6 is a montage of three important physiologic responses in the heart failure milieu. First, regulation of blood flow and cardiac output can be seen as a neurohumoral response. As contractile abnormalities evolve, with stroke volume diminishing and cardiac output decreasing, albeit quite subtly, a variety of neurohumoral responses occur that are centered in activation of the adrenergic nervous system. Increased epinephrine and norepinephrine secretion will cause, generally, an increase in inotropic effects with resulting augmentation of cardiac flow. Cardiac output is inherently related to cardiac contractility, heart rate, and afterload, all of which are controlled, to a great extent, by the adrenergic nervous system. The systemic and tissue renin-angiotensin aldosterone system also plays an important role, as Fig. 32.6 demonstrates. With subtle and sometimes immeasurable changes occurring in renal blood flow, the kidney is stimulated to retain salt and water. Renin and an-

## Cardiac Dysfunction

- **Systolic/contraction abnormalities**
- **Diastolic/relaxation abnormalities**
- **Most patients with combinations of diastolic and systolic abnormalities**

## Pressure/volume Curves in Heart Failure

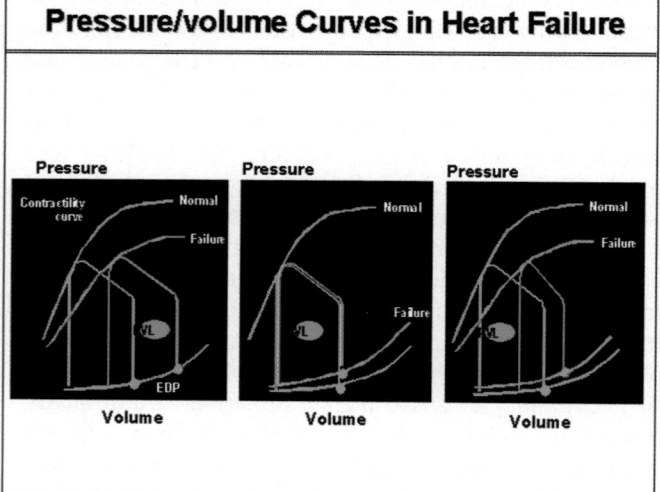

**FIGURE 32.5.** Cardiac dysfunction: systolic and diastolic contractile abnormalities. Modified from Kirklin JK, Young JB, McGiffin DC. Pathophysiology and clinical features of heart failure. In: Heart transplantation. Philadelphia: Churchill Livingstone, 2002.

## Physiologic Responses

- **Sympathetic nervous system up-regulation**
- **Renin-angiotensin-aldosterone release**
- **Inflammation alterations with a shift to proinflammatory cytokine cascades**

### Plasma TNFα Levels in Patients with NYHA Class I-IV Heart Failure*

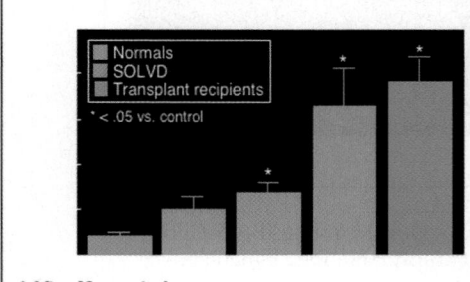

- Normals
- SOLVD
- Transplant recipients

* < .05 vs. control

\* After Mann et al.

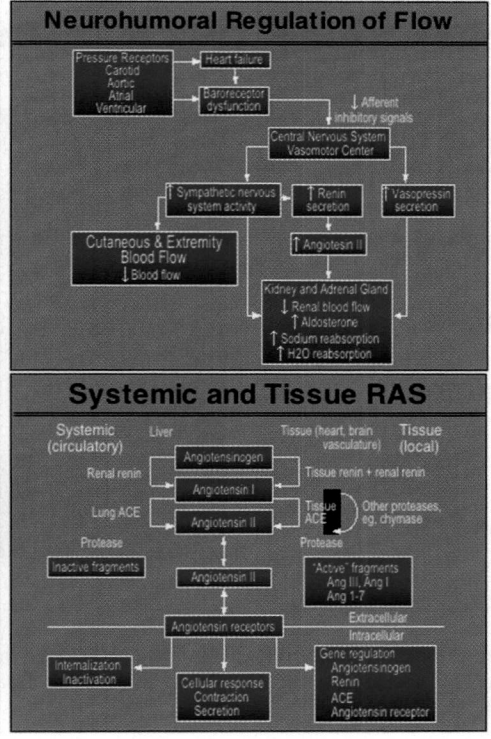

**Neurohumoral Regulation of Flow**

**Systemic and Tissue RAS**

**FIGURE 32.6.** Physiologic responses seen with heart failure. Modified from Kirklin JK, Young JB, McGiffin DC. Pathophysiology and clinical features of heart failure. In: Heart transplantation. Philadelphia: Churchill Livingstone, 2002.

giotensin production largely regulates this response. Much attention has been focused on the renin-angiotensin aldosterone system because angiotensin-II ultimately results in perpetuation of the cardiac remodeling phenomenon, and, specifically, appears to drive interstitial myocardial fibrosis formation, along with aldosterone secretion. Angiotensin II also causes intense vasoconstriction. Angiotensin-I is cleaved to angiotensin-II by angiotensin-converting enzyme. This process primarily occurs in the lung. We now know that angiotensin-I can be converted to angiotensin-II by a variety of bypass processes, primarily driven by chymase and other proteases in the tissues themselves. Thus, conversion of angiotensin-I to the effector agent, angiotensin-II, can occur locally in the cardiac structures. Obviously, these subtle issues have led to development of therapeutic techniques to modulate production of angiotensin-II and decrease aldosterone secretion. Specifically, angiotensin-converting enzyme inhibitors, aldosterone antagonists, and angiotensin-II, receptor-blocking drugs have become mainstays in treating symptomatic congestive heart failure patients because of their ability to attenuate this aspect of heart failure's pathophysiologic response. The third panel in this montage focuses on tumor necrosis factor (TNF) production and demonstrates findings that noted a stepwise increase in TNF alpha as the heart failure syndrome worsened. Recent attention has focused on this important aspect of heart failure. It is reasonable to believe that inflammation plays a key role in induction and perpetua-

tion of the syndrome. It is now well established that inflammation can drive myocyte hypertrophy, and, perhaps, contribute to worsening interstitial fibrosis. Of course, inflammatory pathways are responsible for healing organ systems, or at least making functional improvements in a damaged system, but the nuances of overactive inflammation networks and proinflammatory versus antiinflammatory pathways are just coming to light. Unfortunately, most adventures with immune modulation to treat heart failure have failed to help.

Circulatory perturbation has been coming into scrutiny in patients with heart failure. Indeed, it is now well known that peripheral flow changes in systemic musculature, for example, lead to a variety of striated muscle cell changes that contribute to the weakness and fatigue states patients with heart failure complain of so bitterly. Therefore, autoregulation of peripheral circulation in heart failure is extraordinarily important. Not only are these systemic difficulties problematic, but autoregulation can increase afterload, which directly decreases the ability of an injured heart to empty. These changes are primarily mediated by barroreceptor function and autoregulatory systems, which cause local secretion of potent vasodilators (nitrous oxide and prostacycline, for example) and vasoconstrictors (endothelin, epinephrine, angiotensin-II, and vasopressin). The humoral factors (epinephrine, angiotensin-II, and vasopressin) compete with the local factors (nitric oxide and prostaglandins) to create a dynamic of vasoconstriction and vasodilation.

| **Clinical Manifestations** | **The Many Faces of Heart Failure** |
|---|---|
| • **Patients with 'at risk' HF diseases (HTN, DM, etc)**<br><br>• **Asymptomatic LVD**<br><br>• **Congestive state**<br><br>• **Low output state**<br><br>• **Cardiogenic shock**<br><br>• **Combinations** | 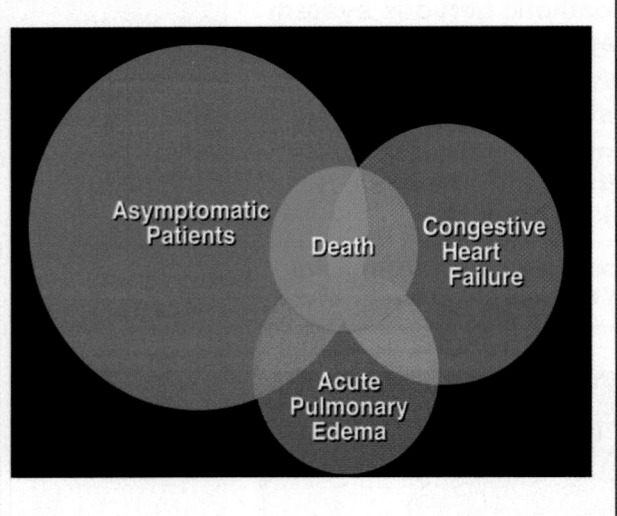 |

**FIGURE 32.7.** Clinical manifestations of heart failure. Modified from Kirklin JK, Young JB, McGiffin DC. Pathophysiology and clinical features of heart failure. In: Heart transplantation. Philadelphia: Churchill Livingstone, 2002.

Figure 32.7 summarizes the clinical manifestations that occur if the heart failure syndrome's pathophysiology proceeds unchecked. A range of conditions exists that extends from asymptomatic left ventricular dysfunction to a frank congestive state (where patients complain of edema, dyspnea syndromes, and problems related to mesenteric congestion), to low cardiac output states (where weakness and fatigue predominate), to frank cardiogenic shock (with hypotension, hypoperfusion of organs, and acidosis). As treatments are employed, patients can move back and forth between these states. Perhaps more frequently, a combination of states exists, such as combined congestive and low output syndromes. All of these states can lead to death. Patients with congestive heart failure can die of either sudden unstable ventricular arrhythmia, without preceding congestive or low output symptoms, or they can have progressive organ dysfunction resulting from chronic circulatory perturbation. The Venn diagram in Fig. 32.7 emphasizes, however, that the majority of patients with heart failure are asymptomatic at any given time. They can be asymptomatic because the syndrome has not progressed to the point at which symptoms manifest, or effective therapies might have been delivered that attenuate their difficulty.

Based on new insights into the pathophysiology of heart failure, a more contemporary definition of the syndrome can be crafted. Heart failure is a shift of the heart's molecular biodynamic paradigm from cellular housekeeping and routine maintenance to cardiac reparation and regeneration, which lead to cellular and organ re-

modeling. This subsequently causes inefficient and abnormal contraction and relaxation dynamics, which then precipitate circulatory perturbation. These changes in peripheral circulation, sometimes subtle and difficult to quantitate, lead to a clinical syndrome with many manifestations. Clinical manifestations of heart failure can be wide and varying, but generally relate to fluid retention states, low output syndromes, arrhythmias, and end organ dysfunction.

**KEY POINTS**

- Heart failure may be defined as failure of normal molecular biodynamic processes, failure of normal cellular responses to signaling hormones or other circulating substances, and failure of the heart with respect to proper filling and emptying. Alternatively, heart failure can be defined by circulatory flow perturbation, sometimes so subtle that it cannot be objectively measured or easily studied.
- Molecular biodynamic alterations lead to differences in cellular membrane receptor expression (up and down regulation of beta-1 and beta-2 adrenergic receptors, for example) and a drive toward myocyte hypertrophy, which leads to anatomic or morphologic remodeling of the heart (cardiac muscle hypertrophy and chamber dilation).

- Systolic left ventricular dysfunction is defined as reduction in contractile capabilities, which translates into a decreased ejection fraction generally measured as a lower stroke volume. The definition of diastolic dysfunction is a higher left ventricular, end diastolic pressure at normal or low left ventricular, end diastolic volume. The vast majority of patients have a combination of systolic and diastolic left ventricular dysfunction when heart failure is present.
- Heart failure is a shift of the heart's molecular biodynamic paradigm from cellular house-keeping and routine maintenance to cardiac reparation and regeneration, which leads to cellular and organ remodeling. This subsequently causes inefficient and abnormal contraction and relaxation dynamics, which then precipitate circulatory perturbation. These changes in peripheral circulation lead to a clinical syndrome with many manifestations.

## REFERENCES

1. Netter FH, Yonkman EF, eds. The heart. the Ciba collection of medical illustrations, vol. 5. A compilation of paintings on the normal and pathologic anatomy and physiology and embryology and disease of the heart. Ciba, 1969.
2. Kirklin JK, Young JB, McGiffin DC. Pathophysiology and clinical features of heart failure. In: Heart transplantation. New York: Churchill Livingstone, 2002.
3. Katz AM. Evolving concepts of heart failure: cooling furnace, malfunctioning pump, enlarging muscle. Parts I and II. J Card Failure 1998;3:329–34 and 4:67–81.
4. Young JB, Mills RM. Pathophysiology in clinical management of heart failure. 2nd ed. Caddo, Oklahoma: Professional Communications Press, 2004.
5. Mann DL, ed. Heart failure. A companion to Braunwald's heart disease. Philadelphia: Saunders (Elsevier), 2004.
6. Francis GS. Pathophysiology of the heart failure clinical syndrome. In: Topol EJ, ed. Textbook of cardiovascular medicine. 2nd ed. Philadelphia: Lippincott William & Wilkins, 2002.
7. Kirklin JK, Young JB, McGiffin DC. Pathophysiology and clinical features of heart failure. In: Heart transplantation. Philadelphia: Churchill Livingstone, 2002.

## QUESTIONS

1. The cardiac cellular response to injury or excessive tension includes which of the following?
   A. Sarcomere slippage
   B. Myocyte hypertrophy
   C. Interstitial fibrosis
   D. Apoptosis
   E. All of the above

2. Cardiac remodeling is characterized by each of the following *except*
   A. Increased cardiac mass
   B. Cardiac chamber dilation
   C. Cardiac hyperplasia
   D. Loss of valve support matrices
   E. Cardiac hypertrophy

3. Cellular death from the process of myocyte condensation without disruption of the cell membrane and fragmentation is referring to which of the following
   A. Apoptosis
   B. Myocyte necrosis
   C. Cellular degradation
   D. Cytoplasm involution
   E. Nuclear exclusion

# Assessment of Cardiomyopathies

*Mark A. Chaney*

## DEFINITION AND CLASSIFICATION OF CARDIOMYOPATHIES

*Cardiomyopathies,* once defined as "heart muscle diseases of unknown cause," are now classified by their dominant pathophysiology or pathogenetic factors. These classifications include dilated cardiomyopathy, hypertrophic cardiomyopathy, restrictive cardiomyopathy, arrhythmogenic right ventricular cardiomyopathy, and unclassified cardiomyopathies (Table 33.1) (1). Some diseases may present with features of more than one type of cardiomyopathy.

## SPECIFIC CARDIOMYOPATHIES

Specific cardiomyopathies describe heart muscle diseases that are associated with cardiac or systemic disorders (1). Ischemic cardiomyopathy for example presents as a dilated cardiomyopathy with impaired contractile performance not explained by the extent of coronary artery disease or ischemic damage. Valvular cardiomyopathy presents with ventricular dysfunction that is out of proportion to the abnormal loading conditions. Hypertensive cardiomyopathy often presents with left ventricular hypertrophy in association with features of dilated or restrictive cardiomyopathy with cardiac failure. Inflammatory cardiomyopathy is defined by myocarditis (diagnosed by established histological, immunological, and immunohistochemical criteria) in association with cardiac dysfunction. Inflammatory myocardial disease may be idiopathic, autoimmune, or infectious, and is involved in the pathogenesis of dilated cardiomyopathy and other cardiomyopathies. Metabolic cardiomyopathy may be caused by a wide variety of etiologies, including endocrine disorders, familial storage diseases, and/or infiltrations, deficiency syndromes, and amyloid diseases, among others. Cardiomyopathy may also be caused by general system disease, muscular dystrophies, and/or neuromuscular disorders. Sensitivity and toxic reactions may also induce cardiomyopathy and include reactions to

alcohol and catecholamines, among others. Finally, peripartal cardiomyopathy may first manifest in the peripartum period.

## DILATED CARDIOMYOPATHY

Dilated cardiomyopathy is characterized by dilation and impaired contraction of the left ventricle or both ventricles (2). It may be idiopathic, familial/genetic, viral and/or immune, alcoholic/toxic, or associated with recognized cardiovascular disease in which the degree of myocardial dysfunction is not explained by the abnormal loading conditions or the extent of ischemic damage. Myocardial his-

▶ **TABLE 33.1. Classification of Cardiomyopathies**

Dilated Cardiomyopathy
- Dilation and impaired contraction
- Left ventricle or both ventricles
- Wide variety of etiologies
- Myocardial histology nonspecific

Hypertrophic Cardiomyopathy
- Left ventricular and/or right ventricular hypertrophy
- Usually asymmetric and involves interventricular septum
- Familial disease with autosomal dominant inheritance etiology is mutations in sarcomeric contractile protein
- Etiology is mutations in sarcomeric contractile protein

Restrictive Cardiomyopathy
- Restrictive filling/reduced diastolic volume
- Either or both ventricles
- Normal or near-normal systolic function/wall thickness
- Idiopathic or associated with other diseases

Arrhythmogenic Right Ventricular Cardiomyopathy
- Progressive fibrofatty replacement of right ventricular myocardium
- Familial disease with autosomal dominant inheritance

Unclassified Cardiomyopathies
- Few that do not fit readily into any group
- May present with features of more than one type

tology is nonspecific. All patients with dilated cardiomyopathy should have their immediate family members screened for the disease because of the high incidence of familial dilated cardiomyopathy (3). Goerss and associates revealed that at least 24% of patients with dilated cardiomyopathy have familial disease and that there appears to be no demonstrable differences in clinical or pathological findings between familial and nonfamilial disease, other than confirmed family history (3). Clinical presentation is usually with heart failure, which is often progressive. Arrhythmias, thromboembolism, and sudden death are common and may occur at any stage. End-diastolic and end-systolic dimensions and volumes are typically increased and all variables of systolic function, such as ejection fraction, stroke volume, and cardiac output are uniformly decreased (Fig. 33.1) (2). While left ventricular mass is uniformly increased, wall thickness varies among patients and typically is within normal limits. Ventricular contractility is usually globally reduced, yet superimposed regional wall motion abnormalities can also be present if substantial coronary artery disease exists. These similar findings occur despite the wide variety of etiologies of dilated cardiomyopathy. Other two-dimensional echocardiographic features of dilated cardiomyopathy include dilation of the mitral valve annulus, leading to incomplete coaption of the anterior and posterior leaflets, causing functional mitral insufficiency, enlarged left and/or right atrial chambers, and apical ventricular thrombi (Fig. 33.2).

Patients with dilated cardiomyopathy exhibit global systolic dysfunction, with some patients having only mild symptoms whereas others exhibit signs of chronic heart failure. Doppler and color-flow imaging provides important hemodynamic information (ejection fraction, fraction area change, stroke volume, cardiac output, and ventricular filling pressures) that can assess management

strategy. Intracardiac pressures (intraatrial, intraventricular, and pulmonary artery) can be assessed with the Bernoulli equation. All four phases of diastole can be assessed by using pulsed wave Doppler interrogation of mitral flow velocity between the valve leaflet tips (Fig. 33.3). Based on the Doppler velocity patterns, diastolic filling abnormalities can be classified into three broad categories. Abnormal relaxation (decreased E/A ratio) is present with decreased preload, myocardial ischemia, and/or the normal effects of aging. Restrictive physiology (increased E/A ratio) is present with left ventricular failure (decreased compliance) and/or volume overload. Pseudonormalization (normal E/A ratio) represents a transition period when diastolic dysfunction (both abnormal relaxation and restrictive physiology coexist) is present yet the E/A ratio is normal. If a patient is suspected of having diastolic dysfunction yet the E/A ratio is normal, one must assess pulmonary venous flow patterns. If true diastolic dysfunction is present, abnormalities of pulmonary venous flow will also be present. If diastolic function is normal, pulmonary venous flow will be normal as well. While analysis of the mitral inflow velocity curve provides useful information regarding diastolic function, mitral inflow is dependent on multiple interrelated factors. To overcome these limitations, other Doppler parameters have been used to assess diastolic function, including pulmonary venous velocity curves, color M-mode, and the response of the mitral inflow to altered loading conditions. Perhaps the most promising of these new techniques of assessing diastolic function is tissue Doppler imaging of mitral annular motion, which has been proposed to correct for the influence of myocardial relaxation on transmitral flows (4).

Patients with dilated cardiomyopathy who are clinically compensated demonstrate a relatively normal stroke volume and cardiac output and an abnormal relaxation

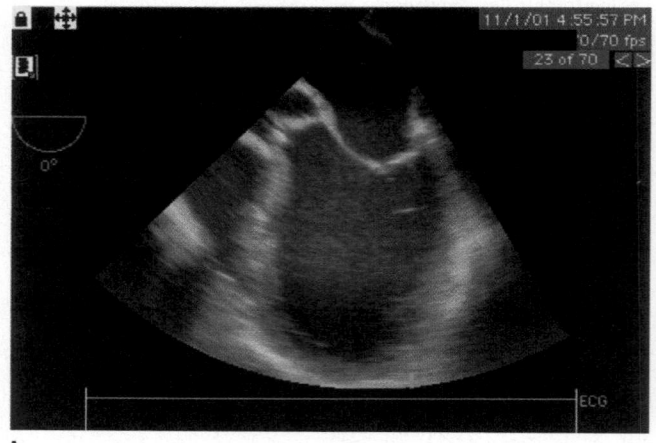
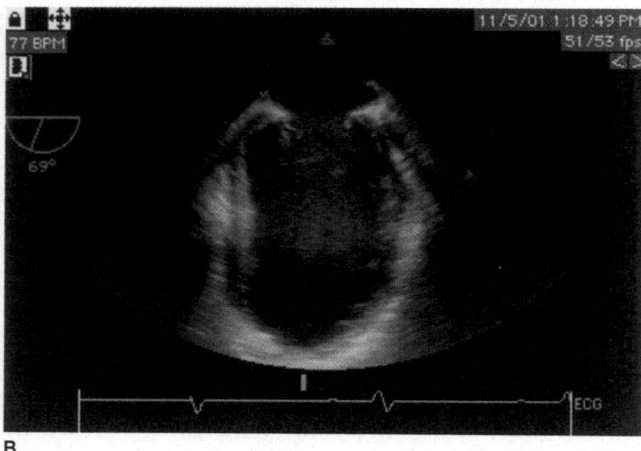

**FIGURE 33.1.** Midesophageal five-chamber view **(A)** and midesophageal mitral commissural view **(B)** of dilated cardiomyopathy, demonstrating increased ventricular dimensions.

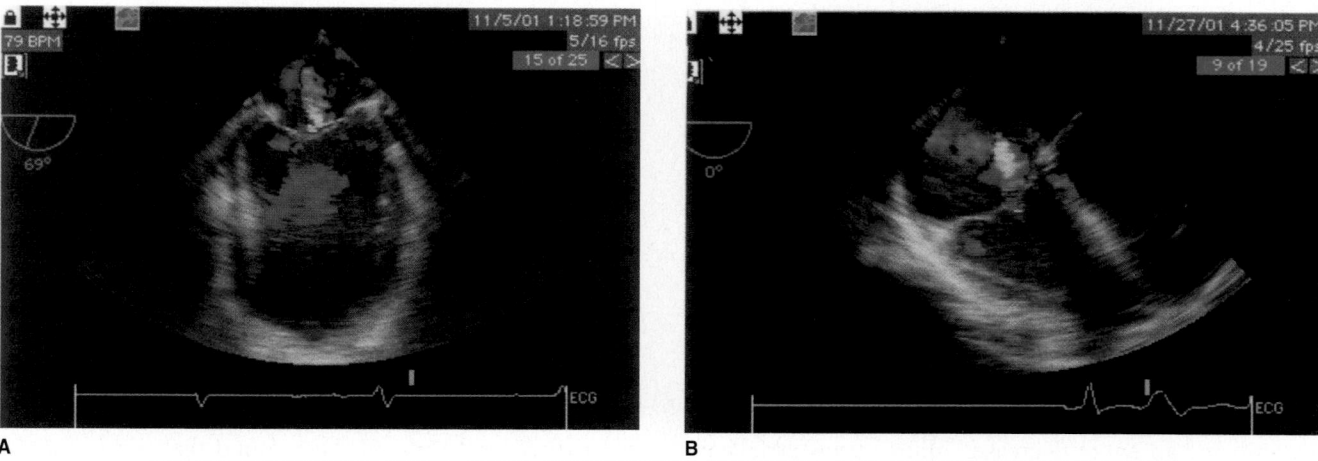

**FIGURE 33.2.** Midesophageal four-chamber view of dilated cardiomyopathy, with color flow Doppler, demonstrating functional mitral insufficiency **(A)** and functional tricuspid insufficiency **(B)**.

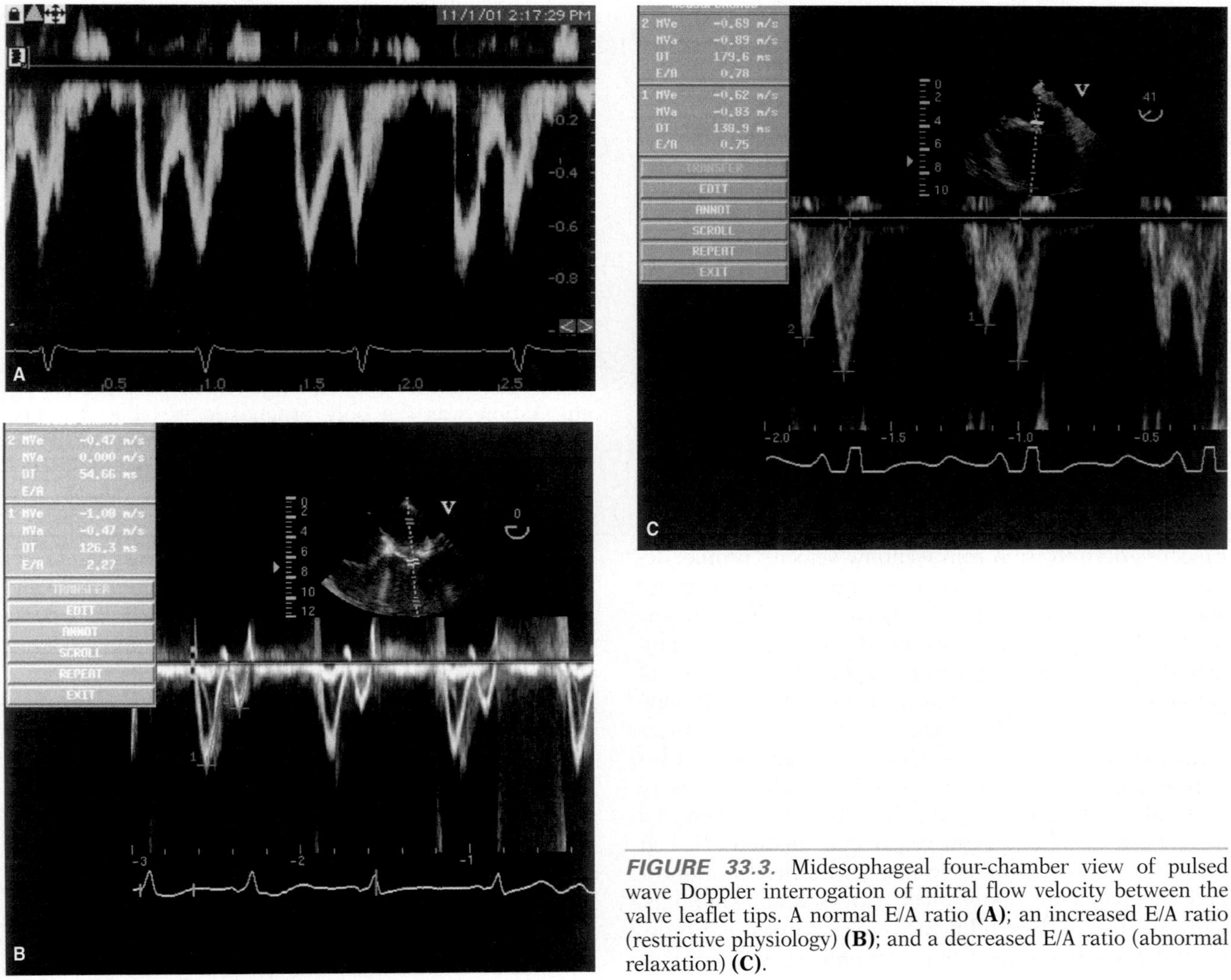

**FIGURE 33.3.** Midesophageal four-chamber view of pulsed wave Doppler interrogation of mitral flow velocity between the valve leaflet tips. A normal E/A ratio **(A)**; an increased E/A ratio (restrictive physiology) **(B)**; and a decreased E/A ratio (abnormal relaxation) **(C)**.

(decreased E/A ratio) inflow profile. When patients begin to decompensate, stroke volume and cardiac output decrease and a restrictive physiology (increased E/A ratio) inflow profile predominates because of decreased left ventricular compliance and increased left ventricular filling pressures (5). St. Goar and associates evaluated patients with idiopathic-dilated cardiomyopathy and severe heart failure who were undergoing cardiac catheterization during evaluation for heart transplantation (5). Simultaneous echocardiographic evaluation revealed that the transmitral flow velocity pattern was characterized by normal peak early filling velocity, low normal isovolumic relaxation time, shortened acceleration and deceleration times of early diastolic flow, decreased early flow velocity integral, and absent or decreased filling during atrial contraction (5). This pattern reflects interaction between elevated transmitral driving pressure and the compromised relaxation and compliance of a left ventricle, functioning on an elevated pressure-volume curve (5). The evolution of diastolic dysfunction from abnormal relaxation to restrictive physiology has been reliably reproduced in animal models of dilated cardiomyopathy (6). Ohno and associates measured left ventricular and left atrial pressures and left ventricular volume, and calculated left ventricular and left atrial stiffness during the development of congestive heart failure produced by rapid pacing in awake, unsedated dogs (6). They revealed that early in congestive heart failure, slowing left ventricular relaxation reduced the maximal early diastolic left atrial-left ventricular pressure gradient, decreasing the peak early filling rate (6). As congestive heart failure progressed, this was overcome by an increase in left atrial pressure that augmented the early diastolic left atrial-left ventricular pressure gradient, increasing peak early filling rate (6). Increasing left ventricular stiffness during the development of congestive heart failure progressively shortened the early filling deceleration time and augmented the early filling deceleration rate (6). These observations suggest that the early filling deceleration time reflects left ventricular stiffness (6). Clinical studies indicate that, of the wide variety of variables derived from mitral inflow velocity profile, deceleration time has the most prognostic value because shorter deceleration time (restrictive physiology) portends a worse prognosis (7,8). Rihal and associates examined the clinical and echocardiographic characteristics of patients with the clinical diagnosis of dilated cardiomyopathy to determine the prognostic implications of these characteristics (7). Patients with severe congestive heart failure had lower indices of systolic function and were more likely to have significant mitral regurgitation and greater left atrial and right ventricular dilation (7). Left ventricular diastolic filling abnormalities were prominent and independently associated with severe symptoms, with a restrictive-type filling pattern (increased E/A ratio, short deceleration time) being common (7). Xie and asso-

ciates confirmed that patients with congestive heart failure with poor prognosis can be identified by a restrictive transmitral flow pattern, female gender, and advanced functional class (8). Of these, the restrictive transmitral flow pattern appears to be the single best predictor of mortality over two years (8). In patients with dilated cardiomyopathy, the deceleration time increases, and the mitral inflow velocity profile becomes less characteristic of restrictive physiology as congestive heart failure symptoms are treated with medication. Improvement in these indices of diastolic dysfunction is associated with a high probability of clinical improvement and survival (9,10). Pinamonti and associates evaluated patients with dilated cardiomyopathy at presentation and after three months of medical treatment (9). They found that persistence of restrictive filling at three months was associated with a high mortality and transplantation rate, whereas patients with reversible restrictive filling had a high probability of clinical improvement and excellent survival (9). Similarly, a retrospective analysis by Lee and associates revealed that, in patients with congestive heart failure, the initial restrictive diastolic filling pattern can be altered to a nonrestrictive filling pattern with medical therapy and a change in diastolic filling to a nonrestrictive pattern is associated with improved survival (10). Another useful prognostic indicator in patients with dilated cardiomyopathy is the status of pulmonary artery pressure as estimated from tricuspid regurgitation velocity (11). Abramson and associates evaluated patients with dilated cardiomyopathy and found that patients exhibiting a high velocity of tricuspid regurgitation (> 2.5 meters/second) had more hospitalizations for congestive heart failure and a higher mortality rate when compared to patients exhibiting a lower velocity of tricuspid regurgitation (≤ 2.5 meters/second) (11). Peak velocity of tricuspid regurgitation was the only prognostic variable that predicted overall mortality, mortality due to myocardial failure, and hospitalization for congestive heart failure (11). Higher tricuspid regurgitation velocities are usually seen in patients with dilated cardiomyopathy and a restrictive physiology mitral inflow velocity profile. The presence of a restrictive physiology mitral inflow velocity profile and high velocity tricuspid regurgitation identifies patients with dilated cardiomyopathy who are at increased risk for development of heart failure and death.

## HYPERTROPHIC CARDIOMYOPATHY

Hypertrophic cardiomyopathy is characterized by left ventricular and/or right ventricular hypertrophy, which is usually asymmetric and involves the interventricular septum. It is a familial disease, with predominately autosomal dominant inheritance. Just as the inheritance of hypertrophic cardiomyopathy is heterogenous, so are the phenotypic manifestations, even in a single family cohort with the same molecular genetic defect. The extent of hypertrophy at any given site can vary greatly and bears importantly on the manifestations of the disease. Mutations in sarcomeric contractile protein genes cause the cardiomyopathy. Typical morphological myocardial changes include myocyte hypertrophy and disarray surrounding areas of increased loose connective tissue. Abnormal thickening of coronary arteries may also occur. Arrhythmias and premature sudden death are common.

Although asymmetric septal hypertrophy is the most common type of morphologic pattern, hypertrophic cardiomyopathy can present with concentric, apical, or free wall left ventricular hypertrophy (12–15). The left ventricular outflow tract becomes narrowed because of the hypertrophied basal septum, providing conditions for dynamic obstruction (Figs. 33.4 and 33.5). The narrowed left ventricular outflow tract increases the velocity of blood flow during systole and produces a Venturi effect. Traditionally, it has been thought that because of the Venturi effect, the mitral valve leaflets and support apparatus are drawn toward the septum during systole (systolic anterior motion), obstructing the left ventricular outflow tract (contact with interventricular septum many occur). However, controversy exists regarding the contribution of the Venturi effect secondary to the increased ejection velocity (13). Most likely, this Venturi effect is the consequence rather than the origin of the left ventricular outflow tract gradient (13). It is believed that the narrow left ventricular outflow tract, caused by the ventricular septal hypertrophy and the anterior displacement of the papillary muscles and mitral leaflets, is important to the development of the obstruction, as is the fact that the mitral leaflets are elongated and coapt in the body of the leaflets, rather than at their tips, as is normal (15). That part of the anterior leaflet distal to the coaptation point is sub-

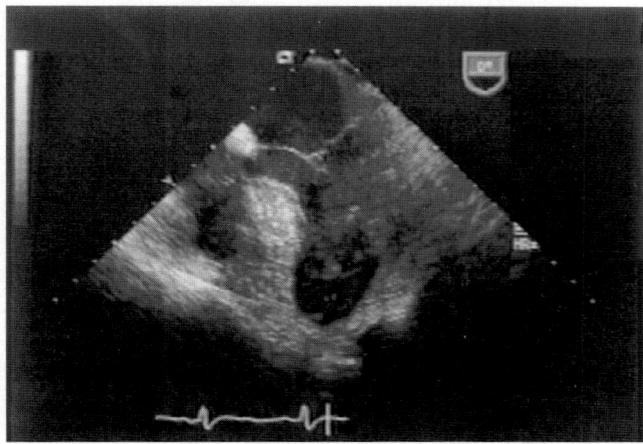

**FIGURE 33.5.** Midesophageal five-chamber view of hypertrophic cardiomyopathy, demonstrating a hypertrophied basal septum, which narrows the left ventricular outflow tract and provides conditions for dynamic obstruction.

jected to Venturi and/or drag forces, resulting in systolic anterior motion and subsequent mitral leaflet-septal contact, causing the subaortic obstruction (Fig. 33.6) (15). The systolic anterior motion of the anterior mitral leaflet also results in a failure of coaptation of the mitral leaflets, and it is through this funnel-shaped interleaflet gap that the mitral regurgitation is directed posteriorly into the left atrium (Fig. 33.7) (15). The obstruction is dynamic, may occur at the papillary muscle (midventricular) level as well as subaortic level, and depends on left ventricular loading conditions, left ventricular size, and left ventricular contractility. Because the left ventricular outflow tract obstruction is dynamic, patients in whom the disease is suspected, who do not have a gradient at rest, should undergo provocation maneuvers with agents such as dobut-

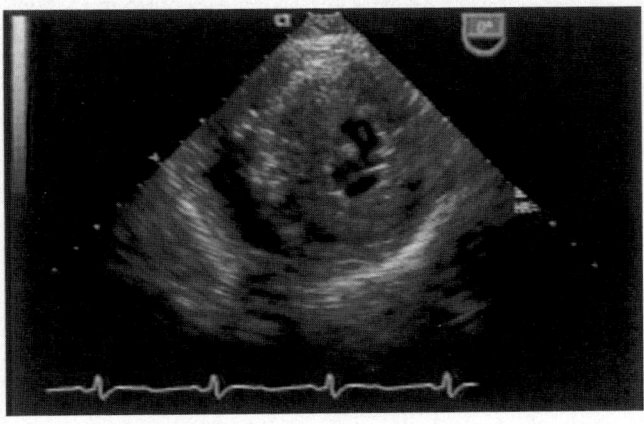

**FIGURE 33.4.** Transgastric mid short-axis view of hypertrophic cardiomyopathy, demonstrating concentric hypertrophy of the left ventricle.

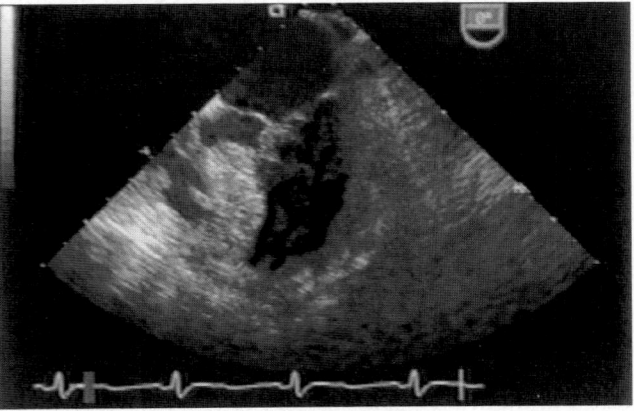

**FIGURE 33.6.** Midesophageal five-chamber view of hypertrophic cardiomyopathy, demonstrating systolic anterior motion of the anterior mitral valve leaflet, resulting in leaflet-septal contact, causing subaortic obstruction.

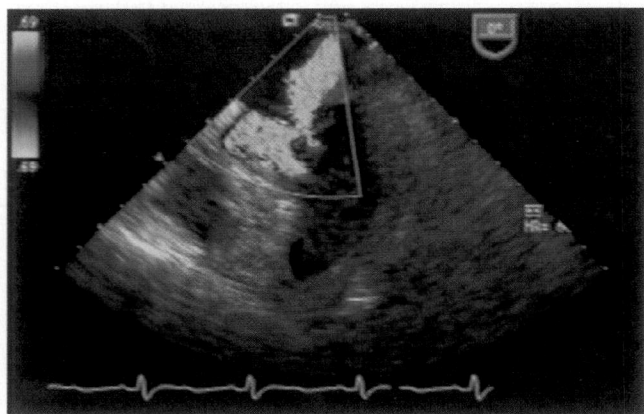

**FIGURE 33.7.** Midesophageal four-chamber view of hypertrophic cardiomyopathy, with color flow Doppler, demonstrating mitral regurgitation directed posteriorly into the left atrium.

amine to determine the severity of the gradient. If pressure gradients of greater than 30 mm Hg at rest are present, the potential for further hypertrophy and deterioration is highly likely (13). Obstruction of the left ventricular outflow tract may cause the aortic valve to close early (premature midsystolic closure). Systolic anterior motion of the mitral valve apparatus distorts mitral valve configuration, resulting in mitral insufficiency. Thus, varying degrees of mitral insufficiency almost invariably accompany the obstructive form of hypertrophic cardiomyopathy.

Two-dimensional echocardiography enables one to establish the diagnosis of hypertrophic cardiomyopathy and provides detailed morphologic characterization. A variable pattern exists regarding morphologic characterization of ventricular hypertrophy. The most common morphologic variety of hypertrophic cardiomyopathy is diffuse hypertrophy of the interventricular septum and anterolateral free wall, followed by basal septal hypertrophy, concentric hypertrophy, apical hypertrophy, and hypertrophy of the lateral wall. Left ventricular systolic function is usually normal to supranormal, with a high ejection fraction. Late in the disease, however, impaired systolic function of both the left and right ventricles, caused by myocardial fibrosis, has been seen with increased frequency (15).

M-mode echocardiography provides useful information in determining asymmetric septal hypertrophy, systolic anterior motion of the mitral valve apparatus, and midsystolic aortic valve closure. However, M-mode findings are not specific for hypertrophic cardiomyopathy because asymmetric septal hypertrophy may occur under other conditions (right ventricular hypertrophy, hypertension) and systolic anterior motion of the mitral valve apparatus may also be observed in other hyperdynamic cardiac conditions.

Continuous wave Doppler is used to assess the degree of left ventricular outflow tract obstruction in patients with hypertrophic cardiomyopathy. Increased flow velocity across the left ventricular outflow tract results in a Doppler spectrum with a characteristic late-peaking (middle to late systole) dagger-shaped appearance (Fig. 33.8). The onset of the pressure gradient is virtually simultaneous with the onset and duration of mitral leaflet-septal contact. The time of onset and duration of mitral leaflet-septal contact in systole determines the magnitude of the pressure gradient and the degree of prolongation of the left ventricular ejection time (the pressure gradient and ejection time become progressively greater as the time of mitral leaflet-septal contact occurs earlier in systole) (15). When there is no additional mitral valve abnormality other than systolic anterior motion, there is a direct relationship between the magnitude of the pressure gradient and the degree of mitral regurgitation (15). Doppler-derived and catheter-derived pressure gradients correlate well (16). Sasson and associates evaluated peak Doppler flow velocity signal for measuring peak pressure gradient with continuous wave Doppler ultrasound and dual catheter pressure recordings across the left ventricular outflow tract (16). They found that peak flow velocity and the characteristic pattern of continuous wave Doppler ultrasound signal accurately reflected the peak magnitude, as well as the timing and contour of the dynamic pressure gradient across the left ventricular outflow tract (r = 0.96) (16). The dynamic nature of left ventricular outflow tract obstruction can be documented in a wide variety of circumstances, such as during a Valsalva maneuver, following amyl nitrite inhalation, or after a meal or ingestion of alcohol.

Patients with the obstructive form of hypertrophic cardiomyopathy frequently have mitral regurgitation. The

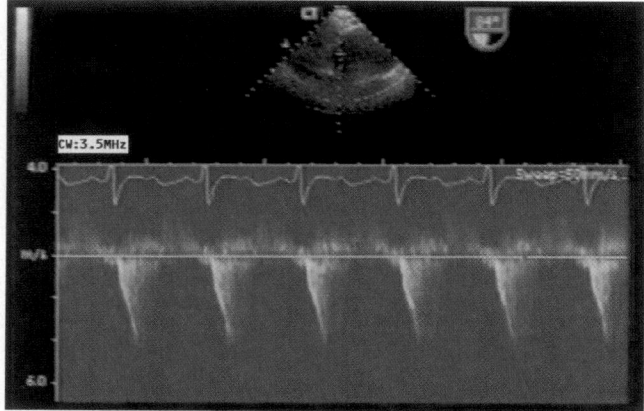

**FIGURE 33.8.** Transgastric long-axis view of hypertrophic cardiomyopathy, with continuous wave Doppler, demonstrating increased flow velocity across the left ventricular outflow tract, resulting in a Doppler spectrum with a characteristic late-peaking (middle to late systole) dagger-shaped appearance.

mitral insufficiency jet is typically directed posterolaterally and occurs after the onset of left ventricular outflow tract obstruction (17). Nishimura and associates revealed a dynamic pattern of the left ventricular outflow tract that consisted of normal-velocity laminar flow during early systole, followed by turbulent flow in midsystole (17). The maximal amount of mitral regurgitation occurred late in systole, after the appearance of turbulent flow in the left ventricular outflow tract (17). The peak velocity detected in the left ventricular outflow tract was positively correlated with the degree of systolic anterior motion of the mitral valve, and patients with higher peak velocities in the left ventricular outflow tract had prolonged ejection times (17). Color-flow imaging is useful in assessing the severity of mitral regurgitation and in separating mitral regurgitation flow from left ventricular outflow tract flow. The peak velocity of the mitral regurgitation jet may also be used to determine the magnitude of the left ventricular outflow tract obstruction via the Bernoulli equation. In about 20% of patients, mitral regurgitation is to a variable extent independent of the systolic anterior motion, in which case, other abnormalities of the mitral valve are present, such as anomalous papillary muscle attachment to the anterior leaflet, mitral valve prolapse, extensive anterior leaflet fibrosis due to repeated mitral leaflet-septal contact, mitral annular calcification, or other rarer abnormalities (15). These independent abnormalities of the mitral valve cause pansystolic mitral regurgitation, which is often anteriorly or centrally directed into the left atrium and is quite different from the late-onset, posteriorly directed mitral regurgitation that is the result of anterior mitral leaflet systolic anterior motion. In a subgroup of patients with hypertrophic obstructive cardiomyopathy, chordal rupture may develop, resulting in severe mitral regurgitation (18).

Patients with hypertrophic cardiomyopathy typically have diastolic dysfunction (abnormal relaxation; decreased E/A ratio) secondary to the hypertrophic myocardium (19). Maron and associates assessed 111 patients representative of the broad clinical spectrum of hypertrophic cardiomyopathy and compared all Doppler indexes of diastolic relaxation and filling to 86 control subjects without heart disease (19). They noted prolongation of isovolumic relaxation and early diastolic peak flow velocity, as well as slower deceleration and reduced maximal flow velocity in early diastole (19). As an apparent compensation for impaired relaxation and early diastolic filling, the atrial contribution to left ventricular filling was increased, as shown by increased late diastolic flow velocity and reduced ratio of maximal flow velocity in early diastole to that in late diastole (19). Abnormal Doppler diastolic indexes were identified with similar frequency in patients with or without left ventricular outflow obstruction, as well as in patients with or without cardiac symptoms (19). Relaxation may be impaired by

the systolic contraction load (outflow obstruction) and perhaps, more importantly, by the reduced relaxation loads (ventricular filling and coronary filling loads) (15). Impaired relaxation may also be initiated by altered myoplasmic calcium regulation and ventricular nonuniformity (15). Late in the evolution of diastolic dysfunction, a restrictive type of diastolic filling defect may become evident, in which a high atrial pressure results in an increased rate and volume of filling during the rapid filling period with reduced filling during atrial systole (15). The mitral valve inflow velocity profile is characterized by a prolonged isovolumic relaxation time, reduced early rapid filling, prolonged deceleration time, and increased atrial filling. Left ventricular filling may be substantially dependent on atrial contraction. Over time, the left ventricle becomes less compliant, and left atrial pressure increases, causing early filling to increase and deceleration time to decrease. Because the deceleration time is markedly prolonged at baseline in patients with hypertrophic cardiomyopathy, the same degree of left atrial pressure increase does not produce similar deceleration time, shortening as it does in patients with dilated cardiomyopathy. Thus, no correlation exists between deceleration time and left ventricular filling pressures in patients with hypertrophic cardiomyopathy (20). Nishimura and associates compared patients with left ventricular systolic dysfunction to patients with hypertrophic cardiomyopathy and demonstrated a significant relation between Doppler echocardiographic variables and mean left atrial pressure in patients with left ventricular systolic dysfunction (20). In this study, the left atrial pressure was directly related to the B/A ratio and inversely related to the deceleration time, yet no such significant relation existed in patients with hypertrophic cardiomyopathy (20). They concluded that because of the complexity and multiple interrelated factors that determine diastolic filling of the left ventricle, these flow velocity curves cannot be used in patients with hypertrophic cardiomyopathy (20). Patients with hypertrophic cardiomyopathy typically demonstrate redistribution of intracavitary flow during isovolumic relaxation due to asynchronous myocardial relaxation, which may lead to erroneous interpretation of mitral inflow velocities and the mitral inflow velocity profile. Not all cases of dynamic left ventricular outflow tract obstruction is due to hypertrophic cardiomyopathy. Patients with basal septal hypertrophy who develop hyperdynamic systolic ventricular function may exhibit dynamic left ventricular outflow tract obstruction (21). Topol and associates identified 21 patients with a syndrome that included severe concentric cardiac hypertrophy, a small left ventricular cavity, and supernormal indexes of systolic function (21). The patients were elderly, hypertensive, predominantly female, and mostly African-American (21). Cardiac function was characterized by excessive left ventricular emptying and abnormal diastolic function as manifested by a prolonged early diastolic filling period and reduced peak diastolic dimension increase (21). In spite of the clinical presentation of heart failure, all of the nine patients receiving either beta-receptor antagonists or calcium-channel blocking agents obtained symptomatic relief, whereas six of twelve patients receiving vasodilator medications had severe hypotensive reactions including one death (21). Following aortic valve replacement for aortic stenosis, patients may develop acute left ventricular outflow tract obstruction as well. Other less common causes of dynamic left ventricular outflow tract obstruction include cardiac amyloidosis, myocardial infarction, and subaortic stenosis, among others.

Interventions that reduce left ventricular contractility, increase peripheral vascular resistance, or both are considered beneficial (13). Interventions that lower peripheral vascular resistance and increase myocardial contractility are thought to be detrimental (13). The occurrence of atrial fibrillation in hypertrophic cardiomyopathy is also associated with clinical deterioration. Beta-blockers are considered the basic treatment for patients with hypertrophic cardiomyopathy (verapamil may serve as an alternative).

Surgical repair of hypertrophic obstructive cardiomyopathy is generally reserved for those individuals who remain refractory to medical therapy (beta-blockers, calcium channel-blockers, amiodarone, etc.). Criteria include an intraventricular gradient at rest of $\geq 30$ mm Hg or $\geq 60$ mm Hg with provocation, and a septum measuring > 18 mm thick (13). Patients should also exhibit typical systolic anterior motion of the mitral valve. Surgical repair is via myectomy, which consists of removing ventricular septal tissue through a transaortic approach (thus, widening the left ventricular outflow tract). Previously, the procedure had been combined with surgery of the mitral valve in some instances, and even selective replacement of the mitral valve by a prosthetic device has been proposed (13). Presently, mobilization of the papillary muscles and readaptation of the mitral valve subvalvular apparatus are favored (13). Intraoperative transesophageal echocardiography is very useful in determining the site of septal contact by the mitral valve leaflet during systolic anterior motion and determining the thickness of the interventricular septum, helping the surgeon decide the extent and depth of the myectomy. The presence of asymmetric septal hypertrophy and severe systolic anterior motion of the mitral valve apparatus predicts a good outcome after septal myectomy (22). McCully and associates evaluated (preoperatively and at one year postoperatively) the clinical and echocardiographic data of 47 patients with hypertrophic cardiomyopathy who underwent isolated septal myectomy (22). While most patients experienced symptomatic improvement at one year, the preoperative echocardiographic variables of asymmetric hypertrophy, severe systolic anterior motion of the mitral leaflet(s), and prolonged isovolumetric relaxation time identified

patients who were most likely to benefit from septal myectomy (22). Evaluation of mitral valve morphology and regurgitation severity is also important because some patients with hypertrophic obstructive cardiomyopathy are prone to develop rupture of the chordae attached to the mitral valve leaflet. Mitral valve repair may be indicated in addition to myectomy if a morphologic abnormality of the mitral valve is present. A rarer finding is right ventricular outflow tract obstruction secondary to hypertrophy. The left ventricular outflow tract gradient may be assessed via the Bernoulli equation or, alternatively, the gradient may be directly measured by inserting a small needle directly into the aorta and left ventricle to measure pressure before and after myectomy. Postoperatively, it is important to determine the severity of residual mitral regurgitation and assess potential complications of myectomy, including ventricular septal defect and/or aortic insufficiency. Other potential complications of myectomy include complete heart block and creation of a coronary artery left ventricular fistula. Commonly, a small shunt may occur between the resected intramyocardial vessel and the left ventricle following myectomy, which should not be misinterpreted as a ventricular septal defect. Systolic anterior motion of the mitral valve apparatus may persist following myectomy even though the left ventricular outflow tract gradient is less. Oftentimes, this persistent systolic anterior motion of the mitral valve apparatus observed within the immediate postoperative period disappears by the time of hospital discharge (23). Park and associates reported that intraoperative transesophageal echocardiography was valuable in detecting (preoperatively) unknown cardiac pathologies in 12%, altering surgical procedure in 4%, and in assessing the result of myectomy, requiring a second pump run, in 5% (23). Transesophageal echocardiography was also useful in identifying the etiology of postoperative left ventricular dysfunction in 7% and intrinsic structural abnormalities of the mitral valve in 19% (23). Residual systolic anterior motion of the mitral valve detected by intraoperative transesophageal echocardiography after septal myectomy resolved in 33% of patients by the time of predischarge transthoracic echocardiography (23).

The beneficial effects of myectomy led to the concept of nonsurgical myocardial reduction, which involves infusion of desiccated alcohol distal to an angioplasty balloon into the first major septal perforator of the left anterior descending coronary artery (producing septal infarction). By the year 2000, more than 1,000 patients had been treated with this technique (13).

## RESTRICTIVE CARDIOMYOPATHY

Restrictive cardiomyopathy is characterized by restrictive filling and reduced diastolic volume of either or both ventricles with normal or near-normal systolic function and wall thickness. Increased interstitial fibrosis may be present. Restrictive cardiomyopathy may be idiopathic or associated with other diseases, such as amyloidosis. Either or both ventricles may be involved. Ventricular systolic function is usually well preserved, yet diastolic pressure is increased, causing increased atrial pressure (with subsequent enlargement). Characteristic two-dimensional echocardiographic findings include normal ventricular cavity size and wall thickness, relatively preserved global systolic function, and atrial enlargement. Pulsed wave Doppler interrogation of mitral (or tricuspid) inflow exhibits a restrictive physiology profile (increased E/A ratio) (24). The differences in the atrial and ventricular filling patterns between restrictive myocardial disease and constrictive pericarditis may serve to distinguish these two disease entities (24). In the presence of restrictive cardiomyopathy, high left atrial pressure results in an increased transmitral pressure gradient, an increased E mitral velocity, and decreased systolic pulmonary venous flow velocity. Because of high ventricular pressure at end diastole, atrial contraction does not contribute substantially to ventricular filling, and the A velocity is decreased. Also, pulmonary venous flow velocity decreases during systole and increases during diastole because of the increased left atrial pressure.

## ARRHYTHMOGENIC RIGHT VENTRICULAR CARDIOMYOPATHY

Arrhythmogenic right ventricular cardiomyopathy, also referred to as right ventricular dysplasia, is caused primarily by progressive replacement of the right ventricular myocardium with fatty and fibrous tissue (25). It is a familial disease, the most common pattern of inheritance being autosomal dominant with variable penetrance (males involved most frequently). The disease is generally discovered during adolescence, but some pediatric cases have been reported. The most striking morphologic feature of the disease is the diffuse or segmental loss of myocardium of the right ventricular free wall by replacement with fat and fibrous tissue. Clinical manifestations vary greatly and include ventricular arrhythmia, congestive heart failure, heart murmur, or sudden death. Characteristic two-dimensional echocardiographic findings include a dilated right ventricle that exhibits poor systolic function. The right atrium sometimes is dilated, which may explain atrial arrhythmias. Left ventricular dilatation and dysfunction may also be observed in some affected individuals. Because of the right ventricular dysfunction, tricuspid regurgitation is also characteristically observed. Clinically, prognosis of arrhythmogenic right ventricular cardiomyopathy depends on both the electrical instability of the diseased myocardium and ventricular dysfunction leading to heart failure. Currently, the

clinical course of affected individuals is not documented sufficiently, even in patients with overt disease and significant ventricular arrhythmia. Natural history of asymptomatic affected family members is also unknown. Therefore, there are no well-established guidelines in the treatment of patients, and the strategies are based largely on local experience gained at different centers.

## KEY POINTS

* Cardiomyopathies are defined as diseases of the myocardium associated with cardiac dysfunction and are classified as dilated cardiomyopathy, hypertrophic cardiomyopathy, restrictive cardiomyopathy, arrhythmogenic right ventricular cardiomyopathy, and unclassified cardiomyopathies.
* Two-dimensional echocardiographic findings characteristic of dilated cardiomyopathy include increased end-diastolic and end-systolic ventricular dimensions and volumes, and decreased ventricular systolic function.
* Doppler and color-flow echocardiographic findings characteristic of dilated cardiomyopathy include either an abnormal relaxation (decreased E/A ratio) or restrictive physiology (increased B/A ratio) mitral inflow velocity profile and varying degrees of mitral and/or tricuspid insufficiency.
* Two-dimensional echocardiographic findings characteristic of hypertrophic cardiomyopathy include left ventricular and/or right ventricular hypertrophy (usually asymmetric) predominantly involving the interventricular septum and systolic anterior motion of the mitral valve apparatus, resulting in mitral insufficiency.
* Doppler and color-flow echocardiographic findings characteristic of hypertrophic cardiomyopathy include increased flow velocity (and pressure gradient) across the left ventricular outflow tract (dagger-shaped appearance of spectral wave form analysis), varying degrees of mitral insufficiency, and an abnormal relaxation (decreased B/A ratio) mitral inflow velocity profile.
* Intraoperative transesophageal echocardiography plays a pivotal role in guiding surgical management of hypertrophic cardiomyopathy (e.g., extent and depth of myectomy, evaluation of mitral valve, assessing postmyectomy left ventricular outflow tract velocity, and pressure gradient) and in assessing potential complications (residual mitral insufficiency, ventricular

septal defect, coronary artery-left ventricular fistula, etc.).

- Characteristic echocardiographic findings of restrictive cardiomyopathy include normal ventricular cavity size and wall thickness, relatively preserved global systolic function, atrial enlargement, a restrictive physiology (increased B/A ratio) mitral inflow velocity profile, and alterations in pulmonary venous flow velocities (decreased systolic, increased diastolic).
- Characteristic echocardiographic findings of arrhythmogenic right ventricular cardiomyopathy include increased end-diastolic and end-systolic right ventricular dimensions and volumes, decreased right ventricular systolic function, and varying degrees of tricuspid insufficiency.

## REFERENCES

1. Richardson P, McKenna W, Bristow M, et al. Report of the 1995 World Health Organization/International Society and Federation of Cardiology Task Force on the Definition and Classification of Cardiomyopathies. Circulation 1996;93:841–2.
2. Corya BC, Feigenbaum H, Rasmussen S, Black MJ. Echocardiographic features of congestive cardiomyopathy compared with normal subjects and patients with coronary artery disease. Circulation 1974;49:1153–59.
3. Goerss JB, Michels VV, Burnett J, et al. Frequency of familial dilated cardiomyopathy. Eur Heart J 1995;16(Suppl):2–4.
4. Ommen SR, Nishimura RA, Appleton CP, et al. Clinical utility of Doppler echocardiography and tissue Doppler imaging in the estimation of left ventricular filling pressures; a comparative simultaneous Doppler-catheterization study. Circulation 2000;102:1788–94.
5. St. Goar FG, Masuyama T, Alderman EL, Popp RL. Left ventricular diastolic dysfunction in end-stage dilated cardiomyopathy: simultaneous Doppler echocardiography and hemodynamic evaluation. J Am Soc Echocardiogr 1991;4:349–60.
6. Ohno M, Cheng CP, Little WC. Mechanism of altered patterns of left ventricular filling during the development of congestive heart failure. Circulation 1994;89:2241–50.
7. Rihal CS, Nishimura RA, Hatle LK, Bailey KR, Tajik AJ. Systolic and diastolic dysfunction in patients with clinical diagnosis of dilated cardiomyopathy; relation to symptoms and prognosis. Circulation 1994;90:2772–9.
8. Xie GY, Berk MR, Smith MD, Gurley JC, DeMaria AN. Prognostic value of Doppler transmitral flow patterns in patients with congestive heart failure. J Am Coll Cardiol 1994;24:132–9.
9. Pinamonti B, Zecchin M, Di Lenarda A, Gregori D, Smagra G, Camerini F. Persistence of restrictive left ventricular filling pattern in dilated cardiomyopathy: an ominous prognostic sign. J Am Coll Cardiol 1997;29:604–12.
10. Lee DC, Oh JK, Osborn SL, Mahoney DW, Seward JB. Repeat evaluation of diastolic filling pattern after treatment of congestive heart failure in patients with restrictive diastolic filling: implication for long-term prognosis (abstract). J Am Soc Echocardiogr 1997;10:431.
11. Abramson SV, Burke JF, Kelly JJ, et al. Pulmonary hypertension predicts mortality and morbidity in patients with dilated cardiomyopathy. Ann Intern Med 1992;116:888–95.
12. Roberts R, Sigwart U. New concepts in hypertrophic cardiomyopathies, part I. Circulation 2001;104:2113–16.
13. Roberts R, Sigwart U. New concepts in hypertrophic cardiomyopathies, part II. Circulation 2001;104:2249–52.
14. Ommen SR, Tajik AJ. Hypertrophic cardiomyopathy; from bedside to bench . . . and now back again? (editorial). Circulation 2001;104:126–27.
15. Wigle ED, Rakowski H, Kimball BP, Williams WG. Hypertrophic cardiomyopathy; clinical spectrum and treatment. Circulation 1995;92:1680–92.
16. Sasson Z, Yock PG, Hatle LK, Alderman EL, Popp RL. Doppler echocardiographic determination of the pressure gradient in hypertrophic cardiomyopathy. J Am Coll Cardiol 1988;11:752–6.
17. Nishimura RA, Tajik AJ, Reeder GS, Seward JB. Evaluation of hypertrophic cardiomyopathy by Doppler color flow imaging: initial observations. Mayo Clin Proc 1986;61:631–9.
18. Zhu WX, Oh JK, Kopecky SL, Schaff HV, Tajik AJ. Mitral regurgitation due to ruptured chordae tendineae in patients with hypertrophic obstructive cardiomyopathy. J Am Coll Cardiol 1992;20:242–7.
19. Maron BJ, Spirito P, Green KJ, Wesley YE, Bonow RO, Arce J. Noninvasive assessment of left ventricular diastolic function by pulsed Doppler echocardiography in patients with hypertrophic cardiomyopathy. J Am Coll Cardiol 1987;10:733–42.
20. Nishimura RA, Appleton CP, Redfield MM, Ilstrup DM, Holmes DR, Tajik AJ. Noninvasive Doppler echocardiographic evaluation of left ventricular filling pressures in patients with cardiomyopathies: a simultaneous Doppler echocardiographic and cardiac catheterization study. J Am Coll Cardiol 1996;28:1226–33.
21. Topol EJ, Traill TA, Fortuin NJ. Hypertensive hypertrophic cardiomyopathy of the elderly. N Engl J Med 1985;312:277–83.
22. McCully RB, Nishimura RA, Bailey KR, Schaff HV, Danielson GK, Tajik AJ. Hypertrophic obstructive cardiomyopathy: preoperative echocardiographic predictors of outcome after septal myectomy. J Am Coll Cardiol 1996;27:1491–6.
23. Park SH, Click RL, Freeman WK, et al. Role of intraoperative transesophageal echocardiography in patients with hypertrophic obstructive cardiomyopathy (abstract). J Am Coll Cardiol 1995;25:82A–83A.
24. Izumi S, Miyatake K, Beppu S, et al. Doppler echocardiographic features of the atrial and ventricular filling modes and their significance in restrictive myocardial diseases. J Cardiol 1990;20:311–19.
25. Fontaine G, Gallais Y, Fornes P, Hebert JL, Frank R. Arrhythmogenic right ventricular dysplasia/cardiomyopathy. Anesthesiology 2001;95:250–4.

## QUESTIONS

1. Cardiomyopathies:
   A. Are defined as diseases of the myocardium associated with cardiac dysfunction
   B. Encompass a wide variety of etiologic factors
   C. Encompass a wide variety of pathophysiologies
   D. All of the above

2. Characteristic echocardiographic findings associated with dilated cardiomyopathy include:
   A. Dagger-shaped appearance of Doppler spectral waveform analysis
   B. Varying degrees of mitral and/or tricuspid insufficiency
   C. Normal end-diastolic and end-systolic ventricular dimensions and volumes
   D. Normal ventricular systolic function

3. Characteristic echocardiographic findings associated with hypertrophic cardiomyopathy include:
   A. Increased end-diastolic and end-systolic ventricular dimensions and volumes
   B. A restrictive physiology (increased E/A ratio) mitral inflow velocity profile
   C. Systolic anterior motion of the mitral valve apparatus
   D. Decreased ventricular systolic function

4. For what purpose would intraoperative transesophageal echocardiography during surgical management of hypertrophic cardiomyopathy be of benefit?

   A. Guidance of extent and depth of myectomy
   B. Evaluation of the mitral valve apparatus
   C. Detecting potential complications
   D. All of the above

5. Characteristic echocardiographic findings associated with restrictive cardiomyopathy include:
   A. Decreased ventricular systolic function
   B. Increased flow velocity (and pressure gradient) across the left ventricular outflow tract
   C. Decreased systolic pulmonary venous flow velocity
   D. Decreased diastolic pulmonary venous flow velocity

# Surgical Considerations in Nontransplant Surgery for Congestive Heart Failure

*Indu Deglurkar, Katherine J. Hoercher, and Patrick M. McCarthy*

The ever-increasing incidence of heart failure, coupled with poorly met demands for donor hearts, has led to the evolution of alternative surgical and device management strategies in end-stage heart failure. Medically treated patients with ischemic cardiomyopathy have a five-year survival of 28%. The most common surgical procedures currently employed in heart failure patients are discussed in this chapter. The selection of the appropriate operation in a patient is a complex decision-making process, rigorously based on pathophysiologic considerations. In this population, all factors affecting surgical risk should be carefully evaluated preoperatively and surgery should be recommended when definite benefits in survival and quality of life can be reasonably predicted. The current treatment options in patients with compensated heart failure include coronary revascularization, mitral valve repair, left ventricular reconstruction, mechanical assist device, and cell therapy (under evaluation). Patients with heart failure may require a combination of procedures, including revascularization, mitral repair, LV reconstruction, and eventually regenerative cell therapy to address all the pathophysiologic components creating the clinical picture. These procedures, combined with optimal medical therapy, help improve survival and avoid or postpone cardiac transplantation.

## CABG IN PATIENTS WITH SEVERE LV DYSFUNCTION

Ischemic cardiomyopathy is the most common cause of heart failure (1,2). Congestive heart failure affects 5.5 million people in the United States with an annual incidence of 550,000. Myocardial dysfunction occurs due to loss of myocytes. At a cellular level, there is loss of myofibrils and disorganization of structural proteins within the myocyte. Fibrosis occurs with loss of the geometrical shape of the

heart (3–5). The sequelae of coronary artery disease are outlined in Fig. 34.1.

The clinical presentation in these patients can be stable or unstable angina, arrhythmia, or heart failure. Evaluation includes assessment of symptoms, presence or absence of angina, NYHA class, episodes of heart failure, and comorbid factors (pulmonary, renal, peripheral, and cerebrovascular disease). Coronary angiography determines the extent of disease, adequacy of distal targets, the patency of prior grafts and the presence of left ventricular aneurysm by LV angiogram that may require concomitant resection, any valvular regurgitation, and the degree of left ventricular dilatation. Myocardial viability tests with nuclear medicine tracer techniques (such as thallium,

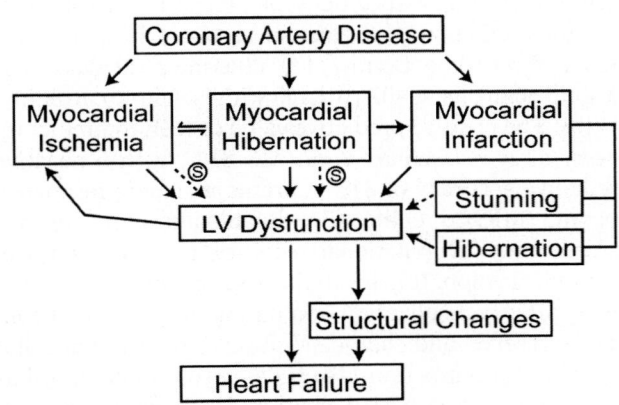

ⓢ *Myocardial Stunning*

**FIGURE 34.1.** Sequelae of coronary artery disease. Except for infarcted myocardial tissue, all other states are potentially reversible with appropriate and timely treatment. Redrawn with permission from Rahimtoola SH. Am J Cardiol 1995;75:16E–22E.

PET, and SPECT scan), echocardiography (resting and dobutamine stress echo), and MRI can be performed to assess the viability and extent of reversibility of the ischemic myocardium. Some studies have suggested that for significant improvement in heart failure symptoms, functional status, and LV function to occur after CABG, the myocardium should have at least 20% viability (6,7).

Positron emission tomography (PET) using perfusion (Rubidium-82 or $^{13}$N-ammonia)/metabolic [F-18 deoxyglucose (FDG) or carbon-11 acetate] tracers is considered the "gold standard" method for detecting viability (7). It has been shown that a region showing high FDG uptake relative to myocardial blood flow (perfusion/metabolic mismatch) represents ischemic, stunned, or hibernating myocardium, whereas myocardial scar represents decreased perfusion at rest with corresponding decreased metabolism (perfusion/metabolic match). The average positive and negative predictive accuracy of PET for predicting improved function after revascularization is 82% and 83%, respectively, with an overall predictive accuracy of 82% (8–10). The improvement in global LV function and symptomatic improvement is directly related to the number of viable myocardial segments. The presence of perfusion/metabolic mismatch can identify patients at increased risk for future cardiac morbidity and mortality.

Dobutamine stress echocardiography (DSE) can be used to identify viability and helps in differentiating between stunned and hibernating myocardium (11–14). A uniphasic response indicates myocardial stunning, is denoted by augmentation of segmental wall motion with low doses of dobutamine, and increases with higher doses. The reduction of augmentation with higher doses is indicative of ischemia and hibernation and is termed a biphasic response. DSE has been found to have an overall accuracy of 86%, a specificity of 91%, and sensitivity of 68% for prediction of segmental recovery. It is also predictive of outcome. Bonow (15). illustrated the data from 15 studies involving 402 patients with ischemic cardiomyopathy. The positive predictive value of DSE to predict recovery after revascularization was 83%, with a negative predictive accuracy of 81%. Cardiac magnetic resonance imaging (MRI) is a clinically valuable alternative to PET in predicting LV functional recovery, following surgical revascularization. It helps in the assessment of tissue perfusion after recanalization, evaluation of myocardial contractile reserve, and characterization of myocardial cellular membrane function (16). Low-dose dobutamine has been combined with MRI for the identification of residual myocardial viability in patients with ventricular dysfunction. The overall accuracy of low-dose dobutamine MRI is 93% compared to 90% by PET (17–19). Cine MRI with a gadolinium-based contrast agent to determine the transmural extent of myocardial viability has been used. New modalities to detect hibernating myocardium include $^{99m}$Tc-sestamibi, perfusion imaging, nuclear magnetic resonance spectroscopic imaging, and ultrasonic tissue characterization.

Revascularization in these high-risk patients should be expeditiously performed. Meticulous myocardial protection and complete revascularization are crucial for good postoperative outcomes.

Several studies have shown that CABG can be performed in high-risk patients with severely impaired LV function (EF < 30%) with low operative mortality, which rivals that of cardiac transplantation. In the past, perioperative mortality after CABG in patients with EF < 25% has been reported to be between 10% and 37%, but more recent reports indicate mortalities between 2.5% and 8%. At Yale University, 188 patients with LVEF < 30% underwent CABG. The mortality in the elective group was 2.8% with 1-, 3-, and 5- year survival of 88%, 77%, and 60% respectively. The functional class improved from 3.1 to 1.4, and LVEF improved from 23.3% to 33.2%.

At the Cleveland Clinic, 1,062 patients underwent primary CABG with or without associated mitral valve surgery and LV reconstruction. The study analyzed the perioperative morbidity, mortality, and late survival. The three groups consisted of CABG (Group I, 728 patients), CABG and mitral valve surgery (Group II, 168 patients), and CABG with LV reconstruction (Group III, 166 patients). The median length of in-hospital stay was 8, 12, and 11 days, respectively. The in-hospital mortality was 2.6%, 3.6%, and 1.2% and overall survival at 1 year, 3 years, and 5 years was 91%, 81%, and 72% in all three groups.

Another recently published prospective study by Shah et al. (20) included 57 patients with a mean age of 67 years and LVEF < 35% who underwent CABG. The majority of these patients were in NYHA Functional Class III–IV. The 1-, 5-, and 10-year survival rates were 83%, 56%, and 24%. Short-term and event-free survival was independently and positively correlated with large reversible perfusion defects in preoperative thallium scans.

Ascione and colleagues (21) compared on-pump (n = 176) and off-pump (n = 74) techniques and analyzed the early and midterm outcomes in patients with severe LV dysfunction. The 30-day, 1-year, and 3-year mortality rate was 97%, 92%, and 87% in the on-pump group. In the off-pump group it was 92%, 85%, and 73%, respectively. Although the mortality in the off-pump group was higher than in the on-pump group, the differences were not statistically significant.

Improved myocardial protection techniques, such as use of the internal mammary artery, platelet inhibitors, angiotensin-converting enzyme inhibitors, statins, beta-blockers, diuretics, intraaortic balloon pumps, and defibrillators in appropriate patients, have contributed immensely to improved outcomes following revascularization. Recent evidence from the SOLVD (Studies of Left

Ventricular Dysfunction) database shows that of the 5,410 patients with LVEF < 35%, 35% of these patients had undergone previous CABG and the all-cause mortality in this group was 26% less at 3 years than the group who had not had bypass surgery. In a selected group of patients with advanced left ventricular dysfunction caused by an ischemic myocardium, CABG may preserve the remaining viable myocardium, provide relief of symptoms, and offer survival of > 60% after 5 years (22).

# VALVE SURGERY IN DILATED CARDIOMYOPATHY

## Mitral Valve Repair

Functional mitral regurgitation frequently occurs with dilated cardiomyopathy because of annular dilatation. The mitral valve apparatus consists of the annulus, leaflets, chordae tendinae, and papillary muscles. The relationship of these components to one another and with the LV wall is a crucial determinant of left ventricular function. Displacement of the papillary muscles occurs with decreased coaptation of the leaflets with or without restricted leaflet motion. This leads to increased left ventricular volume overload and worsens the LV dilatation and MR. The mitral leaflets remain anatomically normal on echocardiography. In ischemic mitral regurgitation, infarction of the papillary muscles may occur and subsequent elongation or rupture may occur. The other mechanism that can cause MR is asynergy of the papillary muscle, or the ventricle that results in mitral regurgitation, located in the commissural area of the same side as the asynergy (23). Recently, real-time, three-dimensional echocardiography (24) has been used to study the geometric differences of the mitral apparatus between ischemic and dilated cardiomyopathy with significant mitral regurgitation. The angles between the annular plane and each leaflet (anterior A$\alpha$, posterior P$\alpha$) were measured. The pattern of deformation from the medial to the lateral was asymmetrical in ICM-MR and symmetrical in DCM-MR. The clinical implications of these need to be studied. It is now a well-recognized fact that there is increased impetus to perform valve repair with an undersized ring rather than by replacement, although this still largely depends on the skill and experience of the surgeon. The repair may also include an "edge-edge" approximation of the anterior and posterior mitral leaflets in the midportion, creating a double orifice of the mitral valve, thus decreasing regurgitation (25).

Several groups have now reported the outcomes of mitral repair in patients with severe LV dysfunction. Bolling and colleagues (26,27) studied 150 patients with end-stage cardiomyopathy and severe MR who underwent mitral annuloplasty. The ejection fraction was < 25%, and all patients were in NYHA Class III-IV. Valve repair was per-

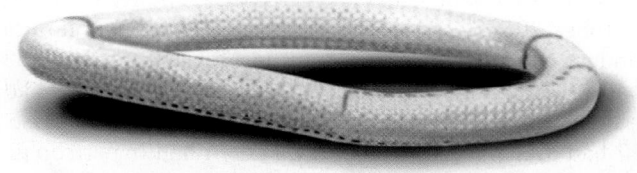

**FIGURE 34.2.** Asymmetric mitral annuloplasty ring (Carpentier-McCarthy-Adams IMR Etlogix ring) for Type IIIb MR. The ring has a reduced AP diameter, dipped P3 region, and reduced P2-P3 curvature.

formed with an undersized flexible annuloplasty ring (Figs 34.2 and 34.3). The operative mortality was 5% (7 patients), and there were 27 late deaths. Mean follow-up was for 45 months (2–83 months). There was an improvement in both the functional class (Class I-II) and in the ejection fraction. The 1-, 2-, 3-, and 5-year actuarial survival following mitral repairs in patients with severe LV dysfunction was 82%, 71%, 68%, and 51%, respectively.

At the Cleveland Clinic (28) between 1990 and 1998, 44 patients with mitral regurgitation and LVEF < 35% underwent mitral repair. The 1-, 2-, and 5-year survival rates were 89%, 86%, and 67%, respectively. The average length of in-hospital stay was 9 days. Heart failure and sudden death accounted for 62% of the late deaths. Freedom from readmission for heart failure was 88%, 82%, and 72% at 1, 2, and 5 years.

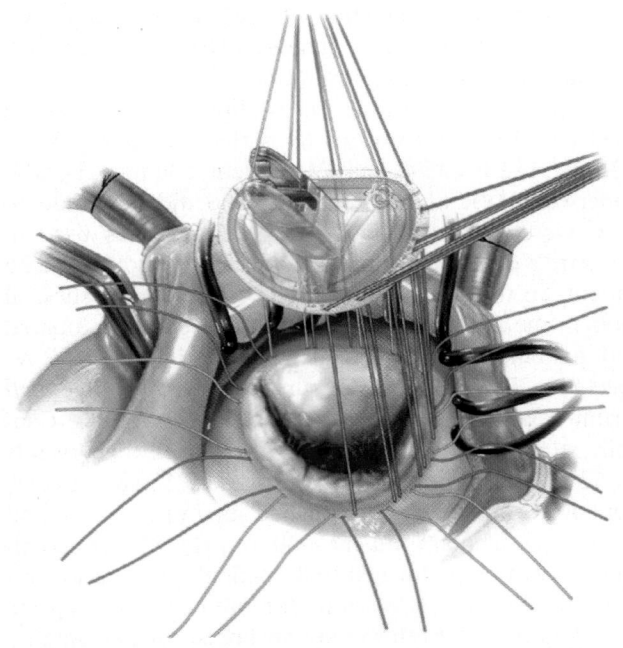

**FIGURE 34.3.** Surgical implantation of the Carpentier-McCarthy-Adams mitral annuloplasty ring.

At the Cleveland Clinic (25), between January 1997 and October 2001, 224 patients with end-stage heart failure underwent mitral repair using the Alfieri stitch and 188 had concomitant annuloplasty. Of these, 143 patients had ischemic cardiomyopathy, 31 had myxomatous disease, 27 had dilated cardiomyopathy, and 14 had hypertrophic obstructive cardiomyopathy. Preoperative MR was graded between III–IV. The in-hospital mortality was 2%. During the first three months, absence of MR declined to 40%, and prevalence of 3+ MR increased to 14%. Survival at 5 years was 65%. However, results indicate that there is a significant late recurrence of mitral regurgitation in patients with ischemic cardiomyopathy. Fourteen patients (12 within 2 years) required mitral valve replacement and 7 required heart transplantation. The reasons attributed to the failure in this group were progressive annular dilatation, ventricular remodeling, and the use of a flexible ring for the annuloplasty.

## Aortic Valve Surgery

Aortic valve disease can manifest with angina, dyspnea, palpitations, syncope, or sudden death. Echocardiographic data should be interpreted with caution in patients with aortic stenosis and low transvalvar gradient, because it is difficult to determine whether there is true aortic stenosis or underlying cardiomyopathy with mild to moderate aortic stenosis. Stress echo and cardiac catheterization help in confirmation of the severity of stenosis. Patients with AR who present with advanced LV dysfunction pose a difficult management problem. Aortic valve surgery may be safely performed with an acceptable clinical outcome in patients with severe ventricular dysfunction and severe aortic stenosis (AS) (low transvalvular gradient) or aortic regurgitation.

At the Cleveland Clinic Foundation (29,30), between 1990 and 1998, a group of 68 patients with an AVA < $0.75 cm^2$, LVEF < 35%, and AV gradient < 30 mm Hg, who underwent AVR and 89 patients who did not undergo AVR, were evaluated. Propensity analysis was used to compare a cohort of 39 patients in the AVR group and 56 patients in the control group. The 1- and 4-year survival rates in the AVR group were 82% and 78% as compared with patients in the control group with 41% and 15%, respectively. The predictors of survival were AVR, age, and serum-creatinine levels. Between 1985 and 1995, Connolly et al., from the Mayo Clinic, reported their results on 52 patients who had a mean age of 71 years; underwent AVR with AS; and who had an LVEF < 35% and mean transvalvular gradient < 30 mm Hg (31). Concomitant CABG was performed in 32 patients. The perioperative mortality was 21%, with 10 more deaths during the follow-up period. In this study, advanced age and smaller prosthesis size were significant predictors of hospital mortality by university analysis. An international multi-

member study by Blackstone et al. (32) quantified the relationship between prosthesis-patient size and long-term survival after AVR. 13,258 patients who had undergone AVR were followed for 15 years. The study showed that prosthesis-patient size down to 1.1 $cm^2/m^2$ did not reduce intermediate or long-term survival after AVR. However, prosthesis-patient size under 1.2 $cm^2$ increased the 30-day mortality by 1% to 2%. These results were more pronounced with mechanical valves. Similarly, AV replacement in patients with chronic AR with severe LV dysfunction (33–35) has shown improved survival when compared with patients who have undergone AVR before 1990. At the Cleveland Clinic, 34 patients with a mean age of 56.4 years underwent AVR after 1990. Several of these patients were listed for cardiac transplantation. There was no perioperative mortality in this group. The 1-year and 5-year survival rates were 97% and 84%, respectively. These results are quite comparable to the outcomes of patients undergoing AVR with moderately impaired or good LV function. Therefore, an aggressive approach to the management of aortic valve disease with severely impaired left ventricular function is recommended.

## LEFT VENTRICULAR RECONSTRUCTION

### Partial Left Ventriculectomy

Partial left ventriculectomy (PLV) was first introduced by Dr. Randas Batista, a Brazilian cardiac surgeon, as an alternative to cardiac transplantation for patients with medically refractory heart failure and dilated cardiomyopathy. The operation was devised based on the Law of LaPlace, which states that wall stress is directly proportional to ventricular pressure and radius and inversely proportional to wall thickness. The goal of the procedure is to reduce the diameter of the LV in order to restore the volume/mass/diameter relationship of the heart and eliminate mitral regurgitation. The resultant decrease in LV wall stress, end diastolic volume, and end systolic volume, would improve ejection fraction and cardiac index and ameliorate symptoms of heart failure.

The criteria for patient selection have been unclear with various groups performing this operation for ischemic, idiopathic dilated cardiomyopathy, Chagas disease, etc. The operation has been performed in nontransplant and transplant centers. Therefore, all patients did not have access to mechanical device assistance or cardiac transplantation in the event of complications, which may explain, in part, the varying outcomes in different centers.

Significant issues exist regarding the amount of myocardium to be resected, heterogenous involvement of the myocardium with the disease, papillary muscle resection, mitral valve repair, and suture line buttressing. The posterolateral wall of the ventricle between the anterolateral and posteromedial papillary muscles is excised. Mitral valve repair or replacement is performed in conjunction with PLV. Early postoperative complications include cardiogenic shock, ventricular rupture, hemorrhage, and ventricular arrhythmias.

In the combined US (SUNY, Buffalo)—Brazilian experience in 120 patients with end-stage heart disease, the 30-day mortality was 22%. Mean follow-up was 9 months, and the one- and two-year survival rates were 66% and 55%, respectively. Angelini et al., from the UK, reported their series of 14 patients had an in-hospital survival of 78.5% (36).

The largest single center experience in the US has been reported by Franco-Cereceda and McCarthy from the Cleveland Clinic (37,38). Between May 1996 and December 1998, PLV was performed in 62 patients (95% transplant candidates) with a mean age of 54 years, mean LVEF of 17.2%, LV end diastolic dimension (LVEDD) of 8.3 cm, and LVEDV of 319 mL. All patients were either in class IV NYHA (60%) or class III (40%), with 42% of patients requiring inotropic or mechanical support. The postoperative LVEF improved to 32.7%, with a decrease in the LVEDD of 5.8 cm and LVEDV of 143 mL. Twenty-five of the 53 (47%) returned to Class II or I after surgery. The perioperative mortality was 1.9%, with 15% of the patients requiring LVAD support. Survival at 1 and 3 years was 80% and 60%. Most of the late deaths reported have been due to arrhythmias or progressive heart failure. The excellent results reported by this group are partly due to the availability of LVAD and cardiac transplantation as a safety net for failed procedures. Based on the above findings, the Society of Thoracic Surgeons (39) issued a position paper that recommended that institutions performing this procedure have extensive experience in all forms of heart failure management to provide all patient options, which include modern drug therapy, cardiac transplantation, and mechanical left ventricular assistance. PLV is now largely abandoned.

## Ischemic LV Reconstruction

Acute transmural infarction leads to cicatrisation, followed by remodeling of the ventricle. The infarcted areas may be akinetic or dyskinetic (aneurysmal). A dyskinetic segment results from a transmural infarction, causing thinning of the ventricular wall and paradoxical movement. An akinetic segment of the myocardium may contain noninfarcted dysfunctional myocardial segments surrounded by a thin rim of viable myocardium. Denton Cooley first performed LV aneurysmectomy on cardiopulmonary bypass in 1958 with excellent symptomatic and survival benefit. However, the resection of the aneurysm with a linear closure causes distortion of the LV geometry.

The different techniques currently used are essentially infarct exclusion procedures (includes the septum) to reconstruct the LV. These include a linear closure by Jatene, a modified linear closure by Mickleborough, a circular closure with a patch by Dor (EVCPP), and a double cerclage closure without a patch by McCarthy. All techniques involve an incision into the diseased segment, an exclusion of the entire diseased segment. A reduction in ventricular cavity size and LV reconstruction has been performed for both akinetic and dyskinetic scars.

Surgery is indicated in patients with angina, heart failure, thromboembolism, or ventricular arrhythmias. At the Cleveland Clinic, LV reconstruction is performed on the beating heart after completing the coronary artery bypass and mitral valve intervention under cardioplegic arrest (40). The LV apex is opened 2 cm lateral to the LAD artery through the thin-walled scar and the ventriculotomy is extended (Fig. 34.4). The LV thrombus is removed and the subendocardial scar is excised down to the border zone where the scar is contiguous with the viable myocardium. Cryolesions are placed at the border zone if the patients have a history of ventricular tachycardia. The border zone is delineated in dyskinetic infarcts but in akinetic hearts, palpation of the beating heart helps to identify the border zone. Two purse-string sutures of 0 polypropylene are placed through the border zone 3 to 5 mm into the scar tissue. The first purse-string suture is tied, reducing the opening by 50% to 70% and creating a neck usually 3 cm to 5 cm. The second purse string is placed 5 mm above the first purse string and tied down. This excludes the infarcted anterior wall and septum, creating an ellipsoidal LV. Horizontal mattress sutures are placed through strips of felt on the LV epicardium, through the LV at the level of the purse-string sutures, then through the septum and out of the LV wall left of the

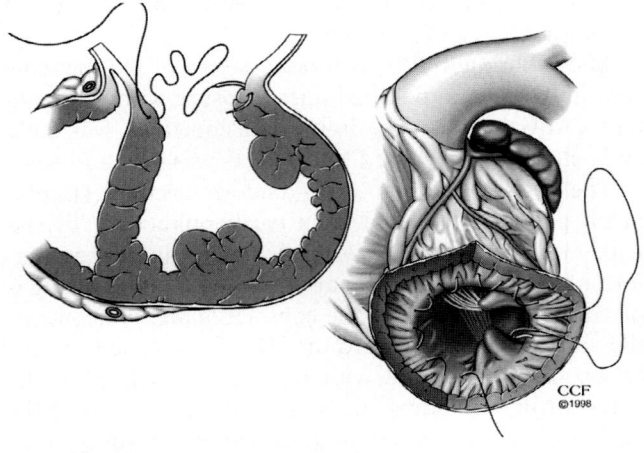

**FIGURE 34.4.** LV reconstruction. The aneurysm is opened 2 cm to the left of the left anterior descending artery. A purse string is placed along the border zone into the scarred tissue.

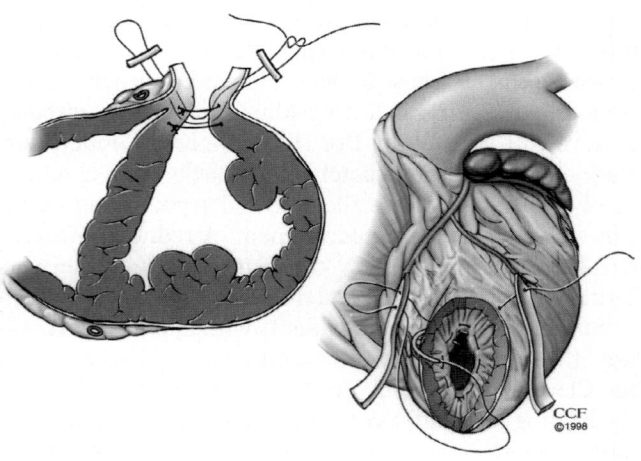

**FIGURE 34.5.** Interrupted horizontal mattress sutures are passed through the felt strips, up to the left of the left anterior descending artery. The cross-sectional view shows the excluded infarct, viable left ventricular myocardium, with the exception of a thin rim of scar at the repair.

LAD (Fig 34.5). The ventriculotomy is oversewn with 2-0 polypropylene to eliminate bleeding. The LV apex is elevated to de-air the heart with an aortic root vent in position. The reconstructed LV chamber consists of viable myocardium apart from the thin rim of scar tissue and no patch.

At the Cleveland Clinic, between January 1997 and August 2002, 224 patients with a mean age of 62 years have undergone this procedure. The majority of the patients were in NYHA Class III–IV with LVEF < 30%. Eighty-five percent had CABG, 43% had mitral valve procedures, and 23% were reoperations. Sixty-nine percent had dyskinetic segments and 31% had akinetic segments. Survival at 30 days, 1, 2, and 3 years was 98%, 92%, 90%, and 86%, respectively. Freedom from adverse events at 1, 2, and 3 years was 89%, 85%, and 83%.

Mickleborough (39) reported a series of 196 patients who underwent a modified linear closure with concomitant CABG in 91%. The in-hospital mortality was 2.6% and actuarial survival at 1 and 5 years was 91% and 84%.

The Dor procedure (42) (endoventricular circular patch plasty) is performed on cardiopulmonary bypass with or without cardioplegia. A ventriculotomy is performed and mural thrombi are removed. A purse string is placed at the junction of the contractile and noncontractile portions of the myocardium. This is tightened and the LV opening is patched with Dacron at the level of the purse string, excluding the nonfunctional portion of the septum. The ventriculotomy is closed with a simple running suture with or without the use of resorcin formol glue.

The RESTORE (**R**econstructive **E**ndoventricular **S**urgery, returning **T**orsion **O**riginal **R**adius **E**lliptical shape to the LV) group consists of an international group of cardiologists and cardiac surgeons, and has studied the outcomes in patients undergoing SAVER (**S**urgical **A**nterior **V**entricular **E**ndocardial **R**estoration) in the dilated remodeled ventricle after myocardial infarction (43). 439 patients underwent the SAVER operation with concomitant CABG (89%), MV repair (22%), and MV replacement (4%). The overall hospital mortality was 6.6%. Intraaortic balloon pump counterpulsation was required in 7.7%, LVAD in 0.5%, and extracorporeal oxygenation in 1.3% of the patients. The LVEF increased from 29 ± 10.4 to 39 ± 12.4%, and the left ventricular systolic volume index decreased from 109 ± 71 to 69 ± 42 ml/m². Survival at 18 months was 89.2% (Fig. 34.6). Risk factors identified in this study at any time after the operation included older age, MV replacement, and lower postoperative ejection fraction.

Dor et al., described their results in both akinetic and dyskinetic scars and showed functional class and ejection fraction with a significantly reduced incidence of ventricular tachycardia. The in-hospital mortality was 10% for the akinetic group and 14% in the dyskinetic group (42).

Following the geometric LV reconstruction there is decreased wall tension with attenuated oxygen requirement of the remote myocardium, improved regional myocardial performance, hemodynamics, and symptomatic improvement. The alteration in shape realigns fiber orientation with improved LVEF, decreased end diastolic and end systolic volumes, and a reduction in LV wall stress.

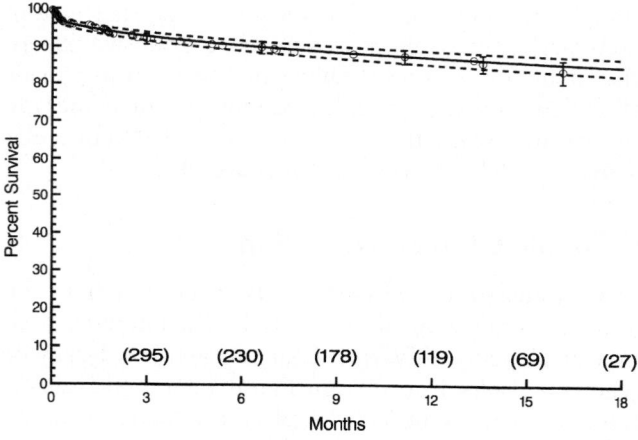

**FIGURE 34.6.** Overall survival after surgical anterior ventricular endocardial restoration. Circles represent a death and the vertical bars are asymmetric confidence limits equivalent to one standard error. The numbers at the foot of the graph represent the number of patients at three month intervals. Reproduced with permission from J Am Coll Cardiol 2001;37: 1199–209.

These findings have been confirmed by real-time three-dimensional echocardiographic study of LV function after infarct exclusion surgery for ischemic cardiomyopathy (44). The most common cause of in-hospital mortality was low cardiac output and late deaths were due to heart failure or sudden death.

## Dynamic Cardiomyoplasty (DCMP)

The first clinical application of cardiomyoplasty as a skeletal muscle assist was performed and reported by Carpentier in 1985. Dynamic cardiomyoplasty (DCMP) has been used as an alternative surgical procedure that combines cardiac and plastic surgery with electrophysiology and bioengineering advances. DCMP has been performed in patients with dilated and ischemic cardiomyopathy, and, in Brazil, it has been performed in end-stage cardiomyopathy due to Chagas disease.

The current criteria to select patients for DCMP are those who are in NYHA Class-III without coronary artery disease, mitral regurgitation, or cardiac dysrhythmias. The LVEF should be at least > 15% and peak $V_{O2}$ > 10 mls/kg/mn. The selection criteria were not refined initially and patients in NYHA Class-IV with dysrhythmias and mitral regurgitation were included. Not surprisingly, this procedure had a prohibitive mortality of 31%. With the current selection criteria the mortality has been as low as 4%.

The surgery involves the mobilization of the latissimus dorsi muscle after severing all the attachments while preserving the neurovascular bundle. The intramuscular stimulation leads are then attached to the muscle flap. A portion of the second rib is excised to create a window through which the muscle flap is passed into the left pleural space with the stimulation electrodes. The humeral tendon is attached to the periosteum of the third rib. The patient is then turned to a supine position and a median sternotomy is performed. Cardiopulmonary bypass is not essential. Epicardial sensing electrodes are placed on the right ventricle and the latissimus dorsi is passed posterior to the heart. The muscle is anchored to the pericardium adjacent to the right atrium and pulmonary artery. The base of the flap is passed to cover as much of the right ventricle as possible. The diaphragmatic and lateral edges of the muscle are sutured without compressing the heart. The myocardial sensing and stimulator leads are attached to the cardiomyostimulator, which is placed in the abdominal pocket.

The muscle conditioning commences two weeks following surgery to allow recovery from ischemia. The pulses delivered (by sensing the R wave) are gradually increased and gradually full contraction of the muscle flap is achieved. The pulse amplitude, duration, sensing threshold, and synchronization ratio can be adjusted.

There have been recent reports of demand stimulation of the LD flap leading to better, event-free survival (45).

The clinical benefit is postulated to be due to systolic augmentation, limitation of ventricular dilatation, reduction of ventricular wall stress, and ventricular remodeling with an active girdling effect (46). The LD muscle consists of mixed Type I (slow twitch) and Type II (fast twitch) fibers. Transformation occurs to convert the Type II into fatigue resistant Type I fibers with a concomitant change in the metabolic pathways.

The lack of survival benefit compared to medical therapy has hindered the acceptance of this procedure. Although there is clinical improvement with improved ejection fraction, functional class, and quality of life, it hasn't been accompanied by a significant improvement in the hemodynamics. Predictors of poor survival are atrial fibrillation, NYHA Class-IV, high PCWP, pulmonary vascular resistance, and the need for an intraaortic balloon pump. Most of the hospital deaths were due to progressive cardiac failure, sepsis, and multiorgan failure, and most of the late deaths were secondary due to sudden death. Another group from Brazil reported their results in a group of 52 patients who underwent DCMP. A comparison was made between the Chagas group (8 patients) and the nonchagasic group. In the nonchagasic group 1-, 2-, and 5-year survival rates were 79.5%, 67.8%, and 49.9%, whereas the survival rates in the Chagas group were 37.5%, 12.5%, and 0%. This was attributed to a higher prevalence of ventricular arrhythmias and possibly a reactivation of the disease.

The Phase III C-SMART (Cardiomyoplasty-Skeletal Muscle Assist Randomized Trial) began in 1994. Patients were randomized to either the surgical or control group (medically treated). There were problems recruiting the required number of patients (400) for this trial; only 103 patients were enrolled. Fifty-four patients have had DCMP with a mortality of 1.9%. Medtronic Corporation no longer manufactures the Cardiomyostimulator and this operation is no longer performed in the US. It is, however, being performed in Asia and some European countries with the availability of the LD Pace myostimulator. Few patients who have had DCMP have progressed to have cardiac transplantation. Dynamic cardiomyoplasty led to the observation that a dynamic unstimulated cardiomyoplasty (girdling effect) also has clinical benefits and has led to the evolution of novel strategies for end-stage heart failure, such as passive constraint devices (e.g., Acorn Cardiac Support Device or Myosplint).

## EMERGING BIOMEDICAL DEVICES

As it is a recognized fact that the progressive increase in cardiac chamber size with decreased ejection fraction and contractile dysfunction leads to heart failure, passive constraint devices have been designed to counteract these changes.

Two passive mechanical devices have now emerged and are currently in clinical trials in the United States. They are the Acorn Cardiac Support device (ACSD, Acorn Cardiovascular, St. Paul, MN) and the Myosplint (Myocor, Maple Grove, MN).

## Acorn Cardiac Support Device

The Acorn Cardiac Support Device consists of a polyester polymer that is wrapped around the epicardial surface of the ventricles and anchored by stay sutures to the atrioventricular groove (Fig. 34.7).

The ACSD has been implanted on beating and arrested hearts. The multiple filaments in each fiber allow the device to evenly conform to the epicardial surface. An acute reduction of 5% is acceptable. Over a period of time the shape of the ventricle becomes more elliptical rather than spherical.

Preclinical studies in dogs have shown decreased LV end diastolic volumes with improved LVEF and no evidence of constrictive or restrictive physiology (47,48). Postmortem studies showed that the device at 3 months was thinly encapsulated without encroachment into the epicardium. The integrity of the coronary vessels was preserved with a reduction in functional mitral regurgitation.

Globally the ACSD has been implanted in more than 130 patients. The safety and feasibility of the procedure was studied in 48 patients with or without concomitant cardiac surgery. Inclusion criteria were medically optimized patients with dilated ischemic or nonischemic cardiomyopathy in NYHA III, LVEF < 35%, indexed LVEDD > 30 mm/m² and acceptable renal function (creatinine < 3.5 mL/dL). Patients in NYHA class IV, hemodynamically unstable with recent myocardial infarctions or previous cardiac surgery were excluded. The mean intraoperative reduction in left ventricular end diastolic dimension was 4.6% ± 1% with no device-related intraoperative com-

plications. Actuarial survival was 73% at 12 months and 68% at 24 months. Two-year follow up has shown a decrease in the end diastolic dimensions and improved ejection fraction. Randomized clinical trials are underway in Europe, the United States, and Australia (49).

## The Myosplint and Coapsys Device

The Myosplint is an implantable transventricular splint with two epicardial pads adjusted to draw the wall of the LV together, thereby reducing the radius. The three Myosplints reduce the LV wall stress. The splint consists of a 1.4 mm diameter polyethylene, braided splint coated with expanded polytetrafluoroethylene and connected to epicardial pads covered with polyester fabric.

Preclinical studies in dogs with heart failure were found to be safe with no device-related complications. Clinical safety (50) and feasibility studies are underway in Europe and the United States. Schenk and colleagues reported the use of Myosplint in 7 patients in functional Class III-IV, LV end diastolic diameter from 70 to 102 mm. Four of these patients received the Myosplint with concomitant mitral annuloplasty. At 90 days postimplantation there were no device-related complications, such as thromboembolism, bleeding, device instability, or vascular damage. The clinical results in this small series were quite variable; therefore, it is difficult to draw conclusions at this stage.

The Myocor Coapsys device (Myocor, Inc., Maple Grove, MN) is currently under evaluation and was developed to treat patients with functional mitral regurgitation. The device consists of epicardial anterior and posterior pads and a subvalvular chord, which passes through the ventricle. The posterior pad has two heads, an annular head that changes the shape of the mitral annulus and a papillary head that provides leverage at the midpapillary muscle level to change the papillary muscle position. The device is tightened under echocardiographic visualization on the beating heart, until the MR is significantly reduced or eliminated.

At the Cleveland Clinic (51), the Coapsys device has been tested on canine models. Functional MR and heart failure was induced in dogs by rapid ventricular pacing. The Coapsys device was implanted off-pump to reduce the MR. Heart failure was maintained by pacing. The device reduced MR and eight weeks later, after cutting the Coapsys subvalvular chord MR returned in the canine models. Trials are currently underway in the United States.

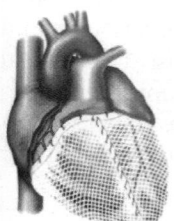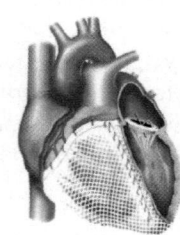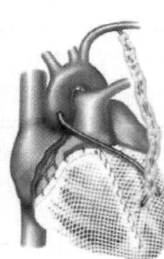

**FIGURE 34.7.** (**Left panel**): Implantation of the cardiac support device (CSD) as the sole surgical procedure. (**Middle**): Surgical implantation of the CSD along with concomitant mitral valve replacement and (**right**) surgical implantation of the CSD along with CABG. Reproduced with permission from Ann Thorac Surg 2003;75:S13–9.

---

**KEY POINTS**

- In the United States, 550,000 patients are diagnosed with heart failure every year.

- Revascularization, valve repair, replacement, and ventricular reconstruction are more commonly performed in this high-risk group with acceptable mortality and morbidity.
- Meticulous myocardial protection with expeditiously performed surgery continues to improve postoperative outcomes in high-risk patients.
- Nontransplant surgical treatment of heart failure negates or postpones the need for cardiac transplantation.

## REFERENCES

1. Rahimtoola SH. From coronary artery disease to heart failure: role of hibernating myocardium. Am J Cardiol 1995;75: 16E –22E.
2. ACC/AHA Task Force Heart Failure Guidelines. Guidelines for the evaluation and management of heart failure report of the American College of Cardiology/American Heart Association Task Force on practice guidelines. J Am Coll Cardiol 1995;26(5):1376–98.
3. Saraste A, Pulkki K, Kallajoki M, Henricksen K, Parvinen M, Voipio-Pulkki L. Apoptosis in human acute myocardial infarction. Circulation 1997;95:320–3.
4. Weisman HF, Bush DE, Mannisi JA. Cellular mechanisms of myocardial infarct expansion. Circulation 1988;78:186–201.
5. Gerdes AM, Capasso JM. Structural remodeling and mechanical dysfunction of cardiac myocytes in heart failure. J Mol Cell Cardiol 1995;27:849–56.
6. DiCarli MF, Asgarzadie F, Schelbert HR, et al. Quantitative relation between myocardial viability and improvement in heart failure symptoms after revascularization in patients with ischemic cardiomyopathy. Circulation 1995;92: 3436–44.
7. Ragosta M, Beller GA, Watson DD, Kaul S, Gimple LW. Quantitative planar rest-redistribution [201] TL imaging in detection of myocardial viability and prediction of improvement in left ventricular function after coronary bypass surgery in patients with severely depressed left ventricular function. Circulation 1993;87:1630–41.
8. Tillish J, Brunken R, Marshal R, et al. Reversibility of cardiac wall motion abnormalities predicted by positron tomography. N Engl J Med 1986;314:884–8.
9. Brunken R, Schawaiger M, Grover-McKay M, et al. Positron emission tomography detects tissue metabolic activity in myocardial segments with persistent thallium perfusion defects. J Am Coll Cardiol 1987;10:557–67.
10. Di Carli M, Davidson M, Little R, et al. Value of metabolic imaging with positron emission tomography for evaluating prognosis in patients with coronary artery disease and left ventricular dysfunction. Am J Cardiol 1994;73:527–33.
11. LaCanna G, Alfieri O, Giubbini M, Ferrari R, Visioli O. Echocardiography during infusion of dobutamine for identification of reversible dysfunction in patients with coronary artery disease. J Am Coll Cardiol 1994;23:617–26.
12. Vanverschelde JL, Gerber BL, AM DH, et al. Preoperative selection of patients with severely impaired left ventricular function for coronary revascularization. Role of low-dose dobutamine echocardiography and exercise-redistribution-reinjection thallium SPECT. Circulation 1995;92(Suppl): II37–44.
13. Williams M, Odabashian J, Lytle B, Marwick T. Prediction of viable myocardium in severe left ventricular dysfunction. Follow-up study of dobutamine echocardiography and positron emission tomography. Circulation 1995;92:I-266.
14. Vanverschelde JL, D'Hondt AM, Marwick T, Gerber BL, Wijns W, Melin JA. Head to head comparison of exercise–redistribution-reinjection thallium SPECT and low-dose dobutamine echocardiography for prediction of the reversibility chronic left ventricular ischemic dysfunction. J Am Coll Cardiol 1996;28:432–42.
15. Bonow RO. Identification of viable myocardium. Circulation 1996;94:2674–80.
16. Higgins C. Prediction of myocardial viability by MRI. Circulation 1999;99(6):727–9.
17. Gunning MG, Anagnostopulos C, Knight CJ, et al. Comparison of [201]TL, [99]Tc-Tetrofosmin, and Dobutamine magnetic resonance imaging for identifying hibernating myocardium. Circulation 1998;98(18):1869–74.
18. Pasquet AA, White RD, Zuchowski C, Marwick TH. A one-stop shop for delineation of viable myocardium? Comparison of function and perfusion assessment by resting MRI with Dobutamine echocardiography. Circulation 1998;98(17):I-514.
19. Baer FM, Voth E, Schneider CA, et al. Dobutamine MRI is a reliable alternative to Positron Emission Tomography for the prediction of functional recovery of viable myocardium after successful revascularization. Circulation 1998;98(17):I-513.
20. Shah PJ, Hare DL, Raman JS, et al. Survival after myocardial revascularization for ischemic cardiomyopathy: a prospective ten-year follow up. J Thorac Cardiovasc Surg 2003;126: 1320–7.
21. Ascione R, Narayan P, Rogers CA, Lim KH, Capoun R, Angelini GD. Early and midterm clinical outcome in patients with severe left ventricular dysfunction undergoing coronary artery surgery. Ann Thorac Surg 2003;76(3):793–9.
22. Trachiotis GD, Weintraub WS, Johnston TS, et al. Coronary artery bypass grafting in patients with advanced left ventricular dysfunction. Ann Thor Surg 1998;66:1632–9.
23. Izumi S, Miyatake K, Nimura Y. Mechanism of mitral regurgitation in patients with myocardial infarction: a study using two-dimensional Doppler flow imaging and echocardiography. Circulation 1987;76(4):777–85.
24. Kwan J, Shiota T, Agler DA, et al. Geometric differences of the mitral apparatus between ischemic and dilated cardiomyopathy with significant mitral regurgitation: real time three-dimensional echocardiographic study. Circulation 2003;107: 1135–40.
25. Bhudia SK, McCarthy PM, Smedira NG, Lam B, Rajeshwaran J, Blackstone EH. Edge-to-edge (Alfieri) mitral repair: results in diverse clinical settings. Ann Thorac Surg 2004;77 (5):1598–606.
26. Badhwar V, Bolling S. Mitral valve surgery in the patient with left ventricular dysfunction. Semin Thorac Cardiovasc Surg 2002;14:133–6.
27. Bolling S, Pagani FD, Deeb GM, Bach DS. Intermediate-term outcome of mitral reconstruction in cardiomyopathy. J Thorac Cardiovasc Surg 1998;115:381–88.
28. Bishay ES, McCarthy PM, Cosgrove DM. Mitral valve surgery in patients with severe left ventricular dysfunction. Eur J Cardiothorac Surgery 2000;17:213–21.
29. McCarthy PM. Aortic valve surgery in patients with severe LV dysfunction. Semin Thorac Cardiovasc Surg 2002;14(2): 137–43.
30. Pereira JJ, Lauer MS, Bashir M, et al. Survival after aortic valve replacement for severe aortic stenosis with low transvalvular gradients and severe left ventricular dysfunction. J Am Coll Cardiol 2002;39:1356–63.
31. Connolly HM, Henly WS, Amar KH, et al. Severe aortic stenosis with transvalvular gradient and severe left ventricular dysfunction. Results of aortic valve replacement in 52 patients. Circulation 101:1940–1946, 2000.
32. Blackstone EH, Cosgrove DM, Jamieson EWR. Prosthesis size and long-term survival after aortic valve replacement. 2003;126(3):783–97.
33. Bonow RO, Nikas D, Elefteriades JA. Valve replacement for regurgitant lesions of the aortic or mitral valve in advanced left ventricular dysfunction. Cardiol Clin 1995;13(1): 73–83.

34. McCarthy PM, Kumpati GS, Blackstone EH, Hoercher KH, Smedira NG. Aortic valve surgery for chronic aortic regurgitation with severe LV dysfunction: time for a reevaluation? Circulation 2001;104(17)(Suppl):II-684.

35. Turina J, Milincic J, Seifert B, Turina M. Valve replacement in chronic aortic regurgitation: true predictors of survival after extended follow-up. Circulation 1998;98:II-100–107.

36. Angelini GD, Pryn S, Mehta D, et al. Left-ventricular volume reduction for end stage heart failure. Lancet 1997;350:489 (letter).

37. McCarthy P, Starling S, Wong J. Early results of partial left ventriculectomy. J Thor Cardiovasc Surg 1997;114:P755.

38. Franco-Cereceda A, McCarthy PM, Blackstone EH, et al. Partial left ventriculectomy for dilated cardiomyopathy: Is this an alternative to transplantation? J Thorac Cardiovasc 2001;121(5):879–93.

39. Society Position Paper. LV Reduction Surgery. Ann Thorac Surg 1997;63:909–10.

40. Caldeira C, McCarthy PM. A simple method of left ventricular reconstruction without patch for ischemic cardiomyopathy. Ann Thorac Surg 2001;72:2148–49.

41. Mickleborough LL. Left ventricular reconstruction for ischemic cardiomyopathy. Semin Thorac Cardiovasc Surg 2002; 14(2):144–9.

42. Dor V, Sabatier M, Di Donato M, et al. Efficacy of endoventricular patch plasty in the large postinfarction akinetic scar and severe LV dysfunction: comparisons with a series of large dyskinetic scars. J Thorac Cardiovasc Surg 1998;116(1).

43. Athanasuleas C, Stanley A, Buckberg G, et al. Surgical Anterior Ventricular Endocardial Restoration (SAVER) in the dilated remodeled ventricle after anterior myocardial infarction. JACC 2001;37(5):1199–209.

44. Qin JX, Shiota T, McCarthy PM, et al. Real-time three-dimensional study of left ventricular function after infarct exclusion surgery for ischemic cardiomyopathy. Circulation 2000;102(Suppl III):III-101–6.

45. Chachques JC, Marino J, Lajos P. Dynamic cardiomyoplasty: clinical follow up at 12 years. Euro J Cardiothorac Surg 1997; 12:560–8.

46. Rigatelli G, Barbiero M. Demand stimulation of the lattissimus heart wrap: experience with humans and comparisons with adynamic girdling. Ann Thorac Surg 2003;76(5):1587–92.

47. Chaudhry PA, Mishima T, Sharov VG, et al. Passive mechanical containment prevents ventricular remodeling in heart failure. Ann Thorac Surg 2000;70:1275–80.

48. Chaudhry PA, Anagnostopoulas PV, Mishima T. Acute ventricular reduction with Acorn cardiac support device: effect on progressive left ventricular dysfunction and dilatation in dogs with chronic heart failure. J Card Surg 2001;16:118–26.

49. Oz MC, Konertz WF, Kleber FX, et al. Global surgical experience with the Acorn cardiac support device. J Thorac Cardiovasc 2003;126(4):983–91.

50. Schenk S, Reichenspurner H, Boehm DH, et al. Myosplint implant and shape change procedure: intra- and peri-operative safety and feasibility. J Heart Lung Transplant 2002;21: 680–6.

51. Inoue M, McCarthy PM, Popovic ZB, et al. The Coapsys device to treat functional mitral regurgitation: in vivo long-term canine study. J Thorac Cardiovasc 2004;127(4):1068–77.

## QUESTIONS

1. All of the following are true of myocardial viability tests *except*:
   A. High fluorodeoxyglucose uptake represents myocardial viability.
   B. A uniphasic response with DSE indicates myocardial stunning.
   C. A biphasic response with DSE indicates myocardial viability.
   D. Stunned myocardium does not show functional recovery.
   E. Hibernation indicates viability despite no contraction.

2. The following risk factors increase operative morbidity and mortality, following coronary artery bypass grafting *except*:
   A. Female gender
   B. Diabetes mellitus
   C. Chronic renal failure
   D. Peripheral vascular disease
   E. Complete revascularization

3. All of the following are true of ischemic LV reconstruction *except*:
   A. It can be performed on dyskinetic segments only.
   B. Risk factors include older age group and mitral valve replacement.
   C. Reported perioperative mortality is between 2% and 10%.
   D. Heart failure and sudden deaths are the most common causes of late deaths.
   E. Survival at one year is approximately 90%.

4. All of the following are incremental risk factors for early and late death, following aortic valve replacement *except*:
   A. Age
   B. NYHA functional class
   C. Concomitant CABG
   D. Previous aortic valve replacement
   E. African-American population

# Assessment in Surgical Procedures for Congestive Heart Failure

*Alina M. Grigore, Randall R. Joe, Robert M. Savage, and Nicholas J. Smedira*

## IMPACT OF CONGESTIVE HEART FAILURE ON THE POPULATION

Congestive heart failure (CHF) has been defined as a complex clinical syndrome caused by any structural or functional cardiac disorder that impairs the ability of the ventricles to maintain adequate cardiac output (Table 35.1). In the United States, more than 4.5 million people have CHF, and its prevalence is estimated at 6.8% in people over the age of 65. Additionally, CHF is equally common in men and women (Fig. 35.1), but twice as prevalent in blacks as it is in whites (1,2). It is likely that the

> **TABLE 35.1. Pathophysiology of Heart Failure— from Injury to Clinical Syndrome**

1. Causes
   a. Myocardial injury
      i. ischemia
      ii. toxins
      iii. volume overload
      iv. pressure overload
   b. Genetic perturbation
2. Cardiac remodeling
   a. Myocyte growth
      i. concentric hypertrophy
      ii. eccentric hypertrophy
   b. Interstitial fibrosis
   c. Apoptosis
   d. Sarcomere slippage
   e. Chamber enlargement
3. Clinical heart failure milieu
   a. Pump performance
   b. Circulatory dynamics
   c. Metabolic abnormalities
   d. Symptoms
   e. Physical findings

number of patients with end-stage CHF will grow as the average age of our population rises. (See Chapter 28, Figure 28.1).

## TRENDS IN MANAGEMENT OF PATIENTS WITH CONGESTIVE HEART FAILURE

Congestive heart failure is a complex syndrome in which myocardial injury and the resulting hemodynamic changes perturb many neuroendocrine, humoral, and inflammatory feedback loops. Early in the course of the disease, ventricular contractility is maintained by adrenergic stimulation, activation of renin-angiotensin-aldosterone, and other neurohormonal and cytokine systems (3,4). However, these compensatory mechanisms become less effective over time, so that ventricular dilation and fibrosis occur and cardiac function deteriorates. This produces a

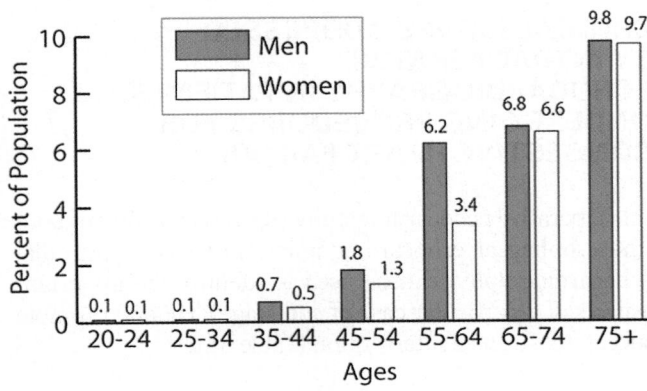

**FIGURE 35.1.** Prevalence of congestive heart failure by age and sex. Zoghbi WA, Enriquez-Sarano M, Foster E. et al. Recommendations for evaluation of the severity of native valvular regurgitation with two-dimensional and Doppler echocardiography. J Am Soc Echocardiogr 2003;16(7):777–802.

chronic state of low perfusion that ends in multisystem failure and death unless adequate circulation is restored.

Strategies for treating end-stage CHF aim to improve quality of life, limit disease progression, and prolong life. Medical therapies, such as angiotensin-converting enzyme inhibitors (ACEI), β blockers, diuretics, inotropic agents, and antiarrhythmics, represent the usual standard of care for CHF management. However, even multidrug regimens may not prevent progression toward end-stage CHF; when this occurs, surgery is the only effective intervention.

Cardiac transplantation is the "gold-standard" surgical treatment for end-stage CHF. While the one-year survival rate after transplantation is 85%, patients in New York Heart Association (NYHA) class IV have a one-year mortality rate of 40%–50% (5,6). Additionally, the small number of donors limits the number of CHF patients who can benefit from cardiac transplantation. Over the past decade, the number of transplant recipients older than 65 years has quadrupled, but the number of donors has remained the same and transplantation waiting times have increased steadily. As a result, even though almost 16,000 people per year could benefit from cardiac transplantation, only 2,400 heart transplantations are actually performed.7 The mismatch between the growing number of cardiac transplant candidates and the limited number of donors has led to increasing use of alternative advanced surgical therapies intended to unload the heart and allow myocardial reverse-remodeling and recovery. Included among these advanced procedures are mechanical ventricular assist device (VAD) implantation, ventricular remodeling procedures in conjunction with revascularization and mitral valvuloplasty (i.e., endoventricular circular patch plasty (ECPP), partial ventriculectomy), newer procedures intended to reduce ventricular dilatation (i.e., external or internal splinting), and total artificial heart (TAH) implantation.

## CRITICAL ISSUES ADDRESSED BY INTRAOPERATIVE ECHOCARDIOGRAPHY IN PATIENTS UNDERGOING PROCEDURES FOR CONGESTIVE HEART FAILURE

Intraoperative echocardiography (IOE) (consisting of both transesophageal echocardiography (TEE) and epicardial echocardiography) can be used to identify the important aspects of a particular case of end-stage CHF and promote successful surgical intervention (Table 35.2).

### Determine the Etiology and Mechanism of CHF

Advanced CHF is caused by a variety of diseases that affect the myocardium. Based on their functional and mor-

phologic features, cardiomyopathies (CMP) can be classified as dilated, hypertrophic, or restrictive. Dilated CMP is the result of viral, bacterial, or parasitic disease of toxic insult. It can also occur in association with pregnancy. Long-term severe myocardial ischemia and chronic regurgitant valvular disease, such as mitral or aortic insufficiency, could also lead to dilated CMP (Figs. 35.2 and 35.3). Hypertrophic CMP is either genetically inherited or is the result of long-standing hypertension or valvular disease, such as aortic stenosis. Infiltrative processes (amyloidosis, hemochromatosis) or inflammatory disease (sarcoidosis) are the most common causes of restrictive CMP. IOE is an important diagnostic tool due to its unique ability to evaluate cardiac morphology and function and to differentiate among various types of CMP (Tables 35.3 and 35.4) (8).

### Assessment of Left and Right Ventricular Function

Assessment of left ventricular (LV) and right ventricular (RV) function is critical to the proper evaluation and perioperative management of patients with end-stage CHF. Using IOE can provide excellent qualitative and quantitative information on RV and LV function.

Dilated CMP is characterized by dilation of both ventricular and atrial chambers associated with systolic heart failure (9). Both motion mode (M-mode) and two-dimensional (2-D) echocardiography can be used for the evaluation of LV systolic function. The high time resolution of M-mode echocardiography enables it to accurately measure ventricular internal dimension and wall thickness. Additionally, placing the M-mode beam at the mitral chordal level to obtain a transgastric longitudinal view of the LV makes it possible to compute LV fractional shorten-

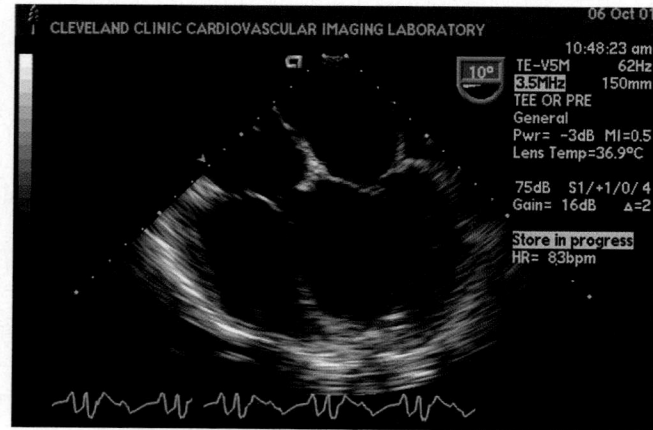

**FIGURE 35.2.** Dilated cardiomyopathy: midesophageal four-chamber view

▶ **TABLE 35.2. Application of Intraoperative Echocardiography During Surgical Procedures for Congestive Heart Failure**

| Surgical Procedure | Critical IOE Issues | Pre-CPB | Post-CPB |
|---|---|---|---|
| LVAD Implantation | RV function<br>Sequelae of CHF<br>　MR, pulmonary HTN<br>　Diastolic dysfunction<br>　Mural thrombi (LA, LV)<br>Potential R → L shunt<br>Potential Ao → LV circuit<br>Cannulation-perfusion<br>LVAD cannula inflow/outflow<br>　Position and function<br>LVAD function<br>　LV volume<br>　Valve competence<br>Complications of CPB | Global RV Fx, RV FAC<br>MR (grade, mechanism)<br>LAA or LV mural thrombi<br>PW of MV Inflow pulm vein<br>　contrast<br>CFD, contrast with valsalva<br>CFD of AV | Global RV Fx, RV FAC<br><br><br>PW of MV and pulmonary vein<br><br><br>CFD of AV<br>TEE and  EPE<br>Apical inflow position<br>　CW, CFD<br>Aortic outflow<br>　Air embolism<br>Hypovolemia, flow < 1.5 m/sec<br>Regurgitant LVAD flow<br>2-D  Asc and descending aorta |
| BI-VAD, ECMO | RV Function<br>Sequelae of CHF<br>　MR, pulmonary HTN<br>　Diastolic dysfunction<br>　Mural thrombi (LA, LV)<br>Potential R → L shunt<br>Potential Ao → LV circuit<br>Cannulation-perfusion<br>LVAD cannula inflow/outflow<br>　Position and function<br>LVAD function<br>　LV volume<br>　Valve competence<br>Complications of CPB cannula positioning<br>　LA, PA, LV, Ao<br>LA thrombus formation | | Global RV Fx, RV FAC<br>PW of MV and pulmonary vein<br>CFD of AV<br>TEE and EPE<br>Apical inflow position<br>　CW, CFD<br>Aortic outflow<br>　Air embolism<br>Hypovolemia, flow < 1.5 m/sec<br>Regurgitant LVAD flow<br>2-D  Asc and descending aorta |
| Dor  Procedure<br>Ventricular Reconstruction<br>　Remodeling LV<br>　CABG<br>　MV Repair | RV function<br>LV function and scar<br>Sequelae of CHF<br>　MR, pulmonary HTN<br>　Diastolic dysfunction<br>　Mural thrombi<br>Potential R → L shunt<br>Embolic source (LA, LV)<br>Cannulation-perfusion strategy<br>Myocardial viability<br>MR severity and mechanism | Global RV Fx, RV FAC, TR<br>RWMA, scar<br><br>MR (severity and mechanism)<br>PWD MW and pulmonary vein<br>Contrast<br>CFD, contrast and valsalva<br><br>EPE<br>Resting RWMA<br>Low-dose dobutamine stress | Global RV Fx, RV FAC<br>PW of MV and pulmonary vein<br>CFD of AV<br>TEE and EPE<br>Apical inflow position<br>　CW, CFD<br>Aortic outflow<br>　Air embolism<br>Hypovolemia, flow < 1.5 m/sec<br>Regurgitant LVAD flow<br>2-D  Asc & descending aorta |
| Revascularization | Myocardial viability | Resting RWM<br>Low-dose dobutamine stress<br>Mitral valve function | Assess for new  RWMA<br>Comprehensive IOE focusing on<br>complications of cannulation,<br>perfusion, myocardial protection,<br>and valve function |
| MV Repair | Mitral regurgitation | MR severity and mechanism<br>Pathoanatomy, annulus size | Success of repair<br>Complications |
| External and Internal<br>　Splinting | Size LV, Systolic LV / RV Fx,<br>MR, diastolic Fx<br>Position of mechanical splints | As above, LV dimensions,<br>LV & RV dimensions, Ej Fx<br>MR mechanism/severity, mitral<br>inflow, pulmonary vein CW | Diastolic function<br>Filling<br>RV function |

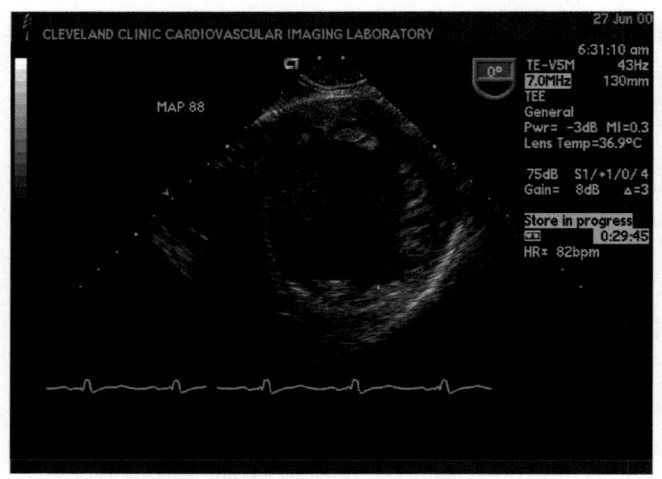

**FIGURE 35.3.** Dilated cardiomyopathy: transgastric midpapillary short-axis view

ing, a rough measurement of LV systolic function with a normal range of 25% to 45%, using the following formula:

$$\text{Fractional shortening (\%)} = (\text{LVID}_d - \text{LVID}_s)/\text{LVID}_d \times 100\%$$

($\text{LVID}_d$ = left ventricular internal diameter at end-diastole; $\text{LVID}_s$ = left ventricular internal diameter at end-systole).

Two-dimensional echocardiography provides both qualitative and quantitative evaluation of systolic ventricular function. Midesophageal four-chamber (ME 4-chamber) and two-chamber (ME 2-chamber) views and the midesophageal long-axis (ME LAX) view, transgastric short-axis (TG SAX) views (basal, midpapillary, and apical), and the transgastric long-axis view (TG LAX) allow assessment of both global and regional ventricular function. Two-dimensional quantitative measures of LV systolic function include ventricular dimensions, volume, stroke volume (SV), cardiac output (CO), ejection fraction (EF), and regional wall motion abnormalities (Figs. 35.4 and 35.5). Left ventricular ejection fraction (LVEF) can be calculated from LV end-systolic volume (LVESV) and end-diastolic volume (LVEDV) as the ratio (LVEDV-LVESV)/LVEDV. Cardiac output can be calculated using the area-length formula across a cardiac valve (most commonly the aortic valve):

$$\text{CO} = 0.785 \times \text{LVOT D}^2 \times \text{LVOT}_{VTI} \times \text{HR}$$

(LVOT = left ventricular outflow tract; D = LVOT diameter; $\text{LVOT}_{VTI}$ = velocity time integral, measured with Doppler spectrum across the aortic valve; HR = heart rate). IOE determination of CO is helpful, even when a pulmonary artery catheter is used, because some patients with dilated CMP present with some degree of tricuspid valve regurgitation, which renders the thermodilution technique inaccurate.

In addition, patients with end-stage CHF often present with coexisting pathology such as acquired left ventricle aneurysm (LVA). LVA is the final expression of transmural infarct expansion and is often accompanied by anterior infarction in the area of the distribution of the left anterior descending coronary artery (Fig. 35.6). Thrombi are frequently detected within aneurysms and are often associated with systemic embolization (Fig. 35.7). Therefore,

▶ **TABLE 35.3. Typical Features of the Three Physiologic Types of Cardiomyopathy**

|  | *Dilated* | *Hypertrophic* | *Restrictive* |
|---|---|---|---|
| LV systolic function | Moderately to severely ↓ | Normal | Normal |
| LV diastolic function | May be abnormal | Abnormal | Abnormal |
| LV hypertrophy | ↑ LV mass due to left ventricular dilation with normal wall thickness | Asymmetric LV hypertrophy | Concentric LV hypertrophy |
| Chamber dilation | All four chambers | Left and right atrial dilation if mitral regurgitation is present | Left and right atrial dilation |
| Outflow tract obstruction | Absent | Dynamic LV outflow tract obstruction may be present | Absent |
| Left ventricular end-diastolic pressure | Elevated | Elevated | Elevated |
| Pulmonary artery pressures | Elevated | Elevated | Elevated |

LV = Left ventricular; ↓ = decreased; ↑ = increased.
From Otto CM. The cardiomyopathies, hypertensive heart disease, post-cardiac-transplant patient and pulmonary heart disease. Textbook of Clinical Echocardiography, Philadelphia: WB Saunders 2000;183–212.

▶ **TABLE 35.4. Echocardiographic Approach to the Patient with a Suspected Cardiomyopathy**

|  | *Qualitative* | *Quantitative* |
|---|---|---|
| 2-D/M-mode imaging | Chamber dimensions | LV-EDV, LV-ESV |
|  | Degree and pattern of LV hypertrophy | LV mass |
|  | Evidence for dynamic outflow tract obstruction |  |
|  | SAM of mitral valve |  |
|  | Aortic valve midsystolic closure |  |
| LV systolic function | Visual estimate of EF | Apical biplane EF |
| Doppler echo | Associated valvular regurgitation | Maximum and mean $\Delta P$ |
|  | Pattern of LV diastolic filling | PA pressures |
|  | Pattern of LA filling (pulmonary venous inflow) |  |
|  | Velocity curve of dynamic outflow tract obstruction |  |
|  | Localization of the level of obstruction |  |

*2-D*, Two-dimensional; *LA,* left atrial; *LV,* left ventricular; *EDV,* end-diastolic volume; *ESV,* end-systolic volume; *SAM,* systolic anterior motion; *ΔP,* pressure gradient; *PA,* pulmonary artery; *EF,* ejection fraction.
Otto CM: The cardiomyopathies, hypertensive heart disease, post-cardiac-transplant patient and pulmonary heart disease. Textbook of Clinical Echocardiography, W.B. Saunders 2000,183-212.

careful echocardiographic assessment is mandatory if cardiopulmonary bypass is to be successful.

Evaluation of RV systolic function is a critical part of the intraoperative management of patients with end-stage CHF. Preexisting pathologic conditions in the RV, such as ischemia, infarction, CMP, and pulmonary hypertension (PHTN) are major risk factors for RV failure. Sometimes, the extent of RV dysfunction becomes apparent only when a sudden increase in venous return challenges an already impaired RV. With dilated CMP, there is an increase in systolic ventricular interaction, making RV systolic performance more dependent on the LV to generate pressure (10). Under these circumstances, sudden LV unloading may depress RV function further.

Two-dimensional/M-mode echocardiography can provide several quantitative and qualitative measurements of RV systolic function. Wall thicknesses over 0.5 cm as measured by M-mode echocardiography are considered abnormal and suggest elevated pulmonary artery pressure, pulmonary valve stenosis, or infitrative CMP. The standard 2-D transesophageal echocardiographic (TEE) views used to evaluate RV function are the ME 4-chamber view, the ME RV inflow-outflow view, the transgastric mid–short-axis (TG mid-SAX) view, and the transgastric right ventricular inflow (TG RV inflow) view. Quantitative assessment of RV function with automated border detection in the midesophageal four-chamber view has been used to calculate RV fractional area change (RVFAC) (11):

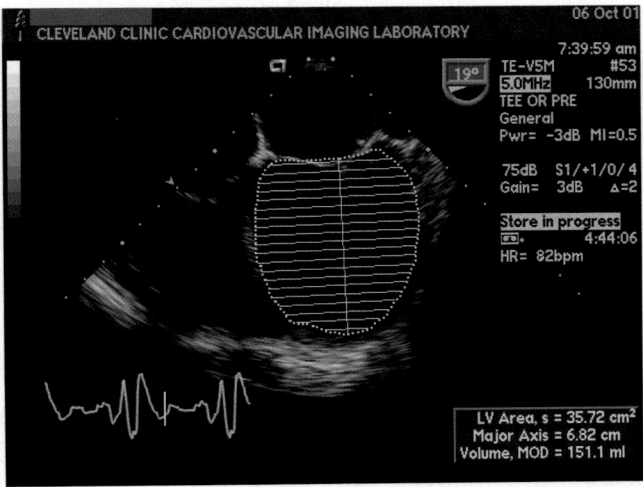

**FIGURE 35.4.** Dilated cardiomyopathy, left ventricle dimensions and volume: midesophageal four-chamber view

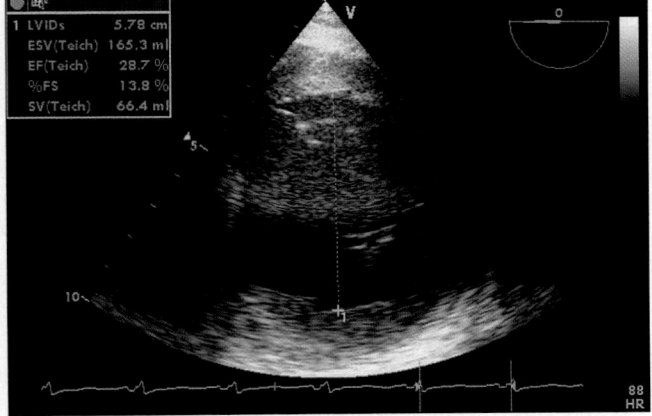

**FIGURE 35.5.** Dilated cardiomyopathy, left ventricle dimension and volume: transgastric short-axis midpapillary view

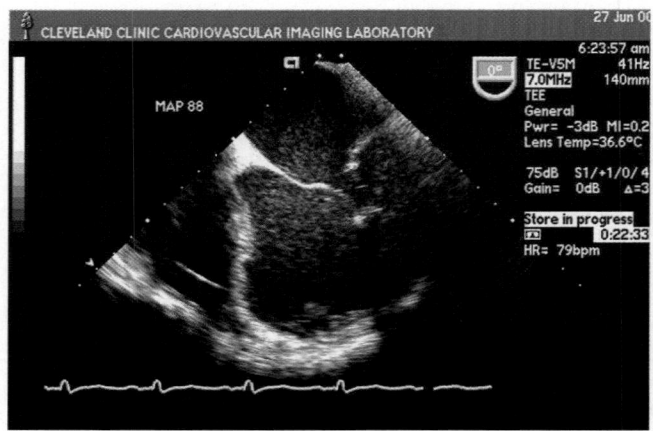

**FIGURE 35.6.** Left ventricular aneurysm: midesophageal four-chamber view

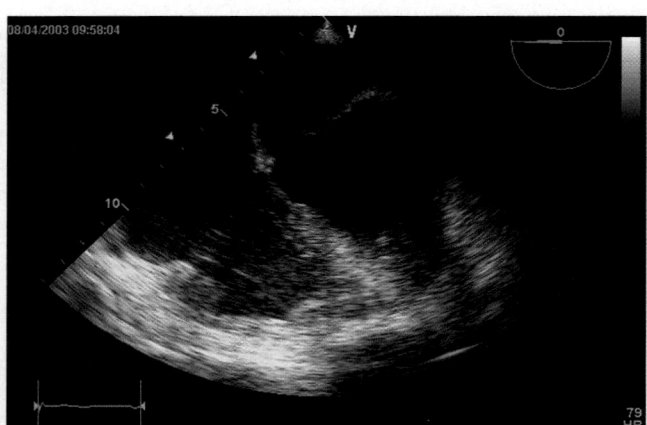

**FIGURE 35.8.** Biventricular failure: midesophageal four-chamber view

$$RVFAC = \text{(end-diastolic area} - \text{end-systolic area)} /$$
$$\text{end-diastolic area} \times 100\%$$

Signs of RV dysfunction include hypokinesis or akinesis of the RV free wall, and RV dilation caused by volume or pressure overload. Normally, the RV end-diastolic cross-sectional area is less than 60% of the LV end-diastolic cross-sectional area. With dilatation, however, the RV changes its shape from triangular to round, with concomitant enlargement of the right ventricular outflow tract (RVOT) and flattening of the bulge in the interventricular septum from right to left can be seen in the ME 4-chamber view and the ME RV inflow-outflow view (Figs. 35.8 and 35.9). With RV pressure overload, a maximal leftward septal shift is noted at end-systole, whereas RV volume overload is associated with a maximum reversed septal curvature in mid-diastole. As RV dilation becomes moderate or severe, the RV replaces the LV in forming the

cardiac apex in the ME 4-chamber view, and the end-diastolic cross-sectional area of the RV may equal or exceed that of the LV. Tricuspid annular plane systolic excursion (TAPSE) may decrease to less than 20 mm, accompanied by impaired RV systolic function (12). At this stage, pulsed wave Doppler (PWD) evaluation of blood flow in the hepatic vein may reveal attenuation of the systolic inflow wave.

Nonetheless, pulmonary artery (PA) pressure estimates remain one of the most important quantitative measures of RV systolic function. As RV dysfunction progresses, dilation of tricuspid valve (TV) annulus occurs, causing varying degrees of tricuspid regurgitation (Fig. 35.10). Measuring the velocity and pressure gradient of the tricuspid regurgitant jet (Fig. 35.11) reveals the gradient between RV and right atrial (RA) pressure and, when added to an estimate of RA pressure (transduced from the central venous line), allows calculation of RV systolic pres-

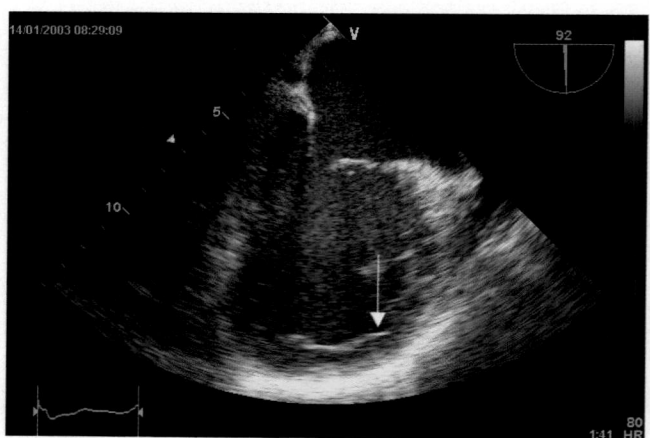

**FIGURE 35.7.** Ventricular thrombus: midesophageal two-chamber view

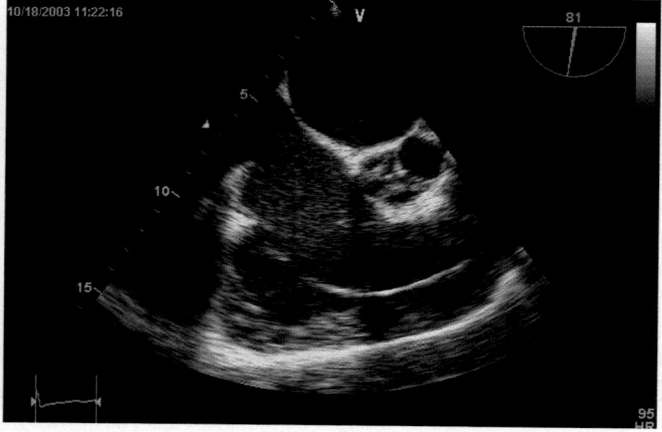

**FIGURE 35.9.** Right ventricular failure: midesophageal right ventricular inflow-outflow view

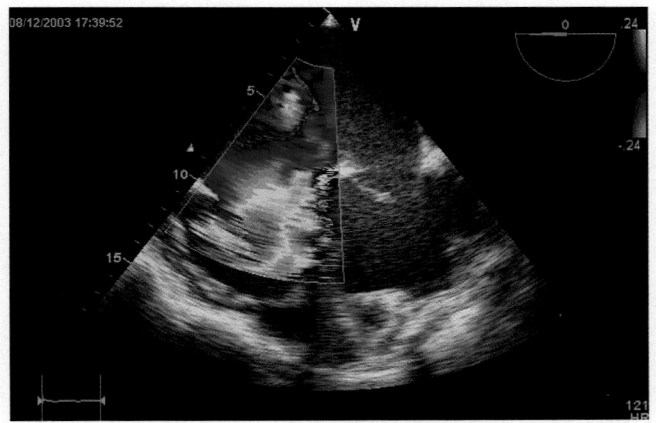

**FIGURE 35.10.** Severe tricuspid regurgitation: midesophageal four-chamber view

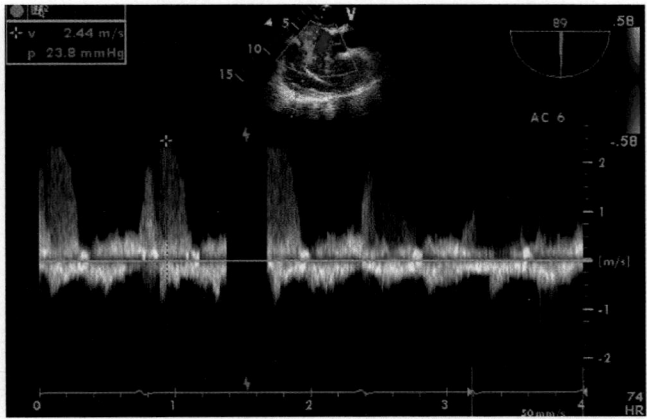

**FIGURE 35.11.** Tricuspid regurgitation, velocity, and pressure gradient

sure (Table 35.5). Right ventricular SV and CO can be measured directly by imaging the RVOT tract and PA in the upper esophageal aortic arch short-axis (UE aortic arch SAX) view (Fig. 35.12). By measuring the diameter (D) of PA annulus and using PWD mode to determine velocity time integral (VTI) across pulmonic valve, right

ventricular SV, and CO can be calculated using the formulas $SV = PA\ D^2 \times 0.785 \times PA_{VTI}$ and $CO = SV \times HR$.

Growing evidence suggests that both systolic and diastolic dysfunction play important roles in the clinical presentation and prognosis of patients with end-stage CHF. Patients with hypertrophic, infiltrative, or primary re-

▶ **TABLE 35.5. Estimation of Intracardiac Pressures**

| Pressure Estimated | Required Measurement | Formula | Normal Valves (mm Hg) |
|---|---|---|---|
| Estimated CVP | Respiratory IVC collapse | > 40% = 5 mm Hg<br>< 40%, (nl RV) = 10 mm Hg<br>0% & RV Dysfx = 15 mm Hg | 5 – 10 |
| RV Systolic(RVSP) | Peak velocity$_{TR}$<br>CVP or measured | $RVSP = 4(V_{TR})^2 + CVP$<br>(No PS) | 16 – 30 |
| RV Systolic (with VSD) | Systemic systolic BP<br>Peak V$_{LV-RV}$ | $RVSP = SBP - 4(V_{LV-RV})^2$<br>(No LVOT Obstruction) | with VSD usually > 50 |
| PA Systolic<br>PASP | Peak velocity$_{TR}$<br>CVP* or measured | $PASP = 4(V_{TR})^2 + CVP$<br>No PS) | 16 – 30 |
| PA Diastolic (PAD) | End diastolic<br>Velocity$_{PR}$<br>CVP* or measured | $PAEDP = 4(V_{PR\ ED})^2 + CVP$ | 0 – 8 |
| PA Mean (PAM) | Acceleration time (AT) to peak V$_{PA}$ | $PAM = (-0.45)\ AT + 79$ | 10 – 16 |
| RV dP/dt | TR spectral envelope<br>$T_{TR(2m/sec)} - T_{TR(1\ m/sec)}$ | $RV\ dP = 4V^2_{TR(2m/sec)} - 4V2_{TR(2m/sec)}$<br>$RV\ dP/dt = dP / T_{TR(2m/sec)} - T_{TR(1\ m/sec)}$ | > 150 mm Hg/msec |
| LA Systolic (LASP) | Peak V$_{MR}$<br>Systolic BP (SBP) | $LASP = SBP - 4(V_{MR})^2$<br>(No LVOT Gradient) | 100 – 140 |
| LA (PFO) | Velocity$_{PFO}$<br>CVP* or measured | $LAP = 4(V_{PFO})^2 + CVP$ | 3 – 15 |
| LV Diastolic (LVEDP) | End diastolic<br>Velocity$_{AR}$<br>Diastolic BP (DBP) | $LVEDP = DBP - 4(V_{AR})^2$ | 3 – 12 |
| LV dP/dt | MR spectral envelope<br>$T_{MR(2m/sec)} - T_{MR(1\ m/sec)}$ | $LV\ dP = 4V2_{TR(2m/sec)} - 4V2_{TR(2m/sec)}$<br>$LV\ dP/dt = dP / T_{MR(2m/sec)} - T_{MR(1\ m/sec)}$ | > 800 mm HG/msec |

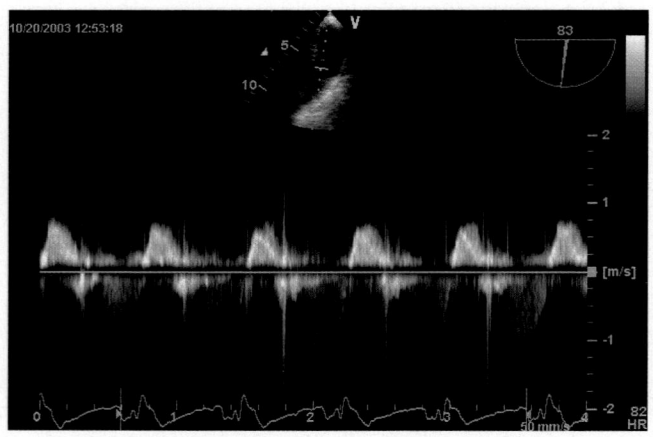

**FIGURE 35.12.** Pulsed wave Doppler of pulmonary artery

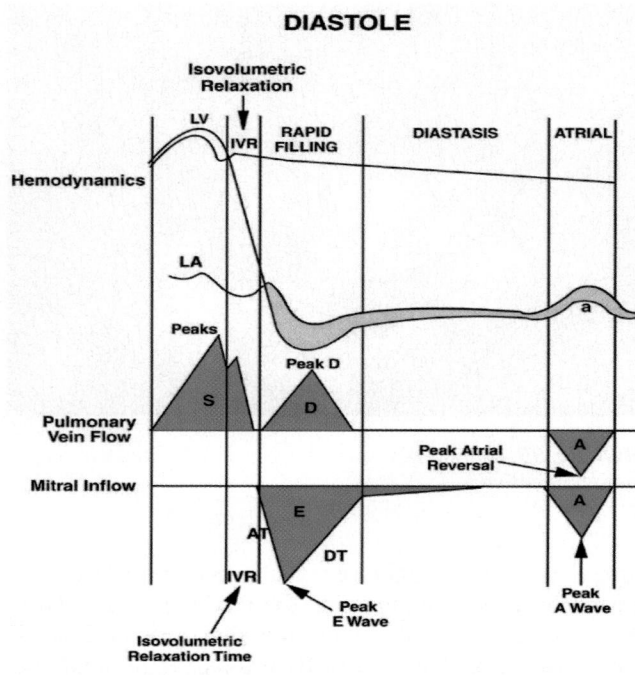

**FIGURE 35.13.** The relationship among left ventricular, left atrial, and aortic pressures

strictive CMP may report symptoms of heart failure despite normal EF, a condition known as diastolic heart failure (13,14). In addition, in patients with preexisting systolic dysfunction, abnormalities in diastolic dysfunction may be significantly related to the severity of cardiac symptoms and prognosis in patients with CHF (15). Diastole is the interval between aortic valve closure and mitral valve closure and can be divided into four phases:

1. Isovolumic relaxation
2. Early rapid diastolic filling
3. Diastasis
4. Late diastolic filling caused by atrial contraction (Fig. 35.13).

Parameters of diastolic function include ventricular relaxation, myocardial compliance, and chamber compliance. Ventricular relaxation is measured by isovolumic relaxation time (IVRT), the rate of pressure decline (dP/dT), and time constant of relaxation ($\tau$). Myocardial compliance is estimated by the ratio of change in volume to change in pressure (dV/dP). Chamber compliance is assessed by measuring early diastolic LV filling (*E* wave), deceleration time (DT), late diastolic LV filling ($A_M$ wave), the $A_P$ wave (reversed) of LA contraction, the *s* wave of the systolic LA filling phase, and the *d* wave of the LA diastolic filling phase.

The earliest stage of abnormal diastolic filling is *impaired relaxation* with inverse E/A ratio as the major Doppler abnormality (Table 35.6). With progression of the disease to moderate diastolic dysfunction, *pseudonormalization of diastolic filling flow* occurs because of impaired myocardial relaxation balanced by elevation of mean LA pressures (Table 35.6). The diagnosis is confirmed by abnormal PV flow or response to Valsalva maneuver. The *restrictive filling pattern* is the most advanced form of diastolic dysfunction that can be associated with either normal or abnormal systolic function. It may accompany advanced infiltrative CMP, such as amyloidosis,

advanced hypertensive disease, or dilated CMP. The hallmark of the disease is elevated LA pressures with increased LV stiffness that causes a large E wave, short DT, a small $A_M$ wave, and a very small s/d ratio on PV PWD trace (Figs. 35.14 and 35.15) (Table 35.7) (16).

## Assessment of Coexisting or Secondary Pathology

Mitral regurgitation (MR) is commonly encountered in CHF as a consequence of dilated cardiomyopathy (17–19). Mitral annular dilation caused by LV dilation and papillary muscle dysfunction are the most common mechanisms behind the development of regurgitation in dilated cardiomyopathy. Abnormal papillary muscle alignment and abnormal leaflet apposition during systole are caused by changes in the shape of the LV chamber during both the systolic and the diastolic periods (20). Color flow Doppler (CFD) imaging has been used to quantitate the severity of MR, whereas PWD is used to measure regurgitant stroke volume and regurgitant fraction (21,22). Tricuspid regurgitation (TR) can be encountered either in isolation or in conjunction with MR. The regurgitant tricuspid jet is usually directed toward the interatrial septum in patients with dilated CMP. RV dysfunction, PHTN, patent foramen ovale (PFO), and aortic regurgitation (AR) are other pathophysiologies that may accompany end-stage CHF.

▶ **TABLE 35.6. Patterns of Diastolic Dysfunction**

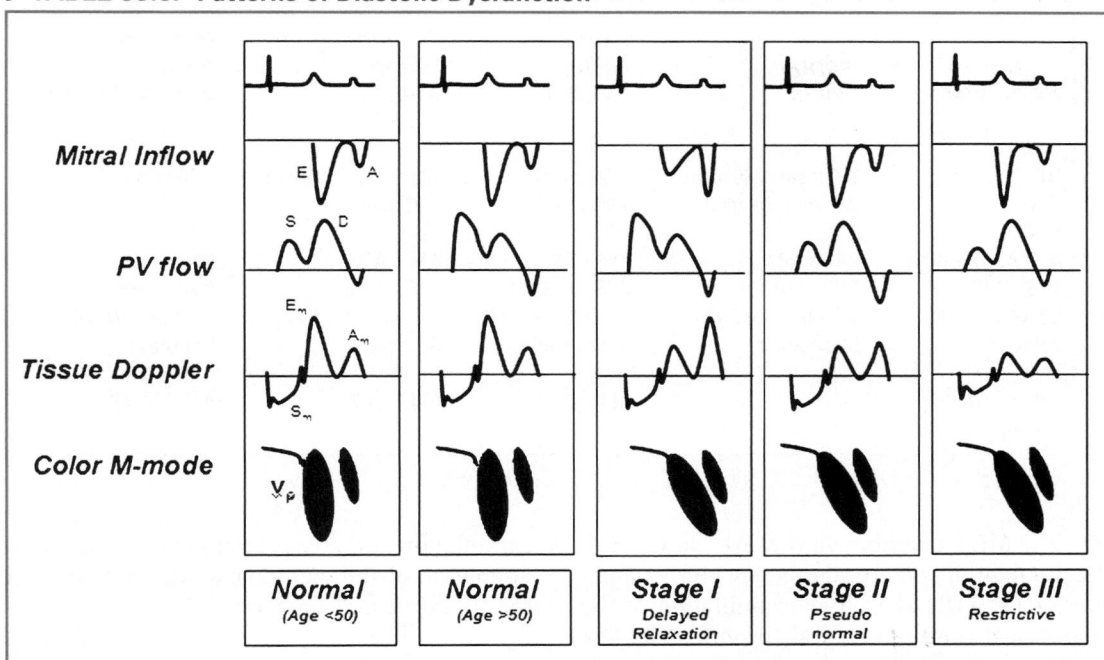

## Standard Intraoperative Echocardiographic Examination

IOE is a key monitoring and diagnostic modality in patients undergoing surgery for heart failure. Standard IOE evaluation usually begins with the ME 4-chamber view. This view provides information about the size of the left and right cardiac chambers; the thickness of ventricular walls and the basal, mid, and apical segments of LV lateral and septal walls; the apical and basal portion of RV free wall; and MV and TV function. PWD assessment of the left upper and lower pulmonary veins (LUPV, LLPV), the right upper pulmonary vein (RUPV), and MV diastolic flow can be used to estimate the severity of MR and the extent of diastolic impairment. Next, the multiplane angle is rotated 30° into the ME AV SAX view, which allows examination of morphology and function of the AV cusps. The ME RV inflow-outflow view is obtained at 60° and provides information about RV diaphragmatic free wall motion, RVOT size, and pulmonary valve (PV) and TV function. The ME mitral commissural view provides information about the A2 scallop of the anterior mitral valve leaflet (AMVL) and the P1 and P2 scallops of the posterior mitral valve leaflet (PMVL) and permits assessment of the severity and direction of the MV regurgitant

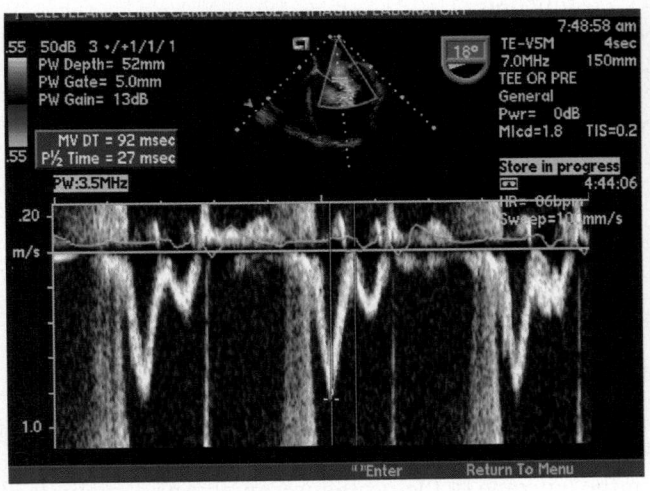

**FIGURE 35.14.** Pulsed wave Doppler: transmitral diastolic flow

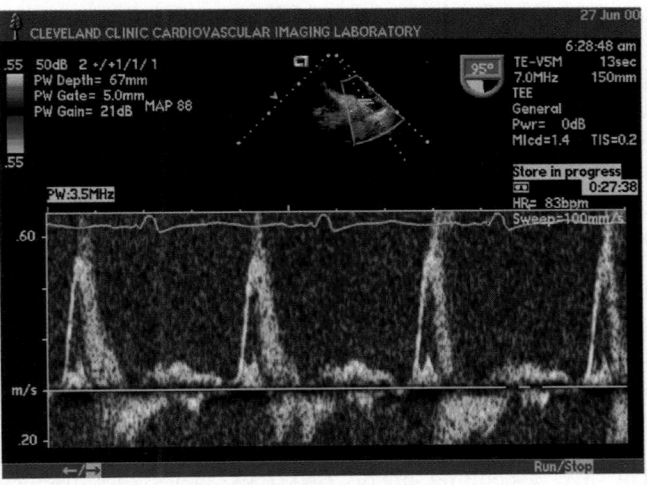

**FIGURE 35.15.** Left upper pulmonary vein pulse wave Doppler: restrictive pattern

▶ TABLE 35.7. Distinguishing the Patterns of Diastolic Dysfunction

| Parameter | Normal Filling | Impaired Filling Stage 1 | Pseudonormal Filling Stage 2 | Restrictive Filling Stages 3 and 4 |
|---|---|---|---|---|
| E Wave | | | | |
| DT | 160 msec–240 msec | > 240 msec | 160 msec–200 msec | < 160 msec |
| IVRT | 70 msec–90 msec | > 90 msec | < 90 msec | < 70 msec |
| E : A | 1–2 | < 1 | 1–1.5 | > 1.5 |
| $A_M : A_P$ Duration | AM ≥ AP | AM > AP | AM < AP | AM << AP |
| PVS : PVD | PVS > PVD | PVS : >> PVD | PVS < PVD | PVS << PVD |
| VE' MA : VA' MA | VE' MA > VA' MA | VE' MA < VA' MA | VE' MA < VA' MA | VE' MA < VA' MA |
| Valsalva | Decreased | Decreased | Reversal | Decreased |
| E : A | | < 1 | | |
| Volume Loading | — | AM < AP | AM << AP | AM <<< AP |
| $A_M : A_P$ Duration | | | | |

jet, if present. The ME 2-chamber view at 90° allows evaluation of the basal, mid, and apical segments of the anterior and inferior LV walls as well as examination of the left atrial appendage (LAA) for mural thrombi. The ME LAX view at 120 shows both basal and midanteroseptal segments, basal and midposterior segments, the left ventricular outflow tract (LVOT), and the aortic valve. The ME bicaval view is the image of choice for evaluating PFO by CFD and contrast study. This view provides information about the size of and blood flow through the RA, the left atrium (LA), and the right lower pulmonary vein (RLPV) using PW Doppler. TG views are obtained by advancing the probe into the stomach and flexing the tip anteriorly. TG basal and mid-SAX views are the views of choice for the examination of LV regional wall motion abnormalities. In addition, the TG basal SAX view provides a short-axis view of the MV that allows further location of the regurgitant jets using CFD. Rotating the multiplane angle 90° to the TG 2-chamber view allows further assessment of the LV anterior and posterior walls, the MV, and the LAA. The TG LAX view at 120° provides a longitudinal view of the AV and allows measurement of pressure gradients across the AV using continuous wave Doppler (CWD) and PWD. Turning the probe to the right and to 120° to the TG RV inflow view allows evaluation of the RV diaphragmatic and free walls, TV function, and RA dimensions. The deep TG LAX view provides a longitudinal view of the LV and AV and allows measurement of AV gradients and calculation of the AV area using CWD and PWD. Atherosclerotic disease in the descending aorta can be detected with the probe in a gastric position and the tip rotated posteriorly into the left descending aortic short-axis (descending aortic SAX) view. A longitudinal view of the descending aorta can be obtained at 90 in the descending aortic long axis (descending aortic LAX) view. The ME ascending aortic SAX/LAX views and upper esophageal (UE) aortic arch LAX/SAX views are used to examine the ascending aorta and should be used to guide cannulation and cross-clamping of the aorta. Doppler examination of the pulmonary valve is best achieved using the UE aortic arch SAX view (23).

## Surgical Procedure-Related Issues

Surgical approaches to end-stage CHF are rapidly becoming more numerous and sophisticated. Substantial advances have been made in myocardial revascularization, mitral valvuloplasty, ventricular remodeling (i.e., ECPP and LV partial resection), ventricular constraint techniques (i.e., Acorn CorCap external splinting, Myosplint internal splinting), mechanical ventricular support, TAH, and heart transplantation. During the period before cardiopulmonary bypass (CBP) is initiated, IOE focuses on the evaluation of

1. RV function, severity of TR, and the potential need for RV mechanical support
2. Baseline LV function
3. Potential sequelae of end-stage-dilated cardiomyopathy, such as LVA, LA mural thrombi, MR, and diastolic dysfunction
4. Potential right-to-left shunting through PFO, which may contribute to hypoxemia
5. The presence of AR or mitral stenosis (MS)
6. The presence of ascending aortic atheroma, which necessitates changing the cannulation strategy and myocardial protection.

This information guides the development of CPB strategy. At the time of separation from CPB, IOE is useful for evaluating the adequacy of deairing of the cardiac chambers. It is also important at that time to establish a comprehensive baseline study for future comparison and to assess LV and RV filling patterns, native valve function, the quality of the valve repair, and the presence of any intracardiac shunts. Given the importance of RV function in the outcome of the procedure, an objective qualitative assessment of RV systolic and diastolic function by RV-

FAC, RV end-diastolic volume (RVEDV), RV dP/dT, TV annulus diameter, and severity of TR is important. These parameters will allow comparison between baseline and postoperative RV performance and dictate postoperative management in the event of acute deterioration of RV function, which is often seen when respiratory insufficiency occurs.

## Transplantation

(Please see Chapter 36, Assessment of Cardiac Transplantation.)

## Complications of Surgical Procedures for CHF

### Right Ventricular Dysfunction

The success of surgical procedures for end-stage CHF depends on postoperative RV performance. Unfortunately, right-sided circulatory failure is a common postoperative complication in patients undergoing surgical procedures for CHF. Patients with end-stage CHF often develop substantial passive pulmonary hypertension secondary to elevated LA and pulmonary venous pressures, a condition that is reversible with LV unloading. When pulmonary disease is also present, irreversible elevated pulmonary vascular resistance (PVR) complicates the clinical picture. RV function is significantly afterload dependent, and the presence of pulmonary congestion in association with high PVR can have a tremendous impact on RV systolic and diastolic performance. RV failure causes dilation, ischemia, and decreased RV contractility. It is associated with decreased pulmonary blood flow and a leftward septal shift that subsequently lowers LV filling pressure and reduces systemic CO. Treatment of RV is difficult (Table 35.8).

IOE plays an important role in the diagnosis and treatment of RV failure. It allows estimation of intracardiac pressures, such as central venous pressure (CVP); RV sys-

tolic pressure; and pulmonary artery (PA) systolic, diastolic, and mean pressures (Table 35.2). In addition, RV afterload can be computed by dividing the mean PA pressure by the CO. RV dP/dT calculation is helpful in assessing the extent of diastolic dysfunction. Optimal mechanical ventilatory settings and mode can be guided by serial measurement of the above-mentioned parameters. Echocardiographic monitoring of the effect of different pharmacological interventions (Tables 35.9 and 35.10) on PVR and RV performance can also be used during the post-CPB and early postoperative period.

### Right-to-Left Shunt

Right-to-left shunt is a condition that may be encountered during the post-CPB period when the RV is dilated and there is TR and increased RA pressure. Distension of RA and elevation of RA pressure increase the pressure gradient across the interatrial septum that can cause the opening of a previously sealed PFO or the unmasking of a previously partially closed PFO. Moreover, when right-to-left shunt is accompanied by severe TR, the regurgitant jet is directed along the interatrial septum, which can amplify the hemodynamic effects of elevated right-side pressure. The bicaval view allows PWD interrogation, measurement of the PFO orifice, and calculation of the shunt volume. Significant right-to-left shunting may be caused by right-side distension and can lead to severe hypoxia, acidosis, and hemodynamic decompensation.

### Hemodynamic Instability

Hemodynamic instability is frequently present during the early post-CPB period and can be caused by LV dysfunction, low systemic vascular resistance (SVR), and hypovolemia. IOE is a helpful tool in differentiating among cardiogenic, vasodilatory, and hypovolemic shock and in assessing the effects of various interventions. Two-dimensional echocardiography and Doppler modalities provide useful information about overall LV contractility, regional wall motion abnormalities, valve function, and adequacy of preload. Transgastric views are extremely helpful in assessing LV loading and contractility as well as calculating CO (SV × HR). Measurements of left ventricular end-diastolic pressure, LVEDV, and LVESV allow calculation of LVEF and may indicate the use of vasoactive therapy. CWD and PWD modes can be used to detect different degrees of diastolic dysfunction that may occur either in isolation or in conjunction with systolic dysfunction (Tables 35.5–35.7). Vasomotor collapse frequently occurs during the post-CPB period, possibly resulting from a CPB-induced systemic inflammatory response, sepsis, anaphylaxis, arginine vasopressin deficiency, or preoperative administration of ACE inhibitors or amiodarone, or intraoperative administration of milrinone or dobutamine. Vasopressin is a useful vasoactive drug for the

▶ **TABLE 35.8. Perioperative Management of Right-Sided Heart Failure Goals**

1. Preserving coronary perfusion through maintenance of systemic blood pressure
2. Optimizing RV preload
3. Reducing RV afterload by decreasing PVR
4. Limiting pulmonary vasoconstriction through optimal ventilation
   a. high inspired oxygen concentration (100% $FiO_2$)
   b. hyperventilation to $PaCO_2$ of 25 mm Hg–30 mm Hg
   c. optimal tidal volumes
   d. correction of acid-base abnormalities
5. Supporting RV function
   a. pharmacological agents
   b. intraaortic balloon pump
   c. RV assist devices

▶ TABLE 35.9. Pulmonary Vasodilator Agents

1. **Phosphodiesteraze-III inhibitors**
   - Inhibition of myocardial type III phosphodiesterase → increase in myocardial cAMP → increase in intracellular Ca2+ influx → positive inotropic effect
   - Unique mechanism of inotropic effects independent of β-receptor stimulation
   - Bypass β-adrenergic receptors in patients with preexisting heart failure
   - Additive effect with cathecholamines
   - Pulmonary vasodilation
   - Coronary vasodilation
2. **B-type natriuretic peptide**
   - Recombinant human B-type natriuretic peptide
   - Site of action: guanylate cyclase receptor of vascular smooth muscle and endothelial cells
   - Effect: increased intracellular cGMP and smooth muscle cell relaxation, dose dependent reduction in PCWP, and systemic arterial pressure in patients with heart failure
   - Increased permeability of vascular endothelium
   - Inhibition of rennin-angiotensin-aldosterone axis
   - Dose: 2g/kg bolus followed by 0.01 μg/kg/min–0.03 μg/kg/min infusion
   - Plasma half-life 18 min
3. **Prostaglandin $I_2$ (PGI$_2$)**
   - Endogenous prostaglandin
   - Synthesized by cyclooxygenase arm of arachidonic acid metabolic pathway
   - Potent vasodilator
   - Inhibits neutrophil activation
   - Stabilized cell membranes
   - Enhances myocardial inotropy by activating adenylate cyclase and increasing intracellular cAMP
4. **Nitric oxide**
   - Selective pulmonary dilator less potent than inhaled prostacyclin
   - Activation of guanylate cyclase
   - Improves ventilation-perfusion distribution
   - No effect on cardiac index and stroke index
   - Complex and expensive technology implied for safe and effective use
   - Could cause rebound pulmonary vasoconstriction with prolonged use
   - Toxic metabolites nitrogen dioxide and methemoglobin
5. **Prostaglandin $E_1$ (PGE$_1$)**
   - Endogenous prostaglandin
   - Synthesized by cyclooxygenase arm of arachidonic acid metabolic pathway
   - Potent pulmonary and systemic vasodilator
   - Cleared from the circulation during its first pass through the lung

▶ TABLE 35.10. Pharmacological Agents

1. Isoproterenol
   - Nonselective beta-adrenergic agonist
   - Positive chronotropic and inotropic agent
   - Pulmonary and systemic vasodilator
2. Dobutamine
   - Beta-adrenergic receptor agonist with minimal alpha-adrenergic receptor agonist activity
   - Positive chronotropic and inotropic agent
   - Pulmonary and systemic vasodilator
3. Epinephrine
   - Alpha- and beta-adrenergic receptor agonist
   - Beta-adrenergic receptor predominance at lower doses
   - Potent RV inotrope
   - Significant arrhytmogenic potential

## INTRAOPERATIVE ECHOCARDIOGRAPHY IN SURGICAL PROCEDURES FOR CHF

### Mitral Valve Repair or Replacement

Mitral valve competence depends on the integrity of all components of the MV apparatus, including the MV annulus, leaflets, chordae tendineae, and papillary muscle, as well as the function of the underlying ventricular myocardium. End-stage CHF is often associated with moderate or severe MR (17–19). The presence of MR in patients with dilated CMP is associated with deterioration of clinical status, diminished response to medical therapy, and reduced survival rate (20,24,25). Thus, MR detection, qualitative and quantitative assessment, and surgical correction (when indicated) is desirable to improve survival and quality of life in patients with end-stage CHF. Annular dilation and change in LV morphology with papillary muscle dysfunction are the most common mechanisms of MR (20).

IOE is extremely helpful in the assessment of the cause and severity of MR. Two-dimensional echocardiography provides information about MV morphology, such as leaflet motion, prolapse or restriction, and leaflet coaptation. Baseline measurements of MV annulus diameter, anterior mitral valve leaflet (AMVL) A3 scallop, and pos-

▶ TABLE 35.11. Arginine Vasopressin

Endogenous peptide with osmoregulatory and vasomotor properties end-organ effect mediated by
- $V_1$ receptor present in vascular smooth muscle
  - ❑ Promotes vasoconstriction by activation of G protein and phospholipase C with release of calcium from sarcoplasmic reticulum
- V2 receptor present in the distal and collecting tubules
  - ❑ Promotes water resorption by increase in intracellular levels of cAMP and activation of protein kinase A

treatment of vasomotor collapse (Table 35.12). The transgastric short-axis view reveals a hyperdynamic LV, decreased LVEDV and LVEDP, elevated CO, and decreased SVR. Hypovolemic shock is characterized by a hyperdynamic LV with adequate contractility, decreased CO, and normal-to-elevated SVR.

▶ TABLE 35.12. **Types of Ventricular Assist Devices (VADs)**

| Type | Device | Length of Support | Position | Ventricular Support | Drive Mechanism |
|------|--------|-------------------|----------|---------------------|-----------------|
| Pulsatile | Abiomed BVS 5000 | Short-term support | Extracorporeal | LV, RV, BV | Atrial and ventricular chambers pneumatically driven |
| | Thoratec VAD | Short- to medium-term support | Extracorporeal | LV, RV, BV | Pneumatically driven sac |
| | HeartMate IP and VE | Long-term as a bridge to transplantation, recovery, or destination therapy (HeartMate VE) | Intracorporeal, abdominal (pre- or intraperitoneal) | LV | Flexible textured polyurethane diaphragm pneumatically or electrically driven |
| | Novacor | Long-term as a bridge to transplantation, or recovery | Intracorporeal, abdominal (pre or intra peritoneal) | LV | Polyurethane pump sac compressed by electrically driven pusher plates |
| | AbioCor TAH | Long-term support | Intracorporeal | BV | Electric |
| Nonpulsatile | Levitronix CentiMag (centrifugal pump) | Short-term | Extracorporeal | LV, RV, BV | Electric |
| | Tandem Heart (centrifugal-flow) | Sort-term | Extracorporeal | LV | Electric |
| | Impella (axial-flow pump) | Short term | Extracorporeal | LV | Electric |
| | Jarvik Flowmaker (axial-flow) | Long-term support | Intracorporeal | LV | Impeller electrically driven |
| | DeBakey LVAD (axial-flow) | Long-term support | Intracorporeal | LV | Electric |
| | HeartMate II (axial flow pump) | Short-term | Intracorporeal | LV | Electric |

*IP,* implantable pneumatic; *VE,* vented electric; *LV,* left ventricle; *VAD,* ventricular assist device; *TAH,* total artificial heart

terior mitral valve leaflet (PMVL) P1 scallop are taken in the ME 4-chamber view. As the multiplane angle is rotated forward to about 60°, into the ME mitral commissural view, the A2 scallop of the AMVL is seen in the middle, with the PMVL P1 scallop on the left and the P3 scallop on the right. The ME 2-chamber view at 90° provides information about the A1 and P3 MV scallops and the ME LAX view shows the A2 and P2 scallops. The ME views should be repeated with CFD, with the color flow sector extended over the LA and over the ventricular portion of MV. Transmitral flow velocity is examined with PWD, with the sample volume placed between the tips of the open MV leaflets, to evaluate the presence and extent of diastolic dysfunction (Fig. 35.14). The TG SAX view visualizes the posteromedial and anterolateral commissures and provides an overall view of the entire MV in the short axis, which allows the detection of leaflet abnormalities and sites where abnormal flows originate. A baseline area of MV can be measured by planimetry in this view. Abnormal motion or fibrosis of papillary muscles can be seen in the TG mid-SAX view. The TG 2-chamber view is extremely useful for assessing the entire MV apparatus

(23). Apical tethering, posterior restriction (secondary to posterolateral infarction), papillary muscle fibrosis, and chordal ribboning are the most common pathologic findings associated with MR in end-stage CHF patients. In addition, 2-D echocardiography allows the measurement of the Lana diameter of greater than 5 mm is considered dilated. The ratio of CFD maximum jet area to LA area has been used to quantify the severity of MR. MR greater than 40% or maximum jet area higher than 8 cm$^2$–10 cm$^2$ is classified as severe, 20%–40% MR is moderate, and MR < 20% is considered mild (26,27).

CFD has certain limitations. In the presence of eccentric jets, maximum jet area is poorly correlated with regurgitant grade because jet impingement on the LA wall produces a smaller color flow area that does not correlate to regurgitant jet size (i.e., the Cowanda effect). In addition, CFD imaging is dependent on the pressure difference between LV and LA, LV systolic function, compliance of LA, gain setting, pulsed repetition frequency, and field depth. Therefore, even though CFD is extremely sensitive in detecting MR, quantitation of the severity of MR is difficult and limited by the significant overlap in jet sizes among patients with mild, moderate, and severe regurgitation (21).

Evaluating pulmonary vein flow with PWD helps to quantify the severity of MR. The systolic component is blunted (s < d) as LA pressure increases, and severe MR causes a systolic flow reversal (28). All four PVs should be carefully examined when there are eccentric jets that may produce flow reversal in only the pulmonary vein at which they are directed. With severe MR, antegrade mitral flow velocity is increased (E-wave peak velocity > 1.5 m/s) and regurgitant jet velocity decreases below 4 m/s because of an increase in LA pressure that reduces the transmitral systolic gradient.

Doppler echocardiographic quantitation of regurgitant stroke volume (MV RV) and regurgitant fraction (MV RF) can also be used to quantify the severity of MR by using continuity equations after measurement of MV annulus diameter (MV D), MV VTI, LVOT diameter (LVOT D), LVOT VTI and calculation of mitral valve stroke volume (MV SV) and LVOT stroke volume (LVOT SV)

$$MV\ RV = MV\ SV - LVOT\ SV$$
$$MV\ SV = 0.785 \times MV\ D^2 \times MV\ VTI$$
$$LVOT\ SV = 0.785 \times LVOT\ D^2 \times LVOT\ VTI$$
$$MV\ RF = MV\ RV/MV\ SV \times 100\%$$

Effective regurgitant orifice (ERO) can be calculated as:

$$MV\ ERO = MV\ RV/MV\ TVI$$

Proximal isovelocity surface area (PISA) is another quantitative method of measuring the severity of MR (Figs. 35.16–35.18). Its advantages are that it is independent of color gain settings and it is not influenced by the eccentricity of the MR jet (29). It is used to calculate MV regurgitant flow rate, volume, and ERO, and is achieved by

- Optimizing color-flow imaging of MR jet
- Expanding the image of the regurgitant MV by using zoom

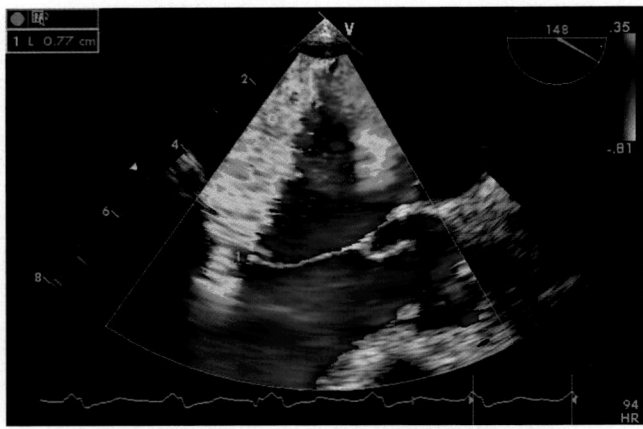

**FIGURE 35.17.** Calculation of PISA: midesophageal long-axis view

- Shifting color flow baseline to 10 cm/sec to 30 cm/sec to set the negative aliasing velocity (Vr)
- Measuring the radius (r) of the proximal isovelocity hemisphere
- Measuring the angle of the isovelocity hemisphere to the leaflets and dividing it by 180°
- Obtaining peak velocity (V) (in cm/s) and TVI of the *mitral regurgitation jet* (in cm)
- Calculating the MR flow rate: flow rate (ml/sec) = $2\pi r^2 \times Vr = 6.28 \times r^2 \times Vr$, in which $2\pi r^2$ is the proximal isovelocity hemispheric surface area at radial distance r from the surface
- Calculating ERO = flow rate/$V_{(MR)}$
- Calculating MV regurgitant volume (ml): MV RV = ERO × MR VTI

A relationship between the severity of MR and PISA radius has been established. A PISA radius of < 2 mm correlates to mild MR, 4 mm–7 mm to mild-to-moderate MR,

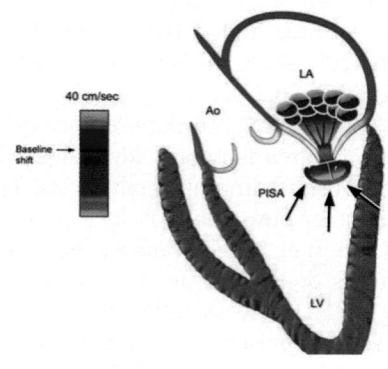

**FIGURE 35.16.** Proximal isovelocity surface area

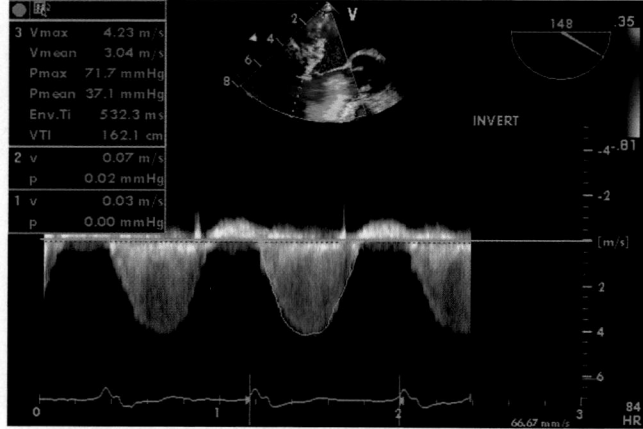

**FIGURE 35.18.** Calculation of PISA: midesophageal long-axis view

7 mm–10 mm to moderate-to-severe MR, and > 10 mm to severe MR (29).

Usually, severe MR is diagnosed if one or more of the following conditions are present: CFD area > 8 cm² or > 40% of LA area, RV > 60 ml, RV > 55%, ERO > 0.35 cm², pulmonary vein systolic flow reversal, dense continuous-wave Doppler signal, decreased maximum velocity of the regurgitant jet (< 3 m/s), increased E velocity (> 1.5 m/s), LV diastolic size > 7 cm, and LA size ≥ 5.5 cm.

Functional mitral regurgitation creates a vicious cycle of increasing volume load, increasing mitral regurgitation, and further LV dilatation. Elevated right-side pressure often occurs in association with severe MV as the result of high pressures in the LA and pulmonary vein. As a result, PHTN, RV dysfunction, TR, and hepatic congestion often accompany severe MR. When MR is associated with severely distorted LV or LVA, alternative surgical procedures for ventricular reconstruction should be considered. Early pre-CPB detection of such conditions can improve postoperative management and surgical outcome.

Intraoperative diagnosis of the cause and severity with MR is crucial for the surgical management of patients with end-stage heart failure. IOE findings, in conjunction with direct examination of the valve, help the surgical team decide among annuloplasty, reconstruction, or replacement of the MV (Fig. 35.19) (30–33). With dilated CMP, the MR jet is typically central because of the symmetrical restriction of the tensor apparatus to the AMVL and PMVL, and the MV annulus is usually > 35 mm, a condition requiring an annuloplasty ring. One may also use an Aliferi repair technique, which involves suturing the A2 and P2 segments of the AMVL and PMVL, resulting in a double-barreled MV orifice with an increased MV leaflet coaptation area (Fig. 35.20). During the post-CPB period and early postoperative care, IOE examination should be focused on the assessment of the quality of valve repair or replacement, RV and LV performance, PHTN, and guiding medical management and the use of vasoactive medication when indicated.

In a cohort of patients with severe MR and LVEF < 25%, Bolling and colleagues performed successful MV reconstruction with undersized flexible annuloplasty rings (Fig. 35.18). In addition, they also performed concomi-

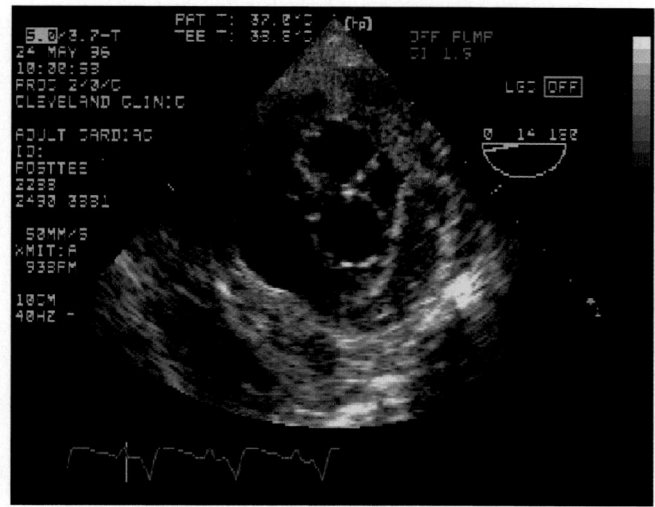

**FIGURE 35.20.** Left ventricular remodeling–Alfieri repair of mitral valve

tant coronary artery bypass grafting and TV repair on several patients (31,32). Actuarial survival rates were 82% at 12 months, 71% at 24 months, and 56% at 5 years. Moreover, the authors reported postoperative improvements in New York Heart Association status and LVEF (31,32).

## Ventricular Reconstruction Surgery

### Partial Left Ventriculectomy (Batista Procedure)

Partial left ventriculectomy is intended to reverse LV dilatation by removing a portion of viable myocardium from the LV lateral free wall. This reduces LV diameter and LV wall stress. Some authors have reported performing concomitant MV repair in 85% of patients who underwent the Batista procedure (33,34).

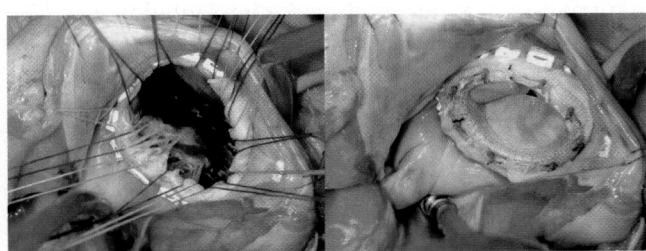

**FIGURE 35.19.** Chordal sparing mitral valve replacement

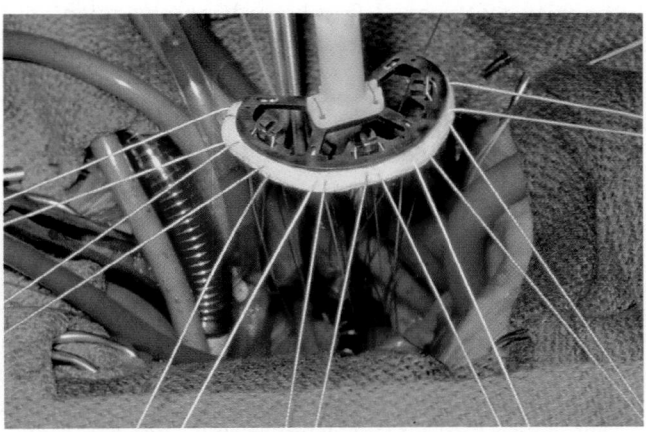

**FIGURE 35.21.** Undersized flexible annuloplasty ring

### Endoventricular Circular Patch Plasty (Dor Left Ventricular Aneurysm Repair)

The Dor procedure, or infarction excision surgery, reduces LV size by surgical reconstruction of ischemic ventricles distorted by dyskinetic or akinetic infarcted myocardium. After coronary revascularization and MV repair (if indicated), endoventricular circular patch plasty (EVCPP) is used to reconstruct the LV. Endocardectomy and cryotherapy are used to prevent ventricular arrhythmia (35).

Patients with severe LV dysfunction, LVEF < 30%, frequent ventricular arrhythmias, and distended LV benefit the most from EVCPP procedures (36). EVCPP (in conjunction with MV repair when indicated) has been shown to improve myocardial ischemia by myocardial revascularization, to diminish ventricular volume, to restore the LV to a more physiologic shape, and to further diminish LVEPD (33). Several studies have reported a significant increase in LVEF, a significant reduction in LV volume, an improvement of NYHA status, a reduction in the rate of ventricular arrhythmias, and an overall 18-month survival rate of 89% in patients who received EVCPP (36–40).

IOE examination of patients undergoing EVCPP should focus on evaluating LV volume and function, assessing the severity of MR, examining myocardial viability issues, and checking for comorbid TR, PHTN, RV dysfunction, and apical thrombus. Myocardial viability can be assessed with IOE stress testing with low-dose dobutamine. Because reducing LV volume is the central aim of this procedure, accurate calculation of LV volume is desirable. LVEF is calculated as (LVEDV-LVESV)/LVEDV. In the presence of LVA, LV is distorted from its symmetrical shape; this limits the usefulness of TEE because the 2-D method assumes that the geometry of the LV is symmetrical. Recent studies found three-dimensional (3-D) echocardiography to be more accurate in estimating LV volume (41). At the present time, 3-D echocardiography has major limitations, mostly related to the system's size, complexity, and low image resolution. However, as the technology advances, 3-D echocardiography might become the method of choice for determining absolute LV volume and EF.

## VENTRICULAR CONSTRAINT TECHNIQUES

Recently, new approaches to treating dilated CMP have evolved. These are designed to unload the heart and promote reverse ventricular remodeling (Fig. 35.22). Some authors have hypothesized that merely limiting remodeling can improve long-term outcomes and quality of life in patients with end-stage CHF.

The Acorn CorCap (for external splinting) is a mesh-like implantable cardiac support device that is positioned

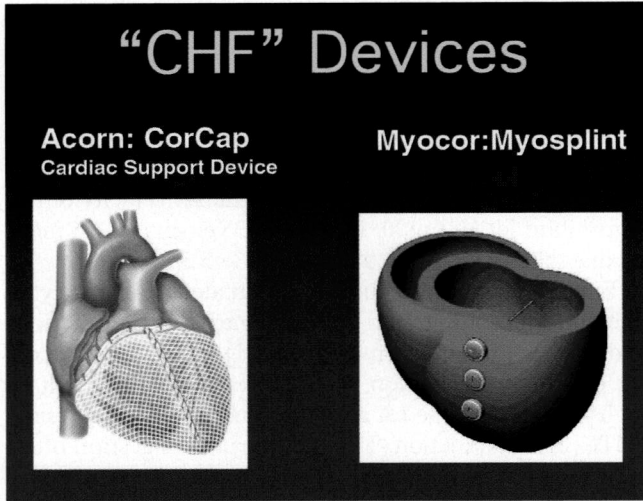

**FIGURE 35.22.** Ventricular constraint devices

around the heart (42). Its purpose is to stop the myocardial remodeling process by reducing LV wall stress and myocyte overstretching—the chief components of postinfarction progressive LV dilation and contractile dysfunction. The mesh-like material of the CorCap has a unique bidirectional compliance that allows the device to conform to the ellipsoidal surface of the heart. When the device is fit snugly, it produces an immediate reduction in the circumference of the heart (42). Candidates for Acorn CorCap implantation are adults with dilated CMP (either ischemic or idiopathic) and LVEF < 35%. MV surgery and myocardial revascularization have been performed concomitantly with the implantation of this device. A large, randomized, multicenter trial is presently underway in Europe and the United States. Patients in this trial have NYHA class III or IV (with or without MR and TR) and dilated cardiomyopathy (ischemic or nonischemic with LVEF < 35% or < 45% in the presence of mild MR), are stable, are on optimal medical management, and have acceptable renal, hepatic, and pulmonary function. Two clinical studies evaluated the initial safety of the device and reported similar results (Fig. 35.23). The Acorn CorCap was shown to improve NYHA functional status, LVEDV, and LVEF at 12 months after surgery (43,44). The authors found no evidence of constrictive physiology. The actuarial survival rate after device implantation was 73% at 12 months and 68% at 24 months (44).

The Myosplint (for internal splinting) is another myocardial restraint device that uses transventricular splints and epicardial pads to constrain the ventricle at the upper, mid, and low ventricular level (Figs. 35.24 and 35.25). This device can be implanted in isolation or in conjunction with MV repair. It is designed to reduce LV wall stress and improve cardiac function by changing LV geometry and reducing LV radius (45). Safety and feasi-

## CorCap Global Implant Trials

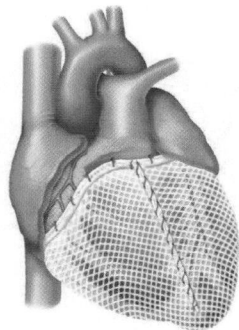

CorCap only
27 pts

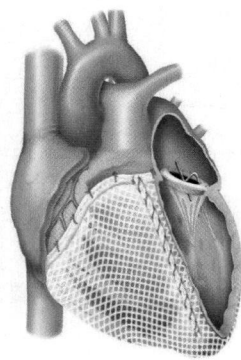

Mitral valve repair/
replacement
59 pts

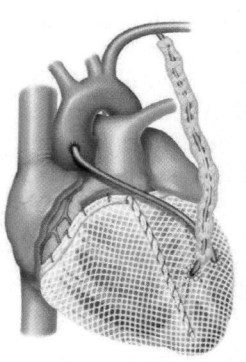

CABG
*(Europe and Asia only)*
25 pts

**FIGURE 35.23.** CorCap global implant trials

bility studies of the device in patients are currently in progress in Europe and United States.

Both the Acorn CorCap and the Myosplint implantation procedures require IOE evaluation similar to that used to guide other surgical approaches for end-stage CHF. In addition, it is necessary to assess the impact of ventricular constraint procedures on systolic and diastolic function. This may be accomplished by determining global ejection fraction using volumetric calculations, global estimation of function, and PWD interrogation of the mitral inflow and pulmonary veins. The appropriate device size is determined by the basal, midpapillary, and apical diameters of LV as measured by IOE. ME SAX views are used to guide the positioning of the device and to confirm its proper placement after surgery (Fig. 35.26). The presence of device-induced constrictive physiology can be evaluated using pressure-volume loop analysis,

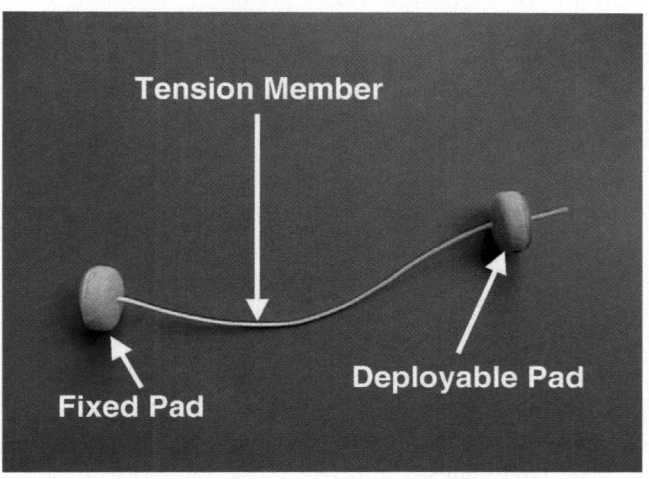

**FIGURE 35.25.** Myosplint epicardial pad and tension member

## Myosplint® Concept

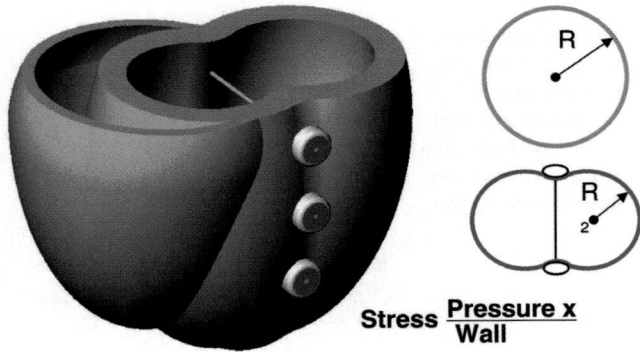

**FIGURE 35.24.** Myosplint concept

## Short Axis TM Positioning

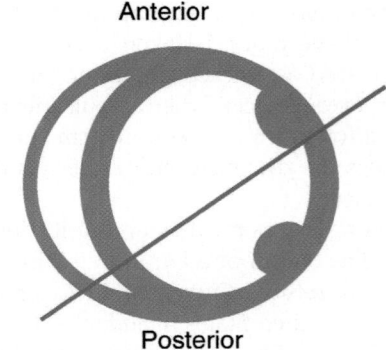

**FIGURE 35.26.** Short-axis tension member positioning

right and left end-diastolic pressures, RA pressure, and RV pressure ratios. Three-dimensional IOE has also been used to demonstrate the impact of ventricular constraint procedures on wall stress and overall LV performance. Given the increasing number of patients who are candidates for ventricular constraint procedures, the outcomes of these surgical interventions will become an expanding area of research and clinical responsibility for the cardiovascular anesthesiologist.

## MECHANICAL CIRCULATORY SUPPORT

Mechanical circulatory support (MCS) includes a wide variety of devices designed to connect to the heart or to be placed within the heart to assume some of the workload and to allow the ventricle to rest, undergo reverse remodeling, and recover some of its contractile function. It has been demonstrated previously that the myocardium is able to repair itself during a period of unloading, after which some patients experience an improvement in quality of life (46,47). Therefore, ventricular assist devices (VADs) have many clinical applications, ranging from temporary support of the ventricle to long-term support, including bridging to heart transplantation. The mismatch between the growing number of cardiac transplant candidates and the limited number of donors has led to a significant increase in the use of mechanical assist devices as bridges to cardiac transplantation (48) or as destination therapy (49).

The latest indications for mechanical assistance include

1. Reversible ventricular dysfunction after cardiac surgery
2. Bridging to heart transplantation
3. Destination therapy for patients who are not transplant candidates.

Compared to medical therapy, left ventricular assist devices (LVADs) can double the 1-year survival rate and triple the 2-year survival rate (50).

Currently, various cardiac assist devices are available for short- and long-term support. VADs may be classified as either nonpulsatile or pulsatile (Table 35.12) depending on the type of blood flow they promote. Alternatively, when the site of the pump is taken into account, VADs may be categorized as extracorporeal or intracorporeal. Most extracorporeal devices, whether pulsatile or nonpulsatile, are used for short- or medium-term support. Nonpulsatile devices are designed with either centrifugal or axial flow patterns.

Pulsatile assist devices provide a pulsatile flow and can generate a cardiac output of 6 L/min to 9 L/min, given an adequate venous return. Currently, FDA-approved pulsatile VADs in the United States include the AbioMed BVS 5000 (Fig. 35.27), the Thoratec VAD System, the Novacor LVAS (Fig. 35.28), and the Heartmate (Figs. 35.24 and

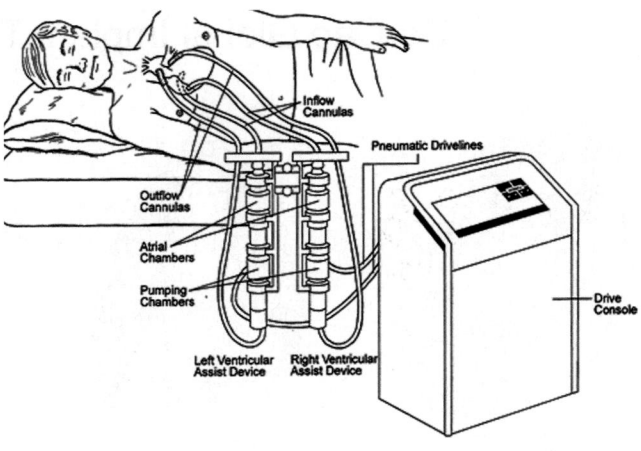

**FIGURE 35.27.** The ABIOMED BVS 5000

35.30). The Heartmate VE (vented electric) is the only mechanical device approved by the FDA for long-term destination therapy. Nonpulsatile pumps generate continuous axial flow and have the advantage of being small, silent, valveless, and fully implantable. By working in concert with the heart, they improve the position of the left ventricle on the Frank-Starling curve. The Jarvik 2000 Flowmaker and the DeBakey VAD can produce high flow rates by generating virtually all of the cardiac output. They can also operate at lower speeds, allowing the LV to assume some of the workload. The Jarvik 2000 Flowmaker is an intraventricular device that is implanted at the left ventricular apex, with the outflow cannula placed in the descending thoracic aorta. The Flowmaker is the only continuous axial flow device approved by the FDA for long-term ventricular support as a bridge to heart transplantation.

The use of mechanical assist devices as bridges to cardiac transplantation has been found to improve the survival rates and outcomes of patients with decompensated

A. Outflow conduit
B. Pump / Drive unit
C. Inflow conduit
D. Percutaneous lead
E. Reserve power pack
F. Electronic controller
G. Primary power pack

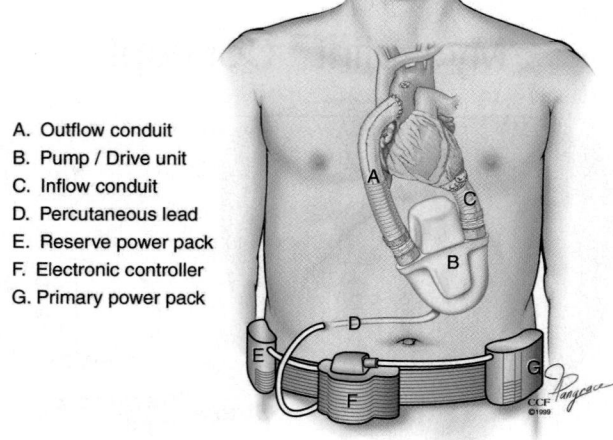

**FIGURE 35.28.** Novacor LVAS

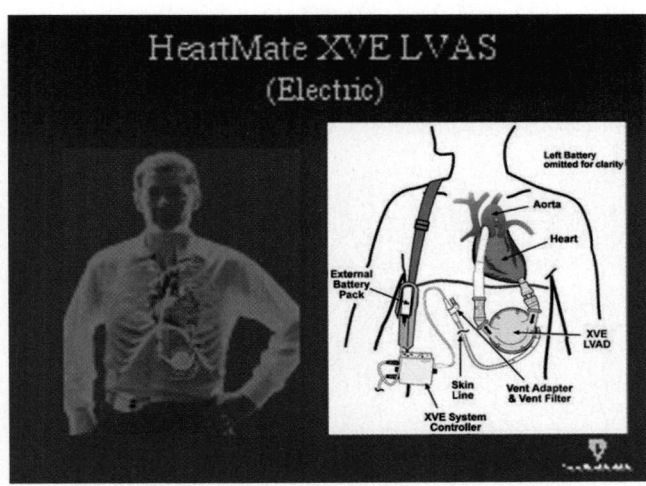

**FIGURE 35.29.** HeartMate XVE LVAS Electric

heart failure (46–49). In addition, long-term LVAD support has proven to be superior to optimal medical treatment in patients with end-stage CHF who are not candidates for heart transplantation (49). Thus, mechanical assistance has become an important tool in the surgical management of patients with failing hearts.

Echocardiography has proven to promote successful outcomes for VAD recipients. Ideally, echocardiographic assessments should be performed before, during, and after VAD implantation (Table 35.2).

## Assessment Before Cardiopulmonary Bypass (CPB) Is Initiated for VAD Implantation

During the pre-CPB period, a careful examination for intracardiac shunts is mandatory. Right-to-left shunting of

unoxygenated blood through a PFO, atrial septal defect (ASD), or ventricular septal defect (VSD) may lead to systemic desaturation and paradoxical embolization when the LVAD is activated (50,51). With a right VAD (RVAD), left-to-right shunting will produce excessive pulmonary blood flow, deceased systemic blood flow leading to hypotension, pulmonary edema, and cardiogenic shock. The bicaval view allows detection of ASD when color-flow mapping and rapidly agitated saline contrast injection are used (Figs. 35.31 and 35.32).

Right ventricular function is the most important factor in the postoperative management and outcome of patients with VADs. RV dysfunction can occur in 20% of patients with isolated LVAD support (52). LVAD inflow is dependent on LA filling pressures and, subsequently, on RV performance. With passive, reversible PHTN and normal transpulmonary pressure gradients, LVAD support will reduce PA pressure and RV afterload, leading to an improvement in RV performance. In the presence of fixed, irreversible PHTN, LVAD support will cause an acute increase in the preload and no change in the afterload of an already impaired RV. Therefore, RV function, severity of TR, and the potential need for biventricular VAD (BiVAD) support should be carefully assessed during the pre-CPB period. The ME 4-chamber view, the RV inflow-outflow view, and TG SAX/LAX RV inflow views can be used to assess RV function (Figs. 35.8–35.10, 35.11, 35.12, 35.17). RVFAC can be calculated using the automated border detection technique described previously (11).

Valvular abnormalities need to be diagnosed and corrected before VAD support is initiated. With regard to the aortic valve, aortic regurgitation (AR) has been found in 22% of patients undergoing LVAD placement. Activation of the pump can increase the pressure gradient across the incompetent aortic valve and cause regurgitant flow from the aorta to the LV, leading to continuous shunting of

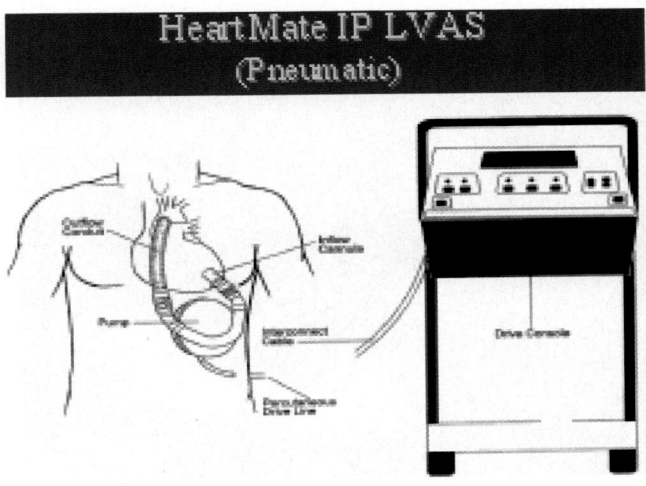

**FIGURE 35.30.** HeartMate IP LVAS-Pneumatic

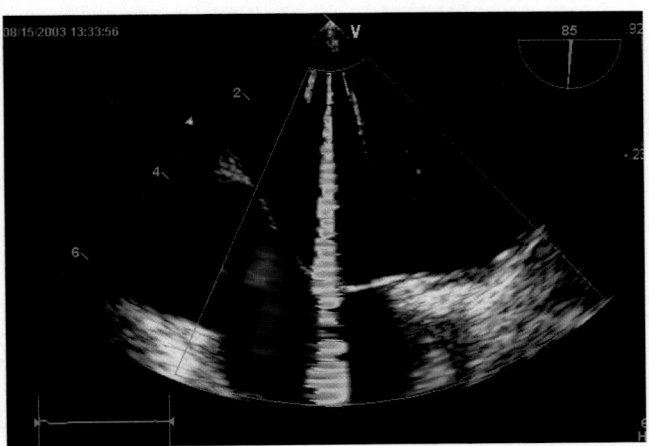

**FIGURE 35.31.** Patent foramen ovale: bicaval view

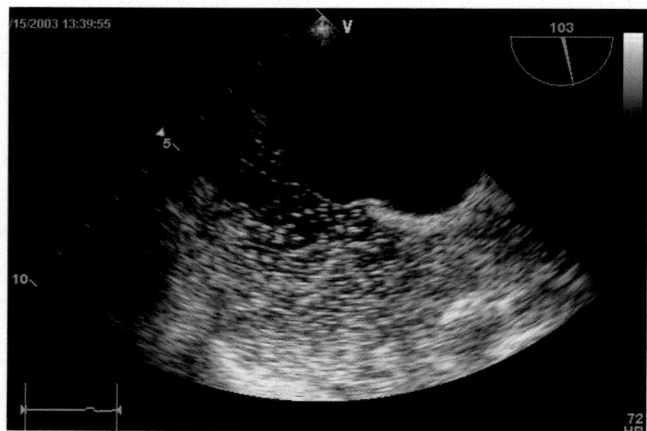

**FIGURE 35.32.** Contrast study: bicaval view

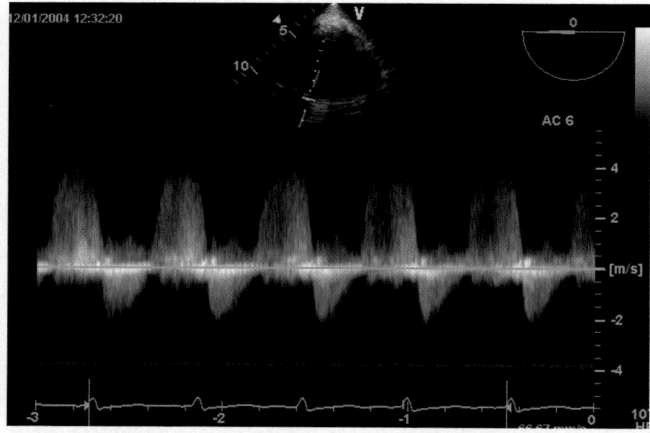

**FIGURE 35.34.** Aortic insufficiency and CWD: deep transgastric long-axis view

blood through the device. This condition prevents LV decompression and decreases the total device output, systemic perfusion, and CO (Figs. 35.33, 35.34) (11). Moderate to severe AR mandates valve replacement.

Mitral stenosis (MS) should be identified during the pre-CPB period because it can severely impair LVAD inflow and cause hemodynamic instability when LVAD support begins. Additionally, mitral regurgitation (MR) is frequently encountered in the LVAD patient population. MR usually improves with LVAD decompression and has only a minor impact on LVAD output (Fig. 35.35).

Tricuspid regurgitation (TR) is often encountered in conjunction with RV dysfunction. Twenty-five percent of patients undergoing LVAD implantation have preexisting TR, and another 19% develop it when the pump is activated. TR can affect thermodilution CO measurements (11). In patients with passive PHTN, the severity of TR decreases with LVAD support. Color-flow mode and Doppler measurements are used to assess the severity of TR (Fig. 35.11).

LV or LA appendage (LAA) thrombi are potential sequelae of end-stage dilated CMP. Their presence should be ruled out before CBP begins to reduce the risk of serious thromboembolic events during or after surgery (Fig. 35.7).

The aortic cannulation site should be evaluated for the presence of atheroma using the ME ascending aortic LAX view or epiaortic scanning. Cannulating a severely diseased aorta, particularly in the presence of mobile plaques, increases the risk of thromboembolic events and poor outcome. The descending aorta should also be scanned for atherosclerotic plaques with mobile components because intraaortic balloon pumps (IABP) are frequently used during the postoperative period, which could dislodge plaques and cause organ embolization.

### Weaning from CPB and Assessment After CPB

Adequate deairing of the VAD and the cardiac chambers is the most critical step in weaning patients from CPB.

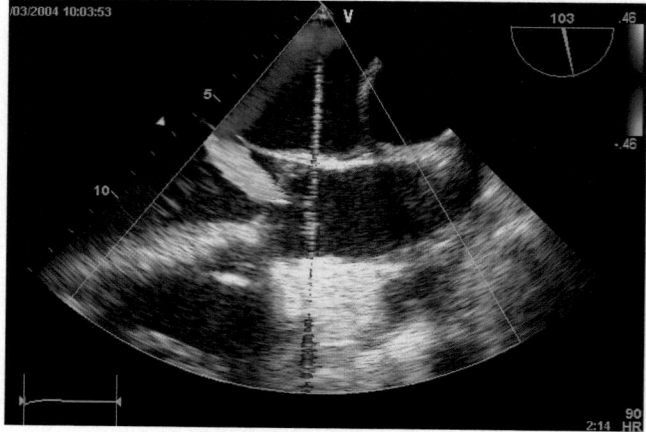

**FIGURE 35.33.** Aortic insufficiency: ME LAX view

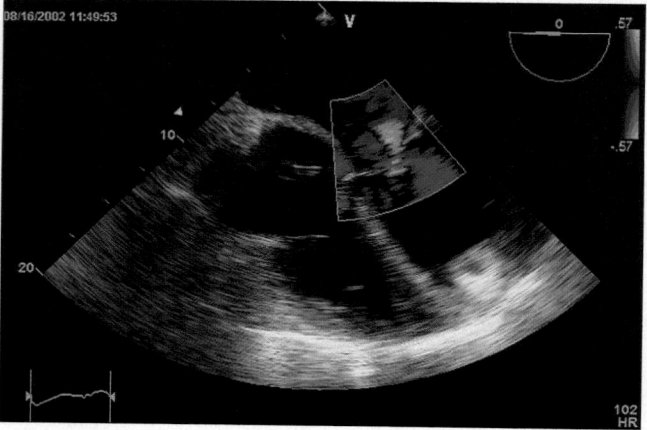

**FIGURE 35.35.** LVAD, MR: ME 4-chamber view

The ME LAX view is used to assess the efflux of microair emboli from the LVAD into the ascending aorta. When a significant amount of air is noted in the ascending aorta, the graft can be reclamped and the aorta vented.

LVAD inlet and outlet cannulas must be assessed for their position and patency. The inflow cannula is evaluated in the ME 4-chamber view, the ME 2-chamber view, and the ME LAX views (Figs. 35.36 and 35.37). CFD mode and Doppler examination are used to assess flow through the LVAD and measure the LV-LVAD inflow gradient (Figs. 35.38–35.40). If the inlet is partially obstructed, high-velocity aliased flow at the cannula orifice will be noted in association with LV distension and an elevated LV-LVAD gradient. The outlet cannula can be visualized in the ME LAX views (Fig. 35.41). CFD mode and Doppler analysis can also be used to assess LVAD output. Different flow patterns are seen with pulsatile and continuous flow devices. With chest closure, LVAD inlet and outlet obstruction can occur; reassessment of flow pattern is advisable at that point.

Adequacy of LV decompression should be also assessed in the ME 4-chamber, ME 2-chamber, TG SAX/LAX, and deep TG views. The supported ventricle should be relatively empty, with the interventricular septum slightly deviated toward the decompressed chamber. Mitral valve and LVAD inlet flow patterns can be used to adjust the pump flow rates to achieve the desired loading conditions (Fig. 35.40).

Ruling out the presence of PFO during the post-CPB period is also important. Activating the pump when the RV is distended can increase the pressure gradient across the interatrial septum, which may cause iatrogenic PFO. Reinstitution of CBP for PFO closure is recommended because PFO can cause significant shunting and systemic desaturation that can complicate the clinical picture and postoperative management.

Successful weaning from bypass depends on adequate RV function. Once the deairing process is complete, the

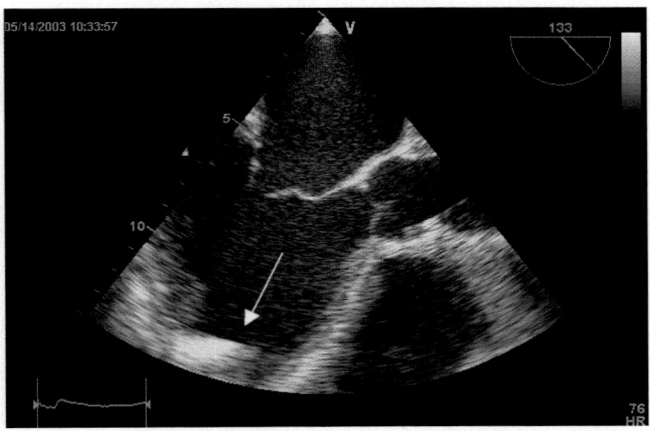

**FIGURE 35.37.** LVAD inflow cannula: ME LAX view

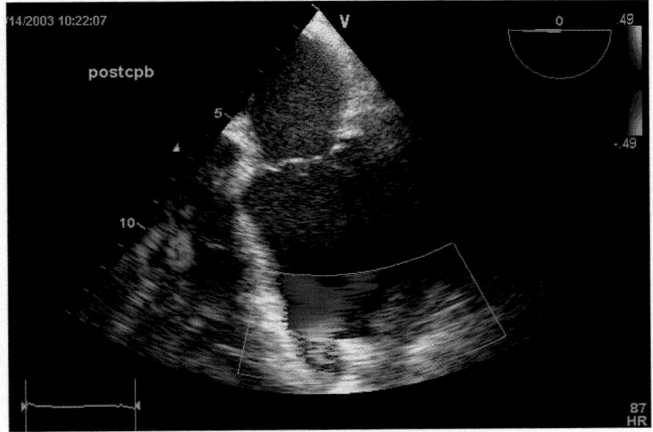

**FIGURE 35.38.** LVAD color flow Doppler of inflow cannula: ME 4-chamber view

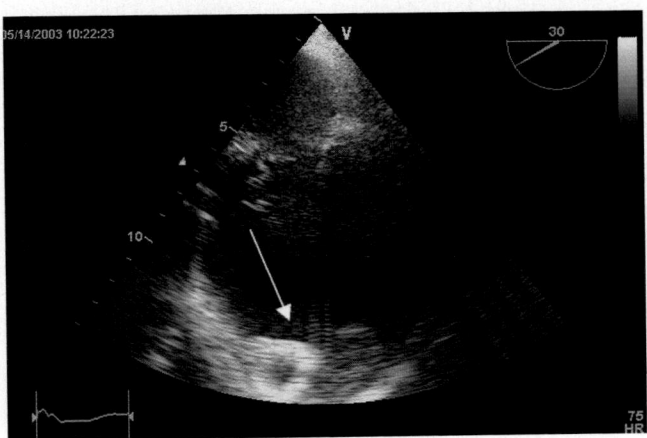

**FIGURE 35.36.** LVAD inflow cannula: ME 2-chamber view

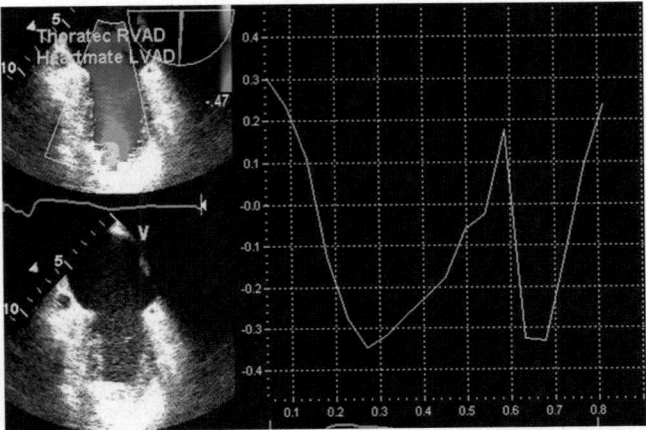

**FIGURE 35.39.** LVAD inflow cannula biphasic flow: ME 2-chamber view

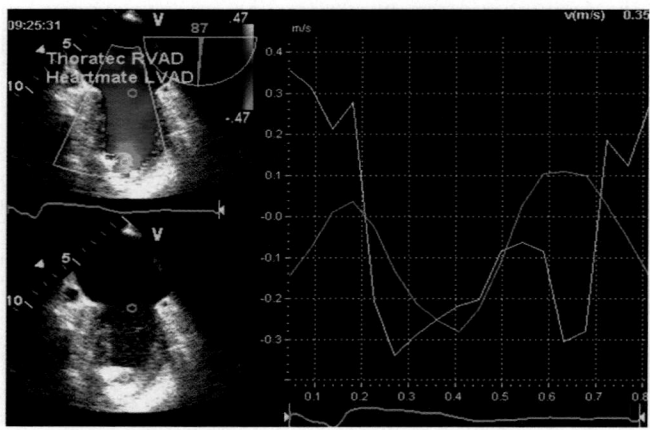

**FIGURE 35.40.** LVAD mitral valve and inflow cannula flow: ME 2-chamber view

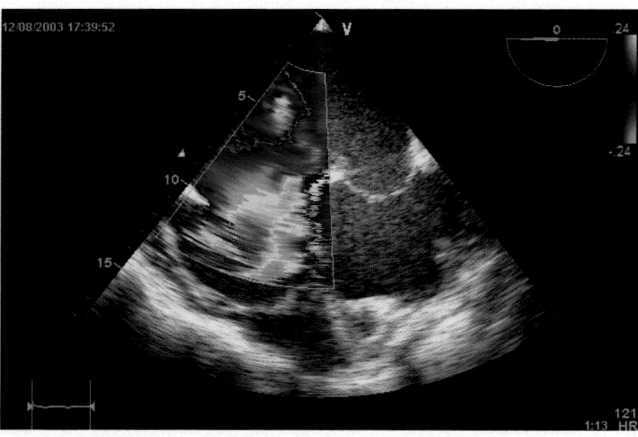

**FIGURE 35.42.** LVAD, severe TR: ME 4-chamber view

pump is started at a low rate of output and RV function is assessed. In patients with fixed PHTN, the RV distends, causing acute severe TR, decreased LV preload, and the collapse of the LV (Fig. 35.42). Additionally, air can be trapped in the cardiac chambers as the result of increased negative pressure generated by the empty device, leading to air embolism of the coronary and systemic circulation. Additionally, the inflow cannula can become obstructed when LVAD preload decreases. Under these circumstances, pharmacological and mechanical RV support is indicated (Tables 35.9 and 35.10).

The AbioMed BVS 5000 and the Thoratec VAD System have been approved by the FDA for short- and medium-term RV support, respectively (Table 35.12, Fig. 35.27). Levitronix CentriMag, a new centrifugal mechanical assist device, is currently being tested for short-term support of both right and left ventricles (Fig. 35.43). These devices can be used for either isolated RV support or biventricular support, according to the patient's needs. Additionally, these devices can be used in conjunction with any LVAD

designed for long-term support (Table 35.12). Midesophageal 4-chamber and ME bicaval views are used to assess the position and patency of right VAD (RVAD) inflow cannulas and to examine blood flow in the superior vena cava. Inadequate RA decompression with leftward deviation of interatrial septum may occur if the RVAD inflow cannula is positioned incorrectly (Fig. 35.44). Proper repositioning of the cannula restores adequate right-side decompression. In patients undergoing BiVAD support, IOE is valuable for confirming the adequate loading of both right and left chambers. The goal of volume management and adjustment of the pump flow rates is to keep the interatrial and interventricular septa close to the midline.

Biventricular mechanical support is important for the management of acute or chronic severe biventricular heart failure (Table 35.13). IOE issues are similar to those previously described for LVAD and RVAD implantation. Echocardiography can ensure that the loading conditions of both right and left chambers are adequate. Optimal

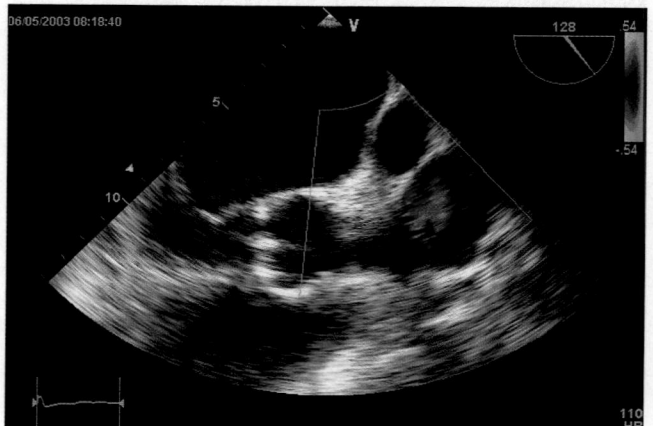

**FIGURE 35.41.** LVAD outflow cannula: ME LAX view

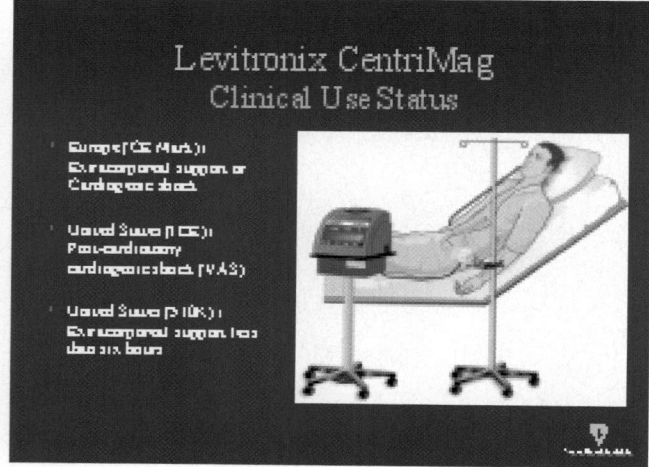

**FIGURE 35.43.** Levitronix CentriMag

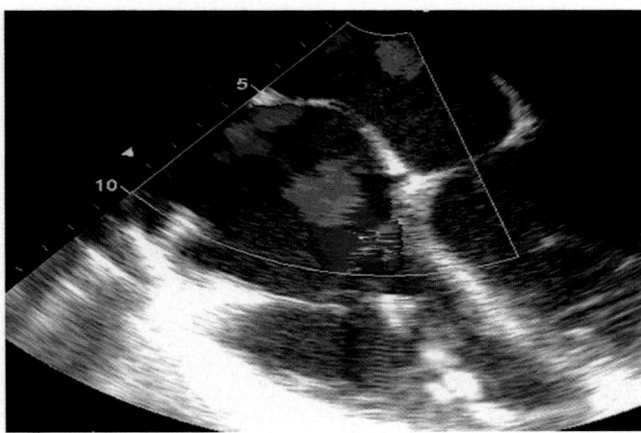

**FIGURE 35.44.** Malposition of RVAD inflow cannula, distended RA: ME 4-chamber view

**▶ TABLE 35.14. Inclusion and Exclusion Criteria for the AbioCor™ Total Artificial Heart**

**Inclusion Criteria**
Age > 18 years
Ineligibility for cardiac transplantation
Optimized medical management (OMM)
High likelihood of dying within next 30 days while on OMM
Acceptable device fitting evaluation
Biventricular failure
Inability to be weaned from a temporary mechanical circulatory assist device

**Exclusion Criteria**
Heart failure with significant potential for reversibility
Chronic dialysis
Irreversible liver failure
Blood dyscrasia
Suspected or active systemic infection
Positive serum pregnancy test result
Severe peripheral vascular disease
Transient ischemic attack or stroke secondary to atherosclerosis
Psychiatric illness (including drug or alcohol abuse)

preload and pump flow rates are achieved when both interatrial and interventricular septa are in the midline position. Doppler analysis of blood flow in the pulmonary veins as well as hepatic vein, inferior vena cava, and SVC provides additional information for assessing the volume status of the patient. As clinicians have gained experience over the years with the management of patients with Bi-VADs, the medical management of these patients has improved. This has led to better outcomes for patients with biventricular failure who require biventricular support as a bridge to heart transplantation. In a recent study,

**▶ TABLE 35.13. Biventricular Support**

**Precardiotomy Shock**
Acute myocardial infarction
Viral myocarditis
Rheumatic pancarditis
Intractable arrhythmia
Spontaneous coronary dissection
Failed Coronary angioplasty

**Postcardiotomy Shock**
Coronary artery bypass grafting
Postinfarction ventral septal defect
Postinfarction mitral regurgitation
Aortic or mitral valve procedures
Left ventricular remodeling procedures
Right ventricular failure
Acutely failed transplant

**Chronic Conditions**
Cardiomyopathies
Chronic rejection
Infiltrative disorders
Nontransplant candidates

Samuels L. Biventricualar mechanical replacement. Surg Clin N Am 2004:84;309–21.

Magliato and colleagues reported a 59% rate of survival to transplantation of patients on biventricular support and a 90% posttransplant survival rate (53). Nonetheless, with the advent of new technologies, TAH may become a better alternative for the treatment of biventricular failure.

### The Total Artificial Heart

Unfortunately, LVAD support is not feasible for patients with certain conditions, including biventricular failure, severe pulmonary hypertension, or any history of malignancy. The AbioCor replacement heart is the first completely implantable total artificial heart (TAH) (54–57).

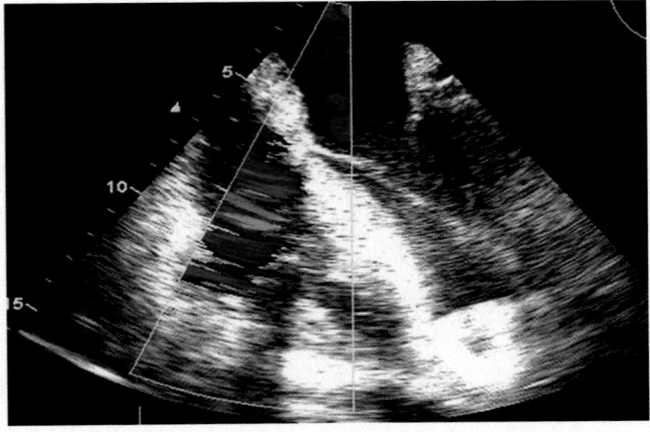

**FIGURE 35.45.** RVAD inflow cannula, decompressed RA: ME 4-chamber view

The first phase of a multicenter trial of this device is currently underway. Recipients are patients with severe, irreversible, inotrope-dependent biventricular failure manifested in many or all organ systems. These patients have no potential for myocardial recovery and are not candidates for other therapies, including transplantation. Many are already receiving pharmacologic or mechanical circulatory support and have overt changes in the hepatic, renal, and coagulation systems. As a group, their predicted 30-day mortality is higher than 70%. Specific inclusion and exclusion criteria for the trial are listed in Table 35.14 (55). Although the AbioCor TAH is used in patients who are not eligible for heart transplantation, supported patients may eventually become heart transplant candidates if their conditions improve sufficiently.

The AbioCor is made primarily of titanium and a proprietary polyurethane. The device is designed to fit inside the body and operate without penetrating the skin so that the recipient can remain mobile (Figs. 35.46 and 35.47). The internal components of the AbioCor system consist of a thoracic unit, an internal transcutaneous energy transfer (TET) coil, a controller, and a battery (4). The thoracic unit (blood pump) weighs approximately 2 pounds and comprises 2 artificial ventricles, 4 valves, and a motor-driven hydraulic pumping system. The hydraulic pumping system uses pressure to move blood between the chambers, from the artificial right ventricle to the lungs, and from the artificial left ventricle to the systemic circulation. The pump's motor rotates at 6000 rpm to 8000 rpm, producing sufficient hydraulic fluid pressure to compress the diaphragm around the blood chamber and eject the blood. A miniaturized electronics package, which is im-

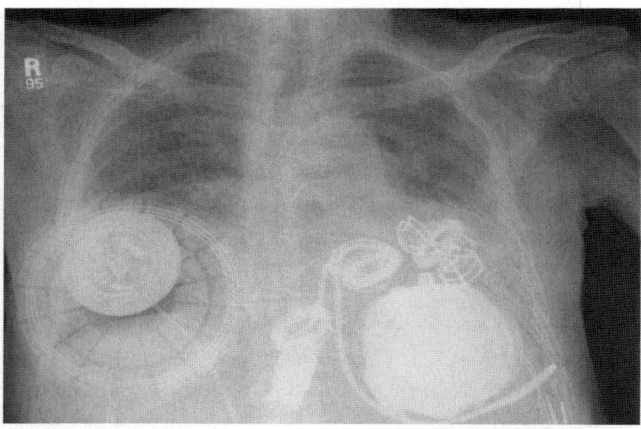

**FIGURE 35.47.** Chest x-ray of the AbioCor in situ

planted in the patient's abdomen, monitors and controls the pump rate, the right-left hydraulic fluid balance, and the speed of the hydraulic motor. A unique feature of the AbioCor is the right-left flow balancing mechanism that compensates for the natural right-left flow imbalance and eliminates the need for an external vent or internal compliance chamber.

The AbioCor TAH uses the TET system to provide external power and radiofrequency communication to control the implanted device. An internal rechargeable battery, also positioned within the abdomen, functions as a backup power source. The internal battery is continually recharged with power received through the TET, and it can provide up to 30 minutes of tether-free operation while disconnected from the main power source. Therefore, unlike many LVAD systems, this system does not require any percutaneous connections, either electrical or mechanical. The external components include a computer console, the external TET coil, and battery packs. The computer receives information about pump performance through the radiofrequency communication system.

IOE has an important role in the perioperative management of TAH recipients. Failure to recognize and correct a PFO can result in postimplantation systemic desaturation because the negative pressures generated in the device may shunt venous blood into the systemic circulation. Both CFD and contrast techniques are helpful in ruling out the presence of PFO (Figs. 35.48 and 35.49). Evaluation of baseline pulmonary flow velocities from all four PVs is important for the detection of pulmonary flow obstruction during the post-CPB period, at the time of chest closure, and during early postoperative care (Fig. 35.50); this obstruction may require repositioning of the device. IOE is also helpful in assessing the adequacy of deairing of the native atria when CPB is discontinued. If further deairing becomes necessary, the aorta is reclamped and

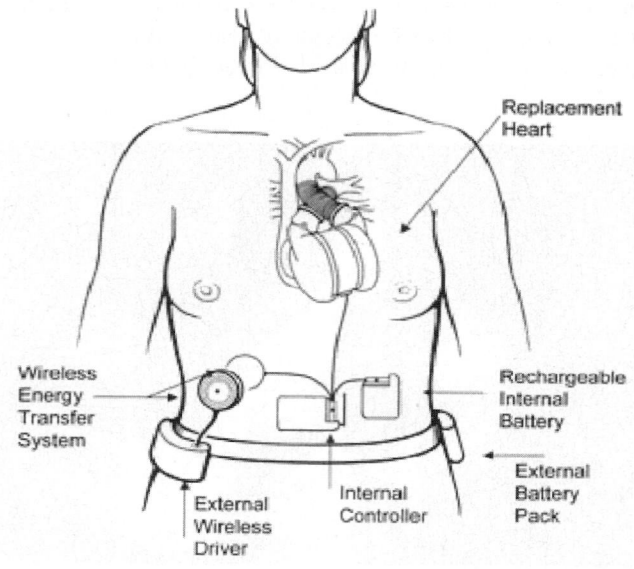

**FIGURE 35.46.** The AbioCor total artificial heart system

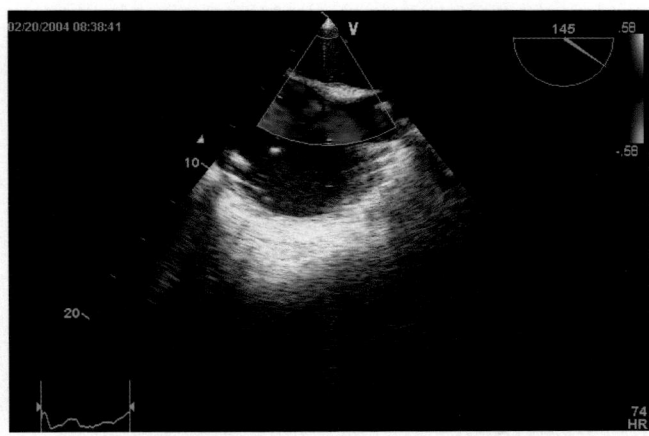

**FIGURE 35.48.** Color flow Doppler of interatrial septum: bicaval view precardiopulmonary bypass

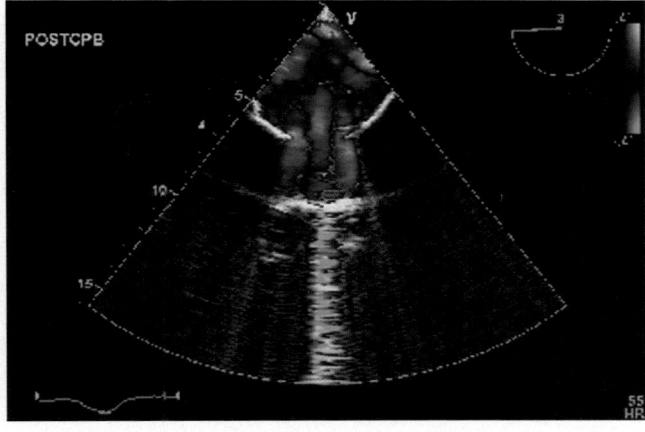

**FIGURE 35.51.** Flow across left polyurethane valve

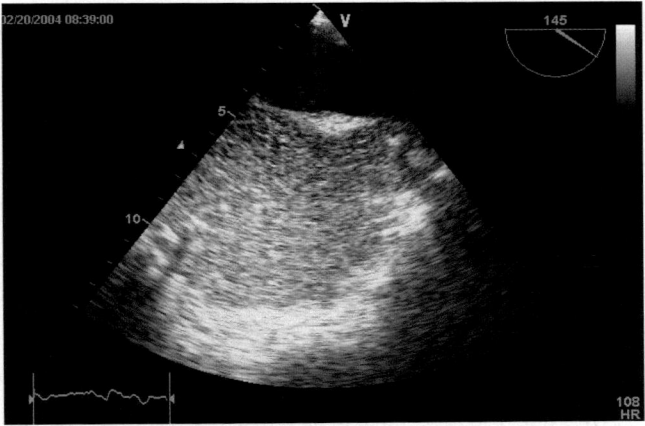

**FIGURE 35.49.** Contrast study: bicaval view precardiopulmonary bypass

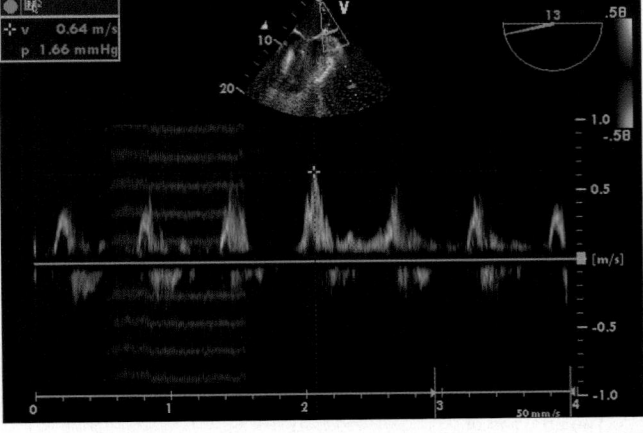

**FIGURE 35.50** Pulse wave Doppler of left lower pulmonary vein: midesophageal 4-chamber view precardiopulmonary bypass

CPB is re-established with the TAH turned off. During the post-CPB period, IOE provides useful information about blood flow across the right and left polyurethane valves into the device and through the outflow conduit and inferior vena cava (Figs. 35.51–35.52) (58). Because TAH recipients do not need inotropic support, vasoactive therapy can be directed at the peripheral (both systemic and pulmonary) circulation. However, adequate volume must be maintained because the negative pressures generated in the TAH make it possible for air to enter through the new suture line if preload is very low.

Early results from the trial of the AbioCor system have demonstrated excellent function of all device components. Nine of the first 11 patients survived the TAH implantation procedure. Additionally, the system has allowed for patient mobility; 5 of 9 recipients are ambulatory, and 3 of these have taken out-of-hospital excursions.

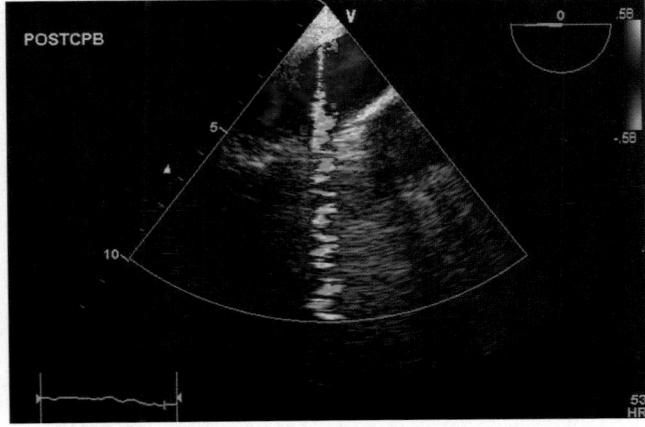

**FIGURE 35.52.** Flow through the outflow conduit

## CONCLUSION

CHF has proven to be one of the greatest challenges in medicine, and it will continue to be in the next century. At present, the treatment of heart failure is a specialty in itself. The best treatment currently available is a combination of medical and surgical therapy. Patient with end-stage CHF have complex, highly individual diseases, and establishing specific and uniform criteria for treatment selection is impractical. As a result, IOE has become an invaluable tool for the diagnosis of heart failure, the selection of appropriate surgical procedures, and the overall perioperative management of heart failure patients. Surgical therapies for end-stage CHF are constantly evolving and will continue to improve as existing treatments are refined and new ones are developed.

## KEY POINTS

- In the United States, more than 4.5 million people have CHF, and its prevalence is estimated at 6.8% in people over the age of 65. It is likely that the number of patients with end-stage CHF will grow as the average age of our population increases.
- Congestive heart failure is a complex syndrome in which myocardial injury and the resulting hemodynamic changes alter many neuroendocrine, humoral, and inflammatory feedback loops.
- Strategies for treating end-stage CHF include medical therapies such as angiotensin-converting enzyme inhibitors (ACEI), beta-blockers, diuretics, inotropic agents, and antiarrhythmics. Multifaceted pharmacologic regimens may not prevent progression toward end-stage CHF and surgical intervention is required.
- Cardiac transplantation is the "gold-standard" surgical treatment for end-stage CHF. While the one-year survival rate after transplantation is 85%. Unfortunately, only 2,400 heart transplants are performed annually. Class IV patients awaiting transplant have a one-year mortality rate of 40% to 50% with an ever expanding mismatch between the number of cardiac transplant candidates and the limited number of donors.
- This mismatch has led to increasing use of alternative surgical therapies, including mechanical ventricular assist devices (VAD), ventricular remodeling procedures in conjunction with revascularization and mitral valvuloplasty (i.e., endoventricular circular patch plasty (ECPP), partial ventriculectomy), newer procedures intended to reduce ventricular dilatation (i.e., external or internal splinting), and total artificial heart (TAH) implantation.
- Critical issues addressed by intraoperative echocardiography in patients undergoing procedures for congestive heart failure include determining the etiology and mechanism of CHF, assessment of ventricular function and coexisting or secondary pathology, surgical procedure-related issue, and the diagnosis of post-CPB bypass complications.

## REFERENCES

1. Givertz MM, Wilson SC, Braunwald E. Clinical aspects of heart failure: high-output failure, pulmonary edema. In Braunwald E, Zipes DP, Libby P, Eds. Heart disease: a textbook of cardiovascular medicine, 6th ed. Philadelphia: WB Saunders, 2001:534–61.
2. Facts about heart failure. US Department of Health and Human Services. NIH publication No 95-923, May 1997.
3. Francis GS, Goldsmith SR, Levine TB, et al. The neurohumoral axis in congestive heart failure. Ann Intern Med 1984;101:370–7.
4. Levine B, Kalman J, Mayer L, Fillit HM, Packer M. Elevated circulating levels of tumor necrosis factor in severe chronic heart failure. N Engl J Med 1990;323:236–41.
5. UNOS Articles, Bylaws and Polices, National Organ Procurement and Transplant Network. Richmond, VA: 1997.
6. The SOLVD Investigators. Effect of enalapril on survival in patients with reduced left ventricular ejection fractions and congestive heart failure. N Engl J Med 1991;325:293–302.
7. Kottke TE, Pesch DG, Frye RL, et al. The potential contribution of cardiac replacement to the control of cardiovascular diseases: a population-based estimate. Arch Surg 1990;125:1148–51.
8. Otto CM. The cardiomyopathies, hypertensive heart disease, post-cardiac-transplant patient and pulmonary heart disease, Textbook of Clinical Echocardiography. Philadelphia: WB Saunders, 2000;183–212.
9. Jessup M, Brozena S. Heart failure. N Engl J Med 2003;348:2007–18.
10. Farrar DJ, Chow E, Brown CD. Isolated systolic and diastolic ventricular interactions in pacing-induced dilated cardiomyopathy and effects of volume loading and pericardium. Circulation 1995;92:1284–90.
11. Scalia GM, McCarthy PM, Savage RM, et al. Clinical utility of echocardiography in the management of implantable ventricular assist devices. J Am Soc Echocardiogr 2000;13:754–63.
12. Hammarstrom E, Wranne B, Pinto FJ, et al. Tricuspid annular motion. J Am Soc Echocardiogr 1991;4:131–9.
13. Zile MR, Brutsaert DL. New concepts in diastolic dysfunction and diastolic heart failure: Part I: diagnosis, prognosis, and measurements of diastolic function. Circulation 2002;105:1387–93.
14. Gaasch WH, Zile MR. Left ventricular diastolic dysfunction and diastolic heart failure. Ann Rev Med 2004;55:373–94.
15. Werner GS, Schaefer C, Dirks R, et al. Prognostic value of Doppler echocardiographic assessment of left ventricular filling in idiopathic dilated cardiomyopathy. Am J Cardiol 1994;73:792–8.
16. Rakowski H, Appleton C, Chan KL, et al. Canadian consensus recommendations for the measurement and reporting of diastolic dysfunction by echocardiography: from the Investigators of Consensus on Diastolic Dysfunction by Echocardiography. J Am Soc Echocardiogr 1996;9:736–60.

17. Johnson RA, Palacios I: Dilated cardiomyopathies of the adult (first of two parts). N Engl J Med 1982;307:1051–8.

18. Lewis JF, Webber JD, Sutton LL, et al. Discordance in degree of right and left ventricular dilation in patients with dilated cardiomyopathy: recognition and clinical implications. J Am Coll Cardiol 1993;21:649–54.

19. Shah PM: Echocardiography in congestive or dilated cardiomyopathy. J Am Soc Echocardiogr 1988;1:20–30.

20. Kono T, Sabbah HN, Stein PD, et al. Left ventricular shape as a determinant of functional mitral regurgitation in patients with severe heart failure secondary to either coronary artery disease or idiopathic dilated cardiomyopathy. Am J Cardiol 1991;68:355–9.

21. Castello R, Lenzen P, Aguirre F, et al. Variability in the quantitation of mitral regurgitation by Doppler color flow mapping: comparison of transthoracic and transesophageal studies. J Am Coll Cardiol 1992;20:433–8.

22. Enriquez-Sarano M, Bailey KR, Seward JB, et al. Quantitative Doppler assessment of valvular regurgitation. Circulation 1993;87:841–8.

23. Shanewise JS, Cheung AT, Aronson S, et al. ASE/SCA guidelines for performing a comprehensive intraoperative multiplane transesophageal echocardiography examination: recommendations of the American Society of Echocardiography Council for Intraoperative Echocardiography and the Society of Cardiovascular Anesthesiologists Task Force for Certification in Perioperative Transesophageal Echocardiography. J Am Soc Echocardiogr 1999;12:884–900.

24. Junker A, Thayssen P, Nielsen B, et al. The hemodynamic and prognostic significance of echo-Doppler-proven mitral regurgitation in patients with dilated cardiomyopathy. Cardiology 1993;83:14–20.

25. Blondheim DS, Jacobs LE, Kotler MN, et al. Dilated cardiomyopathy with mitral regurgitation: decreased survival despite a low frequency of left ventricular thrombus. Am Heart J 1991;122:763–71.

26. Helmcke F, Nanda NC, Hsiung MC, et al. Color Doppler assessment of mitral regurgitation with orthogonal planes. Circulation 1987;75:175–83.

27. Spain MG, Smith MD, Grayburn PA, et al. Quantitative assessment of mitral regurgitation by Doppler color flow imaging: angiographic and hemodynamic correlations. J Am Coll Cardiol 1989;13:585–90.

28. Klein AL, Obarski TP, Stewart WJ, et al. Transesophageal Doppler echocardiography of pulmonary venous flow: a new marker of mitral regurgitation severity. J Am Coll Cardiol 1991;18:518–26.

29. Enriquez-Sarano M, Tajik AJ, Bailey KR, et al. Color flow imaging compared with quantitative Doppler assessment of severity of mitral regurgitation: influence of eccentricity of jet and mechanism of regurgitation. J Am Coll Cardiol 1993;21:1211–9.

30. Carpentier AF, Lessana A, Relland JY, et al. The "physio-ring": an advanced concept in mitral valve annuloplasty. Ann Thorac Surg 1995;60:1177–85.

31. Bolling SF, Pagani FD, Deeb GM, et al. Intermediate-term outcome of mitral reconstruction in cardiomyopathy. J Thorac Cardiovasc Surg 1998;115:381–6.

32. Bolling SF, Smolens IA, Pagani FD. Surgical alternatives for heart failure. J.Heart Lung Transplant 2001;20:729–33.

33. Batista RJ, Verde J, Nery P, et al. Partial left ventriculectomy to treat end-stage heart disease. Ann Thorac Surg 1997;64:634–8.

34. Kass DA. Surgical approaches to arresting or reversing chronic remodeling of the failing heart. J Card Fail 1998;4:57–66.

35. Dor V, Sabatier M, Di Donato M, et al. Efficacy of endoventricular patch plasty in large postinfarction akinetic scar and severe left ventricular dysfunction: comparison with a series of large dyskinetic scars. J Thorac Cardiovasc Surg 1998;116:50–9.

36. Dor V, Sabatier M, Di Donato M, et al. Late hemodynamic results after left ventricular patch repair associated with coronary grafting in patients with postinfarction akinetic or dyskinetic aneurysm of the left ventricle. J Thorac Cardiovasc Surg 1995;110:1291–9.

37. Menicanti L, Di Donato M. The Dor procedure: what has changed after fifteen years of clinical practice? J Thorac Cardiovasc Surg 2002;124:886–90.

38. Di Donato M, Sabatier M, Dor V, et al. Akinetic versus dyskinetic postinfarction scar: relation to surgical outcome in patients undergoing endoventricular circular patch plasty repair. J Am Coll Cardiol 1997;29:1569–75.

39. Athanasuleas CL, Stanley AW, Jr., Buckberg GD, et al. Surgical anterior ventricular endocardial restoration (SAVER) in the dilated remodeled ventricle after anterior myocardial infarction. RESTORE group. Reconstructive Endoventricular Surgery, returning Torsion Original Radius Elliptical Shape to the LV. J Am Coll Cardiol 2001;37:1199–209.

40. Shiota T, McCarthy PM. Volume reduction surgery for end-stage ischemic heart disease. Echocardiography 2002;19:605–12.

41. Qin JX, Jones M, Shiota T, et al. Validation of real-time three-dimensional echocardiography for quantifying left ventricular volumes in the presence of a left ventricular aneurysm: in vitro and in vivo studies. J Am Coll Cardiol 2000;36:900–7.

42. Oz MC. Passive ventricular constraint for the treatment of congestive heart failure. Ann Thorac Surg 2001;71:S185–S187.

43. Konertz, WF, Kleber, FX, Dushe S, et al. Efficacy trends with the Acorn cardiac support device in patients with advanced heart failure. J Heart Fail 2001;7:39.

44. Oz MC, Konertz WF, Kleber FX, et al. Global surgical experience with the Acorn cardiac support device. J Thorac Cardiovasc Surg 2003;126:983–91.

45. Fukamachi K, Inoue M, Doi K, et al. Device-based left ventricular geometry change for heart failure treatment: developmental work and current status. J Card Surg 2003;18 Suppl 2:S43-7.

46. Frazier OH, Benedict CR, Radovancevic B, et al. Improved left ventricular function after chronic left ventricular unloading. Ann Thorac Surg 1996;62:675–81.

47. Bick RJ, Poindexter BJ, Buja LM, et al. Improved sarcoplasmic reticulum function after mechanical left ventricular unloading. Cardiovasc Pathobio 1998;2:159–66.

48. Hunt SA, Frazier OH: Mechanical circulatory support and cardiac transplantation. Circulation 1998;97:2079–90.

49. Rose EA, Gelijns AC, Moskowitz AJ, et al. Long-term mechanical left ventricular assistance for end-stage heart failure. N Engl J Med 2001;345:1435–43.

50. Baldwin RT, Duncan JM, Frazier OH, et al. Patent foramen ovale: a cause of hypoxemia in patients on left ventricular support. Ann Thorac Surg 1991;52:865–7.

51. Shapiro GC, Leibowitz DW, Oz MC, et al. Diagnosis of patent foramen ovale with transesophageal echocardiography in a patient supported with a left ventricular assist device. J Heart Lung Transplant 1995;14:594–7.

52. Santamore WP, Gray LA, Jr. Left ventricular contributions to right ventricular systolic function during LVAD support. Ann Thorac Surg 1996;61:350–6.

53. Magliato KE, Kleisli T, Soukiasian HJ, et al. Biventricular support in patients with profound cardiogenic shock: a single center experience. ASAIO J 2003;49:475–79.

54. Dowling RD, Gray L, Etoch SW, et al. Initial experience with the AbioCor implantable replacement heart system. J Thorac Cardiovasc Surg 2004;127:131–41.

55. Myers TJ, Robertson K, Pool T, et al. Continuous flow pumps and total artificial hearts: management issues. Ann Thorac Surg 2003;75:S79–85.

56. Dowling RD, Gray LA, Etoch SW, et al. Ann Thorac Surg 2003;75:S93–9.

57. Frazier OH. Prologue: Ventricular assist devices and total artificial hearts: A historical perspective. Cardiol Clin 2003;21:1–13.

58. Thielmeier KA, Pank JR, Dowling RD, Gray LA. Anesthetic and perioperative considerations in patients undergoing

placement of totally implantable replacement hearts. Sem Cardiothorac Vasc Anesth 2001;5:335–44.

## QUESTIONS

1. What percent of patients over the age of 65 have congestive heart failure?
   A. 7%
   B. 14%
   C. 21%
   D. 28%
   E. 35%

2. The overall postorthotopic heart transplant 1-year survival rate is
   A. 95%
   B. 90%
   C. 85%
   D. 80%
   E. 75%

3. Hypertrophic cardiomyopathy may be associated with which of the following patterns of diastolic dysfunction:
   A. Normal
   B. Abnormal relaxation
   C. Reversible restrictive physiology
   D. Irreversible restrictive physiology
   E. All of the above

4. The most important determinant of success of surgical procedures for end-stage congestive heart failure is:
   A. LV ejection fraction
   B. Left atrial pressure
   C. Etiology of LV dysfunction
   D. RV function
   E. Hematocrit

5. Which of the following is a contraindication to LVAD implantation?
   A. Moderate aortic regurgitation
   B. Atrial septal defect
   C. Severe mitral regurgitation
   D. Patent foramen ovale
   E. Active systemic infection

# Assessment of Cardiac Transplantation

*Mihai V. Podgoreanu and Joseph P. Mathew*

Although Barnard performed the first human cardiac transplant in 1967, it was only by the early 1980s that it gained widespread acceptance as a realistic therapeutic option for patients with end-stage heart disease. The consistent advancements in donor management, surgical techniques, immunosuppressive therapy, and antibiotic therapy resulted in a dramatic growth of cardiac transplantation in the 1980s, and have led to successful heart-lung and lung transplantation. In 2001, the Registry of the International Society for Heart and Lung Transplantation listed a cumulative total of 57,818 heart transplants and 2,861 heart-lung transplants performed in 211 centers worldwide (1). The annual number of heart transplants reached a plateau in the mid-1990s at approximately 4,500 per year, and has been declining in recent years (1). The limiting factor has been a shortage of suitable donors, further compounded by a tendency to relax the recipient selection criteria in an effort to extend the benefits of transplantation. As of January 2002, the United Network for Organ Sharing national cardiac transplant waiting list (www.unos.org) included 4,119 patients, whereas only 2,197 heart transplants were performed in the U.S. in the year 2000 (2). Although the majority of heart transplant recipients cluster between the ages of 35 and 64 years, 12.4% of all cardiac transplants in the year 2000 were performed in pediatric patients (< 18 years old) and 9.8% in patients 65 years and older, with the recipients being predominantly male (73.3%) and white (83.2%) (2). The most common indications for adult cardiac transplantation are coronary artery disease (46.1%) and cardiomyopathy (45.3%), with valvular heart disease and congenital heart disease contributing only 3.6% and 1.6%, respectively (1). The retransplantation rate in the year 2000 was 3.1% (1,2).

The overall one-year survival for cardiac transplantation is 80%, with a subsequent mortality rate of 4% per year (1). Risk factors for 1- and 5-year mortality in adult heart transplantation have been associated with recipient factors (repeat transplant, ventilator dependence, pul-monary vascular resistance, ischemic or congenital heart disease, ventricular assistance, older age, female gender, risk for primary cytomegalovirus infection, panel reactive antibody, body length, body mass index), medical center factors (volume of heart transplants performed, ischemic time), and donor factors (advanced age, female). Early mortality is most frequently due to primary nonspecific graft failure, intermediate-term deaths are caused by acute rejection or infection, whereas late deaths after cardiac transplantation are most frequently due to allograft vasculopathy, lymphoproliferative or other malignancies, and chronic rejection (1).

The expanding role of transesophageal echocardiography (TEE) in adult cardiac surgery has included its use as a perioperative diagnostic and monitoring technique during cardiac transplantation. There are currently five categories of applications of TEE in the assessment of cardiac transplantation:

1. Cardiac donor screening
2. Intraoperative monitoring in the pretransplantation period
3. Intraoperative evaluation of cardiac allograft function and surgical anastomoses in the immediate posttransplantation period
4. Management of early postoperative hemodynamic abnormalities in the intensive care unit
5. Postoperative follow-up studies of cardiac allograft function

## THE ROLE OF TEE IN CARDIAC DONOR SCREENING

The chronic shortage of ideal donor hearts has led some cardiac transplant centers to liberalize the originally established donor selection criteria (3,4) to include older donors and marginally acceptable hearts, such that, of all the hearts transplanted in the year 2000, 11.5% were harvested from donors > 50 years old (1).

Echocardiography has become an integral component in the evaluation of potential cardiac transplant donors (5). This evaluation should be performed at a time when dosages of intravenous inotropic agents have been lowered to a minimum compatible with adequate blood pressure and cardiac output, and after adequate fluid resuscitation. The echocardiographic assessment allows for the inclusion of donor hearts demonstrating normal function in patients otherwise considered at risk for cardiac injury by clinical criteria (known chest trauma, prolonged hypotension, hemodynamic instability requiring high doses of catecholamines). Additionally, it can circumvent the need for costly and time-consuming direct surgical inspection or cardiac catheterization in potential donors with severely depressed cardiac function (5). However, transthoracic echocardiography (TTE) is technically inadequate in up to 29% of mechanically ventilated brain-dead potential donors (6). In these patients, TEE consistently allows for unobstructed tomographic imaging of the heart, becoming a safe and useful adjunct in the assessment of ventricular function, chamber sizes, valvular structure and function, and septal wall motion and integrity (6).

Brain death is associated with hemodynamic deterioration and biventricular dysfunction, which is usually reversible shortly after transplantation. Studies in potential clinical donors and in experimental animals have suggested that brain death can have major histopathological and functional effects on the myocardium, with very typical focal lesions consisting of petechial subendocardial hemorrhage, contraction bands, and coagulative myocytolysis. Although the mechanism of myocardial injury and contractile dysfunction after brain death remains incompletely understood, it is believed to be caused by a catecholamine excess that occurs during the process of brain death, resulting in cytosolic calcium overload (7–9). Previous studies have shown that segmental wall motion abnormalities and global left ventricular systolic dysfunction [fractional area change (FAC) < 50%] are frequent in brain-dead donors (67.5% and 36%, respectively), improve shortly after heart transplantation, and remain improved 15 months later (4,10), thus suggesting that potential cardiac donors should not be excluded on the basis of segmental wall motion abnormalities. A recent multiinstitutional study, however, identified wall motion abnormalities on the donor echocardiogram as an independent powerful predictor of fatal early graft failure (relative risk of 1.7), especially with increasing donor age and prolonged ischemic time (11). As of yet, the lowest FAC enabling the heart to be transplanted without risk is not known, but one study recommends harvesting and heart transplantation when the FAC is above 35% if there are no other severe cardiac abnormalities (right ventricular failure or valvular dysfunction) (5). One retrospective study suggests that the presence of LVH in the donor

heart increases the incidence of early graft dysfunction (12). Such marginal donor hearts should not be used in high-risk recipients (those on ventilator support, with prior sternotomies, or in renal failure, for example), and should be carefully monitored postoperatively for allograft dysfunction (12b).

## INTRAOPERATIVE MONITORING IN THE PRETRANSPLANTATION PERIOD

The vast majority of patients referred for cardiac transplantation suffers from ischemic or idiopathic cardiomyopathy with a dilated left ventricle and depressed ejection fraction. The currently accepted indications for transplantation, however, include impaired functional status (peak $VO_2$ < 14 ml/kg/min) and/or refractory hemodynamic decompensation, manifested as severe ischemia not amenable to revascularization, or recurrent symptomatic ventricular arrhythmias despite optimal medical management (13). As such, these patients have a relatively fixed low stroke volume and depend on appropriate preload and heart rate to maintain a marginal cardiac output. Due to the characteristics of the end-systolic pressure volume relationship in the myopathic heart, even mild increases in afterload can markedly decrease the stroke volume (14). Sympathetic tone is increased in patients with heart failure, leading to generalized vasoconstriction as well as salt and water retention. The combination of vasoconstriction and ventricular dilation result in a substantial increase in myocardial wall tension. Moreover, in patients with long-standing left-sided cardiac failure, right ventricular impairment may result by a process of ventricular interdependence, independent of neurohumoral or circulatory effects, and can be further compromised by elevations in pulmonary vascular resistance (15). Almost all cardiac transplant candidates will be maintained on a combination of vasodilators for afterload reduction (usually angiotensin-converting enzyme inhibitors, ACE-I), diuretics to minimize volume overload, and antiarrhythmics (usually amiodarone). This combination therapy was associated with a decrease in the overall 1-year mortality, as well as a decrease in the incidence of sudden death in end-stage heart failure (16). The average waiting time for patients at home is currently more than 18 months and continues to lengthen, but patients who develop refractory hemodynamic decompensation will require continued hospitalization for hemodynamic monitoring, prolonged inotropic therapy, or various degrees of mechanical assistance as a bridge to transplantation (intraaortic balloon counterpulsation, uni- or biventricular assist devices). In the United States, priority (Status I) is accorded to hospitalized patients requiring assist devices or intravenous inotropic therapy in intensive care units; all other patients are Status II. In the year 2000, 56.6% of heart transplant recipients were reported to be on life support at the time of transplantation, of which 32.3% were in the intensive care unit (2).

The main goal during the prebypass period is to maintain adequate end-organ perfusion. However, in these patients with end-stage heart failure, cardiovascular decompensation during induction or maintenance of anesthesia can result from multiple mechanisms. Decreases in sympathetic outflow (especially when the renin-angiotensin system is blocked by ACE-I) with resultant hypotension and impaired coronary perfusion, alterations in preload (hypovolemia from exaggerated diuresis), decreases in heart rate (with absent compensatory preload reserve), or increases in pulmonary vascular resistance can be extremely deleterious (14).

In these patients with precarious hemodynamic status, TEE is ideally suited to evaluate and guide intraoperative management decisions in the pretransplantation period. A complete TEE examination will often reveal information not readily available from other sources. Some examples follow.

## Left Ventricular (LV) Volume

Due to a right shift in the left ventricular pressure-volume relationship, the failing heart requires a larger preload to maintain marginal performance. Moreover, superimposed diastolic dysfunction results in a poor correlation between LV filling pressures and volumes, further compounded by the effects of positive-pressure ventilation. Thus, optimization of left ventricular filling is best achieved by monitoring LV volumes under TEE guidance.

## Left Ventricular Contractility

Performed in conjunction with the assessment of LV preload, monitoring global LV systolic function in the pretransplantation period may help achieve hemodynamic stability in the face of reductions in sympathetic outflow associated with induction of anesthesia, by guiding the adjustments in inotropic infusions.

## Intracavitary Thrombus

Particular attention should be paid to the LV apex, the most common site for ventricular thrombus associated with cardiomyopathy or apical infarcts. The left atrial appendage should be inspected for possible thrombi, especially in atrial fibrillation. If intracavitary thrombi are identified, manipulation of the heart should be limited and dissection should proceed with great caution prior to cardiopulmonary bypass to avoid systemic embolization (Fig. 36.1).

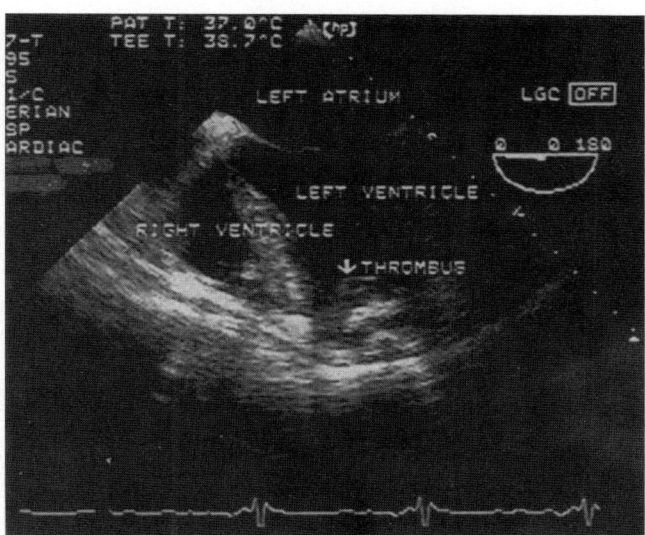

**FIGURE 36.1.** Transesophageal echocardiography image of laminated intraventricular thrombus in the native left ventricular apex. From Quinlan JJ, et al. Anesthesia for heart, lung, and heart-lung transplantation. In Kaplan JA, ed. Cardiac Anesthesia, 4th ed.: Philadelphia: WB Saunders, 1999: 461, with permission.

## Atherosclerosis of the Ascending Aorta and Aortic Arch

Aortic atheroma burden is assessed well by TEE, and should guide aortic cannulation site and cross-clamp placement. The ascending aorta and aortic arch can be assessed in the midesophageal aortic valve long-axis, ascending aortic short-axis and long-axis views, and in the upperesophageal aortic arch long-axis and short-axis views (18). The descending aorta is also assessed for the presence of mobile atheroma, in case an intraaortic balloon pump is required posttransplant. This can be achieved in the descending aortic short-axis and long-axis views (18).

## Right Ventricular Dilation or Hypertrophy

Their presence would be suggestive of long-standing pulmonary hypertension, and should heighten the awareness for possible acute RV dysfunction in the transplanted heart.

## Assessment of Left Ventricular Assist Device (LVAD) Explant

In patients who required mechanical circulatory assistance as a bridge to transplant, microperforations can occur at the time of LVAD explant, during the lengthy dissection onto the inlet cannula and its connections. This can result in air entrainment and subsequent ejection into the aorta (17). TEE monitoring for such an event can be performed in the midesophageal aortic valve long-axis view (18). (See Chapter 35.)

## Hemodynamic Calculations

Most cardiac anesthesiologists agree that a pulmonary artery catheter (PAC) is useful in the hemodynamic evaluation of patients undergoing cardiac transplantation. However, floating the PAC into correct position may be difficult due to cardiac chamber dilation and severe tricuspid regurgitation. Furthermore, PAC placement may be more prone to induce dysrhythmias, resulting in rapid hemodynamic decompensation in these patients with marginal cardiovascular reserve. Consequently, the PAC may be placed in a sterile sheath with the tip advanced to the end of the cordis introducer, during the prebypass period, and subsequently advanced by the surgeon under direct vision before the completion of the right atrial anastomosis. This minimizes the risk of blindly passing the PAC across fresh surgical suture lines. When a PAC cannot be placed, TEE can be used to determine the cardiac output and pulmonary artery pressures in the prebypass period.

The area-length formula can be used to calculate the stroke volume (SV) across a cardiac valve:

$$SV = \text{cross-sectional area (CSA)} \times \text{velocity time integral (VTI)}$$

The SV across a valve can be subsequently used to calculate the cardiac output (CO) if there is no stenosis and/or regurgitation across that valve. Because most of these patients with dilated cardiomyopathies present with various degrees of mitral regurgitation, the aortic valve is usually used for CO measurements. The left ventricular outflow tract (LVOT) diameter is measured from the midesophageal aortic valve long-axis view; the $LVOT_{VTI}$ is measured from the LVOT Doppler spectrum in the transgastric long-axis or deep transgastric long-axis views, which provide windows for continuous wave Doppler interrogation, that is nearly parallel to aortic flow (18). The final formula for CO (in L/min) becomes:

$$CO = 0.785 \, (\text{LVOT diameter})^2 \times LVOT_{VTI} \times \text{heart rate}/1000$$

This TEE determination of CO in the prebypass period should be performed even if the PAC has been successfully advanced into the pulmonary artery, because most of these patients present with various degrees of tricuspid regurgitation, which renders thermodilution cardiac output measurements inaccurate (19).

Doppler echocardiography is an ideal tool for determining pulmonary artery pressures. In the presence of tricuspid regurgitation (TR), the systolic pulmonary artery pressure (PAS) can be calculated using the simplified Bernoulli equation from the peak velocity of the TR jet ($V_{TR}$, measured by continuous wave Doppler in the midesophageal right ventricular inflow-outflow view) (18), and the central venous pressure (CVP) as:

$$PAS = 4 \, (V_{TR})^2 + CVP$$

In the presence of pulmonic regurgitation (PR), the diastolic pulmonary artery pressure (PAD) can be calculated in similar fashion, using the end-diastolic velocity of the PR jet ($V_{PR}$, measured by continuous wave Doppler in the upperesophageal aortic arch short-axis view), and the CVP as:

$$PAD = 4 \, (V_{PR})^2 + CVP$$

As with all Doppler measurements, the ultrasound beam must be parallel to the regurgitant flows or the velocities (hence the PA pressures) will be underestimated.

## Intraoperative Monitoring in the Posttransplantation Period

The pathophysiology of the transplanted heart is dependent upon several factors, including the amount of donor inotropic support, the degree of subclinical myocardial damage, the ischemic time, the myocardial protection during the ischemic interval, cardiac denervation, and the degree of pulmonary hypertension in the recipient.

## Assisting with Venting and De-Airing Maneuvers

Prior to weaning from cardiopulmonary bypass (CPB), TEE is used to detect retained intracardiac air and to assist the de-airing maneuvers. The most common sites of air retention are the right and left upper pulmonary veins, the LV apex, the left atrium, and the right coronary sinus of Valsalva (20). Reports of acute RV dysfunction caused by air embolization to the right coronary artery exist in the literature (21). Detection of echogenic material by TEE in the left atrium or left ventricle after the heart is allowed to fully eject, followed by RV dilatation, loss of contraction, and ST segment changes in inferior leads should raise the suspicion of right coronary air embolus. Full CPB should be reinstituted and the coronary perfusion elevated to allow the dissolution of the coronary embolus. Without the aid of TEE, the real cause of RV dysfunction in this scenario may be missed (see also "Assessment of the Right Ventricle," below).

In the majority of cardiac transplantations, separation from CPB is readily achieved. After separation from cardiopulmonary bypass, TEE allows for the online assessment of biventricular function and flow dynamics across the surgical anastomoses, with important diagnostic and prognostic implications.

## Assessment of the Left Ventricle

The global and segmental LV systolic function should be assessed in the midesophageal four-chamber, two-chamber, and long-axis views, as well as in the transgastric mid short-axis, basal short-axis, and long-axis views (18). To minimize intra- and interobserver variability, the LV fractional area change should always be measured in the transgastric midpapillary muscle short-axis tomographic plane, by manually tracing the endocardial border, or defined with an automated border detection system. Intraoperative TEE assessment of allograft LV systolic function early after separation from cardiopulmonary bypass (CPB), in contrast to routinely measured hemodynamic variables, has been shown to better predict early requirements for inotropic and mechanical support, particularly in patients with longer ischemic times (22).

The following 2D-echocardiographic findings of the LV, which would be considered abnormal in the general population, are characteristic of transplant recipients:

- An increase in LV wall thickness (especially the posterior and septal walls), LV mass, and LV mass index may be observed. It has been hypothesized to represent myocardial edema, resulting from the manipulation and transport of the heart (23–25).
- Paradoxical or flat interventricular septal motion, and decreased interventricular septal systolic thickening compared to normals (31% vs. 44%) (23).
- Because the donor heart is normal in size, it is typically smaller than the original dilated failing heart and, therefore, it is positioned more medially in the mediastinum and tends to be rotated clockwise. This usually necessitates nonstandard transducer locations and angles for echocardiography. Residual fluid accumulations in the posterior pericardial space contribute to the common small postoperative pericardial effusions (30).

## Assessment of LV Diastolic Function

The postischemic condition of the allograft decreases diastolic compliance of both ventricles, necessitating greater than normal filling pressures to adequately preload the heart. The echocardiographic assessment of LV diastolic function in the transplanted heart is complicated by the variability of the Doppler velocity profiles from the atrioventricular valves, which may be observed when the remnant recipient atria retain mechanical activity. This results in asynchronous atrial contractions, modifying the filling patterns of both ventricles (23–27). The beat-to-beat variations in transmitral (and tricuspid) diastolic velocities, assessed by pulsed wave Doppler, relate to the timing of contraction of the recipient atria within the cardiac cycle. Therefore, it is important to locate the recipient P waves within the donor cardiac cycle before making the required Doppler measurements. When the recipient P waves occur between late systole and mitral valve opening, the flow signals should not be used to measure diastolic indices. Recipient P waves occurring during this time frame decrease isovolumic relaxation time and pressure half time, and increase the mitral inflow peak E-wave velocity. If the recipient P waves occur anywhere from late diastole through midsystole, the flow signals may be used (23,24,26) (Table 36.1).

Several studies have demonstrated an abnormal transmitral flow pattern compatible with restrictive diastolic LV dysfunction in orthotopic heart transplant recipients (reduced late maximum flow velocity, increased early-to-late diastolic maximum flow velocity ratio) (25,28). Similarly, an abnormal pulmonary venous flow pattern, characterized by reduced peak flow velocity and reduced time velocity integral in the systolic phase with relatively enhanced flow during the diastolic phase has been observed (22,28). This decreased systolic to diastolic maximum pulmonary venous flow velocity ratio, found despite normal pulmonary capillary wedge pressures and associated with a reduced left atrial area change and a reduced mitral annulus motion is suggestive of left atrial dysfunction (25) secondary to altered atrial anatomy and dynamics

▶ TABLE 36.1. **Mitral Inflow Doppler Velocities**

| *Timing of Recipient Atrial Contraction* | *Peak E-Wave* | *Peak A-Wave* | *Isovolumic Relaxation Time* | *Deceleration Time* |
|---|---|---|---|---|
| Early diastole | Normal | Decreased | Normal | Normal |
| Late diastole | Normal | Increased | Normal | Normal |
| Early systole | Decreased | Normal | Normal | Increased |
| Late systole | Increased | Normal | Decreased | Decreased |
| Overall E/A variability (%) | 28 ± 15 | | | |

Modified from Suriani RJ. Transesophageal echocardiography during organ transplantation. J Cardiothorac Vasc Anesth 1998;12(6):686–98 and Bouchart F, Derumeaux G, Mouton-Schleifer D, et al. Conventional and total orthotopic cardiac transplantation: a comparative clinical and echocardiographical study. Eur J Cardiothorac Surg 1997;12:555–9, with permission.

(29). Beat-to-beat variability of all pulmonary venous flow parameters was found to be higher in transplant recipients than in controls, especially in the systolic phase parameters (25).

Therefore, mitral Doppler inflow analysis alone appears to be inadequate for the assessment of diastolic LV function in heart transplant recipients, as LV diastolic dysfunction cannot be differentiated from atrial dysfunction, and should be therefore corroborated with the analysis of pulmonary venous flow patterns. The assessment is further complicated by the various pacing modalities used in the perioperative period.

## Assessment of the Right Ventricle

### Etiology, Pathophysiology, and Diagnosis of Acute RV Dysfunction

Despite advances in perioperative management, ISHLT registry data show that right ventricular (RV) dysfunction accounts for 50% of all cardiac complications and 19% of all early deaths in patients after heart transplantation (1). Acute RV dysfunction in heart transplant recipients is of multifactorial etiology, resulting either from an increase in pulmonary vascular resistance (PVR) in the recipient, or from a loss of contractility in the donor heart (9,31).

Recipient pulmonary hypertension represents an important risk factor for acute RV failure and for other postoperative morbidity (posttransplant infections, arrhythmias) (31), and is attributed to the inability of the donor RV myocardium to acutely compensate for the recipient's elevated PVR (9). Pulmonary hemodynamic indices represent a spectrum of values associated with postoperative mortality, but this relationship is by no means linear. The literature confirms the absence of threshold hemodynamic values beyond which RV failure is certain to occur and heart transplantation is contraindicated; there are no values below which RV failure is always avoidable (31). Although patients with preoperative fixed pulmonary hypertension are excluded from cardiac transplantation, unfortunately normal preoperative PVR does not rule out the potential for pulmonary hypertension and acute RV failure after heart transplantation, resulting from the effects of cardiopulmonary bypass on the pulmonary circulation, the administration of protamine, or from the simple act of awakening from anesthesia (24,31).

A loss of contractility in the donor heart may be related to the myocardial changes occurring after brain death, which is known to be associated with donor organ dysfunction, cardiovascular deterioration, and metabolic and hormonal changes (7–9). Additionally, adaptation by the donor heart may be impaired by ischemia, reperfusion injury associated with organ preservation, and the deleterious effects that CPB has upon ventricular func-

tion. As mentioned above, acute RV dysfunction can occasionally be caused by air embolization to the right coronary artery (21). This is usually a transient event, and the recovery is uneventful with reinstitution of full CPB.

Irrespective of its etiology, acute RV failure after heart transplantation results in further dilation, ischemia, and decreased contractility. Decreased pulmonary blood flow and leftward shift of the interventricular septum subsequently leads to reduced LV filling and decreased systemic cardiac output.

The complex geometry of the RV, further compounded by the inadequate definition of the RV free wall, makes direct echocardiographic assessment of RV function difficult. Numerous methods of assessing the RV have been developed, including geometry-dependent (i.e., relying on models that assume a specific geometric shape, planimetry), geometry-independent [tricuspid annular plane systolic excursion (TAPSE), Doppler echocardiography, Myocardial Performance Index], quantitative (RV ejection fraction), or qualitative methods (septal curvature, real-time visual assessment) (24,32). (See Chapter 11.)

Planimetry of the RV is performed in the midesophageal four-chamber view or in the transgastric mid short-axis view, with the endocardial border manually traced or defined by an automated border detection system (acoustic quantification, Fig. 36.2). Comparison of serial

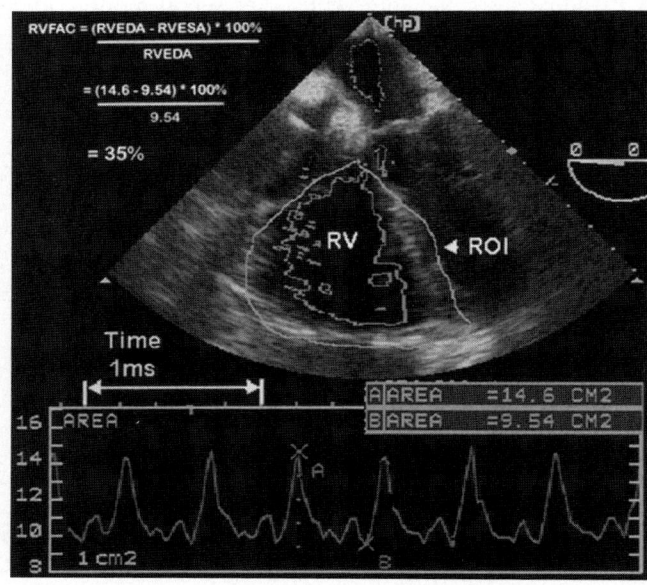

**FIGURE 36.2.** Midesophageal four-chamber view with automatic border detection and region of interest (ROI) around the right ventricle (RV). The area-versus-time curve is used to generate end-diastolic (**A**) and end-systolic (**B**) right ventricular areas (RVEDA, RVESA). The equation is then used to calculate right ventricular fractional area change as a percentage (RVFAC). From Scalia GM, et al. Clinical utility of echocardiography in the management of implantable ventricular assist devices. J Am Soc Echocardiogr 2000;13:757, with permission.

measurements is difficult because of the irregularity of RV anatomy and difficulty in ensuring that the same tomographic plane is obtained during each measurement (24).

The use of tricuspid annular plane systolic excursion (TAPSE) to estimate RV function is based on the concept that, during RV systole, lengthwise shortening of both the interventricular septum and the RV free wall occur. The technique was found to closely correlate with RV ejection fraction (RVEF) as measured by radionuclide angiography (RVEF = 3.2*TAPSE), and attempts to avoid the geometric assumptions involved in extrapolating two-dimensional measurements (i.e., planimetry) to RV volumes (32). TAPSE is measured in the midesophageal four-chamber view as the excursion (in mm) of the junction point of the tricuspid valve with the RV free wall between end-diastole and end-systole.

The maximum acceleration of blood in the pulmonary artery can be used as an index of RV ejection. This can be obtained in the midesophageal ascending aortic short-axis view, where the main pulmonary artery is nearly parallel to the spectral Doppler beam. The maximum acceleration of pulmonary blood flow is defined as the tangent to the upstroke of the velocity profile and is easily measured using the internal calculation software in most echocardiographic machines. Changes in the maximum acceleration of blood in the pulmonary artery have been shown to correlate with changes in the thermodilution RVEF (33).

The RV function can be qualitatively assessed by visually estimating the RV size, the systolic motion of RV free wall, and RVEF, and by examining the interventricular septum for systolic thickening and paradoxical curvature in the midesophageal four-chamber view and in the transgastric mid short-axis view. Normally, the septum bulges from left to right due to the higher left-sided interventricular pressure, but this situation can be reversed during acute RV dysfunction, when the right-sided interventricular pressure exceeds the left ventricular pressure (34). Paradoxical septal shift occurs in late diastole with RV volume overload and at end-systole and early diastole with RV pressure overload (24,35).

### Management of Acute RV Dysfunction

Goals in the treatment of acute RV failure include:

- Preserving coronary perfusion through maintenance of aortic pressure
- Optimizing RV preload
- Reducing RV afterload by decreasing PVR
- Limiting pulmonary vasoconstriction through ventilation with high-inspired oxygen concentrations, increased tidal volume, and optimal PEEP ventilation

Optimizing RV preload should be performed under echocardiographic guidance to avoid overdistending an ischemic RV, and in conjunction with central venous pressure and serial cardiac output measurements. In-

otropes and inodilators are often used to increase RV contractility and decrease PVR. Isoproterenol and phosphodiesterase III inhibitors (milrinone) are the mainstays of therapy, often in combination with alpha-adrenergic agonists (norepinephrine) to maintain systemic vascular resistance and coronary perfusion. Inhaled nitric oxide can be used immediately after heart transplantation to prevent or to treat RV failure, due to its potent, rapidly acting, and selective pulmonary vasodilator properties. Additionally, inhaled nitric oxide can improve hypoxemia by optimizing the ventilation-perfusion relationship.

Intraaortic balloon counterpulsation (IABP) can be employed in patients with LV dysfunction, and may be of benefit in patients with acute RV dysfunction resulting from ischemia, preservation injury, or reperfusion injury. In acute RV failure, RV hypertension and distension may cause reduced coronary blood flow to the RV and impair LV function by reduced filling and altered septal dynamics. In the setting of early postoperative low cardiac output syndrome characterized predominantly by RV failure, IABP placement has been shown to improve hemodynamics and peripheral tissue perfusion (36). The mechanisms involved include improved myocardial perfusion through enhanced coronary filling and improved LV mechanics through afterload reduction. Optimal LV function ultimately indirectly relieves RV dysfunction through reduced RV afterload and PVR (31) and improved ventricular interdependence (36).

The decision regarding RV assist device implantation is dependent upon a stepwise review of overall hemodynamics after the institution of maximal inotropic and vasodilator support. The assessment includes an evaluation of the size and function of both ventricles by TEE, the status of mediastinal bleeding, oxygenation, presence of arrhythmias, and urine output. This assessment usually takes place after several unsuccessful attempts to separate the patient from CPB and approximately one hour after removal of the aortic cross clamp. The observation of a small hyperdynamic LV and a dilated RV by TEE, marginal urine output, arrhythmias, or coagulopathy should prompt the insertion of a RV assist device. The presence of coagulopathy will require ongoing volume resuscitation with blood products, likely resulting in a worsening of pulmonary hypertension, pulmonary edema, and RV failure with its secondary effects on cardiac output and end organ perfusion. Reduction of elevated right-sided pressures following RV assist device implantation is a positive predictor for survival (31). Still, the need for RV mechanical assistance after heart transplantation increases the early mortality to over 50% (37).

### Assessment of the Atria and Atrial Anastomoses

The vast majority of heart transplantation procedures are orthotopic, with heterotopic transplants representing only 0.3% of the procedures performed in the year 2000 (2). Three different orthotopic heart transplantation techniques have been described: standard biatrial, bicaval, and total orthotopic heart transplantation (38). The resultant atrial size and geometry, and the donor-recipient atrial anastomoses are entirely dependent upon the transplantation technique employed. TEE is ideally suited to assess the interatrial septum, atrial free walls, and atrial appendages in the transplanted heart, providing unique information on the sites of atrial anastomoses. This should be performed in the midesophageal four-chamber, two-chamber, and midesophageal bicaval views (18).

In the standard biatrial orthotopic heart transplant technique, originally described by Lower and Shumway, the posterior and lateral portions of the recipient atria and the posterior part of the interatrial septum are left in situ and serve to anchor the corresponding parts of the donor atria. Thus, the size and geometry of both atria are remodeled during the operation (29), and several anatomic and functional abnormalities occur in the recipients. These include biatrial enlargement, asynchronous contraction of the donor and recipient atria, and intraluminal protrusion of the atrial anastomoses, creating distorted "hour-glass" or "snowman" configurations of the new atria (29,38). The atrial suture lines appear prominently as echodense ridges, which give mass-like effects in the atria (24,39,40), are nonmobile and nonpedunculated, and should not be confused with thrombi (Fig. 36.3). These anastomotic protrusions are particularly prominent at the left atrial (LA) free wall and, occasionally, systolic contact between the protruding suture and the posterior mitral leaflet has been reported to occur

(29). Stenotic LA suture lines, causing hemodynamically significant obstruction to blood flow with systemic hypotension and elevated pulmonary artery pressures, have been described in the literature (41–45), and are due to a mismatch of the donor and recipient LA cuff circumferences, worsened by a purse-string effect of the anastomotic suture line. The deformity has been coined *acquired cor triatriatum* (43–45) due to the similarity to the congenital cardiac anomaly in which the LA is subdivided into two chambers by a perforated fibromuscular septum (Fig. 36.4). Occasionally, acquired cor triatriatum can result from an infolding of redundant donor (44) or recipient (45) LA tissue and not the atrial suture line. Intraoperative TEE is clinically crucial in identifying such stenotic suture lines or tissue infoldings, prompting early surgical revision. In the midesophageal four-chamber or two-chamber views, TEE reveals a markedly enlarged atrial remnant with a reduced LV volume, and the suture line protrusion can be measured. Additionally, detection of turbulent flow by color flow Doppler, "fluttering" of the mitral valve leaflets, and elevated transstenotic blood-flow velocities by pulsed wave Doppler confirm the presence of a LA pressure gradient and LV inflow obstruction (43). Failure to identify such LV inflow obstruction may result in unexplained pulmonary hypertension and RV failure in the early postoperative period.

Most heart transplant recipients show some phasic excursion of the interatrial septum during the cardiac cycle. This cyclic septal motion is called "pseudoaneurysm" if a portion of the atrial septum bulges at least 10 mm beyond the atrial septal plane and if the base of the bulging part is at least 15 mm in diameter (46). By

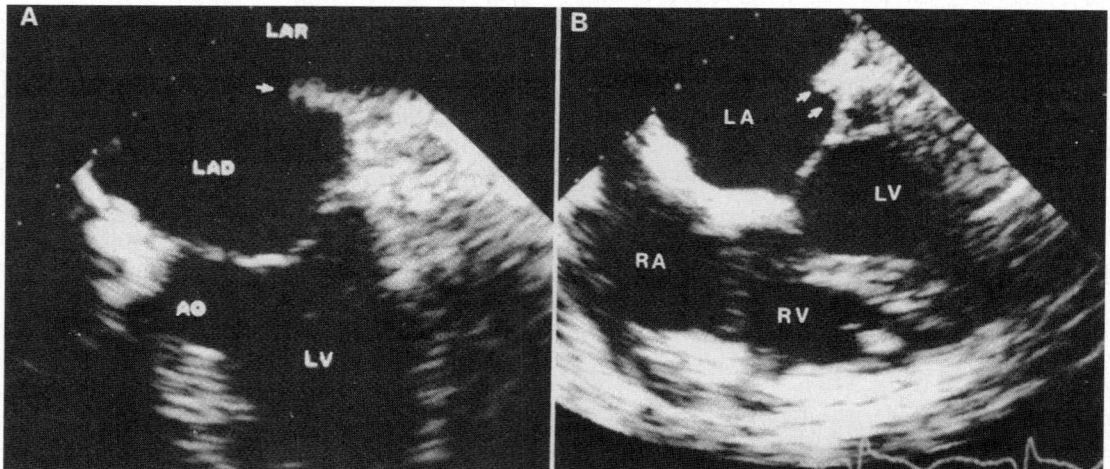

**FIGURE 36.3.** **A:** Prominent suture (*arrow*) between the donor (*LAD*) and recipient (*LAR*) components of left atrium (LA). **B:** Systolic contact (*arrows*) between posterior mitral valve leaflet and suture. *AO*, aortic root; *LV*, left ventricle; *RV*, right ventricle; *RA*, right atrium. From Angermann CE, et al. Anatomic characteristics and valvular function of the transplanted heart: transthoracic versus transesophageal echocardiographic findings. J Heart Transplant 1990;9:333, with permission.

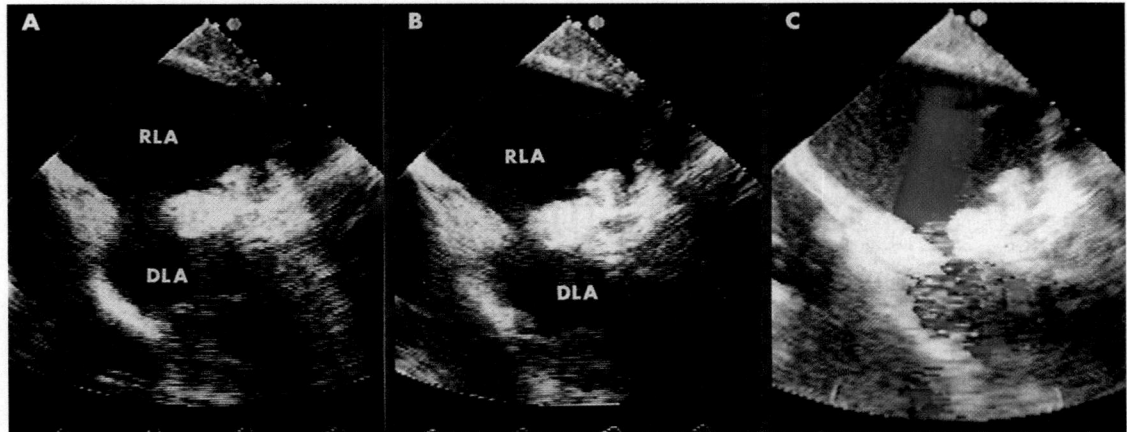

**FIGURE 36.4.** Acquired cor triatriatum. **A:** Intraoperative transesophageal echocardiography (TEE) image of recipient left atrium (*RLA*) and donor left atrium (*DLA*) during systole. **B:** Intraoperative TEE image during diastole shows the dynamic narrowing of the intraatrial channel. **C:** TEE image during diastole with color flow Doppler imaging of the intraarterial channel. From Bjerke RJ, et al. Early diagnosis and follow-up by echocardiography of acquired cor triatriatum after orthotopic heart transplantation. J Heart Lung Transplant 1992;11:1073–7.

these criteria, the incidence of posttransplant atrial septal pseudoaneurysms in one study was 35% (29). The integrity of the interatrial septum should be assessed intraoperatively by using both color flow Doppler and contrast echocardiography (saline microcavitation). Shunts can occur either at the atrial anastomotic site or through a patent foramen ovale (PFO) in the recipient atrial septum. Although uncommon, right-to-left shunting through a PFO that is not apparent preoperatively may become hemodynamically significant postoperatively as the relative pressure difference between the atria changes because of RV dysfunction or tricuspid regurgitation, and can present as refractory postoperative hypoxemia (47). Identification of a left-to-right shunt across the interatrial anastomosis should also prompt surgical repair, as it can contribute to progressive RV volume overload and tricuspid regurgitation (39).

Dissociation of the mechanical performance of recipient and donor atria, a consequence of the persisting independent electrical activity in both atrial components, can be visualized by TEE and has important implications for both left and right heart function. Several studies have reported LA spontaneous echo contrast (SEC) in heart transplant recipients (27,29,39,40,48). The combination of disturbed atrial hemodynamics caused by asynchronous contraction of the atria and atrial enlargement might contribute to slow blood flow within the atrial cavities and explain the relatively high incidence of SEC (25%–55%) despite normal ventricular function in these patients (27,29,39,40). This is usually confined to the donor atrial component and is characterized by multiple microechoes slowly swirling within the enlarged atrial

cavity and disappearing after passage through the mitral valve. SEC is visible at normal gain settings, and the characteristic motion pattern allows clear discrimination from noise echoes or reverberations (29). The importance of diagnosing LA SEC in heart transplant recipients stems from its association with LA thrombi and systemic embolic events on postoperative follow-up studies (29,40,48). In most cases, the thrombi are attached to the atrial free wall underneath the protruding suture in a niche formed after partial removal of the left atrial appendage during transplantation (29,40), but can also be localized on the posterior LA wall or on the suture line (27). Occasionally, protruding suture ends, endocardial tags, or other tissue remnants may have an echocardiographic appearance of thrombus-like structures (Fig. 36.5). Therefore, the presence of LA SEC on intraoperative TEE should prompt postoperative follow-up studies to assess for the presence of atrial thrombi and the need for antiplatelet or anticoagulation therapy.

Previous studies have demonstrated that synchronous atrial contraction is an important compensatory response to RV dysfunction (49). Intact right atrial function may be important in preventing the development of RV failure after orthotopic heart transplantation or in limiting its severity, particularly in patients with elevated pulmonary vascular resistance (38).

In 1990, Reitz (49b) introduced the bicaval anastomotic technique at Stanford University, as a modification of the standard biatrial technique. Using this technique, the donor and recipient superior and inferior venae cavae are anastomosed in an end-to-end fashion, completely avoiding a right atrial suture line. Several reports confirm

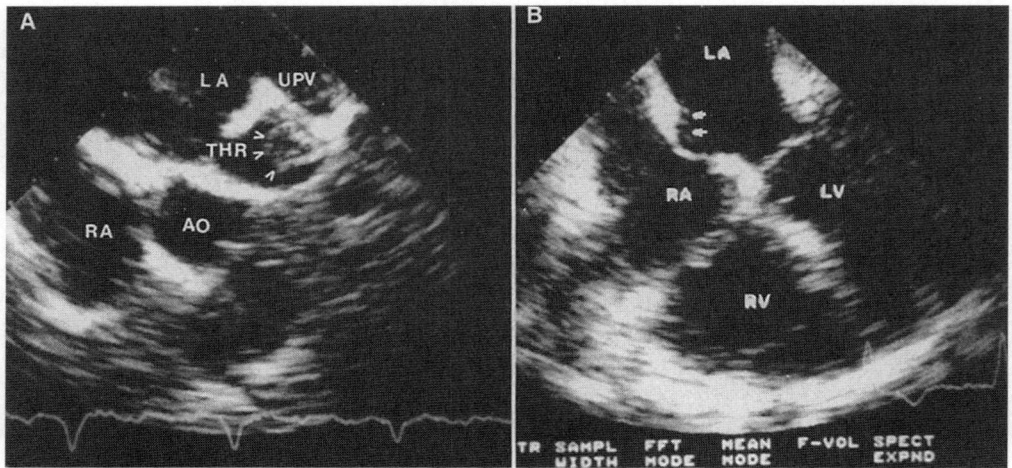

**FIGURE 36.5.** **A:** Atrial thrombus (*THR*) attached to the left atrial (*LA*) free wall. **B:** Small thrombus-like structures (*arrows*) attached to atrial septum. *UPV,* upper pulmonary vein; *RA,* right atrium; *RV,* right ventricle; *LV,* left ventricle; *AO,* aortic root. From Angermann CE et al. Anatomic characteristics and valvular function of the transplanted heart: transthoracic versus transesophageal echocardiographic findings. J Heart Transplant 1990;9:335, with permission.

that the bicaval technique improves atrial function, decreases atrial conduction abnormalities and decreases the incidence of tricuspid regurgitation (50,51). When combined with an everting suture for the left atrial anastomosis, the incidence of left atrial SEC and subsequent left atrial thrombi and systemic embolic events on postoperative follow-up is decreased (48).

In an attempt to further minimize left and right atrial dysfunction and electrophysiologic abnormalities, Dreyfus (51b) and Yacoub (51c) devised a technique of total orthotopic heart transplantation. This technique incorporates the bicaval anastomosis for the implantation of the right atrium and a direct anastomosis between the donor and recipient pulmonary veins to implant the left atrium. Thus, an anatomic replacement of the heart is achieved (38), with normal atrial morphology and normal atrioventricular interactions. When compared to the standard technique, total heart transplantation significantly reduces the incidence of postoperative rhythm disturbances and pacemaker dependence, atrioventricular valve regurgitation (38), and left atrial SEC and thrombi (27).

## Assessment of the Pulmonary Artery (PA) Anastomosis

The main PA anastomosis should be evaluated for stenosis or possible kinking or torsion by 2D-echocardiography, color flow Doppler to detect turbulent flow, and by continuous wave Doppler to measure the pressure gradient across the anastomosis. The main PA can be imaged in the midesophageal RV inflow-outflow or in the midesophageal ascending aortic short-axis views, with the latter offering the best beam alignment for Doppler interrogation (18). Several reports describe PA anastomotic kinking (52) or torsion (53), recognized intraoperatively or early postoperatively, and manifested as elevated RV pressures and high-pressure gradients across the PA anastomoses. The kinking was the result of the excess length of the combined donor and recipient PA segments, whereas PA torsion was related to marked size mismatch between donor and recipient hearts and consequent malalignment of the PA stumps. Occasionally, recipient valve remnants, surface raggedness or protruding suture lines can be identified (41).

## Assessment of the Pulmonary Venous Anastomoses

When the total orthotopic heart transplantation technique is employed, intraoperative TEE assessment of individual pulmonary venous anastomoses should be performed, including pulmonary vein diameter, color flow pattern, and pulsed wave Doppler profile. Identification of hemodynamically significant suture line stenosis or torsion should prompt early surgical revision.

## Assessment of the Atrioventricular Valves

Mild to moderate degrees of mitral and tricuspid regurgitation are commonly found on color flow Doppler imaging after cardiac transplantation. Mitral regurgitation (MR) occurs with an incidence ranging from 48% to 87% depending on the study quoted (29,40,54,55), and is usually mild in severity, with an eccentric jet pointing toward the left atrial free wall. Tricuspid regurgitation (TR), found in 85% of transplant recipients, occurs immediately after heart transplantation, and is usually moderate, with an eccentric jet direction pointing toward the interatrial septum (29,55). We found no association between the incidence and severity of TR immediately after cardiac transplantation and the presence of RV dysfunction (56). Quantification of the severity of TR by color flow Doppler is best achieved using the ratio of the maximum area of the regurgitant jet to the right atrial area (57). This method has been validated in heart transplant recipients, and was found to correlate better with the thermodilution-derived tricuspid regurgitant fraction than the maximum jet area or the maximum jet length (Table 36.2) (58). Still, the area of the color Doppler regurgitant jet may be underestimated because of jet eccentricity.

The etiology of atrioventricular valve regurgitation in the transplanted heart is still controversial, but because no structural valvular abnormalities could be found, it is thought to be caused by the distorted atrial geometry and the tension generated on the muscular parts of the annuli by the enlarged atria (29,55). With the standard biatrial technique, donor-recipient size mismatch is more evident on the right atrial side because the LA anastomosis is performed first, allowing a better degree of adaptation of the LA walls, and might explain the higher incidence of TR in the transplanted heart (55). The severity of posttransplant TR correlates with echocardiographic indices of atrial distortion (recipient to donor atrial area ratio) and the systolic shortening of the tricuspid annulus (55). The significantly reduced incidence of moderate and severe TR with the bicaval anastomotic technique (50,51,59,60), and both TR and MR after total orthotopic heart transplantation (38), further supports this hypothesis. Distortion of the tricuspid annulus may also be caused by a size mismatch of the donor heart and recipient pericardial cavity. In one study, if greater than mild TR was detected by intraoperative echocardiography after discontinuation of CPB, pericardial reduction plasty was performed that successfully prevented TR up to 8 weeks of follow-up (61). Yet other investigators suggested that multivalvular regurgitation observed after heart transplantation might be a result of mild edema of the cardiac structures, as they found a significant LV mass reduction within the first postoperative weeks with a progressive resolution of valvular regurgitation (62). The natural history of these regurgitant lesions varies, but the incidence of severe TR

▶ **TABLE 36.2. Ratio of Jet Area to Right Atrial Area**

Trivial TR < 10%
Mild TR 10%–24%
Moderate TR 25%–49%
Severe TR ≥ 50%

From Chan MCY, Giannetti N, Kato T, et al. Severe tricuspid regurgitation after heart transplantation. J Heart Lung Transplant 2001;20:709–17, with permission.

appears to increase with time, and some patients may require tricuspid valve replacement for refractory symptoms (57).

Rarely, MR secondary to systolic anterior motion (SAM) of the anterior mitral valve leaflet has been reported after heart transplantation (63). This might be caused or aggravated by the common use of the β-adrenergic agonist isoproterenol, with resultant vasodilation, tachycardia, and increased myocardial contractility, along with iatrogenic hypovolemia to prevent graft distension, and increased LV wall thickness observed in the transplanted heart. Intraoperative TEE diagnosis of SAM of the anterior mitral valve leaflet with associated MR is facilitated by the systematic assessment of the mitral valve and left ventricular outflow tract (LVOT) in the midesophageal five-chamber, midesophageal aortic valve long-axis and transgastric long-axis views (18). Characteristic features include SAM of the anterior mitral valve leaflet, mid-systolic notching of the aortic valve, posteriorly directed MR jet, flow turbulence at the site of LVOT obstruction with a dagger-shaped continuous wave Doppler tracing and significant LVOT pressure gradient (> 50 mm Hg). These findings should be managed by optimizing the LV volume, changing the inotrope to one with more α-adrenergic effects (e.g., isoproterenol to dopamine) to decrease the heart rate and increase the afterload, and follow-up echocardiographic assessments of SAM and MR.

## MANAGEMENT OF EARLY POSTOPERATIVE HEMODYNAMIC ABNORMALITIES IN THE INTENSIVE CARE UNIT

TEE has become an invaluable tool in the management of seriously ill intensive care unit patients in whom transthoracic acoustic images may be particularly poor. Particular uses in these circumstances include assessment of biventricular function, anastomotic problems (kinks, torsions, stenoses), valvular abnormalities, sources of systemic emboli, and the exclusion of pericardial fluid. (See Chapters 21 and 23.)

## POSTOPERATIVE FOLLOW-UP STUDIES OF CARDIAC ALLOGRAFT FUNCTION

Echocardiography plays an increasingly important role in the follow-up of recipients after cardiac transplantation as one of the most important potential noninvasive means of diagnosing transplant rejection. Proposed echocardiographic indicators of rejection in cardiac transplantation include:

- Increasing LV mass/LV wall thickness
- Increased myocardial echogenicity
- New or increasing pericardial effusion
- A > 10% decrease in LV ejection fraction

- Restrictive LV filling pattern (> 20% decrease in MV pressure half-time, 20% decrease in isovolumic relaxation time)
- New onset MR

Additionally, two-dimensional echocardiography may be utilized to guide transvenous endomyocardial biopsies and prevent inadvertent damage to the tricuspid valve and its supporting apparatus. Dobutamine stress echocardiography has been used in the detection of allograft vasculopathy and has a high negative predictive value for determining future cardiac events and death in heart transplant recipients (64).

## KEY POINTS

- Cardiac transplantation has become the gold standard treatment of advanced heart failure in selected patients during the last 20 years, but the numerical disparity between donors and recipients continues to increase.
- In an effort to expand the donor criteria, transesophageal echocardiography (TEE) is a useful adjunct to transthoracic echocardiography in the screening of brain-dead potential cardiac donors when the latter is technically inadequate.
- In the pretransplantation period, intraoperative TEE is useful in maintaining cardiovascular stability, performing hemodynamic calculations, and monitoring ventricular assist explantation.
- In the posttransplantation period, intraoperative TEE assists with the de-airing maneuvers, the assessment of global and regional left ventricular systolic and diastolic function, the diagnosis and management of acute right ventricular dysfunction, and should be used in the decision to institute mechanical support for the failing allograft; moreover, intraoperative TEE can be used in diagnosing mechanical complications in the transplanted heart by assessing the atrial and pulmonary artery anastomoses.
- It is important to recognize the two-dimensional echocardiographic and Doppler changes characteristic of transplant recipients, to avoid diagnostic errors.
- TEE can be used to manage the hemodynamically unstable heart transplant recipient in the intensive care unit.
- Echocardiography aids in the follow-up assessment of cardiac allograft function as one of the most important noninvasive methods of diagnosing transplant rejection.

## REFERENCES

1. Hosenpud JD, Bennett LE, Keck BM, et al. The registry of the international society for heart and lung transplantation: eighteenth official report-2001. J Heart Lung Transplant 2001;20:805–15.
2. 2001 Annual Report of the U.S. Organ Procurement and Transplantation Network and the Scientific Registry for Transplant Recipients: Transplant Data 1991–2000. Department of Health and Human Services, Health Resources and Services Administration, Office of Special Programs, Division of Transplantation, Rockville, MD; United Network for Organ Sharing, Richmond, VA; University Renal Research and Education Association, Ann Arbor, MI. The data and analyses reported in the 2001 Annual Report of the U.S. Organ Procurement and Transplantation Network and the Scientific Registry of Transplant Recipients have been supplied by UNOS and URREA under contract with HHS. The authors alone are responsible for reporting and interpreting of these data.
3. Livi U, Bortolotti U, Luciani GB, et al. Donor shortage in heart transplantation. Is extension of donor age limits justified? J Thorac Cardiovasc Surg 1994;107:1346–55.
4. Kron IL, Tribble CG, Kern JA, et al. Successful transplantation of marginally acceptable thoracic organs. Ann Surg 1993;217:518–24.
5. Vedrinne JM, Vedrinne C, Coronel B, et al. Transesophageal echocardiographic assessment of left ventricular function in brain-dead patients: are marginally acceptable hearts suitable for transplantation? J Cardiothorac Vasc Anesth 1996;10(6):708–12.
6. Stoddard MF, Longaker RA. The role of transesophageal echocardiography in cardiac donor screening. Am Heart J 1993;125:1676–81.
7. Powner DJ, Hendrich A, Nyhuis A, et al. Changes in serum catecholamine levels in patients who are brain dead. J Heart Lung Transplant 1992;11:1046–53.
8. Shivalkar B, Van Loon J, Wieland W, et al. Variable effects of explosive or gradual increase of intracranial pressure on myocardial structure and function. Circulation 1993;87(1):230–9.
9. Bittner HB, Chen EP, Biswas SS, et al. Right ventricular dysfunction after cardiac transplantation: primarily related to status of donor heart. Ann Thorac Surg 1999;68:1605–11.
10. Seiler C, Laske A, Gallino A, et al. Echographic evaluation of left ventricular wall motion before and after transplantation. J Heart Lung Transplant 1992;11:867–74.
11. Young JB, Hauptman PJ, Naftel DC, et al. Determinants of early graft failure following cardiac transplantation, a 10 year multi-institutional, multi-variable analysis. J Heart Lung Transplant 2001;20:212.
12. Aziz S, Soine LA, Lewis SL, et al. Donor left ventricular hypertrophy increases risk for early graft failure. Transpl Int 1997;10:446–50.
12b. Mudge GH, Goldstein S, Addonizio LJ, et al. 24th Bethesda conference: Cardiac transplantation. Task Force 3: Recipient guidelines/prioritization. J Am Coll Cardiol 1993;22(1):21–31.
13. Dinardo J. Anesthesia for heart, heart-lung and lung transplantation. In Anesthesia for cardiac surgery, 2nd ed. New York: Appleton & Lange, 1998:201–39.
14. Bove A, Santamore W. Ventricular interdependence. Prog Cardiovasc Dis 1981;23:363–88.
15. Stevenson W, Stevenson L, Middlekauff H, et al. Improving survival for patients with advanced heart failure: a study of 737 consecutive patients. J Am Coll Cardiol 1995;26:1417–23.
16. Dickstein M. Anesthesia for heart transplant. Semin Cardiothorac Vasc Anesth 1998;2:131–9.
17. Scalia GM, McCarthy PM, Savage RM, et al. Clinical utility of echocardiography in the management of implantable ventricular assist devices. J Am Soc Echocardiogr 2000;13:754–63.

18. Shanewise JS, Cheung AT, Aronson S, et al ASE/SCA guidelines for performing a comprehensive intraoperative multiplane transesophageal echocardiography examination: recommendations of the American Society of Echocardiography Council for Intraoperative Echocardiography and the Society of Cardiovascular Anesthesiologists Task Force for certification in perioperative transesophageal echocardiography. Anesth Analg 1999;89:870–84.

19. Heerdt P, Pond C, Blessios G, et al. Inaccuracy of cardiac output determination by thermodilution during acute tricuspid regurgitation. Ann Thorac Surg 1992;53:706–8.

20. Orihashi K, Matsuura Y, Hamanaka Y, et al. Retained intracardiac air in open heart operations examined by transesophageal echocardiography. Ann Thorac Surg 1993;55(6):1467–71.

21. Donica SK, Saunders CT, Ramsay MA. Right ventricular dysfunction during cardiac transplantation: an essential role for transesophageal echocardiography. J Cardiothorac Vasc Anesth 1992;6(6):775–6.

22. Kaye DM, Bergin P, Buckland M, et al. Value of postoperative assessment of cardiac allograft function by transesophageal echocardiography. J Heart Lung Transplant 1994;13:165–72.

23. Homans D, Ulstad V. Echocardiography in heart transplantation. In: Letourneau JG, Day DL, Ascher NL, eds. Radiology of organ transplantation. St. Louis: Mosby Year Book, 1991: 308–21.

24. Suriani RJ. Transesophageal echocardiography during organ transplantation. J Cardiothorac Vasc Anesth 1998;12(6):686-94.

25. Spes CH, Tammen AR, Fraser AG, et al. Doppler analysis of pulmonary venous flow profiles in orthotopic heart transplant recipients: a comparison with mitral flow profiles and atrial function. Z Kardiol 1996;85:753–60.

26. Valantine HA, Appleton CP, Hatle LK, et al. Influence of recipient atrial contraction on left ventricular filling dynamics of the transplanted heart assessed by Doppler echocardiography. Am J Cardiol 1987;59:1159–63.

27. Bouchart F, Derumeaux G, Mouton-Schleifer D, et al. Conventional and total orthotopic cardiac transplantation: a comparative clinical and echocardiographical study. Eur J Cardiothorac Surg 1997;12:555–9.

28. St. Goar FG, Gibbons R, Schnittger I, et al. Left ventricular diastolic function—Doppler echocardiographic changes soon after cardiac transplantation. Circulation 1990;82:872–8.

29. Angermann CE, Spes CH, Tammen A, et al. Anatomic characterstics and valvular function of the transplanted heart: transthoracic versus transesophageal findings. J Heart Lung Transplant 1990:9:331–8.

30. Weitzman LB, Tinker WP, Krozon I, et al. The incidence and natural history of pericardial effusion after cardiac surgery; an echocardiographic study. Circulation 1984;69:506–11.

31. Stobierska-Dzierzek B, Awad H, Michler RE. The evolving management of acute right-sided heart failure in cardiac transplant recipients. J Am Coll Cardiol 2001;38:923–31.

32. Kaul S, Tei C, Hopkins JM, et al. Assessment of right ventricular function using two-dimensional echocardiography. Am Heart J 1984;107:526–31.

33. Dickstein ML, Jackson DT, Dephia E, et al. Validation of maximum acceleration of pulmonary blood flow as an index of right ventricular function in the dog, in Proceedings of the Fourteenth Annual Meeting of the Society of Cardiovascular Anesthesiologists, Boston, May 3–6, 1992:191.

34. Ellis J, Lichtor J, Feinstein S, et al. Right heart dysfunction, pulmonary embolism, and paradoxical embolization during liver transplantation. Anesth Analg 1989;68:777–82.

35. Louis EK, Rich S, Levitsky S, et al. Doppler echocardiographic demonstration of the differential effects of right ventricular pressure and volume overload on left ventricular geometry and filling. J Am Coll Cardiol 1992;19:84–90.

36. Arafa OE, Geiran OR, Andersen K, et al. Intraaortic balloon pumping for predominantly right ventricular failure after heart transplantation. Ann Thorac Surg 2000;70:1587–93.

37. Barnard SP, Hasan A, Forty J, et al. Mechanical ventricular assistance for the failing right ventricle after cardiac transplantation. Eur J Cardiothorac Surg 1995;9:297–9.

38. Magliato KE, Trento A. Heart transplantation—surgical results. Heart Failure Rev 2001;6:213–9.

39. Polanco G, Jafri SM, Alam M, et al. Transesophageal echocardiographic findings in patients with orthotopic heart transplantation. Chest 1992;101:599–602.

40. Derumeaux G, Mouton-Schleifer D, Soyer R, et al. High incidence of left atrial thrombus detected by transesophageal echocardiography in heart transplant recipients. Eur Heart J 1995;16:120–5.

41. Wolfsohn AL, Walley VM, Masters RG, et al. The surgical anastomoses after orthotopic heart transplantation: clinical complications and morphologic observations. J Heart Lung Transplant 1994;13:455–65.

42. Ulstad V, Braunlin E, Bass J, et al. Hemodynamically significant suture line obstruction immediately after heart transplantation. J Heart Lung Transplant 1992;11:834–6.

43. Bjerke RJ, Ziady GM, Matesic C, et al. Early diagnosis of acquired cor triatriatum after orthotopic heart transplantation. J Heart Lung Transplant 1992;11:1073–7.

44. Oaks TE, Rayburn BK, Brown ME, et al. Acquired cor triatriatum after orthotopic cardiac transplantation. Ann Thorac Surg 1995;59:751–3.

45. Law Y, Belassario A, West L, et al. Hypertrophied native atrial tissue as a complication of orthotopic heart transplantation. J Heart Lung Transplant 1997;16:922–5.

46. Hanley PC, Tajik AJ, Hynes JK, et al. Diagnosis and classification of atrial septal aneurysm by two-dimensional echocardiography: report of 80 consecutive cases. J Am Coll Cardiol 1985;6:1370–82.

47. Ouseph R, Stoddard MF, Lederer ED. Patent foramen ovale presenting as refractory hypoxemia after heart transplantation. J Am Soc Echocardiogr 1997;10:973–6.

48. Riberi A, Ambrosi P, Habib G, et al. Systemic embolism: a serious complication after cardiac transplantation avoidable by bicaval technique. Eur J Cardiothorac Surg 2001;19:307–12.

49. Goldstein JA, Harada A, Yagi Y. Hemodynamic importance of systolic ventricular interaction, augmented right atrial contractility and atrioventricular synchrony in acute right ventricular dysfunction. J Am Coll Cardiol 1990;16:181–9.

49b. Reitz BA. Heart and lung transplantation. In: Baumgartner WA, Reitz BA, Achuff SC, eds. Heart and heart-lung transplantation. Saunders: Philadelphia, PA, 1990.

50. Deleuze PH, Benvenuti C, Mazucotelli JP, et al. Orthotopic cardiac transplantation with direct caval anastomosis: is it the optimal procedure? J Thorac Cardiovasc Surg 1995; 109:731–7.

51. Leyh R, Jahnke AW, Kraatz EG, et al. Cardiovascular dynamics and dimensions after bicaval and standard cardiac transplantation. Ann Thorac Surg 1995;59:1495–1500.

51b. Dreyfus G, Jebara V, Mihaileanu S, et al. Total orthotopic heart transplantation: an alternative to the standard technique. Ann Thorac Surg 1991;52(5):1181–4.

51c. Yacoub M, Mankad P, Ledingham S. Donor procurement and surgical techniques for cardiac transplantation. Semin Thorac Cardiovasc Surg 1990;2:153–61.

52. Dreyfus G, Jebara VA, Couetil JP, et al. Kinking of the pulmonary artery: a treatable cause of acute right ventricular failure after heart transplantation. J Heart Lung Transplant 1990;9:575–6.

53. De Marchena E, Futterman L, Wozniak P, et al. Pulmonary artery torsion: a potentially lethal complication after orthotopic heart transplantation. J Heart Lung Transplant 1989; 8:499–502.

54. Stevenson LW, Dadourian BJ, Kobashigawa J. Mitral regurgitation after cardiac transplantation. Am J Cardiol 1987;60:119–22.

55. De Simone R, Lange R, Sack FU, et al. Atrioventricular valve insufficiency and atrial geometry after orthotopic heart transplantation. Ann Thorac Surg 1995;60:1686–93.

56. Lombard FW, Swaminathan M, Podgoreanu MV, et al. The association of tricuspid regurgitation with right ventricular dysfunction after cardiac transplant surgery. Anesth Analg 2002;93:SCA66.

57. Chan MCY, Giannetti N, Kato T, et al. Severe tricuspid regurgitation after heart transplantation. J Heart Lung Transplant 2001;20:709–17.

58. Mugge A, Daniel WG, Herrmann G, et al. Quantification of tricuspid regurgitation by Doppler color flow mapping after cardiac transplantation. Am J Cardiol 1990;66(10):884–7.

59. Blanche C, Valenza M, Czer LSC, et al. Orthotopic heart transplantation with bicaval and pulmonary venous anastomoses. Ann Thorac Surg 1994;58:1505–9.

60. Aziz TM, Burgess MI, Rahman AN, et al. Risk factors for tricuspid valve regurgitation after orthotopic heart transplantation. Ann Thorac Surg 1999;68(4):1247–51.

61. Haverich A, Albes JM, Fahrenkamp G, et al. Intraoperative echocardiography to detect and prevent tricuspid valve regurgitation after heart transplantation. Eur J Cardiothorac Surg 1991;5(1):41–5.

62. Cladellas M, Abadal ML, Pons-Llado G, et al. Early transient multivalvular regurgitation detected by pulsed Doppler in cardiac transplantation. Am J Cardiol 1986;58(11):1122–4.

63. Chatel D, Paquin S, Oroudji M, et al. Systolic anterior motion of the anterior mitral leaflet after heart transplantation. Anesthesiology 1999;91:1535–7.

64. Akosah KO, Olsovsky M, Kirchberg D, et al. Dobutamine stress echocardiography predicts cardiac events in heart transplant recipients. Circulation 1996;94(suppl 9):283–8.

## QUESTIONS

1. All of the following are characteristic two-dimensional echocardiographic changes in the left ventricle of transplant recipients *except*:
   A. Septal wall motion abnormalities
   B. Residual posterior pericardial effusion
   C. Altered mediastinal anatomy requiring non-standard TEE transducer locations and angles
   D. Decreased LV wall thickness, LV mass, and LV mass index

2. Which of the following statements regarding the assessment of left ventricular diastolic function in the transplanted heart is true?
   A. Transmitral Doppler velocity profiles should be interpreted as usual in the transplanted heart.
   B. Diastolic indices should be measured in transmitral flow signals generated by recipient P waves occurring in late systole.
   C. Recipient P waves occurring from late diastole through midsystole result in decreased isovolumic relaxation time and pressure half-time.

   D. Transmitral Doppler inflow analysis should be corroborated with pulmonary vein flow analysis to differentiate LV diastolic dysfunction from left atrial dysfunction.

3. Which of the following echocardiographic findings supports an indication for right ventricular assist device (RVAD) implantation in a transplanted heart?
   A. An under-filled, hypocontractile right ventricle
   B. A dilated, hypocontractile RV after administration of protamine in a patient with no preexisting pulmonary hypertension
   C. A small hyperdynamic LV, dilated RV and paradoxical interventricular septal shift, associated with marginal urine output, arrhythmias, or coagulopathy
   D. An acutely dilated, hypocontractile RV associated with electrocardiographic ST segment changes following TEE detection of echogenic material in the left heart

4. Which of the following statements regarding intraoperative TEE detection of left atrial spontaneous echo contrast (SEC) in the transplanted heart is false?
   A. It represents slow blood flow within the atria, caused by a combination of asynchronous contraction and atrial enlargement.
   B. Because it is not associated with systemic embolic events, further postoperative follow-up or therapy are not indicated.
   C. It is characterized by multiple swirling micro-echoes visible at normal gain settings, confined to the donor atrial component, and disappearing after passage through the mitral valve.
   D. The incidence of SEC is highest with the standard bi-atrial orthotopic heart transplant technique.

5. Characteristics of tricuspid regurgitation in transplant recipients include all of the following, *except*:
   A. A ratio of the maximum area of the regurgitant jet to the right atrial area greater than 30% constitutes severe TR.
   B. Regurgitation is not associated with the incidence and severity of RV dysfunction.
   C. Occurs with high frequency immediately after heart transplantation, is usually moderate, with an eccentric jet pointing toward the interatrial septum.
   D. The incidence and severity of TR is reduced with bicaval anastomotic technique.

# Decision Making in Interventional Cardiovascular Medicine and Noncardiac Surgery

# SECTION VII

# Decision Making in Interventional Cardiovascular Medicine and Noncardiac Surgery

# Chapter 37

# Assessment in Cardiac Intervention

*Ivan P. Casserly, E. Murat Tuzcu, Patrick L. Whitlow, Mario Garcia, and Robert M. Savage*

Although many challenges remain in the field of percutaneous coronary intervention (PCI), the lessons learned over the last three decades have generally made these procedures very safe. More than one million PCIs are performed annually in the United States. During this time, noncoronary cardiac intervention in adult patients was restricted largely to the treatment of aortic, mitral, and pulmonic stenosis, using balloon valvuloplasty techniques. However, over the last 10 years, the field of noncoronary cardiac intervention has rapidly evolved and its scope has extended well beyond the treatment of stenotic valves.

There is no doubt that the dominant force behind these new developments is the proliferation of new technologies. In concert with these developments has come the realization that surgical therapies can be replaced by effective endovascular alternatives. In fact, a number of the newer endovascular technologies have been initiated by cardiothoracic surgeons, seeking to replicate their surgical techniques, using endovascular devices. This burgeoning field presents a tremendous opportunity to offer novel and alternative therapies, but significant challenges, too. Compared with coronary artery disease, the disease states being treated during noncoronary cardiac intervention vary significantly, which necessitates a multidisciplinary approach to patient management. Another challenge is the requirement for high quality echocardiographic imaging during preprocedural evaluation, the procedure itself (Table 37.1), and the postprocedural management of these patients. Although the development of intracardiac echocardiography (ICE) has provided some autonomy for the interventionalist during some procedures, a successful noncoronary cardiac intervention program cannot be built without the support and expertise offered by our echocardiographer colleagues.

In this chapter, the principle noncoronary cardiac interventions that are currently performed by cardiac interventionalists requiring echocardiographic guidance are described. Some of these are well-established techniques with good clinical data supporting their efficacy. Others

are at an early stage of development and, while holding great promise, further study is required before they can gain widespread acceptance.

## PERCUTANEOUS AORTIC VALVE REPLACEMENT

For patients with acquired calcific aortic stenosis, aortic valve replacement is the treatment of choice, providing effective symptomatic relief and a survival benefit (1). However, some patients are not deemed operative candidates due to the presence of serious comorbid conditions that predict high operative mortality. The introduction of percutaneous balloon aortic valvuloplasty (PBAV) in the mid-1980s offered a new therapeutic option for these patients. While the short-term outcomes of PBAV were encouraging, long-term follow-up demonstrated near 100% resteno-

▶ **TABLE 37.1. Utility of Various Echocardiographic Imaging Modalities During Noncoronary Cardiac Intervention**

| Procedure | Echocardiographic technique | | |
|---|---|---|---|
| | TTE | TEE | ICE |
| Alcohol Septal Ablation | ++++ | − | − |
| ASD Closure | − | ++++ | ++++ |
| PFO Closure | − | ++ | ++ |
| Aortic Valve Replacement | − | ++ | ++ |
| Mitral Valve Repair | − | ++++ | − |
|    Annuloplasty | − | ++++ | +++ |
|    Edge-to-Edge Repair | | | |
| LAA Exclusion | − | ++++ | +++ |
| Pericardiocentesis | ++++ | ++ | |
| Myocardial Biopsy | ++++ | − | +++ |
| Mitral Balloon Valvuloplasty | ++++ | ++++ | − |

TTE, transthoracic echo; TEE, transesophageal echo; LAA, left atrial appendage; ++++, vital for the procedure; ++, helpful for the procedure; −, not helpful/not required for the procedure.

sis rates at 2 years (2). PBAV is currently used only to provide palliation or to serve as a bridge toward aortic valve replacement. The limitation of PBAV has provided the impetus to develop percutaneous aortic valve replacement techniques for the treatment of patients with severe aortic stenosis not amenable to surgical valve replacement.

Following ex vivo and animal testing of a variety of valve bioprostheses and techniques, Cribier et al. performed the first percutaneous transcatheter implantation of an aortic valve prosthesis (Percutaneous Valve Technologies, Inc., Fort Lee, NJ) in April 2002 (3). The valve consists of three bovine (subsequently changed to equine) pericardial leaflets that are sutured to a stainless steel stent frame (14 mm long, 21 mm–23 mm diameter) (Fig. 37.1a), which in turn is mounted on a commercially available Z-MED II (NuMED, Inc., Hopkinton NY, USA; 30 mm long, 23 mm diameter) balloon valvuloplasty catheter (Fig. 37.1b). In brief, the prosthesis is introduced over a continuous wire loop (360 cm stiff guidewire) extending from the femoral vein to the right atrium, across the septum into the left atrium, mitral valve, left ventricle, aorta, and femoral artery. To prepare for valve placement, BAV is performed (23 mm balloon). Currently, a 24Fr sheath in the femoral vein is required to allow delivery of the aortic valve prosthesis, which is positioned at the midsection of the native aortic valve, using the valvular calcifications as a marker. Rapid and full inflation of the balloon followed by rapid deflation results in delivery of the valve prosthesis (Fig. 37.2). To date, a total of 14 such procedures have been performed in 12 patients with functional class IV symptoms and two patients with cardiogenic shock (unpublished data). Successful implantation of the prosthesis was achieved in 12 patients (86%). Successful implantation is associated with an impressive reduction of the mean aortic gradient (44 ± 13 to 5 ± 0.5 mm Hg) and increase in aortic valve area (0.5 ± 0.1 to 1.7 ± 0.1 cm$^2$). There was one procedural death, and four late noncardiac deaths. The latter finding is not surpris-

ing, given the clinical context in which device implantation is performed in these patients.

All of these procedures are performed under TEE guidance, and both TTE and TEE are essential in the accurate follow-up of these patients. During the procedure, TEE is most helpful in assessing outcome following implantation of the prosthesis. TEE allows measurement of the stent diameter, which should be between 21 and 23 mm, and assessment of stent geometry, which should ideally be circular. TEE is also helpful in assessing paravalvular regurgitation, which reflects failure of apposition of the prosthesis with the native calcific valve. Severe paravalvular regurgitation ($\geq$ +3) was present in one-third of patients immediately following placement of the aortic prosthesis. Follow-up TEE and TTE allow assessment of the prosthetic leaflets, valvular and paravalvular regurgitation, planimetry of the aortic valve area, aortic valve gradients, and left ventricular function.

## MITRAL VALVE REPAIR

Percutaneous catheter-based approaches to the management of functional and structural mitral regurgitation (MR) in human subjects are at an early stage of development but represent a potentially dramatic advance (5). Functional MR has a complicated pathogenesis, but is felt to result from mitral annular dilatation and altered ventricular geometry, which causes incomplete leaflet coaptation. The resultant mitral regurgitation begets further LV dysfunction and mitral annular dilatation, setting up a vicious perpetuating spiral of progressive mitral regurgitation and left ventricular failure. Surgical repair generally involves a ring- or suture-based mitral annuloplasty, which reshapes the annulus and promotes leaflet coaptation. Several groups have attempted to mimic this strategy, using percutaneous methods by exploiting the relationship of the coronary sinus and great cardiac vein with

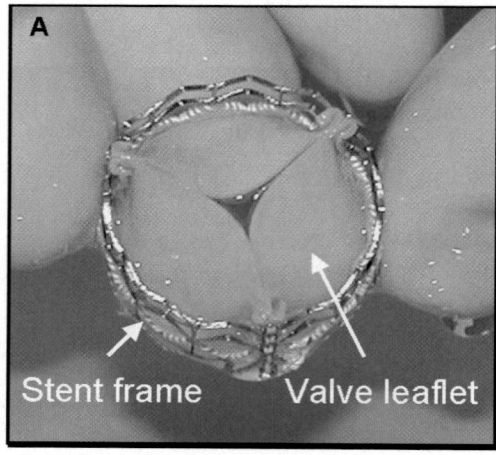

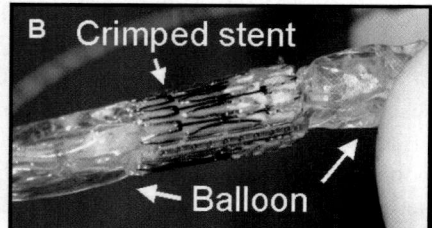

**FIGURE 37.1. A:** Appearance of prosthetic aortic heart valve when expanded. Valve consists of three leaflets attached to a metal stent. **B:** Appearance of valve when crimped onto balloon for delivery into patient via femoral sheath. Reproduced with permission from Eltchaninoff H, et al. J Interv Cardiol 2003;16(6):515–21.

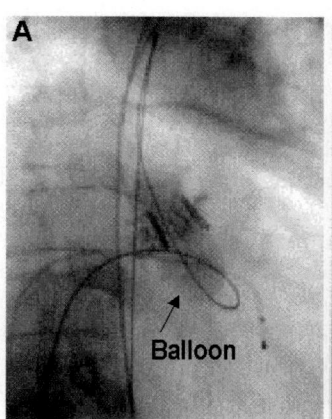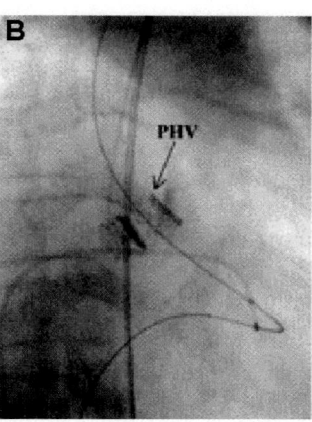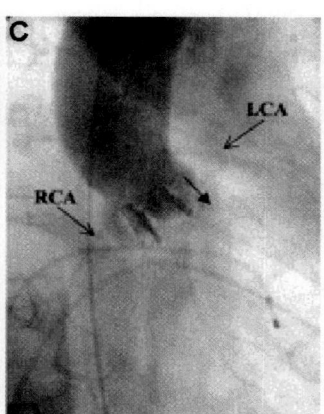

*FIGURE 37.2.* **A:** The prosthetic aortic valve is deployed by inflation of the 23 mm balloon on which the stent valve is delivered. **B:** Appearance of prosthetic valve following deployment. **C:** Aortography following placement of prosthetic aortic valve demonstrating patent right and left coronary arteries above the prosthesis. Reproduced with permission from Cribier A et al. Circulation 2002;106:3006–8.

the posterior aspect of the mitral annulus (Fig. 37.3). Although different types of device are in development (C-Cure, ev3/Mitralife, Santa Rosa, CA, USA; Viacor, Inc., Wilmington, MA), in essence, they each consist of a metal constraint device that is inserted into the coronary sinus, using the internal jugular venous access site. The goal is to apply tension on the underlying annulus, resulting in a ~25% reduction in annular diameter. TEE guidance during the procedure is essential to monitoring the annular diameter and the associated change in mitral regurgitation. Published data has been limited to small animal studies, where insertion of the device was associated with an impressive reduction in mitral annular diameter (4.17 ± 0.14 to 3.24 ± 0.11 cm) and severity of mitral regurgitation, and a consistent improvement in hemodynamic assessments (cardiac output, pulmonary capillary wedge pressure) (6). While this therapy is promising, both short- and long-term clinical data are required. The complexity of functional MR mandates a clear demonstration of effi-

cacy in human subjects before acceptance of the technique. Additionally, a number of safety concerns exist including coronary sinus perforation and thrombosis, coronary ischemia secondary to impingement on the circumflex artery, and arrhythmias. These complications were not seen in the early human experience of a group in Venezuela, but given the small sample size, caution is still warranted (unpublished data).

Structural MR is caused by pathology of the valve leaflets or supporting structures (i.e., chordae, papillary muscles). Since the early 1990s, Alfieri has championed the double-orifice technique of surgical mitral repair for more complicated cases of structural mitral regurgitation with excellent clinical outcomes (7). Most commonly, the technique involves suturing the middle scallops of the anterior and posterior mitral leaflets, and is used to treat bileaflet or anterior leaflet prolapse (7). In a further imitation of a surgical technique, St. Goar et al. have reported an endovascular edge-to-edge technique using a V-shaped, polyester-covered metal clip for repair of structural MR (Evalve, Inc., Redwood City, CA) (Fig. 37.4) (8). The procedure is outlined in Figs. 37.5 and 37.6. In summary, using the femoral venous access site, and transseptal puncture, a steerable guiding catheter is placed in the left atrium above the mitral valve. The V clip is attached to the delivery catheter, then advanced through the guide and opened in the left atrium. The opened clip crosses the mitral valve perpendicular to the line of leaflet coaptation and in the same vertical plane as the middle scallops of the anterior and posterior leaflets. Once in the left ventricle and below the free edges of the leaflets, the clip is retracted and the leaflets grasped. A thorough 2–D and color Doppler echocardiographic assessment is performed to confirm adequate placement with complete or near-complete elimination of mitral regurgitation. If device placement is unsatisfactory, the device may be released and redeployed until successful placement is achieved. The importance of TEE guidance during each step of this procedure cannot be overempha-

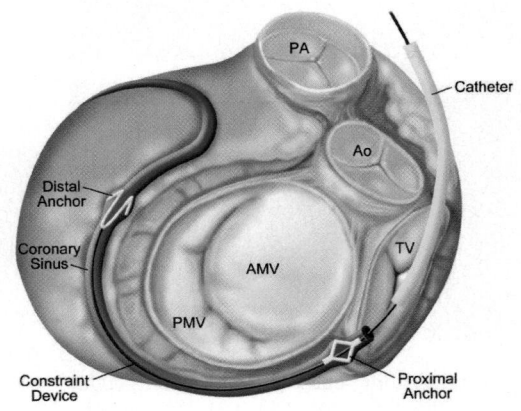

*FIGURE 37.3.* Schematic of percutaneous mitral annular reduction technique for treatment of functional mitral regurgitation. A metal constraint device is positioned in coronary sinus opposite the posterior aspect of the mitral valve.

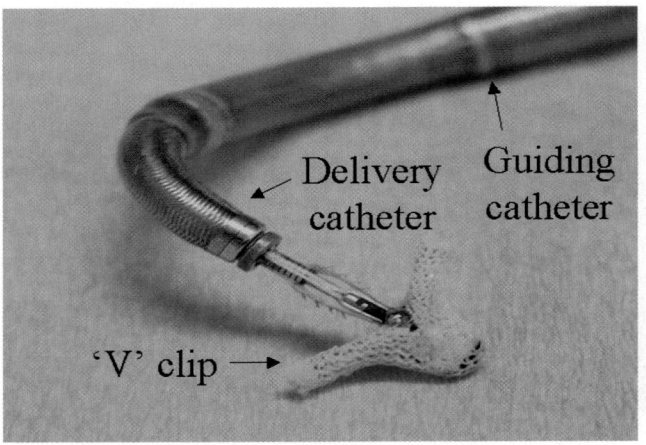

**FIGURE 37.4.** Polyester covered metal V-shaped clip used to perform percutaneous edge-to-edge repair of mitral valve.

sized (Fig. 37.6). Published data with this device is only available from animal studies but is encouraging (8). To date, the device has been placed in eight human subjects, with an effective reduction of MR in six, and no major adverse clinical events (unpublished data). The technical expertise required by both the interventionalist and echocardiographer for this procedure is significantly greater than that for the mitral annular reduction technique. Clearly, this technique is in its infancy, and a much larger body of safety and efficacy data are required before the technique can be applied in clinical practice. It is likely that the ultimate success of percutaneous treatments for structural MR will be determined by the ability to use endovascular techniques to treat both the structural defect *and* mitral annular dilatation, as currently practiced by cardiothoracic surgeons during most surgical repairs. While current technologies offer some promise toward that end, their niche will initially be restricted to nonsurgical candidates. Beyond this patient

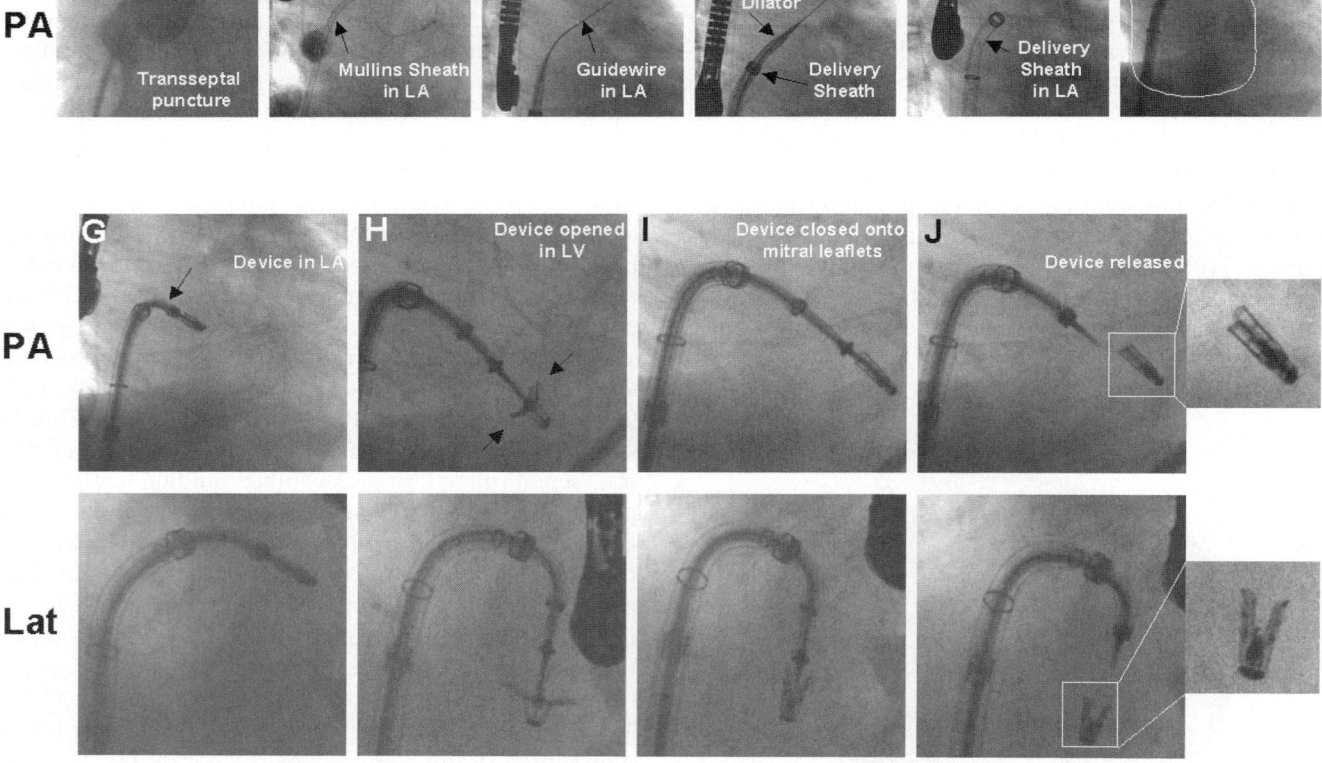

**FIGURE 37.5.** Fluoroscopic procedural images from patient undergoing endovascular edge-to-edge repair of mitral valve using E-valve system. **A–F:** Following transseptal puncture **(A)**, a Mullins sheath is placed in the left atrium **(B)**. A stiff guidewire is placed in the left atrium and the Mulllins sheath is exchanged for a 24 Fr guide **(C–E)**. The device is advanced through the guide into the left atrium **(G),** opened **(H),** advanced across the mitral valve, retracted against the mitral valve, and then closed, grasping the leaflets **(G–I).** Once adequate device placement is determined by echocardiography, the device is released **(J).**

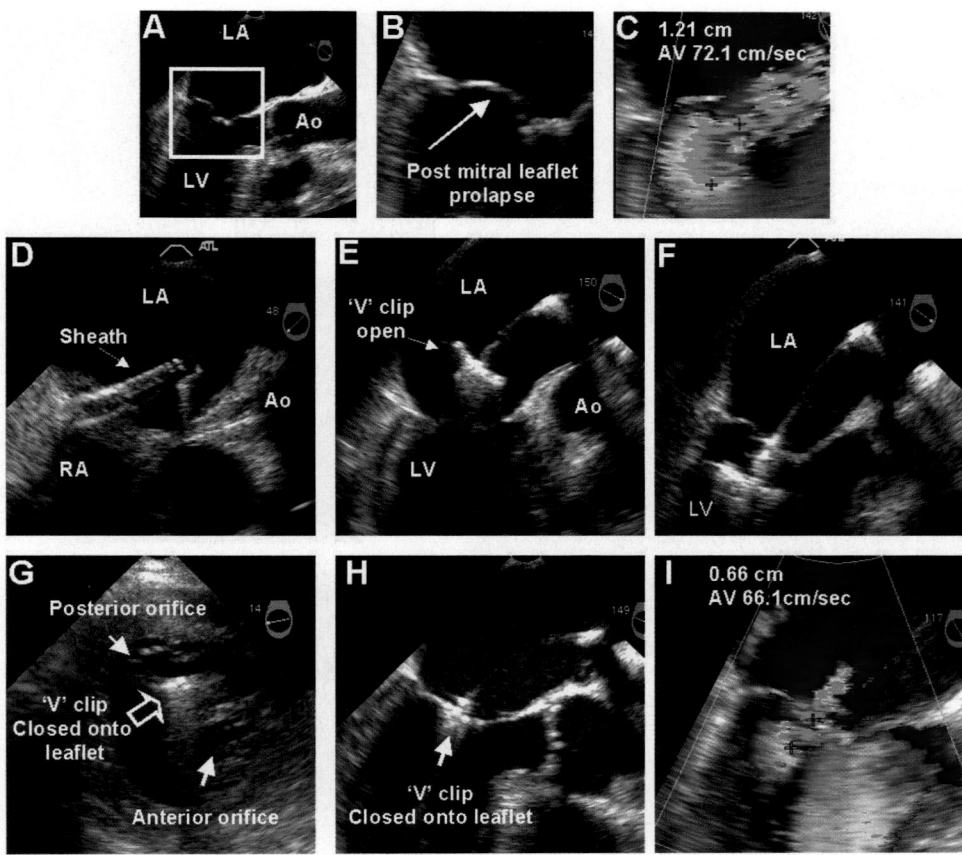

**FIGURE 37.6.** TEE images from same patient described in Figure 37.5. **A–C:** Images demonstrating prolapse of the posterior mitral leaflet and associated anteriorly directed mitral regurgitation at baseline. **D:** Guide catheter in left atrium. **E–F:** Device opened in left atrium and advanced into left ventricle. **G–H:** Transgastric **(G)** and esophageal **(H)** views demonstrating appearance of mitral valve, following capture of the middle scallops of the anterior and posterior mitral leaflets by the V clip. **I:** Color Doppler of mitral flow following device placement.

group, the burden of proof will rest heavily on percutaneous techniques to prove their equivalency or superiority to established surgical techniques.

## NONSURGICAL SEPTAL REDUCTION FOR HYPERTROPHIC CARDIOMYOPATHY

Significant left ventricular outflow tract (LVOT) obstruction is present in 10% of patients with hypertrophic cardiomyopathy (HCM), and is believed to contribute significantly to symptoms of angina, dyspnea on exertion, and syncope (9). Until the early 1990s, surgical myectomy was the only therapeutic option for patients who were refractory to medical therapy. At this time, observational data regarding implantation of DDD pacemakers in these patients showed some promise, but subsequent randomized studies failed to demonstrate any objective improvement in functional status, and this therapy has largely been abandoned (10,11). In 1995, Sigwart reported a novel therapeutic approach that involved the injection of absolute alcohol into the first septal perforator branch, producing a circumscribed myocardial infarction involving the portion of septum in contact with the anterior mitral

leaflet during the typical systolic anterior motion (SAM) of the leaflet observed in HCM (Fig. 37.7) (12). Clinical outcomes were impressive, and subsequent larger series, involving hundreds of patients, demonstrated an early and sustained reduction in LVOT gradient (~90%), and resolution or effective relief of symptoms in > 90% of patients during long-term follow-up (13,14).

The majority of operators use TTE guidance for alcohol septal ablation procedures. The critical function of TTE guidance is to help select the target septal perforator, supplying the area of septum in contact with the anterior mitral leaflet during SAM. This is sometimes challenging because of the tremendous interindividual variation in the number, distribution, and overlap in distribution of the septal perforator branches. Following inflation of a balloon in the selected perforator branch, an echo contrast agent is injected through the balloon lumen (diluted 1:8 with saline). Imaging from the apical and parasternal views allows a determination of the myocardium perfused by the septal perforator branch (Fig. 37.7D). In some patients, this procedure may have to be repeated with the balloon in various branches or sub-branches to confirm the optimal location for injection of alcohol. By more effective localization of the targeted myocardium, the use of myocardial contrast echocardiography (MCE)

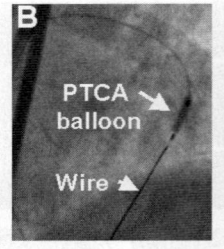

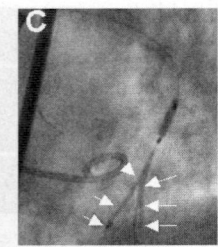

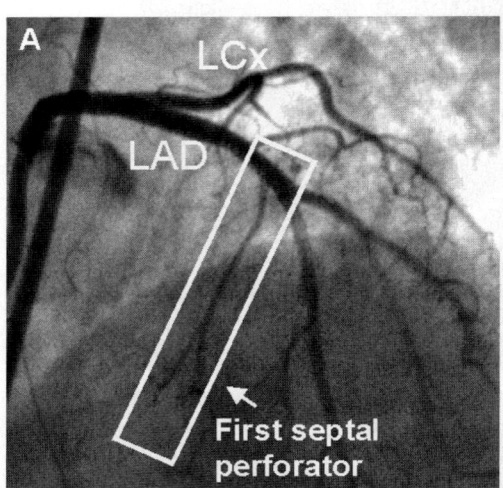

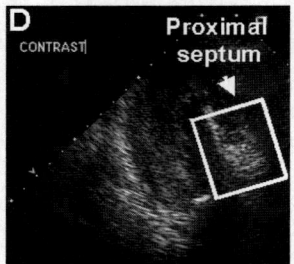

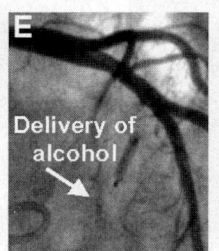

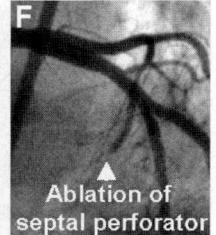

**FIGURE 37.7. A:** Angiogram of left coronary artery demonstrating location of the first septal perforator branch of the left anterior descending artery. **B:** The septal perforator branch is wired and a balloon positioned in the proximal portion of the vessel. **C:** Injection of contrast through the balloon demonstrates anatomy of first septal perforator branch. **D:** Echo contrast injection through the balloon confirms that the selected septal perforator branch perfused the proximal septum and is an appropriate target for alcohol ablation. **E:** Absolute alcohol is injected through the balloon. **F:** Final appearance of the perforator branch following alcohol ablation. *LAD,* left anterior descending artery; *LCx,* left circumflex artery; *PTCA,* percutaneous transluminal coronary angioplasty.

during alcohol ablation has been associated with improved hemodynamic results, despite a reduction in the total infarct size (13). The safety of the procedure is improved by identifying perforator branches whose perfusion distribution involves the posterior free wall and papillary muscles, making them unsuitable targets. Additionally, the incidence of complete heart block, which occurred in 20% to 40% of patients in an early series, has been reduced to 5% to 10% in a series using MCE

guidance (15). TTE may also be used to monitor the effects of the procedure on the LVOT gradient at rest and during provocation (e.g., amyl nitrate, post-PVC), and to document the resolution or improvement in SAM and the associated posteriorly directed mitral regurgitation (Fig. 37.8). In summary, TTE and MCE make alcohol septal ablation a safer and more effective procedure. They should be regarded as mandatory components of the technique.

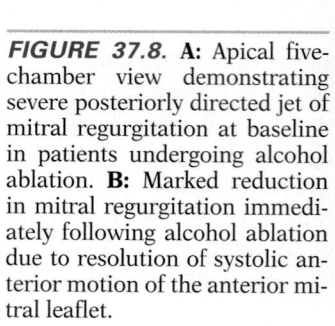

**FIGURE 37.8. A:** Apical five-chamber view demonstrating severe posteriorly directed jet of mitral regurgitation at baseline in patients undergoing alcohol ablation. **B:** Marked reduction in mitral regurgitation immediately following alcohol ablation due to resolution of systolic anterior motion of the anterior mitral leaflet.

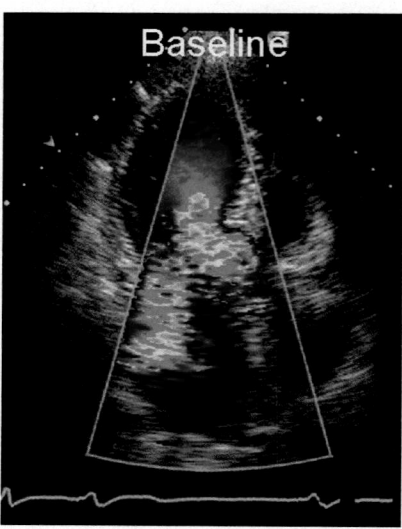

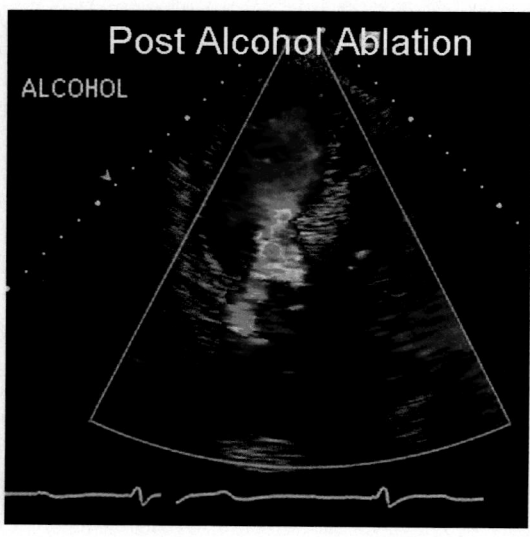

## PFO/ASD CLOSURE

Mills and King performed the first nonoperative ASD closure in 1976, using a double-umbrella device (16). Although further attempts to develop more user-friendly devices were made by individual investigators, the procedure did not gain acceptance until the development of the Clamshell device in the late 1980s. Despite the initial technical limitations of this device (metal arm fractures and high rates of residual shunting), it formed the basis for further generations of similar devices and other novel devices that have been successfully employed in 40,000 percutaneous ASD closures (secundum-type). The late 1980s also saw an appreciation of the role of patent foramen ovale (PFO) in cryptogenic stroke due to paradoxical embolism (17). Many of these same ASD closure devices were applied in PFO closure, and other specific devices for PFO closure were developed.

The ASD/PFO closure devices currently in use are double-disc devices, with right and left atrial disc components that oppose the atrial septum, and a central connecting waist element that rests in the PFO or ASD joining the discs (Fig. 37.9). The discs are composed of a metal frame (most commonly nitinol) that supports a fabric. Both components are important in promoting the formation of a thrombotic layer on the surface of the device with subsequent endothelialization of the device surfaces, which results in closure of the defect. In the United States, the CardioSEAL/STARFlex and Amplatzer PFO/ASD occluder devices represent the majority of the devices used. The basic technique for ASD/PFO closure utilizing the former devices is illustrated in Fig. 37.10. Essentially, the defect is crossed with a diagnostic catheter, which facilitates the placement of a supportive wire in the pulmonary vein. Over this wire, a delivery sheath is placed in the left atrium. Through this sheath, the device attached to a

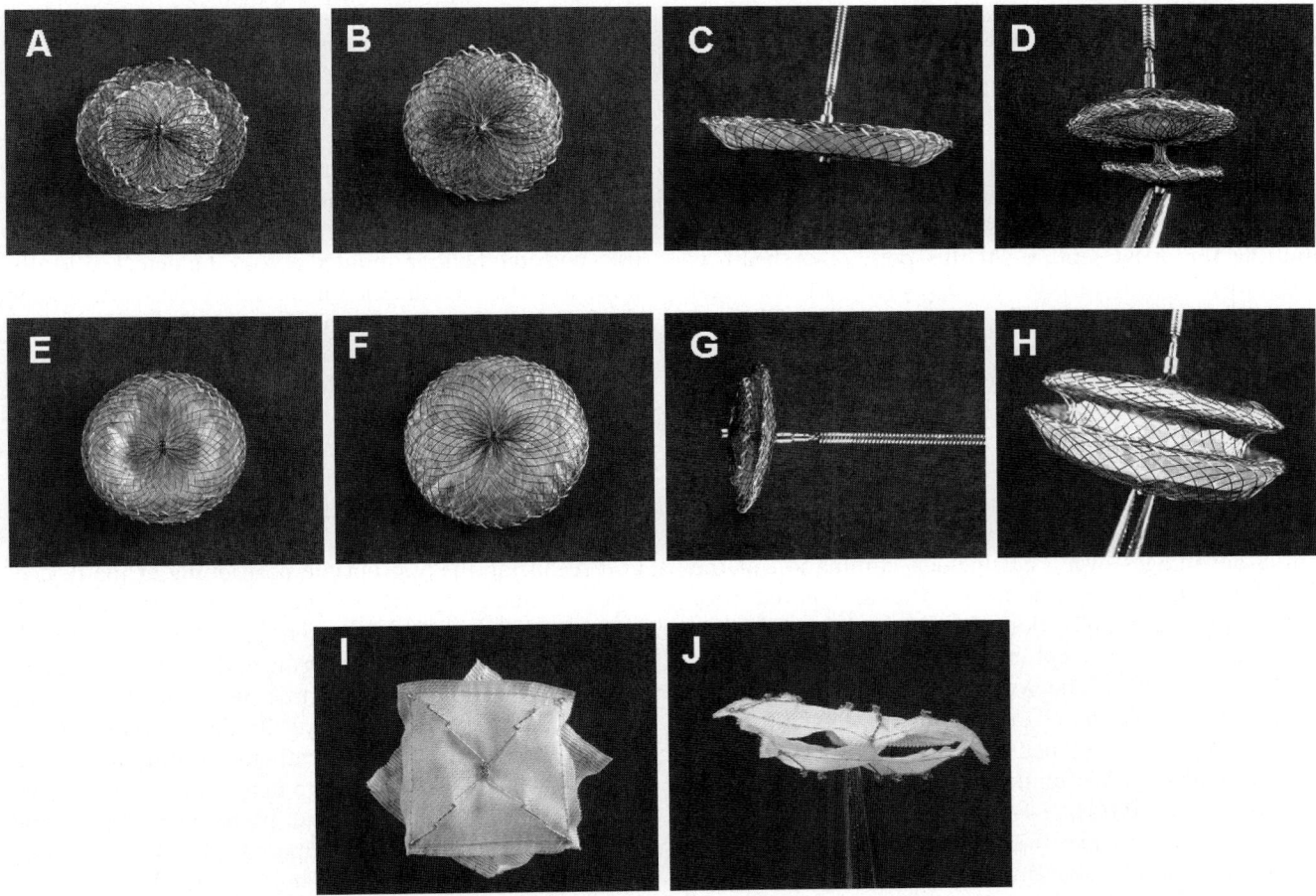

*FIGURE 37.9.* Sample of PFO/ASD devices most commonly used in the United States. **A–D:** Amplatzer PFO occluder device as viewed from left atrial side **(A),** right atrial side **(B),** in side profile **(C),** and in side profile with both atrial components pulled apart to demonstrate the waist portion of the device **(D). E–F:** Amplatzer ASD occluder device as viewed from left atrial side **(E),** right atrial side **(F),** in side profile **(G),** and in side profile with both atrial components pulled apart to demonstrate the waist portion of the device **(H). I–J:** CardioSEAL device in en-face view **(I)** and in side profile **(J).**

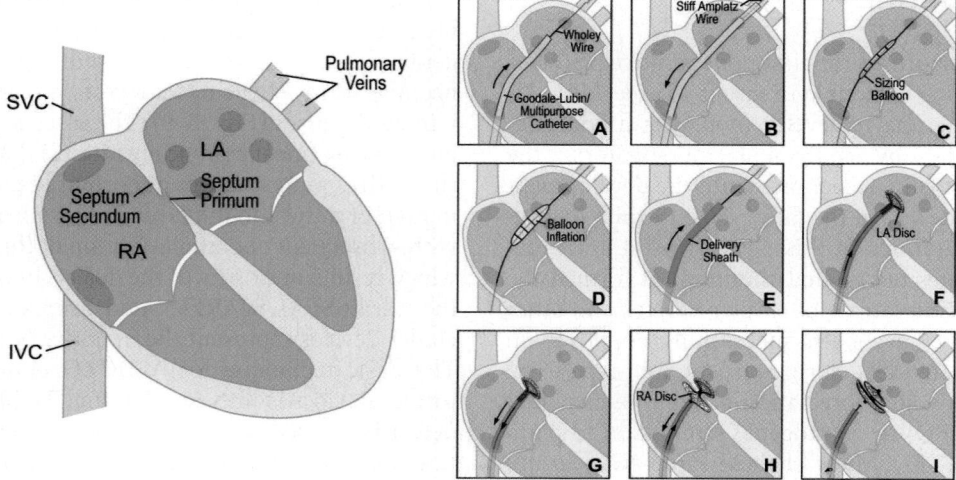

**FIGURE 37.10.** Schematic illustration of the technique used to perform percutaneous patent foramen ovale/atrial septal defect closure (device illustrated is Amplatzer PFO device). **A–B:** A catheter is used to cross the defect and a supportive wire is positioned in the pulmonary vein. **C–D:** The size of the defect is determined using a sizing balloon inflated across the defect. **E:** The delivery sheath is positioned in the left atrium. **F–H:** The left and right atrial components of the device are deployed across the defect. **I:** The device is released by detaching the device from the delivery catheter. Reproduced with permission from Casserly I, et al. Percutaneous Patent Foramen Ovale and Atrial Septal Defects. In: Manual of peripheral vascular intervention. Lippincott Williams & Wilkins.

delivery catheter is passed and the left atrial disc is deployed in the left atrium. Withdrawal of the sheath and delivery catheter together results in the left atrial disc abutting the atrial septum. At this point, the sheath is withdrawn, which results in deployment of the right atrial disc. Detachment of the delivery catheter from the device results in final release of the device. The use of adjunctive imaging modalities during percutaneous PFO/ASD closure is variable, both with respect to usage and the type of adjunctive imaging utilized. TEE and intracardiac echo (ICE) are the best imaging modalities to guide these procedures. ICE is a relatively new imaging modality that is performed by the interventionalist. Potential advantages over TEE include elimination of the need for sedation or general anesthesia required with TEE, improved visualization of the inferoposterior portion of the interatrial septum, and greater autonomy for the interventionalist. The system consists of a 10Fr ultrasound catheter (Acunav™) transducer that is interfaced with the Sequioa™, Aspen™, or Cypress™ ultrasound imaging platforms. Within the catheter tip, there is a multifrequency 5.0–10 MHz, 64–element vector, phased array transducer that provides high-resolution 2D and Doppler imaging (including color Doppler). The catheter is introduced through an 11Fr sheath in the femoral vein and positioned in the right atrium to visualize the right and left atria and atrial septum.

For ASD closure, adjunctive TEE or ICE during percutaneous closure is essential (Fig. 37.11). Prior to closure, the stretch balloon diameter of the defect is determined by both fluoroscopy and echo (Fig. 37.11E). This is a critical measurement because it determines the device size to use. With the balloon inflated across the defect, it is also imperative to examine the remainder of the septum using 2D imaging and color Doppler to ensure the absence of additional defects, which may be present in up to 15% of cases (Fig. 37.11F). Although fluoroscopy and tactile sensation are usually adequate to determine the appropriate location for deployment of the right and left atrial components of the device, echo guidance provides additional confirmation. Following deployment of the device and prior to release, TEE or ICE provides invaluable information regarding the appropriate positioning of the device. To be confident of device stability, it is imperative to visualize the atrial septum between both the right and left atrial components superoanterior and inferoposterior to the defect. The importance of this step is underscored by the inability to reliably retrieve the device following detachment from the delivery catheter. Additionally, echo guidance allows the operator to determine if adjacent vital structures (e.g., right upper pulmonary vein, mitral valve, coronary sinus, and superior/inferior vena cava) are impinged by the device. This is particularly relevant in the closure of large ASDs where the left atrial disc diameter approaches the diameter of the atrial septum.

For PFO closure, adjunctive imaging is very helpful but probably not essential, provided the patient has had a preprocedural TEE to adequately assess the interatrial

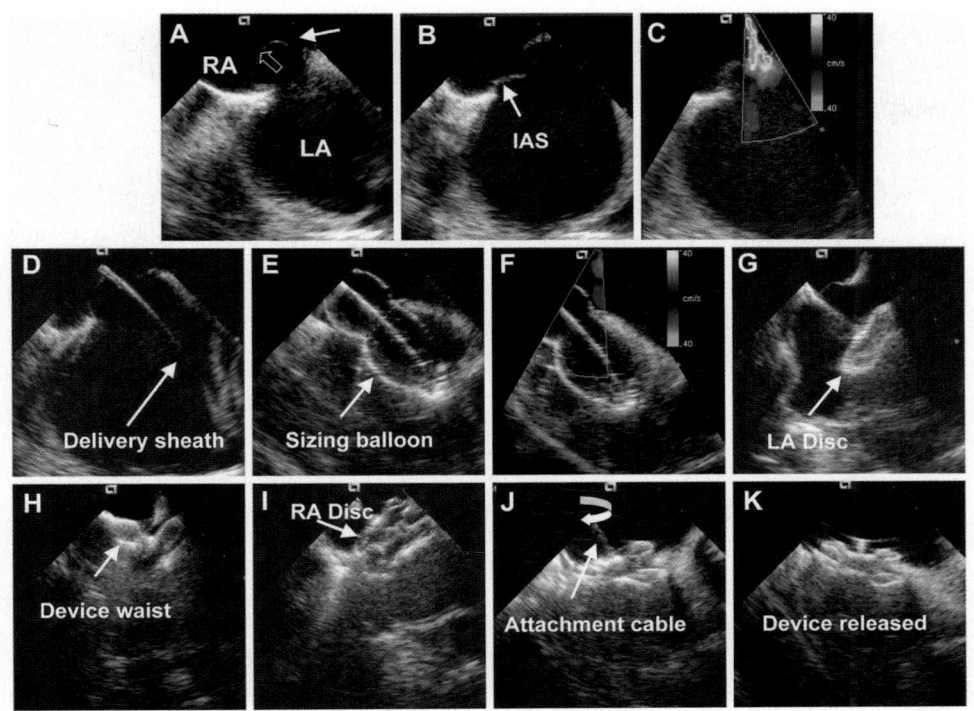

FIGURE 37.11. Series of images obtained using intracardiac echocardiography (ICE) during closure of a secundum type ASD with an Amplatzer ASD occluder. **A–C:** Baseline images demonstrating mobile interatrial septum (*open arrow*) with secundum type ASD. **D:** Delivery sheath is positioned in the left atrium. **E:** Sizing balloon positioned across defect with measurement of waist diameter. **F:** Color flow of septum during balloon inflation to examine for additional defects. **G–I:** Deployment of right and left atrial components of the device across the defect. **J–K:** Device is detached from delivery cable by counterclockwise rotation of cable. Reproduced with permission from Casserly I, et al. Percutaneous Patent Foramen Ovale and Atrial Septal Defects. In: Manual of peripheral vascular intervention. Lippincott Williams & Wilkins.

septum and that the operator has an adequate procedural experience. The presence of a long interatrial tunnel and an associated atrial septal aneurysm is generally an indication to use a larger device for PFO closure. Adjunctive imaging certainly provides reassurance of appropriate device placement prior to release of the device, and is always useful where untoward events occur during the procedure. For example, occasionally, the right atrial component of the device becomes entangled in a prominent eustachian valve or Chiari network. A steerable catheter can be used to displace these structures under echo guidance.

## LEFT ATRIAL APPENDAGE OCCLUSION

Atrial fibrillation (AF) is associated with a 3– to 5–fold increase in stroke risk in patients aged 50 to 90 years (18). Due to the increased prevalence of atrial fibrillation with age (reaching ~10% in octogenarians), the percentage of strokes attributable to AF also increases with age, reaching 23.5% in persons aged 80 to 89 years (18). With the decline in rheumatic valvular disease in developed countries, the majority of AF is now related to nonvalvular etiologies. In patients with nonvalvular AF, the left atrial appendage (LAA) is the location of left atrial thrombus in ~90% of cases (Fig. 37.12) (19). While oral anticoagulation with warfarin (achieving an INR 2–3) has demonstrated efficacy in reducing the risk of stroke in this population (20), issues related to maintenance of a therapeutic INR and bleeding complications limit the efficacy and application of this therapy. This is underscored by a 1996 survey in which the utilization rate for warfarin in patients with atrial fibrillation who met criteria for anticoagulation was only 33% (21). This highlights the need for alternative therapies to prevent stroke from embolization of LAA thrombus in the group of patients who is currently inadequately treated.

Since the late 1940s, surgeons have performed exclusion of the LAA during mitral valve surgery in patients with mitral stenosis in an effort to reduce the risk of subsequent stroke (22). More recently, thoracoscopic closure techniques have been reported for isolated LAA exclusion (23). However, a less invasive endovascular approach is required if the strategy of LAA exclusion is to be applied to a broader population of AF patients. To this end, two endovascular LAA exclusion devices have been developed that are at different stages of clinical testing [Percutaneous Left Atrial Appendage Transcatheter Occlusion device, PLAATO™, Appriva Medical; WATCHMAN® left atrial appendage filter system (24,25)] (Fig. 37.13). The basic technique is similar for both devices, and current protocols mandate TEE guidance during the procedure. Prior to the procedure, TEE is also required to document the absence of LAA thrombus, which is a contraindication to device implantation. Following a transseptal puncture, a specially designed 12Fr delivery sheath is positioned in the LAA appendage. An angiogram of the appendage in orthogonal views, together with TEE measurements of the diameter of the LAA ostium, allows a

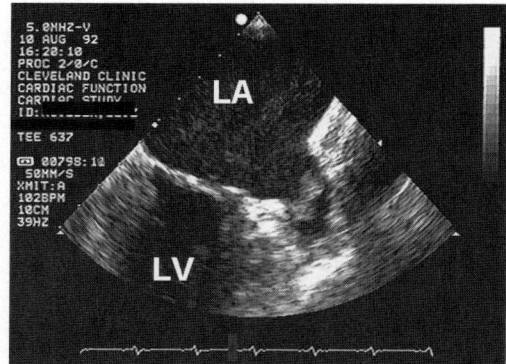
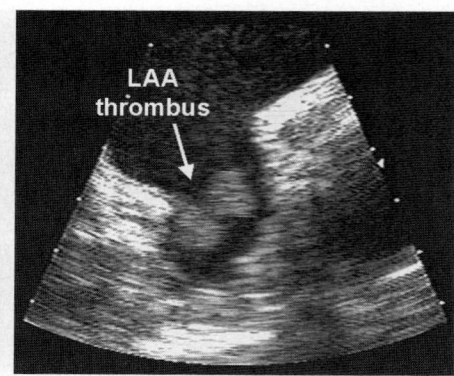

**FIGURE 37.12.** TTE image from patient with left atrial appendage thrombus.

determination of the device size to be used (Fig. 37.14). Generally, the device size chosen is 20% to 40% larger than the LAA orifice diameter. The diameter of the LAA orifice can vary markedly, and enlarges significantly in patients with atrial fibrillation. In a postmortem study of 220 patients, the maximal and minimal diameters of the ostium varied from 5 mm to 27 mm and 10 mm to 40 mm, respectively (26). Although the device shapes and designs differ, they both consist of a self-expandable nitinol metal frame and a covering membrane material (ePTFE in the PLATTO device, and PET in the WATCHMAN device). The device is delivered through the sheath and released into the appendage. Following angiographic and TEE confirmation of appropriate device position and adequate sealing of the appendage, the device is detached from its delivery catheter. At a small number of centers in the US and Europe, operators have used the Amplatzer ASD occluder device in a small group of patients for LAA exclusion (n = 16) with adequate outcomes (27).

In a 103–patient registry of the PLAATO device, successful implantation was achieved in 98% of cases (unpublished data). In follow-up, there were two strokes at 6 months, and three nonprocedure/nondevice-related deaths within the first year (unpublished data). Clinical experience with the WATCHMAN device is limited to a registry of 38 patients from Germany. Successful implantation was achieved in 30 patients (79%), which likely reflects a learning curve with the technique, and the need to refine the device and associated equipment (unpublished data). Clinical follow-up with this device is forthcoming.

In the short term, these devices will be strictly reserved for patients who have contraindications to long-term anticoagulant therapy and are deemed at high risk for stroke from atrial fibrillation (presence of one or more of the following risk factors: hypertension, heart failure, history of TIA/stroke, diabetes mellitus, and clinical coronary artery disease). Broader application will require that these devices be tested in a head-to-head fashion against

ePTFE occlusion membrane

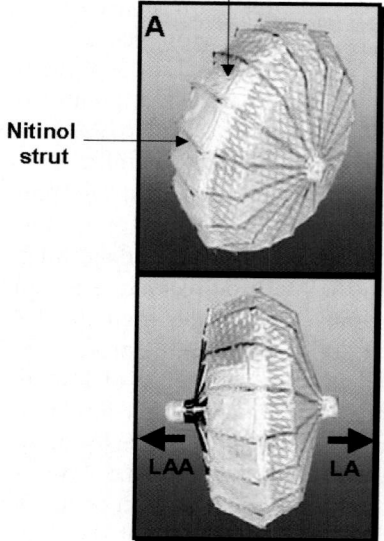

Nitinol strut

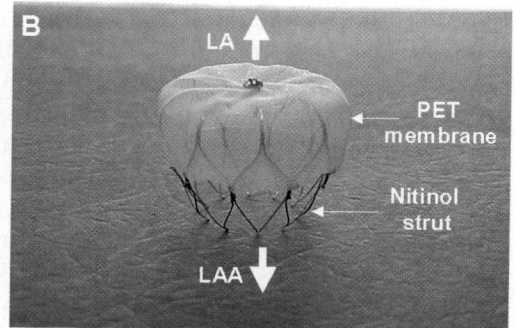

**FIGURE 37.13.** Illustration of the PLAATO (percutaneous left atrial appendage transcatheter occlusion) **(A)** and WATCHMAN devices **(B)** under investigation for percutaneous left atrial appendage occlusion. Reproduced with modification from Sievert H, et al. Circulation 2002;105 (16):1887–9.

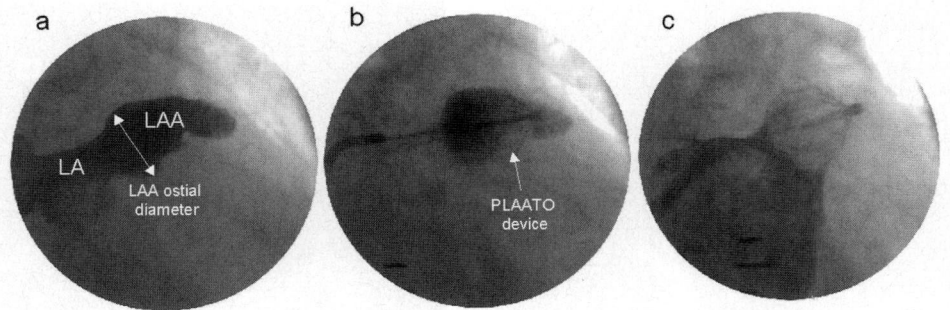

**FIGURE 37.14.** Angiography of left atrial appendage and left atrium during implantation of left atrial appendage (*LAA*) occlusion device. **A:** Baseline LAA angiogram allows determination of the diameter of LAA ostium. **B:** Injection of contrast through a lumen in the device documents stagnation of contrast distal to the sealing surface of the device. **C:** Angiography in left atrium following release of device documents sealing of the appendage. Reproduced with permission from Sievert H, et al. Circulation 2002;105:1887–9.

warfarin for patients who are warfarin-eligible. Such studies are necessary to determine if percutaneous LAA exclusion offers any advantages over oral anticoagulation, or if any subgroups (e.g., high-risk groups) benefit from this more invasive approach to stroke prevention in AF patients.

## PERICARDIOCENTESIS FOR CARDIAC TAMPONADE

The echocardiographic diagnosis of cardiac tamponade in the presence of a large pericardial effusion is established by specific criteria (Fig. 37.15A). These include left or right atrial wall inversion, RV diastolic inversion, hepatic plethora (Fig. 37.15B), and respiratory variation in the flow and volume of the hepatic vein (Fig. 37.15C), and cardiac chambers. The use of echocardiography to guide pericardiocentesis has been previously reported and validated by Armstrong et al. (45). The procedure is performed with the patient in the supine position with the effusion localized by TEE or TTE. The puncture site is chosen based on direct distance to the pericardial effusion and vicinity of vital structures (RV, RA, coronary arteries, and internal mammary artery). The most frequent approach is subcostal; however, it may also be parasternal or apical. The advance of the aspiration needle is guided and monitored echocardiographically. Between 1996 and 2002, 450 echo-guided pericardiocenteses were performed at the Cleveland Clinic. Complications included pneumothorax (1), vasovagal reaction (2), RV puncture (3), and pneumopericardium (1). There were no iatrogenic procedure-related deaths. The success of the procedure was monitored echocardiographically (Fig. 37.15D).

## MYOCARDIAL BIOPSY

Endocardial biopsy is a diagnostic intervention, which is used most commonly to establish the clinical course of rejection following orthotopic heart transplantation. However, as illustrated in Fig. 37.16, it is also used diagnostically in patients with cardiac masses, infiltrative cardiac disease, restrictive cardiomyopathy, chemotherapy-induced cardiomyopathy, and other diagnostic dilemmas involving the heart (cardiac sarcoid and amyloid) (46–49). Endomyocardial biopsy has been associated with perforation of the right atria and ventricle, and trauma to the tricuspid valve. Tricuspid regurgitation following myocardial biopsy has been reported in up to 85% of heart transplant recipients and is associated with traumatic flail (8% to 15%), perforated leaflets, and RV dysfunction secondary to pulmonary hypertension (50–52). To reduce the incidence of complications associated with this necessary diagnostic, the first reported use of echo-guided endomyocardial biopsy was reported in 1988 (52). Pandian et al. have utilized ICE to guide endomyocardial biopsy (49).

## MITRAL BALLOON VALVULOTOMY

The value of TEE in patients with mitral stenosis undergoing percutaneous valvuloplasty has long been established in the diagnosis of LAA thrombi, grading the severity of mitral stenosis and regurgitation, and assessing the results of balloon valvuloplasty (53). Wilkins et al. first reported the ability of an echocardiocardiographic score to predict the long-term course of patients undergoing percutaneous valvuloplasty (54). While it is understood that the scoring parameters are influenced by instrument set-

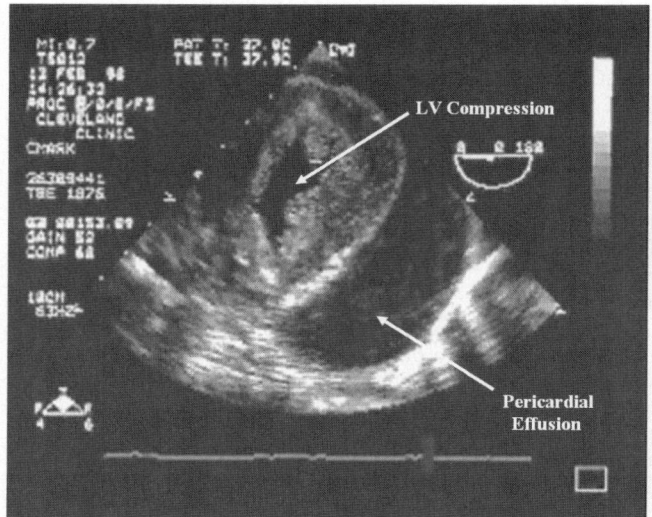

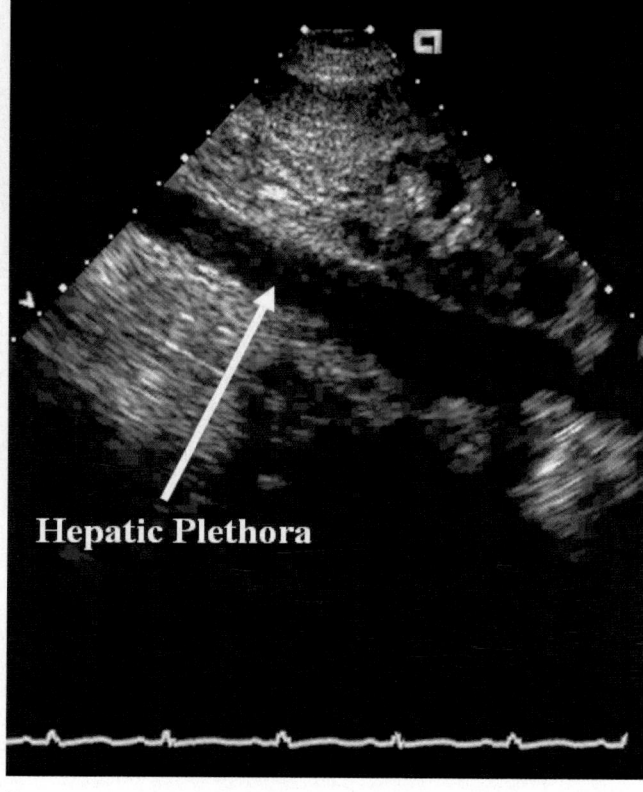

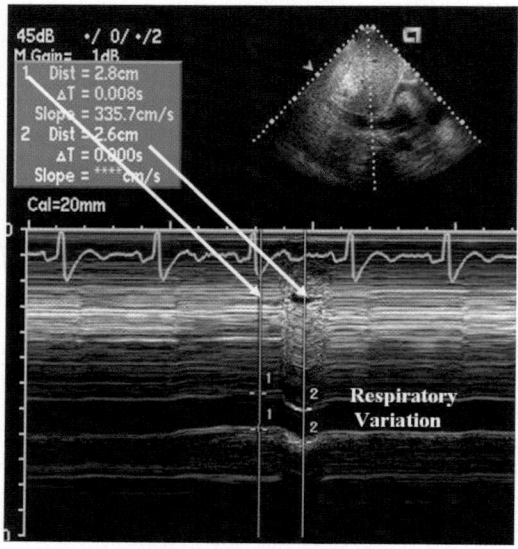

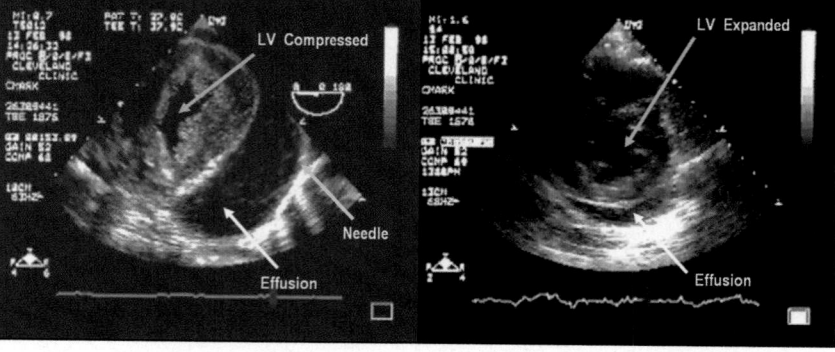

**FIGURE 37.15.** TTE and TEE are utilized in the diagnosis of cardiac tamponade and the guidance of percutaneous pericardiocentesis. **A:** The pericardial effusion and ventricular compression associated with cardiac tamponade are noted. **B:** Hepatic vein engorgement is consistent with the diagnosis of tamponade. **C:** M-mode echo demonstrates the respirator dependence on mediastinal blood flow. **D:** Comparison of effusion during the pericardiocentesis and postpericardiocentesis.

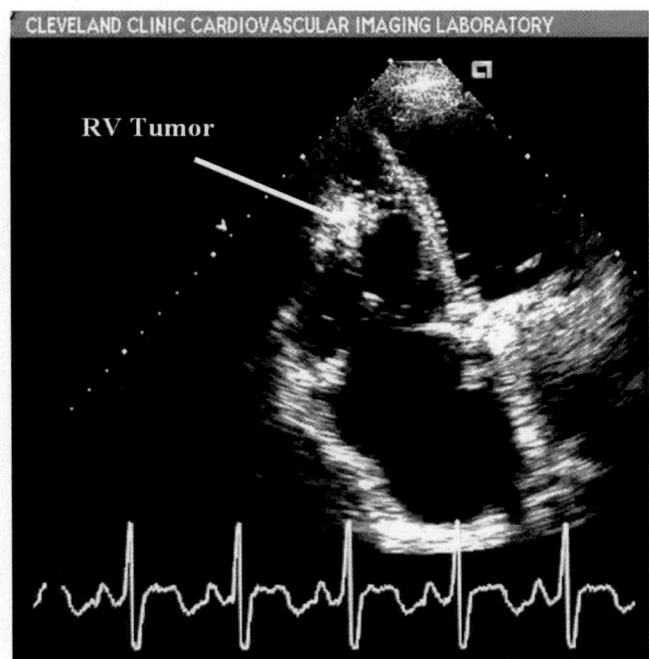

**FIGURE 37.16.** RV tumor demonstrated using apical four-chamber TTE.

tings (gain, wall filter, intensity, and resolution) and transducer frequency, TEE has proven a useful adjunct in the evaluation of the qualitative assessment of rheumatic mitral disease. For anesthetized patients undergoing balloon dilatation of stenotic mitral valves, TEE has provided diagnostic guidance in the baseline assessment of the severity or stenosis and regurgitation, positioning of the balloon, and the serial evaluation of the results of the intervention (Fig. 37.17). Frequently repeated inflations are required as determined by persistence of a significant gradient in the presence of insignificant regurgitation. Ramondo compared the success of performing TEE-guided balloon valvuloplasty with the traditional fluoroscopy-guided procedure. As determined by the absence of significant complications (cardiac tamponade, large residual atrial shunting, and severe mitral regurgitation) and a satisfactory MV area, 96% of the echo-monitored procedures were successful, whereas only 40% of the procedures conducted without echocardiographic control achieved a satisfactory final result (55).

## CONCLUSION

The current definition of noncoronary cardiac intervention extends well beyond the traditional realm of treating stenotic cardiac valves. This is an exciting field that is likely to expand in the coming decades in the same way that PCI has over the last three decades. The use of

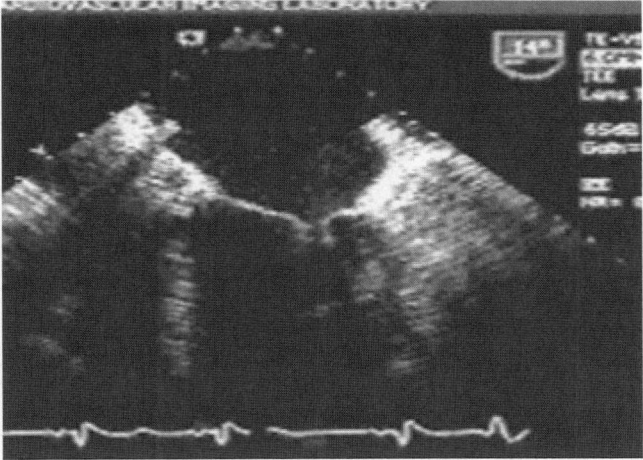

A

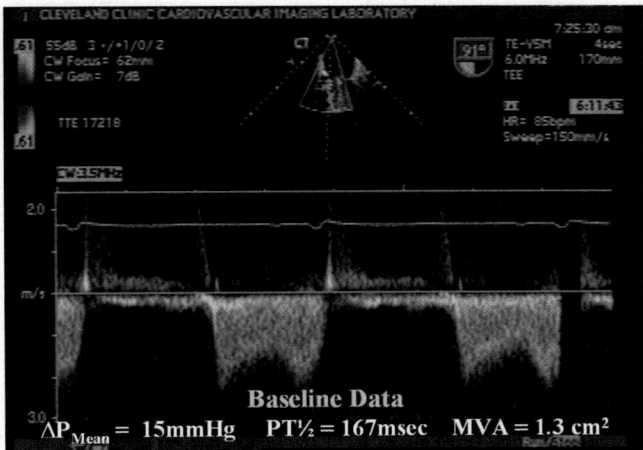

**Baseline Data**
$\Delta P_{Mean}$ = 15mmHg    PT½ = 167msec    MVA = 1.3 cm²

B

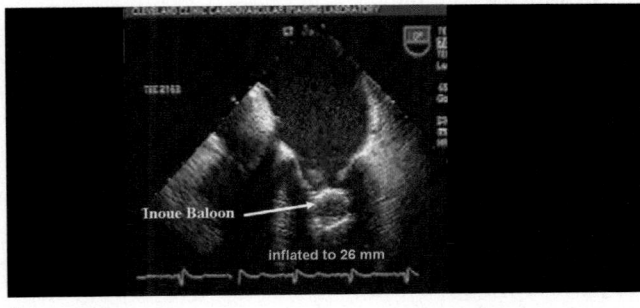

C

**FIGURE 37.17.** TEE is utilized to successfully guide the Inoue balloon valvuloplasty procedure **A:** ME four-chamber TEE image plane, demonstrating rheumatic MS with a spilitability score of 7. **B:** Baseline transvalvular gradient and pressure half time. **C:** Inoue balloon positioned across MV. *(continued)*

echocardiographic support at all stages of patient management is essential for appropriate patient selection, successful procedural outcome, and adequate surveillance following the procedure.

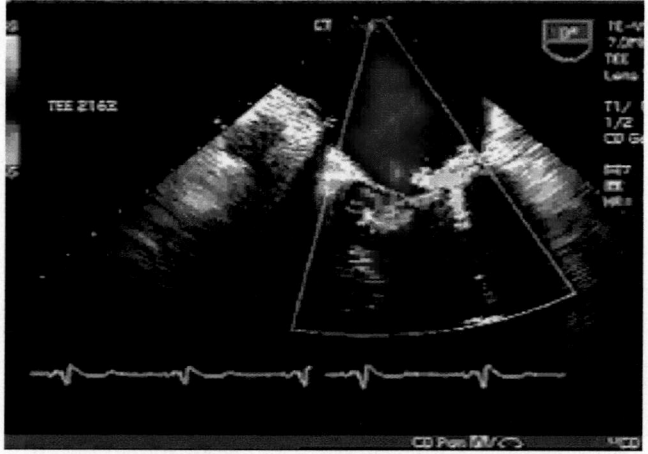

D

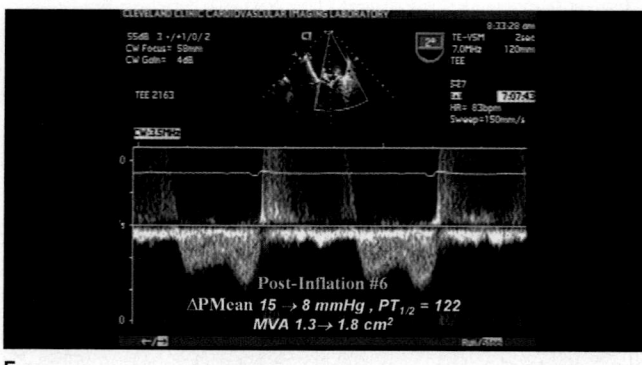

E

**FIGURE 37.17.** *(Continued)* **D:** Resulting MR with two jet directions. **E:** Reduced pressure gradient and pressure half time. Postballoon valvuloplasty. Initial pressure half time may not be as accurate due to LA and LV compliance changes associated acutely with the procedure.

## KEY POINTS

• Percutaneous cardiac intervention has traditionally involved myocardial revascularization. Experience with percutaneous aortic and mitral balloon valvuloplasty, electrophysiologic procedures, and PFO closure demonstrated the potential for other noncoronary applications.

• With the cumulative experience of more than one million percutaneous cardiac interventions annually, other noninvasive approaches to cardiac disease include the management of shunt closure (ASD, PDA, VSD), LAA closure, valvular disease (pulmonic and aortic valve replacement, MV repair), septal reduction in HOCM, and major vascular intervention (carotid and aortic stenting).

• Echocardiography has been utilized to successfully facilitate the safe implementation of new interventional procedures. TTE and TEE hastens the learning curve for the inventional specialist and enables the immediate diagnosis of complications related to the procedure.

• The use of echocardiographic guidance in the newer interventional procedures is essential for appropriate patient selection, successful procedure outcome, and patient safety. Incorporating echocardiography with the collaborative and interdisciplinary management of patients undergoing cutting edge approaches to cardiovascular disease will enable a realistic determination of the full capabilities of these new and exciting developments.

## REFERENCES

1. Schwarz F, Baumann P, Manthey J, et al. The effect of aortic valve replacement on survival. Circulation 1982;66(5):1105–10.
2. Cribier A, Eltchaninoff H, Letac B. Advances in percutaneous techniques for treatment of aortic and mitral stenosis. In: Topol EJ, ed. Textbook of interventional cardiology, 4th ed. Philadelphia:Elsevier Science, 2003:941–53.
3. Cribier A, Eltchaninoff H, Bash A, et al. Percutaneous transcatheter implantation of an aortic valve prosthesis for calcific aortic stenosis: first human case description. Circulation 2002;106(24):3006–8.
4. Eltchaninoff H, Tron C, Cribier A. Percutaneous implantation of aortic valve prosthesis in patients with calcific aortic stenosis: technical aspects. J Interv Cardiol 2003;16(6):515–21.
5. Condado JA, Velez-Gimon M. Catheter-based approach to mitral regurgitation. J Interv Cardiol 2003;16(6):523–34.
6. Kaye DM, Byrne M, Alferness C, Power J. Feasibility and short-term efficacy of percutaneous mitral annular reduction for the therapy of heart failure-induced mitral regurgitation. Circulation 2003;108(15):1795–7.
7. Alfieri O, Maisano F, De Bonis M, et al. The double-orifice technique in mitral valve repair: a simple solution for complex problems. J Thorac Cardiovasc Surg 2001;122(4):674–81.
8. St Goar FG, Fann JI, Komtebedde J, et al. Endovascular edge-to-edge mitral valve repair: short-term results in a porcine model. Circulation 2003;108(16):1990–3.
9. Kimmelstiel CD, Maron BJ. Role of percutaneous septal ablation in hypertrophic obstructive cardiomyopathy. Circulation 2004;109(4):452–6.
10. Maron BJ, Nishimura RA, McKenna WJ, Rakowski H, Josephson ME, Kieval RS. Assessment of permanent dual-chamber pacing as a treatment for drug-refractory symptomatic patients with obstructive hypertrophic cardiomyopathy. A randomized, double-blind, crossover study (M-PATHY). Circulation 1999;99(22):2927–33.
11. Nishimura RA, Trusty JM, Hayes DL, et al. Dual-chamber pacing for hypertrophic cardiomyopathy: a randomized, double-blind, crossover trial. J Am Coll Cardiol 1997;29(2):435–41.
12. Sigwart U. Non-surgical myocardial reduction for hypertrophic obstructive cardiomyopathy. Lancet 1995;346(8969):211–4.

13. Ruzyllo W, Chojnowska L, Demkow M, et al. Left ventricular outflow tract gradient decrease with non-surgical myocardial reduction improves exercise capacity in patients with hypertrophic obstructive cardiomyopathy. Eur Heart J 2000;21(9): 770–7.

14. Lakkis NM, Nagueh SF, Dunn JK, Killip D, Spencer WH, 3rd. Nonsurgical septal reduction therapy for hypertrophic obstructive cardiomyopathy: one-year follow-up. J Am Coll Cardiol 2000;36(3):852–5.

15. Seggewiss H, Faber L. Percutaneous septal ablation for hypertrophic cardiomyopathy and mid-ventricular obstruction. Eur J Echocardiogr 2000;1(4):277–80.

16. Mills NL, King TD. Nonoperative closure of left-to-right shunts. J Thorac Cardiovasc Surg 1976;72(3):371–8.

17. Lechat P, Mas JL, Lascault G, et al. Prevalence of patent foramen ovale in patients with stroke. N Engl J Med 1988; 318(18):1148–52.

18. Kannel WB, Wolf PA, Benjamin EJ, Levy D. Prevalence, incidence, prognosis, and predisposing conditions for atrial fibrillation: population-based estimates. Am J Cardiol 1998; 82(8A):2N–9N.

19. Blackshear JL, Odell JA. Appendage obliteration to reduce stroke in cardiac surgical patients with atrial fibrillation. Ann Thorac Surg 1996;61(2):755–9.

20. Hart RG, Halperin JL, Pearce LA, et al. Lessons from the Stroke Prevention in Atrial Fibrillation trials. Ann Intern Med 2003;138(10):831–8.

21. Stafford RS, Singer DE. Recent national patterns of warfarin use in atrial fibrillation. Circulation 1998;97(13):1231–3.

22. Madden J. Resection of the left auricular appendix. JAMA 1948;140:769–72.

23. Odell JA, Blackshear JL, Davies E, et al. Thoracoscopic obliteration of the left atrial appendage: potential for stroke reduction? Ann Thorac Surg 1996;61(2):565–9.

24. Nakai T, Lesh MD, Gerstenfeld EP, Virmani R, Jones R, Lee RJ. Percutaneous left atrial appendage occlusion (PLAATO) for preventing cardioembolism: first experience in canine model. Circulation 2002;105(18):2217–22.

25. Sievert H, Lesh MD, Trepels T, et al. Percutaneous left atrial appendage transcatheter occlusion to prevent stroke in high-risk patients with atrial fibrillation: early clinical experience. Circulation 2002;105(16):1887–9.

26. Al-Saady NM, Obel OA, Camm AJ. Left atrial appendage: structure, function, and role in thromboembolism. Heart 1999;82(5):547–54.

27. Meier B, Palacios I, Windecker S, et al. Transcatheter left atrial appendage occlusion with Amplatzer devices to obviate anticoagulation in patients with atrial fibrillation. Catheter Cardiovasc Interv 2003;60(3):417–22.

28. Blackshear JL, Johnson WD, Odell JA, et al. Thoracoscopic extracardiac obliteration of the left atrial appendage for stroke risk reduction in atrial fibrillation. J Am Coll Cardiol 2003;42(7):1249–52.

29. Crystal E, Lamy A, Connolly SJ, et al. Left Atrial Appendage Occlusion Study (LAAOS): a randomized clinical trial of left atrial appendage occlusion during routine coronary artery bypass graft surgery for long-term stroke prevention. Am Heart J 2003;145(1):174–8.

30. Pennec PY, Jobic Y, Blanc JJ, Bezon E, Barra JA. Assessment of different procedures for surgical left atrial appendage exclusion. Ann Thorac Surg 2003;76(6):2168–9.

31. Bartel T, Konorza T, Arjumand J, et al. Intracardiac echocardiography is superior to conventional monitoring for guiding device closure of interatrial communications. Circulation 2003;107(6):795–7.

32. Bolling SF, Pagani FD, Deeb GM, Bach DS. Intermediate-term outcome of mitral reconstruction in cardiomyopathy. J Thorac Cardiovasc Surg 1998;115(2):381–6; discussion 387–8.

33. Chant H, McCollum C. Stroke in young adults: the role of paradoxical embolism. Thromb Haemost 2001;85(1):22–9.

34. Chen FY, Adams DH, Aranki SF, et al. Mitral valve repair in cardiomyopathy. Circulation 1998;98(19 Suppl):II124–7.

35. Garcia-Fernandez MA, Perez-David E, Quiles J, et al. Role of left atrial appendage obliteration in stroke reduction in patients with mitral valve prosthesis: a transesophageal echocardiographic study. J Am Coll Cardiol 2003;42(7): 1253–8.

36. Halperin JL, Fuster V. Patent foramen ovale and recurrent stroke: another paradoxical twist. Circulation 2002;105(22): 2580–2.

37. Job FP, Ringelstein EB, Grafen Y, et al. Comparison of transcranial contrast Doppler sonography and transesophageal contrast echocardiography for the detection of patent foramen ovale in young stroke patients. Am J Cardiol 1994; 74(4):381–4.

38. Katz ES, Tsiamtsiouris T, Applebaum RM, Schwartzbard A, Tunick PA, Kronzon I. Surgical left atrial appendage ligation is frequently incomplete: a transesophageal echocardiographic study. J Am Coll Cardiol 2000;36(2):468–71.

39. Khairy P, O'Donnell CP, Landzberg MJ. Transcatheter closure versus medical therapy of patent foramen ovale and presumed paradoxical thromboemboli: a systematic review. Ann Intern Med 2003;139(9):753–60.

40. Koelling TM, Aaronson KD, Cody RJ, Bach DS, Armstrong WF. Prognostic significance of mitral regurgitation and tricuspid regurgitation in patients with left ventricular systolic dysfunction. Am Heart J 2002;144(3):524–9.

41. Lamy C, Giannesini C, Zuber M, et al. Clinical and imaging findings in cryptogenic stroke patients with and without patent foramen ovale: the PFO-ASA Study. Atrial Septal Aneurysm. Stroke 2002;33(3):706–11.

42. Levine MN, Raskob G, Landefeld S, Kearon C. Hemorrhagic complications of anticoagulant treatment. Chest 2001;119(1 Suppl):108S–121S.

43. McGaw D, Harper R. Patent foramen ovale and cryptogenic cerebral infarction. Intern Med J 2001;31(1):42–7.

44. Overell JR, Bone I, Lees KR. Interatrial septal abnormalities and stroke: a meta-analysis of case-control studies. Neurology 2000;55(8):1172–9.

45. Armstrong G, Cardon L, Vilkomerson D, et al. Localization of needle tip with color Doppler during pericardiocentesis: in vitro validation and initial clinical application. J Am Soc Echocardiog 2001;14(1):29–37.

46. Lynch M, Clements SD, Shanewise JS, et al. Right-sided cardiac tumors detected by transesophageal echocardiography and its usefulness in differentiating the benign from the malignant ones. Am J Cardiol 1997;79(6):781–4.

47. Keefe DL. Anthracycline-induced cardiomyopathy. Semin Oncol 2001;28(4 Suppl 12):2–7.

48. Shammas RL, Movahed A. Sarcoidosis of the heart. Clin Cardiol 1993;16(6):462–72.

49. Pandian NG, Hsu TL. Intravascular ultrasound and intracardiac echocardiography: concepts for the future. Am J Cardiol 1992;69(20):6H-17H.

50. Reddy SCB, Rath GA, Ziady GM, et al. Tricuspid flail leaflets after orthotopic heart transplant: a new complication of endomyocardial biopsy. J Am Soc Echocardiol 1993;6:223–6.

51. Williams MJA, Lee MY, DiSalvo TG, et al. Biopsy-induced flail tricuspid leaflet and tricuspid regurgitation following orthotopic cardiac transplantation. Am J Cardiol 1996;77: 1339–44.

52. Miller LW, Labovitz AJ, McBride LA, Pennington DG, Kanter K. Echocardiography-guided endomyocardial biopsy. Circulation 1988;78(suppl III):III-99–III-102.

53. Miche E, Bogunovic N, Fassbender D, et al. Predictors of unsuccessful outcome after percutaneous mitral valvotomy including a new echocardiographic scoring system. J Heart Valve Dis 1996;5:430–5.

54. Wilkins GT, Weyman AE, Abascal VM, et al. Percutaneous balloon dilatation of the mitral valve: an analysis of echocardiographic variables related to outcome and the mechanism of dilatation. Br Heart J 1988;60:299–308.

55. Ramondo A, Chirillo F, Dan M, et al. Value and limitations of transesophageal echocardiographic monitoring during percutaneous balloon mitral valvotomy. Int J Cardiol 1991; 31(2):223–33.

## QUESTIONS

1. The use of balloon valvuloplasty in patients with aortic stenosis is indicated in each of the following clinical situations *except*:
   A. Definitive management of calcific aortic stenosis
   B. Palliative treatment in higher risk patients
   C. Bridge to aortic valve replacement
   D. Short-term management in high-risk patients

2. TEE guidance of percutaneous aortic valve replacement is useful for which of the following?
   A. Positioning of the device for deployment
   B. Aortic valve gradient
   C. Aortic valve area
   D. Paravalvular regurgitation
   E. All of the above

3. Percutaneous approaches to MV repair are for which of the following MV disorders?
   A. Severe rheumatic mitral stenosis
   B. MR secondary to apical tethering (Type IIIb with/without type I)
   C. Segmental myxomatous flail PMVL
   D. Multiple segmental flail PMVL height 2.1 cm
   E. Rheumatic mitral regurgitation

4. The Alfieri repair is used for which of the following?
   A. Type IIIb mechanisms of MR
   B. Type I mechanisms of MR
   C. Failed MV repair
   D. Type IIIa MR
   E. Type II mechanism of MR

5. Complications of alcohol septal reduction of HOCM include each of the following *except*:
   A. VSD
   B. Heart block
   C. Septal infarct
   D. Mitral leaflet perforation
   E. All of the above

## Chapter 38

# Assessment for Noncardiac Surgery

*Albert C. Perrino, Jr. and Scott T. Reeves*

The introduction of commercial TEE systems in the mid-1980s was greeted with considerable enthusiasm by cardiac anesthesiologists recognizing the potential this technology offered to better monitor and diagnose patients undergoing coronary artery bypass and valve surgeries. As cardiac surgery remained the focus of intraoperative TEE, there was a strong undercurrent to explore its applications in noncardiac procedures. Limited availability of echocardiographic systems and clinicians trained in TEE initially slowed the growth of TEE in noncardiac procedures. However, as these limitations abated new applications for TEE emerged in each corridor of the OR. As will be presented in this chapter, the breadth of TEE use in current surgical practice is remarkable. Its use specific to vascular, general, orthopedic, and liver transplantation surgeries will receive detailed attention. Moreover, the ability of TEE to provide a rapid diagnosis in a patient not responding to standard therapies is a universal application warranting TEE availability to most anesthetized patients. Accordingly, the TEE evaluation for the hemodynamically unstable patient is presented independent of surgical procedure.

## INDICATIONS

In common with other intraoperative monitoring devices, the indications for TEE remain only partially defined. Clarifying the indications for TEE is not a trivial concern given the expense incurred and trained personnel required to perform an intraoperative TEE examination (1,2). Unfortunately, well-conducted outcome trials examining the effectiveness of TEE during noncardiac surgery are lacking and unlikely to be forthcoming. Several parties have attempted to provide guidance in this gray area. Most notable among these are the 1996 practice guidelines published from a consensus conference of the American Society of Anesthesiologists and the Society of Cardiovascular Anesthesiologists Task Force on TEE (3).

Their recommendations are divided into three categories based on the strength of supporting evidence and/or expert opinion that TEE improves clinical outcomes. Category I indications are supported by the strongest evidence or expert opinion; TEE frequently is useful in improving clinical outcomes in these settings and often is indicated. Category II indications are supported by weaker evidence and expert consensus; TEE may be useful in improving clinical outcomes in these settings but appropriate indications are less certain. Category III indications have little scientific or expert support and appropriate indications are uncertain. As is true for each of these categories but particularly germane for Category III, the lack of supporting evidence is often owing to the absence of relevant studies rather than to existing evidence of ineffectiveness. Unfortunately, yet appropriately given the paucity and expense of outcome trials, these guidelines are based largely on opinion and mostly refer to the care of cardiac surgical patients. Subsequent clinical trials and technological advances will undoubtedly lead to changes in the indications for intraoperative TEE.

Although most relevant to cardiac surgery, the ASA/SCA practice guidelines have important implications to noncardiac surgery as well. Without controversy is the Category I indication for intraoperative evaluation of acute persistent and life-threatening hemodynamic disturbances in which ventricular function and its determinants are uncertain and have not responded to treatment. This is the all too common scenario of employing TEE as a rescue diagnostic tool. Its sister Category II indication is for perioperative use in patients with increased *risk* of hemodynamic disturbances. Here, TEE is recommended as a preemptive monitoring tool to avoid life-threatening disturbances and to optimize organ perfusion. *Together, these indications remain, by far, the most frequent reasons for the use of intraoperative TEE during noncardiac surgery.* Although the task force notes that direct evidence was lacking to support these indications, expert opinion agreed that TEE was of clear benefit to diagnose the hemodynamic problem and to suggest appropriate therapy. This opinion has been confirmed by a series of clinical trials conducted subsequent to the Task Force deliberations and provides direct evidence for an expanded use of TEE monitoring during noncardiac surgery.

To investigate the use and impact of transesophageal echocardiography, Suriani et al. from Mount Sinai Medical Center, reviewed 123 TEE examinations performed during noncardiac surgery (4). The exams were classified as consultative when performed by a consultant (55 points) and nonconsultative (68 points) when performed by the attending anesthesiologist. The impact of TEE was rated as major if TEE was used to treat a life-threatening event, it changed surgical and/or anesthetic management, or led to further evaluation in the postoperative period. Lesser impacts were rated as minor or limited. They judged TEE as having an impact on care in 81% of the patients, and in 15% the impact was major. Their elderly ASA 3 and 4 patients particularly benefited from TEE during noncardiac surgery. This study confirmed that TEE in patients undergoing noncardiac surgery is efficacious in rapidly disclosing new findings and information during periods of hemodynamic instability.

Kolev and colleagues (5) further studied the current role played by intraoperative TEE and examined the impact of the ASA/SCA category-based TEE indications. The study included 224 patients from seven western European countries. In this group of patients who also were monitored with radial and pulmonary arterial catheters, TEE was the most important guiding factor in 25% of interventions. Not surprisingly, TEE use for Category I indications were associated with the most frequent changes in management. Noteworthy is that these practitioners used TEE most frequently for Category II indications, suggesting the growing acceptance of TEE as a monitor of cardiovascular function. Schmidlin examined the use of TEE at the University Hospital in Zurich, Switzerland, and found that in 123 vascular surgery cases TEE led to changes in drug or fluid therapy in 32% of patients and a new diagnosis in 9% (6).

The impact of TEE on noncardiac surgery has also been widely examined in Canadian practice (7–10). Denault from the Notre Dame Hospital in Montreal examined the records of 214 patients. The indications for TEE slightly favored Category I (37%) versus Categories II (31%) and III (27%) (9). They noted that TEE led to a change in management, either surgical or medical, in 40% of patients. The modifications in case management, in order of frequency, were

1. Change in medical therapy
2. Confirming or invalidating a diagnosis
3. Unplanned surgical reinterventions
4. Substitute for pulmonary artery catheter
5. Positioning of intravascular devices

They concurred with the findings of prior studies regarding the value of TEE in Category I patients, but also demonstrated substantial impact of TEE in Categories II and III patients in the perioperative period. Remarkably, the authors concluded that the impact of TEE in the noncardiac setting was even more important than that they had observed in cardiac surgery.

These observational studies provide strong support for the value of TEE in noncardiac surgeries and suggest outcome trials to further clarify its role and indications. Two recent outcome studies, first by Sinclair (11) and subsequently by TJ Gan and colleagues (12), have demonstrated that goal-directed fluid management guided by echocardiography improves outcomes in a cohort of patients undergoing a variety of noncardiac procedures. *These results give objective support to the many case reports and observational studies of the value of echocardiography as a monitor of fluid management and cardiovascular performance* (13). *In the authors' opinion the body of evidence for its application in this regard now warrants this indication as a promotion to Category I status.*

In summary, these data on noncardiac surgery patients show TEE's value both as a diagnostic tool and as an intraoperative monitor over and above that achievable with radial and pulmonary arterial catheters. This data is not dissimilar to that observed in the ICU setting where at least one-third of noncardiac surgery ICU patients' care is altered by TEE examination independent of the presence of a pulmonary arterial catheter (14,15). While much of the early attention on TEE was focused on its ability to detect myocardial ischemia (16–18) the above studies reveal that in current practice TEE's add-on value exists in its ability to monitor fluid status and global ventricular function.

## APPROACH

### Optimization of Ventricular Performance during Noncardiac Surgery

The principles underlying optimization of ventricular performance using TEE remain guided by the Frank-Starling relationship (19,20). Figure 38.1 demonstrates the classical Frank-Starling curvilinear relationship, showing that increases in left ventricular end-diastolic volume (LVEDV) result in a progressively greater stroke volume. An increase in contractility, such as that which occurs with the addition of an inotrope, will shift the curve upwards, resulting in increasing stroke volume for any given LVEDV. Increases in afterload on the other hand have an inverse relationship to stroke volume as depicted in Figure 38.1.

The remarkable longevity of this approach stems from its ability to incorporate both diastolic (e.g., preload) and systolic functions. As these functions are co-dependent, it

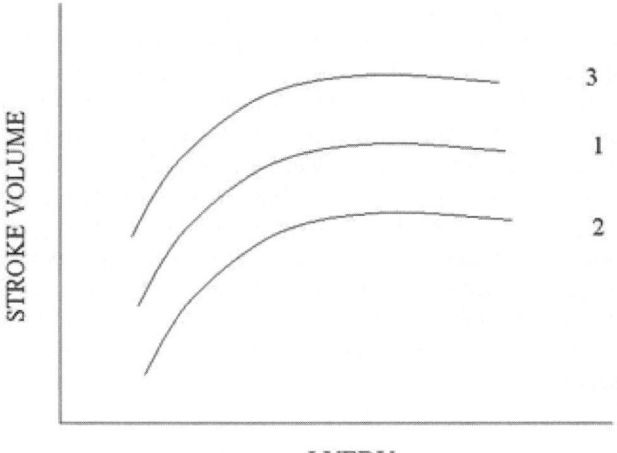

**FIGURE 38.1.** Frank-Starling Relationship: Demonstrates the effect of increasing left ventricular end-diastolic volume (*LVEDV*), i.e., (1) preload on resulting stroke volume in the normal heart, (2) failing heart, and (3) heart exposed to an inotrope.

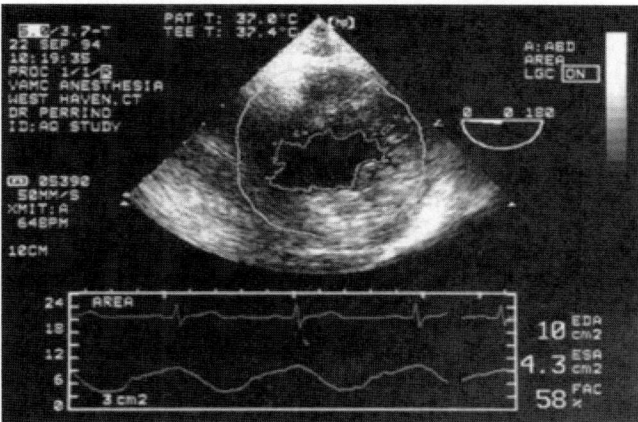

**FIGURE 38.2.** Automated Border Detection has identified the endocardial-blood interface (inner tracing) in this TG SAX view and provides continuous digital waveform display of LV cavity areas and calculation of LV end-diastolic area (*EDA*), end systolic area (*ESA*), and fractional area change (*FAC*). From Perrino et al. Anesthesiology Vol 83, No. 2, August 1995.

is unsatisfactory to attempt to understand the state of cardiac functioning by an independent examination of these factors. For example, although the left ventricular end-diastolic area (LVEDA) has many advantages in assessing preload compared to PA pressures, in itself it is of limited value (21). An intraoperative LVEDA of 12 cm$^2$ is no more sufficient to determine that fluid status is "normal" or ideal than knowing that the PADP is 10 mm HG. The broad diversity in cardiac function and pathology, as well as the effects of surgery and anesthetics, preclude such assessments in the OR. Consequently, the value of the Frank-Starling relationship is that it provides an iterative approach to optimizing the relationship between preload and systolic output for the particular case at hand. The necessary parameters for deriving the Frank-Starling relationship, preload and stroke volume, are easily monitored intraoperatively with TEE.

### Assessing Preload

As a measure of preload, TEE is superb for both quantitative assessment and monitoring the adequacy of preload throughout surgery (22–26). By far the most popular approach to measure LV preload is by determination of the LVEDA from the TG midpapillary SAX view. Although LVEDV is considered the ideal measurement, the time-consuming imaging and calculations required make LVEDV currently an unacceptable measurement for intraoperative use. The LVEDA has been validated to accurately track changes in intraoperative fluid status and is simply calculated from manual tracings of still frame echoes at end-diastole or from the output of an automated border detection system such as Acoustic Quantifi-

cation (27). The border detection algorithm provides beat-to-beat quantitative measures of LV end-diastolic and end-systolic areas as well as the ejection fraction (Figs. 38.2 and 38.3). This system is particularly well suited for noncardiac surgery because there is little interference from the surgical procedure. In contrast, the surgical exposure and cardiac manipulations that occur in

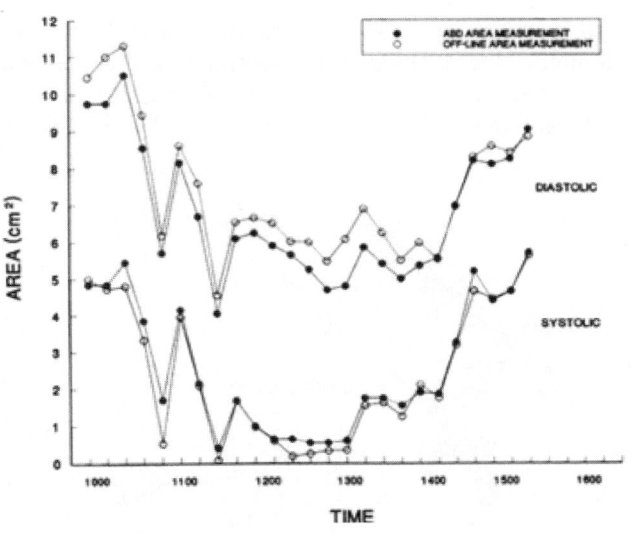

**FIGURE 38.3.** Changes in left ventricular end-diastolic area and end-systolic area by automated border detection and by off-line echocardiographer review in a patient who underwent repair of a hip fracture. Automated measurements accurately tracked the loss in preload secondary to hemorrhage and its recovery following resuscitative therapy. From Perrino et al. Anesthesiology Vol 83, No. 2, August 1995.

open chest procedures often produce repeated disruptions in border detection limiting the use of acoustic quantification for cardiac surgery.

Normal values for LVEDA are typically 12–18 cm²; however preexisting cardiac disease, acute alterations in ventricular compliance, and increased metabolic demands alter the pressure-volume relationship of the ventricle and often the optimal intraoperative LVEDA will exceed normal. For these reasons, we strongly advise against using a single parameter, in this case LVEDA, in isolation as the basis for clinical fluid management. Rather, by using LVEDA measures of preload combined with matched Doppler measurements of stroke volume, the clinician can derive an intraoperative Starling curve for the patient and effectively titrate fluid, inotropic, and vasoactive therapy to optimize cardiovascular status.

## Assessing Stroke Volume

Due to the challenges in obtaining LV volumes with 2-D echoes, Doppler techniques are preferred for stroke volume determination. In using the Doppler approach, it is important not to confuse blood flow velocity, which is the speed at which blood travels and expressed as cm/sec, with stroke volume, which is the amount of blood that travels in a single cycle, expressed as cm³/cycle. Stroke volume (SV) is calculated as the time velocity integral (TVI) multiplied by the cross-sectional area (CSA) of the conduit:

$$SV = TVI \times CSA$$

To perform an echocardiographic determination of volumetric flow, a Doppler measurement of the instantaneous blood-flow velocities and a 2-D measurement of cross-sectional area are obtained (Fig. 38.4). The instantaneous velocities during systole are traced from the spectral display and the echocardiographic system's internal software package calculates the time velocity integral (TVI cm) (Fig. 38.5). Conceptually, the time velocity integral represents the cumulative distance, commonly referred to as the stroke distance, that the red cells traveled during the systolic ejection phase. By multiplying the stroke distance by the CSA (cm²) of the conduit (e.g., aorta, mitral valve, or pulmonary artery) through which the blood traveled, the stroke volume (cm³) is obtained (28–34). Cardiac output, which expresses volumetric flow in cm³/min, is determined from the product of SV and heart rate.

### Echocardiographic Techniques for Stroke Volume Measurement (Table 38.1)

SV and CO measurements using TEE are best measured at the left ventricular outflow tract or at the aortic valve (31,33,34). Multiplane TEE offers excellent windows at these sites for both Doppler blood flow measurements and 2-D echocardiographic measurements of CSA. Several clinical studies have confirmed that the CO measurements obtained by TEE compare favorably to those obtained by thermodilution (33,34).

LVOT or transaortic valvular flows are most reliably obtained from the TG LAX and the deep TG LAX views, as blood flow will be near parallel to the ultrasound beam (Fig. 38.5). It is critical to carefully interrogate blood flow through minor alterations in probe position and multiplane angle to obtain the optimal Doppler spectral signal. The maximal velocity profile associated with a dense spectral signal is sought.

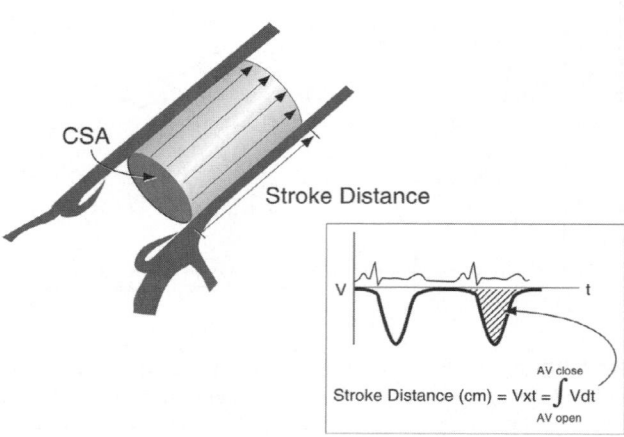

**FIGURE 38.4.** Stroke volume determination. Volumetric flow can be determined from a combination of area and velocity measurements. From Perrino, Reeves eds., A Practical Approach to TEE, Lippincott, 2002.

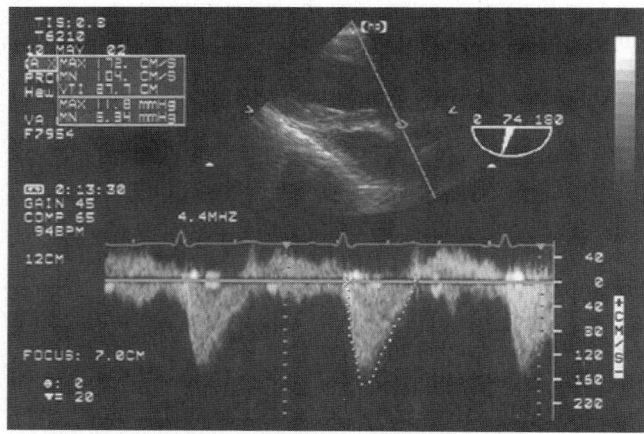

**FIGURE 38.5.** TG Long-axis view is displayed with CW Doppler directed through aortic valve orifice. The outer envelope of the spectral signal is traced, providing a stroke distance calculation. Heart rate is 94/min. Stroke volume = 2.5 cm² × 27.7 cm = 69.2 cc. Cardiac output = 69.2 cc × 94/min = 6505 cc/min. From Perrino, Reeves eds. Practical Approach to TEE, Lippincott, 2002.

▶ **TABLE 38.1.** TEE Measurements of Stroke Volume

| Stroke volume approaches | Doppler view | Doppler system | CSA view | CSA measurement |
|---|---|---|---|---|
| LVOT | TG LAX or deep TG LAX | PW | ME LAX | $\pi(\text{Diameter}/2)^2$ |
| Transaortic Valve | TG LAX or deep TG LAX | CW | ME AV SAX | Planimetry of valve leaflets during midsystole |
| Pulmonary Artery | UE aortic arch SAX or TG 110° | PW or CW | UE aortic arch SAX or TG 110° | $\pi(\text{Diameter}/2)^2$ |

The CSA of the LVOT is best obtained from the ME LAX view. The CSA is calculated from a measurement of the LVOT diameter as: $CSA_{lvot} = \pi(\text{diameter}/2)^2$. For transaortic valve stroke volume calculation, the CSA of the aortic valve is approximated by planimetry of the equilateral triangle-shaped orifice observed in midsystole (33). The aortic valve is viewed in cross section from the ME AV SAX window, and frame-by-frame review is used to capture the valve in midsytole.

### Right Heart Stroke Volume Calculation (Table 38.1)

Alternatively right-sided flows and diameters can be analyzed from the main pulmonary artery (MPA) or the mitral valve (MV). PW or CW Doppler analysis proceeds after the main pulmonary artery is imaged from the UE aortic arch SAX view or from the right ventricular outflow tract imaged from transgastric windows at 110–150 degree rotation of the transducer and rightward turn of the TEE probe (Fig. 38.6). In all cases the maximal velocity profile is sought. Measurement of flow across the mitral valve is accomplished by placing the sample volume at the level of the mitral annulus to obtain the transmitral time velocity integral, which is then multiplied by the mitral valve annulus. Compared to measures from the LVOT or ascending aorta, the diameters of the MPA and MV have greater fluctuation during the cardiac cycle (31) and these measurements are less reliable compared to those from the LVOT and aortic valve (35). In addition, the mitral valve orifice is not circular and its size changes during diastole.

*Generation of the Frank-Starling Curve:* Boluses of IV fluids are administered until a satisfactory end point is achieved (e.g., stroke volume does not increase by 10% with a 3 cc/kg fluid bolus) while avoiding distension of the left ventricle. Great care must be utilized when volume challenging a depressed ventricle. Also, it must be remembered that the *right* ventricle may become distended prior to achieving the desired end point and without left ventricular distension (36).

### Alternative Approaches to Optimizing Fluid Status

Many echocardiographers prefer to use visual estimates of LVEDA to monitor preload with TEE rather than more quantitative approaches (26,38). Reich et al. demonstrated that experienced echocardiographers are able to detect reductions in blood volume from cine-loop video recordings with high sensitivity (80–95%) and specificity (80%). The accuracy of real-time visual estimates of LV dimensions has more recently been challenged (38). We recommend the use of quad screen review to assist these qualitative assessments. Having a baseline TG mid-SAX view displayed improves comparative judgments of fluid status and ventricular performance during the course of surgery (39) (Fig. 38.7).

Another useful echocardiographic marker for inadequate preload is cavity obliteration in the end-systolic frame (Fig. 38.8). Commonly referred to as "kissing papillaries," this finding is suggestive of hypovolemia but is not specific as decreases in vascular resistance and increases in inotropy also affect end-systolic volumes (40,41). When

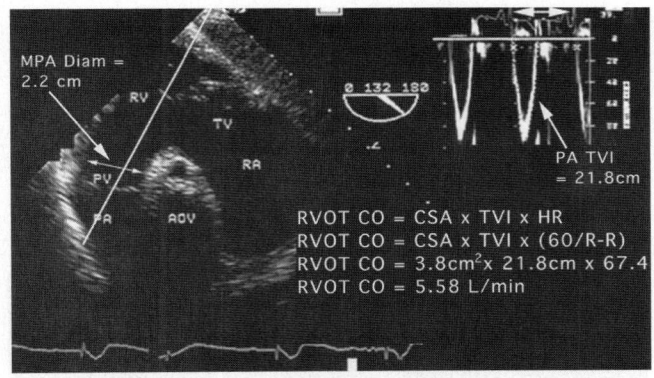

**FIGURE 38.6.** Calculation of Cardiac Output: Right Ventricular Outflow Tract Approach. *Left:* TG right ventricular inflow/outflow view. The Doppler beam is aligned as close to parallel with blood flow through the RVOT and the diameter is measured at the site where the pulse wave sample volume is placed. In this case, the MPA diam = 2.2 cm. *Right:* Using pulsed wave Doppler, the RVOT time velocity integral is obtained and the $(D/2)^2$ formula calculates a cross-sectional area of 3.8 cm$^2$. When multiplied by the TVI and the heart rate, CO is calculated to be 5.58 L/min. *RVOT,* right ventricular outflow tract; *PA,* pulmonary artery; *RV,* right ventricle; *TV,* tricuspid valve; *RA,* right atrium; *PV,* pulmonic valve; *Aov,* aortic valve; *CO,* cardiac output; *Diam,* diameter; *TVI,* time velocity integral; *R-R,* time interval between two 'R' on the electrocardiogram; *cm,* centimeter. From Perrino, Reeves eds. Practical Approach to TEE, Lippincott, 2002.

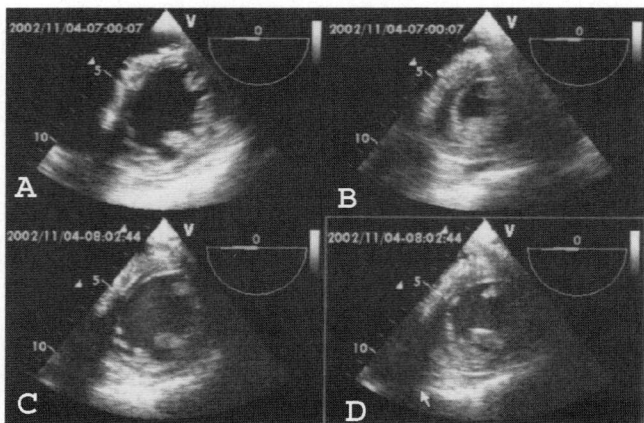

**FIGURE 38.7.** Quad screen display of LV end-diastolic frames (*left*) and end-systolic frames (*right*) in a patient undergoing abdominal aortic aneurysm resection. The **top pair** show LV dimensions prior to placement of the aortic cross clamp and the **bottom pair** are images taken during aortic cross clamping. The significant increase in LV end-systolic area during cross clamping is easily appreciated.

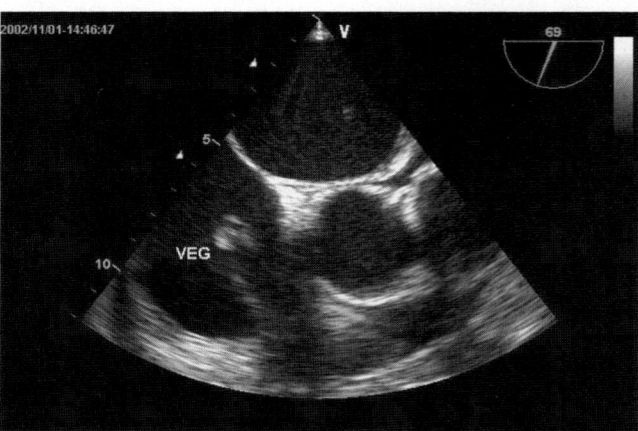

**FIGURE 38.9.** Patient with cardiac pacemaker developed intermittent capturing during the course of surgery. TEE demonstrated a large vegetation on pacemaker lead.

systolic cavity obliteration is observed, additional data from diastolic views and hemodynamic calculations are necessary to complete the diagnosis.

### Completing the Exam

In addition to optimizing fluid status the echocardiographic exam should also include a standard intraoperative examination of regional wall motion, valvular function, and a survey for unexpected pathology (e.g., patent foramen ovale, thrombus) (Fig. 38.9) (Table 38.2). More advanced quantitative assessments of hemodynamics, such as cavitary pressures, are not routinely required un-

less indicated by the patient's condition or pathology in the routine examination (42). Using the approach outlined, the TEE evaluation provides a superior evaluation of cardiac function to that of a PA catheter and the cause of an acute hemodynamic disturbance is rapidly achieved.

## SPECIFIC INDICATIONS

### Vascular Surgery

Major abdominal and peripheral vascular surgeries are associated with greater cardiac morbidity and overall mortality than other forms of noncardiac surgery (43–46). Cardiac events such as unstable angina, congestive heart failure, myocardial infarction, and cardiac death have been reported to occur in 5–18% of patients

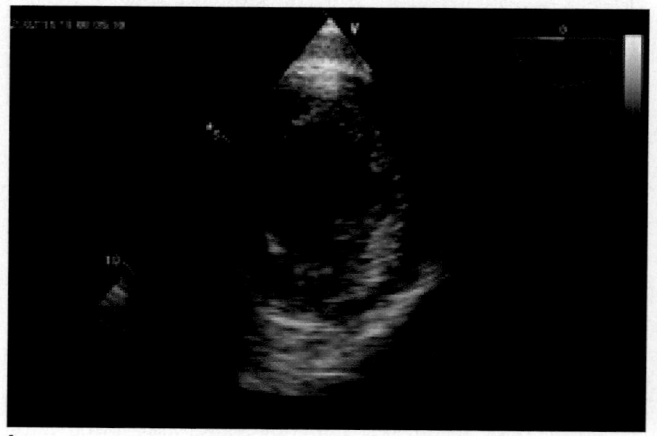

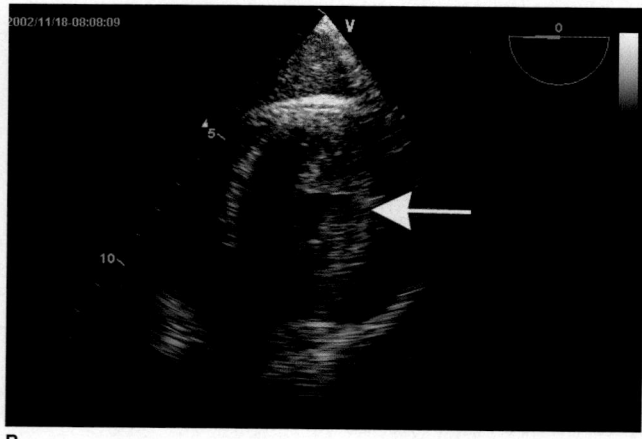

**A**                                                                                   **B**

**FIGURE 38.8. A:** Baseline TG SAX end-systolic frame. **B:** Later in the procedure, treatment with IV nitrates leads to systolic cavity obliteration. Note that the two papillary muscles abut (*arrow*), leading to the common descriptor "kissing papillaries."

▶ TABLE 38.2. Common Echocardiographic Presentations
of Hemodynamic Instability During
Noncardiac Surgery

| Etiology | LVEDA | LVEF | RVEF | RWMAs | MR |
|---|---|---|---|---|---|
| Decreased Contractility | ↑ | ↓ | ↓ | ↑ | — or ↓ |
| Decreased Preload | ↓ | ↑ | ↑ | — | — |
| Decreased LV Afterload | ↓ | ↑ | — or ↑ | — or ↑ | ↓ |
| Ischemia | ↑ | ↓ | — or ↓ | ↑ | — or ↑ |
| Acute Mitral Regurgitation | — or ↑ | — or ↑ | — | ↓ or ↑ | ↑ |
| Increased RV Afterload | ↓ | — | ↓ | ↑ | — |

↑ = increase, ↓ = decrease, — = little change

undergoing peripheral vascular or carotid artery surgery, and up to 25% of patients undergoing major abdominal surgery. Accordingly, the use of TEE is most evident in vascular surgery amongst the noncardiac procedures.

Vascular disease is often a systemic process and there is a strong association between peripheral vascular disease and coronary artery disease (46). Given the association between ischemia and cardiac morbidity, several investigators have examined the value of intraoperative TEE ischemia monitoring on outcome of vascular surgery. These studies provide little support that outcome is improved by TEE indicators of ischemia. Roizen et al. found that 55% of patients undergoing aortic reconstruction experienced new RWMAs at the time of aortic clamping (47). The incidence was highest with supraceliac cross clamping and not evident for infrarenal cross clamping. However, only one patient suffered an MI. Krupski et al. examined the incidence of perioperative cardiac ischemic events in 140 patients undergoing major abdominal or infrainguinal vascular operations (48,49). In contrast to ECG abnormalities, which were similar between the two groups, TEE suggested ischemia more commonly in the aortic procedures (26% versus 10%). However, the patients having peripheral vascular surgery had worse outcome and there was no correlation between TEE ischemia and perioperative outcomes. London et al.'s study of 156 high-risk patients undergoing various vascular and noncardiac surgical procedures corroborates the limited value of TEE ischemia monitoring in a study (50). Again, new SWMA detected by TEE correlated poorly with postoperative outcome. More recently, the same research group confirmed that regional wall motion abnormalities identified by TEE during vascular and noncardiac surgeries had little incremental clinical value in identifying patients at high risk for perioperative ischemic outcomes (51).

The lack of value of TEE ischemia monitoring can be attributed to several factors. TEE is a more sensitive de-

tector of ischemia than ECG or PA catheters (52). Many of the episodes of intraoperative ischemia detected by TEE may be minor and short-lived and may not contribute to postoperative morbidity. The specificity of TEE indicators of ischemia may also be reduced during surgery as alterations in loading conditions, contractility, and conduction are commonplace and can produce wall motion abnormalities in the absence of ischemia.

Aortic reconstructive surgery involving a period of aortic cross clamping followed by unclamping is associated with substantial stress to the cardiovascular system. In contrast, more peripheral procedures such as carotid endarterectomy and lower extremity bypass produce more subtle alterations in cardiovascular physiology (53,54). TEE has been shown to be superior to alternative clinical monitors in assessing the cardiovascular status during the acute challenges during aortic reconstruction (48,55,56). Roizen et al. used TEE to demonstrate the dramatic stresses incurred during suprarenal aortic cross clamping (47). Marked elevations in LV end-systolic and end-diastolic dimensions and a corresponding fall in LVEF substantiated the decrease in LV performance. These findings were not reliably detected with PA catheter monitoring. Gillepsie et al. further corroborated the limited utility of PA catheter monitoring during aortic surgery (55). This group found poor agreement between PA occlusion pressures and TEE estimates of LV volume during the period of infrarenal aortic cross clamping and following its release in their study of 22 patients. These investigations clearly support the use of TEE to obtain reliable information of LV filling and systolic function during the dynamic setting of aortic cross clamping (Fig. 38.7). Catheter data is less reliable and less useful due to the acute alterations in LV compliance seen during aortic reconstructive surgery.

New applications of TEE in vascular surgery continuously emerge. Areas of importance include the use of TEE for spinal cord imaging, imaging of the spinal arteries, and imaging of visceral arteries (57–59). The ability to image the celiac, mesenteric, and renal arteries may provide important data in real-time evaluation of the surgical approach (e.g., assess perfusion, position cross clamp) (60). Similarly, TEE has been reported to confirm deployment and function of endovascular stents used during endovascular repair of aortic aneurysms (61).

## Laparoscopic Surgery

Laparoscopic surgical approaches are being advanced to treat a broad range of pathologies. Although initially introduced for short-duration procedures in low-risk patient groups (gynecology, appendectomy), they are increasingly employed in procedures of greater complexity involving patients with comorbid conditions, such as colonic resections and aortic aneurysm repair. TEE will be increasingly called upon to assist the intraoperative management of these cases and to serve as an emergency diagnostic tool in the advent of untoward complications. Unique to laparoscopic procedures, the intraoperative echocardiographer needs to be cognizant of the unique physiological alterations incurred by intraoperative pneumoperitoneum.

### Physiologic Implication of Pneumoperitoneum

Abdominal $CO_2$ insufflation and the subsequent increase in abdominal pressure during laparoscopic surgery can cause severe changes in hemodynamics. Notably, TEE has played a leading role in the clinical studies that have led to our current understanding of the cardiovascular sequelae of pneumoperitoneum. Pneumoperitoneum results in a marked increase in systemic vascular resistance and afterload (62–68). The increase in afterload is attributed to humoral factors such as vasopressin release and direct effects of increased intraabdominal pressure on the aorta and venous systems. Preload is typically increased due to compression of the splanchnic vessels that shifts blood from the abdomen to the thorax. Ejection fraction often remains preserved or modestly decreased in healthy patients, however those with preexisting cardiovascular disease show more pronounced impairment of cardiac function (64,69,70). An ominous finding by several of these investigators was ventricular distension in the face of decreased ejection fraction and elevated afterload. Of particular concern was that routine monitoring of blood pressure and heart rate did not detect the marked impairment in cardiac performance seen in these studies.

The patient position used to facilitate the procedure (e.g., Trendelenburg, lithotomy) can further impact cardiac performance. Reverse Trendelenburg is commonly used in upper abdominal procedures to facilitate operative exposure. This positioning mitigates the increases in preload seen with abdominal insufflation. In lower abdominal procedures, lithotomy and/or Trendelenburg positions are preferred. In combination with abdominal insufflation they have the opposite effect and can lead to potentially dangerous elevations in preload in the face of increased afterload. These conditions have resulted in severe cardiac impairment in patients with preexisting heart disease (64,71).

Additional factors regarding the echocardiographic evaluation during laparoscopic surgery include the subtle effects of hypercapnia caused by absorbed $CO_2$, decreased hepatic blood flow secondary to pressure effects of pneumoperitoneum, as well as the dramatic consequences of trocar injury to a major blood vessel and carbon dioxide embolism (72–74). TEE is useful in monitoring for each of these complications. It is the technique of choice to diagnose the cause of sudden cardiac collapse during laparoscopic surgery, allowing rapid differentiation of acute hemorrhage versus $CO_2$ embolic events (75). TEE is also useful in preventing such complications. Tupperainen et al. has demonstrated that head down positioning and pneumoperitoneum have a more negative influence on the filling of the left side of the heart than on the filling of the right side and that pressure reversal (right atrial pressure exceeds left atrial pressure) occurs in systole during the expiratory cycle of mechanical ventilation (74). The increase in right atrial versus left atrial pressure places the patient at risk for systemic gas embolism. Tupperainen and his group used TEE to monitor intraatrial septal motion to detect reversal of pressures and to direct fluid therapy to reverse this process.

In summary, TEE is the preferred technique for assessing cardiovascular responses during laparoscopic surgery. It is of proven value both as a rescue diagnostic tool and as an intraoperative monitor. *As a preemptive monitor, TEE is indicated for those patients with preexisting cardiac disease undergoing more complicated procedures.* Routine monitoring of heart rate and blood pressure alone has been shown to be insufficient to alert the clinician of ventricular distension and marked falls in ejection fraction and cardiac index. TEE reliably detects these abnormalities and has been shown to guide therapeutic intervention (69). The use of PA monitoring is complicated during laparoscopic surgery by the variations in patient positioning and transmission of insufflation pressures to the thoracic cavity (76). Further, TEE is the only clinical device that can diagnose each of the variety of events that can compromise cardiac function during laparoscopic surgery. As laparoscopic surgery offers significant advantages in *postoperative* recovery, there is a clear trend towards utilizing this approach in older and sicker patients with coexisting cardiovascular disease. TEE offers a means to ensure the *intraoperative* success of these procedures.

## Orthopedic Surgery

TEE has been widely applied in orthopedic surgeries. *At this point, three major intraoperative complications, namely bone cement implantation syndrome, thromboembolism, and hemorrhage, are the primary indications for TEE.*

### Bone Cement Implantation Syndrome

One of the most feared complications of total hip arthroplasty is bone cement implantation syndrome (77–81). Pressurization of the medullary cavity during reaming and insertion of the cemented femoral prosthesis causes the extrusion of marrow fat, air, and thrombi into the femoral venous channels. Subsequently these materials embolize to the pulmonary vasculature, resulting in increased pulmonary vascular resistance and right heart failure. The syndrome is characterized by systemic hypotension, pulmonary hypertension, and oxygen desaturation. Intraoperative cardiac arrest and lethal pulmonary embolism can result (82–85) (Fig. 38.10). In a review of several studies intraoperative cardiac arrest occurred in 0.6 to 10% of cases (86). Postoperatively these patients experience respiratory and hemodynamic complications.

TEE has played a major role in investigations that have defined the role of surgical maneuvers and the importance of embolization of intramedullary debris in the bone cement syndrome. TEE examinations first demonstrated the temporal association between embolic phenomenon and clinical symptoms of the bone cement syndrome. *The major periods at risk for embolization are during reaming, insertion of the femoral prosthesis, and in more than half of cases, upon reduction of the hip joint.* It is believed that significant amounts of embolic material extruded into the femoral vessels during the prosthesis insertion may not proceed centrally immediately because the femoral vein is distorted by surgical positioning such that venous return is obstructed. With hip relocation the obstruction is relieved and embolism occurs (83).

Most embolic events during THA appear to be clinically benign and their effects short-lived. Two factors have been identified that increase the risk of serious complications during total hip arthroplasty. The first is the amount of emboli present. TEE assessment of embolization is quantified using a four-grade scoring system (Fig. 38.11 and Table 38.3).

Koessler and colleagues demonstrated a nearly immediate cause and effect relationship between embolic events graded 2 and 3 and hypotension, hypoxemia, and decreases in end-tidal $CO_2$ (87). The second factor recognized is that morbidity from the bone cement implantation syndrome is increased in patients with preexisting disease (87,88).

*We feel that in patients undergoing cemented total hip arthroplasty who are compromised, debilitated, or elderly the use of TEE should be considered.* When properly diagnosed and treated, the mortality rate from pulmonary embolism can be reduced significantly. TEE also plays an important role in evaluating the effectiveness of new surgical approaches geared at reducing the embolic load.

### Total Knee Arthroplasty

In patients undergoing total knee arthroplasty intraoperative complications from pulmonary embolic events are

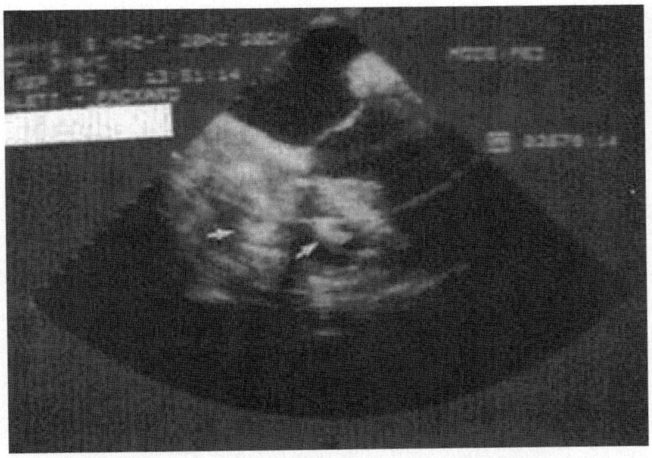

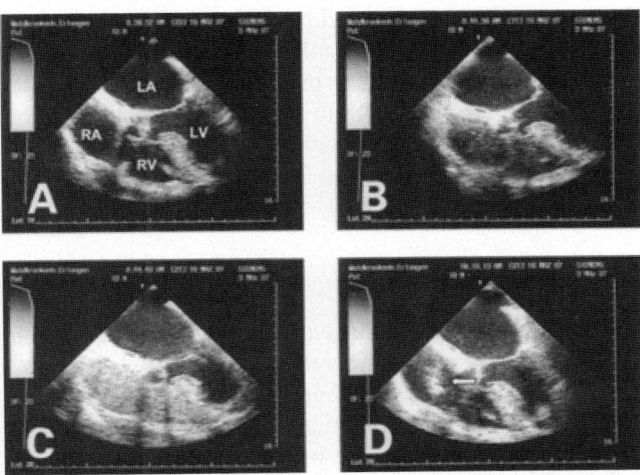

**FIGURE 38.10.** Large grade 3 emboli in this patient undergoing revision total hip arthroplasty resulted in fatal pulmonary embolism. From Urban MK, Sheppard R, Gordon M, et al. Right ventricular function during revision total hip arthroplasty. Anesth Analg 1996;82:1225–29, with permission.

**FIGURE 38.11.** Display of embolic patterns seen during orthopedic surgery. **A:** Grade 0. **B:** Grade 1. **C:** Grade 2. **D:** Grade 3. See Table 38.2 for details. From Koessler MJ, Fabiani R, Hamer H, et al. The clinical relevance of embolic events detected by transesophageal echocardiography during cemented total hip arthroplasty: A randomized clinical trial. Anesth Analg 2001;92:49–54.

▶ **TABLE 38.3. Grading Scale of Embolic Patterns During Orthopedic Surgery**

| Grade 0 | No emboli or small echogenic particles |
|---------|-----------------------------------------|
| Grade 1 | A few fine emboli |
| Grade 2 | A cascade of fine emboli or embolic masses with a diameter of < 5 mm, and the right atrium is opacified with echogenic material |
| Grade 3 | Fine emboli mixed with large embolic masses with a diameter > 5 mm or serpentine emboli |

unusual. Although they were believed to only occur following tourniquet deflation, recent evidence supports their occurrence even while a tourniquet is inflated (89–91). Two patterns of echogenic materials are observed: a miliary pattern or one in which large discrete particles are superimposed on a miliary pattern (89,91). The large particles most likely represent thrombus. An elevated risk for thrombus formation is a result of pneumatic compression of the femoral artery and vein, which produces venous stasis, acidosis, and endothelial disruption. The miliary pattern most likely represents cold blood and air. Kato used TEE to show that grade 3 echogenic findings caused hypotension and decreases in $PaO_2$ (91). In addition to mechanical obstruction of the pulmonary vasculature, increases in pulmonary arterial resistance may result from neurohumoral substances, such as serotonin released from the platelets adhering to the embolus (92). Thus, in addition to examining the extent of the embolic load, the echocardiographer should carefully observe for TEE findings of increased pulmonary vasculature resistance such as a leftward shift of the interatrial septum. An additional clinical caveat in the intraoperative examination of embolic load is to distinguish whether the material originated from the surgical site or from intravenous fluid administration. The ME bicaval view allows visualization of both the IVC and SVC inflow to the right atrium to better determine the source of embolic material.

## Neurosurgery

Utilization of transesophageal echocardiography during neurosurgery is gaining increasing popularity. It is most useful in evaluating and monitoring for the occurrence of venous air embolism in patients undergoing craniotomy in the sitting position. The incidence of venous air embolism (VAE) in the sitting position ranges from 25 to 45%, with early studies indicating a mortality rate approaching 93% without appropriate treatment (93). Early diagnosis and prompt treatment of venous air embolism fortunately dramatically decreases its morbidity and mortality.

Bunegin, using a flexible silastic model cast of the human right atrium, has demonstrated that a multiorifice catheter located in the upper quadrant of the right atrium can achieve optimal aspiration of air (94). The placement of the multiorifice air aspiration catheter is most commonly performed with EKG guidance. However, this can be problematic in up to 10% of patients secondary to the failure to find the characteristic EKG P wave complex changes. TEE guided placement of an air aspiration catheter at the junction of the right atrium-superior vena cava junction is a quick and easy method to learn (95). Figure 38.12 demonstrates a bicaval TEE view with the air aspiration catheter properly positioned at the juncture of the right atrium and superior vena cava.

The advantages of using TEE for sitting craniotomies include (a) the ability to detect venous air embolism as small as 1 millimeter in diameter, which may heighten the vigilance of the anesthesia neurosurgical team to the possibility of a larger VAE occurring in the future; (b) the ability to detect paradoxical air embolism through a patent foramen ovale; (c) the ability to provide online monitoring of cardiac function; and (d) rapid localization and placement of an air aspiration catheter (95).

## Orthotopic Liver Transplantation

Transesophageal echocardiography is becoming a common diagnostic tool in patients undergoing orthotopic liver transplantation (OLT). TEE is primarily utilized to evaluate left ventricular (LV) filling and function. Postreperfusion syndrome (PRS) is a frequent finding during liver transplantation and is defined as a decrease in the arterial pressure 30% below the patient's preoperative value lasting for at least one minute and occurring

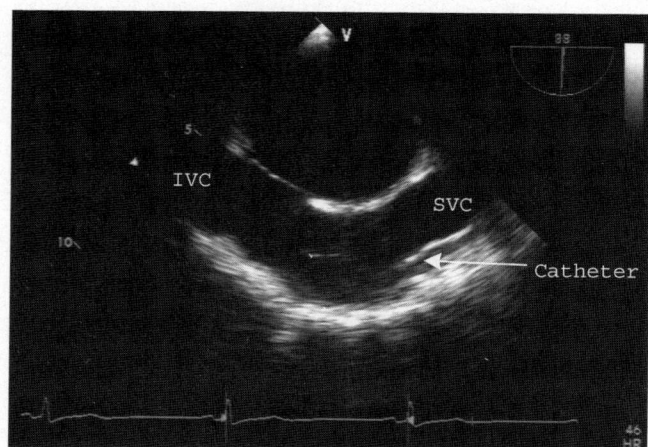

***FIGURE 38.12.*** Bicaval view demonstrating the junction of the superior vena cava (*SVC*) and of the inferior vena cava (*IVC*) with the right atrium. Proper positioning of a multiorifice air aspiration catheter is demonstrated.

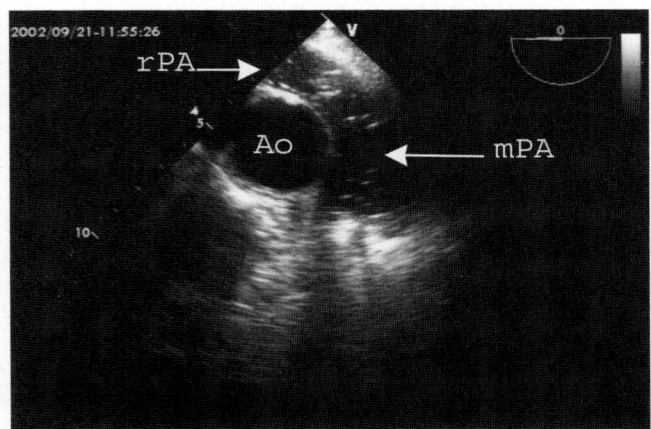

**FIGURE 38.13.** Air embolism; Midesophageal ascending aorta (*Ao*) SAX view demonstrating the bifurcation of the main pulmonary artery (*mPA*) and the right pulmonary artery (*rPA*). Note the multiple small echo lucent air bubbles within the pulmonary artery.

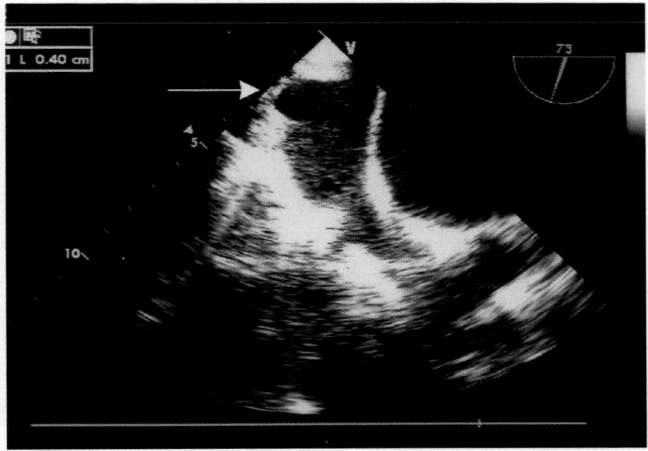

**FIGURE 38.15.** IVC stenosis. A markedly narrowed post liver transplant IVC-right atrial junction is noted with the *arrow*. It measured 4 mm in diameter

during the first five minutes after reperfusion (96). The primary culprit appears to be a drop in LV preload. To effectively treat PRS, TEE guided administration of volume is often necessary to assure adequate LV filling. Air or thrombotic embolisms originating from the newly inserted donor liver are additional ideologies proposed for postreperfusion syndrome (97). Both air and thrombus can be readily seen with transesophageal echocardiography (Fig. 38.13).

The liver is seen as a homogeneous structure in the right upper quadrant of the abdomen (Fig. 38.14). Evaluation of hepatic venous flow is a common occurrence in patients undergoing evaluation for tricuspid regurgitation and cardiac tamponade. The inferior vena cava can also be evaluated. Following liver transplantation, infe-

rior vena cava stenosis and/or thrombus can occur in 2% to 5% of patients (98). As demonstrated in Figure 38.15, the IVC-right atrial junction can easily be visualized. Color flow Doppler imaging in the same patient (Fig. 38.16) demonstrates marked turbulence in the suprahepatic IVC with a narrow jet streaming into the right atrium consistent with an elevated pressure gradient. The presence of IVC stenosis can result in both early and late liver transplant failure (98).

## Other Liver Pathology

TEE monitoring is frequently employed in patients also undergoing circulatory arrest for extensive IVC tumor resection. Figure 38.17 demonstrates a renal cell carcinoma

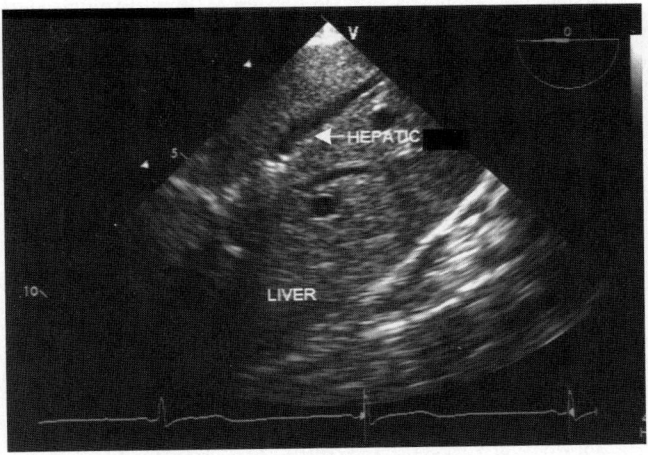

**FIGURE 38.14.** Normal liver. Normal homogenous appearing liver is demonstrated with TEE. A hepatic vein (*hepatic*) is shown.

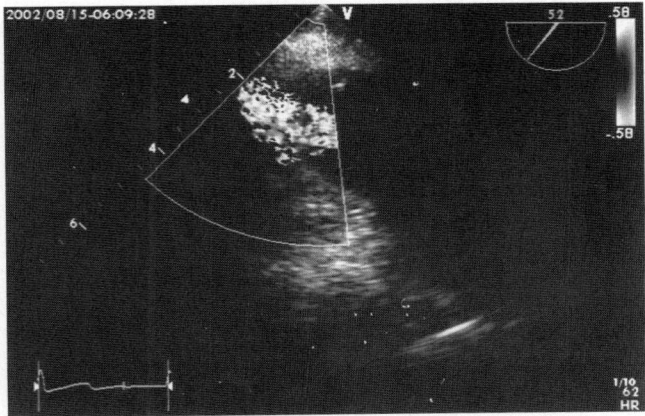

**FIGURE 38.16.** Doppler IVC stenosis. Black and white Doppler of the same patient as figure IVC stenosis. Note the marked turbulence of the suprahepatic IVC with a narrow jet streaming into the right atrium consistent with an elevated pressure gradient.

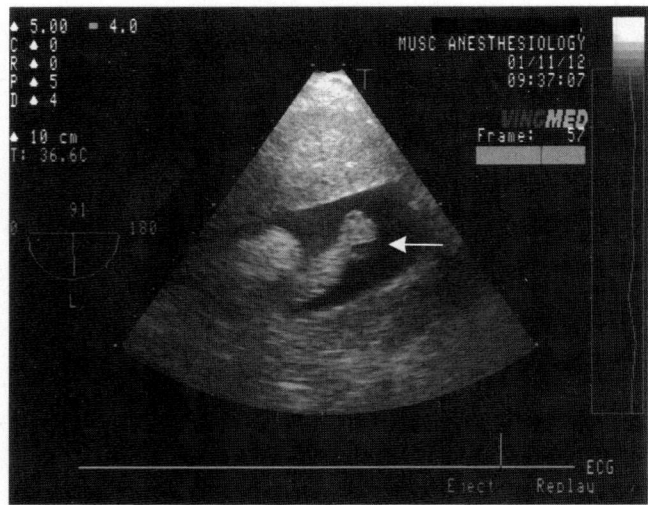

**FIGURE 38.17.** IVC tumor. Demonstrates dilated inferior vena cava with the presence of metastatic renal cell carcinoma (*arrow*).

involving the inferior vena cava that was removed via circulatory arrest.

## CONCLUSION

TEE has a multitude of indications for noncardiac surgeries where it serves as both a rescue diagnostic tool and a monitor of cardiovascular status. As the surgical patient population becomes increasingly elderly with associated co-morbidities, TEE will be all the more important in the management of these cases.

### KEY POINTS

- The value of TEE during noncardiac surgery is well established.
- The most common indications for TEE during noncardiac surgery are as a rescue technique in the hemodynamically unstable patient and as a monitor in patients at risk for cardiovascular complications.
- Assessments of preload and systolic function are the most valued functions of intraoperative TEE during noncardiac surgery.
- Quantitative assessments of ventricular function are preferred to visual estimates.
- The increasingly elderly and high-risk patient population undergoing vascular, laparoscopic, orthopedic, neurosurgical, and hepatic procedures warrants expanded use of TEE.

## REFERENCES

1. Shanewise JS, Cheung AT, Aronson S, et al. ASA/SCA guidelines for performing a comprehensive multiplane transesophageal echocardiography examination. Anesth Analg 1999;89:870–84.
2. Hall RI. Do we all need to have TEE capability? Can J Anesth 1996;43:201–5.
3. American Society of Anesthesiologists and the Society of Cardiovascular Anesthesiologists Task Force on Transesophageal echocardiography. Practice guidelines of perioperative transesophageal echocardiography. Anesthesiology 1996;84:986–1006.
4. Suriani RJ, Neustein S, Shore-Lesserson L, et al. Intraoperative transesophageal echocardiography during noncardiac surgery. J Cardiothorac Vasc Anesth 1998;12:274–80.
5. Kolev N, Brase R, Swanvelder M, et al. The influence of transesophageal echocardiography on intraoperative decision-making. Anaesthesia 1998;53:767–73.
6. Schmidlin D, Bettex D, Bernard E, et al. Transesophageal echocardiography in cardiac and vascular surgery: implications and observer variability. Br J Anaesth 2001;86:497–505.
7. Lambert AS, Mazer CD, Duke PC. Survey of the members of the cardiovascular section of the Canadian Anesthesiologists' Society on the use of perioperative transesophageal echocardiography—a brief report. Can J Anesth 2002;43L:94–296.
8. Jacka MJ, Cohen MM, To T, et al. The use of and preferences for the transesophageal echocardiogram and pulmonary artery catheter among cardiovascular anesthesiologists. Anesth Analg 2002;94:1065–71.
9. Denault AY, Couture P, McKenty S, et al. Perioperative use of transesophageal echocardiography by anesthesiologists: impact in noncardiac surgery and in the intensive care unit. Can J Anesth 2002;49:287–93.
10. Cujec B, Sullivan H, Wilanski S, et al. Transesophageal echocardiography. Experience of a Canadian centre. Can J Cardiol 1989 Jun-Aug 5 (5):255–62.
11. Sinclair S, James S, Singer M. Intraoperative intravascular volume optimization and length of hospital stay after repair of proximal femoral fracture: randomized controlled trial. BMJ 1997;315:909–12.
12. Gan TJ, Soppitt A, Maroof M, et al. Goal-directed intraoperative fluid administration reduces length of hospital stay after major surgery. Anesthesiology 2002;97:820–6.
13. Ashidagawa, M, Ohara M, Koide Y. An intraoperative diagnosis of dynamic left ventricular outflow tract obstruction using transesophageal echocardiography leads to the treatment with intravenous disopryamide. Anesth Analg 2002;94:310–2.
14. Poelaert JI, Trouerbach J, DeBuyzere M, et al. Evaluation of transesophageal echocardiography as a diagnostic and therapeutic aid in a critical care setting. Chest 1995;107:774–9.
15. Fontes ML, Bellow W, Ngo L, et al. Assessment of ventricular function in critically ill patients: limitations of pulmonary artery catheterization. Institution of the McSPI research group. J Cardiothorac Vasc Anesth 1999;13:3521–27.
16. Eisenberg MJ, London MJ, Leung JM, et al. for the study of Perioperative Ischemia Research Group. Monitoring of myocardial ischemia during noncardiac surgery: a technology assessment of transesophageal echocardiography and 12-lead electrocardiography. JAMA 1992;268:210–16.
17. Ellis JE, Shah MN, Briller JE, et al. A comparison of methods for the detection of myocardial ischemia during noncardiac surgery. Automated ST segment analysis systems, electrocardiography, and transesophageal echocardiography. Anesth Analg 1992;75:764–72.
18. Gewertz BL, Kremser PC, Zarins CK, et al. Transesophageal echocardiographic monitoring of myocardial ischemia during vascular surgery. J Vasc Surg 1987;5:607–13.
19. Guyton AC, Hall JE, eds. Textbooks of Medical Physiology, 9th ed. Philadelphia: W.B. Saunders Company, 1996:115–16.
20. Reeves ST, Perrino AC, Jr. Role of transesophageal echocardiography in noncardiac surgery. Refresher courses in Anesthesiology, Volume 30, 2002.

21. Hansen RM, Viquerat CE, Matthay MA, et al. Poor correlation between pulmonary arterial wedge pressure and left ventricular end-diastolic volume after coronary artery bypass graft surgery. Anesthesiology 1986;64:764–70.
22. Cheung AT, Savino JS, Weiss SJ, et al. Echocardiographic and hemodynamic indexes of left ventricular preload in patients with normal and abnormal ventricular function. Anesthesiology 1994; 81(2): 376–87.
23. Matsumoto M, Oka Y, Strom J, et al. Application of transesophageal echocardiography to continue intraoperative monitoring of left ventricular performance. Am J Cardiol 1980;46:95–105.
24. Schiller NB, Shah PM, Crawford NM, et al. for the American Society of Echocardiography Committee on standards, subcommittee on Quantitation of Two-dimensional Echocardiograms: Recommendations for quantitation of the left ventricle by two-dimensional echocardiography. J Am Soc Echocardiogr 1989;2:358–67.
25. Poormans G, Schupfer G, Roosens C, et al. Transesophageal echocardiographic evaluation of the left ventricle. J Cardiothorac Vas Anesth 2000;14:588–98.
26. Reich DL, Konstadt SN, Nejat M, et al. Intraoperative transesophageal echocardiography for the detection of cardiac preload changes induced by transfusion and phlebotomy in pediatric patients. Anesthesiology 1993;79:10–15.
27. Perrino AC Jr., Luther MA, O'Connor TZ, et al. Automated echocardiographic analysis. Examination of serial intraoperative measurements. Anesthesiology. 1995; Aug 83(2): 285–92.
28. Savino JS, Troianos CA, Aukburg S, Weiss R, Reichek N. Measurements of pulmonary blood flow with transesophageal two-dimensional and Doppler echocardiography. Anesthesiology 1991;75:445–51.
29. Gorcsan J III, Diana P, Ball BS, Hattler BG. Intraoperative determination of cardiac output by transesophageal continuous wave Doppler. Am Heart J 1992;123:171–6.
30. Maslow AD, Haering J, Comunale M, et al. Measurement of Cardiac Output by Pulsed Wave Doppler of the Right Ventricular Outflow Tract. Anesth Analg 1996;83:466–71.
31. Stewart WJ, Jiang L, Mich R, Pandian N, Guerrero JL, Weyman AE. Variable effects of changes in flow rate through the aortic, pulmonary, and mitral valves on valve area and flow velocity: Impact on quantitative Doppler flow calculations. J Am Coll Cardiol 1985;6:653–62.5.
32. Muhiudeen IA, Kuecherer HF, Lee E, Cahalan MK, Schiller NB. Intraoperative Estimation of Cardiac Output by Transesophageal Pulsed Doppler Echocardiography. Anesthesiology 1991;74:9–14.
33. Darmon PL, Hillel Z, Mogtader, Mindich B, Thys D. Cardiac Output by Transesophageal Echocardiography Using Continuous-wave Doppler across the Aortic Valve. Anesthesiology 1994;80:796–805.
34. Perrino AC, Harris SN, Luther MA. Intraoperative determination of cardiac output using multiplane transesophageal echocardiography: A comparison to thermodilution. Anesthesiology 1998;89:350–7.
35. Ebeid MR, Ferrer PL, Robinson B, Weatherby N, Gebland H. Doppler echocardiographic evaluation of pulmonary vascular resistance in children with congenital heart disease. J Am Soc Echocardiogr 1996;9:822–831.
36. Swenson JD, Harkin C, Pace NL, et al. Transesophageal echocardiography: An objective tool in defining maximum ventricular response to intravenous fluid therapy. Anesth Analg 1996;83:1149–53.
37. Berquist BD, Lung JM, Bellows WH. Transesophageal echocardiography in myocardial revascularization. I. Accuracy of intraoperative real-time interpretation. Anesth Analg 1996;82:1132–38.
38. Mathew JP, Fontes ML, Garwood S. Transesophageal echocardiography interpretation: a comparative analysis between cardiac anesthesiologists and primary echocardiographers. Anesth Analg 2002:94;302–9.
39. Cahalan MK, deBruijn NP, Clements F, eds. Detection of intraoperative myocardial ischemia with two-dimensional transesophageal echocardiography in intraoperative use of echocardiography. Philadelphia: J.B. Lippincott Company 1991.
40. Leung JM, Levine EH. Left ventricular end-systolic cavity obliteration: An estimate of intraoperative hypovolemia. Anesthesiology 1994;81:1102–09.
41. Daggubati RB, Khanal S, Fallahtafti M, et al. Effect of dobutamine stress on left ventricular systolic and diastolic functions in patients with moderate to severe left ventricular dysfunction. J Am Soc Echocardiogr 1998;11:787–91.
42. Maslow A, Bert A, Schwartz C, et al. Transesophageal echocardiography in the noncardiac surgical patient. International Anesthesiology Clinics 2002;V40;1;73–132.
43. Bode RH Jr., Lewis K, Zarich S, et al. Cardiac outcome after peripheral vascular surgery: Comparison of general and regional anesthesia. Anesthesiology 1996;84:3–13.
44. Gersh BJ, Rihaul CS, Rooke TW, et al. Evaluation and management of patients with both peripheral vascular and coronary artery disease. J Am Coll Cardiol 1991;18:203–14.
45. Mangano DT. Perioperative cardiac morbidity. Anesthesiology 1990;72:153–84.
46. Hertzer NR, Bevan EG, Young JR, et al. Coronary artery disease in peripheral vascular patients. A classification of 1000 coronary angiograms and results of surgical management. Ann Surg 1984;199:223–33.
47. Roizen MF, Beaupre PN, Alpert RA, et al. Monitoring with two-dimensional transesophageal echocardiography: Comparison of myocardial function in patients undergoing supraceliac, suprarenal-infraceliac, or infrarenal aortic occlusion. J Vasc Surg Anesth 1984;1:300–5.
48. Krupski WC, Layug EL, Reilly LM, et al. Comparison of cardiac morbidity between aortic and infrainguinal operations. Study of perioperative ischemia (SPI) research group. J Vasc Surg 1992;15:354–63.
49. Krupski WC, Layug EL, Reilly LM, et al. Comparison of cardiac morbidity rates between aortic and infrainguinal operations: Two-year follow-up. Study of J Vasc Surg 1993;18: 609–15.
50. London MJ, Tubau JF, Wong, MG, et al. For the Society of Perioperative Research Group. The "natural history" of segmental wall-motion abnormalities in patients undergoing noncardiac surgery. Anesthesiology 1990;73:644–55.
51. Eisenberg MJ, London MJ, Leung JM, et al. For the study of perioperative ischemia research group. Monitoring for myocardial ischemia during noncardiac surgery: A technology assessment of transesophageal echocardiography and 12-lead electrocardiography. JAMA 1992;268:210–16.
52. London MJ, Perrino AC, Reeves S, eds. A Practical Approach to TEE. Diagnosis of myocardial ischemia. Philadelphia: Lippincott Williams & Wilkins; 2003.
53. Gelman S. The pathophysiology of aortic cross-clamping and unclamping. Anesthesiology 1995;82:1026–60.
54. O'Connor CJ, Rothenberg DM. Anesthetic consideration for descending thoracic aortic surgery: Part I. Cardiothorac Vasc Anesth 1995;9:581–88.
55. Gillespie DI, Connelly GP, Arkoff HM, et al. Left ventricular dysfunction during infrarenal abdominal aortic aneurysm repair. Am J Surg 1994;168:144–7.
56. Iafrate MD, Gordon G, Staples MH, et al. Transesophageal echocardiography for hemodynamic management of thoracoabdominal aneurysm repair. Am J Surg 1993;166:179–85.
57. Godet G, Couture P, Ionanidis G, et al. Another application of two-dimensional transesophageal echocardiography; spinal cord imaging. A preliminary report. J Cardiothorac Vasc Anesth 1994;8:14–18.
58. Voci P, Tritapepe L, Testa G, et al. Imaging the anterior spinal artery by transesophageal color Doppler ultrasonography. J Cardio Thorac Vasc Anesth 1999;13:586–7.
59. Orihashi K, Matsuura Y, Sueda T, et al. Abdominal aortas and visceral arteries visual visualized by transgastric echocardiography: Technical considerations. Hiroshima J Med Sci 1997;46:151–7.
60. Garwood S, Davis E, Harris SN. Intraoperative transesophageal ultrasonography can measure renal blood flow. J Cardiothorac Vasc Anes 2001;15:65–71.

61. Moskowitz DM, Kahn RA, Konstadt SN, et al. Intraoperative transesophageal echocardiography as an adjuvant to fluoroscopy during endovascular thoracic aortic repair. Eur J Vasc Endovasc Surg 1999;17:22–7.

62. Myre K, Buanes T, Smith G, et al. Simultaneous hemodynamic and echocardiographic changes during abdominal gas insufflation. Surg Laparosc Endosc 1997;7:415–19.

63. Mann G, Boccara G, Poouzeratte, et al. Hemodynamic monitoring using esophageal Doppler ultrasonography during laparoscopic cholesystectomy. Can J Anaesth 1999;46:15–20.

64. Harris SN, Ballantyne GH, Luther MA, et al. Alterations of cardiovascular performance during laparoscopic colectomy: A combined hemodynamic and echocardiographic analysis. Anesth Analg 1996;76:1067–71.

65. Joris JL, Noirot DP, Legrand MJ, et al. Hemodynamic changes during laparoscopic cholecystectomy. Anesth Analg 1993;76:1067—71.

66. Cunningham AJ, Turner J, Rosenbaum S, et al. Transesophageal echocardiographic assessment of haemodynamic function during laparoscopic cholecystectomy. Br J Anaesth 1993;71:621–5.

67. Dorsay DA, Greene FL, Baysinger CL. Hemodynamic changes during laparoscopic cholecystectomy monitored by transesophageal echocardiography. Surg Endosc 1995;9:128–34.

68. Gannendahl P, Odeberg S, Brodin LA, et al. Effects of posture and pneumoperitoneum during anaesthesia in the indices of left ventricular filling. Acta Anaesthesiol Scand 1996;40:160–6.

69. Irwin MG, Ng JKF. Transesophageal acoustic quantification for evaluation of cardiac function during laparoscopic surgery. Anaesthesia 2001;56:623–9.

70. Hein HAT, Joshi GP, Ramsay MAE, et al. Hemodynamic changes during laparoscopic cholecystectomy in patients with severe cardiac disease. J Clin Anesth 1997;9:261–5.

71. Rist M, Hemmerling TM, Rauh R, et al. Influence of pneumoperitoneum and patient positioning on preload and splanchnic blood volume in laparoscopic surgery of the lower abdomen. 2001;13:244–9.

72. Sato K, Kawamura T, Wakusawa R. Hepatic blood flow and function in elderly patients undergoing laparoscopy. Anesth Analg 2000;90:1198–1202.

73. Yacoub OF, Cardona I Jr., Coveler LA, et al. Carbon dioxide embolism during laparoscopy. Anesthesiology 1982;57:533–5.

74. Tupperainen T, Makinen J, Salonen M. Reducing the risk of systemic embolism during gynecologic laparoscopy—effect of volume preload. Acta Anaesthesiol Scand 2001;46:37–42.

75. Nagase K, Terazawa, E, Ueda N, et al. Hemorrhagic shock during laparoscopic cholecystectomy detected by transesophageal echocardiography. Masui 1998;47:358–61.

76. D'Angelo AJ, Kline RG, Chen MHM, et al. Utility of transesophageal echocardiography and pulmonary artery catheterization during laparoscopic assisted abdominal aortic aneurysm repair. Surg Endosc 1997;11:1099–101.

77. Orsini EC, Byrick RJ, Mullen JBM, et al. Cardiopulmonary function and pulmonary microemboli during arthroplasty using cemented or non-cemented components J Bone Joint Surg 1987;69:822–31.

78. Patterson BM, Healey JH, Cornell CN, et al. Cardiac arrest during hip arthroplasty with a cemented long-stem component. J Bone Joint Surg 1991;73:271–7.

79. Murphy P, Edelist G, Byrick RJ, et al. Relationship of fat embolism to hemodynamic and echocardiographic changes during cemented arthroplasty. Can J Anaesth 1997;44:1293–300.

80. Wheelwright EF, Byrick RJ, Wigglesworth DF, et al. Hypotension during cemented arthroplasty: Relationship to cardiac output and fat embolism. J Bone Joint Surg Br 1993;75:715–23.

81. Byrick RJ. Cement implantation syndrome: A time-limited embolic phenomenon. Can J Anaesth 1997;44:107–11.

82. Patterson BM, Healey JH, Cornell CN, et al. Cardiac arrest during hip arthroplasty with a cemented long-stem component. J Bone Joint Surg 1991;73:271–7.

83. Urban MK, Sheppard R, Gordon M, et al. Right ventricular function during revision total hip arthroplasty. Anesth Analg 1996;82:1225–9.

84. Duncan JA. Intraoperative collapse or death related to the use of acrylic cement in hip surgery. Anaesthesia 1989;44:149–53.

85. Chen H, Wong C, Ho, S, et al. A lethal pulmonary embolism during percutaneous vertebroplasty. Anesth Analg 2002;95:1060–2.

86. Woo R, Minster GJ, Fitzgerald RH Jr., et al. Pulmonary fat embolism in revision hip arthroplasty. Clin Orthop 1995;319:41–53.

87. Koessler MJ, Fabiani R, Hamer H, et al. The clinical relevance of embolic events detected by transesophageal echocardiography during cemented total hip arthroplasty: A randomized clinical trial. Anesth Analg 2001;92:49–55.

88. Johnson C, Lewis KD, Steen SN, et al. Transesophageal echocardiography in the anesthetic management of total hip arthroplasty. Acta Anaesthesiol Sin 2001;39:135–8.

89. Parmet JL, Horrow JC, Singer R, et al. Echogenic emboli upon tourniquet release during total knee arthroscopy: Pulmonary hemodynamic changes and embolic composition. Anesth Analg 1994;79:940–5.

90. McGrath BJ, Hsia J, Epstein B. Massive pulmonary embolism following tourniquet deflation. Anesthesiology 1991;74:618–20.

91. Kato N, Nakanski K, Yoshino S, et al. Abnormal echogenic findings detected by transesophageal echocardiography and cardiorespiratory impairment during total knee arthroscopy with tourniquet. Anesthesiology 2002;97:1123–8.

92. Gurewich V, Cohen ML, Thomas DP. Humoral factors in massive pulmonary embolism: An experimental study. Am Heart 1968;76:784–94.

93. Gottlieb JD, Ericsson JA, Sweet RB. Venous air embolism: A review. Anesth Analg 1965;44:773–9.

94. Bunegin L, Albin MS, Helsel PE, et al. Positioning the right atrial catheter: A model for reappraisal. Anesthesiology 1981;55:343–8.

95. Reeves ST, Bevis LA, Bailey BN. Positioning a right atrial air aspiration catheter using transesophageal echocardiography. J Neurosurgical Anesthesiology 1996;8(2):123–5.

96. De La Morena G, Acosta F, Villegas M, et al. Ventricular function during liver reperfusion in hepatic transplantation: A transesophageal echocardiographic study. Transplantation 1994;58(3): 306–10.

97. Ellis JE, Lichtor JL, Feinstein SB, et al. Right heart dysfunction, pulmonary embolism, and paradoxical embolization during liver transplantation. A transesophageal two-dimensional echocardiographic study. Anesth Analg 1989;68(6):777–82.

98. Bjerke RJ, Mieles LA, Borsky BJ, et al. The use of transesophageal ultrasonography for the diagnosis of inferior vena caval outflow obstruction during liver transplantation. Transplantation 1992;54(5):939–41.

## QUESTIONS

1. During orthopedic surgery, Grade 3 embolization is characterized by:
   A. Fine emboli mixed with large embolic masses with a diameter > than 5 mm or serpentine emboli
   B. A few fine emboli
   C. Large amounts of air upon aspiration of right atrium
   D. Rightward bulging of interatrial septum

2. Which of the following is *not* associated with decreased preload?
   A. Low LVEDA
   B. High ejection fraction
   C. "Kissing papillaries"
   D. Pneumoperitoneum

3. Echocardiographic exam of stroke volume at the aortic valve level utilizes each of the following *except*:
   A. TG LAX view
   B. CW Doppler
   C. ME AV SAX
   D. Planimetry of circular orifice of aortic valve during end-systole

4. Intraoperative TEE is useful during liver transplantation to evaluate the following:
   A. LV filling and function
   B. the etiology of post-reperfusion syndrome
   C. air embolism
   D. All of the above

## Chapter 1

1. B. The PRF is affected by the depth of the imaging. This is a method of eliminating aliasing with pulse wave Doppler.
2. C. Decreasing pulse duration is one method to improve axial resolution.
3. D. Beam width is the major determinate of lateral resolution.
4. C. Mitral inflow VTI needs to be measured at the mitral valve leaflet tips. Pulse wave Doppler provides the VTI at a specific location and is thus the correct answer.
5. C. Anything that will make image acquisition simpler will improve temporal resolution.

## Chapter 2

1. B. Only analog signals have a continuous range, typically represented as a series of sine waves. A theoretical advantage of analog data is its ability to provide, in theory, an infinite spectrum of data. Digital representations consist of values measured at discrete intervals, typically a power of two (e.g., 2, 4, 8, 16, 32).
2. C. The size of an image is given by the number of pixels and the number of bits for each pixel. An 8-bit pixel (series of 8 "zeros" and/or "ones") can encode 256 values ($2^8$). A 16-bit pixel is needed to encode 65,536 colors. Thus, $1200 \times 800 \times 16 = 15,360,000$ bits, or when divided by 8—1,920,000 bytes.
3. A. Cardiac ultrasound imaging equipment obtains initial analog data from the imaging transducer, where ultrasonic acoustic reflections stimulate a piezoelectric crystal to produce electrical analog impulses that are sent to a computer board.

## Chapter 3

1. B. Resolution is the ability to distinguish two objects that are close to one another. The resolution of an image is no greater than 1 to 2 wavelengths. The shorter the wavelength, the more compressions and rarefractions there are per unit of time; therefore, the resolution is better. Frequency is indirectly proportional to wavelength. The shorter the wavelength the higher the frequency and the better the resolution. Higher frequencies, however, sacrifice penetration.
2. C. Refraction is the deflection of ultrasound waves from a straight path and can occur as the waves pass through a medium with different acoustic impedance. When an ultrasound wave is refracted, the transducer assumes it has returned from the original scan line and therefore places the image along the original path rather than its actual location.
3. D. Range ambiguity occurs because of increased pulse repetition frequency. With a high pulse repetition frequency, a second signal is sent out before the first signal is received. The transducer cannot discriminate between the returning pulses, that is, whether they represent the first, second, or even later pulses. Decreasing the depth decreases the pulse repetition frequency.
4. A. The Eustachian valve is an embryological remnant of the sinus venosus. It is a thin, elongated structure located at the junction of the IVC and the right atrium. While the Eustachian valve is not pathologic, it can be confused with a cardiac thrombus or mass.

## Chapter 4

1. D. Axial resolution is the ability to distinguish two structures that are close to each other along the direction of beam propagation, as two separate structures. Axial resolution can be optimized by increasing the transducer frequency, which decreases the wavelength, and therefore shortens the pulse duration. The pulse duration can also be shortened by using transducers with broad frequency bandwidths, which include a greater mixture of high and low frequencies compared to narrow bandwidths. Consequently, broad bandwidth transducer pulses are more likely to preserve higher frequencies as ultrasound waves penetrate through tissue, and therefore have greater sensitivity than narrow frequency bandwidths. Finally, the use of damping material in the construction of transducers minimizes piezoelectric crystal ringing and vibration thereby producing shorter pulse duration. Thus, axial resolution can be improved by assuring a short pulse duration using an appropriately dampened transducer with a high frequency and broader frequency bandwidth. (See "The Impact of Ultrasound Instrumentation on Image Generation and Display.")
2. C. Lateral resolution describes the ability of a transducer to resolve two objects that are adjacent to each other and perpendicular to the beam axis. Lateral resolution also refers to the ability of the beam to detect single small objects across the width of the beam. In general, lateral resolution is most optimal when the ultrasound beam width is narrow. Lateral resolution may therefore be improved by increasing the frequency (i.e., shortening the wavelength). Increasing the transducer aperture diameter may also improve lateral resolution by lengthening the near field depth at the expense of a wider proximal near field. Increasing the ultrasound signal amplitude (i.e., POWER) increases the detection of echoes at the beam margins thus effectively increasing beam width and decreasing lateral resolution. Lateral resolution can also be improved by focusing the transducer. Thus, lateral resolution is an important variable in determining ultrasound image quality, and is ultimately influenced by transducer size, shape, frequency, and focusing. (See "The Impact of Ultrasound Instrumentation on Image Generation and Display.")
3. A. Temporal resolution refers to the ability to rapidly display moving structures and distinguish closely spaced events in time. Temporal resolution is related to the time required to generate one complete frame and is therefore directly related to the frame rate. Assuming preservation of scan line density and spatial resolution, the temporal resolution and frame rate can be improved only by reducing depth or sector size. Alternatively, for a given depth and sector size, using a higher frequency transducer with decreased tissue penetration will also permit an increased frame rate and improved temporal resolution. Thus, temporal resolution is dependent upon depth, sector scan angle, scan line density, and transducer frequency. (See "The Impact of Ultrasound Instrumentation on Image Generation and Display.")

## Chapter 5

1. D. The left fibrous trigone extends from the base of the left coronary cusp and is adjacent to the anterior mitral valve leaflet. Identification of the left fibrous trigone is essential in mitral valve surgery due to the necessity of anchoring the annuloplasty ring anteriorly.
2. C. This anterior portion of the mitral annulus has minimal shape change during the cardiac cycle and is less prone to

dilation because of its rigid structure. Its margins are defined surgically by two dimples raised at the border of the right and left trigones when lifting the anterior leaflet. The anterior annulus is more rigid than the posterior annulus such that annular dilatation occurs posteriorly in pathologic conditions such as idiopathic cardiomyopathy.

3. D. The annuli fibrosi of the mitral annulus becomes thinner and poorly defined as it extends posteriorly from the left and right trigones. This portion of the annulus is poorly supported and is prone to dilation in pathologic states. The posterior leaflet of the mitral valve attaches to this portion of the annulus. Dilation of the annular attachment of the posterior leaflet creates increased tension on the middle scallop of the posterior leaflet explaining the 60% occurrence of chordal tears in the middle scallop of the posterior leaflet.

4. B. The Society of Cardiovascular Anesthesiologists and the American Society of Echocardiography have developed a 16-segment model of the LV based on the recommendations of the Subcommittee on Quantification of the ASE Standards Committee. This model divides the LV into three levels: basal, mid, and apical. The basal and mid levels are each divided circumferentially into six segments and the apical into four segments. The apical segments are the anterior, inferior, septal, and lateral.

5. B. There are two chordae attaching to the ventricular surface of the anterior leaflet, which is by far the thickest and largest of the chordae to the mitral valve. They have been called strut or stay chordae. One arises from the anterior papillary muscle and attaches to A1/A2 area of the anterior leaflet; one arises from the posterior papillary muscle and attaches to the A2/A3 portion of the anterior leaflet.

## Chapter 6

1. A. The deep transgastric long-axis view allows the ultrasound beam to be aligned reasonably parallel to the flow through the LVOT and the AV for accurate Doppler measurements of these velocities. Midesophageal views of the AV provide better 2-D images of the valve. The LV is usually foreshortened in the deep transgastric long-axis view. The diameter of the LVOT is usually best measured in the midesophageal AV long-axis view. The transgastric two-chamber view usually shows the mitral chordae most clearly.

2. E. Four-chamber views show the septal and lateral walls. Two-chamber views show the inferior and anterior walls. Transgastric short-axis views show the six segments at the basal or mid levels of the LV including the posterior segment.

3. C. Four- and two-chamber views cut across the mitral valve obliquely. The mitral commissural view transects the MV along the intercommissural plane and the long-axis view through the middle of the anterior and posterior leaflets.

4. B. Eight views are needed to provide a basic perioperative TEE exam to detect markedly abnormal ventricular filling or function, extensive myocardial ischemia or infarction, large air embolism, severe valvular dysfunction, large cardiac masses or thrombi, large pericardial effusions, and major lesions of the great vessels.

## Chapter 7

1. C. The recommendations refer to clinical problems rather than to individual patients, who often have more than one potential reason for performing TEE. Thus, although a patient may not necessarily require perioperative TEE because of a Category III indication (e.g., cardiomyopathy), the same patient may need TEE because of coexisting hemodynamic problems (Category I). See "Practice Guidelines."

2. B. The AHA/ACC guidelines utilize the following classification system for indications.
**Class I:** Conditions for which there is evidence and/or general agreement that a given procedure or treatment is useful and effective.
**Class II:** Conditions for which there is conflicting evidence and/or a divergence of opinion about the usefulness/efficacy of a procedure or treatment.
**Class III:** Conditions for which there is evidence and/or general agreement that the procedure/treatment is not useful/ef-

fective and in some cases may be harmful. See "Practice Guidelines."

3. E. Published reports have indicated that TEE facilitates the placement of intravascular catheters during port-access surgery, the detection of regurgitation after minimally invasive valve surgery, the diagnosis of new regional wall motion abnormalities (RWMA) during coronary artery clampings, and air embolism after termination of CPB following "open heart" procedures. See "Indications for Specific Lesions or Procedures: Minimally Invasive Cardiac Surgery."

4. D. In a recent review of 7,200 adult cardiac surgical patients, Kallmeyer et al. reported on the safety of intraoperative transesophageal echocardiography. They observed no mortality and a morbidity of only 0.2 %. Most complications were related to probe insertion or manipulation that resulted in oropharyngeal, esophageal, or gastric trauma. See "Complications."

## Chapter 8

1. B. There is an increased risk of esophageal perforation when a TEE probe is placed in a patient with a history of an esophageal stricture. All of the other choices are relative contraindications. See Table 8.2. Procedures and Chemicals That Damage TEE Probes.

2. C. Antibiotic prophylaxis is not required for procedures with a low risk of induced bacteremia. Therefore, endocarditis prophylaxis is not needed prior to or during TEE exams, except in patients at high risk for developing endocarditis. See "Safety" and "Infection."

3. C. The duration of the disinfecting process of the TEE probe should be at least 20 minutes to eliminate bacterial and viral contaminants. See "Infection."

## Chapter 9

1. E. An increased emphasis on outcomes research has come in response to the following factors: unexplained variability in practice patterns across geographic areas, economics of health care and the need for cost containment, competition within the health-care sector, and a greater need for accountability.

2. B. Outcomes research primarily focuses on effectiveness. Effectiveness can be thought of as the utility of a health-care intervention in routine clinical practice.

3. E. See "Data Sources." Outcomes research may incorporate a variety of methodologies and approaches to collecting, examining, and analyzing data. Data sources include results from randomized clinical trials, quasiexperimental designs, effectiveness trials, cohort or case-control designs, and/or data from observational databases.

4. E. See "Data Sources." Randomized controlled trials are the strongest trial design for internal consistency. The goal of the randomized controlled trial is to reduce variability and bias, controlling for known and unknown confounding variables. Key design elements in the randomized controlled trial allow for a clarification of differences in outcome due to treatment rather than specific differences in the patient population.

5. E. See "Effectiveness Trials." Effectiveness trials differ significantly from randomized controlled trials in that they are population based, often retrospective, and are significantly less restrictive. Effectiveness trials can provide practical information about patients seen in routine clinical practice. Because of the lack of randomization, risk adjustment strategies are used to control for influential variables in assessing the effectiveness of the health-care intervention.

6. D. See "Performance Measures of Diagnostic Imaging Tests." Tests that seek to exclude or rule out disease and tests that seek to discover disease require a high sensitivity. Those tests that seek to confirm or rule in a target disorder require a high specificity.

## Chapter 10

1. A. Leftward bowing of the interatrial septum in midsystole is a normal echocardiographic finding. Normally, due to higher left-sided pressures, the interatrial septum bulges toward the right atrium. During passive mechanical expiration, right

atrial pressure transiently exceeds left atrial pressure, and the atrial septum momentarily bows towards the left atrium. This midsystolic atrial reversal occurs when the corresponding pulmonary artery occlusion pressure (PAOP) is ≤ 15 mm Hg. A rightward midsystolic bowing or absence of the leftward bowing of the interatrial septum indicates PAOP > 15 mm Hg with a sensitivity of 89%, specificity of 95%, and a positive predictive value = 0.97. As a general guideline, an E/Ea > 10 predicts a mean PCWP > 15 mm Hg with a 92% sensitivity and 80% specificity.

2. E. The deep transgastric long-axis view is not normally a part of a comprehensive exam of the left ventricle. Although the left ventricle can be seen in this view, often it is foreshortened. This view allows for measurements of the flow velocities of the LVOT and the aortic valve using pulsed or continuous wave Doppler because there is good alignment of these structures to the Doppler interrogation beam.

3. C. Echocardiography can be used to noninvasively measure meridional and circumferential wall stress. Meridional stress acts on the long axis of the LV; the circumferential stress acts on the short-axis of the LV. Meridional wall stress can be calculated using noninvasive BP and myocardial area measured with M-mode. The normal left ventricle resembles the ellipsoid model in which circumferential stress at the end of systole is 2.57 times higher than meridional stress. In a dilated failing heart, the left ventricle gradually begins to resemble a sphere, and the meridional and circumferential stress gradually equalizes to a ratio of 1.

4. D. Sinus tachycardia may cause the systolic and diastolic waves to fuse. The peak systolic to diastolic filling ratio increases with sinus tachycardia because the diastolic filling period is shortened. In patients with atrial fibrillation, systolic forward flow is diminished or absent, and diastolic flow is the main contributor to left atrial filling. In the presence of low left atrial pressure, the biphasic nature of the S wave becomes more prominent because of the temporal dissociation of atrial relaxation and mitral annular motion. With TEE, the biphasic systolic wave is commonly seen. The descent of the S wave corresponds with the V wave in the left atrial pressure tracing. The second large flow velocity is the diastolic wave prompted by the antegrade flow of blood from the pulmonary veins into the left ventricle during early diastole. It coincides with the Y descent of the left atrial pressure tracing during early ventricular filling.

5. D. Cross-sectional area can be calculated by measuring the LVOT diameter in the midesophageal long-axis view using the equation AVA = $\pi \times (D/2)^2$. The cross-sectional area can also be calculated by measuring the length of each side of the aortic valve seen in the aortic valve short-axis view using the equation AVA = $0.433 \times S^2$. The transgastric long-axis view can be used to obtain the spectral envelope for measuring the velocity time integral used in the stroke volume calculation. The spectral envelope obtained from the pulmonary artery is not equivalent to that from the aorta in the transgastric long-axis view. The cardiac output derived from measuring the spectral envelope at the pulmonary artery only correlated modestly with cardiac output measured by the thermodilution method (r = 0.65).

## Chapter 11
1. A.
2. D.
3. D.
4. C.
5. A.

## Chapter 12
1. A, D. Regional wall assessment is based on two factors, assessment of endocardial wall motion and systolic myocardial thickening. Regional assessment involves grading endocardial motion with a scale from 15, 1 representing normal myocardium and 5 indicating dyskinetic myocardium.
2. B. While complete visualization of all aspects of the myocardium is ideal, the definition of myocardial function may be based on endocardial wall motion or systolic wall thickening. Grading (15) is dependent on the degree of endocardial motion toward the center of the LV cavity during systole, and the presence of myocardial thickening. Therefore, while it is essential to view the endocardial border, in order to quantitiate its movement in toward the center of the cavity, it is not as essential to view the entire epicardial layer, as one can obtain a qualitative idea of wall thickening by viewing the mid and endocardial layers.

3. D. Foreshortening is the result of improper alignment of the ultrasound beam with the long axis of the image. The result is an oblique view of the chamber resulting in a thicker slice of the myocardium. Therefore, the wall can appear to be thickening when it is not.

4. C. There is significant data associating persistent severe SWMA with myocardial ischemia and postoperative morbidity. However, hypokinetic myocardial segments are not as clearly associated with poor outcome. Transient abnormalities unaccompanied by hemodynamic or electrocardiographic evidence of ischemia may not represent clinically significant myocardial ischemia. Nonischemic causes of RWMA include tethering of the normal myocardium adjacent to abnormally perfused areas, increased afterload in the setting of previously ischemic or scarred myocardium, and conduction delays. Furthermore, it also has been shown that a change in myocardial wall motion by two or more degrees (normal to severely hypokinetic or akinetic) is much more reproducible than a stepwise change of 1 (normal to mildly hypokinetic or mildly hypokinetic to severely hypokinetic).

## Chapter 13
1. D. As the name indicates, pseudonormal stage of mitral inflow resembles normal mitral inflow. This is only the case for mitral inflow. Other measures of diastolic dysfunction include pulse wave Doppler of pulmonary venous flow, Doppler tissue imaging of the mitral valve annulus, or mitral velocity flow propagation. These measurements do not have the same "pseudonormalization" issues. Consequently, adding one of these measurements in assessing diastolic function can help differentiate between a normal and pseudonormal mitral inflow pattern. The accuracy of staging diastolic function is increased with using at least two different measures of diastolic dysfunction.

2. A. Diastolic dysfunction is present in virtually every case of systolic dysfunction but systolic dysfunction is not always present when there is diastolic dysfunction. Therefore, diastolic dysfunction is much more prevalent than systolic dysfunction.

3. D. Mitral inflow pattern is preload dependent. Increase in preload will change stage 1 pattern of diastolic dysfunction (abnormal relaxation) to stage 2 (pseudonormal) or 3 (restrictive) pattern. Inversely, the patient who has restrictive or pseudonormal pattern will change towards stage 1 (abnormal relaxation) with diuresis.

4. B. In restrictive cardiomyopathy there is always lowering of the Em velocity, whereas in constrictive cardiomyopathy the Em velocity can be normal except if the measurement is done in an area of myocardial scarring.

5. C. The thickened and often calcified pericardium or pericardial scarring leads to constrictive physiology. Transthoracic pressures are not transmitted transmurally through this thickened scan consequently causing greater respiratory gradients between intramyocardial pressures and thoracic pressures leading to greater variations in venous return during the respiratory cycle.

## Chapter 14
1. B. The standard nomenclature adopted by the Society of Cardiovascular Anesthesiologists and the American Society of Echocardiography divides both the anterior and posterior leaflets into 3 segmental regions. The anterior mitral leaflet regions are labeled A1, A2, and A3. The posterior mitral leaflet regions are P1, P2, and P3.

2. D. The reversed systolic flow pattern detected with pulsed wave Doppler in the pulmonary veins is a highly specific marker for detecting a large regurgitant orifice area. The

listed results for the continuous wave Doppler, the peak E wave velocity and the color Doppler area measurements are consistent with mild degrees of mitral regurgitation.

3. A. The width of the mitral regurgitant jet at its vena contracta is an accurate marker for severe mitral regurgitation. A width of greater than or equal to 0.5 centimeters is associated with severe mitral regurgitation.

4. B. The pressure half-time measures the rate of decline in the atrioventricular pressure gradient and can be quantitatively related to the severity of mitral stenosis. A pressure half-time of 300 milliseconds is associated with severe degrees of mitral stenosis.

5. D. Potential sources of error should be identified prior to applying the pressure half-time method in the evaluation of the severity of mitral stenosis. Alterations in left atrial or left ventricular compliances, rapid heart rates, and severe aortic insufficiency all influence the accuracy of the pressure half-time method.

## Chapter 15

1. A. Patients with left ventricular dysfunction are unable to generate the high transaortic velocities and high aortic valve gradients characteristic of aortic stenosis. For a given valve area, patients with a lower ejection fraction will generate a lower gradient and valvular velocity; that is why B and D are wrong. Reduced cusp separation is a qualitative sign of stenosis, but a determination of valve area (answer A) is required to quantify the severity of stenosis.

2. B. An examination of Figure 15.13 explains the answer to this question. Cath lab gradients are typically reported as peak-to-peak gradients, which are not "true" gradients, but rather the difference between peak pressures. A peak instantaneous gradient such as the one derived by using echocardiography is usually greater than the difference between peak pressures. The presence of aortic insufficiency may result in increased flow during systole because of the diastolic regurgitant volume, but this does not account for the different gradients obtained by the two techniques.

3. D. Color flow, continuous wave, and pulsed wave Doppler are used to quantify the severity of aortic insufficiency. Color flow Doppler applied to the aortic valve short-axis view is useful for identifying the location of the coaptation defect. However, two-dimensional echocardiography is the one answer that provides definitive information regarding the etiology of the valve dysfunction. Examples would include a dilated root and annulus, prolapsing leaflet, a calcific or rheumatic valve in which the leaflets do not fully open and do not completely close, and endocarditis. The diagnosis of all of these conditions is made with two-dimensional echocardiography. See "Echocardiographic Evaluation of Aortic Insufficiency."

4. D. The aortic valve regurgitant velocity deceleration slope increases with the severity of aortic regurgitation and decreased left ventricular compliance. A deceleration slope of 5 m/sec indicates severe aortic insufficiency. A patient with a competent aortic valve would not be expected to have a regurgitant velocity slope. See "Echocardiographic Evaluation of Aortic Insufficiency."

## Chapter 16

1. C. The PV can be viewed easily via a transgastric approach. It is embryologically derived from the same structure as the aortic valve, namely, the aortic and pulmonary trunks after partition of the bulbis cordis and the truncus arteriosus. In a similar manner to the AV, the tips of the PV leaflets may have nodules, known as the nodulus arrantii. The Ross procedure involves replacement of the aortic valve with the native PV, and subsequent placement of a PV homograft in the pulmonic position. TEE is especially useful in this setting to evaluate the relative sizes of the aortic annulus and the PV. In this way, the long-term consequences of mechanical valves are avoided.

2. A. Tricuspid regurgitation can be either pathologic or a normal finding. Its incidence increases with age, being found in

up to 93% of patients over the age of 70. Differentiating benign TR from pathologic TR involves assessing the degree of regurgitation, the turbulence of the jet, and the peak velocity of transtricuspid flows. Likewise, the peak velocity of the regurgitant jet may be used to estimate the peak pressure in the main pulmonary artery. TR is graded by evaluation of hepatic venous flow patterns, as well as the degree of extension of the color-flow jet into the right atrium.

3. C. Carcinoid heart disease results from chronic exposure to vasoactive amines secreted by the primary tumors, most often from hepatic metastases of primary gastrointestinal tumors. As such, involvement primarily occurs in the right sided cardiac structures, most specifically on the ventricular side of the TV and the arterial side of the PV. The primary tumors are slow-growing, and in those with cardiac involvement death most often follows progressive cardiac failure. TEE may be used to assess results of medical therapy. The TV often develops a mixed picture of TS and TR, with fixed immobile valves.

4. C. Valvular stenosis often involves fusion of the leaflets along their commissures. Right atrial enlargement may result from obstruction to flow through either TS or PS. The degree of stenosis is proportional to the peak velocity of the regurgitant jet. The leaflets in both TS and PS develop doming as well as leaflet thickening and restricted motion. It is rare for rheumatic disease to involve either the TV or the PV.

## Chapter 17

1. C. The tracheobronchial tree is interposed between the esophagus and the aorta blocking the echo penetration of the distal aorta.

2. B. Aortic dissections can cause coronary ischemia by shearing a coronary ostium, can cause AI by disrupting a leaflet, and pleural and pericardial effusion with blood or by causing CHF.

3. A. This is the accepted normal value.

4. D. Cannulation is performed in the distal ascending aorta and this is poorly seen by TEE. Epiaortic scanning is the only reliable means to interrogate this portion of the aorta.

## Chapter 18

1. B. "Profile" describes the height from the base of the prosthetic valve to the top of the supporting struts. Low profile mechanical valves include tilting disk valves and bileaflet valves. Bileaflet valves have the advantage of being less obstructive to flow, with flow occurring across three orifices. See "Low Profile Valves."

2. C. Stentless porcine valves are used in the aortic position. They lack the supporting struts used with the Carpentier-Edwards and Hancock valves, thereby giving them a larger effective orifice area and lower pressure gradients. See "Stentless Porcine Valves."

3. D. Perivalvular leaks must be distinguished from the "normal" regurgitant jets seen with many of the prosthetic valve types. Perivalvular leaks can be caused by valve dehiscence, suture fracture, and endocarditis. See "Prosthetic Valve Regurgitation."

4. A. Prosthetic transvalvular gradients are affected by many factors, including size and type of prosthetic valve, time of implantation, anatomic location, flow, and cardiac function. See "Prosthetic Valve Stenosis."

5. D. TEE is considered the best modality for defining anatomic valve abnormalities seen with prosthetic valve endocarditis. TEE is five times more sensitive than transthoracic echocardiography in the detection of prosthetic valve endocarditis. See "Prosthetic Valve Endocarditis."

## Chapter 19

1. D. Most secondary involvement of the heart by malignancy is pericardial (~ 75%).

2. B. Myxomas are the most common primary tumor.

3. C. LV apical thrombi should be visualized in systole and diastole as well as in more than one view to ensure differentiation from artifact and tangential cuts through the LV apex.

## Chapter 20

1. B. The most common type of atrial septal defect is the Secundum type. See "Atrial Septal Defects."
2. D. The degree of aortic override is best seen with the longitudinal plane. See "Tetralogy of Fallot"; Figure 20.7.
3. C. Protein-losing enteropathy is seen after the Fontan procedure. All other answers can occur after the arterial switch operation. See "Transposition of the Great Arteries."

## Chapter 21

1. A. Pruszczyk has proposed that patients have three of the five criteria (listed in the question) of right ventricular pressure overload in order to proceed to transesophageal echocardiography. Answer A is incorrect because a peak velocity of tricuspid valve insufficiency corresponding to a right ventricular to a right atrial pressure gradient of more than 30 mm Hg is required. See "Trauma with Cardiac Complications: Echocardiography Evaluation."
2. D. All of the responses are true except D. It is not uncommon to have a reduction in cardiac output and RV function lasting several weeks following a myocardial contusion. See "Blunt Cardiac Trauma: Myocardial Contusion or Rupture."
3. E. All are correct and are the common 2-D manifestations of cardiac tamponade. The most sensitive 2-D manifestation of cardiac tamponade is right ventricular collapse during diastole in a patient with a pericardial effusion. See "Table 21.2."

## Chapter 22

1. D. VTI and area should be determined at the same time when calculating a Doppler-derived stoke volume. They may be measured during systole in the LVOT or at the aortic valve when determining cardiac output. However, for determination of mitral regurgitant volume, stroke volumes would need to be determined during diastole at the mitral valve and during systole in the LVOT.
2. D. Results using the simplified proximal flow convergence method for determining mitral regurgitation severity correlate well with those obtained using the standard method.
3. C. The primary concern in determining aortic valve area with the continuity equation using TEE is related to the possible underestimation of time-velocity integrals (or peak velocities) in the LVOT and/or aortic valve due to inadequate beam alignment.
4. D. The pressure half-time method overestimates the area of normal prosthetic mitral valves.
5. B. Estimation of RVSP from the systemic systolic blood pressure and the peak velocity across the VSD is not valid in the presence of aortic stenosis or LVOT obstruction (systolic blood pressure will not approximate LV systolic pressure).

## Chapter 23

1. B. *Viable* means capable of living. One definition of myocardial viability is histological because viability is defined by the presence of living myocytes. Viable myocardium may be normal or dysfunctional in the reversible state of acute ischemia, stunning, or hibernation. During myocardial infarction viability is lost. Regional akinesis without recruitable reserve during low-dose dobutamine is consistent with infarcted tissue. See "Definitions."
2. C. Myocardial stunning is the fully reversible mechanical dysfunction that persists up to 24 hours after reperfusion despite restoration of normal or near-normal coronary blood flow (perfusion-contraction mismatch). The diagnosis of stunning requires demonstration of two conditions: reversibility of the contractile abnormality and evidence of normal or near-normal coronary blood flow in the dysfunctional myocardium. Myocardial stunning is caused in part by injurious events during ischemia and reperfusion, so this contractile dysfunction can be considered a form of ischemia-reperfusion injury. See "Myocardial Stunning."
3. D. Myocardial hibernation can be defined as reversible left ventricular dysfunction due to chronic CAD. Patients with hibernating myocardium have normal or slightly reduced myocardial blood flow and limited coronary flow reserve. Hiber-

nating myocardium reveals residual contractile reserve with adrenergic stimulation. Regional and global ventricular function can improve in a hibernating myocardium after revascularization. See "The Clinical Importance of Assessing Myocardial Viability," "Left Ventricular Remodeling After Revascularization," and "Survival Rates."
4. A. The short- and long-term outcome in patients with chronic left ventricular dysfunction after revascularization is strongly affected by the presence of viable myocardium. Coronary revascularization of hibernating myocardium decreases perioperative morbidity and mortality associated with revascularization procedures. After revascularization of hibernating myocardium improvement in regional systolic function is noted and improvement in the ejection fraction correlates with the number of dysfunctional but viable segments. The presence of viable myocardium in the outer layers of the ventricular wall maintains the left ventricular shape and size by preventing infarct expansion with subsequent heart failure. Long-term morbidity and mortality in patients with hibernating myocardium is associated with a low viability index. See "The Clinical Importance of Assessing Myocardial Viability"; Table 25.1.
5. C. Myocardial stunning, that is, reversible postoperative ventricular contractile dysfunction unrelated to a continuing source of ischemia, may follow CABG surgery. Distinguishing ventricular dysfunction caused by acute ischemia or infarction from stunned myocardium remains critical for determining perioperative management strategies (administration of vasoactive drugs, return to cardiopulmonary bypass, and utilization of a mechanical assist device) and long-term prognosis. Improvement in regional function after an ischemic event or acute myocardial infarction may require days or weeks after the initial compromising episode, despite adequate restoration of coronary blood flow. See "The Clinical Importance of Assessing Myocardial Viability."
6. D. In patients with chronic ischemic dysfunction, preoperative low-dose dobutamine echocardiography can predict regional and global improvement in left ventricular function, left ventricular remodeling, and survival after coronary revascularization. Intraoperative low-dose dobutamine echocardiography can predict recovery of regional myocardial function in these patients immediately after CABG surgery. See "Improvement of Global Systolic Function," "Use of Intraoperative Low-Dose Dobutamine Echocardiography," and "Myocardial Contrast Echocardiography."

## Chapter 24

1. A. Jones et al. combined data from 7 studies to evaluate those recurring factors contributing to in-hospital mortality following CABG. In a clinical study of more than 172,000 patients, those variables having the strongest correlation included:
   1. Patient's age
   2. Gender
   3. Previous cardiac surgery
   4. Operation urgency
   5. Ventricular ejection fraction
   6. Characterization of coronary anatomy [left main > 50% stenosis, number of vessels with > 70% stenosis]
   Of these variables, age, urgency of procedure, and reoperation were the most strongly correlated with patient mortality following CABG surgery.
2. B. The diagnosis of a central mitral regurgitant jet may help guide the surgical team in the repair of the type IIIb mechanism of mitral valve dysfunction CF. However, the presence of a protruding and mobile plaque in the ascending aorta is indicative of a high risk of type I postoperative neurologic dysfunction. Such findings would direct the surgical team to consider an alternative site of cannulation (axillary or femoral) and evaluation of the cross clamp site with epiaortic echo, and/or consideration of the use of circulatory arrest or off pump CABG. A deceleration time of < 120 msec has been associated with a poorer long-term prognosis in patients with congestive heart failure.

3. A. The National Center for Health Statistics and Centers for Disease Control and Prevention estimate that the number of individuals over the age of 65 will be more than 50,000,000 by the year 2020. Eleven percent of females and 17.7% of males in the age group have clinically significant coronary artery disease. Unless there is a significant decline in the incidence or management of diabetes, and hypertension, the health-care system will be confronted with this rapidly expanding patient population.

4. (A, B, and C). Patients with coronary artery disease and significant aortic regurgitation present the surgical team with challenges for myocardial protection. Strategies may include the direct administration of cardioplegia using handheld devices that engage the coronary ostia, retrograde cardioplegia via the coronary sinus, and venting of the LV during periods when the aorta is not cross clamped.

5. (A, B, D, and E). Patients with ischemic heart disease may have mitral regurgitation as a result of structural abnormalities of the components of the mitral valve apparatus. This may be due to a number of mechanisms, including eccentric remodeling of the LV with bileaflet tethering (symmetric IIIb with central MR), an inferoposterior or anterolateral infarct with systolic restriction of the PMVL (asymmetrical IIIb) with an override of the AMVL and posteriorly directed MR jet, an infracted papillary muscle with focal prolapse (type II) or rupture papillary muscle (type II), and chronic enlargement of the MV annulus (type I). Transient ischemia may produce global or regional dysfunction creating either apical tethering or restriction of the PMVL. In elderly patients with extensive mitral annular calcification, the patient may even exhibit diastolic and systolic restriction of the MV leaflets producing a Type IIIa mechanism. While mitral annular calcification has been associated with elevated LDL cholesterol, coronary artery disease, and significant atheroma of the aorta, MACa++ is not a manifestation of ischemic heart disease.

## Chapter 25

1. C. The functional subset of annular dilatation or restrictive leaflet motion was found to have the worst five-year survival rate (43%) compared to ruptured chordae or papillary muscle (76%). The predictor of worse long-term outcome indicated that the pathophysiology may be the major determinate of survival rather than the type of surgical intervention (12–14,34,39).

2. A. The blood supply to the posterior medial papillary muscle is either the right coronary artery or the obtuse marginal artery in 63% of patients and more than one vessel in 37% of patients. It has been observed and concluded that papillary muscle dysfunction paradoxically decreases ischemic MR because the inferiobasal ischemia reduces leaflet tethering and improves coaptation (21,23,28–30,40).

3. D. Research indicates that ring implantation reliably prevents delayed leaflet coaptation after acute ischemia, and also preserves papillary-annular distances, which invariably increase after induction of ischemia. Ring annuloplasty also preserved tethering distance and prevented disturbances in the geometry of the mitral and valve leaflets (30,31,33,40,42,48).

## Chapter 26

1. B. OPCAB is performed without CPB and therefore avoids its adverse effects. Positioning of the heart and occluding the coronary arteries during OPCAB can produce hemodynamic changes. Some concern still exists about the quality of anastomoses performed on a beating heart. OPCAB requires heparin because coronary arteries are temporarily occluded during graft construction. OPCAB does not decrease the number of grafts a patient may need. There tends to be fewer grafts constructed in OPCAB because of the technical difficulties in grafting some areas of the heart without CPB.

2. D. OPCAB allows revascularization of the heart without manipulating the aorta and would seem to be of greatest benefit in a patient with an atherosclerotic ascending aorta. Patients with vessels that are technically difficult to find or graft are particularly challenging OPCAB candidates. Patients with MR may tolerate the manipulation required for OPCAB less well and would need CPB if the mitral valve needs to be repaired or replaced.

3. A. The transgastric mid short-axis view does not include the mitral valve or a good look at the right ventricle and shows only the six mid-level segments of the LV. Usually when the heart is displaced for OPCAB, it is separated from the diaphragm, making transgastric views unobtainable. Some midesophageal views can usually be obtained even after displacement because the echo window to the LV is through the left atrium.

4. E. Baseline wall motion abnormalities rarely improve in the operating room during OPCAB. Most, but not all patients having OPCAB develop a transient wall motion abnormality during graft construction that resolves quickly once flow is restored. Persistence of a new wall motion abnormality after the chest is closed may be due to a problem with the graft supplying this area.

## Chapter 27

1. C. In cases of mitral valve prolapse, the regurgitant jet generally travels opposite to the prolapsing leaflet. See "Introduction: Primary Mitral Valve Disease."

2. D. The most common cause of tricuspid regurgitation is functional, with no structural abnormality of the leaflets. See "Tricuspid Valve: Functional Tricuspid Regurgitation."

3. E. The mitral chordae have several functions. Third order chordae insert into the annulus and maintain ventricular geometry. They may be important to maintenance of ventricular function. See "Structure and Anatomy: The Chords."

4. B. Posterior leaflet prolapse is the most common finding in patients coming to surgery for degenerative mitral valve disease. It is easily and reliably repaired. See "Pathology: Mitral Valve."

5. A. SAM occurs in about 5% of patients having mitral valve repair for degenerative disease. It is associated with excess leaflet tissue and a narrow left ventricular outflow tract. It can be prevented by the use of sliding leaflet repair. See "Pathology: Mitral Valve."

## Chapter 28

1. E. Risk factors for an unsuccessful repair include mitral annular calcification, a central regurgitant MR jet, rheumatic mitral disease, and a mechanism involving the AMVL, a central MR jet, and more than three segments. Greater than 94% of abnormal mitral valves are repaired which have a primary mechanism involving the PMVL.

2. D. While a CF Doppler MJA of 5 cm² warrants further evaluation, CF Doppler should not be used as a stand-alone determinant of severity of MR. The VC diameter of 0.3 is consistent with mild to moderate MR. The PISA calculated ROA of 0.3 cm² is consistent with moderate MR and is the most quantitative estimate of significant MR among the answers provided.

3. D. Post MV repair SAM and LVOTO is associated with a ratio of AMVL:PMVL of < 1.0, a C-sept distance of < 2.6 cm, PMVL height > 1.5 cm, and pre-CPB SAM with an LVOT gradient. While a septal thickness may be associated with other findings (reduced C-sept distance), it is not an established factor of post-CPB SAM with LVOTO.

4. D. Ling et al. documented that 90% of these patients either have surgery or die within 10 years of their initial diagnosis. With an aging population with less severe forms of myxomatous disease, the degenerative process of aging will make these patients more vulnerable to acute rupture of chordae and flail MV segments.

5. C. Both Carpentier and David have reported the ability to successfully repair the younger patient presenting with acute rheumatic valvulitis associated with AMVL prolapse due to chordal elongation. While older patients with MS and lower splitability scores may undergo debridement of the valve and

ring annuloplasty, their long-term durability (freedom from reoperation or other cardiac events) is not as good.

## Chapter 29
1. A. For both tricuspid and bicuspid aortic valves, the most repairable lesion is isolated-leaflet prolapse. Aortic root enlargement is the next most common mechanism of aortic insufficiency.
2. D. The Ross procedure is a more difficult operation when compared to the allograft and has similar resistance to infection. However, it is ideal in infants and young children as it has the potential to grow. The allograft is known to calcify and rapidly fail in infants and young children.
3. C. For most valve replacements the size of the annulus is determined. However, for stented valve it is the sinotubular junction diameter that determines which valve to use.

## Chapter 30
1. C. Rheumatic valve. Rheumatic valves, whether stenotic or regurgitant or both, are those most likely to result in recurrence and failure. Regurgitant lesions in general, especially those associated with prolapse, are those most amenable to repair. Decalcification procedures associated with stenotic valves are also prone to early failure.
2. D. The distal anastomotic site of the aortic homograph usually cannot be visualized secondary to its location near the trachea. Due to its proximity to the aortic valve, the mitral valve, especially the anterior leaflet, should always be inspected after every aortic valve procedure.
3. D. The stentless valve does not have the support required to be placed in a dilated aortic root. Therefore, if the STJ diameter exceeds the annulus diameter by 10%, a root replacement or an aortoplasty should be considered.
4. B. Paravalvular thickening can be quite extensive following stentless valve placement. This is acceptable provided it does not result in regurgitation or interfere with leaflet mobility. Most mild paravalvular leaks (< 3 mm) have been shown to diminish after the addition of protamine and the remainder is nearly completely resolved at follow-up echo up to 3.

## Chapter 31
1. B. Aneurysm is defined as a localized or diffuse aortic dilatation of more than 50% normal diameter. Dilatation develops from weakening of the aortic wall and is progressive. It must include all three layers of the wall or it is considered a pseudoaneurysm.
2. C. Most segments of the thoracic aorta can be clearly imaged with multiplane transesophageal echocardiography (TEE) as the aorta descends along the esophagus. Two blind spots, the distal ascending aorta and the proximal aortic arch, occur due to the intervening trachea and left main stem bronchus. Epiaortic scanning may be useful during surgery in order to visualize these two areas (57).
3. A. Chest x-ray will often reveal larger aneurysms as an enlarged mediastinum, aortic knob or as tracheal deviation. Smaller aneurysms are often entirely missed by chest films. The gold standard for evaluation of size and location remains angiography. Computed tomography and magnetic resonance imaging are replacing more invasive angiography as diagnostic tools. No studies have been performed to compare the accuracies of these techniques.
4. D. TEE is becoming an alternative to CT, MRI, and angiography, particularly if aortic dissection is suspected. The portability and rapidity of TEE diagnosis makes it the diagnostic modality of choice if the patient is unstable. At least 7 studies involving between 50 and 100 patients have reported on the sensitivity and specificity of TEE in the diagnosis of dissection (32). The sensitivity was high, between 97%–100% and the specificity ranged from 77%–100%. A series of 110 patients compared TTE, TEE, CT, and MRI (33). Sensitivities were low for TTE (59%) as compared to the other three imaging modalities, TEE (98%), CT (94%), and MRI (98%). The specificities were TTE (83%), TEE (77%), CT (87%), and MRI (98%). Due to the outstanding accuracy of MRI the au-

thors of this study recommended MRI as the initial diagnostic procedure in stable patients and TEE in unstable patients.

## Chapter 32
1. E. The hallmark of the cardiac response to injury or excessive tension is myocyte growth and hypertrophy, interstitial fibrosis, apoptosis, sarcomere slippage, and cardiac chamber enlargement. This remodeling process is generally characterized by increased cardiac mass and cardiac chamber dilation. As the heart dilates, loss of mitral valve support matrices frequently produces impaired leaflet coaptation with steadily worsening mitral insufficiency. This process, then, contributes to further alteration of myocyte loading conditions. A mechanical disadvantage cycle beginning with structural signaling processes coupling to humoral perturbation to drive hypertrophy and dilatation of the heart.
2. C.
3. A. Apoptosis, or programmed cell death, seems to be regulated via changes in expression of 7Fas ligand-activated genes. This may be the direct consequence of increased tumor necrosis factor levels, which stimulate Fas ligand. Premature cell senescence created by apoptosis up-regulation is enhanced in the heart failure setting, and this will produce cell drop-out. Counter-regulatory forces attempting to balance the development of detrimental hypertrophy and remodeling include release of atrial naturietic factors and nitric oxide. These processes may be linked to increased bradykinin levels. Apoptosis seemingly is particularly important in perpetuating detrimental cardiac remodeling and the heart failure response.

## Chapter 33
1. D. Cardiomyopathies, once defined as "heart muscle diseases of unknown cause," are now classified by their dominant pathophysiology or pathogenetic factors. These classifications include dilated cardiomyopathy, hypertrophic cardiomyopathy, restrictive cardiomyopathy, arrhythmogenic right ventricular cardiomyopathy, and unclassified cardiomyopathies. Some diseases may present with features of more than one type of cardiomyopathy. This information is found in the "Definition and Classification of Cardiomyopathies" section.
2. B. Characteristic echocardiographic findings associated with dilated cardiomyopathy include dilation and impaired contraction of one or both ventricles (with varying degrees of mitral and/or tricuspid insufficiency). Dagger-shaped appearance of the Doppler spectral wave form analysis is associated with hypertrophic cardiomyopathy. See "Dilated Cardiomyopathy."
3. C. Characteristic echocardiographic findings associated with hypertrophic cardiomyopathy include left ventricular and/or right ventricular hypertrophy (usually asymmetric and involving the interventricular septum) along with systolic anterior motion of the mitral valve apparatus. Ventricular dimensions and volumes are typically normal and ventricular systolic function is usually normal to supranormal. Diastolic dysfunction is often present (decreased E/A ratio). See "Hypertrophic Cardiomyopathy."
4. D. During surgical management of hypertrophic cardiomyopathy, intraoperative transesophageal echocardiography may be of benefit regarding guidance of extent and depth of myectomy, evaluation of the mitral valve apparatus, and detecting potential complications. See "Hypertrophic Cardiomyopathy" section.
5. C. Characteristic echocardiographic findings associated with restrictive cardiomyopathy include restrictive filling/reduced diastolic volume of either or both ventricles along with normal or near-normal systolic function/wall thickness. Pulmonary venous flow velocity decreases during systole and increases during diastole because of the increased left atrial pressure. Increased flow velocity (and pressure gradient) across the left ventricular outflow tract is characteristic of hypertrophic cardiomyopathy. See "Restrictive Cardiomyopathy."

## Chapter 34

1. D. Stunned myocardium occurs when myocardium becomes ischemic and then flow is reestablished by thrombolysis, angioplasty, or CABG. Full recovery is expected. However, during this period the patient may require inotropic or circulatory support.
2. E. Incomplete revascularization increases morbidity and mortality. Female gender, diabetes mellitus, and peripheral vascular disease cause a 1.2-fold–1.5-fold increase and chronic renal failure causes a 1.5-fold–1.9-fold increase in morbidity and mortality.
3. A. Ischemic LV reconstruction can be performed on both akinetic and dyskinetic segments.
4. E. The late mortality is increased following AVR in the African-American population. The exact reasons are unclear but compliance with anticoagulation therapy, genetic factors predisposing to hypertension, and socioeconomic factors have been implicated.

## Chapter 35

1. A. 7%
2. C. 85%
3. E. All of the above
4. D.
5. E. Correctable cardiac lesions are not absolute contraindications to LVAD implantation. Systemic infections are a contraindication to LVAD implantation related to the difficulty in effectively treating a systemic infection in the presence of a mechanical device.

## Chapter 36

1. D. There are many 2D-echocardiographic findings of the LV, which would be considered abnormal in the general population, that are characteristic of transplant recipients, including an increase in LV wall thickness (especially the posterior and septal walls), observation of LV mass and LV mass index, paradoxical or flat interventricular septal motion, and decreased interventricular septal systolic thickening compared to normal (31% vs. 44%) (23). Because the donor heart is normal in size, it is typically smaller than the original dilated failing heart and, therefore, it is positioned more medially in the mediastinum and tends to be rotated clockwise, which usually necessitates using nonstandard transducer locations and angles for echocardiography. Residual fluid accumulations in the posterior pericardial space contribute to the common small postoperative pericardial effusions (30).
2. D. The echocardiographic assessment of LV diastolic function in the transplanted heart is complicated by the variability of the Doppler velocity profiles from the atrioventricular valves, which may be observed when the remnant recipient atria retain mechanical activity. This results in asynchronous atrial contractions, modifying the filling patterns of both ventricles (23–27). The beat-to-beat variations in transmitral (and tricuspid) diastolic velocities, assessed by pulsed-wave Doppler, relate to the timing of contraction of the recipient atria within the cardiac cycle. Therefore, it is important to locate the recipient P waves within the donor cardiac cycle before making the required Doppler measurements. When the recipient P waves occur during late systole to mitral valve opening, the flow signals should not be used to measure diastolic indices. Recipient P waves occurring during this period decrease isovolumic relaxation time and pressure half-time, and increase the mitral inflow peak E-wave velocity. If the recipient P waves occur anywhere from late diastole through midsystole, the flow signals may be used (23,24,26).
3. C. The decision regarding RV assist device implantation is dependent upon a stepwise review of overall hemodynamics after the institution of maximal inotropic and vasodilator support. The assessment includes an evaluation of the size and function of both ventricles by TEE, the status of mediastinal bleeding, oxygenation, presence of arrhythmias, and urine output. This assessment usually takes place after several unsuccessful attempts to separate the patient from CPB

and approximately 1 hour after removal of the aortic cross-clamp. The observation of a small hyperdynamic LV and a dilated RV by TEE, marginal urine output, arrhythmias, or coagulopathy should prompt the insertion of a RV assist device. The presence of coagulopathy will require ongoing volume resuscitation with blood products, likely resulting in a worsening of pulmonary hypertension, pulmonary edema, and RV failure with its secondary effects on cardiac output and end organ perfusion.
4. B. The combination of disturbed atrial hemodynamics caused by asynchronous contraction of the atria and atrial enlargement might contribute to slow blood flow within the atrial cavities and explain the relatively high incidence of spontaneous echo contrast (SEC) (25%–55%) despite normal ventricular function in heart transplant recipients (27,29,39,40). This is usually confined to the donor atrial component and characterized by multiple microechoes visible at normal gain settings slowly swirling within the enlarged atrial cavity and disappearing after passage through the mitral valve, which allows clear discrimination from noise echoes or reverberations (29). The importance of diagnosing LA SEC in the heart transplant recipients stems from its association with LA thrombi and systemic embolic events on postoperative follow-up studies (29,40,48). In most cases, the thrombi are attached to the atrial free wall underneath the protruding suture in a niche formed after partial removal of the left atrial appendage during transplantation, but can also be localized on the posterior LA wall or on the suture line (27,29,40). Therefore, the presence of LA SEC on intraoperative TEE should prompt postoperative follow-up studies to assess for the presence of atrial thrombi and the need for antiplatelet or anticoagulation therapy. The incidence of left atrial SEC and subsequent left atrial thrombi and systemic embolic events on postoperative follow up is decreased by using the bicaval (48) or total orthotopic (27) anastomotic techniques.
5. A. Tricuspid regurgitation (TR), found in 85% of transplant recipients, occurs immediately after heart transplantation, and is usually moderate, with an eccentric jet direction pointing toward the interatrial septum (29,55). There is no association between the incidence and severity of TR immediately after cardiac transplantation and the presence of RV dysfunction (56). Quantification of the severity of TR by color flow Doppler is best achieved using the ratio of the maximum area of the regurgitant jet to the right atrial area (57) (< 10% trivial, 10%–24% mild, 25%–49% moderate, 50% severe). The severity of posttransplant TR correlates with echocardiographic indices of atrial distortion (recipient to donor atrial area ratio) and the systolic shortening of the tricuspid annulus (55). The significantly reduced incidence of moderate and severe TR with the bicaval anastomotic technique, and both TR and MR after total orthotopic heart transplantation (38), further supports this hypothesis.

## Chapter 37

1. A. With a 100% restenosis rate at two years, balloon valvuloplasty for aortic stenosis is not indicated in the long-term management of patients with aortic stenosis. Because of a higher incidence of stroke, it has a limited palliative application in patients with severe stenosis who may require other life saving surgical intervention or symptomatic palliation.
2. E. TEE permits the guidance of the percutaneous device to an optimal position for deployment. In addition to determining the size of the device used, it permits a rapid assessment of the results of the procedure (aortic valve area and gradient) and identification of potential complications (paravalvular regurgitation, aortic dissection, LV dysfunction, and segmental LV dysfunction).
3. E. Percutaneous mitral valvuloplasty was first performed in patients with rheumatic MS utilizing balloon valvuloplasty. More recently, percutaneous devices have been developed that reduce the annular diameter through coronary sinus stinting, A-P splinting, and edge-to-edge leaflet attachment

(clip or suture). The FDA has approved the use of multiple clip devices in patients with more than focal segmental MV disease. Calcification and valvular fibrosis (type IIIa) mechanisms of regurgitation are current contraindications for percutaneous MV repair.

4. D. The Alfieri repair is predominantly utilized in patients with apical tethering (with or without annular dilatation). However, it has also been successfully employed in failed MV repairs, and myxomatous MV disease (flail or prolapse). Rheumatic restriction of leaflet motion is less amenable to success of the Alfieri repair.

5. C. Under TTE guidance, percutaneous alcohol reduction of the hypertrophied septum associated with HOCM has been successful in initially reported series. However, there are a number of associated and potential complications related to the extent and specificity of administration of the alcohol. Because the procedure is intracoronary, leaflet perforation is not an associated complication.

## Chapter 38

1. A. Table 38.3 summarizes the grading scale of embolic patterns and Grade 3 is the most severe pattern including large embolic masses or sempentine emboli. See "Orthopedic Surgery."

2. D. With pneumoeritoneum preload is typically increased due to compression of the splanchnic vessels that shifts blood from the abdomen to the thorax. See "Assessing Stroke Volume, Alternative Approaches to Optimizing Fluid Status"; "Laparoscopic Surgery."

3. D. Planimetry of the triangular orifice seen during midsystole provides the best estimate of mean systolic aortic valve area. See "Echocardiographic Techniques for Stroke Volume Measurement."

4. D. TEE is an extremely useful tool for management of the liver transplantation patient providing assessment of LV function, identification of the cause of postperfusion syndrome, including the detection of air or thrombotic embolisms originating from the newly inserted donor liver. See "Orthotopic Liver Transplantation."

# INDEX

# APPENDIX

# Summary Tables

## CHARTS AND GRAPHS

**Normal TEE Measurements**
Stanton K. Shernan and Eric Kraenzler

**Severity Assessment of Valve Dysfunction**
John Apostalakis, Maged Argalious, Greg Pitas, and Jia Lin

**Estimation of Hemodynamic Pressures**
Jack Shanewise, Brian Johnson, and Andra Duncan

**Diastolic Function**
Gardar Sigurdsson, Daryl Atwell, and Brian Johnson

**Grading of Aortic Disease and Neurologic Dysfunction**
Dominique Prud' homme, Pierre Devilliers, and Jay Weller

**Table 1. Normal TEE Measurements**

Reference Values for Normal Adult Transesophageal
Echocardiographic Measurements Indexed to Body Surface Area

| Parameter | Mean ± SD (mm/m²) | Range (mm/m²) |
|---|---|---|
| Right pulmonary artery diameter[1] | 10 ± 1 | 7–12 |
| Left upper pulmonary vein diameter | 6 ± 1 | 5–10 |
| Left atrial appendage | | |
| Length | 16 ± 3 | 10–23 |
| Diameter | 9 ± 3 | 5–17 |
| Superior vena cava diameter | 8 ± 1 | 4–11 |
| Right ventricular outflow tract diameter[2] | 15 ± 2 | 10–20 |
| Left Atrium[3] | | |
| Antero-posterior diameter | 21 ± 4 | 13–33 |
| Medial-lateral diameter | 22 ± 4 | 13–33 |
| Right atrium[3] | | |
| Antero-posterior diameter | 22 ± 3 | 16–28 |
| Medial-lateral diameter | 21 ± 3 | 16–32 |
| Tricuspid annular diameter[3] | 16 ± 3 | 11–24 |
| Mitral annular diameter[3] | 17 ± 2 | 11–22 |
| Coronary sinus diameter | 4 ± 1 | 2–6 |
| Left ventricle[4] | | |
| Antero-posterior diameter (diastole) | 25 ± 3 | 19–31 |
| Medial-lateral diameter (diastole) | 24 ± 4 | 11–30 |
| Antero-posterior diameter (systole) | 16 ± 4 | 10–25 |
| Medial-lateral diameter (systole) | 15 ± 4 | 11–24 |
| Aortic root diameter[2] | 16 ± 2 | 12–23 |
| Descending thoracic aorta diameter | | |
| Proximal | 12 ± 2 | 9–17 |
| Distal | 11 ± 2 | 8–15 |

[1]Right pulmonary artery diameter measured in midesophageal ascending aorta short-axis view.
[2]Aortic root and right ventricular outflow tract diameters measured in the midesophageal right ventricular inflow/outflow tract view.
[3]Atrial (end-systole) and both mitral and tricuspid annular (mid-diastole) diameters measured in the midesophageal four-chamber view.
[4]Left ventricular dimensions measured in transgastric mid short-axis view.
Reprinted with permission from Cohen G, White M, Sochowski R, Klein A, Bridge P, Stewart W, Chan K. Reference values for normal adult transesophageal measurements. J Am Soc Echocardiogr 1995;8:221–30.

Published in Savage and Aronson: Comprehensive Textbook of Intraoperative Transesophageal Echocardiography, Lippincott Williams & Wilkins, 2005.

**Table 2. Normal TEE Measurements**

Reference Values for Normal Adult Transesophageal
Echocardiographic Measurements Absolute (Nonindexed)

| Parameter | Mean ± SD (mm) | Range (mm) |
|---|---|---|
| Right pulmonary artery diameter[1] | 17 ± 3 | 12–22 |
| Left upper pulmonary vein diameter | 11 ± 2 | 7–16 |
| Left atrial appendage | | |
|     Length | 28 ± 5 | 15–43 |
|     Diameter | 16 ± 5 | 10–28 |
| Superior vena cava diameter | 15 ± 3 | 8–20 |
| Right ventricular outflow tract diameter[2] | 27 ± 4 | 16-36 |
| Left atrium[3] | | |
|     Antero-posterior diameter | 38 ± 6 | 20–52 |
|     Medial-lateral diameter | 39 ± 7 | 24–52 |
| Right atrium[3] | | |
|     Antero-posterior diameter | 38 ± 5 | 28–52 |
|     Medial-lateral diameter | 38 ± 6 | 29–53 |
| Tricuspid annular diameter[3] | 28 ± 5 | 20–40 |
| Mitral annular diameter[3] | 29 ± 4 | 20–38 |
| Coronary sinus diameter | 6.6 ± 1.5 | 4–10 |
| Left ventricle[4] | | |
|     Antero-posterior diameter (diastole) | 43 ± 7 | 33–55 |
|     Medial-lateral diameter (diastole) | 42 ± 7 | 23–54 |
|     Antero-posterior diameter (systole) | 28 ± 6 | 18–40 |
|     Medial-lateral diameter (systole) | 27 ± 6 | 18–42 |
| Aortic root diameter[2] | 28 ± 3 | 21-34 |
| Descending thoracic aorta diameter | | |
|     Proximal | 21 ± 4 | 14–30 |
|     Descending | 20 ± 4 | 13–28 |

[1]Right pulmonary artery diameter measured in midesophageal ascending aorta short-axis
   view.
[2]Atrial (end-systole) and both mitral and tricuspid annular (mid-diastole) diameters measured
   in the midesophageal four-chamber view.
[3]Aortic root and right ventricular outflow tract diameters measured in the midesophageal right
   ventricular inflow/outflow tract view.
[4]Left ventricular dimensions measured in transgastric mid short-axis view.
Reprinted with permission from Cohen G, White M, Sochowski R, Klein A, Bridge P, Stewart W,
   Chan K. Reference values for normal adult transesophageal measurements. J Am Soc
   Echocardiogr 1995;8:221–30.

Published in Savage and Aronson: Comprehensive Textbook of Intraoperative Transesophageal
Echocardiography, Lippincott Williams & Wilkins, 2005.

**Table 3A. Intraoperative Assessment of AR Severity**

Qualitative and Semiquantitative Assessment

| Parameter | Utility/Advantages | Limitations | Mild | Moderate | Severe |
|---|---|---|---|---|---|
| **Two-Dimensional Imaging** | | | | | |
| LV size (At end diastole) | Simple<br>LV enlarged in chronic AR<br>Normal LV excludes significant chronic AR | Enlarged in other conditions<br>Normal in acute | Normal (chronic) | Variable | Dilated (chronic) |
| Aortic leaflets | Simple<br>Abnormal in severe<br>Flail denotes severe | Inaccurate<br>Anatomic defect not reflective of severity | Variable | Variable | Abnormal (flail coaptation defect) |
| **Doppler** | | | | | |
| CF Doppler jet diameter in LVOT (Aliasing velocity 50–60 cm/sec) | Simple<br>Quick screen<br>Mechanism evaluation | Inaccurate for eccentric jets | Small | Medium | Large (central)<br>Variable (eccentric) |
| PW Doppler Diastolic flow (Reversal descending aorta) | Simple | Stiff aorta<br>Brief reversal is normal | Brief early diastolic reversal | Variable | Holodiastolic reversal |
| CW Doppler spectral density | Simple<br>Faint or incomplete—mild AR | Qualitative<br>Moderate-severe overlap | Faint | Variable | Dense |
| CW Doppler jet pressure half-time (m/sec) | Simple<br>Semiquantitative | Dependent on aortic-LV gradient | Slow > 500 | Medium 500–200 | Steep < 200 |

Zoghbi WA, Enriquez-Sarano M, Foster E, et al. Recommendations for evaluation of the severity of native valvular regurgitation with two-dimensional and Doppler echocardiography. J Am Soc Echocardiogr 2003;16(7):777–802, modified with permission.

Published in Savage and Aronson: Comprehensive Textbook of Intraoperative Transesophageal Echocardiography, Lippincott Williams & Wilkins, 2005.

**Table 3B. Intraoperative Assessment of AR Severity**

Quantitative AR Assessment

| Parameter | Utility/Advantages | Limitations | Mild | Mild to Moderate | Moderate to Severe | Severe |
|---|---|---|---|---|---|---|
| Vena contracta width (cm) | Simple<br>Quantitative<br>Identifies mild or severe | Multiple jets<br><br>Small error = large<br>  % error | < 0.3 | 0.3–0.60 | | > 0.6 |
| Jet width/LVOT width (%) (Aliasing velocity 50–60 cm/sec) | Simple, very sensitive,<br>  quick screen for AR | Eccentric jets | < 25 | 25–45 | 46–64 | > 65 |
| Jet CSA/LVOT CSA (%) | Simple<br>Sensitive quick screen<br>  for AR | Inaccurate (eccentric<br>  jets) | < 5 | 5–20 | 21–59 | > 60 |
| Regurgitant Volume (cc/beat) | Quantitative<br>Valid with multiple or<br>  eccentric jets<br>Estimates severity and<br>  volume overload | Combined<br>  MR and AR | < 30 | 30–44 | 45–59 | > 60 |
| PISA Proximal Flow Convergence (PFC) | Quantitative<br>Provides severity | Limited by $Ca^{++}$<br>Multiple jets<br>Inaccurate<br>  eccentric jets | **Mild** | **Mild to Moderate** | **Moderate to Severe** | **Severe** |
| Regurgitant Volume (cc/beat) | Quantitative | Maximum | < 30 | 30–44 | 45-59 | ≥ 60 |
| Regurgitant fraction (%) | Quantitative | Maximum | < 30 | 30–39 | 40–49 | ≥ 50 |
| ROA ($cm^2$) | Quantitative | Maximum RVA | < 0.10 | 0.10–0.19 | 0.20–0.29 | ≥ 0.30 |

Zoghbi WA, Enriquez-Sarano M, Foster E, et al. Recommendations for evaluation of the severity of native valvular regurgitation with two-dimensional and Doppler echocardiography. J Am Soc Echocardiogr 2003;16(7):777–802, 2003, modified with permission.

Published in Savage and Aronson: Comprehensive Textbook of Intraoperative Transesophageal Echocardiography, Lippincott Williams & Wilkins, 2005.

**Table 4. Intraoperative Assessment of AS Severity**

| Parameter | Utility/Advantages | Limitations | Mild | Moderate | Severe |
|---|---|---|---|---|---|
| **Two-Dimensional Imaging** | | | | | |
| M mode<br>Maximum cusp<br>separation | Simple | Qualitative<br>Cursor must be<br>perpendicular | > 20 mm | 10–20 mm | < 10 mm |
| Aortic valve leaflets | Simple | Qualitative estimation | ≤ 1 leaflet<br>immobility | 2 leaflet<br>immobility | 3 leaflet<br>immobility |
| Planimetered valve<br>area<br>Normal = 3 − 4 cm² | Simple | Inaccurate with $Ca^{++}$<br>Image plane must be<br>perpendicular | 2.0–1.5 cm² | 1.5–0.75 cm² | < 0.75 cm² |
| **Doppler** | | | | | |
| CW Doppler<br>peak velocity<br>(Assume nl CO) | Simple<br>Little inducible error | Increased with AR | 2.5 m/sec ≤ | 2.5–4.5 msec | > 4.5 m/sec |
| CW Doppler<br>mean gradient<br>(Assume nl CO) | Simple<br>Little inducible error | Cardiac output<br>dependent | < 20 mm Hg* | 30 − 50 mm Hg* | > 50 mm Hg* |
| Continuity equation<br><br>$\text{AoV Area} = \dfrac{TVI_{LVOT} \times Area_{LVOT}}{TVI_{AoV}}$ | Accurate<br><br>May use<br>LVOT as<br>reference with AR | Squared diameter<br>(introduces large error)<br>Regurgitation in<br>reference valve<br>LVOT obstruction | 2.0–1.5 cm² | 1.5–0.75 cm² | ≤ 0.75 cm² |
| Dimensionless index<br>$TVI_{LVOT} / TVI_{AV}$ | Simple<br>Less inducible error | Less quantitative | | | < 0.25 |

*If gradient < 30 mm Hg with poor LVC function, dobutamine may clarify even with AR; gradient > 50 mm Hg suggestive of significant AS.

Published in Savage and Aronson: Comprehensive Textbook of Intraoperative Transesophageal Echocardiography, Lippincott Williams & Wilkins, 2005.

**Table 5A. Intraoperative Assessment of MR Severity**

Qualitative and Semiquantitative Assessment

| Parameter | Utility/Advantages | Limitations | Mild | Moderate | Severe |
|---|---|---|---|---|---|
| **Two-Dimensional Imaging** | | | | | |
| LA size | LAE with chronic MR Normal LA size (no significant chronic MR) | Enlarged other conditions Severe acute (normal) | Normal | Variable | LAE |
| LV size | | | Normal | Variable | Enlarged (chronic) |
| MV apparatus | Flail or ruptured PM— severe MR | Limited to flail and ruptured PM | Normal or abnormal | Normal or abnormal | Flail leaflet/ Ruptured PM |
| **Doppler** | | | | | |
| CF Doppler maximum jet area (MJA) (Aliasing velocity 50–60 cm/sec) | Efficient screen for (mild or severe) Mechanism evaluation | Technical (wall filter, power, aliasing velocity, color gain, frequency) Load dependent Wall impingement underestimates by 60% | < 4 cm$^2$ | Variable | > 8 cm$^2$ PFC present Wall jet Circumferential LA jet |
| PW Doppler | Quantitative dominance excludes severe | Dependent on load, diastolic fx, MVA, a fib Indirect indication | A Dominant | Variable | E Dominant E > 1.2 m/sec |
| PW Doppler PV flow | Systolic reversal (severe MR) | Increased LAP, a fib, need R and L PV to call severe | S > D | S ≤ D | Systolic flow reversal |
| CW Doppler spectral density | Simple | Qualitative | Faint | Dense | "V" wave cut off sign |
| CW Doppler contour | Simple | Qualitative | Parabolic | Variable | Early peak Triangular |

Zoghbi WA, Enriquez-Sarano M, Foster E, et al. Recommendations for evaluation of the severity of native valvular regurgitation with two-dimensional and Doppler echocardiography. J Am Soc Echocardiogr 2003;16(7):777–802, modified with permission.

Published in Savage and Aronson: Comprehensive Textbook of Intraoperative Transesophageal Echocardiography, Lippincott Williams & Wilkins, 2005.

## Table 5B. Intraoperative Assessment of MR Severity

**Quantitative MR Assessment**

| Parameter | Utility/Advantages | Limitations | Mild | Moderate | Severe |
|---|---|---|---|---|---|
| Vena contracta width (cm) | Good eccentric jets; Simple; Quantitative | Not useful for multiple jets; Cannot add diameters | < 0.3 cm | 0.3–0.69 cm | ≥ 0.7 cm |

| PISA Proximal flow convergence (PFC) (Aliasing velocity 50–60 cm/s) | PFC indicates ≥ mod | Eccentric jets; Multiple jets | Mild | Mild to Moderate | Moderate to Severe | Severe |
|---|---|---|---|---|---|---|
| Regurgitant RVol (l/beat) | Quantitative | Peak flow rate | < 30 | 30–44 | 45–59 | ≥ 60 |
| Regurgitant RF (%) | Quantitative | Peak flow rate | < 30 | 30–39 | 40–49 | ≥ 50 |
| ROA (cm²) | Quantitative | Peak ROA (estimates mean ROA) | < 0.20 | 0.20–0.29 | 0.30–0.39 | ≥ 0.40 |

Zoghbi WA, Enriquez-Sarano M, Foster E, et al. Recommendations for evaluation of the severity of native valvular regurgitation with two-dimensional and Doppler echocardiography. J Am Soc Echocardiogr 2003;16(7):777–802, modified with permission.

## Table 5C. Intraoperative Assessment of MR Severity

Proximal Flow Convergence Radius and Severity of MR
$V_{aliasing}$ = 40 cm/sec or 1/12 (0.8) peak $V_{MR}$

| Grade | PISA Radius | ROA r²/2 (peak) | Regurgitant Volume (peak) |
|---|---|---|---|
| Mild | 6.2 mm | < 0.2 cm² | < 30 cc |
| Moderate | 6.3–7.6 mm | 0.20–0.29 cm² | 30–44 cc |
| Moderate to Severe | 7.7–8.8 mm | 0.30–0.39 cm² | 45–59 cc |
| Severe | > 8.9 mm | > 0.40 cm² | > 60 cc |

## Table 6. Qualitative Assessment of Mitral Stenosis

Echocardiographic Splitability Index

| Grade | Mobility | Leaflet Thickening | Subvalvular | Calcification |
|---|---|---|---|---|
| 1 | Tips restricted | Normal 4–5 m | < 1/3 below leaflet | Single area of brightness |
| 2 | Base to mid normal | Mid normal; edges (5–8 mm) | 1/3 of chordae thickened | Scattered areas on leaflet margins |
| 3 | Base normal | Throughout leaflet (5–8 mm) | 2/3 of chordae thickened | Bright to mid leaflet portion |
| 4 | Minimal or no movement | Marked throughout > 8–10 mm | All of chordae thick to PM | Bright throughout leaflet |

Wilkins GT, Weyman AE, Abascal VM, et al. Percutaneous balloon dilatation of the mitral valve: an analysis of echocardiographic variables related to outcome and the mechanism of dilatation. Br Heart J 1988;60:299–308.

Published in Savage and Aronson: Comprehensive Textbook of Intraoperative Transesophageal Echocardiography, Lippincott Williams & Wilkins, 2005.

**Table 7. Assessment of MV Stenosis Severity**

| Parameter Two-Dimensional imaging | Utility/Advantages | Limitations | Mild | Moderate | Severe |
|---|---|---|---|---|---|
| LA size (LAE > 45 mm AP diameter exclude LAA thrombi) | Simple | Nonspecific | Nl excludes chronic MS | | > 60 mm in chronic MS |
| Spontaneous contrast | Simple | Nonspecific | Usually absent | May be present | Present |
| Planimetered MV area | Simple | Inaccurate with Ca++ or previous commissurotomy | 1.5–2.0 cm$^2$ | 1.0–1.5 cm$^2$ | ≤ 0.9 cm$^2$ |
| **Doppler** | | | | | |
| CF Doppler Proximal flow convergence (Aliasing velocity 50–60 cm/sec) | Simple, screen Presence excludes normal valve | Nondiagnostic Present following MVrep MVR | Not present | Usually present | Always present Absence excludes |
| **PW Doppler PV flow** | | | | | |
| CW Doppler peak gradient | Simple Minimal | Severe AR decreases Heart rate dependent Dependent on LA-LV compliance | | | |
| CW Doppler mean gradient* | Simple Minimal inducible error | Severe AR decreases Heart rate dependent Dependent on LA-LV compliance | < 6 mm Hg | 6–12 mm Hg | > 12 mm Hg |
| CW Doppler Pressure half-time* $MVA = 220 / PT_{1/2}$ (Use longer slope if two present) | | Severe AR decreases $PT_{1/2}$ Heart rate dependent Dependent on LA-LV compliance | < 150 msec | 150–220 msec | > 220 msec |
| CW Doppler Deceleration time* $MVA = 759 / DT$ $PT_{1/2} = 0.29 \times DT$ (Use longer slope if two present) | Simple Minimal inducible error | Severe AR decreases Heart rate dependent Dependent on LA-LV compliance | < 517 msec | 517–759 msec | > 759 msec |
| Continuity equation* $MVA = \dfrac{Area_{LVOT} \times TVI_{LVOT}}{TVI_{MV}}$ | Accurate | Time consuming | 1.5–2.0 cm$^2$ | 1.0–1.5 cm$^2$ | ≤ 0.9 cm$^2$ |
| Proximal isovelocity* surface area $MVA = 2 \pi r^2 \times V_{Aliasing}/Peak$ $V_{MS} \times \alpha°/180°$ | Accurate | Funnel angle, Subvalve stenosis Time consuming | 1.5–2.0 cm$^2$ | 1.0–1.5 cm$^2$ | ≤ 0.9 cm$^2$ |

*With atrial fibrillation, average 5 consecutive diastoles

Published in Savage and Aronson: Comprehensive Textbook of Intraoperative Transesophageal Echocardiography, Lippincott Williams & Wilkins, 2005.

**Table 8. Intraoperative Assessment of TR Severity**

| Parameter | Utility/Advantages | Limitations | Mild | Moderate | Severe |
|---|---|---|---|---|---|
| **Two-Dimensional Imaging** | | | | | |
| RA/RV/IVC size<br>RA diameter<br>< 4.6 cm<br>RV diameter<br>< 4.3 cm | RAE and RVE (chronic)<br>Normal excludes<br>significant chronic TR | Not specific<br>Normal in<br>acute TR | Normal | Variable | Usually dilated |
| Tricuspid valve structure | Flail or poor coaptation (significant) | Nonspecific | Normal | Variable | Flail poor coaptation |
| **Doppler** | | | | | |
| CF Doppler<br>Max jet area<br>Nyquist limit<br>50–60 cm/sec | Screen for<br>< mild<br>> moderate | Technical factors<br>Loading<br>Underestimates<br>(eccentric jets) | < 5 cm$^2$ | 5–10 cm$^2$ | > 1 0 cm$^2$ |
| PW Doppler<br><br>Hepatic vein flow | Simple | Blunting multiple causes | Systolic dominance | Systolic blunting | Systolic reversal |
| CW Doppler<br>Jet density-contour | Simple<br>Readily available | Qualitative,<br>complementary data | Soft parabolic | Dense variable contour | Dense triangular with early peaking |
| **Quantitative** | | | | | |
| CF Doppler<br>Vena contracta<br>diameter<br>(VCD) (cm) | Simple<br>Quantitative<br>Distinguishes mild<br>from severe | Directs<br>need of further<br>confirmation | Not defined | < 0.7 | > 0.7 |
| PISA radius (cm)<br>Baseline shift with<br>Nyquist 28 cm/sec | Quantitative | Validation lacking | < 0.5 | 0.6–0.9 | > 0.9 |

Zoghbi WA, Enriquez-Sarano M, Foster E, et al. Recommendations for evaluation of the severity of native valvular regurgitation with two-dimensional and Doppler echocardiography. J Am Soc Echocardiogr 2003;16(7):777–802, modified with permission.

Published in Savage and Aronson: Comprehensive Textbook of Intraoperative Transesophageal Echocardiography, Lippincott Williams & Wilkins, 2005.

**Table 9. Intraoperative Assessment of TS Severity**

| Parameter | Utility/Advantages | Limitations | Mild | Moderate | Severe |
|---|---|---|---|---|---|
| **Two-Dimensional Imaging** | | | | | |
| Tricuspid valve (thickness, reduced mobility, Ca++) | Simple | Nonspecific | Normal | Normal or abnormal | Abnormal |
| RA size | Simple | Nonspecific | | | >4 cm |
| RV size RV diameter < 4.3 cm RV ED area ≤ 35.5 cm² | Increased in chronic significant PR normal size excludes significant PR | Nonspecific | Normal | Normal or dilated | Dilated |
| **Doppler** | | | | | |
| Color flow Proximal flow convergence (Nyquist limit 50–60 cm/s) | Simple screen | Qualitative Poor correlation with severity of PR | | | |
| Continuous wave Jet density and deceleration | Simple Qualitative | Slow deceleration rate caused by PR and left right shunt | Faint Steep deceleration | Dense Variable deceleration | Dense Delayed deceleration |
| Continuous wave velocity Peak gradient Mean gradient | Simple Minimal inducible error | Correct alignment Compliance RA RV Flow and HR dependent | < 1 m/sec < 4 mm Hg < 2 mm Hg | 1–2.5 m/sec 4–25 mm Hg 2–7 mm Hg | > 2.5 m/sec > 25 mm Hg > 7 mm Hg |
| CW Doppler (TVA 5 190/PT$_{1/2}$) | Simple | Inaccurate with Abn Compliance (RA, RV) PR reduces PT$_{1/2}$ and overestimates area | | | > 190 ms |

Hatle L. Noninvasive assessment of valve lesions with Doppler ultrasound. Herz 1984;9(4):213–21.
Fawzy ME, Mercer EN, Dunn B, et al. Doppler echocardiography. In the evaluation of tricuspid stenosis. Eur Heart J 1989;985–90.

Published in Savage and Aronson: Comprehensive Textbook of Intraoperative Transesophageal Echocardiography, Lippincott Williams & Wilkins, 2005.

**Table 10. Intraoperative Assessment of PR Severity**

| Parameter | Utility/Advantages | Limitations | Mild | Moderate | Severe |
|---|---|---|---|---|---|
| *Two-Dimensional Imaging* | | | | | |
| Pulmonic valve | | | Normal | Variable | Abnormal |
| RV size<br>RV diameter<br>< 4.3 cm<br>RV ED area<br>≤ 35.5 cm² | Simple<br>RV enlargement (sensitive for chronic significant)<br>Normal excludes significant chronic | Nonspecific | Normal | Variable | Dilated (except acute) |
| Paradoxical septal motion (volume overload pattern) | Simple sign of severe PR | Not specific for PR | Normal | Variable | Flail and poor coaptation |
| *Doppler* | | | | | |
| Color flow Doppler Jet size | Simple | Poor correlation with severity of PR | Small < 10 mm length | Variable | Large |
| Vena contracta Nyquist limit 50–60 cm/s | Simple | Not validated | < small | Variable | Wide origin |
| CW Doppler Jet density and deceleration | Simple | Qualitative | Faint Slow deceleration | Variable density and deceleration | Dense Steep deceleration Short |
| *Quantitative* | | | | | |
| Pulmonic systolic flow compared to systemic | Quantitative | Time consuming | Slight increase | Intermediate | Great increase |

Zoghbi WA, Enriquez-Sarano M, Foster E, et al. Recommendations for evaluation of the severity of native valvular regurgitation with two-dimensional and Doppler echocardiography. J Am Soc Echocardiogr 2003;16(7):777–802, modified with permission.

Published in Savage and Aronson: Comprehensive Textbook of Intraoperative Transesophageal Echocardiography, Lippincott Williams & Wilkins, 2005.

**Table 11. Estimation of Hemodynamic Pressures**

| Pressure Estimated | Required Measurement | Formula | Normal Values (mm Hg) |
|---|---|---|---|
| *Estimated CVP* | Respiratory IVC collapse (spontaneously breathing) | $\geq 40\% = 5$ mm Hg<br>$< 40\%$, (nl RV) $= 10$ mm Hg<br>None (RV Dysfx) $= 15$ mm Hg | 5–10 mm Hg |
| *RV systolic (RVSP)* | Peak velocity$_{TR}$<br>CVP estimated or measured | $RVSP = 4(V_{TR})^2 + CVP$<br>(No PS) | 16–30 mm Hg |
| *RV systolic (with VSD)* | Systemic systolic BP<br>Peak $V_{LV\text{-}RV}$ | $RVSP = SBP - 4(V_{LV\text{-}RV})^2$<br>(No AS or LVOT obstruction) | usually $> 50$ mm Hg |
| *PA systolic (PASP)* | Peak velocity$_{TR}$<br>CVP estimated or measured | $PASP = 4(V_{TR})^2 + CVP$<br>(No PS) | 16–30 mm Hg |
| *PA diastolic (PAD)* | End diastolic Velocity$_{PR}$<br>CVP estimated or measured | $PAEDP = 4(V_{PR\ ED})^2 + CVP$ | 0–8 mm Hg |
| *PA mean (PAM)* | Acceleration time (AT) to peak $V_{PA}$ (in m/sec) | $PAM = (-0.45)\,AT + 79$ | 10–16 mm Hg |
| *RV dP/dt* | TR spectral envelope<br>$T_{TR\,(2\,m/sec)} - T_{TR\,(1\,m/sec)}$ | $RV\ dP = 4V^2_{TR(2\,m/sec)} - 4V^2_{TR(2\,m/sec)}$<br>$RV\ dP/dt = dP\,/\,T_{TR(2\,m/sec)} - T_{TR(1\,m/sec)}$ | $> 150$ mm Hg/ms |
| *LA systolic (LASP)* | Peak $V_{MR}$<br>Systolic BP (SBP) | $LASP = SBP - 4(V_{MR})^2$<br>(No AS or LVOT obstruction) | 3–15 mm Hg |
| *LA (PFO)* | Velocity$_{PFO}$<br>CVP estimated or measured | $LAP = 4(V_{PFO})^2 + CVP$ | 3–15 mm Hg |
| *LV diastolic (LVEDP)* | End diastolic Velocity$_{AR}$<br>Diastolic BP (DBP) | $LVEDP = DBP - 4(V_{AR})^2$ | 3–12 mm Hg |
| *LV dP/dt* | MR spectral envelope<br>$T_{MR\,(2\,m/sec)} - T_{MR\,(1\,m/sec)}$ | $LV\ dP = 4V^2_{MR(3\,m/sec)} - 4V^2_{MR(1\,m/sec)}$<br>$LV\ dP/dt = dP\,/\,T_{MR\,(3\,m/sec)} - T_{MR\,(1\,m/sec)}$ | $> 800$ mm Hg/ms |

Published in Savage and Aronson: Comprehensive Textbook of Intraoperative Transesophageal Echocardiography, Lippincott Williams & Wilkins, 2005.

# DIASTOLE

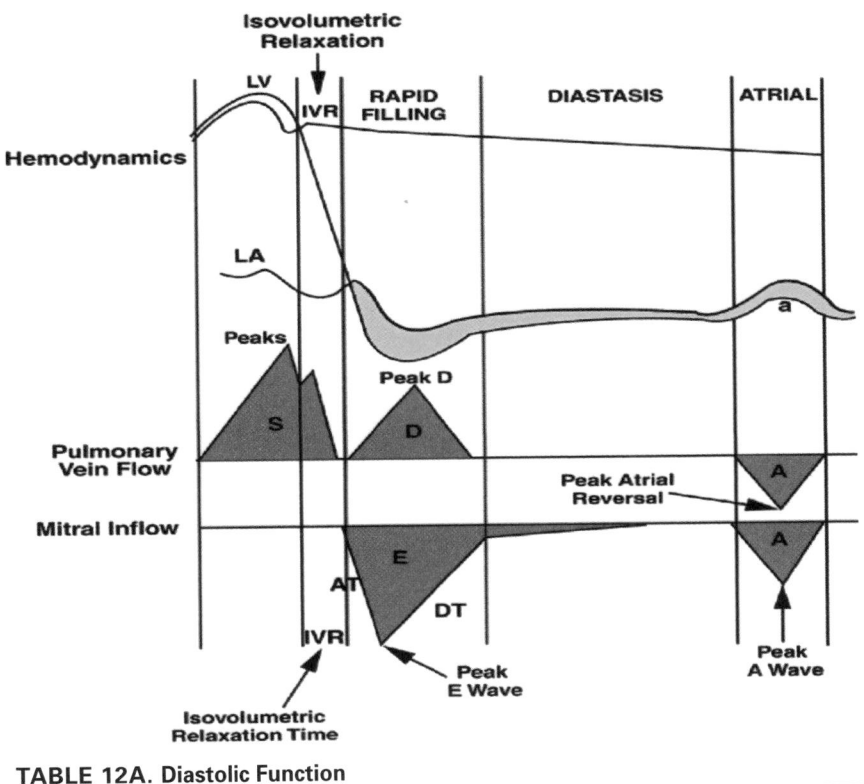

**TABLE 12A.** Diastolic Function

**Table 12B. Assessment of Diastolic Function**

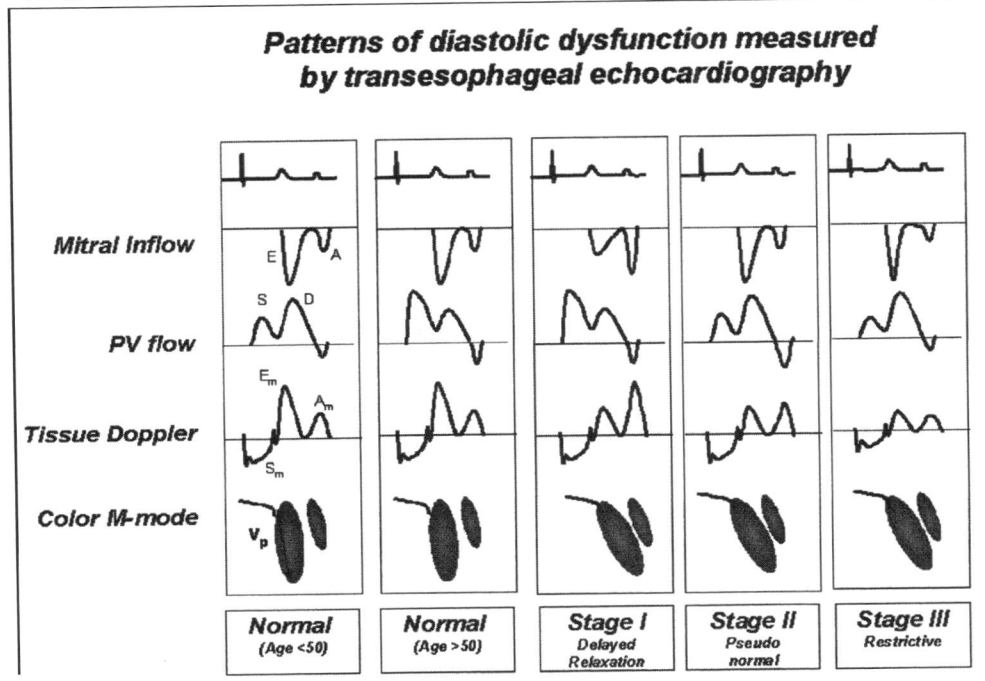

Published in Savage and Aronson: Comprehensive Textbook of Intraoperative Transesophageal Echocardiography, Lippincott Williams & Wilkins, 2005.

## Table 12B. Assessment of Diastolic Function

|  | Normal (age 21–49) | Normal (age > 50) | Stage I (delayed relaxation) | Stage II (pseudonormal filling) | Stage III (restrictive filling) |
|---|---|---|---|---|---|
| E/A | > 1 | > 1 | < 1 | 1–2 | > 2 |
| DT (ms) | < 220 | < 220 | > 220 | 150–200 | < 150 |
| IVRT (ms) | < 100 | < 100 | > 100 | 60–100 | < 60 |
| S/D | < 1 | ≥ 1 | ≥ 1 | < 1 | < 1 |
| AR (cm/s) | < 35 | < 35 | < 35 | ≥ 35 | ≥ 25 |
| Em (cm/s) | > 10 | > 8 | < 8 | < 8 | < 8 |
| Vp (cm/s) | > 55 | > 45 | < 45 | < 45 | < 45 |

## Table 12C. Assessment of Diastolic Function

|  | Where Measured | Method | Preload Dependence | Pitfalls |
|---|---|---|---|---|
| Mitral inflow | Tip of mitral valve leaflets | Pulsed Doppler | +++ | Mitral valve disease, atrial arrhythmias |
| Pulmonary venous flow | Ostium of pulmonary vein | Pulsed Doppler | +++ | Mitral valve disease, atrial arrhythmias |
| Tissue doppler | Lateral or medial mitral valve annulus | Pulsed Doppler | + | Myocardial scarring |
| Color M-mode | Left ventricular inflow | Color M-mode | + | Aortic valve regurgitation |

## Table 13. Aortic Atheroma Grading and Stroke

| Grade | Atheroma Characterization | Stroke 1 Week* |
|---|---|---|
| I | Normal | 0 |
| II | Intimal Thickening | 0 |
| III | Protrudes < 5 mm | 5.6% |
| IV | Protrudes > 5 mm | 10.5% |
| V | Mobile Atheroma | 45.5% |

Katz ES, Tunick PA, Rusinek H, et al. Protruding aortic atheroma predicts stroke in elderly patients undergoing cardiopulmonary bypass; experience with intraoperative transesophageal echocardiography. J Am Coll Cardiol 1992;20:70–77.

Ribakove GH, Katz ES, Galloway AC, et al. Surgical implications of transesophageal echocardiography to grade the atheromatous aortic arch. Ann Thorac Surg 53:758–63,1992.

Tunick PA, Perez JL, Kronzon I: Protruding atheromas in the thoracic aorta and systemic embolization. Ann Int Med 115:423–427,1991.

Hartman GS, Yao FF, Bruefach M. Severity of aortic atheromatous disease diagnosed by transesophageal echocardiography predicts stroke and other outcomes associated with coronary artery surgery: a prospective study anesth analg 1996;83:701–8).

Published in Savage and Aronson: Comprehensive Textbook of Intraoperative Transesophageal Echocardiography, Lippincott Williams & Wilkins, 2005.